Mosby's
Comprehensive
Review of Nursing for the
NCLEX-RN®
Examination

Mosby's
Comprehensive Review of Nursing for the
NCLEX-RN®
Examination

Nineteenth Edition

Editors

†**Dolores F. Saxton,** RN, BSEd, MA, MPS, EdD

Patricia M. Nugent, RN, AAS, BS, MS, EdM, EdD

Professor Emerita
Nassau Community College
Garden City, New York
President, Nugent Books, Inc.

Phyllis K. Pelikan, RN, AAS, BS, MA

Professor Emerita
Nassau Community College
Garden City, New York
President, PKP Books, Inc.

†*Deceased*

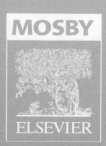

MOSBY
ELSEVIER

11830 Westline Industrial Drive
St. Louis, Missouri 63146

Mosby's Comprehensive Review of Nursing for the NCLEX-RN® Examination   ISBN: 978-0-323-05304-4

Notice

Knowledge and best practice in this field are constantly changing. As new research and experience broaden our knowledge, changes in practice, treatment and drug therapy may become necessary or appropriate. Readers are advised to check the most current information provided (i) on procedures featured or (ii) by the manufacturer of each product to be administered, to verify the recommended dose or formula, the method and duration of administration, and contraindications. It is the responsibility of the practitioner, relying on their own experience and knowledge of the patient, to make diagnoses, to determine dosages and the best treatment for each individual patient, and to take all appropriate safety precautions. To the fullest extent of the law, neither the Publisher nor the Editors assume any liability for any injury and/or damage to persons or property arising out of or related to any use of the material contained in this book.

The Publisher

Previous editions copyrighted 2006, 2003, 1999, 1996, 1993, 1990, 1987, 1984, 1981, 1977, 1973, 1969, 1965, 1961, 1958, 1955, 1951, 1949

NCLEX®, NCLEX-RN®, and NCLEX-PN® are registered trademarks of the National Council of State Boards of Nursing, Inc.

Library of Congress Cataloging-in-Publication Data

Mosby's Comprehensive Review of Nursing for the NCLEX-RN® Examination/editors, Dolores F. Saxton, Patricia M. Nugent, Phyllis K. Pelikan. — 19th ed.
    p. ; cm.
  Includes bibliographical references and index.
  ISBN 978-0-323-05304-4 (pbk. : alk. paper) 1. National Council Licensure Examination for Registered Nurses—Study guides. 2. Nursing—Examinations, questions, etc. 3. Nursing—Outlines, syllabi, etc. I. Saxton, Dolores F. II. Nugent, Patricia Mary, 1944- III. Pelikan, Phyllis K. IV. Title: Comprehensive review of nursing for the NCLEX-RN examination.
  [DNLM: 1. Nursing-Examination Questions. 2. Nursing-Outlines. WY18.2 M8938 2008]
  RT55.M64 2008
  610.76–dc22

2008029429

Managing Editor: Nancy L. O'Brien
Publishing Services Manager: John Rogers
Senior Project Manager: Beth Hayes
Design Direction: Teresa McBryan
Senior Multimedia Producer: David Rushing

Printed in Canada
Last digit is the print number: 9 8 7 6 5 4 3 2 1

Contributing Authors

Mary Ann Hellmer Saul, RNCS, AAS, BS, MS, PhD
Professor
Nassau Community College
Garden City, New York

Barbara A. Vitale, RN, AAS, BSN, MA
Professor Emerita
Nassau Community College
Garden City, New York
President, Professional Resources for Nursing (PRN)

Christina Algiere Kasprisin, RN, MS, EdD
Assistant Professor
University of Vermont College of Nursing and Health Science
Burlington, Vermont

Jane K. Brody, RN, BSN, MSN, PhD
Professor
Nassau Community College
Garden City, New York

Catherine R. Coverston, BS, MS, PhD
Assistant Professor
Brigham Young University
Provo, Utah

Judy S. Green, RN, BA, AAS, MA
Professor Emerita
Nassau Community College
Garden City, New York

Contributing Item Writers

Arline Borella, RN, BSN, CIC
Rogue Community College
Grants Pass, Oregon

Linda Carman Copel, RN, PhD, CS, DAPA
Villanova University College of Nursing
Villanova, Pennsylvania

Jo Elberg, RN, BS, MAE
Iowa Central Community College
Fort Dodge, Iowa

Carmel A. Esposito, RN, BSN, MSN, EdD
Nurse Educator
Follansbee, West Virginia

Carol Flaugher, RN, BSN, MSN
State University of New York at Buffalo School of Nursing
Buffalo, New York

Jane Flickinger, RN, BSN, MSN
Mayo Foundation—Rochester Methodist Hospital
Rochester, Minnesota

Janet T. Ihlenfeld, RN, BSN, MSN, PhD
D'Youville College
Buffalo, New York

Laurie Gaspari Kaudewitz, RN, RNC, BSN, MSN
Heartland Regional Medical Center
Marion, Illinois

Cynthia C. Small, RN, MSN, APRN-BC
Lake Michigan College
Benton Harbor, Michigan

Darlene Sredl, RN, PhD
University of Missouri St. Louis College of Nursing
St. Louis, Missouri

Judy E. White, RNC, BSN, MA, MSN
Sanford University, Ida V. Moffett School of Nursing
Birmingham, Alabama

Reviewers

Jill Espelin, MSN, RN
Clinical Faculty, School of Nursing
University of Connecticut
Storrs, Connecticut

Allison Hale, MSN, RN
Cain, Hale, & Associates
Wilmington, North Carolina

Lynne Tier, MSN, RN, LNC
Associate Professor of Nursing
Florida Hospital College of Health Sciences
Orlando, Florida

Cheryle Whitney, MSN, RN
Nurse Consultant
ciwhitney & associates, L.L.C.
Spring, Texas

With all of our love and appreciation
we dedicate this book to:
Neil Nugent,
Rudy Pelikan,
and
Wendy Ann McNabb

Preface

The information in *Mosby's Comprehensive Review of Nursing for the NCLEX-RN®️ Examination* has been totally reorganized, revised, and updated for this 19th edition. The progression of subject matter in each area reflects the consistent approach that has been used throughout the book. Information presented incorporates the latest knowledge, newest trends, and current practices in the profession of nursing.

The Introduction for Students Preparing for the Licensure Examination provides information about the NCLEX-RN®️ Examination, including the classifications used in the test plan structure. It also reviews clues for answering multiple-choice questions, provides examples of alternate-format items, and discusses the comprehensive tests and how to use this book when studying. Foundations of Nursing Practice, Chapters 1 through 3, discusses factors that influence client needs, the basics of nursing practice, and integral aspects of nursing care. These chapters present information essential to the practice of nursing that is common to all of the clinical areas. Content related to medical, surgical nursing is presented in Chapters 5 through 13; content related to mental health/psychiatric nursing is presented in Chapters 15 through 21; content related to childbearing and women's health nursing is presented in Chapters 23 through 27; and content related to child health nursing is presented in Chapters 29 through 34. Chapters 4, 14, 22, 28, and 35 consist of questions with their answers and rationales that relate to Foundations of Nursing Practice, Medical-Surgical Nursing, Mental Health Nursing, Childbearing and Women's Health Nursing, and Child Health Nursing, respectively.

The medical-surgical, mental health/psychiatric, childbearing and women's health, and child health nursing chapters incorporate information from the basic sciences, nutrition, pharmacology, acute and long-term care, and physical and emotional nursing care. We continue to present the material in the traditional clinical groupings for we still believe that when preparing for a comprehensive examination, the average student will study all of the distinct parts before attempting to put them together. Although we believe that in practice the nursing process is continually evolving rather than remaining a clearly defined step-by-step process, we present the content under the following headings: Assessment/Analysis, Planning/Implementation, and Evaluation/Outcomes. We believe that this grouping avoids needless repetition, recognizes the abilities of our readers, and reflects current practice.

Over 4200 questions have been included in this edition of *Mosby's Comprehensive Review of Nursing for the NCLEX-RN®️ Examination*. Although the majority of the questions are multiple-choice questions, a significant number of questions reflect the new alternate-format questions that appear on the NCLEX-RN®️ examination, such as multiple-response items, ordered-response items, fill-in-the-blank items, illustration items, and chart/exhibit items. For every question in this edition and on the CD-ROM we have provided rationales that state the reason why the correct answer is correct, as well as why the incorrect answers are incorrect.

The questions in Chapters 4, 14, 22, 28, and 35 are grouped according to the chapter in which the content of the question is presented. To further assist the user in studying/reviewing by a specific content area, the questions are also classified according to Client Need, Cognitive Level, Nursing Process, Integrated Process (if applicable), and Reference.

One comprehensive test is included in this textbook and also appears on the Companion CD, along with a second comprehensive test that appears on the Companion CD-ROM. These comprehensive tests provide an opportunity for the test taker to experience testing situations that approximate the NCLEX-RN®. To parallel the NCLEX-RN®, the first 75 questions in each test reflect the minimal testing experience for students taking the NCLEX-RN®. The total number of 265 questions in each test reflects the maximum number of questions that a student can take on the NCLEX-RN®. All of the questions in each comprehensive test have been analyzed as to Client Need, Cognitive Level, Nursing Process, Integrated Processes (if applicable), and Reference.

The Companion CD-ROM contains the 2240 questions from the book, as well as over 1900 additional test questions that can be used in both study and test format. These questions also have been categorized by Client Need, Cognitive Level, Nursing Process, and Integrated Process (if applicable). Whether the test taker answers these questions in a written or computerized format the information being tested remains constant. To reinforce learned information and build confidence in taking a computerized test, we suggest that students practice answering questions on this CD to simulate the computerized NCLEX-RN®.

All of the questions used in this edition have been submitted by outstanding educators and practitioners of nursing. Initially the editorial board reviewed all questions, selecting the most pertinent for inclusion in a mass field-testing project or analysis by a panel of expert nursing educators. Students graduating from baccalaureate, associate degree, and diploma nursing programs in various locations in the United States provided a diverse testing group for the mass field-testing project. The results were statistically analyzed. This analysis, in addition to the input from the panel of expert nursing educators, was used to select questions for inclusion in the book.

We would like to take this opportunity to thank Loren Wilson, executive editor, for her guidance, support, and friendship and Nancy O'Brien, managing editor, for her support, guidance, expert management of this project, and friendship. In addition, we recognize the exemplary contributions of the contributing authors that reflect their dedication and expertise. We especially appreciate our families for their love and encouragement.

We would like to thank the entire Mosby/Elsevier publishing team, especially: Nancy O'Brien, Managing Editor, for her support, professional guidance, expert management of this project, and friendship throughout the years; Teresa McBryan, Design Direction, for her vision, creativity, and use of color in the presentation of this revised, updated, and reorganized edition; and Beth Hayes, Senior Project Manager, for her unfailing ear for the nuance of the English language, her attention to detail throughout the copyediting process, her coordination of illustrations/tables, and her expert consultations and support.

In addition, we recognize the exemplary work of the Contributing Authors, Contributing Item Writers, and Reviewers that reflects their dedication and expertise. We especially appreciate our families for their patience and understanding when the production of this book consumed most of our time and energy.

Patricia M. Nugent
Phyllis K. Pelikan

Contents

UNIT 5   CHILD HEALTH NURSING

29   Foundations of Child Health Nursing, 645

30   Nursing Care of Infants, 650

31   Nursing Care of Toddlers, 681

Introduction for Students Preparing for the NCLEX-RN® Examination

OVERVIEW

The NCLEX-RN® examination is integrated and comprehensive. Nursing candidates are required to answer questions that necessitate a recognition and understanding of the physiologic, biologic, and social sciences, as well as the specific nursing skills and abilities involved in a given client situation.

This text contains objective multiple-choice questions, as well as alternate-format questions such as multiple-response items, ordered-response items, fill-in-the-blank items, illustration items, and chart/exhibit items. To answer the questions appropriately, a candidate needs to understand and correlate certain aspects of anatomy and physiology, the behavioral sciences, basic nursing, the effects of medications administered, the client's attitude toward illness, and other pertinent factors such as legal responsibilities, leadership and management, and critical thinking. Most questions are based on nursing situations similar to those with which candidates have had experiences because they emphasize the nursing care of clients with representative common health problems. Some questions, however, require candidates to apply basic principles and techniques to clinical situations with which they have had little, if any, actual experience.

To prepare adequately for an integrated comprehensive examination, it is necessary to understand the discrete parts that compose the universe of material under consideration. This is one of the major principles of learning that has contributed to the development of *Mosby's Comprehensive Review of Nursing for the NCLEX-RN® Examination*.

Using this principle, the text first presents a review of the Foundations of Nursing Practice and information essential to each of the major clinical areas: medical-surgical nursing, child health nursing, mental health nursing, and childbearing and women's health nursing. Chapters at the end of Foundations of Nursing Practice and at the end of each major clinical area contain questions that test the student's knowledge of principles and theories underlying nursing care in a variety of situations, in a variety of settings, and with a variety of nursing objectives. Each question has rationales for the correct answer and incorrect options as well as a classification of the question that reflects the NCLEX-RN examination test plan. The following descriptions are presented to assist in the understanding of these classifications.

CLASSIFICATION OF QUESTIONS

Each question in both comprehensive tests is classified by the following categories:

CLIENT NEEDS

These categories reflect activities most frequently performed by entry-level nurses.

1. **Safe and Effective Care Environment**

Management of Care: These questions provide or direct nursing activities that promote the delivery of care to clients, family members, significant others, and other health care personnel.

Safety and Infection Control: These questions address the protection of clients, family members, significant others, and health care personnel from health and environmental hazards.

2. **Health Promotion and Maintenance**

These questions provide or direct nursing care of the client, family members, and significant others. They include knowledge of the principles of growth and development, prevention and/or detection of health problems, and interventions to achieve optimum health.

3. **Psychosocial Integrity**

These questions provide or direct nursing care that supports and promotes the emotional, mental, and social well-being of the client, family members, and significant others experiencing stressful events, as well as clients with acute or chronic mental health illness.

4. **Physiological Integrity**

Basic Care and Comfort: These questions address the provision of comfort and support in the performance of the activities of daily living.

Pharmacological and Parenteral Therapies: These questions address the provision of care related to the administration of medications, parenteral therapies, and blood products.

Reduction of Risk Potential: These questions address nursing care that may limit the liklihood of the development of complications or health problems related to existing disorders, treatments, or procedures.

Physiological Adaptation: These questions address the provision and management of nursing care for clients with acute, chronic, or life-threatening physical health problems.

COGNITIVE LEVELS

This category reflects the thinking processes required to answer the question.

Knowledge: These questions require the test taker to recall information from memory. They involve knowledge of facts, principles, generalizations, terminology, and trends, for example.

Comprehension: These questions require the test taker to understand information. They involve the interpretation, paraphrasing, and summarization of information as well as the determination of implications and consequences of information.

Application: These questions require the test taker to use information, principles, or concepts. They involve identifying, manipulating, changing, or modifying information as well as performing mathematical calculations.

Analysis: These questions require the test taker to interpret a variety of information. It involves the recognition of commonalities, differences, and interrelationships among data, concepts, principles, and situations.

INTEGRATED PROCESSES

Integrated processes are fundamental components critical to the practice of nursing. They include the nursing process, caring, communication and documentation, and teaching and learning. Because the nursing process (a scientific problem-solving process that involves critical thinking) is essential to all nursing care, it subsequently is presented in detail.

Caring: These questions reflect interactions between the nurse and client/significant others that demonstrate mutual trust and respect. They include nursing care that provides support, encouragement, hope, and compassion.

Communication and Documentation: These questions involve verbal and nonverbal interactions between the nurse and client, significant others, and members of the health care team. Client status, events, and interventions are communicated and documented according to rights, responsibilities, and standards of care.

Teaching and Learning: These questions include nursing assessments and interventions that relate to the attainment of knowledge, skills, or attitudes that meet client needs.

PHASES OF THE NURSING PROCESS

This category reflects the problem-solving process used by nurses to identify client needs, plan and implement nursing care, and evaluate client responses to care.

Assessment/Analysis: This phase requires the nurse to obtain objective and subjective data from primary and secondary sources, to identify and group significant data, and to communicate this information to other members of the health team. This phase also requires the nurse to interpret data gathered through assessment in order to make nursing decisions. Client and family needs are identified and short-term and long-term goals/outcomes are set.

Planning/Implementation: This phase requires the nurse to design and implement a regimen with the client, family, and other health team members to achieve goals/outcomes set during the assessment/analysis phase. It also requires setting priorities for intervention. The client may be given total care or may be assisted and encouraged to perform activities of daily living or follow the regimen prescribed by the practitioner. In addition, it involves activities such as counseling, teaching, and supervising health team members.

Evaluation/Outcomes: This phase requires the nurse to determine the effectiveness of nursing care. Care is reviewed, the client's response to intervention is identified, and a determination is made as to whether the client has achieved the predetermined outcomes and goals. It also includes appraisal of the client's ability to implement and fulfill the health care plan.

REFERENCE

Each question refers the test taker to the section where the related content concerning the question is within *Mosby's Comprehensive Review of Nursing for the NCLEX-RN® Examination*. This promotes a review of the specific information as it relates to the question as well as permits a more thorough review of related information.

GENERAL CLUES FOR ANSWERING MULTIPLE-CHOICE QUESTIONS

On a multiple-choice test the question and possible answers are called a *test item*. The part of the item that asks the question or poses a problem is called the *stem*. All of the answers presented are called *options*. One of the options is the correct answer; the remaining are incorrect. The incorrect options are called *distractors* because their major purpose is to distract the test taker from the correct answer.

A. Read the question carefully before looking at the answers.
   1. Determine what the question is really asking; look for key words.
   2. Read each answer thoroughly and see if it completely covers the material asked by the question.
   3. Narrow the choices by immediately eliminating answers you know are incorrect.
B. Because few things in life are absolute without exceptions, avoid selecting answers that include words such as *always, never, all, every,* and *none.* Answers containing these key words are rarely correct.
C. Attempt to select the answer that is most complete and includes the other answers within it. An example might be as follows. A stem might ask "A child's intelligence is influenced by:" and three options might be *genetic inheritance*, *environment factors*, and *past experiences*. The fourth option might be *multiple factors,* which is a more inclusive choice and therefore the correct answer.
D. Make certain that the answer you select is reasonable and obtainable under ordinary circumstances and that the action can be carried out in the given situation.
E. Watch for grammatical inconsistencies. If one or more of the options is not grammatically consistent with the stem, the alert test taker can identify it as a probable incorrect option. When the stem is in the form of an incomplete sentence, each option should complete the sentence in a grammatically correct way.
F. Avoid selecting answers that state hospital rules or regulations as a reason or rationale for action.
G. Look for answers that focus on the client or are directed toward feelings.
H. If the question asks for an immediate action or response, all the answers may be correct, so base your selection on identified priorities for action.

I. Do not select answers that contain exceptions to the general rule, controversial material, or degrading responses.

J. Reread the question if the answers do not seem to make sense, because you may have missed words such as *not* or *except* in the statement.

K. Do not worry if you select the same numbered answer repeatedly, because there usually is no pattern to the answers.

L. Mark the number next to the answer you have chosen.

M. Answer every question because on the NCLEX-RN you must answer a question before you move on to the next question.

ALTERNATE-FORMAT ITEMS

In addition to multiple-choice questions the NCLEX-RN includes alternate-format questions. These questions consist of five types: multiple-response items; ordered-response (drag and drop) items; fill-in-the-blank items; illustration items; and chart/exhibit items. The following examples reflect these alternate-response items.

MULTIPLE-RESPONSE ITEM

Multiple-response items pose a question and then include a list of responses that may or may not answer the question. The test taker is directed to indicate all the correct options.

The nurse suspects that a postpartum client is experiencing postpartum depression. Check each assessment that supports this conclusion.

1. _____ Lethargy
2. _____ Somnolence
3. _____ Ambivalence
4. _____ Increased appetite
5. _____ Emotional lability

ORDERED-RESPONSE (DRAG AND DROP) ITEM

Ordered-response items present information or a series of statements and then ask the test taker to place them in order of priority.

A client is receiving an IV piggyback oxytocin (Pitocin) infusion to induce labor. The client experiences three contractions that are 90 seconds long and occur less than 2 minutes apart. List in order of priority the nursing actions that should be taken.

1. _____ Call the physician.
2. _____ Administer oxygen.
3. _____ Interrupt the oxytocin infusion.
4. _____ Document maternal/fetal responses.

FILL-IN-THE-BLANK ITEM

Fill-in-the-blank items involve a calculation that relates to pharmacologic or parenteral therapies. The question presents information and requires the test taker to manipulate the information to solve the problem posed, and then the test taker must record the solution to the problem.

The physician orders an IVPB infusion of 500 mg of an antibiotic to be added to 50 mL of normal saline to be administered qid. The antibiotic is supplied in single-dose vials containing 1 g each. The directions advise that the instillation of 0.8 mL of normal saline will yield 1.2 mL of solution. How much antibiotic solution should be added to the 50 mL of normal saline?

Answer: _____ mL

ILLUSTRATION ITEM

Illustration items pose a question that uses a picture, graph, or diagram. The test taker is asked a question that requires an interpretation or analysis of information presented in the attached illustration.

A client is receiving continuous ECG monitoring while intravenous medication is being administered for a cardiac dysrhythmia. Soon after the client is admitted to the telemetry unit, the nurse reads the illustrated rhythm strip and concludes that the client is experiencing:

1. Atrial flutter
2. Ventricular tachycardia
3. Supraventricular contractions
4. Premature ventricular contractions

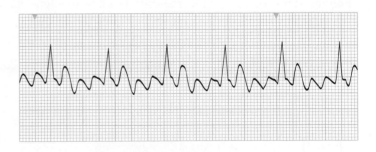

Client name	GPTAL*	Time admitted	Gestational age in weeks	Other	Membrane status†	Time of last exam	Dilation in cm	Effacement	Station
A	1:0000	0200	30	Placenta previa bleeding	Intact	Deferred	Closed by speculum		

Client name	GPTAL*	Time admitted	Gestational age in weeks	Other	Membrane status†	Time of last exam	Dilation in cm	Effacement	Station
B	4:0122	0500	38	VBAC‡	SROM	1430	8	100%	0

Client name	GPTAL*	Time admitted	Gestational age in weeks	Other	Membrane status†	Time of last exam	Dilation in cm	Effacement	Station
C	2:1001	1400	41	Induction	AROM	1400	2	70%	−2

Client name	GPTAL*	Time admitted	Gestational age in weeks	Other	Membrane status†	Time of last exam	Dilation in cm	Effacement	Station
D	3:1102	0400	39	BP 160/96 MgSO₄ and pitocin infusions	AROM	1200	5	90%	−1

Client name	GPTAL*	Time admitted	Gestational age in weeks	Other	Membrane status†	Time of last exam	Dilation in cm	Effacement	Station
E	3:2002	0931	40		AROM	1300	4	80%	−3

*GPTAL, Gravida, parity, term, preterm, living children.
†Intact; SROM, Spontaneous rupture; AROM, artificial rupture.
‡VBAC, Vaginal birth after cesarean.

CHART/EXHIBIT ITEM

Chart/exhibit items present a situation and ask a question. A variety of objective and subjective information is presented about the client in formats such as the hospital record (e.g., laboratory test results, results of diagnostic procedures, progress notes, practitioner orders, medication administration record, health history), physical assessment data, and nurse/client interactions. After analyzing the data presented, the test taker then answers the question. These questions usually reflect the analysis level of cognitive thinking.

The nurse in charge for the 3 PM shift obtains the following information about clients who are in labor to make staff assignments accordingly. Which woman should be assigned the most experienced nurse?

1. A
2. B
3. C
4. D
5. E

COMPREHENSIVE EXAMINATIONS

Mosby's Comprehensive Review of Nursing for the NCLEX-RN® Examination contains two comprehensive examinations on the enclosed Companion CD, consisting of 265 questions each. These tests approximate the NCLEX-RN test plan.

To parallel the NCLEX-RN, the first 75 questions in each examination reflect the minimum testing experience for students taking the NCLEX-RN. The total of 265 questions in each test reflects the maximum number of questions that a student will be asked on the NCLEX-RN. The questions require the test taker to cross clinical disciplines and respond to individual and specific needs associated with given health problems. Rationales are also provided for the correct answers and the incorrect options to these questions. In addition, each question is classified according to client need, cognitive level, integrated process, and nursing process. The purpose of these comprehensive tests is to provide students with an opportunity to simulate the NCLEX-RN experience at the completion of a personalized program review.

HOW TO USE THIS BOOK WHEN STUDYING

A. Start in one area. Study the material covered by the section. Refer to other textbooks to find additional details if you are unsure of a specific fact.

B. Answer the questions following the area. As you answer each question, write a few words about why you think that answer was correct; in other words, justify why you selected the answer. If an answer you provide is a guess, mark the question to identify it. This will permit you to recognize areas that need further review. It will also help you to see how correct your "guessing" can be. Remember, on the licensure examination you must answer every question before moving to the next question.

C. Record the answer by circling the number you believe is correct.

D. Compare your answers with those provided. If you answered the item correctly, check your reason for selecting the answer with the rationale presented. If you answered the item incorrectly, read the rationale to determine why the option you selected was incorrect. In addition, you should review the correct answer and rationale for each item answered incorrectly. If you still do not understand your mistakes, look up the material pertaining to these questions. The Content Area following the answers and rationales informs you of the area within *Mosby's Comprehensive Review of Nursing for the NCLEX-RN® Examination* where you can find related information included in the question. You should carefully review all questions and rationales for items you identified as guesses, because you did not have mastery of the material being questioned.

E. Following the rationales for the correct answer and the incorrect options, you will find that each question in the book is classified according to Client Need, Cognitive Level, Integrated Process, Nursing Process, and Content Area. These areas are described previously in this chapter and should help you to understand the question in relation to the NCLEX-RN examination test plan.

F. After you have completed the area questions, begin taking the comprehensive tests because they will assist you in applying knowledge and principles from the specific clinical area to any nursing situation.

1. Arrange a quiet, uninterrupted time span for each part of a comprehensive test.
2. Avoid spending excessive time on any one question. Most questions can be answered in 1 to 2 minutes.
3. Make educated guesses when necessary.
4. Read carefully and answer the question asked; pay attention to specific details in the question.
5. Try putting questions and answers in your own words to test your comprehension.

G. To help analyze your mistakes on the comprehensive examinations and to provide a data base for making future study plans, worksheets follow each of the comprehensive tests. These worksheets are designed to aid you in identifying and recording errors in the way you apply information and to help you identify and record gaps in knowledge.

H. After completing your worksheets, do the following:

1. Identify the frequency with which you made particular errors. As you review material in class notes or this review book, pay special attention to acquiring information related to content that you found difficult on the tests.
2. Identify the topics you want to review. It might be helpful to set priorities; review the most difficult topics first so that you will have time to review them more than once.

TAKING THE LICENSURE EXAMINATION

The computerized NCLEX-RN is an individualized testing experience in which the computer chooses your next question based on the ability and competency you have demonstrated on previous questions. The minimum number of questions will be 75 and the maximum 265. You must answer each question before the computer will present the next question, and you cannot go back to any previously answered questions. You have a 1 in 4 (25%) chance of selecting the correct answer; go for it! Remember, you do not have to get all the questions correct to pass.

The following are crucial requisites for doing well on the licensure examination:

- A sound understanding of the subject
- The ability to follow explicitly the directions given at the beginning of the test
- The ability to comprehend what is read
- The patience to read each question carefully before deciding how to answer it
- The ability to use the computer correctly to record answers
- The determination to do well
- A degree of confidence

Factors Influencing Client Needs and Nursing Care

CONCEPTS FROM SOCIOLOGY

BASIC CONCEPTS

A. Every human society has institutions for the socialization of its members
   1. Groups establish rules and codes of conduct using a system of rewards and punishment to govern their members, and these become the norms, values, and mores of the group
      a. Reward leads to acceptance as a member of the group
      b. Punishment for antisocial behavior leads to rejection and separation from the group
   2. Role of members includes specified rights, duties, attitudes, and actions
   3. Social boundaries separate one group from another; the nonmembers have, at best, limited social contacts with the members; this causes a segmentation of relationships and provides few rewarding experiences for the nonmembers
   4. Leader's influence is always limited to conditions placed on the leader by the total group
B. A society is a reflection of all the functional relationships that occur among its individual members; participation in society is a major influence on an individual's intellect, creativity, memory, thinking, and feeling
C. Society or a group can change because of conflict among members
   1. This conflict is greatest when there is an absence of certain members, an introduction of new members, or a change in leadership
   2. Ensuing reorganization goes through three stages
      a. Tension: caused by conflict
      b. Integration: during which members learn about "the other's" problem
      c. Resolution: during which a reconstruction of the group's norms and values takes place
   3. Resolution of conflict and the restoring of equilibrium
      a. Occurs when people interact with one another and the group is dynamic
      b. Conflicts are not resolved when groups are rigid with fixed ideas

CULTURE AND HEALTH

A. General influences
   1. Culture defines for its people what is important and what is true and real in the world

2. Ethnocentrism is the belief that one's own culture is generally right or best
3. Age, ethnicity, gender, education, income, and belief system (worldview, religion, or spirituality) make up the sociocultural profile of the client
4. The clients' perceptions of health and illness, their help-seeking behavior, and their treatment adherence depend on their beliefs, social norms, and cultural values
5. When clients face increased stressors, suffering, or pain, their belief systems play an even greater role in their lives
6. Stereotyping, intolerance, stigma, prejudice, discrimination, and racism are common sociocultural stressors

B. Implications for the nurse
   1. Culturally competent nurses are in touch with their own personal and cultural experiences
   2. Nurses must have a holistic perspective to assess the sociocultural context of clients from a different culture
   3. Together, the nurse and the client should agree on the nature of the client's coping responses and set goals and behavioral outcomes within the client's sociocultural context
   4. The degree of compatibility between the client's and the nurse's belief systems often determines a greater satisfaction with treatment, medication compliance, and treatment outcomes
   5. Nurses should expose themselves to cultural diversity and expand their worldviews to enhance cultural competence

SOCIETY AND HEALTH

A. Role of society
   1. Traditionally, societies have placed great emphasis on caring for their members when they are ill
   2. Society's role in health maintenance and the prevention of disease has been given an increased priority
   3. Society's provision for health maintenance includes
      a. Establishment of public health care agencies for the supervision, prevention, and control of disease and illness; the protection of food, water, and drug supplies; the development of public education programs
      b. Awarding scholarships/grants for health education and research

c. Development of unemployment insurance programs and Workers' Compensation insurance

d. Establishment of Social Security and Medicare programs; establishment of social welfare services and Medicaid programs

e. Supervision of medical and hospital insurance programs

B. Health care agency—a bureaucratic subculture of society

1. Employees develop both written and unwritten agency policies that
   a. Set standards of acceptable behavior for both clients and staff
   b. Regulate the hospitalized client's contact with the primary group by limiting visitors
   c. Provide formal delivery of nursing care (e.g., primary nursing, team nursing)
   d. Punish unacceptable behavior by any members of the group, including the client

2. Health care agencies have several functions
   a. Treatment of illness
   b. Rehabilitation
   c. Maintenance of health
   d. Protection of the client's legal rights
   e. Education of health professionals
   f. Education of the general public
   g. Research

C. Delivery of health services is the responsibility of the community

1. Health maintenance and treatment are no longer considered a privilege, but the right of all members of society

2. Members of society become active participants in prevention of illness

3. Community needs influence services provided by health care agencies
   a. More care is being provided in the community setting because of a decreased length of hospitalization in an effort to decrease health care costs
   b. Assisted living facilities are homelike apartments providing limited health care supervision because of an aging population with increased health care needs that family members are unable to meet
   c. Nursing homes and extended care facilities provide skilled nursing care to those who need more extensive health care on a long-term care basis with activities of daily living, subacute needs, and/or rehabilitation needs

GROUPS

A. Group membership helps individuals achieve goals that are not attainable through individual effort

1. Types of groups include social, self-awareness, task-oriented, and therapy

2. Group functional roles include task roles, group-building or maintenance roles, individual or self-serving roles

3. Group content refers to the subject matter or task being addressed

4. Group process refers to what is happening among and to group members while working; it deals with morale, feeling tones, influence, competition, conflict

5. Types of roles assumed by members of the group
   a. Harmonizer: brings other group members into accord while reconciling opposing positions
   b. Questioner: asks questions, seeks information, and gives constructive criticism to other group members
   c. Deserter: talks about irrelevant material; is usually disruptive in some manner
   d. Tension reducer: introduces levity when it is needed and appropriate
   e. Encourager: contributes to the ego of others and is a responsive member
   f. Monopolizer: attempts to control group; does not allow others to talk
   g. Clarifier: restates issues for clarification and then summarizes for the group
   h. Opinion giver: uses own experience to back up opinion or belief
   i. Initiator: proposes ideas or topics for discussion and suggests possible solutions for group discussion
   j. Listener: shows interest in the group by expressions on face or by body language while making little or no comment
   k. Negativist: pessimistic, argumentative, and uncooperative
   l. Energizer: pushes the group into action
   m. Aggressor: hostile and aggressive, verbally attacks other group members

B. Family is the primary group

1. Helps society to establish and maintain its code of behavior

2. Provides individual family members with
   a. Strong emotional ties that occur when members
      (1) Experience sensory stimuli through close contacts
      (2) Learn to care about the emotional and physical well-being of one another
      (3) Are responsive to one another's feelings, acts, and opinions
      (4) Learn empathy by vicariously living the experiences of others
      (5) View selves through others' eyes
   b. A feeling of security by meeting dependent needs
   c. A system of communication: overt (e.g., words) or covert (e.g., body language)
   d. Role identification and intimacy that helps them to internalize the acceptable behavioral patterns of the group
   e. A spirit of cooperation and competition through sibling interaction

3. Changes that have influenced the family's ability to indoctrinate children with the norms of society
   a. Society has progressed from an agrarian culture through the Industrial Revolution to the Computer Age
      (1) Similarly, families have undergone change from extended to nuclear units, with an increase in numbers of blended, single-parent, and same-gender parent households
      (2) New social groups were established to replace the extended family
      (3) Electronic influences (e.g., computers and television) have weakened the structure of the family
      (4) Increased mobility of individuals reduced contact with extended or separated family members
      (5) Participation in individual activities has grown, thereby reducing time for involvement in family activities
   b. Altered male and female role patterns
      (1) Changing status of women: increase in level of education, numbers working outside the home, and role in decision making
      (2) Changing status of men: increase in willingness to assume homemaking responsibilities and shared decision making with women
      (3) Increased partnership in home and financial management has resulted in less stereotyped gender roles
      (4) Increase in numbers of divorced single parents, both male and female, rearing offspring
      (5) Increase in number of financially independent women conceiving a child or children outside of marriage
   c. Factors resulting in a reduction in the size of families
      (1) Choosing to marry in later adulthood
      (2) Delaying the start of a family until later years
      (3) Emphasis on limited population growth
      (4) Dissemination of birth control information
      (5) Legalization of abortions
      (6) Increase in financial cost involved in raising and educating children
C. Peer groups help to establish norms of behavior
   1. Youth learns about society through contact with the peer group, which assists in the rites of passage from the family group to society
   2. Youth develops further self-concept in contact with other youths
   3. Peer group interaction can produce change in its individual members
   4. Members have a strong loyalty to the peer group because of the reciprocal relationships and other rewards the group offers

5. Peer group norms may conflict with family or societal norms
D. Crisis intervention groups
   1. Services
      a. Provide assistance for people in crises; clients' previous methods of adaptation are inadequate to meet present needs
      b. Group focus can be specific (e.g., poison control, drug-addiction centers, and suicide prevention) or general (e.g., walk-in mental health clinics and hospital emergency services)
      c. Some crisis intervention groups provide service over the phone (e.g., poison control, AIDS hotline, and suicide prevention centers); others help those who are physically present (e.g., hospital emergency services and walk-in mental health clinics)
   2. Success factors
      a. Provide help requested by the client or family
      b. Address the immediate problem
      c. Facilitate exploring feelings
      d. Assist the client in perceiving the event realistically
      e. Maximize the client's coping mechanisms
      f. Provide assistance in investigating alternative approaches to solve the problem
      g. Identify support systems
      h. Review how present situation may help in coping with future crises
      i. Provide information about other health resources where the client may receive additional assistance
E. Self-help groups
   1. Services
      a. Organized by clients or their families to provide services that are not adequately supplied by other organizations
      b. Meet the needs of clients and families with chronic problems requiring intervention over an extended time
      c. Focus is usually specific (e.g., Gamblers Anonymous); some deal with a range of problems (e.g., Association for Children with Learning Disabilities)
      d. Some are nonprofit (e.g., Alcoholics Anonymous); others are profit-making organizations (e.g., Weight Watchers International)
      e. Provide help to people who often are not accepted by society (e.g., addicts, child abusers, mentally ill, obese, or brain-injured); many use the 12-step program developed by Alcoholics Anonymous
   2. Success factors
      a. All members are accepted and respected as equals
      b. All members have experienced similar problems
      c. Members feel a decrease in the sense of isolation that has occurred as a result of their problems

d. Members deal with behavior and changes in behavior rather than with underlying causes of the behavior
e. Members have a ready supply of human resources available, such as personal resources, help from peers, and, ultimately, extension of self to others as a role model
f. Each member has identified the problem and wants help in meeting needs—self-motivation
g. Ritual and language may be specific to the group and/or the problems
h. Members retain leadership of the group
i. Group interaction
   (1) Identification with peers—sense of belonging
   (2) Group expectations—self-discipline required of members
   (3) Small steps encouraged and, when attained, reinforced by group
j. As a member achieves success within the group, reinforcement often is received from outside the group
k. Participation in 12-step programs is a lifelong, continuous process; one is never "recovered" but always "recovering" one day at a time
F. Community is a social organization that is considered a secondary group
   1. Relationships among members are usually more impersonal
   2. Individuals participate in a more limited manner or in a specific capacity
   3. The group frequently functions as a means to an end, enables diversified groups to communicate, and helps other groups to identify community problems and possible solutions
   4. The secondary group is usually rather large and meets on an intermittent basis; contacts are usually maintained through correspondence
   5. Leaders of the community facilitate group interaction because they have knowledge of the community and its needs and the skill to stimulate others to act
   6. Secondary groups help establish laws that are necessary to limit antisocial behavior; they provide diversified groups with a common base of acceptable behavior, but they may favor and protect the vested interests of specific groups within the society
G. Health educational groups
   1. Services
      a. Provide health information/support to change behavior
      b. Meet the needs of clients of families adapting to change
      c. Focus is usually specific (e.g., diabetes education group, parenting group, Weight Watchers)
      d. Majority of educational groups are conducted by health care providers and are nonprofit
      e. In-service educational groups are also included in this category

2. Success factors
   a. All members are accepted and respected as equals
   b. All members have the same educational needs and have experienced similar problems (e.g., managing diabetes)
   c. Members experience a decrease in isolation and frustration as knowledge increases
   d. Members have identified the problem and generally are motivated to manage more effectively
   e. Nurse leader is able to educate more people more efficiently using a group format
   f. Members aid each other as they learn together and share information and experiences

HIERARCHY OF NEEDS

(Figure 1-1: Maslow's hierarchy of needs)
A. Need to survive: physiologic needs for such things as air, food, and water
B. Need for safety and comfort: physical and psychologic security
C. Interpersonal needs: social needs for love and acceptance
D. Intrapersonal needs: self-esteem and self-actualization

INDIVIDUAL FACTORS AFFECTING HEALTH

A. Physiologic capacity: All diseases and conditions have a genomic component; genomics refers to the study of genes and their interactions with other genes, the environment, and psychosocial factors

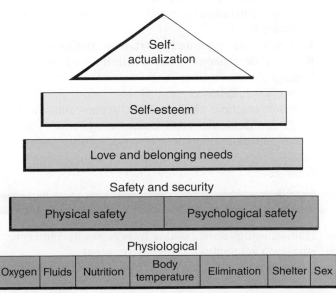

Figure 1-1 Maslow's hierarchy of needs. (Redrawn from Maslow AH: *Motivation and personality*, Upper Saddle River, NJ, 1970, Prentice Hall.)

B. Developmental level
  1. Infant: must adapt to a totally new environment; the stress from the transition from intrauterine to extrauterine living is compounded for the infant with a congenital problem
  2. Child: maturation involves physical, functional, and emotional growth; it is an ever-changing process that produces stress; disabilities provide additional factors that may quantitatively or qualitatively affect maturation
  3. Adolescent: is experiencing a physical, psychologic, and social growth spurt; the individual is asking, "Who am I?" while developing a self-image; limitations provide additional stress during identity formation
  4. Adult: is expected to be independent and productive, to provide for self and family; if one cannot partially or totally accomplish this, additional stress occurs
  5. Older adult: our society tends to value youth and devalue old age; many older adults are experiencing multiple stresses (e.g., loss of loved ones, changes in usual lifestyle, loss of physical vigor, and thought of approaching death) at a time when their ability to adapt is compromised by the anatomic, physiologic, and psychologic alterations that occur during the aging process
C. Intelligence: genetic intellectual potential; amount of formal/informal education; level of intellectual development; and the ability to reason, conceptualize, and translate words into actions
D. Level of self-esteem: attitude that reflects the individual's perception of self-worth; it is a personal subjective judgment of oneself; influenced by loss of independence and changing role
E. Experiential background: knowledge derived from one's own actions, observations, or perceptions; maturation, culture, and environment influence the individual's experiential foundation
F. Level of motivation: internal desire or incentive to accomplish goals
G. Values: factors that are important to the individual
H. Religion: deep personal belief in a higher force than humanity
I. Socioeconomic status
J. Social interaction: ability to clearly communicate needs and desires to others; support systems
K. Stress control: development of varied effective coping skills

STRESS RESPONSE

A. Human beings must be able to perceive and interpret stimuli to interact with the environment
  1. Perception and cognitive functioning are influenced by
    a. Nature of the stimuli
    b. Culture, beliefs, attitudes, and age
    c. Past experiences
    d. Present physical and emotional needs

  2. Personality development is influenced by the ability to perceive and interpret stimuli
    a. Through these processes the external world is internalized
    b. The external world may in turn be distorted by the individual's perceptions
B. Selye's general adaptation syndrome (GAS) is the body's physiologic adaptation to stress; it is a nonspecific response that has three stages: alarm, resistance, and exhaustion
  1. Stress produces wear and tear on the body; it can be internal or external, beneficial or detrimental, and always elicits some response from or change in the individual
  2. Alarm phase: the sympathetic nervous system prepares the body's physiologic defense for fight or flight by stimulating the adrenal medulla to secrete epinephrine and norepinephrine; the adrenocortical hormones (aldosterone and cortisol) are secreted (Figure 1-2: Fight-or-flight response)
    a. Heartbeat is accelerated to pump more blood to the muscles
    b. Peripheral blood vessels constrict to provide more blood to vital organs
    c. Bronchioles dilate, and breathing becomes rapid and deep to supply more oxygen to cells
    d. Pupils dilate to provide increased vision
    e. Liver releases glucose for quick energy
    f. Prothrombin time is shortened to protect the body from loss of blood in the event of injury
    g. Sodium is retained to maintain blood pressure
  3. Resistive stage: When stress continues, the increased secretion of cortisone causes the body to cope with the stress

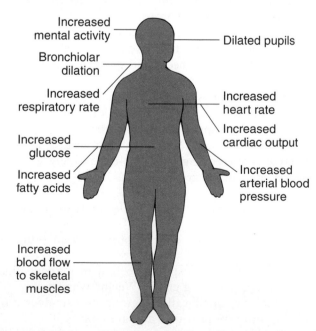

Figure 1-2 Fight-or-flight response. (From Potter PA, Perry AG: *Fundamentals of nursing,* ed 7, St. Louis, 2009, Mosby.)

4. Exhaustion: If the process continues and adaptations are not effective, the last stage is exhaustion and death

C. Local inflammatory response is the body's nonspecific response of tissue to injury or infection
   1. Erythema (redness): histamine is released at the site of injury, causing vasodilation (hyperemia)
   2. Heat: same as for erythema
   3. Edema (swelling): histamine causes increased capillary permeability, allowing fluid, protein, and white blood cells (WBCs) to move into interstitial space
   4. Pain: nerve endings are irritated by chemical mediators (e.g., serotonin, prostaglandin, and kinins) and pressure from edema
   5. Loss of function: this occurs as protective response because of pain

GRIEVING PROCESS

BASIC CONCEPTS

A. Loss is experienced when something of value (e.g., object, person) is changed or gone
   1. Actual: can be validated by others (e.g., death of spouse)
   2. Perceived: experienced internally; cannot be verified by others (e.g., loss of youth)
   3. Anticipatory: occurs before the loss is experienced (e.g., scheduled amputation)

B. Grief is the response to an actual or perceived loss; bereavement is the emotional response to loss; mourning is the behavioral response to loss

THEORISTS: STAGES OF GRIEVING

A. Kübler-Ross: denial, anger, bargaining, depression, acceptance
B. Lindemann: somatic distress, preoccupation with image of the deceased, guilt, hostile reactions, loss of patterns of conduct
C. Engle: shock/disbelief, developing awareness, and restitution/resolution

GRIEVING PROCESS AND NURSING CARE

See Table 1-1

HEALTH-ILLNESS CONTINUUM AND REHABILITATION

A. Health-illness continuum: a concept reflecting the dynamic state of health in which one end of the continuum represents high-level wellness and the other death

B. Rehabilitation
   1. Assists clients in attaining their maximum level of wellness on the continuum after a negative change in health; involves establishing lost function while expanding, maintaining, and supporting the limited remaining function
   2. Focuses on interventions that improve the quality of life rather than saving life
   3. Involves the client, family, health care team, community, and society; not an isolated process
   4. Has social significance because health problems that cause disabilities that are costly both personally and economically affect an increasingly larger number of individuals
   5. Affects more individuals than ever before because of
      a. Advances in technology
      b. Increased survival rates from birth defects, traumatic injuries, and infection
      c. Aging of society and more chronic illness

TYPE OF CONDITION AFFECTING THE CLIENT

A. Acute illness: caused by a health problem that produces signs and symptoms abruptly and runs a short course; this illness may develop into a long-term illness

B. Chronic illness: caused by a health problem that produces signs and symptoms over time and runs a long course
   1. Exacerbation: period when a chronic illness becomes more active and there is a recurrence of pronounced signs and symptoms of the disease
   2. Remission: period when a chronic illness is controlled and signs and symptoms are reduced or not obvious
   3. Progressive degeneration: continuous deterioration or increased impairment of a person's physical state

Table 1-1 Grieving Process and Nursing Care		
Stage of Grieving	Client Response	Nursing Care
Denial, disbelief	Disbelief, intellectualization	Accept response but do not reinforce denial
Anger, hostility	Verbally hostile	Do not become defensive, meet client needs
Bargaining	Seeks to avoid loss, may express feelings of guilt	Listen attentively, refer to spiritual counselor if appropriate
Depression, sadness	Grieves about what may never be, may be verbal or withdrawn	Listen attentively, sit quietly, use touch if appropriate
Acceptance, resolution	Comes to terms with loss, may make future plans, may have decreased interest in people and surroundings	Be quiet but available, help family to accept client's behavior

C. Terminal illness: death is inevitable in the near future (needs are focused on hygiene and physical and emotional comfort)

LEVELS OF PREVENTIVE CARE

A. Primary prevention
1. Interventions aimed at health promotion; precedes disease or disability
2. Examples
   a. Following a heart-healthy diet
   b. Avoiding smoking
   c. Being immunized
   d. Maintaining ideal weight
B. Secondary prevention
1. Interventions directed at diagnosis and prompt intervention; prevents extension of disease or development of complications
2. Examples
   a. Performing monthly self breast and testicular examinations
   b. Getting tuberculosis skin tests
   c. Having a yearly Papanicolaou smear
   d. Scheduling routine tests for glaucoma
C. Tertiary prevention
1. Interventions that minimize the effects of long-term disease or disability; maximizes a person's potential after disease or disability occurs
2. Examples
   a. Adhering to rehabilitation programs after a brain attack or head trauma
   b. Following a cardiac rehabilitation program
   c. Learning to walk after an amputation or joint replacement

Basics of Nursing Practice

NURSING PROCESS

A. Assessment/Analysis
1. Types of data: objective (overt, measurable, detected by use of senses) and subjective (covert, feelings, sensations and symptoms verbalized by client)
2. Sources of data: client (primary); family/friends, health care team members, chart and other documents, textbooks (secondary)
3. Methods of data collection: interviewing, observation of nonverbal cues, congruency between verbal and nonverbal data, physical assessment (observation, palpation, auscultation, percussion) (Figure 2-1: Dimensions for gathering data for a health history)
4. Classification of data: screening, organizing, and grouping/clustering significant defining characteristics and related information
5. Identification of client's problem, concerns, or deficits that can be altered by nursing interventions
B. Planning/Implementation
1. Establish client outcomes
   a. Outcomes are stated as expected changes in the client's behavior, activity, or physical state
   b. Outcomes must be objective, achievable, and measurable, and include a realistic period for accomplishment to determine whether the outcome has been achieved
2. Client, family/significant others, and nurse collaborate with appropriate health care team members to formulate the plan to reach the identified outcome
3. Evidence-based practice
   a. Definition: clinical decision making based on research findings, experience, and client values
   b. Nurses need to evaluate and participate in research that improves the quality of nursing care
   c. Levels of evidence refer to the strength of support for a particular nursing strategy; the levels of support range from systematic review of all relevant randomized controlled trials (RCTs) to reports of a committee of experts
4. Actual administration of the planned care
C. Evaluation/Outcomes
1. Assess client's response to care
2. Compare actual outcome to expected outcome

3. If outcome is not reached, the previous steps must be examined to discover the reason
4. Plan of care may need to be revised
5. Priorities may need to be reordered because process of evaluation is ongoing

COMMUNICATION

BASIC CONCEPTS

A. Need to communicate is universal
B. Through communication, humans maintain contact with reality, validate findings with others to correctly interpret reality, and develop a concept of self in relation to others
C. Validation is enhanced when communication conveys an understanding of feelings
D. Communication is a behavior that is learned through the process of acculturation
E. Communication is the avenue used to make needs known and to satisfy needs

COMMUNICATION PROCESS

A. Requires a sender, message, receiver, and a response
B. Modes of communication
1. Verbal: related to anything associated with the spoken word; includes speaking, writing, the use of language or symbols, and arrangements of words or phrases; hearing is essential to the development of effective speech, because one learns to form words by hearing the words of others; examples include pace, intonation, simplicity, clarity, brevity, timing, relevance, adaptability, credibility, and humor
2. Nonverbal: related to messages sent and received without the use of words and is expressed through appearance, body motions, use of space, nonverbal sounds, personal appearance, posture, gait, facial expression, gestures, and eye contact; more accurately conveys feelings because behavior is less consciously controlled than verbal communication
3. Confusion arises when there is a difference between the verbal and nonverbal message received (lack of congruence in the overt and covert messages)

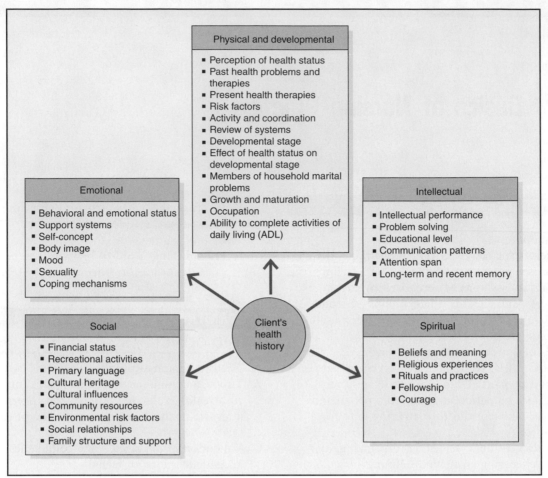

Figure 2-1 Dimensions for gathering data for a health history. (From Potter PA, Perry AG: *Fundamentals of nursing*, ed 7, St. Louis, 2009, Mosby.)

C. Themes of communication: recurring thoughts and ideas that give insight into what a client is feeling and tie the communication together
  1. Content: conversation may appear superficial, but careful attention to the underlying theme helps the nurse identify problem areas while providing insight into the client's self-concept
  2. Mood: emotion or affect that the client communicates to the nurse; includes personal appearance, facial expressions, and gestures that reflect the client's mood and feelings
  3. Interaction: how the client reacts or interacts with the nurse; includes how the client relates and what role is assumed when communicating with the nurse and others
D. Factors affecting the communication process include language, psychosociocultural influences, intellectual development, gender, values and perceptions, personal space (intimate, personal, social, and public), territoriality, roles and relationships, environment, congruence, and interpersonal attitudes
E. Barriers to communication
  1. Variation in culture, language, and education
  2. Problems in hearing, speech, or comprehension: ineffective reception or perception

  3. Refusal to listen to another point of view
  4. Use of selective inattention, which may cause an interruption or distortion of the message
  5. Environmental considerations such as noise, lack of privacy, room temperature
  6. Psychologic or physiologic discomfort, such as anxiety, hunger, pain

THE NURSE-CLIENT RELATIONSHIP

A. Phases in a therapeutic relationship
  1. Preinteraction: this phase begins before the nurse's initial contact with the client
    a. Self-exploration regarding misconceptions and prejudices that are socially learned and acknowledging one's own feelings, fears, personal values, and attitudes should occur before contact; self-awareness is a necessary task before one can establish mutuality with others
    b. Additional tasks of this phase include gathering data about the client and planning for the first interaction with the client
  2. Orientation or introductory: the nurse, who initially is in the role of stranger, establishes a trusting relationship with the client by consistency in

communication and actions; clients are never pushed to discuss areas of concern that are upsetting to them

   a. Introduction of nurse, nurse's role in treatment team, and purpose of meeting need to be clarified

   b. Contract outlining mutually agreed upon goals should be set

   c. Confidentiality issues must be discussed, and client rights must be upheld

   d. Termination begins during the orientation phase

3. Working: the nurse and the client discuss areas of concern, and the client is helped to plan, implement, and evaluate a course of action

   a. Transference and countertransference may become an issue

   b. Anxiety levels may rise, acting-out behaviors can and do occur, and denying is expected; resistance to change can be anticipated, identified, and addressed

   c. Problems should be discussed and resolved

   d. New adaptive behaviors can be learned

4. Termination: the end of the therapeutic relationship between the nurse and the client; the time parameters should be set within the first or second session; meetings spaced farther and farther apart near the end will facilitate termination

   a. Goals and objectives achieved should be summarized

   b. Adaptive behaviors should be reinforced

   c. Feelings and experiences for both client and nurse should be shared

   d. Rejection, anger, regression, or other negative behaviors may be expressed as a means of handling the loss (relationship termination)

B. Fundamental requirements of a therapeutic relationship; recognize that

1. Each client is unique and worthy of respect

2. A client needs to feel accepted

   a. Acceptance is an active process designed to convey respect for another through empathetic understanding

   b. Acceptance of others implies and requires acceptance of self

   c. To be nonjudgmental, one must become aware of one's own attitudes and feelings and their effect on perception

   d. Acceptance requires that clients be permitted and even encouraged to express their feelings and attitudes even though they may be divergent from the general viewpoint; setting limits might be required for inappropriate behavior in a manner that does not reject the client

   e. Acceptance requires a nonjudgmental environment

3. The high stress/anxiety of most health settings is created in part by the health problem itself; treatments and procedures; nontherapeutic behavior of personnel; strange environment; inability to use usual coping skills such as exercise or talking with friends; and change in lifestyle, body image, and/or self-concept

4. Previous patterns of behavior may become inadequate under stress: health problems may produce a change in family or community

5. Health problems may lead to change in self-perception and role identity

6. All behavior has meaning and usually results from the attempt to cope with stress or anxiety

7. Value systems influence behavior

8. Cultural differences are part of an individual

9. The personal meaning of experiences to clients is important

10. Clients have a potential for growth

   a. Clients need to learn about their own behavior in relation to others

   b. Exchanging experiences with others provides a new learning environment and the reassurance that reactions are valid and feelings are shared

   c. Participating in groups increases knowledge of interpersonal relationships and helps individuals to identify strengths and resources

   d. Identification of the client's strengths and resources helps to convey the expectations of growth

11. Behavioral changes are possible only when the client has other defenses to maintain equilibrium

12. Giving information may not alter the client's behavior

13. The use of defense mechanisms needs to be recognized

14. Maintaining confidentiality supports a trusting relationship

15. The use of therapeutic interviewing techniques communicates acceptance and supports expression of feelings

16. Nurses need to recognize and cope with their own anxiety

C. Support therapeutic communication

1. Maintain a nonjudgmental environment

2. Implement actions that support dignity and worth

   a. Maintain eye contact when communicating

   b. Use names rather than labels such as room numbers or diagnoses (e.g., approach the client as a person with difficulties not as a "difficult person")

   c. Provide for privacy

   d. Maintain confidentiality

   e. Be courteous toward the client, family, and visitors

   f. Permit personal possessions when practical

   g. Provide explanations at the client's level of understanding

3. Encourage participation in problem solving and decision making

4. Spend time with the client

5. Foster trust through honesty, consistency, reliability, and competence
6. Answer client call bell immediately

D. Use therapeutic techniques to facilitate communication
1. Reflection of feelings, attitudes, and words helps the client to identify feelings
2. Open-ended questions permit the client to focus on issues
3. Paraphrasing repeats the feeling or thought in similar words to convey that the message was understood or to provide an opportunity for clarification if necessary
4. Silence provides the nurse and client with the necessary time for reflecting about what is being discussed and time to formulate a response
5. Touch conveys caring, but its effectiveness can vary among cultures
6. Clarification is used to ensure that the message was understood as intended
7. Direct questions facilitate collection of objective data but may block expression of feelings; avoid unnecessary probing questions

E. Avoid use of nontherapeutic communication
1. Any overt/covert response that conveys a judgmental (approval or disapproval) or superior attitude
2. Direct personal questions that are probing or invasive
3. Ridicule, which conveys a hostile attitude
4. Talking about one's own problems and not listening, which conveys a self-serving attitude and loss of interest in the client
5. Stereotyping, which devalues the uniqueness of the client
6. Changing the subject, which demonstrates a lack of interest in the client's concerns
7. False reassurance
8. Minimization of concerns
9. Asking for explanations using the word "why"
10. Using clichés
11. Using terms of endearment such as "honey"
12. Defensive responses
13. Giving advice
14. Challenging the client to defend a position/feeling

TEACHING-LEARNING

A. Learning: involves a change in or acquisition of new behavior and takes place within the individual
1. Cognitive: knowledge
2. Psychomotor: skill performance
3. Affective: attitudes, emotions

B. Motivation: desire for change in response to an identified need
1. Intrinsic motivation: motivation that comes from within; preferred to extrinsic motivation
2. Extrinsic motivation: motivation that comes from outside the learner

3. Readiness to learn (physical, emotional, and cognitive)
a. Awareness of health problem and implications
b. Willingness to ask questions
c. Demonstration of indirect health-seeking behaviors
d. Absence of acute distress reactions (e.g., severe anxiety and pain inhibit learning)
4. Culture (e.g., language, values, beliefs)
5. Physical abilities (e.g., vision, hearing)
6. Cognitive ability (e.g., intelligence, developmental level, education)
7. Support systems

C. Teaching: activities that result in learning
1. Involve client and family to individualize teaching plan
2. Exhibit nonjudgmental attitude
3. Build on client's prior knowledge
4. Incorporate multiple strategies that involve multiple senses (e.g., discussion, demonstration, practice, role playing, discovery, audiovisual aids, computer-assisted instruction)
5. Establish short-term achievable learning objectives to maintain motivation
6. Use positive reinforcement; learning by success or positive rewards is preferable to learning by failure or negative consequences
7. Establish an environment conducive for learning (e.g., safe, limited noise, reduced distractions)
8. Evaluate client learning: observation of behavior; written tests; self reports

LEADERSHIP

TYPES OF LEADERSHIP

A. Leadership: influencing the actions of an individual or group toward specific goals; leadership style is affected by
1. Needs of the group members
2. Personality of the leader
3. Cultural climate of the organization

B. Types of leadership
1. Authoritarian or autocratic leader: uses leadership role for power; little communication and interrelating between leader and group; leader sets the goals, plans, makes the decisions, and evaluates the action taken
2. Democratic leader: fair and logical; uses the leadership role to stimulate others to achieve a collective goal; encourages interrelating among members; weaknesses, as well as strengths, are accepted; the contributions of all members are fostered and used; responsibilities for action taken are shared between the leader and the group
3. Emotional leader: reflects the feeling tones, norms, and values of the group
4. Laissez-faire leader: passive and nondirective; assumes participant-observer role and exerts little

control or guidance over group behavior; input and control are minimal

5. Bureaucratic leader: rigid; assumes a role that is determined by formal criteria or rules that are inherent in the organization; the leader is not emotionally involved and avoids interrelating with the group members

6. Charismatic leader: can assume any of the above behaviors, because the group attributes supernatural power to this person or the office and frequently follows directions without question

C. The effective leader modifies style to fit changing circumstances, problems, and people (e.g., autocratic style is appropriate in an emergency situation; democratic style is appropriate when group acceptance and participation are essential; and laissez-faire leadership is appropriate when group members are knowledgeable and capable of self-direction)

PRINCIPLES OF LEADERSHIP

A. Interpersonal influence depends on
  1. Knowledge of human behavior
  2. Sensitivity to others in terms of feelings, values, and problems
  3. Ability to communicate (see Communication)
B. Leader's success is influenced by the ability to respond to group needs and by members' perceptions of effectiveness
  1. The role serves the individual's or the group's needs; some roles are task-oriented and help the group accomplish goals; other roles are more process-oriented and help the group communicate effectively
  2. Power is a leader's source of influence
     a. Positional power: acquired through the position the leader has in the hierarchy of the organization
     b. Professional power: acquired through the knowledge or expertise displayed by the leader and/or perceived by the followers
  3. Leadership moves from one person to another as changes in the situation occur
C. Leadership process requires the use of critical thinking skills associated with problem solving
D. Leader as change agent: movement from goal setting to goal achievement involves change
  1. Need for change should be understood by those effecting the change, as well as those affected by the change
  2. Process of change includes communication, planning, participation, and evaluation by the individual or group affected
  3. Change is more acceptable when it is consistent with beliefs; when it has been planned; when it has not been dictated but follows a sequence of impersonal principles; when it follows a number of

successful rather than unsuccessful series of changes; when it is initiated after other changes have been absorbed rather than during the confusion of a major change; when it does not threaten security; and when the individuals or groups affected have participated in its creation

4. Resistance to change is normal and should be expected and addressed in planning

E. Leadership involves appropriate delegation (assignment of a responsibility/task to a competent subordinate while still retaining accountability); delegation involves "five rights"
  1. Right task: routine, noninvasive tasks (e.g., transferring, bathing, feeding)
  2. Right circumstance: medically stable client; resources available
  3. Right person: delegated task is within the subordinate's scope of practice
  4. Right direction/communication: clear, concise directions
  5. Right supervision/evaluation: monitoring action of subordinate and outcomes; providing feedback

NURSING PRACTICE AND THE LAW
TORTS AND CRIMES IMPORTANT TO NURSES

A. Torts
  1. Violations of civil law against a person or a person's property
     a. Commission: inappropriate action
     b. Omission: lack of appropriate action
  2. Unintentional torts
     a. Negligence: measurement of negligence is "reasonableness"; involves exposure of person or property of another to unreasonable risk for injury by acts of commission or omission
     b. Malpractice: negligence performed in professional practice; any unreasonable lack of skill in professional duties or illegal or immoral conduct that results in injury to or death of the client
     c. Examples of malpractice/negligence include leaving sponges inside a client; causing burns; medication errors; failure to prevent falls; incompetent assessment leading to subsequent inappropriate actions; improper identification of clients; and carelessness in caring for a client's property
  3. Tort is different from crime, but serious tort can be tried as both civil and criminal action
  4. Reasonableness and prudence in actions are usually determining factors in a judgment
  5. Nurses are responsible for their own acts; also, employers may be held responsible under the doctrine of *respondeat superior;* when responsibility is shared, nursing actions must lie within the scope of employment and legislation relating to nursing practice (such as Nurse Practice Acts)

6. Elements essential to prove negligence
   a. Legally recognized duty of care to protect others against unreasonable risk
   b. Failure to perform according to the established standard of conduct and care, which becomes breach of duty
   c. Damage to the client, which can be physical, emotional, and/or mental; no physical harm is necessary to establish liability for an intentional tort
7. Good Samaritan laws protect health care professionals who administer first aid as volunteers in an emergency unless there is gross negligence or willful misconduct; it is expected that the nurse meet a level of care expected of a reasonably prudent professional with the same education
8. Intentional torts occur when a person does damage to another person in a willful, intentional way and without just cause and/or excuse
   a. Assault: mental or physical threat; knowingly threatening or attempting to do violence to another person without actually touching the person; forcing a medication or treatment on a person who does not want it, but without touching the person
   b. Battery: actually touching or wounding a person in an offensive manner with or without the intent to do harm
   c. Fraud: purposeful false presentation of facts to create deception; includes presenting false credentials for licensure or employment
   d. Invasion of privacy: involves privileged communication and privacy
      (1) Encroachment or trespass on another's body includes any unwarranted operation, unauthorized touching, and unnecessary exposure or discussion of the client's case unless authorized
      (2) False imprisonment, even without force or malicious intent, includes the intentional confinement without authorization, as well as the threat of force or confining structures and/or clothing; the charge is not false imprisonment if it is necessary to protect an emotionally disturbed person from harming self or others
      (3) Defamation involves communications, even if true, that cause a lowering of opinion of the person; includes slander (oral) and libel (written, pictured, telecast), both of which are dependent on communication to a third party
B. Crimes
   1. Crime: an intentional wrong that violates societal law punishable by the state; the state is the complainant
      a. Felony: serious crime, such as murder, punishable by a prison term
      b. Misdemeanor: less serious crime that is punishable by a fine and/or a short-term imprisonment

   2. Commission of a crime requires committing a deed contrary to criminal law or failing to act when there is a legal obligation to act
   3. Criminal conspiracy occurs when two or more persons agree to commit a crime
   4. Giving aid to another in the commission of a crime makes the person equally guilty if there is awareness that a crime is being committed
   5. Ignorance of the law is usually not an adequate defense
   6. Search warrants are required before property can be searched
   7. Administration of narcotics by a nurse is legal only when prescribed by a physician; possession or sale of a controlled substance by a nurse is illegal
   8. If a nurse knowingly administers a drug that causes a major disability or death, a crime may be charged

CLIENTS' RIGHTS

A. Clients have the right to choose their own doctor, hospital, or medical insurance based on availability and ability to meet costs free of discrimination; to be given treatment in an emergency; to receive a proper standard of care; to execute informed consent; to decide whether or not to be used for research or teaching; to be treated in confidentiality; to have their personal property protected; and to refuse treatment
B. Statutory restrictions may be imposed on the client's rights (e.g., rights of clients to use specific health resources)
C. The U.S. government has set stringent rules about the use of human subjects in research

Informed Consent

A. Consent is essential for any treatment, except in an emergency in which failure to institute treatment may constitute negligence; routine procedures are covered by a consent signed at admission
B. In an emergency situation, two physicians may sign consent for the client when failure to intervene may cause death or when the common law permits administration of health care to unconscious or mentally incompetent persons in an emergency situation; if family members voice opposition, a court order may be required
C. Essential elements of legally effective consents are that the consent is voluntary, that it authorizes the specific treatment or care and the person giving the treatment or care, and that it is given by a person with the legal and mental capacity to consent based on an informed decision; clients 18 years or older and emancipated minors are legally able to give consent
D. The informed consent must include an explanation of the treatment to be done with a presentation of the advantages and disadvantages and a description of possible alternatives; there must be time for decision making with an absence of undue pressure; the explanation and decision making must occur before sedation is given

Death With Dignity: Legal, Ethical, and Emotional Issues

A. Death with dignity includes two fundamental factors: the individual has control over his or her own life, and the worth of the individual as a unique being is demonstrated through respect even after death

B. Laws must empower clients to have as much control as possible over their care and activities, recognizing that pain, helplessness, and hopelessness lead to despair

C. The ethical/medical problems that exist require the education of an interested public about advance directives through literature distribution and discussions, the use of quality management to include assessment of the appropriate care of terminally ill clients, and an increased availability and accessibility of palliative care services

D. Criteria of death: individual states have increasingly been forced to define death (many using signs of brain death as the indicator) and to define when death occurs

E. Do not resuscitate (DNR) status
   1. All health care agencies are required to have DNR procedures to meet accreditation standards
   2. DNR orders must be included in the client's medical record and periodically updated
   3. Most important factors considered are the client's wishes, the prognosis, the client's ability to cope, and whether CPR will provide benefits sufficient to make it worthwhile
   4. In many states, the right to request a DNR status is mandated within the Patient Care Partnership (previously the Patient's Bill of Rights) and hospitals must also provide education on the issue of DNR to clients and families
   5. A DNR order must be a team decision, and the client and the family must be included in the decision-making process

F. Advance directives
   1. Concepts
      a. Living wills allow clients to state their wish to die in certain situations and not have life prolonged by the use of medications, artificial means, or heroic measures; the living will sets forth the client's wishes regarding health care decisions; it includes which medical procedures are authorized or declined
      b. A health care proxy designates an agent to make health care decisions according to the client's plans or wishes; it includes the power of stopping or not giving treatment necessary for life when the client is unable to do so
   2. Advantages of living wills and health care proxies are that they permit expression of the client's preferences, promote communication between the client and caregivers, foster respect for the client as a person, and support the belief that clients have the right to self-determination

   3. The Client's Self-Determination Act of 1991 mandates that health care agencies receiving Medicare and Medicaid reimbursement advise clients of their right to advance directives

THE NURSE'S RIGHTS AND RESPONSIBILITIES

A. Practice in accordance with standards of the profession

B. Practice after licensure obtained; individual states define scope of professional practice
   1. Independent interventions: nurse-initiated actions based on the nurse's body of knowledge and scope of practice that do not require a physician's order (e.g., teaching, assessment, meeting hygienic needs)
   2. Dependent interventions: physician-initiated interventions or physician-established protocols that require specific nursing responsibilities and technical knowledge (e.g., administration of medications, tube feedings, and dressing changes)
   3. Collaborative interventions: actions the nurse performs that require interaction and coordination with other health professionals (e.g., coordinating intervention from physical therapy and social work to meet the needs of a client before discharge)

C. Intervene to protect clients from incorrect, unethical, and/or illegal actions by any person delivering health care

D. Participate in and promote the growth of the profession and own competence

E. Report any suspected child abuse to the appropriate authority; this reporting is mandatory and does not incur legal jeopardy

F. Code of ethics guides professional practice and reflects moral values of the group (e.g., American Nurses Association [ANA] Code of Ethics for Nurses)
   1. Basic terms: beneficence (promotion of good); nonmaleficence (avoidance of harm); justice (fairness); autonomy (self-determination); fidelity (faithfulness); veracity (truthfulness); accountability (answerable for one's own actions); responsibility (dependable role performance); confidentiality (limiting access to health information to maintain privacy)
   2. Code of ethics is broader and more universal than laws but cannot override laws
   3. Ethical issues become legal issues through court case decisions or by legislative enactment

G. Obtain professional liability insurance

MEDICATION ADMINISTRATION
DRUG EFFECTS

A. Desired effect (therapeutic effect): the action for which the drug is given

B. Adverse effect: a harmful unintended reaction

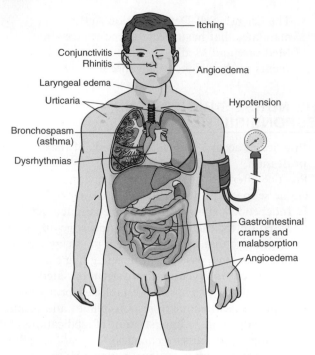

Figure 2-2 Type I hypersensitivity reactions. Manifestations of allergic reactions as a result of type I hypersensitivity include itching, angioedema (swelling caused by exudation), edema of the larynx, urticaria (hives), bronchospasm (constriction of airways in the lungs), hypotension (low blood pressure), and dysrhythmias (irregular heartbeat) because of anaphylactic shock, and gastrointestinal cramping caused by inflammation of the gastrointestinal mucosa. (From McCance KL, Huether SE: *Pathophysiology: the biological basis for disease in adults and children,* ed 5, St. Louis, 2006, Mosby.)

C. Toxic effect: a serious adverse effect that occurs when the plasma concentration of the drug reaches a dangerous, life-threatening level

D. Side effect: a response that is unrelated to the desired action of the drug

E. Cumulative action: the increased activity demonstrated by a drug when repeated doses accumulate in the body and exert a greater biologic effect than the initial dose

F. Drug dependence: the physical or psychologic reliance on a chemical agent resulting from continued use, abuse, or addiction

G. Idiosyncratic response: an individual's unique, unpredictable response

H. Paradoxical reaction: a response that contrasts sharply with the usual, expected response

I. Tolerance: the ability to endure ordinarily injurious amounts of a drug or the lowering of the effect obtained from an established dose that requires raising the dose to a possibly toxic level to maintain the same effect

J. Hypersensitivity: an excessive allergic reaction to an exogenous agent (e.g., drug, food) (Figure 2-2: Type I hypersensitivity reactions)
   1. Anaphylaxis: life-threatening episode of bronchial constriction and edema that obstructs the airway and causes generalized vasodilation, which depletes circulating blood volume; occurs when

an allergen is administered to an individual who has antibodies produced by prior use of the drug
   2. Urticaria: generalized pruritic skin eruptions or giant hives
   3. Angioedema: fluid accumulation in periorbital, oral, and respiratory tissues
   4. Delayed-reaction allergies: rash and fever occurring during drug therapy

K. Drugs and food may interact and alter the therapeutic effect adversely
   1. Antagonistic/inhibiting effect: one drug diminishing the effect of another
   2. Synergistic/potentiating effect: effect of two drugs is greater than either drug alone; often the dose must be reduced

FACTORS INFLUENCING DOSAGE AND RESPONSE

A. Individual factors: age, weight, gender, height, physiologic status, and genetic and environmental factors

B. Therapeutic index (TI) is used as a guide to the safe dosage range (a low TI provides a narrow margin of safety), but the individual factors must be considered

C. Concentration and duration of drug action are affected by
   1. Characteristics of the drug and the rate of absorption, distribution, biotransformation, and excretion
   2. Drug affinity for particular tissues, immaturity of enzymes required for metabolism of the drug, or depressed function of tissues naturally metabolizing or excreting the drug

D. Membrane barriers (e.g., placental or blood-brain) may block or selectively pass the drug from the circulating fluids to protected areas

NURSING RESPONSIBILITIES RELATED TO MEDICATION ADMINISTRATION

A. Recognize that the administration of medications is a dependent function requiring a legally written order that is not blindly followed

B. Make appropriate assessments before administering a drug
   1. Identify the medications the client was taking before admission and compare the list to the medications ordered after admission to the health care agency (drug reconciliation)
   2. Question the client regarding history of allergies
   3. Determine if client is taking any over-the-counter medications or herbal products that may interact with prescribed medications
   4. Establish whether drug is still appropriate based on the client's status
      a. Untoward or toxic manifestations to earlier doses
      b. Compatibility of medications with other medications or substances in the diet
      c. Serum drug levels for attainment of therapeutic level, toxic level, and peak and trough levels

C. Know the common symbols, equivalents, abbreviations, and calculation of dosage; The Joint Commission recommends that the following should not be abbreviated: every day, every other day, right or left eye, both ears or eyes, units, cubic centimeters, morphine sulfate, and magnesium sulfate; subcutaneous can be indicated by the abbreviation Sub-Q or subQ; use a "0" before a decimal point for numbers less than 1

D. Ensure that the right medication is given to the right client at the right time, in the right dose, by the right route; by the right technique, and with the right documentation; use of bar codes or two identifiers such as client's name, birth date, and/or hospital number have reduced incidence of medication errors

E. Teach the client about the therapeutic, side/adverse effects, and any other pertinent information related to the medication regimen; ensure adequate amount of medication is available

F. Recognize the client's right to refuse medication

G. Know common routes
  1. Oral
     a. Most common, convenient, and least expensive
     b. Absorption is slow; may be unpredictable; may cause GI irritation
     c. Preparations include tablets, capsules, pills, powders, or liquids
        (1) Sustained-release or enteric-coated preparations should not be crushed or broken
        (2) Suspensions should be shaken well before pouring
  2. Sublingual: placed under tongue; absorbed rapidly and directly into bloodstream
  3. Parenteral: requires use of sterile technique (Figure 2-3: Sites recommended for subcutaneous injection)
     a. Intradermal: small volume (usually 0.1 mL) under epidermis; most commonly used for allergy and tuberculin testing
     b. Subcutaneous: 0.5 to 2 mL into tissues just below skin
     c. Intramuscular: up to 3 mL into muscle depending on the site; sites include ventrogluteal, dorsogluteal (not generally recommended because of proximity to large blood vessels and the sciatic nerve), vastus lateralis, rectus femoris, and deltoid
     d. Intravenous: given directly into a vein by continuous infusion, bolus (push), or intravenous piggyback (IVPB)

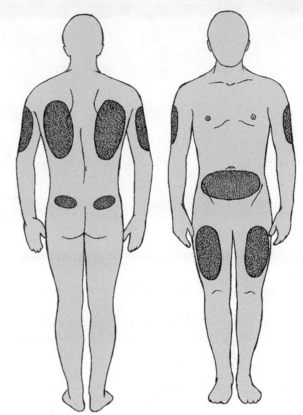

Figure 2-3 Sites recommended for subcutaneous injection. (From Potter PA, Perry AG: *Fundamentals of nursing,* ed 7, St. Louis, 2009, Mosby.)

  4. Transdermal (through the skin) preparations
  5. Inhalation: metered-dose inhaler or nebulizer
  6. Topical preparations for localized effect: skin, body cavities (bladder, eyes, ears, nose, vagina, and rectum); for systemic effect: rectal or nasal

H. Calculate dosage of ordered mediations; use the following formulas for ratio and proportion
  1.
  $$\frac{\text{Ordered dose}}{\text{Supplied dose}} \times \frac{\text{Desired amount}}{\text{Available amount}}$$

  2. Ordered dose:Supplied dose::Desired Amount:Available amount

I. Evaluate client's response to medication

J. Clearly and accurately record and report the administration of medications and client's response; follow standard practice when counting, wasting, or documenting controlled substances

Integral Aspects of Nursing Care

PAIN

OVERVIEW

A. Definition: universally unpleasant emotional and sensory experience that occurs in response to tissue trauma; referred to as the fifth vital sign; subjective

B. Types
1. Acute pain: mild to severe pain lasting less than 6 months; usually associated with specific injury; involves sympathetic nervous system response; this leads to increased pulse rate and volume, rate and depth of respirations, BP, and glucose level; decreased urine production and peristalsis
2. Chronic pain: mild to severe pain lasting longer than 6 months; associated with parasympathetic nervous system; client may not exhibit signs and symptoms associated with acute pain; may lead to depression and decreased functional status

C. Terminology
1. Pain threshold: minimum amount of stimulus required to cause sensation of pain
2. Pain tolerance: maximum pain a client is willing to endure
3. Referred pain: pain experienced in an area different from the site of tissue trauma (Figure 3-1: Common sites of referred pain)
4. Intractable pain: pain not relieved by conventional treatment
5. Neuropathic pain: pain caused by neurologic disturbance; may not be associated with tissue damage
6. Phantom pain: pain experienced in a missing body part
7. Radiating pain: pain experienced at the source and extending to other areas

REVIEW OF PHYSIOLOGY

A. Sensory neurons, nociceptors in the peripheral nervous system, are stimulated by biochemical mediators (e.g., bradykinin, serotonin, histamine, potassium, and substance P) when there is mechanical, thermal, or chemical damage to tissue (viscera do not have special neurons for pain transmission; receptors respond to stretching, ischemia, and inflammation)

B. Pain impulses are transmitted to the spinal column
1. A delta fibers: myelinated, large-diameter neurons
2. C fibers: unmyelinated, narrow-diameter neurons

C. Impulse enters at the dorsal horn and ascends the spinothalamic tract to the thalamus

D. Impulse travels to the basal areas of the brain and to the somatic sensory cortex

E. Endogenous opioids, such as endorphins, are released and bind to receptors to modify pain transmission

F. Gate-control theory suggests that stimulation of the large-diameter fibers can block transmission of painful impulses through the dorsal horn.

NONPHARMACOLOGIC PAIN MANAGEMENT STRATEGIES

A. Acupuncture: insertion of disposable needles into meridians (energy pathways) to change energy flow; may use heat or electric stimulation

B. Acupressure: uses finger pressure on meridians; less invasive but also less effective than acupuncture

C. Aroma therapy: plant oils applied topically or misted (e.g., ginger for arthritis or headaches, lavender to reduce anxiety associated with pain); have shown benefit

D. Distraction: focuses client's attention away from the pain

E. Heat and cold: diminishes pain experience by stimulation of large sensory fibers (gate-control theory); cold also promotes vasoconstriction, which helps reduce edema and promotes local anesthesia; heat also promotes vasodilation, which enhances healing

F. Imagery: calming, peaceful thoughts reduce pain perception

G. Massage: stimulates large-diameter fibers, blocking pain transmission

H. Reflexology: pressure applied to areas on feet, hands, or ears that correspond to specific body organ; may have calming effect through release of endorphins

I. Sequential muscle relaxation: promotes relaxation and decreases anxiety, thereby reducing the painful experience

J. Transcutaneous or percutaneous electric stimulation: stimulation of peripheral sensory nerve fibers blocks transmission of pain impulse

K. Therapeutic touch: use of hands near the body to improve energy imbalances

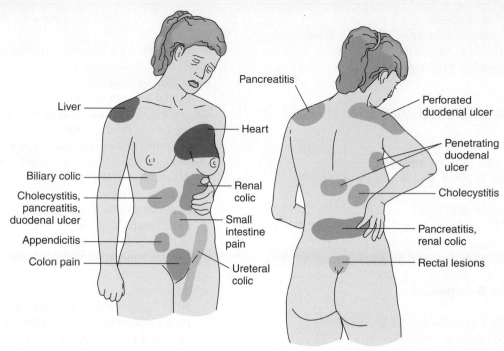

Figure 3-1 Common sites of referred pain. Note that the location of the pain may not be directly over or even near the site of the organ. (From Monahan FD et al: *Phipps' medical-surgical nursing: health and illness perspectives*, ed 8, St. Louis, 2007, Mosby.)

RELATED PHARMACOLOGY
Opioid Analgesics
A. Action
  1. Bind to opiate receptors in CNS
  2. Result in diminished transmission and perception of pain impulse
B. Examples: morphine sulfate, codeine, meperidine (Demerol), hydromorphone (Dilaudid), fentanyl (Sublimaze), propoxyphene (Darvon), hydrocodone (Vicodin); opioids can be administered via oral, buccal, nasal spray, IM, subcutaneous, IV, transdermal, epidural, or rectal routes depending on the drug
C. Major side effects
  1. Respiratory depression
  2. Lethargy
  3. Mental cloudiness
  4. Nausea and vomiting
  5. Hypotension
  6. Constipation
  7. Urinary retention
  8. Euphoria
  9. Allergic reaction
D. Nursing care
  1. Monitor for side effects, especially for respiratory depression (e.g., clinical indicators such as decreased respiratory rate, depth, and O₂ saturation)
  2. Institute measures to support respiratory function, such as turning clients frequently, encouraging coughing and deep breathing
  3. Ensure that an opioid antagonist (nalmefene, naloxone, or naltrexone) is available in case of overdose

  4. Ensure medications are renewed at required intervals
  5. Keep accurate count of opioids
  6. Use measures to promote elimination (e.g., fluids and roughage)
  7. Maintain therapeutic levels of medication
  8. Administer before pain becomes severe; medication less effective when pain is severe
  9. Teach client use of patient-controlled analgesia (PCA) pump (for management of severe pain); infusion pump is programmed for continuous basal dose, client-controlled bolus dose, and lockout time interval, allowing the client to control administration without overdose; may be intravenous, subcutaneous, or epidural
  10. Maintain client safety after administration of opioid analgesia
  11. Instruct client to keep the medication in a secure environment; dispose of excess doses down the toilet
Nonsteroidal Antiinflammatory Drugs (NSAIDs)
A. Action
  1. Act on peripheral nerve endings and decrease inflammatory mediators by inhibiting prostaglandin synthesis
  2. Have analgesic, antiinflammatory, and antipyretic effects
B. Examples: acetylsalicylic acid (aspirin), ibuprofen (Motrin, Advil), naproxen (Naprosyn) (see NSAIDs in under Related Pharmacology in Chapter 11)
C. Major side effects
  1. Gastrointestinal ulceration and bleeding (most common); tarry stools (melena)
  2. Nausea and vomiting

3. Constipation or diarrhea
4. Bone marrow depression and impaired coagulation
5. Visual disturbances, headache
6. Tinnitus (especially with aspirin)
7. Confusion
8. Seizures
9. Hypertension and fluid retention, especially with older adults

D. Nursing care
1. Administer with food or milk
2. Instruct client to drink 6 to 8 glasses of water during therapy
3. Monitor for side effects
4. Monitor CBC
5. Monitor liver and kidney function
6. Avoid use of alcohol or aspirin when taking other NSAIDs

Other Nonopioid Analgesics

A. Action
1. Analgesic effect may be caused by inhibition of CNS prostaglandin synthesis
2. No effect on peripheral prostaglandin synthesis; therefore no antiinflammatory action

B. Example: acetaminophen (Tylenol)

C. Major side effects (few, if therapy is short term; toxicity treated with acetylcysteine)
1. Hemolytic anemia
2. Hepatotoxicity
3. Seizures
4. Coma and death

D. Nursing care
1. Do not crush extended-relief products
2. Monitor CBC
3. Monitor liver function
4. Teach client to avoid alcohol and other over-the-counter products that contain acetaminophen (avoid exceeding the maximum dose of 4 g of acetaminophen daily)
5. Tylenol can be taken concurrently with anticoagulants

General Nursing Care of Clients in Pain

A. Assessment/Analysis
1. Client's description of pain: location; intensity as measured by a numeric rating scale of 0 to 10, Wong-Baker FACES Pain Rating Scale, FLACC Scale (Face, Legs, Activity, Cry, Consolability); character; onset; duration; and aggravating and alleviating factors
2. Associated signs and symptoms: increased vital signs (may be decreased with visceral pain), nausea, vomiting, diarrhea, diaphoresis
3. Nonverbal cues: distraught facial expression, rigid or self-splinting body posture
4. Contributing factors: age (older adults may expect pain or may fear addiction, so they may not complain), culture, past experience,

anxiety, fear, uncertainty (lack of information), fatigue
5. Effect of pain on client's activities of daily living (ADLs)

B. Planning/Implementation
1. Continue to monitor and document client's pain, associated symptoms, and response to pain management interventions
2. Use nonpharmacologic techniques
3. Administer prescribed analgesics and local anesthetics (see Related Pharmacology under Pain and under Perioperative Care)
4. Institute measures to counteract side effects of medications (e.g., increase fiber and fluids to prevent constipation associated with opioids)
5. Provide preoperative and postoperative care for clients requiring surgical intervention for pain management
   a. Rhizotomy: posterior spinal nerve root is resected between the ganglion and the cord, resulting in permanent loss of sensation; the anterior root may be cut to alleviate pain usually associated with lung cancer
   b. Cordotomy: to alleviate intractable pain in the trunk or lower extremities; transmission of pain and temperature sensation is interrupted by creation of a lesion in ascending tracts, percutaneously using an electrode or surgically via laminectomy
   c. Sympathectomy: to control pain of vascular disturbances and phantom limb pain
   d. Dorsal column stimulator and peripheral nerve implant: direct attachment of electrode to sensory nerve; a transmitter attached to the electrode is carried by client so electric stimulation can be administered as needed

C. Evaluation/Outcomes
1. Reports a reduction in pain of equal to or less than 4 on a numeric rating scale
2. Participates actively in ADLs

INFECTION

REVIEW OF PHYSIOLOGY (IMMUNITY)

A. Nonspecific immune response: directed against all invading microbes
1. Body surface barriers: intact skin and mucosa, cilia, and secretion of mucus
2. Antimicrobial secretions: oil of skin, tears, gastric juice, and vaginal secretions
3. Internal antimicrobial agents
   a. Interferon: substance produced within the cells in response to a viral attack
   b. Properdin: protein agent in blood that destroys certain gram-negative bacteria and viruses
   c. Lysozyme: destroys mainly gram-positive bacteria

4. Phagocytes (monocytes, macrophages): cells in the blood that ingest and destroy microbes; part of the reticuloendothelial system
5. Inflammatory response
   a. First stage: release of histamine and chemical mediators (e.g., prostaglandin, bradykinin) leads to vascular dilation and increased capillary permeability, resulting in signs of inflammation: pain, heat, redness, edema, and loss of function
   b. Second stage: exudate production
   c. Third stage: reparative phase
B. Specific immune response: directed against a specific pathogen (foreign protein) or its toxin; may be cell-mediated or humoral
1. Cell-mediated immunity
   a. Occurs within the cells of the immune system
   b. Involves T lymphocytes (T helper, T suppressor, T cytotoxic, lymphokines); each type plays a distinct role in the immune system
   c. Cluster designations: mature T cells carry markers on their surface that permit them to be classified structurally (e.g., CD4 cells associated with AIDS)
   d. Function of cell-mediated immunity
      (1) Protect against most viral, fungal, protozoan, and slow-growing bacterial infections
      (2) Reject histoincompatible grafts
      (3) Cause skin hypersensitivity reactions (e.g., tuberculosis [TB] screening)
      (4) Survey for malignant cells
2. Humoral immunity: concerned with immune responses outside of cell; involves B lymphocytes that differentiate into plasma cells and secrete antibodies
   a. Antigen: any substance, including allergen, that stimulates production of antibodies in the body; typically, antigens are foreign proteins, the most potent being microbial cells and their products
   b. Antibody: immune substance produced by plasma cells; antibodies are gamma globulin molecules; commonly referred to as immunoglobulin (Ig)
   c. Complement-fixation: group of blood serum proteins needed in certain antigen-antibody reactions; both the complement and the antibody must be present for a reaction to occur
   d. Types of immunoglobulins
      (1) Immunoglobulin M (IgM) antibodies: first antibodies to be detected after exposure to an antigen; protection from gram-negative bacteria
      (2) Immunoglobulin G (IgG) antibodies: make up more than 75% of the total immunoglobulins; highest increase in response to subsequent exposure to an antigen; only immunoglobulin that passes the placental barrier

      (3) Immunoglobulin A (IgA) antibodies: present in blood, mucus, and human milk secretions; play an important role against viral and respiratory pathogens
      (4) Immunoglobulin E (IgE) antibodies: responsible for hypersensitivity and allergic responses; cause mast cells to release histamine; protection from parasites
      (5) Immunoglobulin D (IgD) antibodies: help in differentiation of B lymphocytes
C. Types of immunity
1. Active immunity: antibodies formed in the body
   a. Natural active immunity: antibodies formed by the individual during the course of the disease; may provide lifelong immunity (e.g., measles, chickenpox, yellow fever, smallpox)
   b. Artificial active immunity: use of a vaccine or toxoid to stimulate formation of homologous antibodies; revaccination (booster shot) is often needed to sustain antibody titer (anamnestic effect) (Table 3-1: Immunization Schedule—United States 2007)
      (1) Killed vaccines: antigenic preparations containing killed microbes (e.g., pertussis vaccine, typhoid vaccine)

Table 3-1 Immunization Schedule—United States 2007

Vaccine	When to Administer	Dose/Route
Hepatitis B	First dose after birth before discharge Second dose at 4 weeks after first dose Third dose at $\geq$24 weeks	IM
Diphtheria, tetanus, and pertussis (DTaP)	Doses at 2, 4, and 6 months Fourth dose at 15-18 months Fifth dose at $\geq$4-6 years Tetanus and diphtheria toxoids (Td) recommended at 11-12 years and boosters every 10 years	IM
Haemophilus influenzae b (Hib) conjugate vaccine	Dose at 2 and 4 months	IM
Inactivated polio (IVP)	Dose at 2 and 4 months Third dose at 6-18 months Fourth dose at 4-6 years	Sub-Q
Measles, mumps, and rubella (MMR)	First dose at 12-15 months Second dose at 4-6 years	Sub-Q
Varicella (VAR)	First dose at 12-15 months Second dose at 4-6 years	Sub-Q
Pneumococcal (PVC)	Dose at 2, 4, and 6 months Fourth dose at $\geq$12 months	IM or Sub-Q
Influenza	First dose at 6 months Yearly $\geq$59 months	IM
Hepatitis A	Two doses, 6 months apart between 12 and 24 months	IM
Human papillomavirus 2	First dose between 11 and 12 years Second dose 2 months after first dose Third dose 4 months after second dose	IM
Rotavirus vaccine (Rota)	Three doses at 2, 4, and 6 months Do not initiate at $\geq$12 weeks and final dose given before 32 weeks	Oral

(2) Live vaccines: antigenic preparations containing weakened (attenuated) microbes; typically such vaccines are more antigenic than killed preparations (e.g., oral [Sabin] poliomyelitis vaccine, measles vaccine)

(3) Toxoids: antigenic preparations composed of inactivated bacterial toxins (e.g., tetanus toxoids, diphtheria toxoids)

2. Passive immunity: antibodies acquired from an outside source
   a. Natural passive immunity: passage of preformed antibodies from the mother through the placenta to the fetus or colostrum to neonate; during the first few weeks of life the newborn is immune to certain diseases to which the mother has active immunity
   b. Artificial passive immunity: injection of antisera derived from immunized animals or humans; provide immediate protection and also are of value in treatment (e.g., diphtheria antitoxin, tetanus antitoxin)

REVIEW OF MICROBIOLOGY

Pathology of Infection

A. Infection: invasion of the body by pathogenic microorganisms (pathogens) and the reaction of the tissues to their presence and to the toxins generated by them
   1. Pathogenicity: the ability of a microbe to cause disease
   2. Virulence: the degree of pathogenicity
B. Classifications
   1. Extent of involvement
      a. Local infection: limited to one locality of the body (e.g., boil), causing pain, swelling, and erythema; may have systemic repercussions such as fever, malaise, and lymphadenopathy
      b. Focal infection: a local infection from which the organisms spread to other parts of body (e.g., a tooth abscess that seeds organisms into the blood)
      c. Systemic infection: infectious agent is spread throughout the body (e.g., typhoid fever)
   2. Length of infectious process
      a. Acute infection: one that develops rapidly, usually resulting in a high fever and severe sickness; resolves in a short time
      b. Chronic infection: one that develops slowly, with mild but longer-lasting symptoms; sometimes an acute infection can become chronic
   3. Etiology of infectious process
      a. Primary infection: develops after initial exposure to pathogen, unrelated to other health problems
      b. Secondary infection: develops when pathogens take advantage of the weakened defenses resulting from a primary infection (e.g., staphylococcal pneumonia as a sequela of measles)

c. Opportunistic infection: develops when host defenses are diminished because of disease process or therapeutic modalities (e.g., vaginal yeast infection following antibiotic therapy)

C. Chain of infection
   1. Infectious agent
   2. Reservoir: source of almost all pathogens is human or animal
      a. Persons exhibiting symptoms of disease
      b. Carriers: persons who harbor a pathogen in the absence of a discernible clinical disease
         (1) Healthy carriers: those who have never had the disease in question
         (2) Incubatory carriers: those in the incubation phase of a disease
         (3) Chronic carriers: those who have recovered from a disease but continue to harbor pathogens
   3. Portals of exit: route by which microorganisms leave the body; blood and body fluids, skin, mucous membranes, and respiratory, genitourinary, and gastrointestinal tracts
   4. Mode of transmission
      a. Contact transmission (example: *Staphylococcus aureus*)
         (1) Direct: contact between body surfaces
         (2) Indirect: contact between susceptible host and a contaminated intermediate object (e.g., sink faucets)
      b. Droplet transmission (example: common cold) droplets from infected individual are propelled a short distance by coughing, sneezing, talking, or suctioning a client's respiratory secretions
      c. Airborne transmission (example: *Mycobacterium tuberculosis*) small droplet nuclei (5 μm or smaller) or dust particles that contain the pathogen remain suspended in the air for an extended period
      d. Common vehicle transmission (example: typhoid) microorganisms are transmitted by contaminated food, water, or equipment
      e. Vector-borne transmission (example: Rocky Mountain spotted fever) microorganisms are transmitted by vectors such as mosquitoes, flies, ticks, and rats
   5. Portals of entry: same as portals of exit (except skin: intact skin prevents infection)
   6. Susceptible host
      a. Developmental level: extremes of age
      b. Inadequate nutritional status
      c. Coexisting disease
      d. Decreased immune responses
      e. Surgical client; client in ICU

Types of Pathogens

A. Bacteria
   1. Unicellular microbes without chlorophyll
   2. Capsule: a material secreted by the cell, protects it from phagocytosis and increases its virulence (e.g., *Diplococcus pneumoniae*)

3. Spores: the inactive resistant structures into which bacterial protoplasm can transform under adverse conditions; under favorable conditions a spore germinates into an active cell (e.g., *Clostridium tetani*)
4. Examples of medically important bacteria
   a. Eubacteriales: divided into five families based on shape, Gram stain, and endospore formation
      (1) Gram-positive cocci
         (a) Diplococci: occurring predominantly in pairs (e.g., *Diplococcus pneumoniae*)
         (b) Streptococci: occurring predominantly in chains (e.g., *Streptococcus pyogenes*)
         (c) Staphylococci: occurring predominantly in grapelike bunches (e.g., *Staphylococcus aureus*)
      (2) Gram-negative cocci include *Neisseria gonorrhoeae* and *Neisseria meningitidis*
      (3) Gram-negative rods include enterobacteria such as *Escherichia*, *Salmonella*, and *Shigella* species
      (4) Gram-positive rods that do not produce endospores include *Corynebacterium diphtheriae*
      (5) Gram-positive rods producing endospores include *Bacillus anthracis*, *Clostridium botulinum*, and *Clostridium tetani*
   b. Actinomycetales (actinomycetes): moldlike microbes with elongated cells, frequently filamentous (e.g., *Mycobacterium tuberculosis* and *Mycobacterium leprae*)
   c. Spirochaetales (spirochetes): flexuous, spiral organisms (e.g., *Treponema pallidum*)
   d. Mycoplasmatales (mycoplasmas): delicate, nonmotile microbes displaying a variety of sizes and shapes
B. Viruses
1. Obligate intracellular parasite; can replicate only within a cell of another organism; composed of either ribonucleic acid (RNA) or deoxyribonucleic acid (DNA), not both
2. Examples of medically important viruses
   a. Human immunodeficiency virus: AIDS
   b. Hepatitis B virus (HBV): hepatitis type B
   c. Haemophilus influenza virus: influenza
   d. Varicella-zoster virus: chickenpox, herpes zoster, shingles
C. Fungi
1. A saprophytic organism that lives on organic material
2. Molds: fuzzy growths of interlacing filaments called hyphae; reproduce by spores
3. Yeasts: organisms that usually are single-celled and usually reproduce by budding
4. Examples of medically important fungi
   a. *Candida albicans*, a yeast: moniliasis ("thrush")
   b. *Histoplasmosis capsulatum*: histoplasmosis
   c. *Trichophyton rubrum*: tinea pedis ("athlete's foot")

D. Control of microorganisms
1. Medical asepsis (Table 3-2: Precautions to Prevent the Spread of Microorganisms)
   a. Standard precautions (e.g., handwashing, personal protective equipment)
   b. Transmission-based precautions (e.g., airborne, droplet, and contact)
2. Surgical asepsis
3. Disinfection: removal or destruction of pathogens
4. Sterilization: removal or destruction of all microbes
5. Antiseptic: inhibits microbial growth
6. Heat sterilization
   a. Moist heat
      (1) Steam under pressure (autoclave)
      (2) Boiling objects in water; some spores resist boiling
   b. Dry heat
7. Radiation: all types of radiation injurious to microbes
   a. Gamma rays: used to sterilize food and drugs
   b. Ultraviolet light: used to inhibit the microbial population of air in operating rooms, nurseries, and laboratories

RELATED PHARMACOLOGY
Definition of Terms
A. Bactericidal effect: destroys bacteria at low concentrations
B. Bacteriostatic effect: slows reproduction of bacteria
C. Superinfection (secondary infection): emergence of microorganism growth when natural protective flora is destroyed by antiinfective drug
D. Bacterial resistance: a natural or acquired characteristic of an organism, preventing destruction by a drug to which it was previously susceptible
Antibiotics
A. Description
1. Used to destroy bacteria or inhibit bacterial reproduction to control infection
2. Available in oral, parenteral, and topical forms, including ophthalmic and ear drop preparations
B. Antibiotic sensitivity tests: identify antibiotics that are effective against a particular organism
C. Mechanism of action: interferes with or inhibits cell-wall synthesis of RNA or DNA of pathogen
D. Examples
1. Penicillins: broad-spectrum amoxicillin (Amoxil) and penicillin G potassium (Pentids)
2. Cephalosporins: broad-spectrum cefazolin sodium (Ancef, Kefzol) and cephalexin monohydrate (Keflex)
3. Erythromycins: clindamycin HCl (Cleocin), azithromycin (Zithromax), erythromycin (E-Mycin)
4. Tetracyclines: broad-spectrum doxycycline (Vibramycin) and tetracycline (Achromycin, Sumycin)
5. Aminoglycosides: broad-spectrum gentamicin sulfate (Garamycin), neomycin sulfate (Mycifradin), streptomycin sulfate
6. Quinolones: broad-spectrum ciprofloxacin (Cipro) and levofloxacin (Levaquin)

Table 3-2 Precautions to Prevent the Spread of Microorganisms

Category	Indications	Conditions	Room	Gown
STANDARD PRECAUTIONS	Used for all clients regardless of diagnosis when there is contact with: 1. Blood 2. Body fluids 3. Secretions 4. Excretions 5. Nonintact skin 6. Mucous membranes	Used for all clients, particularly those with acquired immunodeficiency syndrome (AIDS) and hepatitis type B	Private room indicated if personal hygiene is inadequate	Indicated if soiling with blood, body fluids, secretions, or excretions is likely (e.g., during client care activities that are associated with splashes of blood); should be impermeable to liquids
Transmission-Based Precautions*				
AIRBORNE PRECAUTIONS	Prevents transmission of droplet nuclei ≤5 μm or dust particles that contain the pathogen; these nuclei and particles remain suspended in the air for an extended period	Tuberculosis, varicella, rubeola	Negative-pressure isolation room with at least six air exchanges per hour Door must be kept closed for negative pressure to be effective	See Standard Precautions
DROPLET PRECAUTIONS	Prevents transmission of particle droplets ≥5 μm that are dispersed by coughing, sneezing, talking, or suctioning; these droplets travel up to 3 feet before settling to the floor or other surfaces	*Haemophilus influenzae* type b in children, meningococci meningitis, *Streptococcus pneumoniae* pneumonia, mycoplasmal pneumonia, streptococcal pharyngitis, scarlet fever, pertussis, rubella, mumps, diphtheria	Private room; clients infected with the same organism may share a room	Don gloves when entering room
CONTACT PRECAUTIONS a. Direct b. Indirect	Prevents transmission of epidemiologically important microorganisms by direct contact with client's skin or indirect contact with contaminated items or surfaces	*Clostridium difficile* enteric infection, enterohemorrhagic *Escherichia coli*, *Shigella*, hepatitis type A, herpes simplex virus, cellulitis, scabies	Private room; clients infected with the same organism may share a room	Don gown when entering room

*Used in addition to standard precautions for clients with documented or suspected infection with highly transmittable or epidemiologically important pathogens.

7. Polymyxin group: polymyxin B sulfate (Aerosporin)
8. Vancomycin: examples: Lyphocin and Vancocin

E. Major side effects
 1. Depressed appetite (altered taste sensitivity)
 2. Nausea, vomiting (normal flora imbalance)
 3. Diarrhea (normal flora imbalance)
 4. Suppressed absorption of a variety of nutrients including fat; protein; lactose; vitamins A, D, K, and B_{12}; and the minerals calcium, iron, and potassium (normal flora imbalance)
 5. Increased excretion of water-soluble vitamins and minerals (normal flora imbalance)
 6. Superinfection (normal flora imbalance)
 7. Allergic reactions, anaphylaxis (hypersensitivity)
 8. Nephrotoxicity (direct kidney toxic effect)
 9. Tetracyclines
  a. Hepatotoxicity (direct liver toxic effect)
  b. Phototoxicity (degradation to toxic products by ultraviolet rays)
  c. Hyperuricemia (impaired kidney function)
  d. Enamel hypoplasia, dental caries, and bone defects in children under 8 years of age (drug binds to calcium in tissue)

10. Aminoglycosides
 a. Ototoxicity (direct toxic effect to auditory [eighth cranial] nerve)
 b. Leukopenia (decreased WBC synthesis)
 c. Thrombocytopenia (decreased platelet synthesis)
 d. Headache, confusion (neurotoxicity)
 e. Peripheral neuropathy (neurotoxicity)
 f. Nephrotoxicity (direct kidney toxic effect)
 g. Respiratory paralysis (neuromuscular blockade)
11. Vancomycin
 a. Ototoxicity (hearing loss)
 b. Nephrotoxicity (kidney damage)
12. Can render oral contraceptives ineffective

F. Nursing care
 1. Assess client for history of drug allergy
 2. Instruct client regarding
  a. How to take the drug (frequency, relation to meals)
  b. Prevention of emergence of resistant strains of microorganisms such as methicillin-resistant *Staphylococcus aureus* (MRSA) by completing prescribed course of therapy
  c. Symptoms of allergic response

Gloves	Mask and Eye	Handwashing	Precautions
Required for touching blood, body fluids, secretions, excretions, contaminated items or surfaces, mucous membranes, and nonintact skin	Required if splashes of blood, body fluids, secretions, or excretions are likely	Required after touching blood, body fluids, secretions, excretions, or contaminated articles whether gloves were worn or not Hands must be washed when gloves are removed, before contact with another client, and before touching a noncontaminated item or surface	Discard items contaminated with blood, body fluids, secretions, or excretions in a biohazard receptacle or handle equipment and remove personal protective equipment in a manner that will prevent transfer of microorganisms. Disinfect and sterilize reusable items. Dispose of used needles and other sharp devices in properly labeled, puncture-resistant container. Never recap used needles. Use ventilation devices instead of mouth-to-mouth resuscitation.
See Standard Precautions	See Standard Precautions Use particulate respirators such as HEPA mask (high-efficiency particulate air filter respirator) when client has a known or suspected diagnosis of tuberculosis People susceptible to varicella or rubeola should not enter the room	See Standard Precautions	See Standard Precautions. Confine client to room; transport only if absolutely essential; during transport have client wear a surgical mask to minimize droplet nuclei dispersal
Don gloves when entering room	Don mask and eye protection equipment when entering room	See Standard Precautions	See Standard Precautions. See Airborne Precautions
Don gloves when entering room; change gloves after contact with substances such as feces or wound drainage that have high concentrations of microorganisms	Don mask and eye protection equipment when entering room	See Standard Precautions	See Standard Precautions. Confine client to room. Transport only if absolutely essential; during transport maintain precautions to limit transmission of microorganisms. If possible, equipment such as a stethoscope or sphygmomanometer should be used only for the infected client

    d. Need to report side effects, including superinfection (vaginal itching, diarrhea, change in cough or sputum, white plaques in mouth); suggest ingestion of yogurt or food supplements containing *Lactobacillus acidophilus* when dairy products cannot be tolerated; suggest nutritional consultation when drug therapy may have an impact on client's nutritional status

    e. Monitor for and promptly report pain, changes in urinary or hearing function

3. Shake liquid suspensions to mix thoroughly

4. Administer most preparations 1 hour before meals or 2 hours after meals for best absorption

5. Administer at equal intervals around the clock to maintain blood levels

6. Assess vital signs during course of therapy

7. Tetracyclines

    a. Avoid use during last half of pregnancy or by children younger than 8 years

    b. Assess for potentiation if client is receiving oral anticoagulants

    c. Teach client to avoid direct sunlight

    d. Advise client to avoid dairy products, antacids, or iron preparations, because they reduce effectiveness

8. Aminoglycosides: assess for potentiation if client is receiving neuromuscular blocking agents, a general anesthetic, or parenteral magnesium; closely monitor renal and neurologic function

9. Vancomycin: peak and trough blood levels need to be assessed because it has a narrow therapeutic range; incompatible with heparin

10. Provide well-balanced diet and adequate fluids

11. Encourage use of alternate form of birth control (vs. birth control pills) during therapy

Antivirals

A. Description

1. Used to provide prophylaxis when exposure to viral infection has occurred; prevent entrance of the virus into host cells

2. Available in oral, parenteral (IV), and topical, including ophthalmic, preparations

B. Examples: acyclovir sodium (Zovirax), amantadine HCl (Symmetrel), and vidarabine (Vira-A)

C. Major side effects
1. CNS stimulation (direct CNS effect)
2. Orthostatic hypotension (depressed cardiovascular system)
3. Dizziness (hypotension)
4. Constipation (decreased peristalsis)
5. Nephrotoxicity (direct kidney toxic effect)
6. Local irritation (direct local tissue effect)
D. Nursing care
1. Assess vital signs during course of therapy
2. Support natural defense mechanisms of client; encourage intake of foods rich in the immune-stimulating nutrients, such as vitamins A, C, and E, and the minerals selenium and zinc
3. Encourage intake of high-fiber foods to reduce potential of constipation
4. Monitor disease symptoms and laboratory data
5. Evaluate client's response to medication

Sulfonamides
A. Description
1. Antiinfective drugs used primarily to treat urinary tract infections; substitute a false metabolite for *para*-aminobenzoic acid (PABA), required in the bacterial synthesis of folic acid
2. Available in oral, parenteral (IM, IV), and topical, including ophthalmic, preparations
B. Examples: sulfisoxazole (Gantrisin) and combination products such as sulfamethoxazole and trimethoprim (Bactrim, Septra)
C. Major side effects
1. Nausea, vomiting; decreased absorption of folacin (irritation of gastric mucosa)
2. Skin rash (hypersensitivity)
3. Malaise (decreased RBCs)
4. Blood dyscrasias (decreased RBCs, WBCs, platelet synthesis)
5. Crystalluria (drug precipitation in acidic urine)
6. Stomatitis (GI irritation)
7. Headache (CNS effect)
8. Photosensitivity (hypersensitivity)
9. Allergic response, anaphylaxis (hypersensitivity)
D. Nursing care
1. Assess client for history of drug allergy
2. Promote increased fluid intake
3. Caution client to avoid direct exposure to sunlight and dehydration
4. Assess vital signs during course of therapy
5. Maintain alkaline urine
6. Administer at routine intervals around the clock to maintain blood levels; obtain blood specimens for peak and trough levels
7. Monitor blood work during therapy; potential for megaloblastic anemia caused by folacin deficiency
8. Assess for potentiation of oral anticoagulant and oral hypoglycemic effects
9. Evaluate client's response to medication
10. Monitor for dysuria and urinary output

Antifungals
A. Description
1. Used to treat systemic and localized fungal infections; destroy fungal cells (fungicidal) or inhibit the reproduction of fungal cells (fungistatic)
2. Available in oral, parenteral (IV), topical, vaginal, and intrathecal preparations
B. Examples
1. Amphotericin B (Fungizone) and nystatin (Mycostatin, Nilstat): disrupts fungal cell membrane permeability
2. Fluconazole (Diflucan): disrupts fungal cell membrane function
3. Griseofulvin (Grisactin): disrupts fungal nucleic acid synthesis
C. Major side effects
1. Nausea, vomiting (irritation to gastric mucosa)
2. Headache (neurotoxicity)
3. Blood dyscrasias (effect on bone marrow)
4. Paresthesia (neurotoxicity)
D. Nursing care
1. Assess vital signs during course of therapy
2. Review proper method of application with client
3. Amphotericin B
   a. Use infusion control device for IV administration
   b. Protect solution from light during IV infusion
   c. Monitor blood work during therapy; potential hypokalemia as well as increased urinary excretion of magnesium
   d. Premedicate with antipyretics, corticosteroids, antihistamines, and antiemetics before IV administration
4. Griseofulvin
   a. Assess for antagonism if client is taking oral anticoagulants
   b. Instruct client to avoid direct exposure to sunlight
5. Evaluate client's response to medication

Antiparasitics
A. Description
1. Used to treat parasitic diseases; interfere with parasite metabolism and reproduction; helminthic (pinworm and tapeworm) as well as protozoal (amebiasis and malaria) infestations respond well to these drugs
2. Available in oral, parenteral (IM, subcutaneous [Sub-Q], IV), vaginal, and rectal preparations
B. Examples
1. Anthelmintics: mebendazole (Vermox) and pyrvinium pamoate (Povan)
2. Amebicides: chloroquine HCl (Aralen) and metronidazole (Flagyl)
3. Antimalarials: chloroquine HCl (Aralen), hydroxychloroquine sulfate (Plaquenil), and quinine sulfate (Quinamm)
4. Antiprotozoal: pentamide isoethionate (NebuPent, Pentacarinat, Pentam 300)
C. Major side effects
1. Anthelmintics
   a. Gastrointestinal irritation (direct tissue irritation)

b. CNS disturbances (neurotoxicity)
c. Skin rash (hypersensitivity)
2. Amebicides
a. Gastrointestinal irritation (direct tissue irritation)
b. Blood dyscrasias (decreased RBCs, WBCs, platelet synthesis)
c. Skin rash (hypersensitivity)
d. Headache (neurotoxicity)
e. Dizziness (CNS effect)
3. Antimalarials
a. Nausea, vomiting (irritation to gastric mucosa)
b. Blood dyscrasias (decreased RBCs, WBCs)
c. Visual disturbances (impairment of accommodation; retinal and corneal changes)
D. Nursing care
1. Administer drug with meals to decrease GI irritability
2. Assess vital signs during course of therapy
3. Monitor blood work during therapy
4. Instruct client regarding proper hygiene to prevent spread of disease
5. Use safety precautions (supervise ambulation) if CNS effects are manifested
6. Antimalarials: encourage frequent visual examinations
7. Antiprotozoals: bronchial constriction could interfere with desired effect of aerosol pentamidine; also assess for side effects of sudden severe hypotension
8. Evaluate client's response to medication
9. Instruct client to report unusual bruising or bleeding

General Nursing Care of Clients at Risk for Infection
A. Assessment/Analysis
1. Obtain history to identify factors affecting chain of infection
2. Obtain baseline vital signs
3. Monitor baseline WBC
4. Review results of culture and sensitivity tests
5. Review medication profile and check for allergies
B. Planning/Implementation
1. Decrease host susceptibility
a. Maintain skin and mucous membranes as first line of defense
b. Reinforce or maintain natural protective mechanisms such as coughing, pH of secretions, resident flora
c. Maintain nutrition/hydration and encourage rest and sleep to promote tissue repair and production of lymphocytes and antibodies
d. Educate client about immunizations
2. Use principles of asepsis
a. Medical asepsis: limits the growth and spread of microorganisms by confining them to a specific area
b. Surgical asepsis
(1) Absence of all microorganisms and spores; prevents microorganisms from entering a specific area
(2) Maintain surgical asepsis

(a) Prevent contact between sterile and nonsterile items
(b) Keep sterile objects within 1-inch border of sterile field
(c) Keep sterile items between waist and shoulder level
(d) Keep sterile field within field of vision
(e) Avoid contact between sterile items and wet porous surface; permeable surface enables contamination by capillary action
(f) Prevent exposure of sterile items to airborne contaminants
(g) Avoid reaching across sterile field
3. Limit or eliminate the microbiologic agent
a. Disinfection and sterilization
b. Administration of antimicrobial agents
c. Use of bacteriocidal agents (e.g., alcohol, povidone-iodine [Betadine])
4. Prevent transmission
a. Employ handwashing techniques
(1) Before client contact; after client contact; after contact with blood, body fluids, secretions, excretions, mucous membranes, or nonintact skin; before and after donning gloves
(2) Use friction, soap, and warm water to loosen and flush microorganisms
b. Use standard precautions (see Table 3-2); used for all clients regardless of diagnosis or presumed infectious status
c. Use transmission-based precautions (see Table 3-2); employed in addition to standard precautions; designed for clients documented or suspected to be infected with highly transmissible or epidemiologically important pathogens; precautions may be combined for diseases that have multiple routes of transmission
d. Correctly dispose of contaminated material
(1) Use impervious bags to dispose of contaminated material
(2) Do not recap or break needles after administering injections; use rigid container for disposal
5. Monitor vital signs: pulse rate—recognize pyrexia increases the work load of the heart; temperature—ensure consistency of measurement (Celsius or Fahrenheit); conversion from one temperature scale to another is accomplished by using the following formulas:
$$F = (\% \times C) + 32$$
$$C = (F - 32) \times \%$$
6. Employ measures to decrease body temperature as prescribed (tepid bath, antipyretics, hypothermia blanket); prevent shivering, which raises the basal metabolic rate (BMR) and thus temperature, pulse rate, and respirations
7. Ensure adequate fluid intake
8. Teach to avoid transmission and autoinnoculation, especially meticulous handwashing

C. Evaluation/Outcomes
1. Complies with medical regimen
2. Establishes health practices that enhance immunity
3. Maintains body temperature within normal range
4. Maintains fluid balance
5. Becomes infection free
6. Remains free from infection

FLUID, ELECTROLYTE, AND ACID-BASE BALANCE

FLUID AND ELECTROLYTE BALANCE

Fluids

A. The average adult contains about 40 L of water, comprising 60% of body weight (may be as high as 80% in infants and as low as 40% in older adults); the volume of fluid in different compartments remains relatively constant
1. Intracellular fluid (ICF) compartment accounts for two thirds of fluid
2. Extracellular fluid (ECF) compartment accounts for one third of fluid
   a. Interstitial compartment: 10 to 12 L
   b. Intravascular compartment: 3 L (plasma)
   c. Small fluid compartments: 1 L (e.g., aqueous humor; serous, cerebrospinal, pleural, and synovial fluid; lymphatic channels)
B. Intake must approximately equal output
1. Water enters the body through the digestive tract by liquids (± 1500 mL) and food (± 1000 mL); it is also formed by the metabolism of foods (± 200 mL)
2. Water leaves the body via the kidneys (± 1500 mL), intestines (± 200 mL), and insensible losses through lungs and skin (± 800 mL)
C. Solutions
1. Substances that dissolve in other substances form solutions
   a. Dissolved substance is called the solute
   b. Substance in which the solute is dissolved is called the solvent
2. Measures of concentration
   a. Osmolality: concentration of solute per kilogram (kg) of water (milliosmoles per kg)
   b. Osmolarity: concentration of solute per liter (milliosmoles per L)
3. Concentrations of solutions
   a. Dilute (hypotonic): small amount of solute in a relatively large amount of solvent (e.g., 0.45% NaCl)
   b. Concentrated (hypertonic): large amount of solute in a relatively small amount of solvent (e.g., 5% dextrose in normal saline)
   c. Isotonic solution: when the osmotic pressures of two liquids are equal, the flow of solvent is equalized and the two solutions are said to be isotonic to each other (e.g., 0.9% sodium chloride, which is normal saline)

Table 3-3 Serum Levels of Major Electrolytes

Ion	Range of Expected Values
Calcium (Ca^{2+})	4.5-5.5 mEq/L (ionized)
	8.5-10.5 mEq/L (total)
Chloride (Cl^-)	97-107 mEq/L
Magnesium (Mg^{2+})	1.5-2.5 mEq/L
Phosphorus (P^-)	1.8-4.6 mEq/L
Potassium (K^+)	3.5-5.0 mEq/L
Sodium (Na^+)	135-145 mEq/L

Major Ions (Electrolytes)

A. When an atom loses or gains an electron, it is no longer neutral but a charged particle called an ion
1. Conducts electric current when dissolved in water
2. Concentration of electrolytes in each fluid compartment remains relatively constant (Table 3-3: Serum Levels of Major Electrolytes)
B. Cations (positively charged ions)
1. Sodium (Na^+)
   a. Most abundant cation in extracellular fluid
   b. Sodium pump in most body cells pumps sodium out of intracellular fluid
   c. Action potential of nervous and muscle fibers requires sodium; sodium is basic to communication between nerves and muscles
   d. Helps to regulate acid-base balance by exchanging hydrogen ions for sodium ions in the kidney tubules; excess hydrogen ions (acid) are excreted
   e. Foods high in sodium include celery, processed foods, snack foods, condiments, smoked meats, and cheese
2. Potassium (K^+)
   a. Most abundant cation of intracellular fluid
   b. Potassium pump brings potassium into cells
   c. Resting polarization and repolarization of nerve and muscle fibers depend on potassium
      (1) If potassium concentration of extracellular fluid rises above normal (hyperkalemia), the force of the contracting heart weakens; with extremely high concentrations, the heart will not contract
      (2) If potassium concentration of extracellular fluid drops below normal (hypokalemia), the resting polarization in nerve and muscle fibers increases, resulting in weakness, eventual paralysis, and a flattened T wave on ECG
   d. Foods high in potassium include bananas, avocados, oranges, dates, apricots, cantaloupe, potatoes, and raisins
3. Calcium (Ca^{2+})
   a. Forms salts with phosphates, carbonate, and fluoride in bones and teeth to make them hard
   b. Required for correct functioning of nerves and muscles
      (1) If calcium concentration rises above normal levels (hypercalcemia), nervous system becomes depressed and sluggish

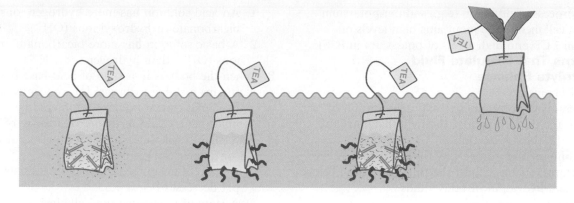

Diffusion
is the passage of particles through a semipermeable membrane. Tea, for example, diffuses from a tea bag into the surrounding water.

Osmosis
is the movement of fluid across a semipermeable membrane from a lower concentration of solutes to a higher concentration of solutes.

Diffusion and **Osmosis**
can occur at the same time.

Filtration
is the passage of fluids through a membrane.

Figure 3-2 Mechanisms of fluid and electrolyte movement. (Modified from Mahan KL, Escott-Stump S: *Krause's food & nutrition therapy,* ed 12, St. Louis, 2008, Saunders.)

    (2) If calcium concentration falls below normal levels (hypocalcemia), nervous system becomes extremely excitable, resulting in cramps and tetany

  c. Required for blood clotting, acting as a cofactor in the formation of prothrombin activator and thrombin

  d. Foods high in calcium include milk, dairy products, canned fish with bones, whole grains, legumes, and leafy green vegetables

 4. Magnesium (Mg^{2+})

  a. Cofactor for many enzymes involved in energy metabolism

  b. Normal constituent of bone

  c. Foods high in magnesium include nuts, soybeans, cocoa, seafood, whole grains, dried beans, and peas

C. Anions (negatively charged ions)

 1. Chloride (Cl^-)

  a. Most abundant anion in extracellular fluid

  b. Helps balance sodium

  c. Major component of gastric secretions

  d. Dietary source of chloride is salt

 2. Bicarbonate (HCO_3^-)

  a. Part of bicarbonate buffer system

  b. Reacts with a strong acid to form carbonic acid and a basic salt; limits drop in pH level (acidosis)

 3. Phosphate (PO_4^{2-})

  a. Part of phosphate buffer system

  b. Functions in cellular energy metabolism: phosphate + ADP → ATP (the energy currency of the cell)

  c. Combines with calcium ions in bone, providing hardness

  d. Involved in structure of genetic material, DNA and RNA

Fluid and Electrolyte Movement

(Figure 3-2: Mechanisms of fluid and electrolyte movement)

A. Osmosis: movement of fluid across a semipermeable membrane from a lesser concentration to a greater concentration of solutes; movement of fluid across the membrane continues until solution concentrations are equal

 1. Pressure forcing the fluid across the membrane is called osmotic pressure; osmotic pressure exerted by large protein molecules such as albumin is also called oncotic pressure

 2. Hypertonic solutions: when one solution has more osmotic pressure (is more concentrated) than another, it draws fluid from the other

 3. Hypotonic solutions: when one solution has less osmotic pressure (is more dilute) than another, it forces fluid into the other

 4. Albumin is most important in the development of the plasma colloid osmotic (oncotic) pressure, which helps control (through osmosis) the flow of water between the plasma and interstitial fluid; during a condition such as starvation, a fall in the albumin level of the blood results in a fall in the plasma colloid osmotic pressure, which leads to edema because less fluid is being drawn by osmosis into the capillaries from the interstitial spaces

B. Diffusion: movement of molecules from an area of higher concentration to an area of lesser concentration

C. Filtration: movement of fluid and solutes from an area of increased hydrostatic pressure to an area with less pressure; higher pressure within the arterial capillary intravascular compartment moves fluid from vessels to interstitial spaces

D. Active transport: movement of molecules across a cell membrane from an area of lower concentration to an area of greater concentration; requires energy to reverse natural process of diffusion (e.g., sodium-potassium pump on cell membrane maintains high levels of sodium in ECF and high levels of potassium in ICF)

Mechanisms That Regulate Fluid and Electrolyte Balance

A. Thirst mechanism
   1. Dryness of the oral mucosa and dehydration of cells in the thirst center of the hypothalamus give rise to the thirst sensation
   2. Stretching of the stomach by fluid and moistening of the oral mucosa cancel the thirst sensation before the actual hydration of body fluids
B. Osmoreceptor system
   1. Cells in hypothalamus synthesize antidiuretic hormone (ADH), which is stored in the posterior pituitary before release into circulation
   2. Osmoreceptors respond to dehydration by increasing the ADH released; this increases water reabsorption in the kidney tubules and decreases urinary output; the opposite occurs with overhydration
C. Aldosterone feedback mechanism
   1. Adrenal cortex secretes the mineralocorticoid hormone aldosterone when extracellular fluid sodium concentrations decrease or potassium concentrations increase; produced in response to renin release by kidneys when renal perfusion is decreased
   2. Aldosterone stimulates kidney tubules to reabsorb sodium; potassium reabsorption decreases as sodium reabsorption increases; occurs during stress, such as surgery
   3. This mechanism helps preserve normal sodium and potassium levels in extracellular fluid
   4. Secondary effects of aldosterone
      a. Chloride conserved with sodium
      b. Water conserved because it is reabsorbed by osmosis as tubules reabsorb sodium
D. Parathyroid regulation of calcium
   1. Parathyroid glands secrete parathormone when extracellular fluid calcium levels decrease
   2. Parathormone stimulates the release of calcium from bone, calcium reabsorption in the small intestine (vitamin D required), and calcium reabsorption in kidney tubules
   3. Increased extracellular fluid calcium levels result in decreased secretion of parathormone
E. Atrial natriuretic peptide (ANP)
   1. Released from atrial muscle cells in response to volume expansion and stretching of atrial wall
   2. Promotes excretion of sodium and water by kidney, and decreases thirst, resulting in decreased blood volume

ACID-BASE BALANCE

Basic Concepts

A. The pH denotes the strength of hydrogen (ions) in a solution

   1. An acid solution has more hydrogen ions (H^+) than bicarbonate or hydroxyl ions (OH^-)
   2. A basic solution has more bicarbonate or hydroxyl ions (OH^-) than hydrogen ions (H^+)
B. When the body is in a state of acid-base balance, it maintains a stable hydrogen ion concentration in the extracellular (intravascular and interstitial compartments) fluid in the narrow range of 7.35 to 7.45 (slightly alkaline); a pH of 7 or less or a pH of 7.8 or greater can result in death
   1. A state of uncompensated acidosis exists if blood pH decreases below 7.35
   2. A state of uncompensated alkalosis exists if blood pH increases above 7.45
C. Certain body fluids have a different pH: gastric juice has a pH of 1 or 2 caused by presence of hydrochloric acid; bile and pancreatic secretions are alkaline; urine may be acidic or alkaline

Acids

A. Acid: a compound that yields hydrogen ions when dissociated in solution
B. Properties of an acid
   1. Acts as an electrolyte in water
   2. Reacts with bases to form water and a salt (neutralization)
   3. In high concentration, destroys body tissues (corrosive)
C. Common acids
   1. Hydrochloric acid: secreted by the parietal cells of the stomach; transforms pepsinogen into pepsin, which is a protein-digesting enzyme of gastric juice
   2. Carbonic acid
      a. One form in which CO_2 is transported in the blood
      b. Part of the bicarbonate buffer system, which is the most important buffer system regulating the pH of body fluids
   3. Acetic acid: vinegar
   4. Lactic acid: builds up in muscle tissue during excessive exercise when there is insufficient oxygen for metabolism of carbohydrates to glucose and water

Bases

A. Base: a compound that combines with an acid to form water and a salt (neutralization)
B. Properties of a base: acts as an electrolyte in water; destroys body tissues (corrosive) in high concentrations
C. Common bases
   1. Magnesium hydroxide: water solution marketed under brand name Milk of Magnesia; antacid, mild laxative
   2. Aluminum hydroxide: component of many antacids
   3. Ammonium hydroxide: commonly used in household cleaners

Salts

A. Salt: the compound (besides water) formed when an acid is neutralized by a base

B. Properties of a salt: acts as an electrolyte in water; is crystalline in nature; "salty" taste
C. Common salts
   1. Sodium chloride: salt of extracellular compartment
   2. Potassium chloride: salt of intracellular spaces
   3. Calcium phosphate: bone and tooth formation
   4. Barium sulfate: when taken internally, outlines internal structures for x-ray studies
   5. Silver nitrate: antiseptic
   6. Ferrous sulfate: treatment of anemia
   7. Sodium bicarbonate: antacid

Mechanisms That Maintain Acid-Base Balance

A. Buffer mechanism: rapid first line of defense (takes seconds)
   1. Combine with relatively strong acids or bases to convert them to weaker acids or bases to prevent marked changes in blood pH levels
   2. Often referred to as a buffer pair because it consists of a weak acid and its basic salt
   3. Bicarbonate buffer system
      a. The most important buffer in body fluids because its components, base bicarbonate (HCO_3^-) and carbonic acid (H_2CO_3), are actively and constantly regulated by the action of the respiratory and urinary systems
      b. When the body is in a state of acid-base balance, blood contains 27 mEq base bicarbonate/L and 1.35 mEq carbonic acid/L; the base bicarbonate/carbonic acid ratio is 20:1
   4. Phosphate buffer system; more important in intracellular fluids, where its concentration is considerably higher
   5. Protein buffer system; hemoglobin, a protein buffer, promotes the movement of chloride across the RBC membrane in exchange for bicarbonate ions
B. Respiratory mechanism: second line of defense (takes minutes)
   1. CO_2 is carried in the body in the forms of carbonic acid and bicarbonate
   2. Controls rate of carbon dioxide exhalation from lungs
      a. When there are increased amounts of CO_2 in the body, the medulla is stimulated to increase the rate and depth of respirations
      b. When there are decreased amounts of CO_2 in the body, the rate and depth of respirations decrease
   3. During body metabolism, CO_2 is produced, which reacts with water to form carbonic acid, resulting in a decrease in pH (as acidity increases, pH decreases)
   4. In the lungs, carbonic acid breaks down into CO_2 and H_2O; increased exhalation of CO_2 results in an increase in pH (as acidity decreases, pH increases)
C. Renal mechanism: third line of defense (takes hours to days)
   1. The kidneys function to increase the blood's sodium bicarbonate content and decrease its carbonic acid content, thereby increasing the base bicarbonate/carbonic acid ratio and blood pH

Table 3-4 Primary and Compensatory Acid-Base Changes

	PRIMARY DISTURBANCE			COMPENSATIONS		
	pH	PCO_2	HCO_3^-	pH	PCO_2	HCO_3^-
Metabolic acidosis	↓	N	↓	↑-N	↓	↓
Metabolic alkalosis	↑	N	↑	↓-N	↑	↑
Respiratory acidosis	↓	↑	N	↑-N	↑	↑
Respiratory alkalosis	↑	↓	N	↓-N	↓	↓

From McCance KL, Huether SE, *Pathophysiology: the biological basis for disease in adults and children*, ed 5, St. Louis, 2006, Mosby.
HCO_3^-, Bicarbonate, N, normal; ↑-N, increase toward normal; ↓-N, decrease toward normal; PCO_2, partial pressure of carbon dioxide; pH, measure of the acidity or alkalinity of a solution.

   2. When there are high levels of hydrogen ions in the body, the kidneys
      a. Secrete hydrogen ions and reabsorb sodium ions
      b. Form ammonia that combines with hydrogen ions to form ammonium ions (NH_4^+); ammonium ions are excreted in the urine in exchange for sodium ions, which are reabsorbed into the blood
   3. When there are low levels of hydrogen ions in the body, the kidneys retain hydrogen ions to form bicarbonate

Acid-Base Imbalances

(Table 3-4: Primary and Compensatory Acid-Base Changes)
A. Respiratory acidosis
   1. Carbonic acid excess; increased retention of carbon dioxide; PCO_2 is greater than 45 mm Hg (hypercapnia)
   2. pH is below 7.35
   3. Common causes
      a. Inadequate ventilation (e.g., dyspnea)
      b. Respiratory obstruction: mechanical (e.g., tumors) or functional (e.g., asthma)
      c. Impaired gas exchange in the alveoli (e.g., emphysema)
      d. Neuromuscular impairment (e.g., spinal cord injury)
   4. Signs of respiratory acidosis: dyspnea, irritability, disorientation, tachycardia, cyanosis, and coma
   5. Compensatory mechanisms
      a. The urinary system excretes increased hydrogen ions to compensate for the respiratory system's inability to blow off CO_2
      b. The urinary system retains sodium to facilitate the body's attempt to increase sodium bicarbonate
      c. The rate and depth of respirations increase; however, this is inefficient because the primary dysfunction involves the respiratory system
      d. With chronic hypoxia, decreased oxygen levels become the stimulant to breathe; normally, elevated carbon dioxide levels stimulate breathing
B. Metabolic acidosis
   1. Base bicarbonate deficit; excess acid other than carbonic acid (a respiratory acid) accumulates

beyond the body's ability to neutralize it; bicarbonate level is below 22 mEq/L

2. pH is below 7.35
3. Common causes
   a. Cellular breakdown with increased ketones: e.g., starvation, terminal cancer, ketoacidosis, dieting
   b. Renal insufficiency: e.g., acute and chronic renal failure
   c. Direct loss of bicarbonate: e.g., loss of intestinal and pancreatic secretions via diarrhea
   d. Lactic acid accumulation from anaerobic metabolism
4. Signs of metabolic acidosis: weakness, headache, disorientation, deep and rapid breathing (Kussmaul's respirations), fruity odor to the breath, nausea and vomiting, and coma
5. Compensatory mechanisms
   a. The respiratory system compensates by hyperventilation in an attempt to blow off CO_2 and raise the pH
   b. The urinary system excretes hydrogen ions and retains bicarbonate

C. Respiratory alkalosis
1. Carbonic acid deficit; hyperventilation blows off excessive CO_2; PCO_2 is less than 35 mm Hg
2. pH is above 7.45
3. Common causes
   a. Hyperventilation related to anxiety/panic
   b. Excessive mechanical ventilation
4. Signs of respiratory alkalosis: deep and rapid breathing, lightheadedness, tingling and numbness, tinnitus, loss of concentration, and unconsciousness
5. Compensatory mechanisms: the urinary system retains hydrogen ions and excretes bicarbonate

D. Metabolic alkalosis
1. Base bicarbonate excess; bicarbonate level is above 26 mEq/L
2. pH is above 7.45
3. Common causes
   a. Loss of gastric juices (e.g., vomiting, nasogastric decompression, lavage)
   b. Excessive ingestion of alkaline drugs (e.g., sodium bicarbonate [baking soda])
   c. Potent diuretics may precipitate hypokalemia: in the presence of hypokalemia, the kidneys conserve potassium and excrete hydrogen, intracellular potassium moves into the interstitial compartment, and hydrogen moves into cells; as a result of these processes, the plasma hydrogen level is decreased and the base bicarbonate level is increased
4. Signs of metabolic alkalosis: muscle hypertonicity (tetany), tingling, tremors, shallow and slow respirations, dizziness, confusion, and coma

5. Compensatory mechanisms for metabolic alkalosis
   a. The respiratory system compensates by decreasing the rate and depth of breathing to retain CO_2 and decrease the pH
   b. The urinary system excretes sodium bicarbonate

General Nursing Care of Clients With Fluid and Electrolyte Problems

A. Assessment/Analysis
1. Obtain history to identify etiology of fluid and electrolyte imbalances (Table 3-5: Fluid/Electrolyte Imbalances: Etiology, Assessments, and Treatments)
2. Monitor vital signs
3. Evaluate skin turgor, hydration, and temperature
4. Auscultate breath sounds
5. Weigh client daily (1 L weighs 1 kg, or 2.2 lb)
6. Monitor intake and output (1 oz = 30 mL)
7. Measure abdominal girth or extremity circumference as necessary
8. Evaluate changes in behavior, energy level, and level of consciousness
9. Review laboratory tests: urinary specific gravity; serum pH and arterial blood gases; serum electrolytes; hematocrit; blood urea nitrogen; creatinine clearance

B. Planning/Implementation
1. Manage fluid and electrolyte intake
   a. Fluids may be encouraged to correct deficit (usually 3000 mL/day); may be restricted to prevent excess
   b. Nutritional intake can be increased or restricted to correct electrolyte disturbances (e.g., sodium, potassium, calcium)
2. Administer intravenous therapy
   a. Fluids
      (1) Dextrose in water
         (a) Provides fluid and limited calories (1 L of 5% dextrose provides 170 calories); may result in negative nitrogen balance if client is not eating
         (b) Used to correct dehydration, ketosis, and hypernatremia
      (2) Dextrose in sodium chloride (NaCl): used to correct fluid loss from excessive perspiration or vomiting and to prevent alkalosis
      (3) NaCl: used to manage alkalosis, fluid loss, and adrenal cortical insufficiency
      (4) Ringer's solution
         (a) Contains sodium, chloride, potassium, and calcium
         (b) Used to correct dehydration from vomiting, diarrhea, or inadequate intake
      (5) Lactated Ringer's solution
         (a) Contains sodium, chloride, potassium, calcium, and lactate
         (b) Lactate is metabolized by the liver and forms bicarbonate

Table 3-5 Fluid/Electrolyte Imbalances: Etiology, Assessments, and Treatments

Fluid/Electrolyte Imbalance	Etiology	Signs and Symptoms	Treatment
Extracellular fluid deficit	Decreased fluid intake Prolonged fever Vomiting Excessive use of diuretics Diabetes insipidus Hemorrhage (acute)	Increased thirst Dry skin and mucous membranes Increased temperature Flushed skin Rapid, thready pulse Decreased BP Increased Hct, Na^+, BUN, and specific gravity	Administration of hypotonic or isotonic fluids Vasopressin injection Transfusions if due to blood loss
Extracellular fluid excess	Heart failure Liver disease Malnutrition (decreased plasma protein) Renal disease Excessive parenteral fluids	Weight gain Crackles Edema Ascites Confusion Weakness Increased BP Bounding pulse Distended neck veins Decreased Hct	Administration of diuretics Fluid restriction Administration of colloids if kidney function normal Dialysis if impaired kidney function
Hypokalemia K^+ <3.5 mEq/L	Diarrhea Vomiting Diabetic acidosis Diuretics (loop or thiazide) Inadequate intake Excess aldosterone	Loss of muscle tone Cardiac dysrhythmias Abdominal distention Vomiting Decreased serum K^+	Parenteral/oral administration of potassium supplement Increased dietary intake of potassium
Hyperkalemia K^+ >5.0 mEq/L	Advanced kidney disease Severe burns or tissue trauma Excessive dosages of potassium Decreased aldosterone K^+-sparing diuretics	Cardiac irregularities Weakness Diarrhea Nausea Irritability Increased serum K^+	Administration of potassium-free fluids Dialysis Potassium-removing resin Diuretics Glucose and insulin
Hyponatremia Na^+ <135 mEq/L	Diuretics Electrolyte-free IV fluids Diarrhea GI suction Excessive perspiration followed by increased water intake	Abdominal cramps Seizures Oliguria Decreased serum Na^+ and specific gravity	Administration of IV solutions containing NaCl Administration of NaCl tablets Fluid restriction
Hypernatremia Na^+ >145 mEq/L	Diabetes insipidus Excess NaCl IV fluid intake Watery diarrhea Water deprivation Insensible fluid loss	Dry, sticky mucous membranes Oliguria Firm tissue turgor Dry tongue Increased serum Na^+ and specific gravity Weakness	Low-Na^+ diet Increased Na^+-free fluid intake
Hypocalcemia Ca^{2+} <4.5 mg/dL (ionized) Ca^{2+} <8.5 mg/dL (total)	Removal of parathyroid glands Administration of electrolyte-free solutions Alkalosis Acute pancreatitis	Tingling of extremities Tetany Cramps Seizures Hyperactive deep tendon reflexes Positive Chvostek's and Trousseau's signs	Oral or parenteral calcium replacement
Hypercalcemia Ca^{2+} >5.5 mg/dL (ionized) Ca^{2+} >10.5 mg/dL (total)	Hyperparathyroidism Prolonged immobility Bone cancer Excessive intake of Ca^{2+} or vitamin D	Flank pain (renal calculi) Deep bone pain Relaxed muscles Decreased deep tendon reflexes Constipation	Correction of primary problem Increased fluid intake Weight-bearing exercises

      (c) Used to correct extracellular fluid shifts and moderate metabolic acidosis

   (6) Plasma expanders

      (a) Used to increase blood volume in trauma or burn victims

      (b) Examples: albumin, plasma, Plasmanate, dextran, and hetastarch

      (c) Need to be administered slowly

  b. Regulation of IV flow rates

   (1) Manual regulation of gravity flow with clamp; the potential energy of fluid in an

IV bag is converted to kinetic energy when it flows through the tubing

Drop rate/min =

$$\frac{mL \text{ to be infused} \times \text{drop factor (drops per 1 mL delivered by tubing)}}{\text{Number of hours} \times 60 \text{ minutes}}$$

   (2) Use of infusion pump or controller: volume control usually is in milliliters per hour (follow manufacturer's instructions when setting desired rate of flow)
  c. Monitor client for complications
   (1) Infiltration
      (a) Catheter is displaced, allowing fluid to leak into tissues
      (b) Insertion site is pale, cool, and edematous; flow rate decreases
      (c) IV must be removed and restarted in a new site
   (2) Phlebitis
      (a) Vein is irritated by catheter or medications
      (b) Insertion site is red, painful, and warm; flow rate is decreased
      (c) IV must be removed and restarted in a new site; warm compresses are applied to inflammation
   (3) Circulatory overload
      (a) Flow rate exceeds cardiovascular system's capability to adjust to the increased fluid volume
      (b) Client exhibits dyspnea, crackles, distended neck veins, and increased BP
      (c) Rate is decreased to keep the vein open; physician is notified and diuretics administered as prescribed
   (4) Infection
      (a) Change of solution bag every 24 hours because risk for contamination is increased after this time; frequency of tubing and site change is based on agency policy (usually every 3 days)
      (b) Client exhibits signs of inflammation at insertion site, lymphatic streaking, and fever
 3. Administer pharmacologic agents
  a. Diuretics (e.g., thiazide, potassium-sparing, loop, or osmotic diuretics); see Related Pharmacology under Circulatory System in Chapter 6
  b. Electrolyte replacement (e.g., sodium chloride, potassium chloride, calcium gluconate)
  c. Reduce serum K^+ level: sodium polystyrene sulfonate (Kayexalate); insulin to carry K^+ into cells
 4. Provide care (e.g., skin care, safe environment) based on specific clinical findings

C. Evaluation/Outcomes
 1. Maintains fluid balance
 2. Maintains serum electrolyte levels within normal limits
 3. Maintains vital signs within normal limits

PERIOPERATIVE CARE

CLASSIFICATION OF SURGERY

A. Surgery may be classified as elective, diagnostic, urgent (emergency), ablative, palliative, or curative
B. Methods of surgical approaches have advanced to minimize tissue trauma, duration of anesthesia, and postoperative recovery time; and to improve client outcomes
 1. Laparoscopic surgery uses small incisions and fiberoptic instruments to perform surgery that in the past required larger surgical incisions and opening of the operative site; depending on site, may require insufflation of cavity with carbon dioxide to enhance visualization of structures, particularly for abdominal surgery (after abdominal insufflation, client may experience right shoulder or scapular pain postoperatively because of migration of carbon dioxide)
 2. Robotic surgery uses laparoscopic cameras that provide a three-dimensional view and robotic equipment that is manipulated by the surgeon at a surgical console; robotics improves precision and control
C. Ambulatory surgery
 1. Hospital-based out-patient settings
  a. Diagnostic workup several days before surgery
  b. Direct admission to ambulatory surgery
  c. Discharged from the postanesthesia or clinical unit the same day as the surgery is performed; if complications occur, the client is admitted to the hospital
 2. Private surgical offices
  a. Surgical procedures are performed in a private office, which has a surgical suite and surgical staff
  b. Preoperative workup is performed by hospital, physician, or clinic before surgery
  c. In-patient surgical care: client is admitted to the hospital setting for surgical care

RELATED PHARMACOLOGY

General Anesthetics
A. Description
 1. Used in combination to produce varying levels of loss of consciousness, amnesia, anesthesia, analgesia, and/or skeletal muscle relaxation
 2. Depress the CNS through a progressive sequence (four stages)

3. Neuromuscular blocking agents (depolarizing and nondepolarizing muscle relaxants): inhibit transmission of nerve impulses by binding with cholinergic receptor sites, antagonizing action of acetylcholine
4. Available in parenteral (IM, IV) and inhalation preparations
    a. Ultra-short-acting IV barbiturates are useful in the induction of anesthesia because they quickly penetrate the blood-brain barrier
    b. IV and IM nonbarbiturates produce a special type of anesthesia in which the client appears to be awake but dissociated from the environment, resulting in amnesia for the surgical experience
B. Examples
1. Inhalation anesthetics: halothane (Fluothane); nitrous oxide
2. IV barbiturates: high lipoid affinity provides prompt effect on cerebral tissue
    a. Methohexital sodium (Brevital)
    b. Thiopental sodium (Pentothal)
3. IV and IM nonbarbiturates: induce a cataleptic state and produce amnesia for the procedure
    a. Midazolam HCl (Versed)
    b. Combination product: fentanyl (Sublimaze) and droperidol (Innovar)
4. Conscious sedation: uses IV or nasal routes of sedation to depress consciousness but maintains airway and ventilations (e.g., midazolam [Versed], ketamine [Ketalar], and fentanyl [Sublimaze])
5. Neuromuscular blocking agents (depolarizing and nondepolarizing muscle relaxants)
    a. Pancuronium (Pavulon)
    b. Succinylcholine chloride (Anectine)
C. Major side effects
1. Inhalation anesthetics
    a. Excitement and restlessness (initial CNS stimulation)
    b. Nausea and vomiting (stimulation of chemoreceptor trigger zone in medullary vomiting center)
    c. Respiratory distress (depression of medullary respiratory center)
    d. Liver failure: halothane (Fluothane)
    e. Affinity for adipose tissue, resulting in prolonged effects
2. IV barbiturates
    a. Respiratory depression (depression of medullary respiratory center)
    b. Hypotension and tachycardia (depression of cardiovascular system)
    c. Laryngospasm (depression of laryngeal reflex)
3. IV and IM nonbarbiturates
    a. Respiratory failure (depression of medullary respiratory center)

b. Changes in BP: hypertension; hypotension (alterations in cardiovascular system)
    c. Rigidity (enhancement of muscle tone)
    d. Psychic disturbances (emergence reaction in recovery period)
4. Depolarizing muscle relaxants
    a. Hypotension (increased vagal stimulation; increased release of histamine; ganglionic blockade)
    b. Respiratory depression (neuromuscular blockade)
    c. Dysrhythmias (increased vagal stimulation)
D. Nursing care
1. Assess for allergies and other medical problems that could alter the client's response to the anesthetic agents
2. Have O$_2$ and emergency resuscitative equipment available
3. Assess vital signs before, during, and after anesthetic administration
4. Maintain a calm environment during induction of anesthesia
5. Use safety precautions with flammable agents
6. Protect client during this period because of decreased sensory awareness
7. Judiciously administer opioids in the initial postanesthetic period because of potential interaction with anesthetic agent
8. Provide care for the client receiving a depolarizing muscle relaxant
    a. Administer sedation; have emergency resuscitative equipment available
    b. Assess vital signs before, during, and after administration
    c. Administer under direct medical supervision
    d. Maintain airway and oxygenation
9. Maintain side-lying position to prevent aspiration after general anesthesia
10. Restrict oral intake after client has had general anesthesia until ability to swallow has returned

Local Anesthetics
A. Description
1. Used for pain control without rendering the client unconscious; useful for obstetric, dental, and minor surgical procedures; block nerve impulse conduction in sensory, motor, and autonomic nerve cells by decreasing nerve membrane permeability to sodium ion influx
2. Available in topical, spinal, regional, and nerve block preparations; epinephrine may be added to enhance the duration of the local anesthetic effect and to decrease regional bleeding
B. Examples
1. Topical: local infiltration of tissue (e.g., benzocaine; lidocaine HCl [Xylocaine], also used for nerve block; tetracaine HCl [Pontocaine], also used for spinal anesthesia and nerve block)
2. Spinal: injected into the subarachnoid space (e.g., lidocaine HCl [Xylocaine]; procaine HCl [Novocain], also used for nerve block)

3. Epidural: injected into the epidural space of the spinal column (e.g., bupivacaine HCl [Marcaine]; lidocaine HCl [Xylocaine])
4. Nerve block: injected at perineural site distant from desired anesthesia site (e.g., bupivacaine HCl [Marcaine]; chloroprocaine HCl [Nesacaine]; mepivacaine HCl [Carbocaine]; ropivacaine hydrochloride [Naropin])

C. Major side effects
1. Allergic reactions; anaphylaxis (hypersensitivity)
2. Respiratory arrest (depression of medullary respiratory center)
3. Dysrhythmias; cardiac arrest (depression of cardiovascular system)
4. Seizures (depression of CNS)
5. Hypotension (depression of cardiovascular system)

D. Nursing care
1. Assess for allergies and other medical problems that could alter the client's response to the anesthetic agent
2. Have O$_2$ and emergency resuscitative equipment available
3. Assess vital signs before, during, and after anesthetic administration
4. Protect anesthetized body parts from mechanical and/or thermal injury
5. Keep client flat for a specified period (usually 6 to 12 hours) after spinal anesthesia to prevent severe headache; avoid pillows; monitor for hypotension
6. Use safety precautions and maintain bed rest until motor and sensory function returns to lower extremities after spinal anesthesia
7. If local anesthetic is administered along a nerve via a pump for pain control, teach client how to use the pump; monitor for local anesthetic toxicity

Sedatives/Hypnotics

A. Description
1. Used for short-term treatment of clients with situational anxiety and insomnia
2. Act by depressing the CNS; produce sedation in small doses and sleep in larger doses
3. Available in oral, parenteral (IV, IM), and rectal preparations

B. Examples
1. Benzodiazepines: act on many levels of the CNS to produce short-term sedation, anxiolysis, and amnesia; used during diagnostic procedures (conscious sedation); midazolam (Versed), diazepam (Valium), temazepam (Restoril)
2. Barbiturates: depress CNS starting with diencephalon; sodium methohexital (Brevital), pentobarbital sodium (Nembutal), secobarbital (Seconal)
3. Nonbarbiturates: depress CNS and relax skeletal muscles; chloral hydrate (Noctec), hydroxyzine (Vistaril)

C. Major side effects
1. Drowsiness (depression of CNS)
2. Hypotension (depression of cardiovascular system)
3. Dizziness (hypotension)
4. Gastrointestinal irritation (local effect)
5. Skin rash (hypersensitivity)
6. Blood disorders (hematologic alterations)
7. Drug dependence
8. Barbiturates
   a. "Hangover" (persistence of low barbiturate concentration in body caused by decreased metabolism)
   b. Photosensitivity (hypersensitivity)
   c. Excitement in children and older adults (paradoxic reaction)

D. Nursing care
1. Avoid administration with other CNS depressants
2. Caution client to avoid engaging in hazardous activity; avoid concurrent use of alcohol; avoid long-term use
3. Assess for signs of dependence
4. Use safety precautions
5. Implement measures to promote sleep (back rub, warm milk, support bedtime rituals)
6. Instruct client to avoid placing medication within easy reach when in the home to prevent possible excessive intake while drowsy
7. Monitor blood work during long-term therapy
8. Administer controlled substances according to appropriate schedule restrictions

General Nursing Care of Clients During the Preoperative and Intraoperative Periods

A. Assessment/Analysis
1. Obtain history of current health problems and factors that may influence surgery, anesthesia, or recovery
2. Perform physical assessment to identify potential health problems
3. Determine client's understanding of disease and treatment plan
4. Identify client's emotional state and coping skills
5. Obtain comprehensive list of client's medications including herbal and vitamin supplements and over-the-counter agents

B. Planning/Implementation
1. Witness signing of the consent form by the client; the surgeon is responsible for explaining the reasons for and risks of the surgery; if the client appears not to understand, the nurse should inform the surgeon
2. Ensure that the client's identification band is in place and accurate; client verification must be implemented at each step of the preoperative, intraoperative, and postoperative phases of surgery
3. Follow agency policy to ensure that the operative site is identified and marked
4. Explain all procedures to the client and give reasons for them
5. Explain to the client what to expect in the operating room, postanesthesia unit, and/or

intensive care units, including use of anticipated equipment such as PCA pump
6. Allow the client and family time to ask questions about procedures and surgery
7. Allow and encourage the client to vent feelings about diagnosis and surgery
8. Provide a spiritual counselor if desired by the client
9. Provide perioperative teaching about ventilatory function: diaphragmatic breathing, coughing, incentive spirometry, splinting, and turning postoperatively
10. Teach the client physical exercises that will be used to promote circulation after surgery: leg exercises (dorsiflexion, plantar flexion, eversion, inversion), ambulation routines, isometric exercises
11. Inform the client to expect some discomfort after surgery and teach importance of requesting medication for pain or using client-controlled analgesia before pain becomes severe
12. Make certain that the history, physical examination results, recent laboratory tests, and chest x-ray report are entered on the client's record
13. Inform all members of the health care team of the client's allergies and other health problems, and prominently mark the chart
14. Implement preoperative preparation orders (e.g., enemas, douches, intestinal antibiotics for bowel surgery, and preoperative antibiotics)
15. Inform the client of dietary restrictions to prevent aspiration when having general anesthesia. Clients generally should refrain from eating a heavy meal 8 hours before surgery, a light breakfast up to 6 hours before surgery, and clear liquids 2 hours before surgery. Check with the anesthesiologist for specific instructions because some physicians may require clients to be NPO after midnight
16. Provide care for the client on the day of surgery
    a. Before surgery check the client's vital signs and assess overall physical status; record and report any deviations to physician
    b. Before surgery assess the client's emotional status; notify the physician if the client expresses an impending sense of doom
    c. Complete the preoperative checklist: such as presence of consent form, preoperative tests, and identification and allergy bands
    d. Provide hygiene and have the client void
    e. Remove any prosthetics such as dentures, contact lenses, and wigs
    f. Apply antiembolic stockings as ordered
    g. Arrange for insertion of any tubes as ordered: nasogastric tube, indwelling urinary catheter, intravenous line
    h. Administer prescribed preoperative medications as ordered (e.g., antianxiety agents, sedatives, opioid analgesics, anticholinergics)
    i. Provide for client safety after administering medications
17. Provide care for the client in the operative suite
    a. Assume role of client advocate during the intraoperative phase; identify client and operative site
    b. Complete preoperative checklist
    c. Perform skin preps as ordered (e.g., shaving, scrubs used for orthopedic surgery)
    d. Apply monitoring devices as needed
    e. Insert urinary retention catheter if ordered
    f. Allay client's anxiety; ambulatory surgical clients remain aware during most of their stay in the operating room because local anesthetics are frequently used
    g. Position and drape client for surgery
    h. Anesthesia is introduced to produce four stages of anesthesia
       (1) Stage 1: client becomes drowsy and loses consciousness
       (2) Stage 2: stage of excitement; muscles are tense, breathing may be irregular
       (3) Stage 3: depression of vital signs and reflexes; operation begins during this phase
       (4) Stage 4: complete respiratory depression
C. Evaluation/Outcomes
   1. Verbalizes fears concerning operative process
   2. Verbalizes understanding of postoperative interventions
   3. Demonstrates an understanding of preoperative teaching
   4. Remains free from injury

General Nursing Care of Clients During the Postoperative Period
A. Assessment/Analysis
   1. Verify patency of airway and maintain oxygenation
   2. Establish baseline vital signs, breath sounds
   3. Determine level of consciousness
   4. Observe tubes for patency and placement and drainage for characteristics
   5. Inspect dressing if present; mark borders of dressing if bleeding is identified with date and time; observe for frequent swallowing, spitting up, or vomiting of blood with oral or nasal surgery
   6. Determine if client has sufficient urinary output
   7. Assess for signs of wound healing after initial postoperative period
   8. Assess for complications (Figure 3-3: Potential problems in the postoperative period)
B. Planning/Implementation
   1. Provide immediate care in the postanesthesia care unit (PACU)
      a. Maintain airway and breathing (anesthesia depresses respiratory function)
         (1) Keep the artificial airway in place until gag reflex returns; suction client's airway before extubation to clear secretions as needed; after

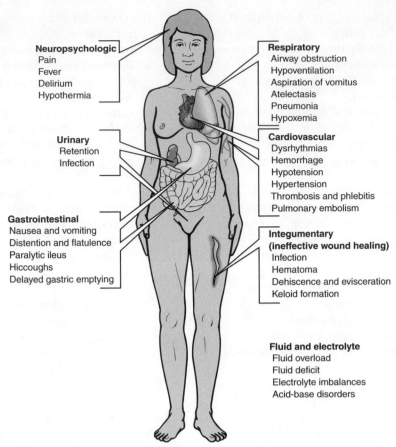

Neuropsychologic
Pain
Fever
Delirium
Hypothermia

Respiratory
Airway obstruction
Hypoventilation
Aspiration of vomitus
Atelectasis
Pneumonia
Hypoxemia

Urinary
Retention
Infection

Cardiovascular
Dysrhythmias
Hemorrhage
Hypotension
Hypertension
Thrombosis and phlebitis
Pulmonary embolism

Gastrointestinal
Nausea and vomiting
Distention and flatulence
Paralytic ileus
Hiccoughs
Delayed gastric emptying

**Integumentary
(ineffective wound healing)**
Infection
Hematoma
Dehiscence and evisceration
Keloid formation

Fluid and electrolyte
Fluid overload
Fluid deficit
Electrolyte imbalances
Acid-base disorders

Figure 3-3 Potential problems in the postoperative period. (From Lewis SL et al: *Medical-surgical nursing: assessment and management of clinical problems*, ed 7, St. Louis, 2007, Mosby.)

extubation assess for respiratory distress (restlessness, confusion, dyspnea, stridor, decreased oxygen saturation, inability to expectorate)

(2) Position client on one side with neck slightly extended to prevent aspiration and accumulation of mucous secretions

(3) Monitor the rate, rhythm, symmetry of chest movement, breath sounds, pulse oximeter, behavior, and color of mucous membranes

(4) Suction artificial airway and the oral cavity as needed to remove secretions

(5) Administer oxygen as ordered or needed; monitor oxygen saturation

(6) Encourage coughing and deep breathing as soon as the client is able to cooperate

b. Circulatory needs: anesthesia and immobilization during surgery may result in circulatory compromise

(1) Monitor the heart rate and rhythm as well as the blood pressure at frequent intervals, approximately every 5 minutes initially and then every 15 minutes

(2) Monitor peripheral circulation by noting the color, temperature, capillary refill

(may not be helpful if client has chronically poor circulation), presence of pulses to ensure tissue perfusion, and motor and sensory function

(3) Monitor for hemorrhage by measuring BP for hypotension, checking pulse rate for tachycardia, and observing and measuring wound drainage; frequent swallowing or expectoration of blood with surgery of the respiratory tract; report signs of hemorrhage immediately

c. Neurologic needs: medications and anesthetic agents depress the CNS

(1) Monitor the client's level of consciousness

(2) Monitor pupillary blink and gag reflexes

(3) Monitor motor and sensory status of extremities

(4) Call client by name; reorient to time, place, and situation

(5) Answer questions as honestly and simply as possible; repeat as needed

d. Wound care

(1) Note the location and size of the wound and the color, odor, amount, and consistency of drainage (Table 3-6: Types of Wound Drainage)

Table 3-6 Types of Wound Drainage

Type	Appearance
Serous	Clear, watery plasma
Purulent	Thick, yellow, green, tan, or brown
Serosanguineous	Pale, red, watery: mixture of clear and red fluid
Sanguineous	Bright red: indicates active bleeding

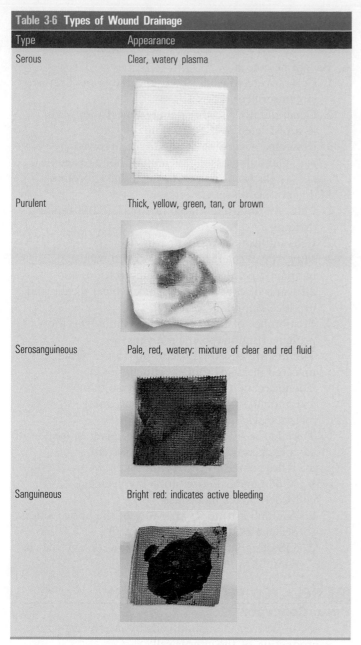

From Potter PA, Perry AG: *Fundamentals of nursing*, ed 7, St. Louis, 2009, Mosby.

    (2) Circle drainage on the dressing and mark time and date to allow for objective assessment

    (3) Reinforce postoperative dressings because surgeons generally perform the first dressing change

    (4) Protect the integrity of the surgical incision: instruct client how to sit up in bed, how to splint the incision, and how to maintain a clean, dry dressing

    (5) Protect client if wound edges separate (dehiscence) or abdominal organs extrude through incision (evisceration); supine position, cover site with sterile towel moistened with normal saline

  e. Care of drains and tubes

    (1) Maintain patency of tubing (e.g., gravity, negative pressure, instillation, or irrigation as indicated)

    (2) Attach tubing to appropriate collection containers; maintain negative pressure in portable wound drainage systems (e.g., empty when half full and compress before closing port; maintain surgical asepsis)

    (3) Monitor drainage for amount and color

  f. Fluid and electrolyte needs

    (1) Maintain IV therapy as ordered

    (2) Record intake and output accurately

    (3) Monitor for electrolyte imbalances

  g. Comfort needs

    (1) Assess the client's pain (e.g., location, intensity, duration, precipitating factors, and effectiveness of pain management)

    (2) Medicate as ordered to reduce pain and increase postoperative activities such as breathing, coughing, and mobility

    (3) Reinforce teaching about how to use PCA

2. Provide ongoing postoperative care

  a. Protect the client from injury

  b. Use pharmacologic and nonpharmacologic measures to manage pain

  c. Turn frequently; encourage deep breathing and coughing and use of incentive spirometer to prevent the development of atelectasis or hypostatic pneumonia; assess for diminished breath sounds in lower lobes

  d. Perform or encourage range of motion and isometric exercises and early ambulation to prevent phlebitis, paralytic ileus, and venous stasis; notify physician of complications

  e. Maintain patency of tubing (e.g., urinary catheter, gastric tube, T-tube, chest tubes, incisional drains) to promote drainage and maintain decompression to reduce pressure on suture line

  f. Use surgical aseptic technique when changing dressings or as necessary when irrigating tubing or emptying portable wound drainage systems to prevent infection

  g. Monitor intake and output to prevent dehydration, electrolyte imbalance, and urinary suppression or retention; encourage client to void; provide privacy

  h. Assess for urinary retention; client must void in 8 to 12 hours after surgery, or a catheter may be inserted

  i. Prevent constipation with fluid, fiber, and exercise; observe for abdominal distention; rectal tube (usually for 30 minutes) or Harris flush may be ordered to relieve flatus

  j. Regulate IV therapy to prevent overload or circulatory collapse; maintain hydration

k. Encourage client to support and splint the incisional site when coughing, moving, or turning to prevent tension on suture line

l. Position client as required by type of surgery to maintain alignment and prevent accumulation of fluid or blockage of the drainage tubes

m. Provide emotional support; assist client to cope with changes in body image

n. Provide for nutritional needs
   (1) Maintain IV therapy to provide water and electrolytes
   (2) Monitor parenteral nutrition (total parenteral nutrition [TPN] and peripheral parenteral nutrition [PPN]) (see Parenteral Replacement Therapy under Gastrointestinal System in Chapter 8)
   (3) Gradually increase oral intake as permitted (see Review of Diets under Gastrointestinal System in Chapter 8)
   (4) Provide for special nutritional needs
       (a) Protein: increased need caused by protein losses and the anabolism of recovery and tissue healing; approximate requirement for adult is 1.2 to 2 g/kg/day
       (b) Calories: adequate amount to supply energy and spare protein for tissue building
       (c) Vitamins and minerals: need for most will be increased after surgery and the nutrition program must be designed to ensure that individual requirements are met; zinc increases the strength of the healing wound (4 to 6 mg/day recommended); vitamin C required for collagen formation (500 to 1000 mg/day recommended)

o. When the ambulatory surgical client is stable, has retained foods, and has voided, reinforce postoperative teaching and discharge planning with client and family members; evaluate understanding of teaching

p. Provide client with discharge instructions and document; include wound care, hydration, nutrition, prevention/management of constipation, exercise, pain management, coughing and deep breathing

C. Evaluation/Outcomes
   1. Avoids respiratory complications
   2. Remains free of clinical indicators of infection
   3. Reports relief of pain
   4. Maintains integrity of surgical incision
   5. Maintains fluid balance
   6. Returns to expected volume of urinary output
   7. Returns to expected pattern of bowel function
   8. Demonstrates ability to care for self
   9. Copes with changes resulting from surgery

NEOPLASTIC DISORDERS
CLASSIFICATION OF NEOPLASMS

A. Benign neoplasia
   1. Cells adhere to each other, and the growth remains circumscribed
   2. Generally not life-threatening unless they occur in a restricted area (e.g., skull)
   3. Classified according to the tissue involved: e.g., glandular tissue (adenoma), bone (osteoma), nerve cells (neuroma), fibrous tissue (fibroma)

B. Malignant neoplasia
   1. Cells are undifferentiated (anaplasia) and rapidly dividing
   2. Cells infiltrate surrounding tissue
   3. May spread (metastasize) by direct extension, lymphatic permeation and embolization, and diffusion of cancer cells by mechanical means and produce secondary lesions
   4. Membranes of malignant cells contain specific proteins (tumor-specific antigens)
   5. Tumors are classified according to the tissue involved (e.g., glandular epithelial tissue [adenocarcinoma], epithelial surface tissue [carcinoma], connective tissue [sarcoma], melanocytes [melanoma])
   6. Tumors are often classified by a universal system of staging classification, the TNM system
      a. T designates a primary tumor
      b. N designates lymph node involvement
      c. M designates metastasis
      d. A number (0 to 4) after any of the above letters designates degree of involvement
      e. TIS designates carcinoma in situ, or one that is noninfiltrating

RELATED PHARMACOLOGY
Basic Concepts

A. Used to destroy malignant cells by interfering with reproduction of the cancer cell
B. Act at specific points in the cycle of cell division (cell-cycle specific) or at any phase in the cycle of cell division (cell-cycle nonspecific)
C. Affect any rapidly dividing cell within the body, thus having the potential for toxicity development in healthy, functional tissue (bone marrow, hair follicles, GI mucosa); to reduce the possibility of toxicity, combination therapy is often used
D. Available in oral, parenteral (IM, Sub-Q, IV), intraarterial, intrathecal, and topical preparations

Alkylating Agents

A. Cell-cycle nonspecific; attack the DNA of rapidly dividing cells
B. Examples
   1. Nitrosourea: carmustine (BCNU)
   2. Nitrogen mustard: chlorambucil (Leukeran), cyclophosphamide (Cytoxan)
   3. Inorganic heavy metal: cisplatin (Platinol)

Vinca Alkaloids

A. Cell-cycle specific; work during "M" phase; interfere with mitosis
B. Examples: vincristine (Oncovin), vinblastine (Velban)

Antibiotics

A. Cell-cycle nonspecific; inhibit DNA and RNA synthesis of rapidly dividing tissue
B. Examples: mitomycin (Mutamycin), plicamycin (Mithracin), doxorubicin liposome (Doxil), doxorubicin (Adriamycin)

Antimetabolites

A. Cell-cycle specific; inhibit protein synthesis in rapidly dividing cells during "S" phase
B. Examples: fluorouracil (5-FU), hydroxyurea (Hydrea), methotrexate (Mexate)

Hormones

A. Tissue-specific; inhibit RNA and protein synthesis in tissues that are dependent on the opposite (sex) hormone for development
B. Examples: androgens, estrogens (estramustine phosphate sodium [Emcyt]), progestins, steroids (prednisone [Meticorten]), hormone antagonists (mitotane [Lysodren]), cortisol antagonist, estrogen antagonist (tamoxifen citrate [Nolvadex]), and leuteinizing hormone–releasing hormone agonist (leuprolide [Lupron])

Monoclonal Antibodies

A. Exogenous antibodies produced in a laboratory by combining specific cancer cells with antibody-producing B cells; may be derived from different sources: mouse (murine), a combination of mouse and human sources (chimeric), or humanized
B. Examples: rituximab (Rituxan) for non-Hodgkin's lymphoma; trastuzumab (Herceptin) for certain types of breast cancer; gemtuzumab ozogamicin (Mylotarg) for leukemia; alemtuzumab (Campath) for B-cell chronic lymphocytic leukemia; ibritumomab tiuxetan (Zevalin) for B-cell non-Hodgkin's lymphoma; cetuximab (Erbitux) for advanced colorectal cancer; bevacizumab (Avastin) for colorectal cancer

Other Immune Agents

A. Involve introduction of noncancerous antigens or other agents into the body to stimulate production of lymphocytes and antibodies
B. Examples
   1. Bacille Calmette-Guérin (BCG) vaccine: provides active immunity
   2. Interferon alfa-2a (Roferon-A), interferon alfa-2b (Intron A): suppresses cell proliferation
   3. Filgrastim (Neupogen): granulocyte colony–stimulating factor

Miscellaneous Agents

A. Leucovorin calcium: a reduced form of folic acid; acts as an antidote to folic acid antagonists
B. Paclitaxel (Taxol): inhibits the reorganization of the microtubule network that is needed for interphase and mitotic cellular functions and causes abnormal bundles of microtubules during cell cycle and multiple esters of microtubules during mitosis

Common Combinations of Neoplastic Agents

A. CAP: cyclophosphamide (Cytoxan), doxorubicin HCl (Adriamycin), cisplatin (Platinol); lung cancer
B. CHOP: cyclophosphamide (Cytoxan), doxorubicin HCl (Adriamycin), vincristine sulfate (Oncovin), prednisone; non-Hodgkin's lymphoma
C. CMF (referred to as CMFP when prednisone is included): cyclophosphamide (Cytoxan), methotrexate (Mexate), fluorouracil (5-FU); breast cancer
D. COPP (referred to as A-COPP when Adriamycin is included): cyclophosphamide (Cytoxan), vincristine sulfate (Oncovin), procarbazine HCl (Matulane), prednisone; Hodgkin's disease
E. FAC: fluorouracil (5-FU), doxorubicin HCl (Adriamycin), cyclophosphamide (Cytoxan); breast cancer
F. MOPP: mechlorethamine HCl (nitrogen mustard, Mustargen), vincristine sulfate (Oncovin), procarbazine HCl (Matulane), prednisone; Hodgkin's disease relapse

Major Side Effects

A. Anorexia, nausea, vomiting, stomatitis (irritation of GI tract; quick uptake by rapidly dividing alimentary tract tissue)
B. Diarrhea (irritation of GI tract; quick uptake by rapidly dividing alimentary tract tissue); Oncovin: constipation, paralytic ileus
C. Bone marrow depression (quick uptake by rapidly dividing myeloid tissue)
D. Blood dyscrasias (neutropenia, anemia, and thrombocytopenia) resulting from bone marrow depression
E. Alopecia (rapid uptake by rapidly dividing hair follicle cells)
F. CNS disturbances (neurotoxicity)
G. Hepatic disturbances (hepatotoxicity)
H. Tumor lysis syndrome: release of large quantities of breakdown products, causing hyperkalemia, hyperuricemia, hyperphosphatemia, and acute kidney failure
I. Kidney failure (direct kidney toxic effect)
J. Cardiomyopathy (irreversible myocardial toxicity, congestive heart failure [CHF], ventricular dysrhythmias)
K. Metabolic abnormalities (hypercalcemia, hyperuricemia)
L. Allergic reactions, anaphylaxis with BCG vaccine

RADIATION

Purpose

A. Diagnosis
B. Treatment: curative, palliative, adjuvant (used in conjunction with chemotherapy or surgery)

Action
A. Disrupts tissue by altering function during DNA synthesis
B. Malignant cells, which rapidly reproduce, are most sensitive to radiation

Examples
A. Alpha particle: fast-moving helium nucleus; slight penetration
B. Beta particle: fast-moving electron; moderate penetration
C. Gamma ray: similar to light ray; high penetration
D. Gold (^{198}Au): effective for ascites; pleural effusions
E. Sodium iodide (^{131}I): effective for thyroid gland
F. Sodium phosphate (^{32}P): effective for erythrocytes
G. Proton therapy: accurately targets tumor, thereby minimizing collateral tissue damage

Methods of Delivery
A. External beam radiotherapy or teletherapy delivers radiation to a tumor by means of an external machine (cobalt or linear accelerator) at a predetermined distance
B. Internal radiation therapy or brachytherapy delivers radiation by systemic, interstitial, or intracavity means
   1. Systemic (metabolized) involves administration by intravenous or oral routes
   2. Interstitial involves implantation of needles, wires, or seeds into the tissue
   3. Intracavity radiation involves placing an implant into a body cavity and may require a surgical procedure

Major Side Effects
A. Localized skin irritation; erythema to moist desquamation
B. Vary based on site and size of treatment field
   1. GI tract: nausea, vomiting, diarrhea, xerostomia, mucositis, dysphagia
   2. Gonads: temporary or permanent sterility
   3. Bone marrow: leukopenia, thrombocytopenia, anemia
   4. Respiratory tract: pneumonitis, cough, dyspnea
   5. Genitourinary tract: cystitis, urethritis
   6. Heart: fibrosis
   7. Excessive tissue sloughing can cause hemorrhage, pain, and/or infection as a result of internal radiotherapy

BONE MARROW TRANSPLANTATION

Purpose
A. Treatment of hematologic cancer
B. Treatment of certain solid tumor recurrences that require ablative chemotherapy, which destroys bone marrow

Types
A. Autologous: bone marrow is removed from the client and reinfused after high-dose chemotherapy
B. Allogeneic: bone marrow from a donor with compatible human leukocyte antigen (HLA); infused after the client's own bone marrow is destroyed by chemotherapy or radiation
C. Syngeneic: bone marrow is obtained from an identical twin
D. Peripheral stem cell transplantation: after stem cell production is stimulated by administration of growth factor, cells are collected by apheresis and reinfused after high-dose chemotherapy

Major Side Effects
A. Infection, fever, chills
B. Venous occlusive disease: vascular injury to liver as a result of high-dose chemotherapy during first 30 days after transplant
C. Graft-versus-host disease: transplanted bone marrow activates an immune response against the recipient's tissue
D. Bone marrow: failure to respond and proliferate limits blood-making capacity, leading to hemorrhage and infection
E. GI: stomatitis, nausea, vomiting, diarrhea
F. Cardiovascular: hypotension, hypertension, tachycardia, chest pain
G. Respiratory: shortness of breath, pneumonia

General Nursing Care of Clients With Neoplastic Disorders
A. Assessment/Analysis
   1. Obtain a description of onset and progression of clinical indicators
   2. Perform physical assessment to determine general state of health and nutrition
   3. Determine client's understanding of disease and treatment plan
   4. Monitor laboratory values such as CBC, electrolytes, levels of tumor-specific antigens
B. Planning/Implementation
   1. Instruct client regarding special measures to limit infection (e.g., avoiding crowds; handwashing; the home environment is safer than the hospital environment, which contains pathogens to which the client is not usually exposed); instruct client to report temperature higher than 100° F (37.7° C)
   2. Use special measures to limit injury (e.g., gentle oral hygiene, use non–alcohol-based mouthwash; move slowly and support joints to prevent pathologic fractures)
   3. Explain side effects that influence appearance and encourage positive adaptations (e.g., purchase of wigs, scarves, hats)
   4. Administer medications to reduce or eliminate nausea, such as antiemetics
   5. Monitor blood values during therapy
      a. WBCs, RBCs, platelets
      b. Tumor markers: alpha fetoprotein—liver, testes; CA-125—GI, ovaries; carcinoembryonic antigen (CEA)—breast, colon, lung; prostate specific antigen (PSA)—prostate
   6. Administer prescribed colony-stimulating factors to increase the production of WBCs

and RBCs: epoetin alfa (Epogen) and filgrastim (Neupogen); administer prescribed platelet transfusions

7. Offer emotional support to client and family; answer questions and encourage verbalization of fears

8. Encourage delegation and organization of activity to conserve the client's decreasing energy

9. Encourage client to enroll in American Cancer Society's "Look Good, Feel Better" program

10. Support natural defense mechanisms of client; encourage intake of foods rich in the immune-stimulating nutrients, especially vitamins A, C, and E, and the mineral selenium, which is found in whole grains and seeds

11. Implement measures to support the patient's nutritional intake (Table 3-7: Nursing Care to Promote Nutritional Intake)

12. Encourage women of childbearing age to use birth control measures while receiving therapy because of mutagenic/teratogenic effects; avoid use of birth control pill

13. Counsel clients regarding use of sperm or ova harvesting if permanent infertility may result

14. Keep client well hydrated (3000 mL/24 hr); monitor I&O

15. Assess client for pain; administer analgesics or antidepressant to control the pain; provide for client comfort

16. Encourage client to become involved in decision making; support client's decisions whenever possible

17. Help client to discriminate between scientifically based therapy versus fraudulent therapy

18. Provide specific care for clients receiving chemotherapy
    a. Monitor IV infusion site for infiltration of chemotherapeutic agent capable of causing tissue necrosis (vesicant)
    b. Follow established protocols for handling chemotherapeutic agents and equipment to minimize exposure of the nurse
    c. Institute protective isolation if WBC count falls below 1000/mm^3
    d. Observe for signs of bleeding; avoid anticoagulants because of decreased platelets
    e. Prevent bleeding: avoid use of rectal thermometers, enemas, IM injections, and razor blades
    f. Monitor renal function for nephrotoxicity
    g. Monitor vital signs; monitor for cardiac toxicity
    h. Encourage client to check with physician before consuming OTC drugs, such as aspirin; avoid alcohol
    i. Follow sterile protocol when accessing an implantable port; use a noncoring needle (Huber) to access port; when not in use, monthly heparinization generally is implemented to maintain port patency

Table 3-7 Nursing Care to Promote Nutritional Intake

Symptom/ Problem	Nursing Care
Nausea	Encourage small, frequent meals
	Avoid high-fat, greasy foods
	Eat cool or room-temperature foods
	Avoid lying flat after eating
	Take medications after meal
Sore mouth or throat	Encourage soft, moist foods
	Avoid spicy or acidic foods
	Experiment with temperature of foods (avoid very hot or very cold foods; cool or room-temperature foods are best)
	Use nutrient- and energy-dense foods to maximize oral intake
Xerostomia (dry mouth)	Encourage foods that are moist or served with a sauce or gravy
	Consume liquids at mealtimes and extra fluids between meals
	Emphasize good oral hygiene: flossing, brushing, and rinsing; regular dental care
	Use fluoride gels or mouthwashes
	Consider prophylactic antifungal therapy
	Chew sugarless gum or suck mints
Difficulty with breathing	Use easy-to-eat foods
	Use nutrient- and energy-dense foods
Diarrhea	Encourage fluid and electrolyte replacement
	Consume low-insoluble and high-soluble fiber diet
	Consider possible benefits from low-lactose diet
	Low-fat diet may be indicated
	Avoid gas-causing foods and beverages
	Avoid caffeine
	Take medications after meal
Constipation	Increase fluid intake
	Increase dietary fiber intake
Inadequate oral intake	Consume nutrient- and energy-dense foods, including nutritional supplements
	Consume small, frequent meals and snacks
	Consider alternative nutrition support or appetite stimulant such as Megace or Marinol
Fatigue	Obtain adequate sleep, relaxation, exercise
	Consume adequate diet, especially foods rich in vitamins B$_{12}$, A, C, folate, and carotene or zinc; inadequate amounts may cause fatigue (Coodley et al, 1993; Tang et al, 1996)
	Avoid caffeine, alcohol, cigarette smoking, and recreational drug use
	Avoid stress and treatment of anxiety or depression
	Identify and manage possible causes for anemia: medications—AZT, Bactrim, dapsone, ganciclovir, interferon, pyrimethamine; other causes of anemia—alcohol abuse, bleeding, Mycobacterium avium complex, tuberculosis, fungal infections, cytomegalovirus
	Check lactic acid levels for indications of mitochondrial toxicity
Body cell mass loss	Consume adequate diet
	Perform resistance exercises
	Correct for testosterone deficiency
	Consider anabolic agents (prescription from physician)

Modified from Mahan LK, Escott-Stump S: *Krause's food, nutrition, & diet therapy,* ed 12, St. Louis, 2008, Saunders.

19. Provide specific care for clients receiving external radiation
    a. Assess skin for erythema or moist desquamation; avoid creams, soaps, powders, cosmetics, perfumes, and deodorants in the area during the treatment periods
    b. Instruct client to wear loose-fitting cotton clothing; protect skin from sunlight

c. Promote the use of gentle detergents (Dreft or Ivory Snow) to wash clothing

d. Avoid during treatment period: sources of heat or cold (heating pads, sunlamps, ice bags, cold weather); salt water; chlorinated pools; shaving hair in treatment field

e. Apply a nonadherent dressing to areas of skin breakdown

f. Reassure others that the client will not be a source of radiation

20. Provide specific care for clients receiving internal radiation

a. Explain the procedures involved and the side effects that may occur

b. Explain the need for isolation; explain to client and visitors that the amount of time visitors can spend in the room and how close they can be to the client will be limited to avoid overexposure to radiation; restrict children and pregnant women from visiting; use dosimeter badge to monitor exposure

c. Inspect the implant for proper positioning and prevent dislodgement of intercavity radiation implants to avoid irradiation of adjacent healthy tissue (e.g., bed rest, urinary retention catheter, low-residue diet, antidiarrheal agents)

d. Use principles of time, distance, and shielding to minimize staff exposure

e. Provide only necessary hygiene while implant is in place

f. Ascertain if body excreta has to be placed in lead containers for disposal when systemic metabolized radiation is used

g. If radiation source becomes dislodged: use long-handled forceps to place in lead container to prevent contamination of environment; immediately inform radiation therapist and radiation safety officer

h. Radiation for prostate cancer: assess for signs of bladder irritability such as nocturia, urgency, dysuria

i. Radiation of cervix: keep supine with head of bed flat or only slightly elevated, urinary catheter, low-residue diet

21. Provide specific care for clients receiving radiation via an unsealed source (IV, orally, or direct instillation into body cavity)

a. Isotope may be excreted in body waste: instruct client to flush toilet several times after each use for several days; additional precautions may be necessary depending on radioisotope used

b. Remove trash when client is discharged

c. Use paper plates and disposable utensils

22. Begin palliative care early in cancer treatment

23. Provide information about and support the choice of hospice care when curative options are exhausted: provide multidisciplinary services to support quality rather than quantity of remaining life (e.g., pain management, spiritual support)

C. Evaluation/Outcomes

1. Remains free from infection

2. Verbalizes feelings about disease and treatment

3. Maintains skin and mucous membrane integrity

4. Maintains body weight within expected range

5. Verbalizes details concerning self-care related to treatment regimen

EMERGENCY SITUATIONS

CONCEPTS RELATED TO FIRST AID

A. Maintain or establish the ABCs: Airway, Breathing, Circulation

B. Provide for physical safety

1. Remove client from immediate danger

2. Control bleeding

3. Avoid unnecessary movement of spinal column or extremities; use neck brace and back board; consider all clients experiencing trauma to have an unstable spine until this is ruled out with a radiograph

4. Monitor level of consciousness

C. Establish priority for care

1. Triage: system of client evaluation to establish priorities and assign appropriate treatment or personnel

2. Determination of priority

a. Emergency situations: greatest risk receives care first

b. Major disasters: classification based on principles to benefit the largest number; those requiring highly specialized care may be given minimal or no care; those requiring minimal care to save their lives or to be available to help others should be treated first; the Simple Triage And Rapid Transport (START) system can be used to categorize clients

(1) Red: critically ill clients that need immediate care

(2) Yellow: injured clients whose medical care needs can be delayed

(3) Green: clients who can ambulate and care for their own injuries

(4) Black: clients with catastrophic injuries who are expected to die

D. Offer psychologic support

1. Reduce panic to prevent its spread

2. Establish and maintain open communication with the client and family to mediate feelings of loss of control

3. Allow contact between the client and family as soon as feasible

SPECIFIC EMERGENCIES

A. Near-drowning
1. Assessment
   a. Possible airway obstruction from bronchospasm
   b. Adventitious or absent breath sounds
   c. Hypoxia, hypercarbia, and acidosis
   d. Possible pulmonary edema
      (1) Saltwater: high osmotic pressure of aspirated water draws additional fluid into alveolar spaces from the vascular bed
      (2) Freshwater: removes surfactant, leading to alveolar collapse
2. Treatment and nursing care
   a. Establish an airway and ventilate with 100% oxygen and positive pressure
   b. Correct the acidosis
   c. Insert a nasogastric tube and decompress the stomach to prevent aspiration of gastric contents
   d. Treat pulmonary edema and hypothermia if present

B. Heatstroke
1. Assessment
   a. Risk factors: advanced age, strenuous exercise in heat, medications such as antipsychotic agents and anticholinergics, which interfere with perspiring
   b. Hot, dry, flushed skin progressing to pallor in late circulatory collapse
   c. Elevation of body temperature greater than 105° F (40.5° C)
   d. Complaints of dizziness, nausea, and headaches
   e. Seizures
   f. Altered level of consciousness
2. Treatment and nursing care
   a. Rapidly reduce temperature: hypothermia blanket or mattress, cool-water baths, and cool enemas
   b. Administer oxygen to meet increased metabolic demands
   c. Institute seizure precautions

C. Hypothermia
1. Assessment
   a. Risk factors: exposure to cold; submersion in cold water; age (older adults and very young)
   b. Local (frostbite): pallor, paresthesia, pain to absence of sensation of involved body part
   c. Systemic: core temperature less than 94° F (34.4° C), weak and irregular pulse, decreased level of consciousness
2. Treatment and nursing care
   a. Monitor core temperature
   b. Continually assess cardiac status and levels of arterial blood gases, electrolytes, glucose, and BUN
   c. Rewarm: systemic—to prevent cardiovascular collapse, core rewarming with heated oxygen and/or irrigations must precede surface rewarming; warm IV fluids according to agency policy; local—controlled rewarming is instituted (98.6° to 104° F) and massage is avoided to prevent further injury
   d. Correct fluid and electrolyte imbalances

D. Terrorism
1. Definition: threat or intentional use of violence to intimidate society to achieve religious or politically motivated goals
2. Types: conventional weapons (bombs, guns); nonconventional weapons (biologic, chemical, radiation)
3. Disaster planning includes: mitigation (minimizing the harmful effects of the disaster), preparedness (having a disaster plan in place), response (provides assistance to meet needs as a result of the situation), and recovery (reconstruction)
4. Nursing responsibilities for nonconventional terrorist acts (follow agency policy associated with exposure to specific agent)
   a. Surveillance: detection and reporting of unusual pattern of clinical indicators (vesicular lesions, vomiting and diarrhea, fever, erythema)
   b. Immunizations: nurses should become immunized first and then administer immunizations to noninfected individuals as available
   c. Isolation: use standard and transmission-based precautions in response to bioterrorism event; use of personal protective equipment may be expanded to include a gas mask if contaminants are aerosolized
   d. Decontamination: remove clothing and jewelry and thoroughly shower individual with soap and water (or bleach solution and rinse after 15 minutes) to remove residual chemical, biologic, or radiation contaminants; contain clothing in plastic bags
   e. Treatment to counteract the agent and to manage clinical indicators: e.g., anthrax (ciprofloxacin); nerve agents (atropine); internal radiation, e.g., radiation-contaminated water (chelating agents); vomiting (IV hydration)

Foundations of Nursing Practice Review Questions With Answers and Rationales

QUESTIONS

1. The nurse is aware that rehabilitation plans for a client who has paraplegia as a result of spinal cord severance:
   1. Should be left up to the client and the client's family
   2. Should be considered and planned for early in the client's care
   3. Are not necessary, because the client will return to former activities
   4. Are not necessary, because the client will probably not be able to work again

2. The nurse provides care to a client who experienced a brain attack. Which statement best reflects a basic concept associated with the rehabilitation of this client?
   1. Rehabilitation needs are best met by the client's family and community resources.
   2. Rehabilitation is a specialty area with unique methods for meeting the client's needs.
   3. Rehabilitation needs, immediate or potential, are exhibited by all clients with a health problem.
   4. Rehabilitation is unnecessary for clients returning to their usual activities following hospitalization.

3. The nurse is caring for an adolescent who is receiving frequent visits from peer group members. The nurse understands that groups are important in the emotional development of an individual because they:
   1. Always protect their members
   2. Are easily identified by their members
   3. Go through the same developmental phases
   4. Identify acceptable behavior for their members

4. The nurse is teaching a client how to use the call bell system. Which level of Maslow's Hierarchy of Needs does this nursing action address?
   1. Safety
   2. Self-esteem
   3. Physiologic
   4. Interpersonal

5. The nurse is supportive of a client receiving long-term rehabilitation in the home rather than in a health care facility. The nurse encourages this because the nurse understands that family is most important in the emotional development of the individual because it:
   1. Provides support for the young
   2. Gives rewards and punishment

   3. Helps one to learn identity and roles
   4. Reflects the mores of a larger society

6. The nurse understands that clients attending Alcoholics Anonymous (AA) meetings will be required to:
   1. Speak aloud at weekly meetings
   2. Maintain controlled drinking after 6 months
   3. Promise to attend at least 12 meetings yearly
   4. Acknowledge their inability to control the problem

7. When caring for a client with a history of alcoholism, the nurse discusses attendance at Alcoholics Anonymous (AA) meetings with the client. Self-help groups such as AA are successful because they rely on the client's need for:
   1. Trust
   2. Growth
   3. Belonging
   4. Independence

8. A nurse manager notices that Latino clients are always assigned to the Latino-American nurse working on the unit, that the other nurses are slow to answer Latino clients' call lights, and that the nurses spend little time with their Latino clients when they are assigned to them. The nurse manager recognizes that these behaviors are reflective of cultural:
   1. Dissonance
   2. Discomfort
   3. Superiority
   4. Insensitivity

9. The nurse manager who works on a unit where the nursing staff members are uncomfortable taking care of clients from cultures that are different from their own should:
   1. Plan a workshop that offers the nurses opportunities to learn about the cultures they might encounter
   2. Relocate the nurses to units where they will not have to care for clients from such a variety of cultures
   3. Assign articles about various cultures so that the nurses become knowledgeable about other cultures
   4. Rotate the nurses' assignments so they have an equal opportunity to care for clients from other cultures

10. To help parents cope with the behavior of young school-age children, the nurse suggests that it would help if they:
    1. Avoid asking specific questions
    2. Give children a list of expectations

3. Be consistent about established rules

4. Allow the children to set up their own routines

11. The nurse in the health clinic is caring for a male college student who was recently diagnosed with asthma. What should be the initial focus of discharge planning?

1. Teaching the student how to make his room allergy-free

2. Referring the student to a support group for individuals with asthma

3. Collaborating with the student and college to ensure a speedy return to school

4. Ensuring that the student understands his disease and the best way to care for it

12. The nurse is held responsible for the commission of a tort. The nurse understands that the best definition of a tort is:

1. The application of force to the person of another by a reasonable individual

2. An illegality committed by one person against the property or person of another

3. Doing something that a reasonable person under ordinary circumstances would not do

4. An illegality committed against the public and punishable by the law through the courts

13. A client is placed on a stretcher and restrained with straps while being transported to the x-ray department. A strap breaks, and the client falls to the floor, sustaining a fractured arm. Later the client states, "The strap was worn just at the very spot where it snapped." The nurse is:

1. Totally and singly responsible for the obvious negligence because of failure to report defective equipment

2. Liable, along with the employer, for misapplication of equipment or use of defective equipment that harms the client

3. Exempt from any lawsuit because of the doctrine of *respondeat superior*

4. Exonerated, because only the hospital, as principal employer, is primarily responsible for the quality and maintenance of equipment

14. A 2-year-old child is admitted with a diagnosis of pneumonia and is given antibiotics, fluids, and oxygen. The child's temperature rises until it reaches 103° F. The nurse calls the physician at the mother's request, but the physician sees no need to change treatment, even though the child has a history of febrile seizures. Although concerned, the nurse takes no further action. Later, the child has a seizure that results in neurologic impairment. Legally:

1. The physician's decision takes precedence over the nurse's concern

2. The nurse's failure to further question the physician placed the child at risk

3. High fevers are common in children; therefore presents little cause for concern

4. The physician is totally responsible for the client's health history and treatment regimen

15. A graduate nurse is preparing to apply to the State Board of Nursing for licensure to practice as a registered professional nurse. The nurse understands that the primary purpose for regulating nursing practice is to protect:

1. The public

2. Practicing nurses

3. The employing agency

4. Professional standards

16. A client with coronary artery disease has a sudden episode of cyanosis and a change in respirations. The nurse starts O_2 administration immediately. In this situation:

1. The symptoms were too vague for the nurse to determine a need for O_2

2. The nurse's observations were sufficient and therefore O_2 can be administered

3. The O_2 had not been ordered and therefore should not be administered

4. The physician should have been called for an order before O_2 administration was started

17. A 15-year-old is taken to the emergency department of the local hospital after stepping on a nail. The puncture wound is cleansed and a sterile dressing applied. The nurse asks if the client has been immunized against tetanus. The reply is affirmative. Penicillin is administered, and the client is sent home with instructions to return if there is any change in the wound area. A few days later, the client is admitted to the hospital with a diagnosis of tetanus. Legally, the:

1. Nurse's judgment was adequate in view of the client's symptoms

2. Assessment by the nurse was incomplete and the treatment was inadequate

3. Nurse should routinely administer immunization against tetanus after such an injury

4. Possibility of tetanus could not have been foreseen, because the client had been immunized

18. When being interviewed for a position as a registered professional nurse, the applicant is asked to identify an example of an intentional tort. Which is an appropriate response?

1. Negligence

2. Malpractice

3. Breach of duty

4. False imprisonment

19. Several recently licensed RNs are discussing whether they should purchase personal professional liability insurance. Which statement best indicates the most accurate understanding of professional liability insurance?

1. "If you have liability insurance, you are more likely to get sued."

2. "Your employer provides you with the liability insurance you will need."

3. "Liability insurance is not available for nursing professionals working in a hospital."

4. "Personal liability insurance can provide representation if your state board files charges against you."

20. A 3-year-old boy with eczema of the face and arms has disregarded the nurse's warnings to "stop scratching—or else!" The nurse finds the toddler scratching so intensely that his arms are bleeding. With great flurry, the nurse ties the toddler's arms to the crib sides, saying "I'm going to teach you one way or another." In this situation, the nurse:
    1. Has used actions that can be interpreted as assault and battery
    2. Has responded to the problem with considerable accountability
    3. Had to protect the toddler's skin and acted the same as any reasonably prudent nurse
    4. Had tried to explain to the toddler and expected the toddler to understand and cooperate

21. When teaching about child abuse, the nurse tells a parent group that the best legal definition of assault is:
    1. Threats to do bodily harm to another person
    2. The application of force to another person without lawful justification
    3. A legal wrong committed by one person against the property of another
    4. A legal wrong committed against the public that is punishable by state law

22. When teaching staff about the legal terminology used in child abuse, the nurse emphasizes that the term battery means:
    1. The application of force to another person without lawful justification
    2. A legal wrong committed by one person against the property of another
    3. Maligning the character of a person while threatening to do bodily harm
    4. Doing something that a reasonable person with the same education or preparation would not do

23. A toddler screams and cries noisily after parental visits, disturbing all the other children. When the crying is particularly loud and prolonged, the nurse puts the crib in a separate room and closes the door. The toddler is left there until the crying ceases, a matter of 30 or 45 minutes. Legally:
    1. The child needed to have limits set to control the crying
    2. The child had a right to remain in the room with the other children
    3. The segregation of the child for more than 30 minutes was too long
    4. The other children had to be considered, so the child needed to be removed

24. A client is admitted with the diagnosis of possible placenta previa. The nurse begins IV fluids, administers oxygen, and draws blood for laboratory tests as ordered. The client's apprehension is increasing, and she asks the nurse what is happening. The nurse tells her not to worry, that she is going to be all right, and that everything is under control. What is the best description of the nurse's statement?
    1. Adequate, because the preparations are routine and need no explanation

2. Incorrect, because only the physician should explain why treatments are being done
3. Proper, because the client's anxieties would be increased if she knew the dangers
4. Questionable, because the client has the right to know what treatment is being given and why

25. What should the nurse do initially when obtaining consent for surgery?
    1. Explain the risks involved in the surgery
    2. Inform the client that obtaining the signature is routine for any surgery
    3. Determine whether the client's knowledge level is sufficient to give consent
    4. Witness the client's signature because this is what the nurse's signature is documenting

26. A client who has been told she needs a hysterectomy for cervical cancer is upset about being unable to have more children. What should the nurse should do?
    1. Evaluate her willingness to pursue adoption.
    2. Encourage her to focus on her own recovery.
    3. Emphasize that she does have two children already.
    4. Ensure that all treatment options have been explored.

27. The family of an older adult who is aphasic complains that the nurse failed to obtain a signed consent before inserting an indwelling catheter to measure hourly output. This is an example of a(n):
    1. Situation that does not need a separate consent form
    2. Routine procedure for the client's benefit, so consent is unnecessary
    3. Treatment without consent of the client, which is an invasion of rights
    4. Inability to obtain consent for treatment because the client was aphasic

28. The spouse of a comatose client who has severe internal bleeding refuses to allow transfusions of whole blood because they are Jehovah's Witnesses. What should the nurse involved in this situation do?
    1. Phone the physician for a special administrative order to give the blood under these circumstances.
    2. Have the spouse sign a treatment refusal form and notify the physician so that a court order can be obtained.
    3. Gently explain to the spouse why the transfusion is necessary, emphasizing the implications of not having the transfusion.
    4. Institute the blood transfusion anyway, because the physician ordered it and the client's survival depends on volume replacement.

29. A client is voluntarily admitted to the psychiatric unit. Later the client develops severe pain in the right lower quadrant and is diagnosed as having acute appendicitis. What should the nurse do when preparing the client for the appendectomy?
    1. Have two nurses witness the operative consent as the client signs it.
    2. Ensure that the surgeon and the psychiatrist sign for the surgery because it is an emergency procedure.

3. Phone the client's next of kin to come in to sign the consent form because the client is on a psychiatric unit.

4. Ask the client to sign the preoperative consent form after the client has been informed of the procedure and required care.

30. In relation to obtaining an informed consent from a 17-year-old adolescent, the nurse should remember that the adolescent:

1. Does not have the legal capacity to give consent
2. Cannot make informed decisions about health care
3. Is able to give voluntary consent when parents are not available
4. Will most likely be unable to choose between alternatives when asked to consent

31. A client with rheumatoid arthritis does not want cortisone even if it is prescribed and informs the nurse. Later, the nurse attempts to administer cortisone ordered by the physician. When the client asks what the medication is, the nurse gives an evasive answer. The client takes the medication and later finds that it was cortisone. The client states an intent to sue. The decision in this suit should take into consideration the fact that the:

1. Nurse should have notified the physician
2. Nurse is required to answer the client truthfully
3. Client has insufficient knowledge to make such a decision
4. Physician's order takes precedence over a client's preference

32. A client using fentanyl (Duragesic) transdermal patches for pain management in late-stage cancer has died. What should the hospice nurse who is caring for this client do?

1. Remove and dispose of the patch.
2. Tell the family to remove and dispose of the patch.
3. Leave the patch in place for the mortician to remove.
4. Have the family return the patch to the pharmacy for accounting.

33. At 11:00 PM, the count of hydrocodone (Vicodin) is incorrect. After several minutes of searching the medication cart and medication administration records, no explanation can be found. Who should the nurse in charge notify next?

1. Nursing unit manager
2. Hospital administrator
3. Quality control manager
4. Physician ordering the medication

34. An intentional tort is committed when the nurse:

1. Miscounts the gauze pads during a client's surgery
2. Divulges private information about the client to the media
3. Causes a burn when applying a warm soak to a client's extremity
4. Fails to monitor the client's blood pressure when administering an antihypertensive

35. Twenty-four hours after a cesarean birth, a client elects to sign herself and her baby out of the hospital because of difficulty at home with her 2-year-old son. Staff members are unable to contact her physician. The client arrives at the nursery dressed and ready to leave and asks that her infant be given to her to dress and take home. What is the most appropriate nursing action?

1. Explain to the client that her infant must remain in the hospital until signed out by the physician.
2. Give the infant to the client to take home, making sure that she receives information regarding care of a 2-day-old infant.
3. Allow the client time with the baby before she leaves, but emphasize that the baby is a minor and legally must remain until orders are received.
4. Tell the client that under the circumstances, hospital policy prevents the staff from releasing the infant into her care, but she will be informed when the infant is discharged.

36. A female client is hospitalized because of severe depression. She refuses to eat, stays in bed most of the time, does not talk with family members, and will not leave her room. The nurse caring for the client attempts to talk to her by asking questions but receives no answers. Finally, in exasperation, the nurse tells the client that if she does not respond, she will be left alone. The nurse is:

1. Assaulting the client and should refrain from saying this
2. Using a system of rewards and punishment to motivate the client
3. Leaving the client alone until the client is ready to talk about the situation
4. Responding to the client's nonverbal behavior that indicates a desire for solitude

37. A newborn is admitted to the nursery. During the newborn assessment the nurse notes that the temperature, pulse, respirations, and other physical characteristics are within the expected range. The nurse records all observations on the baby's chart. The nurse's actions are:

1. Correct, because the nurse met the requirements set forth in the Nurse Practice Act
2. Correct, because the assessment by the nurse is not equivalent to the physician's assessment
3. Incorrect, because making this type of medical diagnosis is not within the purview of the nurse
4. Incorrect, because the initial assessment of the infant's physical status is the responsibility of the physician

38. Nurses are protected from legal action when they:

1. Provide health teaching regarding family planning
2. Offer first aid at the scene of a collision between an automobile and a bus
3. Report incidents of suspected child abuse to the appropriate authorities
4. Administer CPR measures to an unconscious child pulled from a swimming pool

39. A client with a history of emphysema is now terminally ill with cancer of the esophagus. The client is weak,

dyspneic, emaciated, and apathetic. The plan of care includes a soft diet, modified postural drainage, and nebulizer treatments. What should be the priority in the nursing plan of care for this client?
1. Intake and output
2. Diet and nutrition
3. Hygiene and comfort
4. Body mechanics and posture

40. A terminally ill client is visited frequently by her spouse, a 16-year-old daughter, and a 20-year-old son. In view of the client's extreme weakness and dyspnea, the client's nursing plan of care should include:
1. Allowing self-activity whenever possible
2. Encouraging family members to assist with caring for the client
3. Limiting family visiting hours to the evening before the client sleeps
4. Planning necessary care at one time with long rest periods between care

41. When preparing a client for ambulation with crutches, the nurse should recognize the need for further teaching when the client states, "I must practice:
1. Sitting down and standing up."
2. Ambulating several hours a day."
3. Standing and maintaining balance."
4. Doing active exercises on a regular schedule."

42. A nurse educator is presenting information about the Nursing Process to a class of nursing students. The nurse educator states that the Nursing Process can best be defined as the:
1. Implementation of client care by the nurse
2. Steps the nurse employs to meet client needs
3. Activities a nurse employs to identify a client's problem
4. Process the nurse uses to determine nursing goals for the client

43. To utilize the Nursing Process, the nurse must first:
1. Identify goals for nursing care
2. State the client's nursing needs
3. Obtain information about the client
4. Evaluate the effectiveness of nursing actions

44. A nurse explains to a nursing assistant that the interpretation of the data collected about the client represents the:
1. Assessments of the client
2. Health problems of the client
3. Proposed plan of care for the client
4. Actual nursing interventions done for the client

45. The nurse who collaborates directly with the client to establish and implement a plan of care is the:
1. Primary nurse
2. Nurse clinician
3. Clinical specialist
4. Nurse coordinator

46. A newly oriented home health nurse arrives at a client's home. During the visit the nurse plans to check the client's vital signs and obtain a blood sample for an INR. After completion of these tasks, the client asks

the nurse to straighten the blankets on the bed. What is the nurse's most appropriate response?
1. "I would, but my back hurts today."
2. "OK. It will be my good deed for the day."
3. "I would like to, but it is not in my job description."
4. "Of course. I would like to do whatever I can for you."

47. The nurse is planning to review the plan of care for a client. What is the determining factor in the revision of a nursing plan of care?
1. Time available for care
2. Validity of the problem
3. Method for providing care
4. Effectiveness of the interventions

48. A need for cognitive learning becomes apparent when an adolescent, recently diagnosed as having diabetes mellitus, asks the nurse:
1. "What is diabetes?"
2. "What will my friends think?"
3. "How do I give myself an injection?"
4. "Can you show me how the glucose monitor works?"

49. Developing independence is a primary goal for a client with hemiplegia who is frustrated. How can the nurse best motivate the client?
1. Establish long-range goals for the client.
2. Reinforce success in tasks accomplished.
3. Point out errors so they can be corrected.
4. Demonstrate ways the client can regain independence.

50. A client is receiving an antihypertensive drug intravenously for control of severe hypertension. The client's blood pressure is unstable and is 160/94 mm Hg before the infusion. Fifteen minutes after the infusion is started, the blood pressure rises to 180/100 mm Hg. The response to the drug is described as a(n):
1. Allergic response
2. Synergistic response
3. Paradoxical response
4. Hypersusceptibility response

51. The nurse recognizes that the client experiencing an anaphylactic reaction after receiving penicillin indicates that the client has:
1. An acquired atopic sensitization
2. Passive immunity to the penicillin allergen
3. Antibodies to penicillin developed after earlier use of the drug
4. Developed potent bivalent antibodies when the IV administration was started

52. At the conclusion of visiting hours, the mother of a 14-year-old girl scheduled for orthopedic surgery the following day hands the nurse a bottle of capsules and says, "These are for my daughter's allergy. Will you be sure she takes one about 9 tonight?" What is the best response by the nurse?
1. "One capsule at 9 PM? Of course, I will give it."
2. "Did you ask the doctor if she should have this tonight?"

3. "I am certain the doctor knows about your daughter's allergy."

4. "I will ask your daughter's doctor to write an order so I can give this medication to her."

53. The physician orders filgrastim (Neupogen) 5 mcg/kg/day by injection for a client who weighs 132 lb. The vial label reads Neupogen 300 mcg/mL. How many milliliters should the nurse administer?

Answer: _____ mL

54. An infant is to receive thyroxine sodium, 0.35 mg once a day orally. The medication is available in elixir form, 0.25 mg/mL. How much elixir should the nurse administer?

Answer: _____ mL

55. The physician orders 375 mg ampicillin IV every 6 hours. The drug is supplied as 500 mg of powder in a vial. The directions are to mix the powder with 1.8 mL of diluent, which yields 250 mg/mL. How much prepared solution should the nurse administer?

Answer: _____ mL

56. Based on the client's reported pain level, the nurse administering medications decides to administer 8 mg of morphine. The medication available has 10 mg in a syringe. Wasting of the remaining 2 mg of morphine should be done by the nurse responsible for administering the medication and the:

1. LPN on the unit
2. Client's physician
3. Nursing supervisor
4. Nursing assistant assigned to the nurse

57. The nurse is instructing a group of volunteer nurses on the technique of administering the smallpox vaccine. What method should the nurse teach the group to administer the vaccine correctly?

1. Z-track injection
2. Intravenous injection
3. Subcutaneous injection
4. Intradermal scratch injection

58. A client is scheduled to receive phenytoin (Dilantin) 100 mg orally at 6 PM but is having difficulty swallowing capsules. The nurse should:

1. Open the capsule and sprinkle the powder in a cup of water
2. Insert a rectal suppository containing 100 mg of phenytoin
3. Administer 4 mL of phenytoin suspension containing 125 mg/5 mL
4. Obtain a change in the prescribed administration route to allow IM administration

59. What are the desired outcomes that the nurse would expect when administering a nonsteroidal antiinflammatory drug (NSAID)? Select all that apply.

1. ❐ Pain relief
2. ❐ Antipyresis
3. ❐ Anticoagulation
4. ❐ Bronchodilation
5. ❐ Urinary diuresis
6. ❐ Reduced inflammation

60. A pregnant client is now in the third trimester. The client tells the nurse she wants to have general anesthesia for the birth. What is the nurse's best response?

1. "You are worried about too much pain?"
2. "I will tell your doctor about this request."
3. "You don't want to be awake during the birth?"
4. "I can understand that because labor is uncomfortable."

61. When promoting affective learning (developing attitudes) in a client with a newly diagnosed disease, the nurse must first consider the influence of the:

1. Client's past experiences
2. Client's personal resources
3. Total stress of the situation
4. Type of onset of the disease

62. When evaluating the appropriateness of a response by a family member in the developing awareness stage of grief, the most important factor for the nurse to consider is the individual's:

1. Personality traits
2. Educational level
3. Cultural background
4. Past experiences with death

63. Communication is a major component of providing nursing care. The nurse understands that communication is important because it ties people to their:

1. Social surroundings
2. Physical surroundings
3. Materialistic surroundings
4. Environmental surroundings

64. The effectiveness of nurse-client communication is best validated by:

1. Client feedback
2. Medical assessments
3. Health care team conferences
4. Client's physiologic adaptations

65. The nurse on the medical-surgical unit tells other staff members, "That client can just wait for his lorazepam (Ativan); he shouldn't have been drinking anyway." It is important to identify that this nurse is:

1. Exhibiting personal bias
2. Using client acuity to set priorities
3. Aware of the complexity of client care
4. Making decisions based on assessments

66. A client becomes openly hostile when learning that amputation of a gangrenous toe is being considered. What is the best indication that the nurse's interaction has been therapeutic?

1. Increase in physical activity
2. Relaxation of tensed muscles
3. Absence of further outbursts
4. Denial that further discussion is necessary

67. The nursing supervisor sends a recently oriented nursing assistant to help relieve the burden of care on a short-staffed medical-surgical unit. Appropriate duties to delegate to the nursing assistant include:

1. Obtaining routine vital signs and answering call lights
2. Performing range-of-motion exercises and changing sterile dressings

3. Changing linens on occupied beds and documenting client responses to ambulation
4. Caring for clients with transmission-based precautions and changing normal saline infusions

68. While talking with the nurse about the problem of not being able to make friends, a teenager begins to cry. At this time it is most therapeutic for the nurse to:
   1. Sit quietly with the client
   2. Tell the client that crying is not helping
   3. Point out how the client can change this
   4. Suggest that the client play a board game

69. The client has been told to stop smoking by the physician. The nurse discovers a pack of cigarettes in the client's bathrobe. What should be the initial action by the nurse?
   1. Report the situation to the head nurse.
   2. Call the physician to request directions.
   3. Let the client know the cigarettes were found.
   4. Discard the cigarettes without making comments to the client.

70. A client with internal bleeding is in the ICU for observation. At the change of shift an alarm sounds, indicating a fall in BP. What should the nurse do?
   1. Assess the client before resuming the change-of-shift report.
   2. Lower the diastolic pressure limits on the monitor during the change-of-shift report.
   3. Continue the change-of-shift report, but include this information about the fall in blood pressure.
   4. Turn the alarm off to avoid disturbing the other clients, but alert the oncoming nurse to the fall in blood pressure.

71. While awaiting the biopsy report before removal of a tumor, the client reports being afraid of a diagnosis of cancer. What is the best response by the nurse?
   1. "Worrying today is not going to help the situation."
   2. "Let's wait until we hear what the biopsy report says."
   3. "It is very upsetting to have to wait for a biopsy report."
   4. "No operation is done without specimens being sent to the laboratory first."

72. A client is admitted for surgery. Although not physically distressed, the client appears apprehensive and alienated. What is the best action by the nurse?
   1. Explain that everything is all right.
   2. Orient the client to the unit environment.
   3. Give the client a copy of hospital regulations.
   4. Provide reassurance that staff will be available to answer questions.

73. In today's health care delivery system, the nurse as a teacher is confronted with multiple stressors. The major stressor that detracts from the effectiveness of the teaching effort is the:
   1. Extent of informed consumerism
   2. Limited time to engage in teaching
   3. Variety of cultural beliefs that exist
   4. Deficient motivation of adult learners

74. A nurse in a long-term health care setting is assigned to introduce a client who has a Ph.D. to the other clients. The client tells the nurse, "I wish to be called Doctor." What is the nurse's best response?
   1. "Why do you insist on being called Doctor?"
   2. "That's fine; that is how I will introduce you, then."
   3. "All the clients here call one another by their first names."
   4. "I can't do that. Isn't it better if the other clients do not know you are a doctor?"

75. "But you don't understand" is a common statement associated with adolescents. The best response by the nurse when communicating with an adolescent is to say:
   1. "I don't understand."
   2. "I would like to understand; let's talk."
   3. "I do understand. I was a teenager once too."
   4. "I'm not sure I have to. I believe it's you who has to understand."

76. When planning care for assigned clients, what care can the registered nurse on a medical-surgical unit safely delegate to a nursing assistant?
   1. Evaluating the effectiveness of acetaminophen and codeine (Tylenol No. 3)
   2. Obtaining an apical pulse rate before administration of oral digoxin (Lanoxin)
   3. Assisting a client who has patient-controlled analgesia (PCA) to the bathroom
   4. Assessing the wound integrity of a client recovering from an abdominal laparotomy

77. A client is hospitalized with a diagnosis of possible cancer of the pancreas. On admission the client asks the nurse, "Do you think I have anything serious, like cancer?" What is the nurse's best reply?
   1. "What makes you think you have cancer?"
   2. "I don't know if you do, but let's talk about it."
   3. "Why don't you discuss this with your doctor?"
   4. "Don't worry, we won't know until all the test results are back."

78. What type of interview is most appropriate when the nurse talks with a client being admitted to the clinic?
   1. Directive
   2. Exploratory
   3. Problem solving
   4. Information giving

79. A pediatric nurse has received a subpoena in a court case involving a child. To prepare for this experience, the nurse should review the State Nurse Practice Act, the ANA Code for Nurses, and:
   1. Nursing's Social Policy Statement
   2. ANA Standards of Clinical Nursing Practice
   3. References regarding a child's right to consent
   4. The state's law regarding the protection of minors

80. An older adult woman is treated in the emergency department for soft-tissue injuries that the medical team suspects might be caused by physical abuse. The daughter-in-law states that her mother-in-law is forgetful and confused and that she fell. A mini-mental examination indicates that the client is oriented

to person, place, and time, and the client does not comment when asked directly how the bruises and abrasions occurred. The nurse should now:

1. Recommend that the client be admitted for further assessment of the situation
2. Believe the daughter-in-law until further data prove her information to be untrue
3. Act on instinct and report the abuse to the appropriate state agency for investigation
4. Refer the client's record to the hospital ethics committee for analysis and recommendations

81. While taking a nursing history from a client, the nurse promotes communication by:
1. Asking "why" and "how" questions
2. Using broad, open-ended statements
3. Reassuring the client that there is no cause for alarm
4. Asking questions that can be answered by a "yes" or "no"

82. To give nursing care to a newly admitted homosexual client, the nurse must first:
1. Understand the client's emotional conflict
2. Develop rapport with the client's physician
3. Recognize personal feelings toward this client
4. Talk with the client's family or significant other

83. A 35-year-old client is brought to the emergency department for a bee sting. The client has a history of allergies to bees and is having trouble breathing. The nurse is aware that this client could die from:
1. Ischemia
2. Asphyxia
3. Lactic acidosis
4. Antihistamines

84. The nurse understands that the symptoms experienced by a client during an anaphylactic reaction to peanuts are the result of:
1. Increased cardiac output and hypertension
2. Respiratory depression and cardiac standstill
3. Constriction of capillaries and decreased cardiac output
4. Bronchial constriction and decreased peripheral resistance

85. The nurse is aware that standard precautions should be used for self-protection. Identify the nursing interventions that require the nurse to use standard precautions. Check all that apply.
1. ☐ Performing a back rub
2. ☐ Administering the first bath to a newborn
3. ☐ Emptying a portable wound drainage system
4. ☐ Interviewing a client in the emergency department
5. ☐ Obtaining the blood pressure of a client who is HIV-positive

86. The nurse is assigned to change a central line dressing. The nurse knows that the agency policy is to clean the site with Betadine and then clean with alcohol. The nurse recently attended a conference that presented information that alcohol should precede Betadine in a dressing change. In addition, an article in a nursing journal stated that a new product on the market was a more effective antibacterial product than alcohol and Betadine. The nurse has a sample of the new product. How should the nurse proceed?
1. Use the new product sample to perform the dressing change.
2. Cleanse the site with alcohol first and then with Betadine.
3. Follow agency policy unless it is contradicted by a physician's order.
4. Cleanse the site with the new product first and then follow the agency's protocol.

87. Immediately after a storm has passed, the rescue team with which the nurse is working is searching for injured people. A victim lying next to a broken natural gas main is not breathing and is bleeding heavily from a wound on the foot. The nurse's first step should be to:
1. Treat the victim for shock
2. Start rescue breathing immediately
3. Apply surface pressure to the foot wound
4. Remove the victim from the immediate vicinity

88. The nurse is responding to the needs of victims at a collapsed building soon after an earthquake. The principle that guides the nurse's priorities during this disaster is:
1. Hemorrhage necessitates immediate care to save the most lives
2. Those requiring minimal care are treated first so that they can help others
3. Clients with head injuries should be treated first because the care is most complex
4. Children should receive the highest priority because they have the greatest life expectancy

89. A recent immigrant from mainland China is critically ill and dying. When collecting information necessary to meet the emotional needs of a client from this culture, the nurse should ask:
1. "How do you like living in this country?"
2. "When did you come to the United States?"
3. "What family member would you prefer to receive information?"
4. "Do you have a family member who can translate medical information for you?"

90. A client with a terminal illness reaches the stage of acceptance. The nurse can best help the client during this stage by:
1. Allowing the client to cry
2. Encouraging unrestricted visiting
3. Explaining to the client what is being done
4. Being around though not necessarily speaking

91. The nurse is assessing the needs of a client who was just told by the physician that the client's tumor is malignant, that it has already metastasized to several organs, and that the client does not have long to live. The nurse is aware that characteristic behavior in the initial stage of coping with dying includes:
1. Crying uncontrollably
2. Criticizing medical care
3. Refusing to receive visitors
4. Asking for additional medical consultations

92. A client with cancer of the lung says to the nurse, "If I could just be free of pain for a few days, I might be able to eat more and regain strength." In reference to the stages of dying, the client indicates:
    1. Bargaining
    2. Depression
    3. Frustration
    4. Rationalization

93. A client who has reached the point of acceptance in the stages of dying appears peaceful but demonstrates a lack of involvement with the environment. The nurse can best deal with this client by:
    1. Accepting the client's behavior at this point
    2. Ignoring the client's behavior when possible
    3. Joining the client in denial because this is a defense
    4. Pointing out the reality of the situation to the client

94. A 24-year-old college student had a right above-the-knee amputation after trauma sustained in a work-related accident. Upon awakening from surgery the client says, "What happened to me? I don't remember a thing." The nurse's initial response should be:
    1. "Tell me what you think happened."
    2. "You were in a work-related accident this morning."
    3. "An amputation of your leg was necessary because of an accident."
    4. "You sound concerned; you'll probably remember more as you wake up."

95. After being medicated for anxiety, a client says to the nurse, "I guess you are too busy to stay with me." The nurse's best response in this circumstance is:
    1. "I have to see other clients."
    2. "The medication will help you rest soon."
    3. "I have to go now, but I will come back in 10 minutes."
    4. "You will feel better; I will adjust your oxygen mask."

96. A physically ill client is being verbally assertive. What is the most appropriate initial nursing response?
    1. Verbal defense of the staff's actions
    2. Reasonable exploration of the situation
    3. Silent acceptance of the client's behavior
    4. Complete physical withdrawal from the client

97. A client asks the nurse, "Should I tell my husband I was just diagnosed with AIDS?" What is the nurse's most appropriate response?
    1. "This is a decision you alone can make."
    2. "Do not tell him anything unless he asks."
    3. "You are having difficulty deciding what to say."
    4. "Tell him you feel you contracted AIDS from him."

98. After being scheduled for a colostomy, a client is obviously anxious. What is the most effective way for the nurse to help the client?
    1. Administer a prescribed PRN sedative.
    2. Encourage the client to express feelings.
    3. Explain the procedure and postoperative course.
    4. Reassure the client that many people cope with this problem.

99. A client with hemiplegia is staring blankly at the wall and complains of feeling like half a person. Initially the nurse should:
    1. Distract the client from self-pity
    2. Include the client in all decisions
    3. Help the client explore personal feelings
    4. Prevent the client from developing contractures

100. While receiving a preoperative enema a client starts to cry and says, "I'm sorry you have to do this messy thing for me." What is the best response by the nurse?
    1. "I don't mind it."
    2. "You seem to be upset."
    3. "This is part of my job."
    4. "Nurses get used to this."

101. The nurse is teaching a client about a prescribed restricted diet. What is the nurse's best initial comment?
    1. "You can eat only the foods on this list."
    2. "What type of foods do you usually eat?"
    3. "You need to limit the intake of foods on this list."
    4. "Do you understand why you have these food restrictions?"

102. The nurse in the ambulatory preoperative unit identifies that a client is more anxious than most clients. The nurse's best intervention is to:
    1. Attempt to identify the client's concerns
    2. Report the client's anxiety to the surgeon
    3. Reassure the client that the surgery is routine
    4. Provide privacy by pulling the curtain around the client

103. A client is admitted to the hospital with metastatic cancer and is experiencing abdominal pain, a temperature of 100.4° F, and a distended abdomen. The client asks the nurse, "Do you think that I'm going to have surgery?" The statement by the nurse that best helps to establish a therapeutic relationship is:
    1. "You seem concerned about having surgery."
    2. "Some people with your problem have surgery."
    3. "I really don't know. You'll have to ask your doctor."
    4. "Has someone talked to you about your scheduled surgery?"

104. When caring for a client with a portable wound drainage system, the nurse understands that the principle behind its functioning is:
    1. The lumen diameter will determine the rate of fluid flow
    2. Gravity causes liquids to flow down a pressure gradient
    3. Siphonage causes fluids to flow from one level to a lower one
    4. Fluids flow from an area of higher pressure to one of lower pressure

105. It is most important that the nurse observe the client who has had extensive, prolonged surgery for the depletion of which electrolyte?
    1. Sodium
    2. Calcium
    3. Chloride
    4. Potassium

106. When preparing an IV piggyback medication for a client, the nurse is aware that it is essential to:
    1. Use strict sterile technique
    2. Rotate the bag after adding the medication
    3. Use exactly 100 mL of fluid to mix the medication
    4. Change the needle just before adding the medication

107. A nurse administers an intravenous solution of 0.45% sodium chloride. With respect to human blood cells, to which category of fluids does this solution belong?
    1. Isotonic
    2. Isomeric
    3. Hypotonic
    4. Hypertonic

108. Which assessment data should the nurse anticipate when admitting a client with an extracellular fluid excess?
    1. Rapid, thready pulse
    2. Distended jugular veins
    3. Elevated hematocrit level
    4. Increased serum sodium level

109. The nurse is aware that the body's adaptation to excessive fluid losses by a client with diarrhea are evident by a decrease in which clinical indicator?
    1. Pulse rate
    2. Skin turgor
    3. Specific gravity
    4. Body temperature

110. A client complains of vomiting and diarrhea for 3 days. Which assessment most accurately reflects that the client is experiencing a fluid deficit?
    1. A change in body weight
    2. The presence of dry skin
    3. A decrease in blood pressure
    4. An altered general appearance

111. A client is admitted with metabolic acidosis. The nurse understands that two body systems interact with the bicarbonate buffer system to preserve the normal body fluid pH. What two body systems should the nurse assess for compensatory changes?
    1. Skeletal and nervous systems
    2. Circulatory and urinary systems
    3. Respiratory and urinary systems
    4. Muscular and endocrine systems

112. The nurse is reviewing a client's serum electrolytes. Which statement correctly compares blood plasma and interstitial fluid?
    1. Both contain the same kinds of ions.
    2. Plasma exerts lower osmotic pressure than does interstitial fluid.
    3. Plasma contains slightly more of each kind of ion than does interstitial fluid.
    4. The main cation in plasma is sodium, whereas the main cation in interstitial fluid is potassium.

113. The nurse explains to an obese client that the rapid weight loss experienced during the first week after initiating a diet is because of fluid loss. The weight of extracellular body fluid is approximately 20% of the total body weight of an average individual. The nurse understands that the component of the extracellular fluid contributing the greatest portion to this amount is:
    1. Plasma fluid
    2. Interstitial fluid
    3. Fluid in dense tissue
    4. Fluid in body secretions

114. The nurse assesses a client's electrolyte levels. Which electrolyte of intracellular fluid does the nurse identify as the most important?
    1. Sodium
    2. Calcium
    3. Chloride
    4. Potassium

115. The nurse is caring for a client with chronic kidney failure. The nurse understands that ammonia is normally excreted by the kidney to help maintain:
    1. Osmotic pressure of the blood
    2. Acid-base balance of the body
    3. Low bacterial levels in the urine
    4. Normal red blood cell production

116. Which finding best suggests that nursing interventions for a client with an excess fluid volume have been effective?
    1. Clear breath sounds
    2. Positive pedal pulses
    3. Normal potassium level
    4. Increased urine specific gravity

117. The nurse understands that a client with albuminuria has edema because of:
    1. Fall in tissue hydrostatic pressure
    2. Rise in plasma hydrostatic pressure
    3. Rise in tissue colloid osmotic pressure
    4. Fall in plasma colloid oncotic pressure

118. A client is admitted with dehydration as a result of prolonged watery diarrhea. Which intervention ordered by the physician should the nurse question?
    1. Parenteral albumin
    2. Psyllium (Metamucil)
    3. Potassium supplements
    4. Half normal saline solution

119. When the nurse uses the clamp on the administration set to manually adjust the flow of IV fluid into a client by gravity, what change in energy takes place?
    1. Potential energy is converted to kinetic energy
    2. Kinetic energy is converted to potential energy
    3. Chemical energy is converted to kinetic energy
    4. Potential energy is converted to chemical energy

120. Larger than normal amounts of acetoacetic acid have been entering the blood as one of the indirect results of a client's insulin deficiency. The nurse understands the chemical mainly responsible for buffering acetoacetic acid is:
    1. Potassium
    2. Bicarbonate
    3. Carbon dioxide
    4. Sodium chloride

121. For what clinical indicator must the nurse assess the client with gastric lavage or prolonged vomiting?
    1. Decreased serum pH
    2. Increased serum oxygen level
    3. Increased serum bicarbonate level
    4. Decreased serum osmotic pressure

122. A client is in a state of uncompensated acidosis. What is the approximate arterial blood pH the nurse expects the client to have?
    1. 7.20
    2. 7.35
    3. 7.45
    4. 7.48

123. The client with which condition has an increased risk for developing hyperkalemia?
    1. Crohn's disease
    2. Cushing's syndrome
    3. Chronic heart failure
    4. End-stage renal disease

124. The nurse notes that a client's serum potassium level is 5.8 mEq/L. What action should the nurse take first?
    1. Call the laboratory to repeat the test.
    2. Call the cardiac arrest team to alert them.
    3. Obtain an ECG strip and have lidocaine available.
    4. Take the client's vital signs and notify the physician.

125. What clinical indicators should the nurse expect a client with hyperkalemia to exhibit? Check all that apply.
    1. ☐ Tetany
    2. ☐ Seizures
    3. ☐ Diarrhea
    4. ☐ Weakness
    5. ☐ Dysrhythmias

126. The nurse adds potassium chloride 20 mEq to the IV solution of a client with diabetic ketoacidosis. What is the primary purpose for administering this drug?
    1. Treatment of hyperpnea
    2. Prevention of flaccid paralysis
    3. Replacement of excessive losses
    4. Treatment of cardiac dysrhythmias

127. The I&O for a client over an 8-hour period (8 AM to 4 PM) is as follows:
    8 AM: IV with D$_5$W infusing and 900 mL left in bag
    8:30 AM: 150 mL urine voided
    9 AM to 3 PM: 200 mL gastric tube formula and 50 mL water at q3h intervals
    1 PM: 220 mL voided
    3:15 PM: 235 mL voided
    4 PM: IV with 550 mL left in bag
    What is the client's total I&O for the 8-hour period?
    1. Intake 550 mL and output 600 mL
    2. Intake 1650 mL and output 550 mL
    3. Intake 1100 mL and output 605 mL
    4. Intake 1000 mL and output 1155 mL

128. A client with ascites is experiencing shortness of breath. The nurse understands that ascites can be related to which problem?
    1. Portal hypotension
    2. Kidney malfunction
    3. Diminished plasma protein levels
    4. Decreased production of potassium

129. A client is receiving an IV of 5% dextrose in water. Why may this client develop negative nitrogen balance?
    1. Excessive carbohydrate intake
    2. Lack of protein supplementation
    3. Insufficient intake of water-soluble vitamins
    4. Increased concentration of electrolytes in cells

130. An IV of 1000 mL 5% dextrose in water to be infused at 125 mL/hr is started on admission to correct a client's fluid imbalance. The infusion set delivers 15 drops/mL. So that the solution will infuse over an 8-hour period, at how many drops per minute should the nurse set the rate of flow?
    Answer: _____ gtt/min

131. The nurse observes an anxious client hyperventilating and intervenes to prevent:
    1. Cardiac arrest
    2. Carbonic acid deficit
    3. Reduction in serum pH
    4. Excess oxygen saturation

132. An arterial blood gas report indicates the client's pH is 7.25, P$_{CO_2}$ is 35 mm Hg, and HCO$_3^-$ is 20 mEq/L. Which disturbance does the nurse identify based on these results?
    1. Metabolic acidosis
    2. Metabolic alkalosis
    3. Respiratory acidosis
    4. Respiratory alkalosis

133. A client's arterial blood gas report indicates the pH is 7.52, P$_{CO_2}$ is 32 mm Hg, and HCO$_3^-$ is 24 mEq/L. What does the nurse identify as a possible cause of these results?
    1. Airway obstruction
    2. Inadequate nutrition
    3. Prolonged gastric suction
    4. Excessive mechanical ventilation

134. While a client with ascites is receiving albumin, the planned therapeutic effect will be greater if the nurse regulates the infusion to flow:
    1. Slowly, and restricts fluid intake
    2. Rapidly, and withholds fluid intake
    3. Rapidly, and encourages fluid intake
    4. Slowly, and encourages liberal fluid intake

135. What is the reason the nurse administers serum albumin to a client?
    1. Clotting of blood
    2. Formation of red blood cells
    3. Activation of white blood cells
    4. Maintenance of oncotic pressure

136. What is the maximum length of time the nurse allows an IV bag of solution to infuse into the client?
    1. 6 hours
    2. 12 hours

3. 18 hours
4. 24 hours

137. What does the nurse identify as the most likely cause of the infiltration of a client's IV?
1. Excessive height of the IV solution
2. Failure to adequately secure the catheter
3. Lack of asepsis during catheter insertion
4. Infusion of chemically irritating medication

138. What are the clinical indicators that the nurse should identify to conclude that an IV has infiltrated? Check all that apply.
1. ❒ Heat
2. ❒ Pallor
3. ❒ Edema
4. ❒ Decreased flow rate
5. ❒ Increased blood pressure

139. A client has an IV infusion. If the IV infusion infiltrates, what should the nurse do first?
1. Elevate the IV site.
2. Discontinue the infusion.
3. Attempt to flush the tube.
4. Apply a warm, moist compress.

140. A client is to receive 2000 mL of IV fluid in 12 hours. The drop factor is 10 gtt/mL. At how many drops per minute should the flow rate be set?
Answer: _____ gtt/min

141. A client with hypokalemia is placed on a cardiac monitor to evaluate cardiac activity during IV potassium replacement. Before starting the IV, what ECG change is the nurse most likely to identify when observing the monitor?
1. Lowering of the T wave
2. Elevation of the ST segment
3. Shortening of the QRS complex
4. Increased deflection of the Q wave

142. The nurse inadvertently infuses an IV solution containing potassium too rapidly. The physician prescribes insulin added to a 10% dextrose in water solution. What is the rationale for the order?
1. Potassium moves into body cells with glucose and insulin.
2. Increased insulin accelerates excretion of glucose and potassium.
3. Glucose and insulin increase metabolism to accelerate potassium excretion.
4. Increased potassium causes a temporary slowing of pancreatic production of insulin.

143. Which clinical indicator leads the nurse to suspect a client has hypokalemia?
1. Edema
2. Muscle spasms
3. Kussmaul breathing
4. Abdominal distention

144. An intravenous piggyback (IVPB) of cefazolin sodium (Kefzol) 500 mg in 50 mL of 5% dextrose in water is to be administered over a 20-minute period. The tubing has a drop factor of 15 drops/mL. The nurse should regulate the infusion to run at what rate per minute?
Answer: _____ gtt/min

145. A husband spends most of the day with his wife, who is receiving chemotherapy for inoperable cancer, and asks the nurse how he can continue to help her. The nurse should plan to:
1. Assist the couple to maintain open communication
2. Talk with the husband alone to promote venting of feelings
3. Instruct the husband about the action of the various drugs
4. Offer the couple a detailed description of the disease process

146. During admission a client appears anxious and says to the nurse, "The doctor told me I have lung cancer. My father died from cancer. I wish I had never smoked." Which is the nurse's best response?
1. "You are concerned about your diagnosis."
2. "You are feeling guilty about your smoking."
3. "Trust your doctor; it's important you have faith."
4. "There have been improvements in lung cancer therapy."

147. When a disaster occurs, the nurse may have to treat mass hysteria first. The person or persons to be cared for immediately are those experiencing:
1. Panic
2. Coma
3. Euphoria
4. Depression

148. A client with hypothermia is brought to the emergency department. The nurse should explain to the family members that treatment will include:
1. Core rewarming with warm fluids
2. Ambulation to increase metabolism
3. Frequent oral temperature assessment
4. Gastric tube feedings to increase fluids

149. A 72-year-old unresponsive man is admitted to the emergency department after playing tennis on a hot, humid day. The initial nursing assessment reveals that he has hot, dry skin; a respiratory rate of 36 breaths/min; and a heart rate of 128 beats/min. Which is the nurse's initial action?
1. Suction the airway.
2. Remove all clothing.
3. Offer cool oral fluids.
4. Prepare for intubation.

150. The nurse is working in a busy emergency department on a hot summer day and four near-drowning victims are admitted. Which near-drowning victim should the nurse assess for signs of hypovolemia?
1. 72-year-old rescued from a lake
2. 2-year-old rescued from a bath tub
3. 50-year-old rescued from the ocean
4. 17-year-old rescued from a backyard pool

151. What clinical indicator will the nurse most likely identify when assessing a client with pyrexia?
1. Dyspnea
2. Precordial pain
3. Increased pulse rate
4. Elevated blood pressure

152. What action should the nurse include in a care plan to prevent a pulmonary embolus in a client prescribed bed rest?
    1. Limit the client's fluid intake.
    2. Encourage deep breathing and coughing.
    3. Use the knee gatch when the client is in bed.
    4. Teach the client to move the legs when in bed.

153. Immediately after receiving spinal anesthesia a client experiences hypotension as a result of postural changes. To what physiologic change does the nurse attribute the change in BP?
    1. Dilation of blood vessels
    2. Decreased response of chemoreceptors
    3. Decreased strength of cardiac contractions
    4. Interruption of cardiac accelerator pathways

154. A 35-year-old executive secretary is hospitalized for treatment of severe hypertension. The physician orders captopril (Capoten) and alprazolam (Xanax). The client quickly finds fault with the therapeutic regimen and nursing care. The nurse identifies that this behavior is probably a manifestation of the client's:
    1. Denial of illness
    2. Fear of the health problem
    3. Response to cerebral anoxia
    4. Reaction to hypertensive medications

155. A 2-g sodium diet is prescribed for a client with severe hypertension. The client does not like the diet, and the nurse hears the client request that the spouse "Bring in some good home-cooked food." What is the most effective nursing intervention?
    1. Call in the dietitian for client teaching.
    2. Wait for the client's family and discuss the diet with the client and family.
    3. Tell the client that the use of salt is forbidden, because it will raise the BP.
    4. Catch the family members before they go into the client's room and tell them about the diet.

156. A 22-year-old student, whose immunization status is current, asks the nurse which immunizations will be included in the precollege physical. The nurse indicates that the necessary immunizations will include:
    1. MMR
    2. Influenza
    3. Hepatitis C
    4. TDaP booster

157. A 76-year-old female client with COPD is being admitted to a rehabilitation facility and asks the nurse about the pneumococcal vaccine that the nurse is preparing to administer. The nurse responds that because the client received this vaccine at age 65, an immunization will be administered today and then:
    1. Every 2 years
    2. At each annual physical
    3. In September every year
    4. No further doses will be required

158. The nurse is caring for a client with an impaired immune system. When caring for this client, the nurse understands that the blood protein associated with the immune system is:
    1. Albumin
    2. Globulin
    3. Thrombin
    4. Hemoglobin

159. A client who was exposed to hepatitis A is given gamma globulin. The nurse understands that this will provide passive immunity because it:
    1. Increases production of short-lived antibodies
    2. Provides antibodies that neutralize the antigen
    3. Accelerates antigen-antibody union at the hepatic sites
    4. Stimulates the lymphatic system to produce large numbers of antibodies

160. A client is admitted to the emergency department with a contaminated wound. The client is a poor historian, and it is impossible to determine whether the client is immunized against tetanus. Which of the following is the preparation of choice that will permit this client to produce passive immunity for several weeks with minimal danger of allergic reactions?
    1. DTaP vaccine
    2. Tetanus toxoid
    3. Tetanus antitoxin
    4. Tetanus immune globulin

161. A client who is suspected of having tetanus asks the nurse about immunizations against tetanus. What information about the benefits of using tetanus antitoxin should the nurse include in the response to this client? It:
    1. Stimulates plasma cells directly
    2. Provides a high titer of antibodies
    3. Provides immediate active immunity
    4. Stimulates long-lasting passive immunity

162. What clinical indicator is important for the nurse to assess when a client undergoes a submucosal resection (SMR) for a deviated septum?
    1. Occipital headache
    2. Periorbital crepitus
    3. Expectoration of blood
    4. Changes in vocalization

163. The nurse must establish and maintain an airway in a client who has experienced a near-drowning in the ocean. For which potential danger should the nurse assess the client?
    1. Alkalosis
    2. Renal failure
    3. Hypervolemia
    4. Pulmonary edema

164. Which is an independent nursing measure that would be helpful in preventing the accumulation of secretions in a client who had general anesthesia during surgery?
    1. Postural drainage
    2. Cupping the chest
    3. Nasotracheal suctioning
    4. Frequent changes of position

165. In which position should the nurse place a client recovering from general anesthesia?
    1. Supine
    2. Side-lying
    3. High-Fowler
    4. Trendelenburg

166. What is the priority nursing intervention for a client during the immediate postoperative period?
    1. Observing for hemorrhage
    2. Maintaining a patent airway
    3. Recording the intake and output
    4. Checking the vital signs every 15 minutes

167. A client has seeds containing radium implanted in the pharyngeal area. What should the nurse include in the plan of care for this client?
    1. Have the client void every 2 hours.
    2. Maintain the client in an isolation room.
    3. Provide frequent contact for the client to verbalize feelings.
    4. Wear two pairs of gloves when providing hygiene for the client.

168. The nurse in the postanesthesia care unit identifies that after an abdominal cholecystectomy a client has serosanguineous drainage on the abdominal dressing. What should the nurse do?
    1. Change the dressing.
    2. Reinforce the dressing.
    3. Apply an abdominal binder.
    4. Replace the tape with Montgomery straps.

169. Four days after abdominal surgery a client has not passed flatus and there are no bowel sounds. Paralytic ileus is suspected. The nurse understands that this decrease in bowel function is most likely caused by which situation?
    1. Decreased blood supply
    2. Impaired neural functioning
    3. Perforation of the bowel wall
    4. Obstruction of the bowel lumen

170. The physician orders a rectal tube to help a client relieve abdominal distention following surgery. To achieve maximum effectiveness, how long should the nurse leave the tube in place once it is inserted into the rectum?
    1. 15 minutes
    2. 30 minutes
    3. 45 minutes
    4. 60 minutes

171. A client is admitted with diarrhea, anorexia, weight loss, and abdominal cramps. A diagnosis of colitis is made. What symptoms of fluid and electrolyte imbalance caused by this condition should the nurse report immediately?
    1. Skin rash, diarrhea, and diplopia
    2. Extreme muscle weakness and tachycardia
    3. Distended neck veins and auscultatory crackles
    4. Nausea, vomiting, and leg and stomach cramps

172. The nurse understands the emotional aspects of ulcerative colitis more readily by identifying the stress-related functions of which body systems?
    1. CNS and hypothalamus
    2. Sympathetic nervous system and pancreas

3. Autonomic nervous system and adrenal glands
    4. Thyroid gland and sympathetic nervous system

173. A 68-year-old client with arthritis has increased the intake of ibuprofen (Motrin) to abate joint discomfort. After several weeks on the regimen the client became increasingly weak. The physician identifies that the client is severely anemic and admits the client to the hospital. When performing an admission assessment, the nurse should expect the client to have a history of which clinical indicator?
    1. Constipation
    2. Recent melena
    3. Clay-colored stools
    4. Painful bowel movements

174. The nursing plan includes that before discharge a client with diabetes mellitus will know how to self-administer insulin, adjust the insulin dosage, understand the diet, and test the serum for glucose level. The client progresses well and is discharged 5 days following admission. Legally the:
    1. Nurse was properly functioning as a health teacher
    2. Visiting nurse should do health teaching in the client's home
    3. Family members also should have been taught to administer the insulin
    4. Physician was responsible and the nurse should have cleared the care with the physician

175. The nurse understands that the main reason sink faucets in a client's room are considered contaminated is that:
    1. They are not in sterile areas
    2. They are opened with dirty hands
    3. Large numbers of people use them
    4. Water encourages bacterial growth

176. When the nurse washes the hands before and after caring for a client, the nurse understands that the most important aspect of handwashing is:
    1. Time
    2. Soap
    3. Water
    4. Friction

177. The nurse is applying a dressing to a client's surgical wound using sterile technique. While engaging in this activity, the nurse accidentally places a moist sterile gauze pad on the cloth sterile field. The nurse understands that the sterile field is now contaminated because of:
    1. Dialysis
    2. Osmosis
    3. Diffusion
    4. Capillarity

178. The nurse is preparing to change a client's dressing. Which statement best explains the basis of surgical asepsis as it relates to this procedure?
    1. Keep the area free of microorganisms.
    2. Confine microorganisms to the surgical site.
    3. Protect self from microorganisms in the wound.
    4. Keep the number of opportunistic microorganisms to a minimum.

179. When assessing an obese client, the nurse identifies dehiscence and evisceration of the abdominal surgical wound. After placing the client in the low-Fowler's position with the knees slightly bent and encouraging the client to lie quietly, what should the nurse do next?
    1. Notify the physician.
    2. Obtain the client's vital signs.
    3. Reinsert the protruding organs.
    4. Cover the wound with a sterile towel moistened with saline.

180. The nurse is caring for a client with a portable wound drainage system and identifies that the collection container is half full. After emptying the collection container, what should the nurse do next?
    1. Irrigate the suction tube with sterile saline.
    2. Encircle the drainage present on the dressing.
    3. Clean the drainage port with an alcohol wipe.
    4. Compress the container before closing the port.

181. The nurse is informed that a client with a large surgical incision is being transferred from the intensive care unit to the surgical unit. What medication does the nurse anticipate the physician will order for this client?
    1. Vitamin A
    2. Mephyton
    3. Ascorbic acid
    4. Vitamin B_{12} complex

182. During the initial physical assessment of a newly admitted client with a pressure ulcer, the nurse identifies that the client is dehydrated and the skin is dry and scaly. The nurse immediately applies emollients to the client's skin and reinforces the dressing on the pressure ulcer. Legally:
    1. The nurse should have instituted a plan to increase activity
    2. The nurse provided supportive nursing care for the well-being of the client
    3. No treatment should have been instituted for the client until the physician's orders were received
    4. Debridement of the pressure ulcer should have been done by the nurse before the dressing was applied

183. An emaciated older adult develops a large pressure ulcer after refusing to change position for extended periods of time. The family is very upset, blames the nurses, and threatens to sue. The decision in this suit would take into consideration the fact that:
    1. The client should be turned every hour
    2. Pressure ulcers frequently occur in older clients
    3. Nurses are not responsible to the client's family
    4. The nurse should uphold the client's right not to be moved

184. The physician suspects that a client with a melanoma also has primary cancerous lesions in the connective tissue. The nurse understands that these lesions are classified as:
    1. Sarcomas
    2. Carcinomas
    3. Collagenomas
    4. Osteoblastomas

185. A client expresses concern about being exposed to radiation therapy because it can cause cancer. When assisting the client to understand the treatment, the nurse should emphasize the:
    1. Dosage of radiation utilized
    2. Extent of the body irradiated
    3. Physical condition of the client
    4. Nutritional environment of the cells

186. A client who is to receive radiation therapy for cancer says to the nurse, "My family said I will get a radiation burn." Which is the best response by the nurse?
    1. "It will be no worse than a sunburn."
    2. "A localized skin reaction usually occurs."
    3. "Daily application of an emollient will prevent the burn."
    4. "They must have had experience with radiation therapy."

187. The nurse applies an ice pack to a client's leg for 20 minutes. Which clinical indicator helps the nurse determine the effectiveness of the cold application?
    1. Local anesthesia
    2. Peripheral vasodilation
    3. Depression of vital signs
    4. Decreased viscosity of blood

188. A homeless person is brought to the emergency department after prolonged exposure to cold weather. The nurse should assess the client for hypothermia, which is manifested by:
    1. Stupor
    2. Erythema
    3. Increased anxiety
    4. Rapid respirations

189. A client complains of severe pain 2 days after surgery. Which initial action should the nurse take after assessing the character of the pain?
    1. Have the client rest
    2. Take the client's vital signs
    3. Administer the prn analgesic
    4. Document the client's complaint

190. Electric stimulation by the use of a peripheral nerve implant or dorsal column stimulator is used in the management of a client's intractable pain. What discharge instructions should the nurse give the client after surgery?
    1. Tub baths should not be taken.
    2. Analgesics will no longer be necessary.
    3. The transmitter must be worn externally.
    4. The device may interfere with the television remote control.

191. A client with intractable pain in the upper torso is admitted to the hospital. The nurse understands that the client may be a candidate for surgery to control the pain. Which surgery should the nurse expect to schedule?
    1. Rhizotomy
    2. Rhinotomy

3. Cordotomy

4. Chondrectomy

192. After abdominal surgery a client complains of pain. What action should the nurse take first?
    1. Reposition the client.
    2. Monitor the vital signs.
    3. Administer the ordered analgesic.
    4. Determine the characteristics of the pain.

193. A client with an inflamed sciatic nerve is to have a conventional transcutaneous electrical nerve stimulation (TENS) device applied to the painful nerve pathway. When operating the TENS unit, which nursing action is appropriate?
    1. Maintain the same dial settings every day.
    2. Turn the machine on several times a day for 10 to 20 minutes.
    3. Adjust the TENS dial until the client experiences relief of pain.
    4. Apply the color-coded electrodes anywhere it is comfortable for the client.

194. The nurse is caring for a client following radium insertion for cancer of the cervix. Which client response identified by the nurse is indicative of a radium reaction?
    1. Pain
    2. Nausea
    3. Excoriation
    4. Restlessness

195. Radium inserted in the vagina of a client is now being removed. Which safety precaution should the nurse employ when assisting with the radium removal?
    1. Cleaning the radium in ether or alcohol
    2. Ensuring that long forceps are available for use
    3. Handling the radium carefully, wearing foil-lined rubber gloves
    4. Charting the date and hour of removal and the total time of treatment

196. The nurse checking the perineum of a client with a radium implant for cervical cancer finds the packing protruding from the vagina. The immediate action by the nurse is to report this situation to the physician at once because the packing:
    1. Must be removed
    2. Has become radioactive
    3. Prevents excessive loss of blood
    4. Decreases trauma to normal tissue

197. The nurse is caring for a client who has a radium implant for cancer of the cervix. What should the nurse do?
    1. Restrict visitors to a 10-minute stay.
    2. Store urine in a lead-lined container.

3. Wear a lead apron when giving care.

4. Avoid giving IM injections into the gluteal muscle.

198. A client has a radium implant for cancer of the cervix. Which information is important for the nurse to teach the client during the presentation of the discharge instructions?
    1. Limiting daily fluid intake
    2. Continuing a low-residue diet
    3. Returning for medical follow-up care
    4. Taking daily multivitamin supplements

199. A client has corrective surgery for a bladder laceration. Which nursing intervention takes priority during this client's postoperative period?
    1. Turning frequently
    2. Raising side rails on the bed
    3. Providing range-of-motion exercises
    4. Massaging the back three times a day

200. A 67-year-old woman, who has cancer of the breast, decided to have a lumpectomy followed by chemotherapy. After receiving chemotherapy for several weeks she comes to the clinic and states, "I don't feel well." The nurse reviews the medications the client is receiving, checks the client's laboratory results, and obtains the client's vital signs. What should the nurse conclude is the client's priority need based on the information collected?
    1. Promoting rest
    2. Avoiding injury
    3. Preventing infection
    4. Maintaining fluid balance

CLIENT CHART
Medications
cyclophosphamide (Cytoxan)
doxorubicin (Adriamycin)
fluorouracil (5-FU)
Laboratory Results
RBC: 4.2 µL
WBC: 3000 µL
Hb: 12.5 g/dL
Hct: 39%
Platelets: 190,000 µL
Vital Signs
Temperature (oral): 99.8° F
Pulse: 88 beats/min
Resp: 24 breaths/min
Blood pressure: 126/88 mm Hg

ANSWERS AND RATIONALES

1. 2 To promote optimism and facilitate smooth functioning, all rehabilitation should begin on admission to the hospital.
1 The client and family often are unaware of the options available in the health care system; the nurse should be available to provide the necessary information and support. 3 Because paralysis is permanent, alterations in the client's lifestyle are required. 4 Rehabilitation helps a client adjust lifestyle to compensate for paralysis.
Client Need: Management of Care; **Cognitive Level:** Comprehension; **Nursing Process:** Planning/Implementation; **Reference:** Ch 2, Nursing Process

2. 3 All nursing intervention aims to assist an individual in maximizing capabilities and coping with modifications in lifestyle.
1 All resources that can be beneficial to client rehabilitation, including the private physician and acute care facilities, should be utilized. 2 Rehabilitation is a commonality in all areas of nursing practice. 4 Rehabilitation is necessary to help clients return to a previous level of functioning.
Client Need: Management of Care; **Cognitive Level:** Application; **Nursing Process:** Planning/Implementation; **Reference:** Ch 1, Health-Illness Continuum and Rehabilitation

3. 4 Learning from others occurs in a group setting and is reinforced by group acceptance of the norms.
1 One member of a group can be the target of hostility. 2 A group member may not be easily identified. 3 Groups do not go through the same developmental phases as individuals.
Client Need: Psychosocial Integrity; **Cognitive Level:** Application; **Nursing Process:** Assessment/Analysis; **Reference:** Ch 1, Groups

4. 1 The use of a call bell system enables the client to communicate with the staff and supports safety and security, which is a second level need.
2 Self-esteem involves intrapersonal needs, the fourth level of basic needs. 3 Physiologic needs include air, food, water, etc. and represent the first level of needs. 4 Interpersonal needs involve love and belonging, third-level needs.
Client Need: Safety and Infection Control; **Cognitive Level:** Application; **Integrated Process:** Teaching/Learning; **Nursing Process:** Planning/Implementation; **Reference:** Ch 2, The Nurse-Client Relationship

5. 3 Socialization, values, and role definition are learned within the family and help develop a sense of self. Once established in the family, the child can more easily move into society.
1 Although true, it is not as important as identity and roles in relation to emotional development. 2, 4 This is a small aspect of the family's influence.
Client Need: Psychosocial Integrity; **Cognitive Level:** Comprehension; **Integrated Process:** Communication/Documentation; **Nursing Process:** Planning/Implementation; **Reference:** Ch 1, Groups

6. 4 A major premise of AA is that to be successful in achieving sobriety, clients with alcohol abuse problems must acknowledge their inability to control the use of alcohol.
1 There are no rules of attendance or speaking at meetings, although both actions are strongly encouraged. 2 This is not part of AA; this group strongly supports total abstinence for life. 3 There are no rules of attendance at meetings; the member is strongly encouraged to attend as often as possible.
Client Need: Psychosocial Integrity; **Cognitive Level:** Comprehension; **Nursing Process:** Planning/Implementation; **Reference:** Ch 1, Groups

7. 3 Self-help groups are successful because they support a basic human need for acceptance. A feeling of comfort and safety and a sense of belonging may be achieved in a nonjudgmental, supportive, sharing experience with others.
1, 2 AA would probably not meet this need. 4 On the contrary, AA meets dependency needs rather than focusing on independence.
Client Need: Psychosocial Integrity; **Cognitive Level:** Comprehension; **Integrated Process:** Caring; **Nursing Process:** Planning/Implementation; **Reference:** Ch 1, Groups

8. 2 Cultural discomfort occurs when a person is uncomfortable with those from another culture.
1 There is no clash of cultures being exhibited in this situation. 3 There are no data to support this conclusion; ethnocentrism is the belief in the inherent superiority of the group to which one belongs. 4 The nurses are sensitive to those of another culture, but they are not addressing it positively.
Client Need: Psychosocial Integrity; **Cognitive Level:** Analysis; **Integrated Process:** Caring; **Nursing Process:** Evaluation/Outcomes; **Reference:** Ch 1, Culture and Health

9. 1 A workshop provides an opportunity to discuss the topic of culture, which should include identification of one's own feelings; also, it provides an opportunity for the participants to ask questions.
2 This is not feasible or desirable; clients from other cultures are found in all settings. 3 Although this would provide information, it does not promote a discussion about the topic. 4 This would probably increase tension on the unit.
Client Need: Management of Care; **Cognitive Level:** Application; **Integrated Process:** Teaching/Learning; **Nursing Process:** Planning/Implementation; **Reference:** Ch 1, Culture and Health

10. 3 Because of a short attention span and distractibility, consistent limit setting is crucial toward providing an environment that promotes concentration, prevents confusion, and minimizes conflicts.

1 Questions are appropriate as long as the answers are not judgmental. **2** A list of expectations may be overwhelming. It is better to set priorities. **4** Parents need to assist children with routine tasks; children this age may not be concerned with time frames.
Client Need: Health Promotion and Maintenance; **Cognitive Level:** Application; **Integrated Process:** Communication/ Documentation; **Nursing Process:** Planning/Implementation; **Reference:** Ch 1, Individual Factors Affecting Health

11. **4** Understanding the disease and the details of care are essential for the client to become self-sufficient at home.

   1 Although this is important, it is not the priority; a perceived understanding of the need for specific interventions must be expressed before there is a readiness for learning. **2** This is premature and not the priority; this may be done eventually. **3** Although this is important, it is not the priority; involving the college should be the clients' decision.
   Client Need: Health Promotion and Maintenance; **Cognitive Level:** Analysis; **Integrated Process:** Teaching/Learning; **Nursing Process:** Evaluation/Outcomes; **Reference:** Ch 2, Teaching-Learning

12. **2** An individual is held legally responsible for actions committed against another individual or an individual's property.

   1 This is battery, which involves physical harm.
   3 This is the definition of negligence. **4** This is the definition of a crime.
   Client Need: Management of Care; **Cognitive Level:** Comprehension; **Nursing Process:** Assessment/Analysis; **Reference:** Ch 2, Torts and Crimes Important to Nurses

13. **2** Using a stretcher with worn straps is negligent; this oversight does not reflect the actions of a reasonably prudent nurse.

   1 The hospital shares responsibility for safe, functioning equipment. **3, 4** The nurse is responsible for his or her own actions and must ascertain the adequate functioning of equipment.
   Client Need: Management of Care; **Cognitive Level:** Analysis; **Nursing Process:** Evaluation/Outcomes; **Reference:** Ch 2, Torts and Crimes Important to Nurses

14. **2** It is the nurse's responsibility to foresee potential harm and prevent risks by acting as an advocate.
   1 This is not acceptable as a rationale for inaction.
   3 High temperatures are common in children but are nonetheless a valid cause for concern. **4** The nurse and physician share interdependent roles in the assessment and care of clients.
   Client Need: Management of Care; **Cognitive Level:** Analysis; **Nursing Process:** Evaluation/Outcomes; **Reference:** Ch 2, The Nurse's Rights and Responsibilities

15. **1** Each state or province protects the health and welfare of its populace by regulating nursing practice.

   2 Although the members of the profession can also benefit from a clear description of their role, this is not the primary purpose of the law. **3** The employing agency does assume responsibility for its employees and therefore benefits from maintenance of standards,

but this is not the purpose of the law. **4** Professional standards are established by the profession to ensure quality care for the public.
Client Need: Management of Care; **Cognitive Level:** Comprehension; **Nursing Process:** Planning/Implementation; **Reference:** Ch 2, The Nurse's Rights and Responsibilities

16. **3** The Nurse Practice Act states that nurses diagnose and treat human responses to actual or potential health problems. Administration of oxygen in an emergency situation is within the scope of nursing practice.

   1, 2, 4 Because the client's symptoms reflect an immediate need for oxygen, postponement of treatment could result in further deterioration of the client's condition.
   Client Need: Management of Care; **Cognitive Level:** Analysis; **Nursing Process:** Evaluation/Outcomes; **Reference:** Ch 2, The Nurse's Rights and Responsibilities

17. **2** The nurse's data collection was not adequate because no questions were asked concerning the date of the previous tetanus inoculation. The nurse failed to support the life and well-being of a client.

   1 The nurse's assessment was not thorough in regard to determining the date of immunization. **3** This is not an independent function of the nurse. **4** It was essential to determine when the client was last immunized; for a "tetanus-prone" wound, like a puncture from a rusty nail, some form of tetanus immunization usually is given.
   Client Need: Management of Care; **Cognitive Level:** Analysis; **Nursing Process:** Evaluation/Outcomes; **Reference:** Ch 2, Torts and Crimes Important to Nurses

18. **4** False imprisonment is a wrong committed by one person against another in a willful, intentional way without just cause and/or excuse.

   1 Negligence is an unintentional tort. **2** Malpractice, which is professional negligence, is classified as an unintentional tort. **3** Breach of duty is an unintentional tort.
   Client Need: Management of Care; **Cognitive Level:** Comprehension; **Nursing Process:** Planning/Implementation; **Reference:** Ch 2, Torts and Crimes Important to Nurses

19. **4** Personal liability insurance will represent a nurse before the State Board of Nursing, whereas employee liability insurance will not.

   1 A nurse can be sued whether or not the nurse has liability insurance. **2** Employer liability insurance will represent the nurse in charges related to employment, not charges brought by the State Board of Nursing.
   3 Liability insurance is available for all nurses.
   Client Need: Management of Care; **Cognitive Level:** Analysis; **Nursing Process:** Evaluation/Outcomes; **Reference:** Ch 2, Nurse's Rights and Responsibilities

20. **1** Assault is a threat or an attempt to do violence to another, and battery means touching an individual in an offensive manner or actually injuring another person.

   2 The nurse's behavior demonstrates anger and does not take into account the growth and developmental

needs of this age-group. **3** Although the behavior (scratching) needs to be decreased, this can be done with mittens so as not to immobilize a child of this age. **4** A 3-year-old does not have the capacity to understand cause (scratching) and effect (bleeding).
Client Need: Management of Care; **Cognitive Level:** Analysis; **Nursing Process:** Evaluation/Outcomes; **Reference:** Ch 2, Torts and Crimes Important to Nurses

21. **1** Assault is a threat or an attempt to do violence to another.
    2 This is the definition of battery. **3** Assault implies harm to persons, rather than property. **4** This definition is too broad to describe assault.
Client Need: Management of Care; **Cognitive Level:** Comprehension; **Integrated Process:** Teaching/Learning; **Nursing Process:** Planning/Implementation; **Reference:** Ch 2, Torts and Crimes Important to Nurses

22. **1** Battery means touching in an offensive manner or actually injuring another person.
    2 Battery refers to harm against persons instead of property. **3** Battery refers to actual bodily harm rather than threats of physical or psychologic harm. **4** This is the definition of negligence.
Client Need: Management of Care; **Cognitive Level:** Comprehension; **Integrated Process:** Teaching/Learning; **Nursing Process:** Planning/Implementation; **Reference:** Ch 2, Torts and Crimes Important to Nurses

23. **2** Legally, a client cannot be locked in a room (isolated) unless there is a threat of danger involved either to the client or to other clients.
    1 This is a reaction to separation from the parent, which is common at this age. **3** The child should never be isolated. **4** Crying, although irritating, will not harm the other children.
Client Need: Management of Care; **Cognitive Level:** Analysis; **Nursing Process:** Evaluation/Outcomes; **Reference:** Ch 2, Torts and Crimes Important to Nurses

24. **4** The client's rights are violated. All clients have the right to a complete and accurate explanation of treatment.
    1 All interventions should be explained because they are not routine to the client. **2** The Patient Care Partnership (formerly The Patient's Bill of Rights) states that the client should be informed. **3** When administering treatment, the nurse is responsible for explaining to the client what the treatment is and why it is being done.
Client Need: Management of Care; **Cognitive Level:** Analysis; **Nursing Process:** Evaluation/Outcomes; **Reference:** Ch 2, Clients' Rights

25. **2** Informed consent means the client must comprehend the surgery, the alternatives, and the consequences.
    1 This explanation is not within nursing's domain. **3** Although this is true, it does not determine the client's ability to give informed consent. **4** Although this is true, the nurse should first assess the client's knowledge of the surgery.

Client Need: Management of Care; **Cognitive Level:** Application; **Integrated Process:** Teaching/Learning; **Nursing Process:** Evaluation/Outcomes; **Reference:** Ch 2, Clients' Rights

26. **4** Although a hysterectomy may be performed, conservative management may include cervical conization and laser treatment that do not preclude future pregnancies; clients have a right to be informed by their physician of all treatment options.
    1 This currently is not the issue for this client.
    2, 3 This negates the client's feelings.
Client Need: Management of Care; **Cognitive Level:** Application; **Integrated Process:** Communication/Documentation; **Nursing Process:** Planning/Implementation; **Reference:** Ch 2, Clients' Rights

27. **1** This is considered a routine procedure to meet basic physiologic needs and is covered by a consent signed at the time of admission.
    2 The need for consent is not negated because the procedure is beneficial. **3, 4** This treatment does not require special consent.
Client Need: Management of Care; **Cognitive Level:** Analysis; **Integrated Process:** Communication/Documentation; **Nursing Process:** Evaluation/Outcomes; **Reference:** Ch 2, Clients' Rights

28. **2** The client is unconscious. Although the spouse can consent, there is no legal power to refuse a treatment for the client unless previously authorized to do so by a power of attorney or a health care proxy; the court can make a decision for the client.
    1, 4 This alternative is without legal basis, and the nurse could be held liable. **3** Explanations are not effective at this time and will not meet the client's needs.
Client Need: Management of Care; **Cognitive Level:** Analysis; **Integrated Process:** Communication/Documentation; **Nursing Process:** Planning/Implementation; **Reference:** Ch 2, Clients' Rights

29. **4** Because the client is not certified as incompetent, the right of informed consent is retained.
    1 The client can sign the consent, and the client's signature requires only one witness. **2, 3** Because there is no evidence of incompetence, the client should sign the consent.
Client Need: Management of Care; **Cognitive Level:** Application; **Integrated Process:** Communication/Documentation; **Nursing Process:** Planning/Implementation; **Reference:** Ch 2, Clients' Rights

30. **1** An individual is legally unable to sign a consent until the age of 18 years. The only exception is the emancipated minor, a minor who is self-sufficient or married.
    2 Although the adolescent may be capable of intelligent choices, 18 is the legal age of consent. **3** Parents or guardians are legally responsible under all circumstances unless the adolescent is an emancipated minor. **4** Adolescents have the capacity to choose, but not the legal right in this situation.
Client Need: Management of Care; **Cognitive Level:** Comprehension; **Integrated Process:** Communication/Documentation;

Nursing Process: Planning/Implementation; **Reference:** Ch 2, Clients' Rights

31. **2** The client has a right to know what medication is being administered (informed consent).
    1 The physician should be notified only after the nurse has interviewed the client to determine the reasons for the decision. **3** This cannot be determined from the situation described; the client should be questioned about the reasons for refusing the drug. **4** The client has a right to refuse treatment; this right takes precedence over the physician's order.
    Client Need: Management of Care; **Cognitive Level:** Analysis; **Integrated Process:** Communication/Documentation; **Nursing Process:** Evaluation/Outcomes; **Reference:** Ch 2, Clients' Rights

32. **1** The nurse needs to remove and dispose of the patch in a manner that protects self and others from exposure to the fentanyl.
    2, 3 This is not the responsibility of nonprofessionals because they do not know how to protect themselves and others from exposure to the fentanyl. **4** It is unnecessary to return a used fentanyl patch for accounting purposes.
    Client Need: Basic Care and Comfort; **Cognitive Level:** Application; **Nursing Process:** Planning/Implementation; **Reference:** Ch 2, Clients' Rights

33. **1** Controlled substance issues for a particular nursing unit are the responsibility of that unit's manager.
    2 The responsibility flows from the staff of a nursing unit to the nurse manager and from there up the line of responsibility depending on the table of organization for the institution. **3** There is no direct flow of accountability from the nurse manager to the quality control manager. **4** There is no direct responsibility to physicians regarding issues of nursing unit management.
    Client Need: Safety and Infection Control; **Cognitive Level:** Application; **Integrated Process:** Communication/Documentation; **Nursing Process:** Planning/Implementation; **Reference:** Ch 2, Nursing Responsibilities Related to Medication Administration

34. **2** This is an invasion of privacy, an intentional tort.
    1, 3, 4 This is an example of professional negligence (malpractice).
    Client Need: Management of Care; **Cognitive Level:** Analysis; **Nursing Process:** Planning/Implementation; **Reference:** Ch 2, Torts and Crimes Important to Nurses

35. **2** When the client signs herself and the baby out of the hospital, she is legally responsible for her infant and must be given the baby.
    1, 3, 4 The baby belongs to the mother and can leave with the mother when she signs them out.
    Client Need: Management of Care; **Cognitive Level:** Application; **Integrated Process:** Communication/Documentation; **Nursing Process:** Planning/Implementation; **Reference:** Ch 2, Clients' Rights

36. **1** The nurse's response really is a threat by attempting to put pressure on the client to speak or be left alone.

2 This is not reward and punishment, which is used in behavior modification therapy. **3** Clients in emotional crisis should not be left alone. **4** The client is depressed and should not be left alone.
Client Need: Management of Care; **Cognitive Level:** Analysis; **Nursing Process:** Evaluation/Outcomes; **Reference:** Ch 2, Torts and Crimes Important to Nurses

37. **1** The Nurse Practice Act requires nurses to diagnose human responses.
    2 Assessment should not differ if done by the nurse. **3** This is physical assessment, not medical diagnosis, and is within the nurse's role. **4** The nurse is capable of independently making a physical assessment.
    Client Need: Management of Care; **Cognitive Level:** Analysis; **Integrated Process:** Communication/Documentation; **Nursing Process:** Evaluation/Outcomes; **Reference:** Ch 2, The Nurse's Rights and Responsibilities

38. **3** The reporting of possible child abuse is required by law, and the nurse's identity can remain confidential.
    1 The nurse is functioning in a professional capacity and therefore can be held accountable. **2, 4** Although the Good Samaritan Act protects health professionals, the nurse is still responsible for acting as any reasonably prudent nurse would in a similar situation.
    Client Need: Management of Care; **Cognitive Level:** Comprehension; **Nursing Process:** Planning/Implementation; **Reference:** Ch 2, The Nurse's Rights and Responsibilities

39. **3** Because the client's condition is terminal, the nursing priority should be directed toward providing comfort.
    1, 2, 4 Although these are important aspects of nursing care, provision of comfort retains the priority in the care of a dying client.
    Client Need: Basic Care and Comfort; **Cognitive Level:** Application; **Integrated Process:** Caring; **Nursing Process:** Planning/Implementation; **Reference:** Ch 1, Type of Condition Affecting the Client

40. **2** Because family members are old enough to understand the client's needs, they should be encouraged to participate in the care.
    1 Self-care increases oxygen utilization, thereby increasing fatigue and dyspnea. **3** This deprives the client of a support system. **4** Overworking the client causes undue fatigue; frequent rest periods are indicated.
    Client Need: Psychosocial Integrity; **Cognitive Level:** Application; **Integrated Process:** Caring; **Nursing Process:** Planning/Implementation; **Reference:** Ch 1, Type of Condition Affecting the Client

41. **2** Practicing ambulation without proper preparation (e.g., ambulation techniques and strengthening the involved muscle groups) is not helpful in the rehabilitation process and could exhaust the client.
    1 Because different muscle groups are utilized, the client must be instructed about simple maneuvers; transfer from a sitting to a standing position must be accomplished before ambulation. **3** Balance is

essential to prevent falls. **4** The muscles used for crutch walking are different from those used in normal ambulation; therefore they must be strengthened by active exercises before ambulation. **Client Need:** Health Promotion and Maintenance; **Cognitive Level:** Application; **Integrated Process:** Teaching/Learning; **Nursing Process:** Evaluation/Outcomes; **Reference:** Ch 2, Teaching-Learning

42. **2** The nursing process is a step-by-step process that scientifically provides for a client's nursing needs.
1, 3, 4 This is only one step in the nursing process.
Client Need: Management of Care; **Cognitive Level:** Comprehension; **Integrated Process:** Teaching/Learning; **Nursing Process:** Planning/Implementation; **Reference:** Ch 2, Nursing Process

43. **3** The first step in problem solving is data collection.
1 Goals are set after nursing needs are established.
2 Nursing needs are based on assessment.
4 Evaluation is the last phase of the nursing process.
Client Need: Management of Care; **Cognitive Level:** Knowledge; **Nursing Process:** Assessment/Analysis; **Reference:** Ch 2, Nursing Process

44. **2** An actual or potential client health problem is based on the analysis and interpretation of the data collected during the assessment phase of the nursing process.
1, 4 The plan of care includes nursing actions to meet client needs. The needs must first be identified before nursing actions are planned and implemented.
3 Assessments are made before data analysis, which then leads to the identification of the client's health problem or need.
Client Need: Management of Care; **Cognitive Level:** Comprehension; **Integrated Process:** Teaching/Learning; **Nursing Process:** Planning/Implementation; **Reference:** Ch 2, Nursing Process

45. **1** The primary nurse provides or oversees all aspects of care, including assessment, implementation, and evaluation of that care.
2 A clinician is an expert teacher or practitioner in the clinical area. **3** A clinical specialist is a title given to a specially prepared nurse for one very specific clinical role. It requires a master's degree level of education. **4** The nurse coordinator oversees all the staff and clients on a unit and coordinates care.
Client Need: Management of Care; **Cognitive Level:** Comprehension; **Nursing Process:** Planning/Implementation; **Reference:** Ch 1, Society and Health

46. **4** Helping the client to meet physical needs is within the role of the nurse; arranging blankets on the client's bed is an appropriate intervention.
1 The nurse's comfort needs should not take precedence over the client's needs; the nurse should not assume responsibility for the role of care provider if incapable of providing care. **2** It is not a good deed but fulfills the expected role of the nurse; this response sounds grudgingly compliant. **3** This is within the nurse's job description.

Client Need: Management of Care; **Cognitive Level:** Application; **Integrated Process:** Caring; **Nursing Process:** Planning/ Implementation; **Reference:** Ch 2, The Nurse-Client Relationship

47. **4** When a plan does not effectively produce the desired outcome, the plan should be changed.
1 Time is not relevant in care plan revision. **2** Client response to care is the determining factor, not the original health problem. **3** Various methods may have the same outcome; effectiveness is most important.
Client Need: Management of Care; **Cognitive Level:** Comprehension; **Nursing Process:** Evaluation/Outcomes; **Reference:** Ch 2, Nursing Process

48. **1** Acquiring knowledge or understanding aids in developing concepts, rather than skills or attitudes, and is a basic learning task in the cognitive domain.
2 Values and self-realization are in the affective domain. **3, 4** Skills acquisition is in the psychomotor domain.
Client Need: Health Promotion and Maintenance; **Cognitive Level:** Analysis; **Integrated Process:** Teaching/Learning; **Nursing Process:** Assessment/Analysis; **Reference:** Ch 2, Teaching-Learning

49. **2** Success is a basic motivation for learning. People receive satisfaction when a goal is reached.
1 Progress toward long-range goals is often not readily apparent and may be discouraging.
3 Constructive criticism is an important aspect of client teaching; but if not tempered with praise, it is discouraging. **4** This is an important part of teaching, but it will not necessarily motivate the client.
Client Need: Health Promotion and Maintenance; **Cognitive Level:** Application; **Integrated Process:** Teaching/Learning; **Nursing Process:** Planning/Implementation; **Reference:** Ch 2, Teaching-Learning

50. **3** A paradoxical response to a drug is directly opposite the desired therapeutic response.
1 An allergic response is an antigen-antibody reaction. **2** A synergistic response involves drug combinations that enhance each other. **4** This is a response to a drug that is more pronounced than the common response.
Client Need: Pharmacological and Parenteral Therapies; **Cognitive Level:** Comprehension; **Nursing Process:** Evaluation/ Outcomes; **Reference:** Ch 2, Drug Effects

51. **3** Hypersensitivity results from the production of antibodies in response to exposure to certain foreign substances (allergens). Earlier exposure is necessary for the development of these antibodies.
1 This is not a sensitivity reaction to penicillin; hay fever and asthma are atopic conditions. **2** It would be an active immune response. **4** Antibodies have been developed in a prior exposure to penicillin.
Client Need: Pharmacological and Parenteral Therapies; **Cognitive Level:** Comprehension; **Nursing Process:** Evaluation/ Outcomes; **Reference:** Ch 2, Drug Effects

52. **4** By law, a nurse cannot administer medications without a prescription from a legally licensed individual.

1, 2 The nurse gives only ordered medications. **3** The nurse should not assume that the physician is aware of the problem.

Client Need: Pharmacological and Parenteral Therapies; **Cognitive Level:** Application; **Integrated Process:** Communication/Documentation; **Nursing Process:** Planning/Implementation; **Reference:** Ch 2, Nursing Responsibilities Related to Medication Administration

53. **Answer: 1 mL**

When 132 pounds is converted to kilograms, it equals 60 kg; the physician has ordered 5 mcg/kg, or 5 times 60 equals 300 mcg; this amount is contained in 1 mL, as indicated on the vial label.

Client Need: Pharmacological and Parenteral Therapies; **Cognitive Level:** Application; **Nursing Process:** Planning/Implementation; **Reference:** Ch 2, Nursing Responsibilities Related to Medication Administration

54. **Answer: 1.4 mL**

(0.35 mg/X mL) = (0.25 mg/1 mL)

0.25 mg × X mL = 0.35 mg × 1 mL

0.25X = 0.35

X = 0.35 ÷ 0.25 = 1.4 mL

Client Need: Pharmacological and Parenteral Therapies; **Cognitive Level:** Application; **Nursing Process:** Planning/Implementation; **Reference:** Ch 2, Nursing Responsibilities Related to Medication Administration

55. **Answer: 1.5 mL**

(375 mg/250 mg) = (X mL/1 mL)

250X = 375

X = 375 ÷ 250

X = 1.5 mL

Client Need: Pharmacological and Parenteral Therapies; **Cognitive Level:** Application; **Nursing Process:** Planning/Implementation; **Reference:** Ch 2, Nursing Responsibilities Related to Medication Administration

56. **1** The wasting of controlled substances should be witnessed by two licensed personnel according to federal regulations; this can be done by an RN or LPN.

2 Federal regulations do not require the participation by the client's physician in this situation. **3** Although the nursing supervisor is licensed and could perform this function, it would not be an efficient use of this individual's expertise. **4** A nursing assistant is not a licensed person who can take responsibility for the wasting of controlled substances.

Client Need: Pharmacological and Parenteral Therapies; **Cognitive Level:** Application; **Nursing Process:** Planning/Implementation; **Reference:** Ch 2, Nursing Responsibilities Related to Medication Administration

57. **4** The vaccination is scratched into the skin using a bifurcated needle.

1 An intramuscular injection using the Z-track technique would administer the vaccine too deeply. **2** This is unsafe and ineffective. **3** This would administer the vaccine too deeply.

Client Need: Pharmacological and Parenteral Therapies; **Cognitive Level:** Application; **Integrated Process:** Teaching/Learning; **Nursing Process:** Planning/Implementation; **Reference:** Ch 2, Nursing Responsibilities Related to Medication Administration

58. **3** When an oral medication is available in a suspension form, the nurse should use it for clients who cannot swallow capsules.

1 Because a palatable suspension is available, it is a better alternative than opening the capsule. **2** The route of administration cannot be altered without physician approval. **4** Intramuscular injections should be avoided because of risks for tissue injury and infection.

Client Need: Pharmacological and Parenteral Therapies; **Cognitive Level:** Analysis; **Nursing Process:** Planning/Implementation; **Reference:** Ch 2, Nursing Responsibilities Related to Medication Administration

59. **1** ☒ Prostaglandins accumulate at the site of an injury, causing pain; NSAIDs inhibit COX-1 and COX-2 (both are isoforms of the enzyme cyclooxygenase), which inhibit the production of prostaglandins, thereby contributing to analgesia.

2 ☒ NSAIDs inhibit COX-2 which is associated with fever, thereby causing antipyresis.

3 ❏ This is an adverse effect, not a desired outcome; NSAIDs can impair platelet function by inhibiting thromboxane, an aggregating agent, resulting in bleeding.

4 ❏ NSAIDs do not cause bronchodilation.

5 ❏ NSAIDs do not cause urinary diuresis; reversible renal ischemia and renal insufficiency in clients with heart failure, cirrhosis, or hypovolemia can be a potential adverse effect of NSAIDs.

6 ☒ NSAIDs inhibit COX-2 which is associated with inflammation, thereby reducing inflammation.

Client Need: Pharmacological and Parenteral Therapies; **Cognitive Level:** Comprehension; **Nursing Process:** Evaluation/Outcomes; **Reference:** Ch 3, Nonsteroidal Antiinflammatory Drugs (NSAIDS)

60. **3** Paraphrasing encourages the client to express the rationale for this request.

1 This is making an assumption without enough information. **2** Although this request would be forwarded to the physician, the reason for the choice of general anesthesia should be explored. **4** This statement may raise the client's anxiety.

Client Need: Psychosocial Integrity; **Cognitive Level:** Application; **Integrated Process:** Communication/Documentation; **Nursing Process:** Assessment/Analysis; **Reference:** Ch 2, The Nurse-Client Relationship

61. **1** Past experiences have the most meaningful influence on present learning.

2-4 Although these considerations affect learning, their influence is not as great as past experiences.

Client Need: Psychosocial Integrity; **Cognitive Level:** Application; **Integrated Process:** Teaching/Learning; **Nursing Process:** Assessment/Analysis; **Reference:** Ch 2, Teaching-Learning

62. **3** In this stage the degree of anguish experienced is influenced by cultural background.
   1 Although these factor, enter into the grief process, they are is not as important as culture. **2** This is not directly related. **4** While past experience is important, it is not as significant as culture.
   Client Need: Psychosocial Integrity; **Cognitive Level:** Application; **Integrated Process:** Caring; **Nursing Process:** Assessment/ Analysis; **Reference:** Ch 1, Culture and Health

63. **1** Without some form of communication there can be no socialization.
   2-4 People interact with other social beings, not with inanimate objects.
   Client Need: Psychosocial Integrity; **Cognitive Level:** Comprehension; **Integrated Process:** Communication/ Documentation; **Nursing Process:** Assessment/Analysis; **Reference:** Ch 2, Communication; Basic Concepts

64. **1** Feedback permits the client to ask questions and express feelings and allows the nurse to verify client understanding.
   2 Medical assessments do not necessarily include nurse-client relationships. **3** Team conferences are subject to all members' evaluations of a client's status. **4** Nurse-client communication should be evaluated by the client's verbal and behavioral responses.
   Client Need: Psychosocial Integrity; **Cognitive Level:** Comprehension; **Integrated Process:** Communication/ Documentation; **Nursing Process:** Assessment/Analysis; **Reference:** Ch 2, Communication; Basic Concepts

65. **1** When nurses make judgmental remarks and client needs are not placed first, the standards of care are violated and quality of care is compromised.
   2 There is no information about client acuity to come to this conclusion. **3** The statement does not reflect any information about complexity of care. **4** Assessments should be objective, not subjective and biased.
   Client Need: Psychosocial Integrity; **Cognitive Level:** Comprehension; **Integrated Process:** Communication/ Documentation; **Nursing Process:** Evaluation/Outcomes; **Reference:** Ch 2, The Nurse-Client Relationship

66. **2** Relaxation of muscles and facial expression are examples of nonverbal behavior; nonverbal behavior is a better index of feelings because it is less likely to be consciously controlled.
   1 Increased activity may be an expression of anger or hostility. **3** Clients may suppress verbal outbursts despite feelings and become withdrawn. **4** Refusing to talk may be a sign that the client is just not ready to discuss feelings.
   Client Need: Psychosocial Integrity; **Cognitive Level:** Analysis; **Integrated Process:** Communication/Documentation; **Nursing Process:** Evaluation/Outcomes; **Reference:** Ch 2, The Nurse-Client Relationship

67. **1** These are universal activities that all nursing assistants (NAs) are taught to perform regardless of the setting; these activities are within the job description of NAs.
   2 Although NAs may perform range-of-motion exercises, they do not have the credentials or expertise to perform sterile dressing changes. **3** Although NAs may change linens on occupied beds, they cannot document client responses in medical records. **4** Although NAs may care for clients with transmission-based precautions, they may not change intravenous solutions.
   Client Need: Management of Care; **Cognitive Level:** Application; **Nursing Process:** Planning/Implementation; **Reference:** Ch 2, Principles of Leadership

68. **1** Sitting quietly with the client gives the message that the nurse cares and accepts the client's feelings.
   2 This is negating feelings and the client's right to cry when upset. **3** Helping the client explore reasons is more therapeutic than giving advice. **4** This, in effect, closes the door on any further communication of feelings.
   Client Need: Psychosocial Integrity; **Cognitive Level:** Application; **Integrated Process:** Caring; **Nursing Process:** Planning/Implementation, **Reference:** Ch 2, The Nurse-Client Relationship

69. **3** An honest nurse-client relationship should be maintained so that trust can develop.
   1 Although other health care team members may need to be informed eventually, the initial action should concern only the nurse-client relationship. **2, 4** This does nothing to establish communication about feelings or motivation behind behavior.
   Client Need: Psychosocial Integrity; **Cognitive Level:** Application; **Integrated Process:** Communication/Documentation; **Nursing Process:** Planning/Implementation; **Reference:** Ch 2, The Nurse-Client Relationship

70. **1** The cause of the alarm should be investigated and appropriate intervention instituted if necessary; after the client's needs are met, then other tasks can be accomplished.
   2, 4 The alarm indicates that the client's BP is decreased; it should not be ignored. Alarms should always remain on and should not be changed for the convenience of the nurse. **3** An alarm should never be ignored, and the client's status takes priority over the change-of-shift report.
   Client Need: Management of Care; **Cognitive Level:** Application; **Nursing Process:** Planning/Implementation; **Reference:** Ch 2, Nursing Process

71. **3** This recognizes that the client's feelings of anxiety are valid.
   1, 2 This does not recognize the client's concerns and may inhibit the expression of feelings. **4** This is not true and does not recognize the client's concerns.
   Client Need: Psychosocial Integrity; **Cognitive Level:** Application; **Integrated Process:** Caring; **Nursing Process:** Planning/ Implementation; **Reference:** Ch 2, Nurse-Client Relationship

72. **2** Orienting the client to the hospital provides knowledge that may reduce the strangeness of the environment.
   1 This may be false reassurance, because no one can guarantee that everything will be all right. **3** This

would be part of orienting the client to the unit. **4** This implies that staff members are available only if the client has specific questions.
Client Need: Psychosocial Integrity; **Cognitive Level:** Application; **Integrated Process:** Caring; **Nursing Process:** Planning/Implementation; **Reference:** Ch 2, The Nurse-Client Relationship

73. **2** Because of the variety of factors vying for the nurse's time, efficient use of the time available for teaching is essential to meet the standards of care and legal responsibilities of the nurse.
1 The increased awareness and knowledge of health issues by consumers may provide a foundation on which the teaching plan may be built; informed consumerism should be viewed as a positive, not a negative. **3** Assessing clients' cultural beliefs is part of the initial and continuing assessment of clients; this should not cause additional stress during teaching. **4** Generally, adults are motivated, independent learners and the nurse teacher should be a facilitator of learning.
Client Need: Health Promotion and Maintenance; **Cognitive Level:** Comprehension; **Integrated Process:** Teaching/Learning; **Nursing Process:** Evaluation/Outcomes; **Reference:** Ch 2, Teaching-Learning

74. **2** The client has the right to make this decision, and the staff should accept the client's wishes.
1 The client is a doctor, and the nurse's statement attacks the client's self-concept. **3** The informality of using first names is not encouraged unless it is the client's choice. **4.** The nurse can and should honor the client's request.
Client Need: Psychosocial Integrity; **Cognitive Level:** Application; **Integrated Process:** Caring; **Nursing Process:** Planning/Implementation; **Reference:** Ch 2, The Nurse-Client Relationship

75. **2** This response attempts to open the communication process.
1 Restating only serves to entrench each communicant's position and does little to open the flow of communication. **3** This shifts the focus away from the client. **4** This is authoritative and closes down the flow of communication.
Client Need: Psychosocial Integrity; **Cognitive Level:** Application; **Integrated Process:** Caring; **Nursing Process:** Planning/Implementation; **Reference:** Ch 2, The Nurse-Client Relationship

76. **3** This activity does not require professional nursing judgment and is within the job description of nursing assistants.
1, 4 Evaluating human responses to health care interventions requires the expertise of a licensed professional nurse. **2** This activity requires a professional nursing judgment to determine whether or not the medication should be administered.
Client Need: Management of Care; **Cognitive Level:** Application; **Nursing Process:** Planning/Implementation; **Reference:** Ch 2, Principles of Leadership

77. **2** The nurse should demonstrate to the client a recognition of the verbalized concern and a willingness to listen.

1 The client did not state this as the diagnosis; this response puts the client on the defensive. **3** Avoiding the question indicates that the nurse is unwilling to listen. **4** This cuts off communication and denies feelings.
Client Need: Psychosocial Integrity; **Cognitive Level:** Application; **Integrated Process:** Caring; **Nursing Process:** Planning/Implementation; **Reference:** Ch 2, The Nurse-Client Relationship

78. **1** The first step in the problem-solving process is data collection so that client needs can be identified. A direct approach obtains specific information needed during the initial interview.
2 This would be too broad because in a nondirective interview the client controls the subject matter. The nurse needs to be direct to collect specific information such as allergies, current medication, and health history. **3, 4** This is premature.
Client Need: Management of Care; **Cognitive Level:** Comprehension; **Integrated Process:** Communication/Documentation; **Nursing Process:** Assessment/Analysis; **Reference:** Ch 2, The Nurse-Client Relationship

79. **2** These guidelines govern safe nursing practice; nurses are legally responsible to perform according to these guidelines.
1 This explains what the public can expect from nurses, but it is not used to govern nursing practice. **3, 4** There are no data in the question that indicate this information is necessary.
Client Need: Management of Care; **Cognitive Level:** Comprehension; **Nursing Process:** Planning/Implementation; **Reference:** Ch 2, The Nurse's Rights and Responsibilities

80. **1** The client needs to be kept safe; this action ensures additional time for assessment to rule out the possibility of abuse.
2 This would form a coalition with the daughter-in-law and would not be in the client's best interest. The nurse must be objective. **3** Not all states require the reporting of elder abuse; further assessment is needed to rule out abuse. **4** This is inappropriate; this situation presents a legal, not ethical, issue.
Client Need: Management of Care; **Cognitive Level:** Analysis; **Integrated Process:** Caring; **Nursing Process:** Planning/Implementation; **Reference:** Ch 2, The Nurse's Rights and Responsibilities

81. **2** Open-ended statements provide a milieu in which people can verbalize their problems rather than be placed in a situation of forced response.
1 This can be threatening to the client, who may not have the answer to these questions. **3** False reassurance is detrimental to the nurse-client relationship and does not promote communication. **4** Direct questions do not open or promote communication.
Client Need: Management of Care; **Cognitive Level:** Application; **Integrated Process:** Communication/Documentation; **Nursing Process:** Assessment/Analysis; **Reference:** Ch 2, The Nurse-Client Relationship

82. 3 Nurses must actively try to understand their own feelings and prejudices because these will affect the ability to assess a client's behavior objectively.
1 Understanding a client's emotional conflict can be accomplished only after dealing with one's own feelings. **2** The health team members should work together for the benefit of all clients, not just this client. **4** Information from significant others is beneficial, but only after nurses are able to deal with their own feelings.
Client Need: Psychosocial Integrity; **Cognitive Level:** Application; **Integrated Process:** Caring; **Nursing Process:** Assessment/Analysis; **Reference:** Ch 2, The Nurse-Client Relationship

83. 2 Hypersensitivity can result in anaphylaxis; edema of the respiratory system can result in respiratory obstruction and respiratory arrest, causing asphyxia.
1 This is unrelated to anaphylaxis. **3** This is associated with excessive exercise. **4** Antihistamines may reverse the effects of histamine, which contributes to an anaphylactic reaction.
Client Need: Physiological Adaptation; **Cognitive Level:** Comprehension; **Nursing Process:** Assessment/Analysis; **Reference:** Ch 2, Drug Effects

84. 4 Hypersensitivity to a foreign substance can cause an anaphylactic reaction. Histamine is released, causing bronchial constriction, increased capillary permeability, and dilation of arterioles. This decreased peripheral resistance is associated with hypotension and inadequate circulation to major organs.
1 Vasodilation causes hypotension. **2** These are the problems that result from bronchial constriction and vascular collapse. **3** Arterioles dilate, capillary permeability increases, and eventually vascular collapse occurs.
Client Need: Physiological Adaptation; **Cognitive Level:** Comprehension; **Nursing Process:** Assessment/Analysis; **Reference:** Ch 2, Medication Administration, Drug Effects

85. 1 ☐ Standard precautions generally are not required because the nurse should not be coming in contact with body secretions.
2 ☒ Standard precautions should be used because the newborn is covered with amniotic fluid and maternal blood.
3 ☒ Standard precautions should be used because the nurse may be exposed to blood and interstitial fluid that is contained in the portable wound drainage system.
4 ☐ Standard precautions are not necessary when conducting an interview because it is unlikely that the nurse will come in contact with the client's body secretions.
5 ☐ Standard precautions are not necessary when obtaining the blood pressure of a client, even if the client is HIV-positive.
Client Need: Safety and Infection Control; **Cognitive Level:** Application; **Nursing Process:** Planning/Implementation; **Reference:** Ch 3, Types of Pathogens

86. 3 Agency policy determines procedures; if the procedure is out of date or problematic, the nurse should contact the physician for a change in orders.
1, 4 The nurse cannot use the sample without a physician's order. **2** The nurse would be risking liability if the agency policy is not followed unless the order is changed by the physician.
Client Need: Management of Care; **Cognitive Level:** Analysis; **Nursing Process:** Planning/Implementation; **Reference:** Ch 2, The Nurse's Rights and Responsibilities

87. 4 The first action should be to remove the victim from a source of further injury.
1 Preventing further injury and reestablishing breathing are the priorities. **2** Breathing is the priority once further injury is avoided. **3** This would be treated after the victim is moved from danger and patency of the airway is verified.
Client Need: Safety and Infection Control; **Cognitive Level:** Application; **Nursing Process:** Planning/Implementation; **Reference:** Ch 3, Concepts Related to First Aid

88. 2 The goal in a disaster, when need exceeds resources, is to benefit the largest number of people; helping those who need less care first benefits the largest number by not tying up personnel and by making these victims available to serve others.
1, 3, 4 This is not the priority in a disaster.
Client Need: Safety and Infection Control; **Cognitive Level:** Application; **Nursing Process:** Planning/Implementation; **Reference:** Ch 3, Concepts Related to First Aid

89. 3 Studies have demonstrated that people from mainland China, Greece, and Ethiopia view honesty about diagnosis and prognosis as heartless, uncalled for, and even harmful to the client; if the client chooses the family, then family members can decide what is most appropriate to share with the client based on the client's cultural background and beliefs.
1, 2 This information is not as necessary as data collected from another option. **4** Translation should be done by a person outside the family because a family member may relate medical information with bias.
Client Need: Psychosocial Integrity; **Cognitive Level:** Application; **Integrated Process:** Caring; **Nursing Process:** Planning/Implementation; **Reference:** Ch 1, Concepts from Sociology

90. 4 The nurse's presence communicates concern and provides an opportunity for the client to initiate communication; silence is an effective interpersonal technique that permits the client to direct the content and extent of verbalizations without the nurse imposing on the client's privacy.
1 Crying, part of depression, usually ceases when the individual reaches acceptance. **2** During acceptance the client may decide not to have visitors, preferring time for reflection. **3** Detached from the environment, the client may find that the details of various hospital procedures lose significance.
Client Need: Psychosocial Integrity; **Cognitive Level:** Application; **Integrated Process:** Caring; **Nursing Process:** Planning/Implementation; **Reference:** Ch 1, Grieving Process

91. **4** Seeking other opinions to disprove the inevitable is a form of denial employed by individuals having illnesses with a poor prognosis.

1 If the client is crying, the client is aware of the magnitude of the situation and is past the stage of denial. **2** Criticism that is unjust is often characteristic of the stage of anger. **3** This is common during the depression experienced as one moves toward acceptance.

Client Need: Psychosocial Integrity; **Cognitive Level:** Comprehension; **Integrated Process:** Caring; **Nursing Process:** Assessment/Analysis; **Reference:** Ch 1, Grieving Process

92. **1** Bargaining is one of the stages of dying in which the client promises some type of desirable behavior to postpone the inevitability of death.

3 Frustration is a subjective experience, a feeling of being thwarted, but not one of the stages of dying. **2** Classified as the fourth stage of dying, depression represents the grief experienced as the individual recognizes the inescapability of fate. **4** Rationalization is a defense mechanism in which attempts are made to justify or explain an unacceptable action or feeling, not a stage of the dying process.

Client Need: Psychosocial Integrity; **Cognitive Level:** Analysis; **Integrated Process:** Caring; **Nursing Process:** Assessment/Analysis; **Reference:** Ch 1, Grieving Process

93. **1** The client is in acceptance; detachment is a coping mechanism often needed by the client, especially when facing a devastating illness, and should be accepted by the nurse.

2 Ignoring the behavior does not convey a willingness to listen and denies the client's feelings. **3** The client is past the denial phase and is in acceptance. **4** Coping mechanisms are needed by the client as psychologic protection and must not be taken away until the client is able to replace one coping mechanism for another.

Client Need: Psychosocial Integrity; **Cognitive Level:** Application; **Integrated Process:** Caring; **Nursing Process:** Planning/Implementation; **Reference:** Ch 1, Grieving Process

94. **2** This is truthful and provides basic information that may prompt recollection of what occurred; it is a starting point.

1 This ignores the client's question; avoidance may increase anxiety. **3** This is too blunt for the initial response to the client's question; the client may not be ready to hear this at this time. **4** This ignores the client's question; the client has indicated no memory of what happened.

Client Need: Psychosocial Integrity; **Cognitive Level:** Application; **Integrated Process:** Caring; **Nursing Process:** Planning/Implementation; **Reference:** Ch 2, The Nurse-Client Relationship

95. **3** The response demonstrates that the nurse cares about the client and will have time for the client's special emotional needs. Such an approach allays anxiety and reduces emotional stress.

1 This indicates a lack of interest in the client and is not therapeutic. **2** This statement does not respond to the client's need and cuts off communication. **4** This is false reassurance and not therapeutic.

Client Need: Psychosocial Integrity; **Cognitive Level:** Application; **Integrated Process:** Caring; **Nursing Process:** Planning/Implementation; **Reference:** Ch 2, The Nurse-Client Relationship

96. **3** At this time the client is using this behavior as a defense mechanism. Quiet acceptance can be an effective interpersonal technique, since it is nonjudgmental. Eventually, limits may need to be set to address the behavior if it becomes more aggressive or hostile.

1 The nurse may be the target of a broad array of emotions; by focusing on only behaviors that affect the nurse, the full scope of the client's feelings are not considered. **2** During periods of overt hostility, perceptions are altered, making it difficult to evaluate the situation rationally. **4** Withdrawal signifies nonacceptance and rejection.

Client Need: Psychosocial Integrity; **Cognitive Level:** Application; **Integrated Process:** Caring; **Nursing Process:** Planning/Implementation; **Reference:** Ch 2, The Nurse-Client Relationship

97. **3** This promotes an exploration of the client's dilemma; this response encourages further communication.

1 Although this is true, this response is not supportive and abandons the client. **2** It is inappropriate for the nurse to give advice. **4** It is inappropriate for the nurse to give advice; the nurse is directing the client to be judgmental.

Client Need: Psychosocial Integrity; **Cognitive Level:** Application; **Integrated Process:** Caring; **Nursing Process:** Planning/Implementation; **Reference:** Ch 2, The Nurse-Client Relationship

98. **2** Open communication lines are always important in relieving anxiety and reducing stress, which might interfere with postoperative recovery.

1 This does not acknowledge the client's feelings and does not deal with the source of the anxiety. **3** Learning is limited when anxiety is too high. **4** Reassurances do not allow for open communication and deny emotions.

Client Need: Psychosocial Integrity; **Cognitive Level:** Application; **Integrated Process:** Caring; **Nursing Process:** Planning/Implementation; **Reference:** Ch 2, The Nurse-Client Relationship

99. **3** Because of the profound effect of paralysis on body image, the nurse should provide the client with an environment that permits exploration of feelings without judgment, punishment, or rejection.

1 Attempts to distract the client may be interpreted as denial of the client's feelings and will not resolve the underlying conflict. **2, 4** This is an important part of nursing care, but it is not related to the client's feelings.

Client Need: Psychosocial Integrity; **Cognitive Level:** Application; **Integrated Process:** Caring; **Nursing Process:** Planning/Implementation; **Reference:** Ch 2, The Nurse-Client Relationship

100. 2 The nurse should pick up all clues to client anxiety and allow for verbalization. This response recognizes the client's feelings.

1, 4 This response negates the client's feelings and presents a negative connotation. 3 This response focuses on the task rather than on the client's feelings.

Client Need: Psychosocial Integrity; **Cognitive Level:** Application; **Integrated Process:** Caring; **Nursing Process:** Planning/Implementation; **Reference:** Ch 2, The Nurse-Client Relationship

101. 4 This question may validate the client's understanding; the response may indicate the need for further teaching or that the client understands; understanding and accepting the need for restrictions will increase adherence to the diet.

1 These are authoritarian approaches that should be avoided. 2 Assessing the client's food preferences and teaching about diets would follow an assessment of the client's understanding about the need for a specific diet; the client must understand the need for and the benefits of the diet before there is a readiness for learning.

Client Need: Health Promotion and Maintenance; **Cognitive Level:** Application; **Integrated Process:** Teaching/Learning; **Nursing Process:** Evaluation/Outcomes; **Reference:** Ch 2, Teaching-Learning

102. 1 The nurse needs to assess the situation before planning an intervention.

2 This is premature; more information is needed. 3 This minimizes concerns and cuts off communication. 4 The nurse needs more information; pulling the curtain may make the client feel isolated, which could increase anxiety.

Client Need: Psychosocial Integrity; **Cognitive Level:** Application; **Integrated Process:** Caring; **Nursing Process:** Assessment/Analysis; **Reference:** Ch 2, Nursing Process

103. 1 This statement is open-ended and encourages the client to verbalize concerns.

2, 3 This cuts off communication. 4 Nothing in the situation indicates that surgery is planned; this response could increase anxiety.

Client Need: Psychosocial Integrity; **Cognitive Level:** Application; **Integrated Process:** Caring; **Nursing Process:** Planning/Implementation; **Reference:** Ch 2, Nurse-Client Relationship

104. 4 A portable wound drainage system has negative pressure; fluid flows down the pressure gradient from the client to the collection device.

1 Although true, this is not what causes the fluid to drain. 2 This is Newton's law of gravity, which is not the physical principle underlying the functioning of a portable wound drainage system. 3 Siphonage is not the principle underlying the functioning of a portable wound drainage system; it is the force of atmospheric pressure on the surface of a liquid.

Client Need: Reduction of Risk Potential; **Cognitive Level:** Comprehension; **Nursing Process:** Planning/Implementation; **Reference:** Ch 3, General Nursing Care of Clients During the Perioperative Period

105. 4 Release of adrenocortical steroids (cortisol) by the stress of surgery causes renal retention of sodium and excretion of potassium.

1 Although sodium may be depleted by nasogastric suction, retention by the kidneys generally balances this loss. 2, 3 This is not depleted by surgery or urinary excretion.

Client Need: Physiological Adaptation; **Cognitive Level:** Comprehension; **Nursing Process:** Evaluation/Outcomes; **Reference:** Ch 3, Acid-Base Balance

106. 1 Because IV solutions enter the body's internal environment, all solutions and medications using this route must be sterile to prevent the introduction of microbes.

2 The medication can be mixed with the IV solution in many ways; sterility takes priority. 3 The amount and type of solution depend on the medication; sterility takes priority. 4 The needle does not have to be changed if sterility is maintained.

Client Need: Pharmacological and Parenteral Therapies; **Cognitive Level:** Application; **Nursing Process:** Planning/Implementation; **Reference:** Ch 2, Nursing Responsibilities Related to Medication Administration

107. 3 Hypotonic solutions are less concentrated (contain less than 0.85 g of sodium chloride in each 100 mL) than body fluids.

1 Isotonic solutions are those that cause no change in the cellular volume or pressure, because their concentration is equivalent to that of body fluid. 2 This relates to two compounds that possess the same molecular formula but that differ in their properties or in the position of atoms in the molecules (isomers). 4 Hypertonic solutions contain more than 0.85 g of solute in each 100 mL.

Client Need: Pharmacological and Parenteral Therapies; **Cognitive Level:** Comprehension; **Nursing Process:** Planning/Implementation; **Reference:** Ch 3, Fluid and Electrolyte Balance

108. 2 Because of fluid overload in the intravascular space, the neck veins become visibly distended.

1, 3 This occurs with a fluid deficit. 4 If sodium causes fluid retention, its concentration is unchanged; if fluid is retained independently of sodium, its concentration will be decreased.

Client Need: Physiological Adaptation; **Cognitive Level:** Analysis; **Nursing Process:** Assessment/Analysis; **Reference:** Ch 3, General Nursing Care of Clients With Fluid and Electrolyte Problems

109. 2 Skin tugor will decrease because of a decrease in interstitial fluid.

1 The pulse rate will increase to oxygenate the body's cells. 3 Specific gravity will increase because of the greater concentration of waste particles in the decreased amount of urine. 4 The temperature will increase, not decrease.

Client Need: Physiological Adaptation; **Cognitive Level:** Analysis; **Nursing Process:** Assessment/Analysis; **Reference:** Ch 3, Acid-Base Balance

110.   1 Dehydration is most readily and accurately measured by serial assessments of body weight; 1 L of fluid weighs 2.2 lb.
2 Although dry skin may be associated with dehydration, it also is associated with aging.
3 Although hypovolemia will eventually result in a decrease in blood pressure, it is not an accurate, reliable assessment because there are many other causes of hypotension. 4 This is too general and not an accurate assessment to determine fluid volume deficit.

Client Need: Physiological Adaptation; **Cognitive Level:** Analysis; **Nursing Process:** Assessment/Analysis; **Reference:** Ch 3, Acid-Base Balance

111.   3 Increased respiration blows off carbon dioxide, which decreases the hydrogen ion concentration and the pH rises (less acidity). Decreased respiration results in CO_2 buildup, which increases hydrogen ion concentration and the pH falls (more acidity). The kidneys either conserve or excrete bicarbonate and hydrogen ions, which helps to adjust the pH. The buffering capacity of the renal system is greater than that of the pulmonary system, but the pulmonary system is quicker to respond.
1, 4 These two systems do not maintain the pH.
2 Although the circulatory system carries fluids and electrolytes to the kidneys, it does not interact with the urinary system to regulate plasma pH.

Client Need: Physiological Adaptation; **Cognitive Level:** Comprehension; **Nursing Process:** Assessment/Analysis; **Reference:** Ch 3, Acid-Base Balance

112.   1 Blood plasma and interstitial fluid are both part of the extracellular fluid and are of the same ionic composition.
2 The osmotic pressure is the same. 3 The composition is the same. 4 The main cation of both extracellular fluids is sodium.

Client Need: Physiological Adaptation; **Cognitive Level:** Comprehension; **Nursing Process:** Assessment/Analysis; **Reference:** Ch 3, Acid-Base Balance

113.   2 Interstitial fluid constitutes about 16% of body weight, which is 10 to 12 L in an adult male of 68 kg (150 lb).
1 Plasma is 4% of body weight. 3 This is part of the intracellular component. 4 This is derived from extracellular fluid and is calculated as part of the 20% of the total body weight.

Client Need: Physiological Adaptation; **Cognitive Level:** Comprehension; **Nursing Process:** Assessment/Analysis; **Reference:** Ch 3, Acid-Base Balance

114.   4 The concentration of potassium is greater inside the cell and is important in establishing a membrane potential, a critical factor in the cell's ability to function.
1 Sodium is the most abundant cation of the extracellular compartment. 2 Calcium is the most

abundant electrolyte in the body; 99% is concentrated in the teeth and bones and only 1% is available for bodily functions. 3 Chloride is an extracellular anion.

Client Need: Physiological Adaptation; **Cognitive Level:** Comprehension; **Nursing Process:** Assessment/Analysis; **Reference:** Ch 3, Acid-Base Balance

115.   2 The excreted ammonia combines with hydrogen ions in the glomerular filtrate to form ammonium ions, which are excreted from the body. This mechanism helps rid the body of excess hydrogen, maintaining acid-base balance.
1, 4 This is not affected by excretion of ammonia.
3 Ammonia is formed by the decomposition of bacteria in the urine; ammonia excretion is not related to the process and does not control bacterial levels.

Client Need: Physiological Adaptation; **Cognitive Level:** Comprehension; **Nursing Process:** Assessment/Analysis; **Reference:** Ch 3, Acid-Base Balance

116.   1 Excess fluid can move into the lungs, causing crackles; clear breath sounds support that care was effective.
2 While it may make palpation more difficult, excess fluid will not diminish pedal pulses. 3 A normal potassium level can be maintained independently of fluid excess correction. 4 Increased specific gravity indicates the urine is concentrated, suggesting that the body is retaining fluid.

Client Need: Physiological Adaptation; **Cognitive Level:** Analysis; **Nursing Process:** Evaluation/Outcomes; **Reference:** Ch 3, Acid-Base Balance

117.   4 Because the plasma colloidal oncotic pressure (COP) is the major force drawing fluid from the interstitial spaces back into the capillaries, a drop in COP caused by albuminuria results in edema.
1 Hydrostatic tissue pressure is unaffected by alteration of protein levels; colloidal pressure is affected. 2 Hydrostatic pressure is influenced by the volume of fluid and the diameter of the blood vessel, not directly by the presence of albumin. 3 The osmotic pressure of tissues is unchanged.

Client Need: Physiological Adaptation; **Cognitive Level:** Analysis; **Nursing Process:** Assessment/Analysis; **Reference:** Ch 3, Acid-Base Balance

118.   1 Albumin is hypertonic and will draw additional fluid from the tissues into the intravascular space.
2 This will absorb the watery diarrhea, giving more bulk to the stool. 3 This is appropriate because diarrhea causes potassium loss. 4 This is a hypotonic solution, which can correct dehydration.

Client Need: Pharmacological and Parenteral Therapies; **Cognitive Level:** Analysis; **Nursing Process:** Planning/Implementation; **Reference:** Ch 3, Acid-Base Balance

119.   1 The fluid in an IV bag hung over a person lying down possesses potential energy. When that fluid is allowed to drip into the person intravenously, its potential energy is then converted to kinetic energy (energy of motion).
2 Energy is not being stored in this action; rather, stored energy is converted to energy of motion.

3 No chemical reaction occurs when fluid drips into a vein. **4** No chemical reaction or formation of new substances occurs when fluid drips into a vein.
Client Need: Pharmacology and Parenteral Therapies; **Cognitive Level:** Comprehension; **Nursing Process:** Assessment/Analysis; **Reference:** Ch 3, Acid-Base Balance

120. **2** Sodium bicarbonate is a base and one of the major buffers in the body.
1 Potassium, a cation, is not a buffer; only a base can buffer an acid. **3** Carbon dioxide is carried in aqueous solution as carbonic acid (H_2CO_3); an acid does not buffer another acid. **4** Sodium chloride is not a buffer; it is a salt.
Client Need: Physiological Adaptation; **Cognitive Level:** Comprehension; **Nursing Process:** Assessment/Analysis; **Reference:** Ch 3, Acid-Base Balance

121. **3** Excessive loss of gastric fluid results in excessive loss of hydrochloric acid and can lead to alkalosis; the HCl is not available to neutralize the sodium bicarbonate ($NaHCO_3$) secreted into the duodenum by the pancreas. The intestinal tract absorbs the excess bicarbonate and alkalosis results.
1 Gastric lavage will lead to alkalosis, which is associated with increased pH. **2** Gastric lavage will not affect this. **4** Gastric lavage may lead to dehydration, which would increase osmotic pressure.
Client Need: Physiological Adaptation; **Cognitive Level:** Comprehension; **Nursing Process:** Assessment/Analysis; **Reference:** Ch 3, Acid-Base Balance

122. **1** The pH of blood is maintained within the narrow range of 7.35 to 7.45. When there is an increase in hydrogen ions, the respiratory, buffer, and renal systems attempt to compensate to maintain the pH. If compensation is not successful, acidosis results and is reflected in a lower pH.
2, 3 This is within the normal range for pH. **4** This is slightly alkaline.
Client Need: Physiological Adaptation; **Cognitive Level:** Comprehension; **Nursing Process:** Assessment/Analysis; **Reference:** Ch 3, Acid-Base Balance

123. **4** The kidneys normally eliminate potassium from the body; diseases of the kidneys often interfere with this function and hyperkalemia may develop, necessitating dialysis.
1 Crohn's disease leads to diarrhea and potassium loss. **2** With Cushing's syndrome the client will retain sodium and excrete potassium. **3** Heart failure can lead to sodium and water retention, which then cause potassium loss.
Client Need: Physiological Adaptation; **Cognitive Level:** Analysis; **Nursing Process:** Assessment/Analysis; **Reference:** Ch 3, Acid-Base Balance

124. **4** Vital signs monitor cardiorespiratory status; hyperkalemia causes serious cardiac dysrhythmias.
1 A repeat laboratory test would take time and probably reaffirm the original results; the client needs immediate attention. **2** The cardiac arrest team is always on alert and will respond when called for a cardiac arrest. **3** These are insufficient interventions.

Client Need: Physiological Adaptation; **Cognitive Level:** Analysis; **Nursing Process:** Planning/Implementation; **Reference:** Ch 3, Acid-Base Balance

125. **1** ☐ Tetany is caused by hypocalcemia.
  2 ☐ Seizures caused by electrolyte imbalances are associated with low calcium or sodium levels.
  3 ☒ Because of potassium's role in the sodium/potassium pump, hyperkalemia will cause diarrhea.
  4 ☒ Because of potassium's role in the sodium/potassium pump, hyperkalemia will cause weakness.
  5 ☒ Because of potassium's role in the sodium/potassium pump, hyperkalemia will cause cardiac dysrhythmias.
Client Need: Physiological Adaptation; **Cognitive Level:** Application; **Nursing Process:** Assessment/Analysis; **Reference:** Ch 3, Acid-Base Balance

126. **3** Once treatment with insulin for diabetic ketoacidosis is begun, potassium ions reenter the cell, causing hypokalemia; therefore potassium, along with the replacement fluids, is generally supplied.
1 Potassium would not correct this. **2** Flaccid paralysis would not occur in diabetic ketoacidosis; potassium replaces that which has reentered the cell after insulin therapy. **4** Knowing the relationship of insulin and potassium, the nurse should recognize that treatment with KCl is prophylactic, preventing any development of dysrhythmias.
Client Need: Pharmacological and Parenteral Therapies; **Cognitive Level:** Comprehension; **Nursing Process:** Planning/Implementation; **Reference:** Ch 3, General Nursing Care of Clients With Fluid and Electrolyte Problems

127. **3** Intake 1100 mL and output 605 mL. Intake includes 350 mL of IV fluid, 600 mL of NGT feeding, and 150 mL of water via NGT, for a total intake of 1100 mL; output includes voidings of 150, 220, and 235 mL for a total output of 605 mL.
2 This intake is too much and the output is too little. **4** This intake is too little and the output is too much. **1** Both the intake and output are too little.
Client Need: Physiological Adaptation; **Cognitive Level:** Application; **Nursing Process:** Planning/Implementation; **Reference:** Ch 3, General Nursing Care of Clients With Fluid and Electrolyte Problems

128. **3** The liver manufactures albumin, the major plasma protein. A deficit of this protein will lower the osmotic (oncotic) pressure in the intravascular space, leading to a fluid shift.
1 The enlarged liver compresses the portal system, causing increased, rather than decreased, pressure. **2** The kidneys are not the primary source of the pathologic condition. It is the liver's ability to manufacture albumin, which maintains the colloid oncotic pressure. **4** Potassium is not produced by the body, nor is its major function the maintenance of fluid balance.

Client Need: Physiological Adaptation; **Cognitive Level:** Comprehension; **Nursing Process:** Assessment/Analysis; **Reference:** Ch 3, Fluid and Electrolyte Balance

129. **2** IV fluids do not provide proteins required for tissue growth, repair, and maintenance; therefore tissue breakdown occurs to provide the essential amino acids.

1 Each liter provides approximately 170 calories, which is insufficient to meet minimal energy requirements; tissue breakdown will result. **3** Weight loss is caused by insufficient nutrient intake; vitamins do not prevent weight loss. **4** An infusion of 5% dextrose in water may decrease electrolyte concentration.

Client Need: Physiological Adaptation; **Cognitive Level:** Comprehension; **Nursing Process:** Evaluation/Outcomes; **Reference:** Ch 3, General Nursing Care of Clients With Fluid and Electrolyte Problems

130. **Answer:** 31 drops per minute.

Amount to be infused (125 mL) times the drop factor (15 gtt/mL) divided by 1 hour (60 minutes) equals 31 gtt/min.

Client Need: Pharmacological and Parenteral Therapies; **Cognitive Level:** Application; **Nursing Process:** Planning/Implementation; **Reference:** Ch 3, General Nursing Care of Clients With Fluid and Electrolyte Problems

131. **2** Hyperventilation causes excessive loss of carbon dioxide, leading to carbonic acid deficit and respiratory alkalosis.

1 The client may experience dysrhythmias but will lose consciousness and begin breathing regularly; cardiac arrest is unlikely. **3** Hyperventilation causes alkalosis; the pH is increased. **4** This cannot occur; the usual oxygen saturation of hemoglobin is 95% to 98%.

Client Need: Physiological Adaptation; **Cognitive Level:** Analysis; **Nursing Process:** Planning/Implementation; **Reference:** Ch 3, Acid-Base Balance

132. **1** A low pH and low bicarbonate level are consistent with metabolic acidosis.

2, 4 The pH indicates acidosis. **3** The CO_2 concentration is within normal limits, which is inconsistent with respiratory acidosis.

Client Need: Physiological Adaptation; **Cognitive Level:** Analysis; **Nursing Process:** Assessment/Analysis; **Reference:** Ch 3, Acid-Base Balance

133. **4** The high pH and low carbon dioxide level are consistent with respiratory alkalosis, which can be caused by aggressive mechanical ventilation.

1 This causes carbon dioxide buildup, which leads to respiratory acidosis. **2** This causes excess ketones, which can lead to metabolic acidosis. **3** This causes loss of hydrochloric acid, which can lead to metabolic alkalosis.

Client Need: Physiological Adaptation; **Cognitive Level:** Analysis; **Nursing Process:** Evaluation/Outcomes; **Reference:** Ch 3, Acid-Base Balance

134. **1** Albumin acts to elevate the BP to normal levels when it is administered slowly and oral fluid

intake is restricted. It causes fluid to move from the interstitial spaces into the circulatory system so it can be eliminated by the kidneys. Administration should not exceed 5 to 10 mL/min.

2 Rapid administration could cause circulatory overload; fluid is restricted, not withheld. **3** Rapid administration could cause circulatory overload; high fluid intake would limit the shift of fluid from the interstitial to the intravascular compartment, interfering with the optimal effects of the drug. **4** Oral fluids are restricted to facilitate the optimal effects of the drug, which shifts fluids from the interstitial spaces to the intravascular compartment.

Client Need: Physiological Adaptation; **Cognitive Level:** Application; **Nursing Process:** Planning/Implementation; **Reference:** Ch 3, General Nursing Care of Clients With Fluid and Electrolyte Problems

135. **4** Blood albumin, a protein, establishes the plasma colloid osmotic (oncotic) pressure because of its high molecular weight and size.

1 Blood clotting involves blood protein fractions other than albumin; for example, prothrombin and fibrinogen are within the alpha- and beta-globulin fractions. **2** Red blood cell formation (erythropoiesis) occurs in red marrow and can be related to albumin only indirectly; albumin is the blood transport protein for thyroxine, which stimulates metabolism in all cells, including those in red bone marrow. **3** Albumin does not activate WBCs; WBCs are activated by antigens and substances released from damaged or diseased cells.

Client Need: Physiological Adaptation; **Cognitive Level:** Comprehension; **Nursing Process:** Planning/Implementation; **Reference:** Ch 3, Fluid and Electrolyte Balance

136. **4** After 24 hours there is increased risk for contamination of the solution and the container should be changed.

1-3 It is unnecessary to change the bag this often.

Client Need: Pharmacological and Parenteral Therapies; **Cognitive Level:** Comprehension; **Nursing Process:** Planning/Implementation; **Reference:** Ch 3, General Nursing Care of Clients With Fluid and Electrolyte Problems

137. **2** Infiltration is caused by catheter displacement, allowing fluid to leak into the tissues.

1 This will affect the flow rate, not cause infiltration. **3** This can lead to infection and phlebitis, not cause infiltration. **4** This can lead to phlebitis, not cause infiltration.

Client Need: Pharmacological and Parenteral Therapies; **Cognitive Level:** Application; **Nursing Process:** Evaluation/Outcomes; **Reference:** Ch 3, General Nursing Care of Clients With Fluid and Electrolyte Problems

138. **1** ☐ Heat is associated with phlebitis; the accumulation of room temperature IV fluid in the tissue makes the site feel cool.

2 ☒ The accumulation of fluid in the tissues between the surface of the skin and the blood vessels makes the skin appear pale.

3 ☒ The accumulation of fluid in the interstitial compartment causes swelling.

4 ☒ As the needle/catheter is dislodged from the vein, the drip rate of the IV slows or ceases.

5 ☐ This is a sign of circulatory overload; with an infiltration, the IV fluid does not increase the intravascular fluid volume.

Client Need: Pharmacological and Parenteral Therapies; **Cognitive Level:** Application; **Nursing Process:** Evaluation/Outcomes; **Reference:** Ch 3, General Nursing Care of Clients With Fluid and Electrolyte Problems

139.   2 When an IV infusion is infiltrated, it should be removed to prevent swelling of the tissues and pain.

1 Elevation does not change the position of the IV cannula; the infusion must be discontinued. 3 This would add to the infiltration of fluid. 4 Soaks may be applied, if ordered, after the IV is removed.

Client Need: Pharmacological and Parenteral Therapies; **Cognitive Level:** Application; **Nursing Process:** Planning/Implementation; **Reference:** Ch 3, General Nursing Care of Clients With Fluid and Electrolyte Problems

140.   Answer: 28 drops per minute.

Solve the problem by using the following formula: (amount to be infused × drop factor)/(amount of time, in minutes); (2000 × 10)/(12 × 60) = 20,000/720 = 27.77; 27.77 must be rounded up to 28 drops/min.

Client Need: Pharmacological and Parenteral Therapies; **Cognitive Level:** Application; **Nursing Process:** Planning/Implementation; **Reference:** Ch 3, General Nursing Care of Clients With Fluid and Electrolyte Problems

141.   1 Hypokalemia causes a flattening of the T wave of the ECG because of its effect on muscle function.

2 Hypokalemia causes a depression of the ST segment. 3 Hypokalemia causes a widening of the QRS complex. 4 Hypokalemia does not cause a deflection of the Q wave.

Client Need: Physiological Adaptation; **Cognitive Level:** Application; **Nursing Process:** Assessment/Analysis; **Reference:** Ch 3, Fluid and Electrolyte Balance

142.   1 Potassium follows insulin into the cells of the body, thereby raising the intracellular potassium level and preventing fatal dysrhythmias.

2 Insulin does not cause excretion of these substances. 3 Potassium is not excreted as a result of this therapy; it shifts into the intracellular compartment. 4 The potassium level has no effect on pancreatic insulin production.

Client Need: Pharmacological and Parenteral Therapies; **Cognitive Level:** Analysis; **Nursing Process:** Planning/Implementation; **Reference:** Ch 3, General Nursing Care of Clients With Fluid and Electrolyte Problems

143.   4 Hypokalemia diminishes the magnitude of the neuronal and muscle cell resting potentials. Abdominal distention results from flaccidity of intestinal and abdominal musculature.

1 This is a sign of sodium excess. 2 This is a sign of hypocalcemia. 3 This is a sign of metabolic acidosis.

Client Need: Physiological Integrity; **Cognitive Level:** Application; **Nursing Process:** Assessment/Analysis; **Reference:** Ch 3, Fluid and Electrolyte Balance

144.   Answer: 38 drops per minute.

Solve the problem by using the following formula: (50 × 15) = 750/20 = 37.5; 37.5 is rounded up to 38 drops/min.

Client Need: Pharmacological and Parenteral Therapies; **Cognitive Level:** Application; **Nursing Process:** Planning/Implementation; **Reference:** Ch 3, General Nursing Care of Clients With Fluid and Electrolyte Problems

145.   1 Clients and their families need to maintain honest, open interpersonal communication to allow sharing of concerns and to promote future problem solving.

2 The spouse should be encouraged to share feelings with the client. 3 The spouse may want to know this, but it will not help meet the general needs of both the client and the spouse. 4 While an understanding of the disease is important, details will not assist the significant other in maintaining an active role in the situation.

Client Need: Psychosocial Integrity; **Cognitive Level:** Application; **Integrated Process:** Documentation/Communication; **Nursing Process:** Planning/Implementation; **Reference:** Ch 3, General Nursing Care of Clients With Neoplastic Disorders

146.   1 This recognizes and acknowledges the client's concerns without assuming a specific feeling is involved; it allows the client to set the framework for discussion and express self-identified feelings.

2 This is an assumption by the nurse; the data presented are not specific enough to come to this conclusion. 3, 4 This avoids the client's concerns and cuts off communication.

Client Need: Psychosocial Integrity; **Cognitive Level:** Analysis; **Integrated Process:** Caring; **Nursing Process:** Planning/Implementation; **Reference:** Ch 3, General Nursing Care of Clients With Neoplastic Disorders

147.   1 People in panic could initiate the panic reaction in those who appear to be in control.

2 Comatose individuals will not cause panic in others. 3 Euphoric individuals would not adversely affect others. 4 Depressed people will be calm and not affect others.

Client Need: Management of Care; **Cognitive Level:** Application; **Nursing Process:** Planning/Implementation; **Reference:** Ch 3, Concepts Related to First Aid

148.   1 Core rewarming with heated oxygen and administration of warmed PO or IV fluids is the preferred method of treatment.

2 The client would be too weak to ambulate. 3 Oral temperatures are not the most accurate assessment of core temperature because of environmental influences. 4 Warmed oral feedings are advised; gastric gavage is unnecessary.

Client Need: Reduction of Risk Potential; **Cognitive Level:** Application; **Integrated Process:** Teaching/Learning; **Nursing Process:** Planning/Implementation; **Reference:** Ch 3, Specific Emergencies

149. 2 Clothing insulates body heat; clothing must be removed before rapid cooling methods are employed to reduce body temperature.

1 This scenario does not provide data that indicate the need for suctioning. **3** Offering oral fluids is contraindicated because the client is unresponsive. **4** Although intubation may become necessary, it is not the initial action; also, this scenario does not provide data that indicate the need for intubation.

Client Need: Reduction of Risk Potential; **Cognitive Level:** Application; **Nursing Process:** Planning/Implementation; **Reference:** Ch 3, Specific Emergencies

150. 3 The high osmotic pressure of the saltwater draws fluid from the vascular space into the alveoli, causing hypovolemia.

1, 2, 4 This would involve aspiration of hypotonic freshwater, which causes fluid to move into the vascular system, leading to fluid overload.

Client Need: Physiological Adaptation; **Cognitive Level:** Analysis; **Nursing Process:** Assessment/Analysis; **Reference:** Ch 3, Specific Emergencies

151. 3 The pulse rate increases to meet increased tissue demands for oxygen in the febrile state.

1 Fever may not cause difficulty in breathing. **2** Pain is not related to fever. **4** Blood pressure is not necessarily elevated in fever.

Client Need: Physiological Adaptation; **Cognitive Level:** Application; **Nursing Process:** Assessment/Analysis; **Reference:** Ch 3, General Nursing Care of Clients at Risk for Infection

152. 4 The client who is prescribed bed rest must do exercises such as dorsiflexion of the feet to prevent venous stasis and thrombus formation.

1 Limiting fluid intake may lead to hemoconcentration and subsequent thrombus formation. **2** This improves pulmonary function rather than prevents venous stasis. **3** This actually promotes venous stasis by compressing the popliteal space.

Client Need: Reduction of Risk Potential; **Cognitive Level:** Application; **Nursing Process:** Planning/Implementation; **Reference:** Ch 3, General Nursing Care for Clients During the Postoperative Period

153. 1 Paralysis of the sympathetic vasomotor nerves after administration of a spinal anesthetic results in dilation of blood vessels, which causes a subsequent drop in blood pressure.

2 These receptors are sensitive to pH, oxygen, and carbon dioxide tension; they are not related to postural hypotension and are not affected by spinal anesthesia. **3** The strength of cardiac contractions is not affected by spinal anesthesia and postural hypotension. **4** The cardiac accelerator center neurons in the medulla regulate heart rate; they are not related to postural hypotension and are not affected by spinal anesthesia.

Client Need: Reduction of Risk Potential; **Cognitive Level:** Comprehension; **Nursing Process:** Evaluation/Outcomes; **Reference:** Ch 3, Perioperative Care, Local Anesthetics

154. 2 Clients adapting to illness frequently feel afraid and helpless and strike out at health team members as a way of maintaining control or denying their fear.

1 There is no evidence that the client denies the existence of the health problem. **3** Although disorders such as brain attacks and atherosclerosis, which are associated with hypertension, may lead to cerebral anoxia, there is insufficient evidence to support this conclusion in this situation. **4** Capoten (an antihypertensive) is a renin-angiotensin antagonist that reduces blood pressure and does not cause behavioral changes; Xanax reduces anxiety and may cause transient hypotension, not hypertension.

Client Need: Psychosocial Integrity; **Cognitive Level:** Application; **Nursing Process:** Assessment/Analysis; **Reference:** Ch 1, Grieving Process

155. 2 Clients' families should be included in dietary teaching; families provide support that promotes adherence.

1 The dietitian is a resource person who can give specific, practical information about diet and food preparation once the client has a basic understanding of the reasons for the diet. **3** Foods high in sodium will also have to be restricted; this teaching is inadequate. **4** The client should be included in his or her own care; the client will ultimately assume the responsibility.

Client Need: Health Promotion and Maintenance; **Cognitive Level:** Application; **Integrated Process:** Teaching/Learning; **Nursing Process:** Planning/Implementation; **Reference:** Ch 2, Teaching-Learning

156. 1 Individuals born after 1957 should receive one additional dose of measles, mumps, and rubella (MMR) vaccine if they are students in post-secondary educational institutions; MMR should not be given to a pregnant woman, and pregnancy should be avoided for 4 weeks after vaccination.

2 The influenza vaccine is unnecessary; people who are 22 years of age are not considered in the high-risk age-groups. **3** Currently there is no vaccine for hepatitis C. **4** An additional tetanus/diphtheria vaccine (DTaP) is not recommended for people in the 22-year-old age-group.

Client Need: Health Promotion and Maintenance; **Cognitive Level:** Analysis; **Integrated Process:** Teaching/Learning; **Nursing Process:** Planning/Implementation; **Reference:** Ch 3, Review of Physiology (Immunity)

157. 4 In 2004 the Centers for Disease Control and Prevention recommended that adults be immunized with pneumococcal vaccine at age 65 or older with a single dose of the vaccine; if the pneumococcal vaccine was given before 65 years of age, revaccination should occur 5 years after the initial vaccination.

1 The pneumococcal vaccine should not be administered every 2 years. **2, 3** The pneumococcal vaccine should not be administered annually.

Client Need: Health Promotion and Maintenance; **Cognitive Level:** Application; **Integrated Process:** Teaching/Learning; **Nursing Process:** Planning/Implementation; **Reference:** Ch 3, Review of Physiology (Immunity)

158. **2** The gamma-globulin fraction in the plasma is the fraction that includes the antibodies.

1 Albumin helps regulate fluid shifts by maintaining plasma oncotic pressure. **3** Thrombin is involved in clotting. **4** Hemoglobin carries oxygen.

Client Need: Physiological Adaptation; **Cognitive Level:** Comprehension; **Nursing Process:** Assessment/Analysis; **Reference:** Ch 3, Review of Physiology (Immunity)

159. **2** Gamma globulin, an immune globulin, contains most of the antibodies circulating in the blood. When injected into an individual, it prevents a specific antigen from entering a host cell.

1, 4 This does not stimulate antibody production. **3** This does not affect antigen-antibody function.

Client Need: Health Promotion and Maintenance; **Cognitive Level:** Comprehension; **Nursing Process:** Assessment/Analysis; **Reference:** Ch 3, Review of Physiology (Immunity)

160. **4** Tetanus immune globulin (TIG) provides antibodies against tetanus; it is used if the client has never received tetanus toxoid or has not received it for more than 10 years. It confers passive immunity.

1 DTaP vaccine—diphtheria and tetanus toxoid (Td) combined with pertussis vaccine—produces active, not passive, immunity; in addition, DTaP is not usually given to adults; Td is used. **2** Administration of this substance would produce active immunity. **3** Although this substance provides passive immunity, the risk for a hypersensitivity reaction is high and therefore TIG is preferred.

Client Need: Health Promotion and Maintenance; **Cognitive Level:** Analysis; **Nursing Process:** Planning/Implementation; **Reference:** Ch 3, Review of Physiology (Immunity)

161. **2** Tetanus antitoxin provides antibodies, which confer immediate passive immunity.

1 Antitoxin does not stimulate production of antibodies. **3** It provides passive, not active, immunity. **4** Passive immunity, by definition, is not long-lasting.

Client Need: Health Promotion and Maintenance; **Cognitive Level:** Application; **Integrated Process:** Teaching/Learning; **Nursing Process:** Planning/Implementation; **Reference:** Ch 3, Review of Physiology (Immunity)

162. **3** After a submucosal resection (SMR), hemorrhage from the area is frequently detected by vomiting of blood that has been swallowed.

2 Crepitus would be caused by leakage of air into tissue spaces; it is not usually a complication of SMR. **1** Headaches in the back of the head would not be a complication of a submucosal resection. **4** The nerves and structures involved with speech are not within the operative area. However, the sound of the voice is altered by the presence of nasal packing and edema.

Client Need: Physiological Adaptation; **Cognitive Level:** Application; **Nursing Process:** Evaluation/Outcomes; **Reference:** Ch 3, General Nursing Care of Clients During the Postoperative Period

163. **4** This may occur because of the high salt content of the aspirated ocean water, which raises its osmotic pressure; additional fluid from the surrounding tissues will be drawn into the lung, causing pulmonary edema.

1 Hypoxia and acidosis may occur after a near-drowning. **2** This is not a sequela of near-drowning. **3** Hypovolemia occurs because fluid is drawn into the lungs by the hypertonic saltwater.

Client Need: Physiological Adaptation; **Cognitive Level:** Analysis; **Nursing Process:** Assessment/Analysis; **Reference:** Ch 3, Specific Emergencies

164. **4** This minimizes pooling of respiratory secretions and maximizes chest expansion, which aids in the removal of secretions; this maintains the airway and is an independent nursing function.

1, 2 This is part of pulmonary therapy that requires a physician's order. **3** This will remove secretions once they accumulate in the upper airway, not prevent their accumulation.

Client Need: Physiological Adaptation; **Cognitive Level:** Application; **Nursing Process:** Planning/Implementation; **Reference:** Ch 3, General Nursing Care of Clients During the Postoperative Period

165. **2** Turning the client to the side promotes drainage of secretions and prevents aspiration, especially when the gag reflex is not intact. This position also brings the tongue forward, preventing it from occluding the airway in the relaxed state.

1 The risk for aspiration is increased when this position is assumed by a semialert client. **3** This increases the risk for aspiration; this position may flex the neck in an individual who is not alert, interfering with respirations. **4** This position is not generally used for a postoperative client because it interferes with breathing.

Client Need: Physiological Adaptation; **Cognitive Level:** Application; **Nursing Process:** Planning/Implementation; **Reference:** Ch 3, General Nursing Care of Clients During the Postoperative Period

166. **2** Maintenance of a patent airway is always the priority, because airway obstruction impedes breathing and may result in death.

1, 3, 4 This is important in the client's postoperative care; however, a patent airway is the priority.

Client Need: Physiological Adaptation; **Cognitive Level:** Application; **Nursing Process:** Planning/Implementation; **Reference:** Ch 3, General Nursing Care of Clients During the Postoperative Period

167. **2** During radiation therapy with radium implants the client is placed in isolation so that exposure to radiation by family and staff will be decreased.

1 This is unnecessary; a full bladder will not disrupt the seeds. **3** Excess exposure to radiation is hazardous to personnel. **4** Gloves will not protect the nurse from radiation.

Client Need: Physiological Adaptation; **Cognitive Level:** Application; **Nursing Process:** Planning/Implementation; **Reference:** Ch 3, Radiation

168. **2** The nurse should anticipate drainage and reinforce the surgical dressing as needed.

1 Changing a dressing at this time unnecessarily increases the risk for infection. **3** An abdominal binder is rarely ordered, and it would interfere with assessment of the dressing at this time. **4** Montgomery straps are used when frequent dressing changes are anticipated; they are not appropriate at this time.

Client Need: Reduction of Risk Potential; **Cognitive Level:** Application; **Nursing Process:** Evaluation/Outcomes; **Reference:** Ch 3, General Nursing Care of Clients During the Postoperative Period

169. **2** Paralytic ileus occurs when neurologic impulses are diminished, as from anesthesia, infection, or surgery.

1 Interference in blood supply would result in necrosis of the bowel. **3** Perforation of the bowel would result in pain and peritonitis. **4** Obstruction of the bowel would initially cause increased peristalsis and bowel sounds.

Client Need: Reduction of Risk Potential; **Cognitive Level:** Application; **Nursing Process:** Evaluation/Analysis; **Reference:** Ch 3, General Nursing Care of Clients During the Postoperative Period

170. **2** A rectal tube promotes maximum benefits in 30 minutes. This allows adequate time for gas to escape.

1 This is not adequate time to permit removal of flatus. **3, 4** After 30 minutes the release of flatus is minimal.

Client Need: Reduction of Risk Potential; **Cognitive Level:** Comprehension; **Nursing Process:** Planning/Implementation; **Reference:** Ch 3, General Nursing Care of Clients During the Postoperative Period

171. **2** Potassium, the major intracellular cation, functions with sodium and calcium to regulate neuromuscular activity and contraction of muscle fibers, particularly the heart muscle. These adaptations develop with hypokalemia.

1 These symptoms do not indicate an electrolyte imbalance. **3** These symptoms would indicate fluid excess, which does not generally occur in colitis. **4** Nausea and vomiting might occur with prolonged potassium deficit; however, this is not an early sign; leg and abdominal cramps occur with potassium excess, not deficit.

Client Need: Physiological Adaptation; **Cognitive Level:** Analysis; **Nursing Process:** Assessment/Analysis; **Reference:** Ch 3, Fluid and Electrolyte Balance

172. **3** The parasympathetic nervous system (a branch of the autonomic nervous system) causes increased GI motility and secretions. The adrenal cortex releases glucocorticoids, which also stimulate the GI tract, increasing the acidity of the secretions.

1, 4 They do not affect involuntary muscles of the colon. **2** The stress function of the pancreas is not directly related to the intestines but is related to glycogen release from the liver. The sympathetic nervous system decreases GI motility.

Client Need: Physiological Adaptation; **Cognitive Level:** Application; **Nursing Process:** Assessment/Analysis; **Reference:** Ch 1, The Stress Response

173. **2** Ibuprofen (Motrin) irritates the GI mucosa and can cause mucosal erosion, resulting in bleeding; fatigue occurs in response to a reduction in the number of RBCs precipitated by the bleeding; bleeding in the upper GI tract causes melena (tarry stools), which occurs when hemoglobin is exposed to the digestive process.

1 This usually is related to immobility, a low-fiber diet, and inadequate fluid intake, not the data listed in this situation. **3** This is related to biliary problems, not GI bleeding. **4** This is related to hemorrhoids, not GI bleeding.

Client Need: Pharmacological and Parenteral Therapies; **Cognitive Level:** Application; **Nursing Process:** Evaluation/Outcomes; **Reference:** Ch 3, Pain, Related Pharmacology

174. **1** The Nurse Practice Act states that the nurse will do health teaching and administer nursing care supportive to life and well-being.

2 The teaching was essential before discharge. **3** The client is responsible for self-care. **4** Health teaching is an independent nursing function.

Client Need: Management of Care; **Cognitive Level:** Analysis; **Integrated Process:** Teaching/Learning; **Nursing Process:** Evaluation/Outcomes; **Reference:** Ch 2, The Nurse's Rights and Responsibilities

175. **2** Unwashed hands are considered contaminated and are used to turn on sink faucets. The use of foot pedals or a paper towel barrier prevents recontamination of washed hands.

1 They are not considered contaminated for this reason; areas cannot be sterile. **3** It is unrelated to the number of people, but rather to being touched by contaminated hands. **4** Although bacterial growth is facilitated in moist environments, this is not why sink faucets are considered contaminated.

Client Need: Safety and Infection Control; **Cognitive Level:** Application; **Nursing Process:** Assessment/Analysis; **Reference:** Ch 3, Infection Review of Microbiology

176. **4** Soap helps by reducing the surface tension of water, but friction is necessary for the removal of microorganisms.

1 Although this aspect of handwashing is important, without friction it has minimal value. **2** Although soap reduces surface tension, without friction it has minimal value. **3** Although water flushes some microorganisms from the skin, without friction it has minimal value.

Client Need: Safety and Infection Control; **Cognitive Level:** Application; **Nursing Process:** Assessment/Analysis; **Reference:** Ch 3, General Nursing Care of Clients at Risk for Infection

177. 4 When a sterile surface becomes wet, microorganisms from the unsterile surface below the sterile field will be drawn up, contaminating the sterile field; the absorption of fluids by gauze results from the adhesion of water to the gauze threads; the surface tension of water causes contraction of the fiber, pulling fluid up the threads.

1 This is separation of substances in solution utilizing their differing rates of diffusion through a membrane. 2 This refers to movement of water through a semipermeable membrane. 3 This is movement of molecules from high to low concentration.

Client Need: Safety and Infection Control; **Cognitive Level:** Analysis; **Nursing Process:** Planning/Implementation; **Reference:** Ch 3, General Nursing Care of Clients at Risk for Infection

178. 1 Surgical asepsis means that practices are employed to keep a defined site or objects free of all microorganisms.

2, 3 This would apply to personal protective equipment and medical asepsis. 4 This would apply to medical asepsis.

Client Need: Safety and Infection Control; **Cognitive Level:** Application; **Nursing Process:** Planning/Implementation; **Reference:** Ch 3, General Nursing Care of Clients at Risk for Infection

179. 4 This covering will not adhere to the wound and it will protect the area until the physician arrives.

1 This is not the priority; the client has needs that must be met first. 2 Although this would eventually be done, it is not the priority. 3 This is contraindicated because it could injure delicate tissues and organs.

Client Need: Reduction of Risk Potential; **Cognitive Level:** Application; **Nursing Process:** Planning/Implementation; **Reference:** Ch 3, General Nursing Care of Clients During the Postoperative Period

180. 4 The Jackson-Pratt or Hemovac is compressed before closing the port to reestablish the negative pressure necessary to provide suction.

1 Portable wound drainage systems are not irrigated because this will increase the risk of instilling microorganisms into the wound. 2 This does not need to be done when emptying the device; a portable wound drainage system usually removes excess drainage before it leaks onto the dressing. 3 The nurse should avoid touching the port because it is sterile.

Client Need: Physiological Adaptation; **Cognitive Level:** Application; **Nursing Process:** Planning/Implementation; **Reference:** Ch 3, General Nursing Care of Clients During the Postoperative Period

181. 3 Vitamin C (ascorbic acid) plays a major role in wound healing. It is necessary for the maintenance and formation of strong collagen, the major protein of most connective tissues.

1 Vitamin A is important for the healing process; however, vitamin C cements the ground substance of supportive tissue. 2 Phytonadione (Mephyton) is vitamin K, which plays a major role in blood coagulation. 4 Vitamin B_{12} is needed for RBC synthesis and a healthy nervous system.

Client Need: Pharmacological and Parenteral Therapies; **Cognitive Level:** Analysis; **Nursing Process:** Assessment/Analysis; **Reference:** Ch 3, General Nursing Care of Clients During the Postoperative Period

182. 2 According to the Nurse Practice Act, a nurse may independently treat human responses to actual or potential health problems.

1 Activity is prescribed by the physician. 3 Providing supportive care is an independent, not dependent, function of the nurse. 4 Surgical wound debridement is performed by the physician.

Client Need: Management of Care; **Cognitive Level:** Analysis; **Nursing Process:** Evaluation/Outcomes; **Reference:** Ch 2, The Nurse's Rights and Responsibilities

183. 1 Reasonably prudent behavior in dealing with a client such as this is to change the client's position at least every hour to relieve pressure on tissues and promote circulation. The nurse was negligent in not doing this.

2 Although pressure ulcers may occur, nursing care must include preventive measures. 3 The family is included in the health team. 4 When a capable client refuses necessary health care, the nurse should provide health teaching to promote compliance with the treatment plan. If the client makes an informed decision after an explanation, then the client's rights must be respected; however, a document absolving health professionals of liability also must be signed.

Client Need: Management of Care; **Cognitive Level:** Analysis; **Nursing Process:** Planning/Implementation; **Reference:** Ch 2, The Nurse's Rights and Responsibilities

184. 1 A sarcoma is defined as a malignant tumor with cells that resemble those of the supportive (connective) tissues of the body.

2 Carcinoma refers to a malignant neoplasm of epithelial tissue. 3 Although collagen is the substance used to form the connective tissue, the term collagenoma is incorrect. 4 These are benign tumors of the bone.

Client Need: Physiological Adaptation; **Cognitive Level:** Knowledge; **Nursing Process:** Assessment/Analysis; **Reference:** Ch 3, Classification of Neoplasms

185. 1 Radiation in controlled doses is therapeutic. When uncontrolled or in excessive amounts, it is carcinogenic.

2 Therapeutic doses are helpful regardless of the size of the area being treated. 3 This does not affect the outcome of radiation therapy. 4 This does not influence radiation's effect.

Client Need: Physiological Adaptation; **Cognitive Level:** Application; **Integrated Process:** Teaching/Learning; **Nursing Process:** Planning/Implementation; **Reference:** Ch 3, Radiation

186. 2 Radiodermatitis occurs 3 to 6 weeks after the start of treatment.

1 The word burn should be avoided because it may increase anxiety. 3 Emollients are contraindicated; they may alter the calculated x-ray route and injure

normal tissue. **4** This response does not address the client's concern.
Client Need: Physiological Adaptation; **Cognitive Level:** Application; **Integrated Process:** Teaching/Learning; **Nursing Process:** Planning/Implementation; **Reference:** Ch 3, Radiation

187. **1** Cold reduces the sensitivity of receptors for pain in the skin. In addition, local blood vessels constrict, limiting the amount of interstitial fluid and its related pressure and discomfort.

2 Local blood vessels constrict. **3** Local cold applications do not depress vital signs. **4** Local cold applications do not directly affect blood viscosity.
Client Need: Basic Care and Comfort; **Cognitive Level:** Application; **Nursing Process:** Evaluation/Outcomes; **Reference:** Ch 3, Nonpharmacologic Pain Management Strategies

188. **1** Stupor may occur with hypothermia because of slowed cerebral metabolic processes.

2 Pallor, not erythema, would be present as a result of peripheral vasoconstriction. **3** Drowsiness occurs; the client is unable to focus on anxiety-producing aspects of the situation. **4** Respirations would be decreased.
Client Need: Physiological Adaptation; **Cognitive Level:** Application; **Nursing Process:** Assessment/Analysis; **Reference:** Ch 3, Specific Emergencies

189. **2** Immediately before administration of analgesia, an assessment of vital signs is necessary to determine whether any contraindications to the medication exist (e.g., hypotension, a respiratory rate of 12 breaths/min or less).

1 Pain prevents both psychologic and physiologic rest. **3** Before administration, the nurse must check the physician's orders, the time of the last administration, and the client's vital signs. **4** A complete assessment including vital signs should be done before documenting.
Client Need: Reduction of Risk Potential; **Cognitive Level:** Application; **Nursing Process:** Planning/Implementation; **Reference:** Ch 3, General Nursing Care of Clients in Pain

190. **3** Electrodes are attached to sensory nerves or over the dorsal column; a transmitter is worn externally and, by electric stimulation, may be used to interfere with the transmission of painful stimuli as needed.

1 Clients may bathe when the transmitter is disconnected. **2** The client may need analgesics in conjunction with the transmitter. **4** The device should not interfere with a remote control apparatus.
Client Need: Basic Care and Comfort; **Cognitive Level:** Application; **Integrated Process:** Teaching/Learning; **Nursing Process:** Planning/Implementation; **Reference:** Ch 3, General Nursing Care of Clients in Pain

191. **1** A rhizotomy is the resection of posterior nerve roots to eliminate nerve impulses associated with severe pain from the thoracic area (as in lung cancer).

2 A rhinotomy is an incision into the nose. **3** A cordotomy is the surgical interruption of

pain-conducting pathways in the spinal cord. **4** A chondrectomy is the surgical excision of cartilage.
Client Need: Basic Care and Comfort; **Cognitive Level:** Analysis; **Nursing Process:** Planning/Implementation; **Reference:** Ch 3, General Nursing Care of Clients in Pain

192. **4** The exact nature of the pain must be determined to distinguish whether this is pain caused by the surgery or is from some other cause.

1-3 This should be done later, but the first action would be to determine the nature of the pain.
Client Need: Basic Care and Comfort; **Cognitive Level:** Application; **Nursing Process:** Assessment/Analysis; **Reference:** Ch 3, General Nursing Care of Clients in Pain

193. **3** The voltage or current is adjusted on the basis of the degree of pain relief experienced by the client.

1 This may provide too little or too much stimulation to achieve the desired response. **2** This is true of the pain suppressor TENS unit, not the conventional units. **4** The electrodes should be applied either on the painful area or immediately below or above the area.
Client Need: Basic Care and Comfort; **Cognitive Level:** Application; **Nursing Process:** Planning/Implementation; **Reference:** Ch 3, Nonpharmacologic Pain Management Strategies

194. **1** Pain may indicate a toxic effect.

2, 3 This is an expected side effect of internal radiotherapy. **4** This is associated with the need to maintain position, not with radium itself.
Client Need: Physiological Adaptation; **Cognitive Level:** Application; **Nursing Process:** Evaluation/Outcomes; **Reference:** Ch 3, Radiation

195. **2** Radium must be handled with long-handled forceps because distance helps limit exposure.

1 A nurse does not clean radium implants. **3** This does not provide adequate shielding from the gamma rays emitted by radium. **4** The amount and duration of exposure are important in assessing the effect on the client; however, this will not affect safety during removal.
Client Need: Physiological Adaptation; **Cognitive Level:** Application; **Nursing Process:** Planning/Implementation; **Reference:** Ch 3, General Nursing Care of Clients With Neoplastic Disorders

196. **4** Packing maintains a radium implant in its correct placement; correct placement minimizes the effect on normal tissue.

1 The packing must be readjusted or replaced to protect normal tissue from radiation damage. **2** This is not true. **3** There should be no active bleeding with radium implants; cellular sloughing is expected.
Client Need: Management of Care; **Cognitive Level:** Comprehension; **Integrated Process:** Communication/Documentation; **Nursing Process:** Planning/Implementation; **Reference:** Ch 3, General Nursing Care of Clients With Neoplastic Disorders

197. **1** Restriction of each visitor to a 10-minute stay minimizes the risk for exposure. Some institutions will not allow visitors while an implant is in place.

2 The urine is not radioactive. **3** Lead aprons are not effective shields against rays emitted by internal sources of radiation. **4** Radium implants will not affect the location of IM injections.

Client Need: Reduction of Risk Potential; **Cognitive Level:** Application; **Nursing Process:** Planning/Implementation; **Reference:** Ch 3, General Nursing Care of Clients With Neoplastic Disorders

198. **3** Before discharge it is important for the nurse to instruct the client to follow through with medical care at specified intervals.

1 Fluids are not reduced unless other cardiac or renal pathology is present. **2** A low-residue diet is indicated to avoid pressure from a distended colon only when the implant is in place; the radium implant is removed before discharge. **4** If diet is adequate, multivitamins are unnecessary.

Client Need: Management of Care; **Cognitive Level:** Application; **Integrated Process:** Teaching/Learning; **Nursing Process:** Planning/Implementation; **Reference:** Ch 3, General Nursing Care of Clients With Neoplastic Disorders

199. **1** Frequent position changes are important to ensure proper urinary drainage; gravity promotes flow, which prevents obstruction.

2 This is not a priority unless the client is sedated. **3** Range of motion would be of minimal importance, because the client would be able to move without limitation. **4** Back care is necessary but is not the priority.

Client Need: Physiological Adaptation; **Cognitive Level:** Application; **Nursing Process:** Planning/Implementation; **Reference:** Ch 3, General Nursing Care of Clients During the Postoperative Period

200. **3** The prevention of infection is the priority because an infection can be life-threatening for a client who is immunocompromised. Chemotherapeutic medications depress the bone marrow, causing leukopenia. This client's white blood cell count is below the expected range of 3100 to 10,000/mm^3 for an older female adult. While the elevation in the client's temperature, pulse, and respirations may be related to the direct effects of the chemotherapeutic agents, they also may reflect that the client is resisting a microbiologic stress.

1 Although a balance between rest and activity is important, it is not the priority. While chemotherapeutic medications depress the bone marrow and cause anemia, this client's red blood cell count is within the expected range of 4.0 to 5.0 million/mm^3 for an older female adult. The client's hemoglobin level is within the expected range of 11.5 to 16.0 g/dL. **2** Even though preventing injury is important, it is not the priority. Although chemotherapeutic medications depress the bone marrow, causing thrombocytopenia, this client's platelet count is within the expected range of 150,000 to 400,000/mm^3 for an adult. **4** While maintaining fluid balance is important, it is not the priority. The client's hematocrit is within the expected range of 38% to 41% for an older female adult, indicating that the client is not dehydrated. The client's blood pressure is not decreased, which occurs with dehydration. Although chemotherapeutic medications may cause nausea, vomiting, and diarrhea, the client did not indicate that these occurred.

Client Need: Reduction of Risk Potential; **Cognitive Level:** Analysis; **Nursing Process:** Assessment/Analysis; **Reference:** Ch 3, General Nursing Care of Clients With Neoplastic Disorders

CHAPTER 5

Growth and Development of the Adult

THE YOUNG ADULT (AGE 20 TO 44 YEARS)

DATABASE

A. Physiologic development
1. Physical maturation occurs
2. Muscle strength and coordination peak
3. Biorhythms become established
4. Sexuality
   a. Established sex drive remains high for men
   b. Female sex drive reaches a peak during later phase of young adulthood
   c. Physiologically optimal period for childbearing
5. Basal metabolic rate (BMR) decreases at a rate of 2% to 4% per decade after 20 years of age
B. Psychosocial development
1. Mental abilities reflect formal operations (see Growth and Development in Chapter 34, Nursing Care of Adolescents
2. Resolving the developmental crisis of intimacy versus isolation and beginning to resolve the developmental crisis of generativity versus stagnation
3. Establishing new family relationships and parenting patterns
4. Establishing the self in, and advancing in, a chosen occupation
C. Common health problems: accidents, AIDS, STDs, cancer involving the reproductive organs, hypertension, suicide, alcoholism, spousal abuse, fertility regulation, periodontal disease, unbalanced diet, obesity, and intimacy problems

General Nursing Care of Young Adults

A. Assessment/Analysis
1. Obtain history of drug and alcohol use, sexual practices, and family relationships
2. Determine baseline height, weight, and dietary history
3. Measure vital signs to establish baseline
4. Question client about health practices related to cancer prevention and detection
B. Planning/Implementation
1. Encourage attendance at safety programs to promote accident prevention (e.g., defensive driving)
2. Increase public awareness of problems and availability of crisis counseling, support groups, and other community resources (e.g., hot lines, Alcoholics Anonymous, family planning clinics)
3. Teach safe sex practices
4. Promote awareness that optimal diet and exercise are essential to achieving and maintaining optimal health; encourage nutritional evaluation and consultation
5. Teach client to use exogenous supplemental vitamins with caution, especially vitamins A, D, and E; higher doses than necessary can cause health problems
6. Teach dietary guidelines following USDA recommendations
   a. Eat a variety of foods
   b. Maintain ideal weight
   c. Avoid too much fat, saturated fat, and cholesterol
   d. Eat diet with adequate vegetables, grain products, and fruit (fruits are low in sodium but high in sugar)
   e. Use salt in moderation
   f. Limit daily intake of alcoholic beverages to no more than one drink for women and two drinks for men
   g. Maintain recommended daily caloric and calcium intake
7. Teach breast and testicular self-examination techniques and encourage regular medical checkups
C. Evaluation/Outcomes
1. Establishes safe health care practices
2. Maintains ideal body weight
3. Maintains blood pressure within expected limits
4. Remains free from infection

THE MIDDLE-AGE ADULT (AGE 45 TO 59 YEARS)

DATABASE

A. Physiologic development
1. Greater diversity in physiologic conditioning resulting from established lifestyle
2. Early clinical findings of aging (e.g., wrinkling, thinning hair, decreased muscle tone, decreased nerve function)

3. Decreased BMR with subsequent weight gain unless caloric intake is reduced
4. Decreased production of sexual hormones
   a. Menopause (see Unit 4, Childbearing and Women's Health Nursing)
   b. Male climacteric; may pass unnoticed, especially in those with high self-esteem; clinical findings may include diminished potency, less forceful ejaculation, thinning and graying hair, fatigue, and depression
B. Psychosocial development
   1. Cognitive abilities enhanced because of motivation and past experiences
   2. Resolving developmental crisis of generativity versus stagnation
   3. Adjusting to changes in family caused by aging parents and growing or returning children
   4. Maintaining satisfactory status of one's career
   5. Accepting physical changes associated with advancing age
   6. Developing social and civic activities that are personally satisfying
C. Health problems: cardiovascular disease, hypertension, alcoholism, sexual dysfunction, presbyopia, unbalanced or inadequate diet, deteriorating vision and hearing, type 2 diabetes, obesity, and depression

General Nursing Care of Middle-Age Adults

A. Assessment/Analysis
   1. Determine cardiovascular status: vital signs, peripheral pulses, peripheral edema, shortness of breath, and chest pain
   2. Measure visual acuity
   3. Obtain history of alcohol use, sexual patterns, and family relationships
   4. Determine baseline height and weight and dietary history
   5. Question client about leisure activities and retirement plans
B. Planning/Implementation
   1. Reinforce importance of regular exercise to prevent cardiovascular and musculoskeletal deterioration
   2. Emphasize dietary changes: reduction of calories, fats, and protein; increased calcium and fiber; encourage individuals to follow USDA recommendations
   3. Stress the need for regular medical evaluations as well as self-evaluations
   4. Encourage attendance at self-help groups to stop substance dependency (e.g., smoking, drinking alcohol, overeating)
C. Evaluation/Outcomes
   1. Maintains ideal body weight
   2. Maintains BP within normal limits
   3. Establishes healthy dietary pattern
   4. Participates in exercise regimen
   5. Develops coping skills to manage stress

THE YOUNG-OLDER ADULT (AGE 60 TO 74 YEARS)

DATABASE

A. Physiologic development
   1. Slowing of reaction time
   2. Loss of sensory acuity
   3. Diminished muscle tone and strength
   4. Increased diversity in health status and function resulting from earlier lifestyle and development of chronic health problems
B. Psychosocial development
   1. Cognitive abilities may be affected by cardiovascular disease
   2. Adjusting to retirement: some individuals experience a loss of self-esteem; others enjoy the freedom to explore other interests
   3. Coping with altered economic status; adjusting to fixed income
   4. Resolving death of parents and possibly spouse
   5. Accepting separation from their children and their families
   6. Resolving developmental crisis of ego integrity versus despair
C. Health problems: cardiovascular disease, cancer, presbyopia, accidents, respiratory disease, osteoporosis/osteoarthritis, hearing loss (especially for high-pitched sounds), unbalanced or inadequate diet, and depression

General Nursing Care of Young-Older Adults

A. Assessment/Analysis
   1. Determine cardiovascular status: vital signs, peripheral pulses, peripheral edema, shortness of breath, history of chest pain, and changes in sensation
   2. Measure visual and auditory acuities
   3. Obtain history relative to warning signs of cancer
   4. Identify coping skills and support systems
B. Planning/Implementation
   1. Encourage individuals to maintain a schedule of regular medical, dental, and visual examinations to prevent or control health problems
   2. Assess living conditions for possible hazards that could cause accidents
   3. Refer widows and widowers to appropriate self-help groups as necessary
   4. Encourage individuals to anticipate and plan for retirement and to develop new interests and support systems
   5. Encourage nutritional assessment and consultation to prevent nutrient deficiencies and to provide for diet modifications with aging
C. Evaluation/Outcomes
   1. Participates in an exercise program
   2. Verbalizes fears to health care providers
   3. Remains free from injury
   4. Maintains satisfying interpersonal relationships

5. Consumes nutritionally adequate diet
6. Maintains therapeutic regimen

THE MIDDLE-OLDER ADULT (AGE 75 TO 84 YEARS) AND OLD-OLDER ADULT (AGE 85+ YEARS)

DATABASE

A. Physiologic development
   1. Diminished sensation (visual and auditory) and diminished reaction time
   2. Increased sensitivity to cold because of decreased subcutaneous tissue, decreased thyroid functioning, and impaired circulation
   3. Decreased enzyme secretion in, and motility of, the GI tract
   4. Decreased glomerular filtration rate
   5. Decreased cardiac output
   6. Arteriosclerotic changes with diminished elasticity of blood vessels
   7. Decreased lung capacity
   8. Demineralization and other degenerative skeletal changes, particularly in weight-bearing bones
   9. Muscle atrophy
B. Psychosocial development
   1. Cognitive abilities not necessarily affected by age, but may be impaired as a result of disease, leading to diminished awareness and increased safety risk
   2. Resolving the developmental crisis of ego integrity versus despair; depends on previous resolution of task of generativity versus stagnation
   3. Adjusting to the death of significant others
   4. Adapting to decreased physical capacity and changes in body image
   5. Adjusting to the economic burden of a fixed income
   6. Recognizing the inevitability of death
   7. Reminiscing increasingly about the past
C. Health problems: cardiovascular disease, cancer, accidents (e.g., falls, automobile collisions), respiratory disease, cerebral vascular insufficiency, malnutrition, and problems with perception (cataracts, glaucoma, hearing loss)

General Nursing Care of Middle-Older and Old-Older Adults

A. Assessment/Analysis
   1. Determine cardiovascular status: vital signs, peripheral pulses, peripheral edema, shortness of breath, history of chest pain, and changes in sensation
   2. Identify neurologic deficits: level of consciousness, orientation, motor function, and sensory function
   3. Identify deteriorating musculoskeletal functioning and effect on quality of life
   4. Determine respiratory function: respiratory rate, rhythm, and depth; use of accessory muscles; breath sounds; vital capacity; and arterial blood gas levels
   5. Review nutritional status: dietary history, body height and weight, skin condition, and serum protein and albumin levels
   6. Assess individual coping ability
   7. Assess resources
B. Planning/Implementation
   1. Encourage client to maintain a schedule of regular medical supervision and exercise
   2. Promote maximal degree of independence
   3. Initiate appropriate referrals for individuals requiring assistance with activities of daily living
   4. Open channels of communication for reality orientation, reminiscing, and emotional support; explain procedures and expectations; reinforce and repeat as necessary
   5. Refer to social services and other resources that can provide economic assistance when necessary
   6. Ensure that prosthetic devices (e.g., dentures, contact lenses, eye prosthetics, hearing aids, braces, limbs) fit comfortably and do not cause irritation; teach proper care of such devices
   7. Encourage following the USDA dietary recommendations; require fewer total calories
C. Evaluation/Outcomes
   1. Performs or assists with self-care activities
   2. Remains free from injury
   3. Uses community resources to maximize independence
   4. Maintains nutritionally adequate diet
   5. Maintains social relationships
   6. Adjusts to changes in functional ability
   7. Maintains therapeutic regimen

Nursing Care of Clients With Circulatory System (Cardiovascular, Blood, and Lymphatic Systems) Disorders

OVERVIEW
REVIEW OF ANATOMY AND PHYSIOLOGY

Blood
A. Volume: males: 5 to 6 L; females: 4.5 to 5.5 L
B. Viscosity: about 5.5 times as viscous as pure water; reflected by hematocrit (percentage of blood volume that is RBCs)
  1. Males: 45% to 52%
  2. Females: 37% to 48%
C. Hematopoiesis
  1. Location: red marrow of vertebrae, sternum, ribs, iliac crests, clavicles, scapulae, and skull
  2. Pluripotential stem cell differentiates into myeloid and lymphoid stem cells
    a. Myeloid stem cells further differentiate into erythrocytes, platelets, neutrophils, monocytes, eosinophils, basophils, and mast cells
    b. Lymphoid stem cells further differentiate into B and T lymphocytes
D. Blood components
  1. Plasma
    a. Water: 3 L in average adult; 90% of plasma
    b. Ions: see Fluid, Electrolyte, and Acid-Base Balance in Chapter 3
    c. Albumin (major plasma protein)
      (1) Acts as a buffer
      (2) Maintains plasma colloid osmotic pressure
    d. Glucose: prime oxidative metabolite
    e. Serum: plasma with fewer or no coagulating proteins
  2. Formed elements
    a. Erythrocytes (RBCs)
      (1) Shape: pliable biconcave disk that maximizes surface area proportional to volume for ease of diffusion of gases
      (2) Number: males: 4.5 to 6.2×10^6/mm^3; females: 4.0 to 5.5×10^6/mm^3
      (3) Formation (erythropoiesis): liver and kidneys secrete proteins that help form erythropoietin, which stimulates erythrocyte production by red marrow
      (4) Principal component is hemoglobin; functions to bind O_2 through iron in heme and CO_2 through globulin portion; can carry both simultaneously

      (5) Erythrocytes live for about 120 days; old or deteriorated ones are removed by reticuloendothelial cells of the liver, spleen, and bone marrow; heme is converted to bilirubin, which is excreted from the liver as part of bile
    b. Leukocytes (WBCs)
      (1) Types
        (a) Granulocytes (polymorphonuclear): neutrophils, eosinophils, and basophils
        (b) Agranulocytes (mononuclear): monocytes that become macrophages in tissue spaces and lymphocytes
      (2) Functions
        (a) Phagocytosis of bacteria by neutrophils and macrophages; phagocytosis of antigen-antibody complexes by eosinophils
        (b) Antibody synthesis: B lymphocytes become plasma cells, which produce most circulatory antibodies
        (c) Destruction of transplanted tissues and cancer cells by T lymphocytes, which form in lymphoid tissue and mature in the thymus
      (3) Leukocytes live for a few hours or days; some T lymphocytes live for many years and provide long-term immunity
    c. Platelets (thrombocytes)
      (1) Number: 150,000 to 500,000/mm^3
      (2) Function in blood coagulation
        (a) Adhere to each other and to damaged areas of circulatory system to limit or prevent blood loss
        (b) Release chemicals that constrict damaged blood vessels
E. Blood groups
  1. There are four blood types: A, B, AB, and O; type indicates antigens on or in the RBC membrane (e.g., type A blood has A antigens; type O blood has no antigens)
  2. Blood can be either Rh-positive or Rh-negative; usually blood does not contain anti-Rh antibodies. However, Rh-negative blood will contain anti-Rh antibodies if the individual has been transfused with Rh-positive blood or has carried an Rh-positive

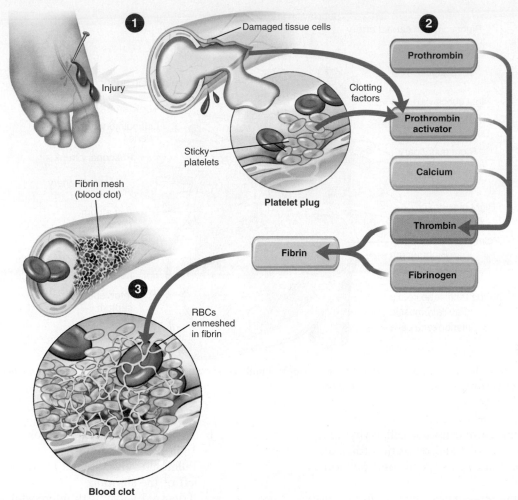

Damaged tissue cells

Injury

Clotting factors

Sticky platelets

Platelet plug

Fibrin mesh (blood clot)

Prothrombin

Prothrombin activator

Calcium

Thrombin

Fibrin

Fibrinogen

RBCs enmeshed in fibrin

Blood clot

Figure 6-1 Blood clotting mechanism. The complex clotting mechanism can be condensed into three basic steps: (1) release of clotting factors from both injured tissue cells and sticky platelets at the injury site (which form temporary platelet plug); (2) series of chemical reactions that eventually result in the formation of thrombin; and (3) formation of fibrin and trapping of blood cells to form a clot. (From Thibodeau GA, Patton KT: *Anatomy and physiology*, ed 6, St Louis, 2007, Mosby.)

fetus without treatment; Rh-positive blood never contains anti-Rh antibodies

3. Plasma: normally contains no antibodies against antigens present on its own RBCs, but does contain antibodies against other A or B antigens not present on its RBCs

4. The potential danger in transfusing blood is that the donor's blood may be agglutinated (clumped) by the recipient's antibodies

F. Hemostasis: process to arrest blood loss (Figure 6-1: Blood clotting mechanism)
   1. Vasoconstriction
   2. Aggregation of platelets: adhere to damaged blood vessel walls, forming plugs
   3. Blood coagulation (clotting): blood becomes gel as soluble fibrinogen is converted to insoluble fibrin
      a. Extrinsic clotting mechanism: trigger is blood contacting damaged tissue
      b. Intrinsic clotting mechanism: trigger is release of chemicals (platelet factors such as thromboplastin) from platelets aggregated at the site of an injury

c. Liver cells synthesize prothrombin, fibrinogen, and other clotting factors; adequate amounts of vitamin K must be present in blood for the liver to make prothrombin; calcium acts as a catalyst to convert prothrombin to thrombin

d. Prothrombin is converted to thrombin, which converts fibrinogen to fibrin; fibrin is an insoluble protein formed from the soluble protein fibrinogen in the presence of thrombin; fibrin appears as a tangled mass of threads in which blood cells become enmeshed

e. When new endothelial cells form, the fibrin clot is destroyed by plasmin, which is formed from plasminogen

Heart

(Figure 6-2: Structures of the heart and course of blood through chambers)

A. Layers
   1. Pericardium (protective covering): parietal and visceral (epicardium) layers create a protective sac that contains a small amount of lubricating fluid that reduces friction

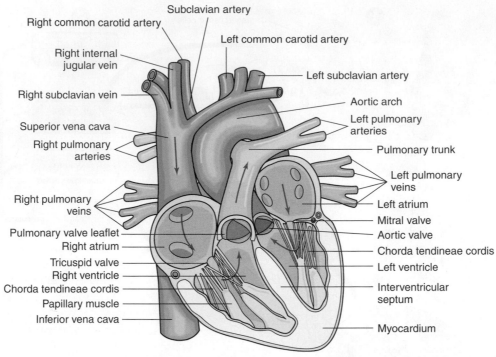

Figure 6-2 Structures of the heart and course of blood through chambers. (From Monahan FD et al: *Phipps' medical-surgical nursing: health and illness perspectives*, ed 8, St Louis, 2007, Mosby.)

2. Myocardium (cardiac muscle cells): rhythmic contraction (systole) and relaxation (diastole) pumps blood through systemic and pulmonary circulation
3. Endocardium (endothelial inner lining of inner chambers and valves)

B. Chambers
1. Right atrium: receives deoxygenated blood from systemic circulation via the vena cava
2. Right ventricle: pumps deoxygenated blood to the pulmonary circulation via the pulmonary artery
3. Left atrium: receives oxygenated blood from the pulmonary circulation via the pulmonary vein
4. Left ventricle: pumps oxygenated blood to the systemic circulation via the aorta

C. Valves
1. Atrioventricular valves between atria and ventricles: tricuspid on right, mitral (bicuspid) on left; valves consist of three parts: flaps or cusps, chordae tendineae, papillary muscles; closure during early systole to prevent backward flow of blood (regurgitation) into atrium causes first heart sound (S_1)
2. Semilunar valves: pulmonic valve between right ventricle and pulmonary arteries, and aortic valve between left ventricle and the aorta; closure at the end of systole to prevent backward flow of blood into ventricles causes second heart sound (S_2)
3. Auscultation for S_1, S_2, murmurs caused by regurgitation of blood through valves, and snaps/clicks caused by stenosis of valves
   a. Apical pulse or mitral valve: fifth intercostal space near left midclavicular line
   b. Aortic valve: second intercostal space on the right of the sternum
   c. Pulmonic valve: second intercostal space on the left of the sternum
   d. Tricuspid valve: fifth intercostal space on the left of the sternum

D. Blood supply to myocardium (heart muscle)
1. Left coronary artery branches to the left anterior descending artery, the circumflex artery, and the right coronary artery
2. Right coronary artery branches mainly to supply the right side of the heart, but also to carry some blood to the left ventricle
3. Greatest flow of blood into myocardium occurs when the heart relaxes, as a result of decreased arterial compression; an increased heart rate shortens diastole, leading to decreased time for myocardial perfusion
4. Relatively few anastomoses exist between the larger branches of the coronary arteries (poor collateral circulation); hence if one of these vessels becomes occluded suddenly, little or no blood can reach the myocardial cells supplied by that vessel; however, collateral circulation can develop slowly over time

E. Conduction system of heart: cardiac muscle cells have the ability to generate impulses that cause contractions (automaticity)
1. Sinoatrial (SA) node: located in the right atrial wall; referred to as the pacemaker of the heart because it inherently generates impulses at the highest rate of 60 to 100/min

2. Atrioventricular (AV) node: located in the base of the right atrium; capable of generating 40 to 60 impulses per minute if SA node is nonfunctional

3. AV bundle of His: originates in the AV node and extends by two branches down the two sides of the interventricular septum (right and left bundle branches); a disruption in conduction here is called a bundle branch block

4. Purkinje fibers: extend from the AV bundles throughout the walls of the ventricles

5. Normally a nerve impulse begins at the SA node and spreads through both atria to the AV node; after a short delay it is conducted by the bundle of His and the Purkinje fibers to the lateral walls of the ventricles; the ventricles can generate 30 to 40 impulses per minute if both the SA and AV nodes are nonfunctional

F. Cardiac output (CO): volume of blood pumped per minute by the ventricles; average for adult at rest is approximately 3 to 5 L/min; calculated by multiplying the stroke volume (SV) times the heart rate (HR)

1. Preload: extent to which left ventricle stretches at the end of diastole as a result of left ventricular end-diastolic volume; Frank-Starling law states when the heart is stretched by an increased returning volume of blood, it contracts more strongly, resulting in an increased stroke volume; subject to physiologic limitations

2. Afterload: arterial resistance that the heart must overcome to eject contents of the left ventricle during systole; an increased afterload caused by systemic vasoconstriction will decrease the stroke volume unless contractility is increased

3. Contractility: force of cardiac muscle contraction; increased by sympathetic nervous system, leading to increased stroke volume; decreased by parasympathetic nervous system; influences ejection fraction (percent of blood volume at the end of diastole that is ejected by ventricular contraction)

4. Heart rate: cardiac contractions per minute; increased by sympathetic nervous system and decreased by parasympathetic nervous system; bradycardia is a rate less than 60 beats/min; tachycardia is a rate greater than 100 beats/min

Blood Vessels

A. Arteries
1. Carry blood away from the heart (all arteries except pulmonary artery carry oxygenated blood)
2. Branch into smaller and smaller vessels called arterioles, which branch into microscopic capillaries
3. Structure: lining (tunica intima) of endothelium; middle coat (tunica media) of smooth muscle, elastic, and fibrous tissues, which permits constriction and dilation; outer coat (tunica adventitia or externa) of fibrous tissue; this firmness makes arteries stand open instead of collapsing when cut

4. Peripheral pulses can be felt wherever an artery lies near the surface and over a firm background such as bone, because of elasticity of arterial walls; sites: radial—at wrist; carotid—along anterior edge of sternocleidomastoid muscle, at level of lower margin of thyroid cartilage; brachial—at bend of the elbow, along the inner margin of the biceps muscle; femoral—in groin; popliteal—behind knee; posterior tibial—behind the medial malleolus; dorsalis pedis—on anterior surface of the foot, just below the bend of the ankle; volume or amplitude of pulse may be absent, thready or diminished, normal or bounding (Figure 6-3: Palpation of the arterial pulses)

5. Pulse deficit: difference between the apical and radial pulses

6. Blood pressure: systolic—pressure within the arteries when the heart is contracting; diastolic—pressure within the arteries when the heart is at rest between contractions; pulse pressure—difference between the systolic and diastolic pressures

B. Veins
1. Carry blood toward the heart (all veins except pulmonary veins carry deoxygenated blood)
2. Branch into venules, which collect blood from capillaries; veins in the cranial cavity formed by the dura mater are called sinuses
3. Structure: same three coats as arteries, but thinner and fewer elastic and muscle fibers, allowing veins to collapse when cut; semilunar valves present in most veins more than 2 mm in diameter to prevent backward flow of blood

C. Capillaries
1. Carry blood from arterioles and unite to form small veins or venules, which in turn unite to form veins
2. Exchange of substances between blood and interstitial fluid occurs in capillaries
3. Structure: only lining coat present (intima); wall only one cell thick to allow for diffusion of gases and small molecules

Regulatory Mechanisms Affecting Circulation

A. Autonomic nervous system
1. Sympathetic nervous system increases heart rate and cardiac contractility, dilates coronary and skeletal blood vessels, and constricts blood vessels supplying the abdominal organs and skin through stimulation of alpha- and beta-adrenergic receptors by catecholamines (epinephrine, norepinephrine, dopamine)
2. Parasympathetic nervous system decreases heart rate and contractility, and causes vasodilation through cholinergic fibers; stimulation of vagus nerve initiates parasympathetic response
3. Baroreceptors in the aortic arch and carotid sinus respond to changes in BP
   a. Increased arterial BP baroreceptors, which then cause a parasympathetic response

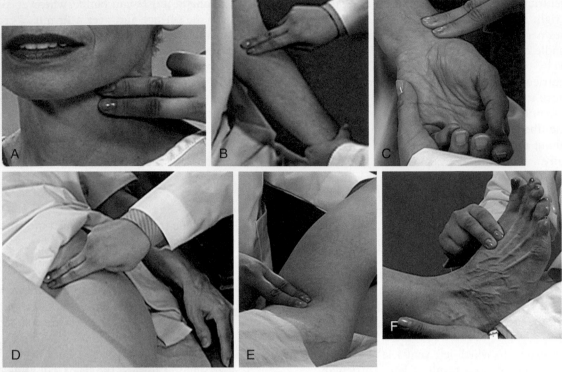

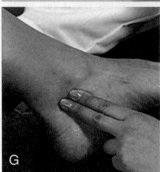

Figure 6-3 Palpation of the arterial pulses. **A,** Carotid. **B,** Brachial. **C,** Radial. **D,** Femoral. **E,** Popliteal. **F,** Dorsalis pedis. **G,** Posterior tibial. (From Seidel HM, Dains JE, Benedict GW: *Mosby's guide to physical examination*, ed 6, St Louis, 2006, Mosby.)

(vasodilation and decreased heart rate and contractility)

   b. Decreased arterial pressure inhibits baroreceptors, resulting in increased sympathetic response (vasoconstriction and increased heart rate and contractility)

  4. Chemoreceptors respond to changes in levels of oxygen and carbon dioxide and changes in pH by stimulation of the autonomic nervous system

B. Renin-angiotensin-aldosterone mechanism: when renal perfusion decreases, this mechanism increases retention of sodium and water to increase blood volume, and causes vasoconstriction; increases BP

C. Intrinsic circulatory regulation: increased blood pressure raises the hydrostatic pressure of plasma, leading to increased filtration of plasma from the circulatory system to interstitial spaces, resulting in reduced venous return, decreased cardiac output, and decreased BP

Lymphatic System

A. Lymph vessels

  1. Structure: lymph capillaries similar to blood capillaries in structure; larger lymphatics similar to veins but are thinner-walled, have more valves, and have lymph nodes along their course

  2. Functions: return fluid and interstitial proteins to the venous system via the thoracic and right lymphatic ducts at the junction between the internal jugular and subclavian veins; interference with the return of proteins to the blood results in edema, caused by the loss of protein and changes in colloid osmotic pressure

B. Lymph nodes

  1. Located throughout the body; usually occur in clusters

  2. Functions: help defend the body against foreign substances (notably, bacteria and tumor cells)

   a. Release lymphocytes into circulation for surveillance

b. Respond to sensitized lymphocytes in proliferation stage: dormant T and B lymphocytes in nodes enlarge, multiply, and differentiate

C. Spleen
1. Location: left hypochondrium, above and behind cardiac portion of the stomach
2. Functions
   a. Reticuloendothelial cells of spleen form macrophages that protect the body from antigens through phagocytosis; removes damaged cells from circulation
   b. Contains B and T lymphocytes essential for humoral and cellular immune responses
   c. Sequesters newly formed reticulocytes until matured erythrocytes; serves as reservoir of erythrocytes and platelets; sympathetic stimulation causes constriction of its capsule, squeezing out an estimated 200 mL of blood into general circulation within 1 minute
   d. Resumes hematopoiesis if bone marrow fails to function

REVIEW OF MICROORGANISMS

A. *Streptococcus pyogenes:* gram-positive streptococcus; the most virulent strain (group A beta hemolytic) causes scarlet fever, septic sore throat, tonsillitis, cellulitis, puerperal fever, erysipelas, rheumatic fever, and glomerulonephritis
B. *Streptococcus viridans:* gram-positive streptococcus; distinguishable from *S. pyogenes* by its alpha hemolysis (rather than beta) of RBCs; the most common cause of subacute bacterial endocarditis

RELATED PHARMACOLOGY
Cardiac Glycosides
A. Description
1. Produce a positive inotropic effect (increased force of contraction) by increasing permeability of cardiac muscle membranes to the calcium and sodium ions required for contraction of muscle fibrils
2. Increase cardiac output by increasing effectiveness of heart pump
3. Produce a negative chronotropic effect (decreased rate of contraction) by an action mediated through the vagus nerve, which slows firing of the SA node and impulse transmission at the AV node
4. Effective in treating heart failure, and atrial flutter and fibrillation
5. Available in oral and parenteral (IM, IV) preparations
6. Initially, loading dose is administered to digitalize the client; after the desired effect is achieved, the dosage is lowered to a maintenance level, which replaces the amount of drug metabolized and excreted each day
B. Examples: digitalis; digoxin (Lanoxin)

C. Major side effects: diarrhea (local effect), nausea, vomiting (malabsorption of all nutrients); bradycardia (increased vagal tone at AV node)
D. Toxicity: premature ventricular complexes (increased spontaneous rate of ventricular depolarization), xanthopsia/yellow vision (effect on visual cones); muscle weakness (CNS effect, neurotoxicity, hypokalemia), blurred vision (CNS effect), anorexia and vomiting (local effect stimulates chemoreceptor zone in medulla); toxicity treated with digoxin immune Fab (Digibind)
E. Nursing care
1. Check apical pulse before administration: withhold dose and notify physician if rate is outside ordered parameters (e.g., less than 50 or 60 beats/min, greater than 110 beats/min)
2. Encourage intake of potassium-rich foods unless potassium supplement is ordered
3. Assess client for signs of impending toxicity (anorexia, nausea, vomiting, dysrhythmias, xanthopsia)
4. Monitor for hypokalemia, which potentiates the effects of digitalis; ECG will indicate depressed T waves with hypokalemia
5. Instruct the client to count radial pulse and record before each administration; notify physician of any side effects; report any changes in heart rate to physician (irregular heartbeats; increased or decreased rate)
6. Digoxin—monitor blood level during therapy (normal serum level: 0.9 to 2.0 ng/mL)

Antidysrhythmics
A. Description
1. Treat abnormal variations in cardiac rate and rhythm; also prevent dysrhythmias
2. Available in oral and parenteral (IM, IV) preparations
B. Examples
1. Class IA antidysrhythmics suppress ectopic foci by increasing the refractory period and slowing depolarization: disopyramide phosphate (Norpace), procainamide HCl (Pronestyl), quinidine preparations (quinidine sulfate, quinidine polygalacturonate [Cardioquin])
2. Class IB antidysrhythmics suppress ventricular dysrhythmias by decreasing automaticity and increasing the ventricular electrical stimulation threshold: lidocaine HCl (Xylocaine), mexiletine (Mexitil), tocainide HCl (Tonocard), phenytoin (Dilantin)
3. Class IB antidysrhythmics slow conduction and increase ventricular refractoriness: flecainide (Tambocor)
4. Class II antidysrhythmics, beta blockers (BBs) or beta-adrenergic blockers, decrease heart rate, contractility, and automaticity by blocking beta-adrenergic receptor sites from catecholamines; decrease myocardial workload and oxygen requirements; indicated for tachydysrhythmias,

hypertension, angina: propranolol (Inderal), metoprolol (Lopressor), atenolol (Tenormin), timolol (Blocadren), nadolol (Corgard), sotalol (Betapace), which also has class III actions

5. Class III antidysrhythmics prolong repolarization; amiodarone (Cardarone) and bretylium (Bretylol) for ventricular tachycardia and fibrillation; ibutilide (Corvert) for atrial flutter and fibrillation

6. Class IV antidysrhythmics, calcium channel blockers or calcium antagonists, block calcium influx into muscle cells during depolarization; control atrial dysrhythmias by decreasing cardiac automaticity and impulse conduction; reduce peripheral vascular resistance in treatment of hypertension: diltiazem (Cardizem), nifedipine (Procardia), verapamil (Calan), amlodipine (Norvasc), felodipine (Plendil)

C. Major side effects: hypotension (decreased cardiac output caused by vasodilation); dizziness (hypotension); nausea, vomiting (irritation of gastric mucosa); heart block (direct cardiac toxic effect, cardiac depressant); heart failure (decreased contractility); anticholinergic effect (decreased parasympathetic stimulation); blood dyscrasias (decreased RBCs, WBCs, and platelet synthesis)

D. Toxicity: diarrhea (GI irritation), CNS disturbances (neurotoxicity), sensory disturbances (neurotoxicity)

E. Nursing care
1. Assess vital signs during course of therapy; monitor drug blood levels
2. Use cardiac monitoring during IV administration; ensure follow-up ECGs
3. Use infusion-control device for continuous IV administration
4. Administer oral preparations with meals to reduce GI irritation
5. Use safety precautions (supervise ambulation, side rails up) when CNS effects are manifested
6. Instruct client to notify physician of any side effects (e.g., changes in heart rate or rhythm, fatigue, weight gain, bleeding)
7. Instruct client to change positions slowly; increase fiber and fluid intake to prevent constipation
8. Use caution when administering beta blockers to clients with diabetes (may mask signs of hypoglycemia), bronchospasm, or heart failure

Cardiac Stimulants

A. Description
1. Increase the heart rate
2. Act by either indirect or direct mechanisms affecting the autonomic nervous system
3. Available in parenteral (IM/IV), endotracheal, and intracardiac preparations

B. Examples
1. Atropine sulfate: suppresses parasympathetic nervous system control at SA and AV nodes by reducing vagal stimulation, thus allowing heart rate to increase

2. Epinephrine HCl (Adrenalin): stimulates the rate and force of cardiac contraction via the sympathetic nervous system
3. Isoproterenol HCl (Isuprel): stimulates beta-adrenergic receptors of the sympathetic nervous system, thus increasing heart rate

C. Major side effects: tachycardia (sympathetic stimulation); headache (dilation of cerebral vessels); CNS stimulation (sympathetic stimulation); cardiac dysrhythmias (cardiovascular system stimulation); atropine: anticholinergic effects (dry mouth, blurred vision, urinary retention as a result of decreased parasympathetic stimulation)

D. Nursing care: assess vital signs during course of therapy; use cardiac monitoring during IV administration; ensure follow-up ECGs

Coronary Vasodilators

A. Description
1. Decrease cardiac work and myocardial oxygen requirements by their vasodilatory action to decrease preload and afterload
2. Nitrates act directly at receptors in smooth muscles, causing vasodilation, which decreases the preload, thus decreasing cardiac workload
3. Calcium channel blockers inhibit the influx of the calcium ion across the cell membrane during depolarization of the cardiac and vascular smooth muscle
4. Effective in the treatment of angina pectoris
5. Available in oral, sublingual tablets and spray, sustained-release buccal, topical (including transdermal), and IV preparations

B. Examples
1. Nitrates (sublingual): nitroglycerin, isosorbide dinitrate (Isordil, Sorbitrate)
2. Nitrates (oral): isosorbide dinitrate (Isordil, Sorbitrate)
3. Nitrates (topical)
   a. Nitroglycerin ointment (Nitro-Bid; Nitrol)
   b. Nitroglycerin transdermal (Nitro-Dur; Transderm-Nitro)
4. Nitrates (IV): nitroglycerin (Nitro-Bid IV, Nitrostat IV)
5. Calcium channel blockers: see class IV antidysrhythmics

C. Major side effects: headache (dilation of cerebral vessels); flushing (peripheral vasodilation); orthostatic hypotension (loss of compensatory vasoconstriction with position change); tachycardia (reflex reaction to severe hypotension); dizziness (orthostatic hypotension)

D. Nursing care
1. Assess for hypotension before administering; if present, withhold drug
2. Encourage client to change positions slowly to avoid orthostatic hypotension and to remain seated after taking sublingual nitroglycerin
3. Instruct client to take sublingual nitroglycerin preparations before angina-producing activities; note slight stinging, burning, tingling under the

tongue that indicate potency of drug; avoid placing the drug in heat, light, moisture, or plastic; store in original amber glass container; obtain a new supply every 3 months; take sublingual preparations every 5 minutes, not to exceed 3 in 15 minutes for chest pain; if pain persists, get emergency care
4. Wear clean gloves when administering topical preparation to prevent absorption
5. Use glass container and tubing supplied by manufacturer when administering IV nitroglycerin preparations; standard tubing can absorb nitroglycerin; titrate using an infusion control pump; monitor BP every 5 to 15 minutes
6. Do not confuse with isosorbide, an osmotic diuretic

Antihypertensives
A. Description
1. Actions
a. Promote dilation of peripheral blood vessels, thus decreasing BP, peripheral vascular resistance, and afterload
b. Reduce cardiac contractility
c. Reduce volume
2. Available in oral, parenteral (IM, IV), and transdermal preparations
B. Examples
1. Angiotensin-converting enzyme inhibitors (ACE inhibitors) stop conversion of angiotensin I to II, blocking vasoconstriction and fluid retention from aldosterone secretion: captopril (Capoten), enalapril maleate (Vasotec), benazepril (Lotensin), lisinopril (Prinivil, Zestril), quinipril (Accupril), fosinopril (Monopril)
2. Angiotensin II receptor blockers block angiotensin II from binding to specific vascular smooth muscle and adrenal gland receptor sites; stop vasoconstriction and fluid retention; similar antihypertensive effect to that of ACE inhibitors but are less likely to cause chronic cough: candesartan (Atacand), irbesartan (Avapro), losartan (Cozaar), valsartan (Diovan)
3. Calcium channel blockers (see class IV antidysrhythmics)
4. Diuretics (see Diuretics)
5. Beta blockers (see class II antidysrhythmics)
6. Alpha$_1$ blockers inhibit effects of norepinephrine by blocking the receptors that control vasomotor tone: doxazosin (Cardura), prazosin (Minipres), terazosin (Hytrin)
7. Alpha-beta blockers combine the effects of alpha$_1$ and beta blockers, leading to vasodilation, decreased contractility, and decreased heart rate: labetalol (Normodyne), carvedilol (Coreg)
8. Central alpha$_2$ agonists decrease sympathetic activity from the CNS: clonidine (Catapres), methyldopa (Aldomet)
9. Direct vasodilators relax the smooth muscles of the arterioles, resulting in decreased peripheral vascular resistance: hydralazine (Apresoline),

minoxidil (Loniten), nitroprusside sodium (Nipride, Nitropress), diazoxide (Hyperstat IV)
C. Major side effects
1. Orthostatic hypotension (loss of compensatory vasoconstriction with position change)
2. Dizziness (orthostatic hypotension); drowsiness (cerebral hypoxia)
3. Cardiac rate alteration: bradycardia caused by sympatholytics (decreased sympathetic stimulation to the heart); tachycardia caused by direct relaxers (reflex reaction to severe hypotension)
4. Sexual disturbances (failure of erection or ejaculation caused by loss of vascular tone)
5. Blood dyscrasias (hemolytic anemia, decreased WBCs, decreased platelet synthesis)
6. Beta blockers can cause bronchospasm and mask hypoglycemia
7. ACE inhibitors can cause a dry cough
D. Nursing care
1. Assess vital signs, especially pulse rate; monitor blood pressure in standing and supine positions; maintain systolic pressure above 80 mm Hg
2. Monitor urinary output during initial titration
3. Protect nitroprusside IV solution from light during administration
4. Instruct client to follow a low-sodium diet; eat foods high in B-complex vitamins; change positions slowly; continue to take medication as prescribed because therapy usually is lifelong; report occurrence of any side effects to physician; avoid engaging in hazardous activities when initially prescribed antihypertensives

Diuretics
A. Description
1. Interfere with sodium reabsorption in kidney
2. Increase urine output, which reduces hypervolemia; decrease preload and afterload
3. Available in oral and parenteral preparations
B. Examples
1. Thiazides interfere with sodium ion transport at loop of Henle and inhibit carbonic anhydrase activity at distal tubule sites: chlorothiazide (Diuril); hydrochlorothiazide (HydroDIURIL); metolazone (Zaroxolyn) is a thiazide-like diuretic
2. Potassium-sparers interfere with aldosterone-induced reabsorption of sodium ions at distal nephron sites to increase sodium chloride excretion and decrease potassium ion loss: spironolactone (Aldactone), triamterine (Dyrenium), amiloride (Midamor)
3. Loop diuretics interfere with active transport of sodium ions in loop of Henle and inhibit sodium chloride and water reabsorption at proximal tubule sites; may be given IV: ethacrynic acid (Edecrin), furosemide (Lasix), bumetanide (Bumex), and torsemide (Demadex)
C. Major side effects: GI irritation (local effect); hyponatremia (inhibition of sodium reabsorption at the kidney tubule); orthostatic hypotension

(reduced blood volume); hyperuricemia (partial blockage of uric acid excretion); dehydration (excessive sodium and water loss); hyperglycemia; Lasix: may cause hearing problems when administered rapidly
1. All diuretics except potassium-sparers: hypokalemia (increased potassium excretion); increased urinary excretion of magnesium and zinc
2. Potassium-sparers: hyperkalemia (reabsorption of potassium at the kidney tubule); hypomagnesemia (increased excretion of magnesium at kidney tubule); increased urinary excretion of calcium
3. Furosemide (Lasix) competes with aspirin for renal excretion sites and can cause aspirin toxicity
4. Thiazides and loop diuretics: may cause hyperglycemia in clients with diabetes
D. Nursing care
1. Maintain intake and output; weigh daily (same time, scale, clothing); assess for signs of fluid-electrolyte imbalance
2. Administer the drug in the morning so that the maximal effect occurs during waking hours
3. Monitor pulse rate and BP; instruct client to change position slowly
4. Encourage intake of foods high in calcium, magnesium, zinc, and potassium (except if taking potassium-sparers)
5. Monitor serum electrolytes and serum glucose levels

Medications to Manage Hypotension in Shock
A. Description
1. Constrict peripheral blood vessels and/or increase cardiac output through alpha- and beta-adrenergic stimulation
2. Elevate BP
3. Available in parenteral (IV) preparations
B. Examples: norepinephrine (Levophed), phenylephrine HCl (Neo-Synephrine), dopamine HCl (Depostat), dobutamine HCl (Dobutrex)
C. Major side effects: hypertension (compression of cerebral blood vessels); headache (increase in BP); GI disturbance (autonomic dysfunction)
D. Nursing care
1. Assess vital signs; monitor BP frequently; titrate IV depending on BP readings to prevent hypertension
2. Assess for IV infiltration; may lead to tissue necrosis; use infusion control pump to administer
3. Monitor peripheral circulation and urinary output

Anticoagulants
A. Description
1. Prevent fibrin formation by interfering with the production of various clotting factors in the coagulation process
2. Prevent platelet aggregation and clot extension
3. Used for prevention and treatment of thrombus and embolus
4. Available in oral and parenteral (Sub-Q, IV) preparations; may be given concurrently until oral medication reaches therapeutic level

B. Examples
1. Heparin sodium administered intravenously or subcutaneously
2. Low-molecular-weight heparin administered subcutaneously: enoxaparin (Lovenox), dalteparin (Fragmin)
3. Warfarin sodium (Coumadin) administered orally
4. Antiplatelet drugs administered orally: aspirin (ASA), ticlopidine (Ticlid), clopidogrel (Plavix)
C. Major side effects: fever, chills, bronchospasm (hypersensitivity); skin rash (hypersensitivity); petechiae, bruising, hemorrhage (interference with clotting mechanisms); diarrhea (GI irritation); thrombocytopenia and other blood dyscrasias; tinnitus and hearing loss (aspirin)
D. Nursing care
1. Monitor blood work during course of therapy, especially coagulation studies
   a. Warfarin derivatives: platelets; international normalized ratio (INR), and prothrombin time (PT); therapeutic INR values should be 2.0 to 3.5; a change in drug regimen requires more frequent INRs because many drugs have interactive effects; therapeutic PT value should be 1.5 to 2 times the normal value
   b. Heparin derivatives: activated partial thromboplastin time (aPTT); therapeutic aPTT value should be 1.5 to 2 times the normal value
2. Assess client for signs of bleeding
3. Have appropriate antidote available: vitamin K for warfarin; protamine sulfate for heparin
4. Avoid intramuscular injections and salicylates with the concomitant administrations of anticoagulants to prevent bleeding
5. Instruct client to carry a medical alert card; immediately report to the physician any signs of bleeding or injury; avoid any medications containing aspirin, alcohol, and herbal supplements such as ginseng, green tea, and St. John's wort; avoid cranberry juice when taking warfarin sodium; use an electric razor and soft toothbrush; follow schedule for coagulation studies
6. Administer subcutaneous heparin in the abdomen; do not aspirate or massage the area

Thrombolytics (Fibrinolytics)
A. Description
1. Convert plasminogen to plasmin, which initiates local fibrinolysis
2. Dissolve occluding thrombi
3. Administered intravenously or intraarterially
4. Initially, loading dose is administered concomitantly with heparin
5. Therapy must be instituted within hours of the onset of myocardial infarction, pulmonary embolism, or acute ischemic brain attack
B. Examples: streptokinase (Streptase); tissue plasminogen activator (t-PA) such as alteplase (Activase), retaplase (Retavase)

C. Major side effects: bleeding, especially GI if there is a history of peptic ulcer disease or cerebral if there is a history of uncontrolled hypertension (increased fibrinolytic activity); allergic reactions (introduction of a foreign protein); low-grade fever (resulting from absorption of infarcted tissue); reperfusion dysrhythmias

D. Nursing care
1. Screen clients carefully for contraindications before initiating therapy; observe for signs of bleeding; monitor PTT and fibrinogen concentration; monitor vital signs and neurologic status
2. Assess for signs of allergic reactions such as chills, urticaria, pruritus, rash, and malaise
3. Keep aminocaproic acid (Amicar), a fibrinolysis inhibitor, available
4. Maintain continuous IV infusion of heparin after thrombolytic therapy

Antianemics
A. Description
1. Promote RBC production; effective in the treatment of anemia caused by chronic kidney disease or chemotherapy, iron deficiency anemia, and nutritional anemias
2. Include colony-stimulating factors that stimulate red blood cell production; iron-containing compounds and vitamin replacements needed for the formation of RBCs
3. Available in oral and parenteral (IM, IV, Sub-Q) preparations

B. Examples
1. Colony-stimulating factors: epoetin (Epogen, Procrit) administered subcutaneously or intravenously three times a week
2. Iron compounds (oral): ferrous gluconate, ferrous sulfate; iron compounds (parenteral): iron dextran (Imferon)
3. Vitamin replacements: cyanocobalamin—vitamin B_{12}, folic acid—vitamin B_9 (Folvite)

C. Major side effects
1. Epoetin: seizures, hypertension, thrombotic events
2. Iron replacements: nausea, vomiting (irritation of gastric mucosa); constipation (delayed passage of iron and stool); black stools (presence of unabsorbed iron in stool); stained teeth (liquid preparations that come into contact with enamel); tissue staining (injectable preparations that leak iron into tissue)
3. Vitamin replacements: local irritation (local tissue effect); allergic reactions, anaphylaxis (hypersensitivity); diarrhea (GI irritation)

D. Nursing care
1. Epoetin
   a. Monitor BP, hematocrit, patency of dialysis shunt if present
   b. Start seizure precautions if precipitous rise in hematocrit level
   c. Do not shake vial; may inactivate drug

2. Iron replacements
   a. Inform client about side effects of therapy
   b. Administer vitamin B_{12} intramuscular injection using Z-track method; administer liquid preparations diluted with water or fruit juice through a straw on an empty stomach, if possible, for optimum absorption; ascorbic acid (vitamin C) increases absorption; encourage oral hygiene
   c. Encourage intake of foods high in iron, vitamin B_{12}, and folic acid; increase high-fiber foods to reduce the potential of constipation
   d. Deferoxamine mesylate (Desferal) is the antidote for iron toxicity

3. Vitamin replacements
   a. Vitamin B_{12}: inform client that this drug cannot be administered orally; therapy is lifelong in pernicious anemia
   b. Folic acid: instruct client about dietary sources of folic acid (fresh fruits, vegetables, and meats)

Antilipidemics
A. Description
1. Improve lipid profile by reducing cholesterol or triglyceride synthesis and/or increasing high-density lipoprotein (HDL) level
2. Used to attain recommended goals for low-density lipoprotein (LDL) levels established by the National Cholesterol Education Program's (NCEP) Adult Treatment Panel (ATP)
   a. Very-high-risk clients: less than 70 mg/dL
   b. High-risk clients: less than 100 mg/dL
   c. Moderately high-risk clients: less than 130 mg/dL with option to set lower goal of less than 100 mg/dL

B. Examples
1. HMG-CoA reductase inhibitors (statins) lower levels of total cholesterol, LDL, and triglycerides; increase HDL levels: pravastatin (Pravachol), lovastatin (Mevacor), simvastatin (Zocor); fluvastatin (Lescol), atorvastatin (Lipitor)
2. Fibrates decrease levels of total cholesterol, LDL, and triglycerides: gemfibrozil (Lopid), clofibrate (Atromid-S), fenofibrate (Tricor)
3. Bile acid sequestrants bind with intestinal bile, preventing absorption and lowering LDL and total cholesterol levels: cholestyramine (Questran), colestipol (Colestid)
4. Nicotinic acid reduces levels of total cholesterol, triglycerides, and LDL; increases HDL levels

C. Major side effects
1. Nausea, vomiting, diarrhea (GI irritation)
2. Musculoskeletal disturbances (direct musculoskeletal tissue effect)
3. Hepatic disturbances (hepatic toxicity)
4. Statins: rhabdomyolysis (potentially fatal skeletal muscle disease)
5. Bile acid sequestrants: constipation
6. Nicotinic acid: facial flushing
7. Reduced absorption of fat and fat-soluble vitamins (A, D, E, K) as well as vitamin B_{12} and iron

D. Nursing care
   1. Encourage adherence to dietary program
      a. Low cholesterol, low fat (especially saturated)
      b. Replace vegetable oils high in polyunsaturated fatty acid with those high in monounsaturated fatty acid, such as olive, avocado
      c. Eat fish high in omega-3 fatty acids several times per week (salmon, tuna)
      d. Increase intake of high-fiber foods, such as fruits, vegetables, cereal grains, and legumes; soluble fiber is particularly effective in reducing blood lipid levels (oat bran, legumes)
   2. Administer statins at hour of sleep to enhance effectiveness; administer other medications with meals to reduce GI irritation
   3. Monitor liver function tests and serum cholesterol, LDL, HDL, triglyceride, hemoglobin, RBC, and fat-soluble vitamin levels
   4. Cholestyramine: mix with full glass of liquid
   5. Lovastatin and gemfibrozil: assess for visual disturbances with prolonged use
   6. Statins: instruct client to report muscle pain, fever, dark urine; may be signs of rhabdomyolysis; monitor creatine kinase (CK) level

Phosphodiesterase Inhibitors
A. Description
   1. Inhibit cyclic adenosine monophosphate phosphodiesterase, leading to increased levels of adenosine monophosphate within the cells
   2. Increase cardiac contractility (inotropic effect) and cardiac output
   3. Cause vasodilation, decreasing peripheral vascular resistance, preload, and afterload
   4. Used for short-term treatment of heart failure; administered intravenously
B. Examples: inamrinone lactate (Inocor), milrinone lactate (Primacor)
C. Major side effects: hypotension, dysrhythmias, nephrogenic diabetes insipidus, hepatotoxicity, anorexia, abdominal cramps, thrombocytopenia
D. Nursing care
   1. Monitor for therapeutic effects: decreased pulmonary capillary wedge pressure (PCWP), resolution of clinical indicators of heart failure (daily weights, intake and output, breath sounds)
   2. Monitor BP and cardiac rhythm
   3. Use infusion control pump to administer; consult with physician for titration based on clinical indicators
   4. Monitor potassium levels, which may be low secondary to diuresis; administer supplements as needed

◼ RELATED PROCEDURES
Angiography (Arteriogram)
A. Definition: an x-ray examination using contrast agent to visualize patency of arteries; angiography may also be done using CT with contrast or MRI

B. Nursing care
   1. Screen client for iodine or shellfish allergy and adequate kidney function to excrete dye
   2. Inform the client of risks (allergic reaction, bleeding, embolus, cardiac dysrhythmia) and to expect sensation of warmth as contrast agent is injected
   3. Administer ordered sedative before procedure
   4. Monitor for indicators of an allergic response such as dyspnea and diaphoresis; be prepared to administer steroids, antihistamines, and epinephrine
   5. Postprocedure care: check injection site for bleeding and inflammation; maintain pressure over insertion site; assess circulatory status of extremities; maintain bed rest; provide hydration; monitor urinary output

Angioplasty
A. Definition
   1. Percutaneous transluminal coronary angioplasty (PTCA) is the introduction of a balloon-tipped catheter into the coronary artery to the stenosis to reduce or eliminate the occlusion by the atheroma (plaque)
      a. Performed via coronary catheterization; heparin infusion is used to prevent thrombus formation
      b. Thrombolytic therapy may be combined with PTCA in some situations
      c. Stents, mesh structural supports, may be inserted fo maintain patency; use of stents requires long-term anticoagulation therapy
      d. If lesions are calcified and cannot be removed by PTCA, an atherectomy may be performed, which mechanically removes the plaque by shaving and retrieving it from the vessel's lumen
      e. Complications include arterial spasm or perforation and thrombus formation; emergency open heart surgery may be necessary; vessel occlusion may occur as a result of the cellular response to the procedure
   2. Percutaneous transluminal angioplasty (PTA) is used to dilate stenotic vessels by stretching the artery wall away from the plaque; used in aorta, iliac, femoral, popliteal, tibial, renal vessels, and arteriovenous dialysis shunts; stent placement generally follows procedure
B. Nursing care: see care for Cardiac Catheterization; administer vasoactive drugs such as calcium channel blockers and nitroglycerin before, during, and after this procedure as ordered; monitor client for angina, dysrhythmias, bleeding, and evidence of restenosis and reocclusion

Blood Transfusion
A. Purpose: restore blood volume after hemorrhage; maintain hemoglobin levels in cases of severe anemia; replace specific blood components

B. Sources of blood for transfusions
   1. Homologous: random collection of blood by volunteer donors
   2. Autologous: donation of a client's own blood before hospitalization; possible when donor's hemoglobin remains higher than 11 g/dL; donations can be saved for 5 weeks
   3. Directed donation: donation of blood by a donor specifically for a client
   4. Blood salvage: a method by which a client's blood is suctioned from a closed body cavity (operative site, trauma site, joint) into a cell-saver machine and processed to be transfused; must be used within 6 hours of collection; contain high levels of potassium
C. Blood components and use
   1. Whole blood: volume replacement for blood loss
   2. Packed RBCs: increase RBC mass
   3. Platelets: increase platelets to prevent bleeding from thrombocytopenia
   4. Fresh frozen plasma: contains plasma, antibodies, clotting factors
   5. Cryoprecipitate: contains factor VIII, fibrinogen, and factor XIII to treat hemophilia
   6. Albumin: volume expander to treat hypoproteinemia
   7. Plasma protein factor: to treat some types of hemophilia
   8. IV gamma globulin: contains IgG antibodies to treat immunodeficiency
D. Nursing care
   1. Obtain and document informed consent
   2. Check that blood or blood components have been typed and cross-matched for compatibility; follow agency policy; two nurses should verify the blood type, Rh factor, client identification and blood numbers, and expiration date
   3. Blood must be hung within 30 minutes of arriving on the unit
   4. Obtain baseline vital signs before administration and monitor them every 5 minutes for 15 minutes and then every 15 minutes during the transfusion
   5. An IV with normal saline infusing through a large-bore Angiocath and a blood administration set containing a filter are used to start the infusion; solutions containing glucose should not be used
   6. Maintain standard precautions when handling blood or IV equipment; assure client that the risk for AIDS is minimal because blood is screened
   7. Invert the container gently to suspend the RBCs within the plasma
   8. Administer at appropriate rate
      a. Platelets, plasma, and cryoprecipitate may be infused rapidly; assess for signs of circulatory overload
      b. Blood transfusions should be completed within 4 hours because potential for bacterial contamination increases over time
      c. Administer slowly for first 10 to 15 minutes to detect transfusion reaction

9. Observe for signs of hemolytic reaction, which generally occur within the first 10 to 15 minutes: shivering; headache; lower back pain as a result of hemoglobin from ruptured erythrocytes blocking kidney tubules; increased pulse rate and respiratory rate; hemoglobinuria; oliguria; hypotension
10. Infuse by gravity or with a controller; ensure that controller will not cause hemolysis of RBCs
11. Observe for signs of febrile reaction, which usually occur within 30 minutes: shaking; headache; elevated temperature; back pain; confusion; hematemesis
12. Observe for allergic reaction: hives; wheezing; pruritus; joint pain
13. If any reaction occurs: stop infusion immediately and replace IV tubing containing blood; maintain patency of the IV with normal saline; send blood to the laboratory; monitor vital signs and I&O frequently; send a urine specimen to the laboratory if a hemolytic reaction is suspected; evaluate hemoglobin and hematocrit, monitor urine output; notify the physician

Bone Marrow Aspiration

A. Definition: puncture to collect tissue from the bone marrow of the sternum or iliac crest; performed to study the cells involved in blood production
B. Nursing care: allay anxiety of the client; pain is brief, only occurs during aspiration (conscious sedation may be used); position the client to expose site; apply pressure for several minutes; monitor for bleeding or infection

Cardiac Catheterization

A. Definition: introduction of a catheter into the heart via a peripheral vessel
   1. Injection of contrast material to visualize chambers, coronary circulation, and great vessels
   2. Withdrawal of blood samples to evaluate cardiac function
   3. Measurement of pressures within chambers and blood vessels (e.g., pulmonary wedge pressure)
B. Nursing care
   1. Inform client of procedure's purpose, its possible complications (e.g., hemorrhage, myocardial infarction, brain attack), and sensations it causes (e.g., urge to cough, nausea, heat); allow time for verbalization of fears
   2. Identify allergies to iodine and adequate kidney function
   3. Keep NPO for 8 to 12 hours before the procedure; administer sedatives as ordered before the procedure
   4. After catheterization: monitor vital signs frequently; cardiac dysrhythmias are more common during the procedure but may occur afterward; assess the puncture site for bleeding (sandbags or ice packs may be ordered if the femoral artery is used); assess the involved extremity for signs of ischemia (e.g., absence of peripheral pulses, changes in sensation, color, and temperature); maintain bed

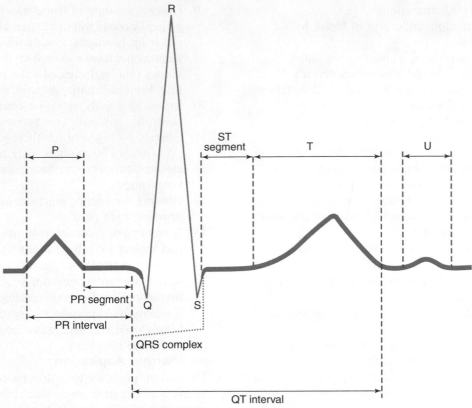

Figure 6-4 Events of the cardiac cycle. (From Ignatavicius DD, Workman ML: *Medical-surgical nursing: critical thinking for collaborative care*, ed 5, St Louis, 2006, Saunders.)

rest for the prescribed number of hours; increase fluids to eliminate dye; keep client in supine position and prevent hip flexion

Cardiac Monitoring

(Figure 6-4: Events of the cardiac cycle)
A. Definition
1. Electric observation of the conductivity patterns of the heart by the use of skin electrodes and a monitoring device; the heart's electric activity is conducted to the surface of the skin by the ionized fluids bathing the cells and tissues
2. Used when danger of dysrhythmias is apparent (e.g., heart disease, surgery, invasive procedures)
3. Conduction from the SA node through the atria causes atrial contraction and gives rise to the P wave; conduction from the AV node down the bundle of His to Purkinje's fibers, which extend to the lateral walls of the ventricles, causes ventricular contraction, which gives rise to the QRS wave; ventricular repolarization is associated with the T wave; late ventricular repolarization is associated with the U wave
4. Holter monitor allows cardiac tracings to be recorded on an ambulatory basis to assess for dysrhythmias
5. Stress test assesses cardiac conduction and function after being stressed (treadmill or bicycle exercise, stimulatory medication)

B. Nursing care
1. Explain the procedure to client and attempt to allay anxiety
2. Prepare the skin on the chest for electrode attachment; cleanse area with alcohol to remove dirt and oils; shave area if necessary
3. Place electrodes on the skin and attach to the monitor cable as indicated: RA (attach to right upper arm or chest); LA (attach to left upper arm or chest); RL (attach to right leg or lower chest [ground]); LL (attach to left leg or lower chest); turn on the monitor scope and set the sensitivity when a clear picture is obtained; set the alarm and readout attachment (if available) so that a record will be made if there is a change in cardiac activity
4. Observe the monitor for signs of normal sinus rhythm: ventricular and atrial rate of 60 to 100 beats/min; regular rhythm; a P wave (representing atrial depolarization) precedes each QRS complex (representing ventricular depolarization); PR interval (representing conduction of an impulse from the SA node through the AV node) is 0.12 to 0.20 second; T wave after each QRS complex (representing repolarization of the ventricles)
5. Intervene immediately when life-threatening dysrhythmias occur; brain damage will occur if client is anoxic for more than 4 minutes

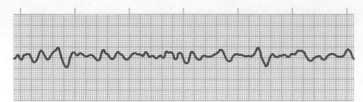

Figure 6-5 Ventricular fibrillation. (From Monahan FD et al: *Phipps' medical-surgical nursing: health and illness perspectives*, ed 8, St Louis, 2007, Mosby.)

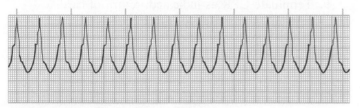

Figure 6-6 Ventricular tachycardia. (From Monahan FD et al: *Phipps' medical-surgical nursing: health and illness perspectives*, ed 8, St Louis, 2007, Mosby.)

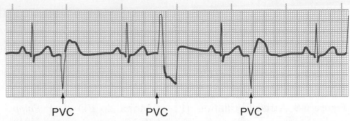

PVC   PVC   PVC

Figure 6-7 Premature ventricular complexes: normal sinus rhythm with multifocal PVCs. (From Monahan FD et al: *Phipps' medical-surgical nursing: health and illness perspectives*, ed 8, St Louis, 2007, Mosby.)

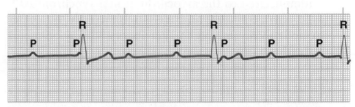

Figure 6-8 Third-degree heart block. (From Monahan FD et al: *Phipps' medical-surgical nursing: health and illness perspectives*, ed 8, St Louis, 2007, Mosby.)

a. Ventricular fibrillation (Figure 6-5: Ventricular fibrillation)
   (1) Repetitive rapid stimulation from ectopic ventricular foci to which the ventricles are unable to respond; ventricular contraction is replaced by uncoordinated twitching; circulation ceases and death ensues
   (2) Defibrillate immediately; inject medications per protocol; institute CPR; document the dysrhythmia and notify the physician
b. Ventricular tachycardia (Figure 6-6: Ventricular tachycardia)
   (1) Series of three or more bizarre premature ventricular complexes that occur in a regular rhythm; this electric activity results in decreased cardiac output and may rapidly convert to ventricular fibrillation
   (2) Administer medications per protocol; administer cardioversion if medications fail; be prepared to administer defibrillation and cardiopulmonary resuscitation; document the dysrhythmia and notify the physician; prepare for possible implantable cardioverter defibrillator (ICD) insertion; monitor vital signs, oxygen saturation, and potassium levels
c. Premature ventricular complexes or beats (Figure 6-7: Premature ventricular complexes)
   (1) Originate in the ventricles and occur before the next expected sinus beat; they can be life-threatening when they occur close to the T wave because cardiac repolarization is disrupted and ventricular fibrillation may ensue
   (2) Administer medications per protocol; document the dysrhythmia and notify the physician; institute oral antidysrhythmics as ordered; monitor vital signs, oxygen saturation, and potassium levels

d. Third-degree atrioventricular block (complete heart block) (Figure 6-8: Third-degree heart block)
   (1) Occurs when there is no electric communication between the atria and ventricles and each beats independently; this activity will not provide long-term adequate circulation, and syncope, heart failure, or cardiac arrest may ensue
   (2) Document the dysrhythmia and notify the physician; administer medications per protocol; prepare for pacemaker insertion (see Cardiac Pacemaker Insertion procedure)
e. Cardiac standstill (asystole)
   (1) Occurs when there is no cardiac activity (flat line on ECG tracing); this terminates in death unless intervention is begun immediately
   (2) Institute cardiopulmonary resuscitation; document the dysrhythmia and notify the physician; cardiac stimulants may be given via IV or intracardiac route; pacemaker insertion may be indicated (see Cardiac Pacemaker Insertion procedure)
f. Atrial fibrillation (Figure 6-9: Atrial fibrillation)
   (1) Results from rapid firing of atrial ectopic foci, between 400 and 700/min; ECG shows no P waves, rather irregular forms; pulse deficit is common; danger from blood pooling in quivering atria leads to emboli
   (2) Administer antidysrhythmics as ordered; anticoagulant may reduce incidence of brain attack until rhythm is controlled; prepare for cardioversion
   (3) Monitor vital signs, O_2 saturation, and potassium levels

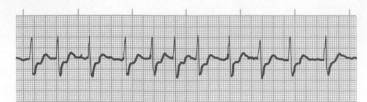

Figure 6-9 Atrial fibrillation. (From Monahan FD et al: *Phipps' medical-surgical nursing: health and illness perspectives*, ed 8, St Louis, 2007, Mosby.)

Cardioversion

A. Definition: elective procedure during which current is administered to the myocardium in a synchronized fashion to depolarize all cells simultaneously, allowing SA node to resume pacemaker function; may be useful in treating tachydysrhythmias, atrial fibrillation, supraventricular tachycardia, and ventricular tachycardia

B. Nursing care
1. Obtain informed consent
2. Maintain NPO, verify patent IV line, administer oxygen, and have suction available
3. Ensure that no one is touching the bed/client when shock is delivered
4. Monitor cardiac status for dysrhythmias for several hours after procedure

Basic Life Support (Cardiopulmonary Resuscitation, CPR) by Health Care Providers

A. Definition: institution of artificial ventilation and circulation with rescue breathing and external cardiac compression

B. Nursing care
1. Assess level of consciousness if found unconscious: shake victim's shoulder and shout, "Are you OK?"; if no response, call for help or activate the EMS system and obtain automated external defibrillator (AED) if available
2. Assess and establish an airway (in less than 10 seconds): use head tilt–chin lift maneuver (jaw thrust without hyperextension of the neck if cervical injury is suspected); determine whether air is being exchanged by looking to see whether the chest is moving, listening for whether air can be heard escaping during exhalation, and feeling whether air can be felt escaping during exhalation
3. Initiate rescue breathing: maintain the head-tilt or jaw-thrust maneuver and pinch the victim's nostrils; give two breaths (each over 1 second); use pocket mask or bag mask if available
4. Assess circulation; take no more than 10 seconds to palpate carotid pulse
5. Deliver external cardiac compressions: ensure that the victim is on a firm surface and in the supine position; place heel of hand over lower half of body of sternum between the nipples, interlock hands, and compress the chest 3.8 to 5 cm (1½ to 2 inches) for an adult

6. Maintain the ventilation/compression ratio: one or two rescuers—2 breaths after every 30 compressions (rate of 100/min); reassess carotid pulse after first five cycles and then every few minutes
7. Defibrillate using AED; part of basic life support (BLS) for health care providers
8. Place client in recovery position if pulse and respirations resume; continue to monitor breathing regularly
9. Terminate CPR as indicated: return of cardiac rhythm and spontaneous respirations; rescuer exhaustion; physician-ordered cessation

Cardiac Pacemaker Insertion

A. Definition: artificial pacemakers replace natural electric stimulation of the heart (SA node) and are indicated in the treatment of the following conditions
1. Third-degree atrioventricular block: impulses from SA node do not stimulate ventricles; atria and ventricles beat independently; slow ventricular rate causes signs and symptoms
2. Second-degree atrioventricular block: intermittent failure of impulse to reach the ventricles
3. Adams-Stokes syndrome: a sudden drop in ventricular rate that causes syncope and temporary loss of consciousness

B. Pacemakers: involve the insertion of an electrode catheter into the heart, which transmits impulses generated by the pacing unit
1. May be temporary and worn externally or may be permanent and surgically placed under the skin
2. On-demand pacing: pacemaker stimulates the heart to contract only if the client's ventricular rate falls below a preset rate; most frequently used
3. Fixed (asynchronous) pacing: pacemaker is set at a constant rate independent of client's intrinsic rhythm
4. Number of leads and parts of the heart stimulated depend on the client's status and needs
5. Universal code using letters indicates details about pacemaker: chambers being paced; chambers being sensed; pacemaker response to sensing; programmability; antitachycardia/defibrillation capability

C. Nursing care
1. Observe the cardiac monitor before, during, and after the procedure to verify pacemaker capture (QRS following pacemaker spike) and observe for dysrhythmias; note stimulation threshold; have emergency medications (e.g., lidocaine, atropine sulfate) available, as well as a defibrillator; ensure electrical equipment is grounded; monitor incision for hematoma and infection
2. Teach the client how to measure pulse rate, to keep a diary of pulse rates, to notify the physician immediately if the rate falls below that set on the pacemaker, and to remain under a physician's

supervision because batteries must be replaced periodically; pacemaker function may be checked by special telephone devices

3. Encourage the client to wear a Medic-Alert bracelet or carry a medical alert card
4. Teach client to avoid high-magnetic fields such as high-tension wires, hand-held screening devices, and MRI; the pacemaker may trigger airport or store alarms, but these will not affect the pacemaker

Nuclear Medicine Procedures

A. Multiple-gated angiographic radioisotope (MUGA) scan or equilibrium radionuclide angiocardiography (ERNA)
   1. Noninvasive test using computer and scintillation camera to study ventricular wall motion
   2. Volume of blood pumped during one ventricular contraction is compared with the total volume in the left ventricle, which yields an ejection fraction
   3. The ejection fraction gives important information on ventricular size and wall motion abnormalities
B. Myocardial perfusion imaging
   1. Intravenous injection of a radioisotope such as thallium or technetium-99m (TC-99m), which is taken up by the heart muscle
   2. Damaged myocardial tissue absorbs the isotope more slowly and retains it for a longer period
   3. The isotope can be injected during and after exercise to determine myocardial perfusion
C. Positron emission tomography (PET) scan
   1. A positron-emitting isotope is administered intravenously to study patency of vessels
   2. Provides detailed information about cardiac circulation
   3. Clients should be encouraged to drink fluids after the test to facilitate excretion of the isotope
D. Magnetic resonance imaging (MRI)
   1. Use of powerful magnetic field and computer to generate images of the heart and large blood vessels
   2. Noninvasive and painless; clients with claustrophobia may require sedation for traditional closed MRIs
   3. Contraindicated for clients with pacemaker or metal implants
   4. All jewelry and transdermal patches that contain an aluminized layer must be removed
   5. Clients should be instructed to lie still and to expect an intermittent thumping sound
E. Nursing care
   1. Review client's medications because some may affect results (e.g., beta blockers)
   2. Monitor client's vital signs before and after test
   3. Determine history of allergies and notify radiologist before test
   4. Offer emotional support to client, who may be apprehensive about test and results; allay client's fears about the use of radioactive substances

Hemodynamic Monitoring With Pulmonary Artery Catheter

A. Definition: catheter used to measure pulmonary capillary wedge pressure (PCWP), pulmonary artery pressure (PAP), and right atrial pressure (central venous pressure)
   1. The double- or triple-lumen catheter with a balloon tip is inserted into a vein and advanced through the superior vena cava into the right atrium and ventricle, then into the pulmonary artery; the catheter is guided further until, when the balloon is inflated, it is wedged in the distal arterial branch
   2. This catheter yields information on the client's circulatory status, left ventricular pumping action, filling pressures, and vascular tone
B. Nursing care
   1. Assist physician with catheter insertion into jugular or subclavian vein using sterile technique; obtain chest x-ray to check for placement and complication of pneumothorax
   2. Observe the insertion site for inflammation
   3. Observe the line for patency and air bubbles
   4. Take readings with client in supine position if possible with transducer at the level of the client's phlebostatic axis (intersection of horizontal line extending from the sternal border of the fourth intercostal space and midaxillary line)
   5. Provide site care; flush unused ports as per policy
   6. Notify the physician if the waveform changes or pressure readings are altered
   7. Ensure that balloon does not remain inflated after wedge pressure determination
   8. Normal readings
      a. Pulmonary capillary wedge pressure: 5 to 13 mm Hg
      b. Pulmonary artery pressure: systolic—16 to 30 mm Hg; diastolic—0 to 7 mm Hg; mean—15 mm Hg
      c. Right atrial pressure: 2 to 6 mm Hg; less than 2 mm Hg suggests low blood volume; greater than 6 mm Hg suggests fluid overload
   9. Keep emergency medications and a defibrillator available

MAJOR DISORDERS OF THE CIRCULATORY SYSTEM (CARDIOVASCULAR, BLOOD, AND LYMPHATIC SYSTEMS)

✦ HYPERTENSION

Data Base

A. Etiology and pathophysiology
   1. Etiology is complex; begins insidiously; changes in arteriolar bed cause increased resistance; increased blood volume may result from hormonal or renal

dysfunction; arteriolar thickening causes increased peripheral vascular resistance; abnormal renin release constricts arterioles
   a. 90% to 95% have an unidentifiable cause (primary hypertension); multiple factors such as the renin-angiotensin-aldosterone mechanism, sympathetic nervous system activity, and insulin resistance may be involved
   b. 5% to 10% have identifiable causes (secondary hypertension), and the pathophysiology is related to the condition causing the rise in pressure; conditions include renovascular disease; primary hyperaldosteronism; Cushing's syndrome; diabetes mellitus; neurologic disorders; dysfunction of thyroid, pituitary, or parathyroid glands; coarctation of the aorta; and pregnancy
2. Risk factors
   a. Stress
   b. Abdominal obesity (apple-shaped body)
   c. Diet (high sodium, low calcium, low magnesium, and low potassium)
   d. Substance abuse (cigarettes, alcohol, cocaine)
   e. Family history
   f. Age
   g. Sedentary lifestyle
   h. Hyperlipidemia (increased LDL and cholesterol levels, decreased HDL level)
   i. African-American heritage
   j. Diabetes mellitus
   k. Renal disease
3. Often asymptomatic; diagnosis requires three assessments of elevated BP on separate occasions
4. Classification of BP
   a. Normal: systolic less than 120 mm Hg and diastolic less than 80 mm Hg
   b. Prehypertension: systolic 120 to 139 mm Hg or diastolic 80 to 89 mm Hg
   c. Stage 1 hypertension: systolic 140 to 159 mm Hg or diastolic 90 to 99 mm Hg
   d. Stage 2 hypertension: systolic greater than 160 mm Hg or diastolic greater than 100 mm Hg
5. Hypertension increases the risk for coronary artery disease, heart failure, myocardial infarction, brain attacks (cerebral vascular accidents [CVAs]), retinopathy, and nephropathy
B. Clinical findings
   1. Subjective: headache (occipital area); light-headedness; tinnitus; easy fatigue; visual disturbances; palpitations
   2. Objective: BP greater than 140/90 mm Hg obtained on three separate occasions; retinal changes; renal pathology (e.g., azotemia); epistaxis; cardiac hypertrophy
C. Therapeutic interventions
   1. Lifestyle modifications recommended by the Joint National Committee on Prevention, Detection,

Evaluation, and Treatment of High Blood Pressure (JNC 7)
   a. Weight control or reduction to attain a body mass index of 18.5 to 24.9 kg/m^2
   b. Dietary Approaches to Stop Hypertension (DASH) eating plan: increased fruits, vegetables, and low-fat dairy products that are rich in calcium and potassium
   c. Sodium restriction (less than 2.4 g daily)
   d. Aerobic exercise at least 30 minutes on most days
   e. Alcohol moderation (no more than 1 drink daily for women, 2 for men)
2. Drug therapy recommended by JNC 7
   a. Prehypertension: only for compelling indications
   b. Stage 1 hypertension: thiazide diuretics for most; may consider angiotensin-converting enzyme inhibitors (ACEIs), ARBs, CCBs, BBs
   c. Stage 2 hypertension: second drug added to thiazide diuretic for most
3. Other interventions: smoking cessation, relaxation modalities such as biofeedback and imagery; antianxiety agent

Nursing Care of Clients With Hypertension
A. Assessment/Analysis
   1. Vital signs with client in both upright and recumbent positions; use proper size BP cuff (width should be 40% of the arm's circumference); avoid errors of parallax when reading sphygmomanometer
   2. Baseline weight
   3. Presence of risk factors and clinical evidence of target organ damage
B. Planning/Implementation
   1. Monitor levels of electrolytes, blood urea nitrogen (BUN), creatinine, lipid profile, and urine for protein
   2. Encourage weight reduction if indicated; weigh daily when there is a threat of heart failure to monitor fluid balance
   3. Teach client to monitor own BP; a BP of 180/120 mm Hg or higher represents a hypertensive emergency; advise client to change position slowly and avoid hot showers to prevent orthostatic hypotension
   4. Support expression of emotions; encourage relaxation techniques
   5. Reinforce that hypertension is not cured, but controlled
   6. Educate the client and family regarding drugs (see Antihypertensives under Related Pharmacology), follow-up care, activity restrictions, smoking cessation, limiting alcohol intake, and diet; note that many salt substitutes contain potassium chloride rather than sodium chloride and may be permitted by the physician if the client has no renal impairment; caution about use of NSAIDs, which can cause hypertension

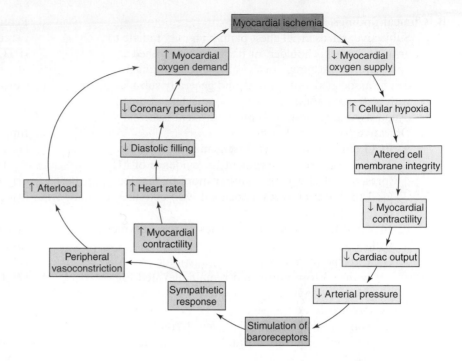

Figure 6-10 Effects of prolonged myocardial ischemia. (From Monahan FD et al: *Phipps' medical-surgical nursing: health and illness perspectives*, ed 8, St Louis, 2007, Mosby.)

C. Evaluation/Outcomes
1. Maintains blood pressure at an acceptable level
2. Understands and adheres to therapeutic regimen
3. Verbalizes need for stress reduction

 CORONARY ARTERY DISEASE (CAD): ISCHEMIC HEART DISEASE (IHD), CORONARY HEART DISEASE (CHD), ATHEROSCLEROSIS, ANGINA PECTORIS, MYOCARDIAL INFARCTION (MI)

Data Base
A. Etiology and pathophysiology
1. Atherosclerosis: deposition of fatty plaques along inner wall of coronary arteries leads to inflammation; macrophages infiltrate the endothelium, causing further damage and the development of atheromas (fibrous caps over fatty deposits); narrowing and possible obstruction occur; also affects peripheral and cerebral vessels
2. Angina pectoris: episodic pain experienced when O_2 supplied by the blood cannot meet the metabolic demands of the muscle. In addition to atherosclerosis, this temporary ischemia may be precipitated by coronary artery spasms, strenuous exercise, heavy meals, hyperthyroidism, exposure to cold, and emotional stress; classified as stable, unstable (preinfarction), intractable, variant (Prinzmetal)
3. Myocardial infarction (MI): acute necrosis of the heart muscle caused by interruption of oxygen supply to the area (ischemia), resulting in altered function and reduced cardiac output

(Figure 6-10: Effects of prolonged myocardial ischemia)
4. Risk factors
   a. Family history
   b. Increasing age
   c. Gender: men; women, especially after menopause (estrogen seems to provide some degree of protection)
   d. Race: risk appears higher in African-Americans
   e. Cigarette smoking (contributes to vasoconstriction, platelet activation, arterial smooth muscle cell proliferation, and reduced oxygen availability)
   f. Hypertension; widened QRS complex (bundle branch block)
   g. Hyperlipidemia: increased total cholesterol; increased LDL; increased ratio of total cholesterol or LDL to HDL; HDL; HDL seems to protect against coronary artery disease (CAD); increased triglycerides
   h. Obesity (particularly abdominal obesity)
   i. Sedentary lifestyle (contributes to obesity and reduced HDL)
   j. Diabetes mellitus, particularly in women
   k. Stress (an innate competitive, aggressive type A personality seems less important than amount of stress and client's psychologic response)
   l. Metabolic syndrome: a cluster of signs including hyperlipidemia, low HDL level, abdominal obesity, increased BP, insulin resistance, increased levels of C-reactive protein, and increased fibrinogen level

B. Clinical findings
  1. Subjective: retrosternal chest pain; pain may radiate to arms, jaw, neck, shoulder, or back; pain described as "pressure," "crushing," or "viselike"; pain of angina can be associated with activity and generally subsides with rest; palpitations; apprehension, feeling of dread; dyspnea; nausea; asymptomatic with silent ischemia
  2. Objective
    a. ECG changes may reveal ischemia (inverted T wave, elevated ST segment) or evidence of MI (presence of Q wave); a Holter monitor may be used to detect changes associated with activities of daily living (ADLs)
    b. Elevated levels of serum enzymes and isoenzymes with MI
      (1) Cardiac troponin T (cTnT) levels increase within 3 to 6 hours and remain elevated for 14 to 21 days; very accurate for assessing myocardial damage
      (2) Cardiac troponin I (cTnI) levels rise 7 to 14 hours after an MI and remain elevated for 5 to 7 days; highly specific for myocardial damage
      (3) Creatinine kinase (CK) levels elevate 3 to 6 hours after infarction, peaking at 24 hours, and returning to normal within 72 hours
      (4) CK-MB levels elevate 4 to 6 hours after pain, peaking within 24 hours, and returning to normal within 72 hours; specific for myocardial damage
      (5) Myoglobin levels elevate in 1 to 3 hours; returning to normal within 12 hours
    c. C-reactive protein (CRP): elevation suggests inflammation of the vascular endothelium and coronary artery calcification
    d. Doppler flow studies
    e. Cardiac nuclear scanning (thallium, MUGA) or echocardiographic studies can help determine extent of vessels involved
    f. Sympathetic nervous system responses: pallor, rapid pulse rate, diaphoresis, vomiting
    g. Signs associated with MI: dysrhythmia, elevated temperature, elevated sedimentation rate, and increased WBCs
C. Therapeutic interventions
  1. Prevention of MI
    a. Supervised exercise program to avoid ischemia but promote collateral circulation and increase HDL; weight control; smoking cessation; dietary restriction of sodium, cholesterol, and total and saturated fat; management of hypertension, hyperlipidemia, and diabetes
    b. Pharmacologic management: nitrates, beta-blocking agents, calcium channel blocking agents, antilipidemics, antiplatelet agents, ACE inhibitors (see Related Pharmacology)
    c. Supplemental O_2 during anginal attack as needed

    d. Percutaneous coronary interventions such as percutaneous transluminal coronary angioplasty (PTCA), coronary artery stent placement, and atherectomy to revascularize myocardium
    e. Coronary artery bypass graft (CABG) if medical regimen not successful
  2. Management of acute MI
    a. Improvement of perfusion
      (1) Administer ASA immediately, often on way to hospital
      (2) Begin beta blocker and IV nitroglycerin
      (3) Thrombolytic therapy within 6 hours of MI; anticoagulants
      (4) ACE inhibitors
      (5) Antidysrhythmics to maintain cardiac function
      (6) Percutaneous coronary intervention
      (7) Intraaortic balloon pump that inflates during diastole and deflates during systole to decrease cardiac workload by decreasing afterload and increasing myocardial perfusion for cardiogenic shock
    b. Promotion of comfort and rest
      (1) Administer analgesics such as IV morphine sulfate to reduce pain, anxiety, and cardiac workload by decreasing preload and afterload
      (2) Oxygen administration to improve tissue oxygenation
      (3) Maintain bed or chair rest to decrease oxygen tissue demands
      (4) Diet therapy may be 2-g sodium diet or clear liquids, depending on presence of nausea
    c. Monitoring client
      (1) Pulse oximetry
      (2) Cardiac monitoring for rate, evidence of ischemia, and dysrhythmias
      (3) Vital signs
      (4) Swan-Ganz catheter
    d. Assessment for complications of MI
      (1) Dysrhythmias
      (2) Cardiogenic shock
      (3) Pulmonary edema caused by acute heart failure
      (4) Thromboembolism
      (5) Extension of MI
      (6) Pericardial effusion and cardiac tamponade

Nursing Care of Clients With Coronary Artery Disease

A. Assessment/Analysis
  1. History of chest, arm, shoulder, neck, jaw pain
  2. Precipitating factors (e.g., exercise, cold)
  3. Risk factors (nonmodifiable and modifiable)
  4. Vital signs
  5. Intake and output (fluid volume overload is dangerous if cardiac output is compromised)
  6. Adventitious breath sounds and dependent edema with impending failure
  7. Restlessness, dyspnea

8. Skin: diaphoresis; pallor; cyanosis
9. If MI is suspected, continuous ECG monitoring to detect changes in rate, rhythm, and conduction of heartbeat; life-threatening dysrhythmias (ventricular fibrillation and ventricular standstill); dysrhythmias such as premature ventricular complexes close to a T wave, ventricular tachycardia, torsades de pointes (a ventricular tachycardia with a prolonged QT interval that is linked to rapid deterioration), and atrial fibrillation

B. Planning/Implementation
1. Teach signs and management of cardiac ischemia (rest; nitrates; emergency care if ineffective)
2. Encourage prophylactic administration of nitrates (see Related Pharmacology)
3. Reinforce need to avoid exertion (e.g., shoveling snow) and exposure to cold; however, emphasize the need for regular exercise approved by physician or participation in cardiac rehabilitation program
4. Support involvement in smoking cessation, weight control, and exercise programs
5. Encourage following dietary program
   a. Low cholesterol, low fat (substitute unsaturated fat for saturated fat), low sodium
   b. Replace vegetable oils high in polyunsaturated fatty acids with those high in monounsaturated fatty acids, such as olive oil and avocado oil
   c. Eat fish high in omega-3 fatty acids several times per week (salmon, tuna)
   d. Follow DASH diet; increase intake of high-fiber foods such as fruits, vegetables, cereal grains, and legumes; soluble fiber is particularly effective in reducing blood lipid levels (oat bran, legumes); low-fat dairy
6. Educate client about medications (see Related Pharmacology)
7. Provide emotional support regarding alteration in lifestyle
8. Care of client after acute MI
   a. Document dysrhythmia and respond per protocol: medication, defibrillation, or CPR
   b. Reduce cardiac demand; administer O_2, analgesics, vasodilators, and other medications as ordered
   c. Recognize risk for sensory overload: orient to unit and equipment; allow time to express feelings; encourage short visits by significant others
   d. Use measures to prevent sequelae to diminished activity: thrombophlebitis, pneumonia, constipation, skin breakdown, deconditioning

C. Evaluation/Outcomes
1. Remains free of chest pain
2. Verbalizes a reduced level of anxiety
3. Adheres to prescribed regimen (dietary, pharmacologic, and exercise)
4. Maintains oxygen saturation at 95% on room air

 INFLAMMATORY DISEASE OF THE HEART: PERICARDITIS, MYOCARDITIS, INFECTIVE ENDOCARDITIS

Data Base
A. Etiology and pathophysiology
1. Pericarditis
   a. Acute or chronic inflammation of the pericardium
   b. May be idiopathic or result from the following: bacterial infection (streptococcal, staphylococcal, gonococcal, meningococcal organisms); viral infection (coxsackievirus, influenza); mycotic (fungal) infection; rickettsial and parasitic infestation; trauma; collagen disease; rheumatic fever; neoplastic disease secondary to lung and breast metastasis; post cardiac surgery
   c. Sequelae: loss of pericardial elasticity or an accumulation of fluid within the sac; heart failure or cardiac tamponade
2. Myocarditis
   a. Inflammation of the myocardium
   b. May result from viral, bacterial, mycotic, parasitic, protozoal, or spirochetal infections or infestations; rheumatic fever; endocarditis; impaired immune system
   c. Sequelae: impaired contractility of the heart caused by the inflammatory process; myocardial ischemia and necrosis; heart failure
3. Infective endocarditis
   a. Inflammation of the inner lining of the heart and valves
   b. May result from *Streptococcus viridans*, bacterial, fungal, or rickettsial infections; rheumatic heart disease; presence of invasive lines or prosthetic valves
   c. Sequelae: structural damage to the valves; pump failure; embolization

B. Clinical findings
1. Subjective: precordial or substernal pain; dyspnea; chills; fatigue and malaise
2. Objective: dysrhythmias; increased cardiac enzymes; fever; positive blood cultures; friction rubs evident on auscultation

C. Therapeutic interventions
1. Oxygen therapy and bed rest
2. Antibiotics to relieve underlying infection; corticosteroids; antidysrhythmics; and nonsteroidal antiinflammatory agents to suppress rheumatic activity
3. Pericardectomy (surgical removal of scar tissue and the pericardium), if indicated
4. Cardiac monitoring

Nursing Care of Clients With Inflammatory Disease of the Heart
A. Assessment/Analysis
1. Signs of shock, heart failure, and dysrhythmias
2. Temperature to obtain baseline data

3. Distention of neck veins
4. Friction rub and murmur
5. Overt and covert indicators of pain

B. Planning/Implementation
1. Maintain a tranquil environment and help the client achieve maximum rest; medicate for discomfort as needed
2. Explain posthospitalization therapy to improve compliance (lifelong doses of antibiotics prophylactically when undergoing invasive procedures)
3. Administer IV antibiotics as ordered
4. Monitor temperature and blood cultures to evaluate antibiotic therapy
5. If surgical intervention is undertaken, care for chest tubes and follow the postoperative chest surgery routine (see Cardiac Surgery)

C. Evaluation/Outcomes
1. Verbalizes pain is relieved
2. Achieves afebrile state
3. Maintains vital signs within normal limits
4. Adheres to therapeutic regimen

❁ HEART FAILURE (HF)

Data Base

A. Etiology and pathophysiology
1. Inability of the heart to meet the oxygen demands of the body
2. Pump failure may be caused by cardiac abnormalities or conditions that place increased demands on the heart such as cardiac muscle disorders, valvular defects (e.g., mitral valve prolapse with regurgitation, aortic stenosis), hypertension, coronary atherosclerosis, hyperthyroidism, obesity, chronic obstructive pulmonary disease (COPD), and circulatory overload
3. Heart failure may be classified as diastolic (impaired ventricular filling) or systolic (impaired ventricular contraction); determined by ejection fraction
4. When one side of the heart "fails," there is essentially a buildup of pressure in the vascular system feeding into that side; signs of right ventricular failure will be evident in the systemic circulation first; those of left ventricular failure are first evident in the pulmonary system, causing pulmonary edema; eventually affects both pulmonary and systemic circulation
5. Decreased cardiac output activates the renin-angiotensin-aldosterone mechanism and sympathetic nervous system, leading to vasoconstriction and retention of sodium and water; increases cardiac workload

B. Clinical findings
1. Left ventricular heart failure
   a. Subjective: dyspnea from fluid within the lungs; orthopnea; fatigue and restlessness; paroxysmal nocturnal dyspnea
   b. Objective: decreased oxygen saturation, crackles; peripheral cyanosis; Cheyne-Stokes respirations; frothy, blood-tinged sputum; dry, nonproductive cough; decreased ejection fraction, dyspnea, decreased urine output
2. Right ventricular failure
   a. Subjective: abdominal pain; fatigue; bloating; nausea
   b. Objective: jugular vein distention (JVD); dependent, pitting edema that often subsides at night when legs are elevated; ankle edema is frequently the first sign of heart failure (HF); ascites from increased hydrostatic pressure within the portal system; hepatomegaly; anorexia; respiratory distress; increased central venous pressure (CVP); diminished urinary output
3. Diagnostic tests
   a. B-type natriuretic peptide (BNP) rises (normal value is <100 pg/mL); produced by the myocardium in response to increased ventricular end-diastolic pressure; functions to promote diuresis and vasodilation to reduce cardiac workload
   b. Echocardiogram to assess ventricular function/hypertrophy
   c. Hemodynamic monitoring for cardiogenic shock
   d. Electrolytes, hematocrit, hemoglobin, BUN, creatinine, complete blood count, thyroid-stimulating hormone; ECGs are done to identify underlying causes

C. Therapeutic interventions
1. Rest in Fowler's or orthopneic position to reduce cardiac workload
2. Morphine sulfate to reduce anxiety and dyspnea
3. Oxygen therapy; in acute ventricular failure endotracheal intubation and a ventilator
4. Decrease cardiac workload with diuretics, vasodilators, ACE inhibitors, angiotensin II receptor blockers, beta blockers, phosphodiesterase inhibitors, and nesiritide (Natrecor), a form of BNP
5. Increase pump performance with digitalis or dobutamine (Dobutrex)
6. Potassium supplements to prevent digitalis toxicity and hypokalemia
7. Hemodynamic monitoring through a multilumen pulmonary artery catheter
8. Sodium-restricted diet to limit fluid retention and promote fluid excretion
9. Paracentesis if ascites exists and is causing respiratory distress
10. Cardiac resynchronization therapy: use of right and left ventricular pacemakers to synchronize contractions and improve cardiac output

Nursing Care of Clients With Heart Failure

A. Assessment/Analysis
1. Baseline vital signs, breath sounds, oxygen saturation (Sao_2)

Table 6-1 Pitting Edema Scale

Scale	Description	Measurement
1+	Barely perceptible pit	2 mm (3/32 in.)
2+	Deeper pit; rebounds in a few seconds	4 mm (5/32 in.)
3+	Deep pit; rebounds in 10-20 seconds	6 mm (1/4 in.)
4+	Deeper pit; rebounds in >30 seconds	8 mm (5/16 in.)

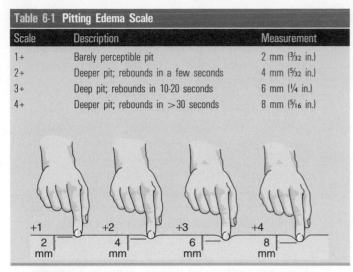

From Monahan FD et al: *Phipps' medical-surgical nursing: health and illness perspectives*, ed 8, St. Louis, 2007, Mosby.

2. Daily weight, extent of pitting edema, circumference of edematous extremities, abdominal girth, jugular vein distention (JVD) (Table 6-1: Pitting Edema Scale)
3. Hemodynamic status (CVP, pulmonary capillary wedge pressure [PCWP])
4. Electrolyte levels (sodium, chloride, potassium)
5. Intake and output

B. Planning/Implementation
   1. Maintain the client in high-Fowler's or orthopneic position; administer supplemental oxygen
   2. Elevate extremities except when the client is in acute distress
   3. Frequently monitor vital signs, breath sounds, JVD, Sao$_2$
   4. Change position slowly and frequently
   5. Monitor intake and output, daily weight, electrolytes
   6. Restrict fluids as ordered
   7. Provide small, frequent, low-sodium meals
   8. Monitor invasive lines
   9. Administer medications as ordered; refer to Cardiac Glycosides, Antihypertensives, Diuretics, and Phosphodiesterase Inhibitors under Related Pharmacology
   10. Collaborate with client to establish balanced schedule of rest and activity

C. Evaluation/Outcomes
   1. Maintains adequate tissue perfusion
   2. Reduces peripheral edema/ascites
   3. Verbalizes understanding of pharmacologic and diet therapy

CARDIAC SURGERY
Data Base
A. Purposes
   1. Correct abnormalities: mitral stenosis or regurgitation; aortic stenosis or insufficiency; coronary occlusion; ventricular aneurysm
   2. Replace failing heart (cardiac transplantation): terminal heart disease with life expectancy of less than 1 year; viral myocarditis; toxic injury to the myocardium; severe coronary heart disease

B. Types of procedures: open or closed heart surgery (when extracorporeal circulation or the heart-lung machine is used, it is called open heart surgery)
   1. Hypothermia may be used to decrease metabolic rate during cardiac surgery
   2. Coronary artery bypass graft (CABG) surgery is done when severe atherosclerotic disease causes ischemia; involves anastomosis of a graft or a segment of a vessel (often the internal mammary artery or the saphenous vein), bypassing the diseased portion of a coronary artery; one or more vessels may be bypassed
   3. Cardiac transplantation involves replacement of the client's diseased heart with one from a compatible donor; requires lifelong antirejection drugs including steroids and immunosuppressants
   4. Surgical removal (ablation) of foci and pathways of dysrhythmias; involves mapping cardiac electrophysiologic function to locate the source of the dysrhythmic foci; surgical resection of the focus is made through a sternotomy
   5. Surgical repair or replacement of valves

Nursing Care of Clients After Cardiac Surgery
A. Assessment/Analysis
   1. Hemodynamic monitoring, vital signs
   2. Airway patency, breath sounds, Sao$_2$
   3. Tubes (indwelling urinary, chest, nasogastric [NG]) to ensure patency and to assess drainage
   4. Incision for signs of hemorrhage or infection
   5. Clinical indicators of complications: MI, HF, cardiac tamponade, cerebral ischemia, bleeding, hypovolemia or fluid overload, dysrhythmias, renal failure

B. Planning/Implementation
   1. Monitor hemodynamic functioning
   2. Evaluate neurologic signs
   3. Monitor temperature closely; rewarm slowly to prevent shivering; fever increases the workload of the heart
   4. Maintain airway; the client will have an endotracheal tube in place postoperatively and require mechanical ventilation; suction secretions as necessary; encourage coughing, deep breathing, and incentive spirometry when artificial airway is removed
   5. Monitor intake and output; weigh regularly
   6. Assess pain (nature, site, duration, type) and provide relief
   7. Monitor arterial blood gases
   8. Maintain an indwelling urinary catheter in place; in addition to output, monitor specific gravity
   9. Care for chest tubes: maintain patency of tubes; avoid kinked tubing; drainage should not be more than 200 mL/hr

10. Administer parenteral therapy, including electrolytes and blood
11. Provide relief of anxiety and fear by staying with the client and explaining procedures; encourage expression of feelings; provide emotional support
12. If saphenous vein has been used, assess leg for signs of impaired circulation, edema, or infection; some edema expected when leg is dependent
13. Monitor client for signs of complications
    a. Hemorrhage that can lead to hypovolemia: decreased BP, increased pulse rate; restlessness, apprehension; lowered CVP; pallor
    b. Cardiac tamponade caused by collection of fluid or blood within pericardium: decreased arterial pressure; elevated CVP; rapid, thready pulse; diminished output
    c. Heart failure: dyspnea; elevated CVP; tachycardia; edema
    d. Myocardial infarction
    e. Renal failure
    f. Thromboembolic event affecting pulmonary, cerebral, or peripheral circulation
    g. Infection
    h. Psychosis resulting from an inability to cope with anxiety associated with cardiac surgery

C. Evaluation/Outcomes
    1. Achieves adequate cardiac output
    2. Verbalizes lower pain levels
    3. Performs self-care activities

VASCULAR DISEASE: THROMBOPHLEBITIS, VARICOSE VEINS, AND PERIPHERAL VASCULAR DISEASE

Data Base

A. Etiology and pathophysiology
    1. Thrombus: a clot composed of platelets, fibrin, clotting factors, and cellular debris attached to the interior wall of an artery or vein
    2. Embolus: a clot or solid particle carried by the bloodstream; may interfere with tissue perfusion in an artery or vein
    3. Arterial disorders involve depriving O_2 to a body part or tissue; this is affected by BP and presence of collateral circulation
        a. Reduced blood flow resulting from atherosclerosis, thrombus, or embolus
        b. Buerger's disease (thromboangiitis obliterans)
            (1) Peripheral circulation impaired by inflammatory occlusions of peripheral arteries; thromboses of arteries may occur
            (2) Incidence is highest in young adult males who smoke
        c. Raynaud's disease
            (1) Spasms of digital arteries thought to be caused by abnormal response of the sympathetic nervous system to cold or

emotional stress; usually bilateral; primarily occurs in young females
            (2) Raynaud's phenomenon is episodic arterial spasm of the extremities secondary to another disease or abnormality
    4. Venous disorders involve a problem with transportation of blood back to the heart from the capillary beds as a result of changes in smooth muscle around vessels, lack of muscular contraction, damage to the intima, incompetent valves
        a. Thrombophlebitis: inflammation of a vein; when associated with clot formation known as deep vein thrombosis; risk factors include immobilization, venous stasis, vessel trauma, oral contraceptive use, pregnancy, obesity, and pelvic surgery
        b. Varicose veins: occur when veins in lower extremities become dilated, congested (increasing hydrostatic pressure), and tortuous as a result of weakness of valves or loss of elasticity of vessel walls; risk factors include family history, prolonged standing, pregnancy, leg trauma, thrombophlebitis

B. Clinical findings
    1. Peripheral arterial disorders
        a. Subjective: paresthesia; aching to severe or burning pain
        b. Objective: pallor or dependent rubor; shiny, cool skin; hair loss; thickened nails; gangrenous ulcers of toes or heel; diminished or absent pulses; and decreased ankle-brachial index
    2. Varicose veins
        a. Subjective: heaviness and fatigue in legs with cramping; usually relieved when legs are elevated
        b. Objective: positive venogram; positive Trendelenburg test is diagnostic of varicose veins; brown skin discoloration from breakdown of hemoglobin and deposition of ferrous sulfate; stasis ulcers; edema
    3. Thrombophlebitis
        a. Subjective: may be asymptomatic until embolus is released and occludes organ; calf pain on dorsiflexion of ankle (Homans' sign) is not a reliable indicator
        b. Objective: edema of one leg; redness and warmth of area along the vein; Doppler studies/flow studies of lower extremities indicate obstruction or decreased flow from the area, suggesting thrombus formation; positive D-dimer assay, which indicates products of fibrin degradation in the blood (normal value is <250 mcg/L)

C. Therapeutic intervention
    1. Peripheral vascular disease
        a. Arterial vasodilators and antiplatelet agents
        b. Sympathectomy to sever the sympathetic ganglia supplying the area; there is local vasodilation with improved circulation
        c. Bypass grafting
        d. Amputation if vascular supply is severely impaired (see Amputation in Nursing Care of Clients With

Neuromusculoskeletal System Disorders in Chapter 11)

2. Varicose veins
   a. Sclerotherapy: injection of a chemical irritant into the vein
   b. Surgical intervention: ligation of the vein above the varicosity and removal of the involved vein; the great saphenous vein may be ligated near the femoral junction (deep veins must be able to accommodate venous flow)
   c. Postoperative early ambulation is essential to prevent formation of thrombi
3. Thrombophlebitis
   a. Prophylactic antiembolytic stockings and exercises to promote venous return
   b. Moist heat as ordered to promote vasodilation
   c. Elevation of extremity to reduce edema
   d. Anticoagulants to prevent recurrence
   e. Vasodilators to prevent vascular spasm
   f. Thrombolytic therapy to dissolve clot
   g. Transvenous filter or thrombectomy

Nursing Care of Clients With Vascular Disease

A. Assessment/Analysis
   1. Risk factors and subjective data
   2. Affected extremity for pulses, color, temperature, and circumference
   3. Mobility of involved extremity
B. Planning/Implementation
   1. Observe frequently for signs of vascular impairment (e.g., pallor, cyanosis, coolness of involved extremities, and amplitude and symmetry of peripheral pulses)
   2. Elevate legs to prevent edema from venous insufficiency; apply antiembolism stockings before arising; apply sequential compression device for clients prescribed bed rest; if thrombophlebitis is suspected, maintain bed rest and notify physician
   3. Instruct the client to avoid cigarette smoking (nicotine constricts vessels), massaging legs, maintaining one position for long periods, and wearing tight clothing that can affect peripheral vessels; reduce weight when indicated; control diabetes, hypertension, and lipid levels; maintain adequate hydration; perform ankle exercises so muscle contractions prevent venous stasis
   4. In arterial disease, keep extremities warm; instruct the client to wear gloves when exposed to cold and apply lubricants to keep skin supple; dependent position of extremity increases arterial flow and relieves pain
   5. Observe for signs of pulmonary embolism (e.g., sudden chest pain, cyanosis, hemoptysis, shock)
   6. Provide specific care if undergoing vascular surgery: monitor for hemorrhage; notify physician if bleeding is suspected; assess neurovascular status of extremity; keep extremity elevated in immediate

postoperative period; allow out of bed as ordered (see care associated with amputation under Amputation in Nursing Care of Clients With Neuromusculoskeletal System Disorders in Chpater 11)
   7. Provide specific care for the client after a vein ligation: elevate the foot of the bed for the first 24 hours; observe for signs of hemorrhage; maintain compression dressings; assist with ambulation
   8. Provide specific care for the client after endarterectomy and bypass grafting
      a. Assess circulation of involved area by checking pulses, color, temperature, mobility, and sensory function
      b. Observe blood pressure frequently because hypotension increases the possibility of thrombus formation; encourage hydration to maintain blood volume and decrease viscosity
      c. Observe for signs of hemorrhage, pain, change in skin color, and alteration of vital signs
      d. Ambulate as ordered; sitting should be avoided after bypass surgery
C Evaluation/Outcomes
   1. Maintains tissue perfusion
   2. Verbalizes reduction in pain

✿ ANEURYSMS

Data Base

A. Etiology and pathophysiology
   1. Distention at the site of a weakness in the arterial wall
      a. Saccular aneurysm: pouchlike projection on one side of the artery
      b. Fusiform aneurysm: entire circumference of the artery wall is dilated
      c. Mycotic aneurysm: tiny weaknesses in arterial walls resulting from infection
      d. Dissecting aneurysm: tear in the inner lining of an arteriosclerotic aortic wall causes blood to form a hematoma between layers of the artery, compressing the lumen
   2. Causes: congenital weakness; syphilis; trauma; atherosclerosis (most common cause of both thoracic and abdominal aortic aneurysms)
   3. Represent surgical emergency if ruptured
   4. Thoracic aortic aneurysms occur most frequently in middle-aged males; abdominal aneurysms between 60 and 90 years
   5. Risk factors include history of hypertension, obesity, stress, hypercholesterolemia, cigarette smoking, familial tendency
B. Clinical findings
   1. Thoracic aortic aneurysm
      a. Subjective: may be asymptomatic; dyspnea; dysphagia; pain resulting from pressure against the nerves or vertebrae
      b. Objective: hoarseness, cough, and aphonia from impingement on laryngeal nerve;

unequal pulses and arterial pressure in upper extremities; trachea may be displaced from midline because of adhesions between trachea and aneurysm
2. Abdominal aortic aneurysm
   a. Subjective: may be asymptomatic; lower back or abdominal pain (severe if aneurysm is leaking); sensory changes in the lower extremities if aneurysm ruptures
   b. Objective: hypertension; pulsating abdominal mass; mottling of the lower extremities and increased abdominal girth if aneurysm ruptures
3. Dissecting aortic aneurysm
   a. Subjective: restlessness; anxiety; severe pain
   b. Objective: diminished pulses; signs of shock
C. Therapeutic interventions
1. Resection/repair of aneurysm and use of vascular graft or endovascular stent
2. Medical treatment is aimed at controlling cardiac output and BP through the use of drugs; elevated pressure increases the risk of rupture

Nursing Care of Clients With Aneurysms

A. Assessment/Analysis
1. History of risk factors
2. Pulsation in abdomen (palpate gently)
3. Severe back or abdominal pain (may indicate impending rupture)
4. Peripheral neurovascular status
B. Planning/Implementation
1. Monitor neurovascular status of extremities
2. Monitor hemodynamic status, vital signs, Sao$_2$, ECG
3. Record I&O, because kidney failure may occur after surgery
4. Administer opioids as ordered to alleviate pain
5. Apply abdominal binders to provide support when the client is coughing, deep breathing, and ambulating
6. Prevent flexion of hip and knees to eliminate pressure on the arterial wall
C. Evaluation/Outcomes
1. Maintains adequate peripheral circulation
2. Identifies ways to modify risk factors

❄ SHOCK

Data Base

A. Etiology and pathophysiology
1. Hypovolemic: occurs when there is a loss of fluid that results in inadequate tissue perfusion; caused by excessive bleeding, diarrhea, or vomiting; fluid loss from fistulas or burns
2. Cardiogenic: occurs when pump failure causes inadequate tissue perfusion; caused by HF, MI, cardiac tamponade
3. Neurogenic: caused by rapid vasodilation and subsequent pooling of blood within the peripheral vessels; caused by spinal anesthesia, emotional stress, drugs that inhibit the sympathetic nervous system, spinal injury

4. Anaphylactic: caused by an allergic reaction that causes a massive release of histamine and subsequent vasodilation
5. Septic (similar to anaphylaxis): reaction to bacterial toxins (generally gram-negative infections) that causes the leakage of plasma into tissues, resulting in hypovolemia
B. Clinical findings
1. Subjective: apprehension; restlessness; paresis of extremities
2. Objective: weak, rapid, thready pulse; diaphoresis; cold, clammy skin; pallor; decreased urine output; progressive loss of consciousness; decreased mean arterial pressure (normal 80 to 120 mm Hg)
C. Therapeutic interventions
1. Correction of the underlying cause
2. Fluid and blood replacement
3. Oxygen therapy, ventilator
4. Vasoconstricting drugs to increase BP
5. Cardiac and hemodynamic monitoring
6. Cardiotonics for cardiogenic shock
7. Adrenergic blockage: prevents effects of prolonged vasoconstriction; causes loss of fluid from vascular compartment
8. Antihistamines such as diphenhydramine (Benadryl) and steroids for anaphylactic shock
9. Antibiotics for septic shock based on blood cultures
10. Elevation of lower extremities to ensure circulation to vital organs
11. Intraaortic balloon pump may be used to augment the failing heart

Nursing Care of Clients in Shock

A. Assessment/Analysis
1. History of causative and risk factors from client
2. Fluid intake and output over the previous 24 hours
3. Signs of covert bleeding: rapid, thready pulse; hypotension; increased respirations; cold, clammy skin
4. Mental status changes: restlessness and confusion to lethargy and decreased level of consciousness
5. Cardiovascular status: ECG, hemodynamic monitoring, peripheral vascular assessment
6. Respiratory status: breath sounds, arterial blood gases, Sao$_2$
B. Planning/Implementation
1. Keep client warm; place in supine position
2. Monitor hemodynamic status and vital signs
3. Monitor urine output and specific gravity
4. Allay client's anxiety
5. Administer intravenous fluids and medications as ordered
6. Monitor oxygen saturation and provide oxygen therapy as indicated
C. Evaluation/Outcomes
1. Maintains stable hemodynamic status
2. Maintains a urine output >30 mL/hour
3. Remains oriented to time, place, and person
4. Maintains adequate cardiac output

✾ ANEMIAS AND BLOOD DISORDERS

Data Base

A. Etiology and pathophysiology
1. Iron deficiency anemia: most common cause is bleeding related to GI bleeding, menstruation, malignancy; other causes include inadequate dietary intake, malabsorption, and increased demand (e.g., pregnancy)
2. Megaloblastic anemia
   a. Folate deficiency: amount of folic acid absorbed or ingested is insufficient to synthesize DNA, RNA, and proteins; associated with alcoholism, malabsorption, pregnancy, lactation
   b. Pernicious anemia: lack of intrinsic factor in the stomach prevents the absorption of vitamin B_{12}, which reduces the number of erythrocytes formed
3. Aplastic (hypoplastic) anemia: bone marrow is depressed or destroyed by a chemical or drug, leading to leukopenia, thrombocytopenia, decreased erythrocytes, and decreased leukocytes (agranulocytosis)
4. Hemolytic anemia: excessive or premature destruction of RBCs; there are many causes, including sickle cell anemia, thalassemia, glucose-6-phosphate dehydrogenase (G-6-PD) deficiency, antibody reactions, infection, and toxins
5. Polycythemia vera: a sustained increase in the number of erythrocytes, leukocytes, and platelets, with an increased viscosity of the blood
6. Thrombocytopenic purpura: appears to result from the production of an antiplatelet antibody that coats the surface of platelets and facilitates their destruction by phagocytic leukocytes
B. Clinical findings
1. Subjective: fatigue, headache, paresthesias, dyspnea, sore mouth with pernicious anemia, gum bleeding and epistaxis with thrombocytopenic purpura
2. Objective
   a. Ankle edema
   b. Dry, pale mucous membranes
   c. Pallor except with polycythemia vera; jaundice with hemolytic anemia
   d. Decreased levels of hemoglobin, erythrocytes, ferritin; increased iron-binding capacity; megaloblastic condition of the blood with iron deficiency anemia
   e. Beefy red tongue, lack of intrinsic factor, positive Romberg's test (loss of balance with eyes closed) with pernicious anemia
   f. Fever, bleeding from mucous membranes; decreased levels of leukocytes, erythrocytes, and platelets with aplastic anemia
   g. Increased hemoglobin level, purple-red complexion with polycythemia vera
   h. Low platelet count, ecchymotic areas, hemorrhagic petechiae with thrombocytopenic purpura
   i. Increased reticulocytes and unconjugated bilirubin levels with hemolytic anemia

C. Therapeutic interventions
1. Improve diet: include ascorbic acid, which enhances iron uptake
2. Supplements: iron, vitamin B_{12}, folic acid
3. Blood transfusions (except for polycythemia vera)
4. Oxygen as needed
5. Epoetin (Epogen, Procrit) to stimulate bone marrow function; bone marrow transplant (BMT); peripheral blood stem cell transplant (PBSCT), immunosuppressive therapy for aplastic anemia
6. Phlebotomy, low-iron diet, radioactive phosphorus, busulfan (Myleran) for polycythemia vera
7. Removal of causative agent; splenectomy may be indicated for hemolytic anemias

Nursing Care of Clients With Anemias and Blood Disorders

A. Assessment/Analysis
1. History of dietary habits, symptoms, and causative agents
2. Status of skin, mucous membranes, and sclera
3. Baseline vital signs
B. Planning/Implementation
1. Teach client about dietary modifications and medication administration; foods high in iron include spinach, raisins, liver
2. Collaborate with client to balance rest and activity
3. Explain the need for prevention of hemorrhage (thrombocytopenia) and phlebotomies (for polycythemia vera)
4. Provide postoperative care if splenectomy is performed; encourage deep breathing and coughing because these actions precipitate pain and may be avoided; assess for abdominal distention that may reflect hemorrhage
C. Evaluation/Outcomes
1. States dietary sources of iron, folic acid, and vitamin B_{12}
2. Verbalizes understanding of long-term need for therapeutic supervision
3. Performs ADLs
4. Remains afebrile and injury-free

✾ DISSEMINATED INTRAVASCULAR COAGULATION (DIC)

Data Base

A. Etiology and pathophysiology
1. Body's response to overstimulation of clotting and anticlotting processes in response to injury or disease; massive amounts of microthrombi affect microcirculation
2. Complicated by hemorrhage at various sites as a result of fibrinolytic response
3. Multiple system failure can occur (circulatory, respiratory, GI, renal, neurologic) from bleeding or thrombosis

B. Clinical findings
  1. Subjective: restlessness, anxiety
  2. Objective
    a. Laboratory tests indicate low fibrinogen level and prolonged prothrombin and partial thromboplastin times, reduced platelets, positive D-dimer assay
    b. Hemorrhage, both subcutaneous and internal; petechiae; signs of organ failure
C. Therapeutic interventions
  1. Relieve the underlying cause
  2. Heparin to prevent the formation of thrombi
  3. Transfusion of blood products
  4. Antifibrinolytic therapy to prevent bleeding may be necessary

Nursing Care of Clients With Disseminated Intravascular Coagulation

A. Assessment/Analysis
  1. History of causative factors (generally septicemia, obstetric emergencies, and septic shock)
  2. Bleeding; abnormal coagulation profile
B. Planning/Implementation
  1. Observe for bleeding; replace fluids
  2. Minimize skin punctures; prevent injury
  3. Monitor for renal, cerebral, and respiratory complications
  4. Provide emotional support
C. Evaluation/Outcomes
  1. Maintains circulation to all tissues
  2. Verbalizes a decrease in fears
  3. Maintains adequate cardiac output

❀ LEUKEMIA

Also see Leukemia in Nursing Care of Preschoolers in Chapter 32

Data Base

A. Etiology and pathophysiology
  1. Incidence highest in children ages 2 to 6; declines until age 35, then increases steadily
  2. Etiology unknown, although genetic factors and exposure to certain toxic substances such as radiation seem to increase the incidence
  3. In general, an uncontrolled proliferation of WBCs; classified according to type of WBC affected
    a. Acute lymphocytic leukemia (ALL): primarily occurs in children
    b. Acute myeloid leukemia (AML): occurs throughout life cycle; incidence increases with age; prognosis is poor with or without chemotherapy; leukocytes are immature and abnormal
    c. Chronic myeloid leukemia (CML): occurs after the second decade; majority have Philadelphia chromosome; results from abnormal production of granulocytic cells
    d. Chronic lymphocytic leukemia (CLL): occurs most commonly in persons 50 to 70 years old;

life expectancy is 2.5 to 14 years; results from increased production of leukocytes and lymphocytes and proliferation of cells within the bone marrow, spleen, and liver
B. Clinical findings
  1. Subjective: malaise, bone pain
  2. Objective: anemia, thrombocytopenia, elevated leukocytes, decreased platelets, petechiae, gingival bleeding, fever, infection
C. Therapeutic interventions
  1. Chemotherapy
  2. Transfusions of whole blood or blood fractions
  3. Analgesics
  4. Bone marrow transplant; peripheral blood stem cell transplantation
  5. Radiation to areas of lymphocytic infiltration
  6. Granulocytic growth factors for neutropenia

Nursing Care of Clients With Leukemia

A. Assessment/Analysis
  1. History of infectious processes
  2. Overt and covert bleeding
  3. Baseline vital signs; observe for signs of anemia, thrombocytopenia, and neutropenia
B. Planning/Implementation
  1. Discuss the importance of follow-up care with the client and family
  2. Provide emotional support for the client and family
  3. Provide specific nursing care related to chemotherapeutic therapy, transfusion, or diagnostic tests
  4. Provide a safe injury-free environment because of increased risk of bleeding
  5. Use appropriate infection control techniques; initiate neutropenic precautions as needed (private room; no flowers, fresh fruit or vegetables)
  6. Pace care to avoid client fatigue and assist as necessary
  7. Provide nutrient-dense food and adequate fluid intake
C. Evaluation/Outcomes
  1. Remains free from bleeding episodes
  2. Verbalizes a decrease in fears
  3. Plans strategies to avoid fatigue
  4. Remains free from infection

❀ LYMPHOMA

Data Base

A. Etiology and pathophysiology
  1. Types
    a. Hodgkin's disease: proliferation of malignant cells (Reed-Sternberg cells) within lymph node(s) usually on one side of the neck; relatively rare with good cure rate; peak incidence in young adult males, second peak when older than 50 years of age
    b. Non-Hodgkin's lymphoma: 95% involves B lymphocytes, which become infiltrated with malignant cells that spread unpredictably; increased

incidence with aging; average age at diagnosis is during sixth decade; becoming increasingly prevalent (sixth most common cancer)
2. Cause is unknown; impaired immune function linked to increased incidence
3. All tissues may eventually be involved, but chiefly lymph nodes, spleen, liver, tonsils, and bone marrow
4. Classification by staging and the presence or absence of systemic symptoms
B. Clinical findings
1. Subjective: pruritus; anorexia; dyspnea and dysphagia caused by pressure from enlarged nodes
2. Objective
   a. Enlarged lymph nodes (generally cervical nodes are involved first)
   b. Diagnosis confirmed by histologic examination of a lymph node
   c. Progressive anemia
   d. Elevated temperature
   e. Enlarged spleen and liver may occur
   f. Pressure from enlarged lymph nodes may cause symptoms of dyspnea, edema, and obstructive jaundice
   g. Thrombocytopenia if spleen and bone marrow involved
C. Therapeutic interventions
1. Radiotherapy
   a. Vital organs must be shielded
   b. Potential side effects: nausea; skin rashes; dry mouth; dysphagia; infections; pancytopenia

2. Chemotherapy: see Related Pharmacology under Neoplastic Disorders, in Chapter 3
3. Bone marrow transplant; peripheral blood stem cell transplantation
4. Surgical intervention includes excision of masses to relieve pressure on other organs

Nursing Care of Clients With Lymphomas
A. Assessment/Analysis
1. Lymph nodes to determine enlargement
2. Temperature for baseline data
3. Liver and spleen to determine enlargement
4. CBC and liver profile for baseline data
B. Planning/Implementation
1. Provide emotional support for the client and family
2. Protect from infection
3. Monitor temperature
4. Observe for signs of anemia; provide adequate rest
5. Examine sclera and skin for signs of jaundice
6. Encourage high nutrient density foods; observe for anorexia and nausea; prevent dehydration
C. Evaluation/Outcomes
1. Remains afebrile
2. Conserves energy
3. Verbalizes feelings related to therapy and prognosis

Nursing Care of Clients With Respiratory System Disorders

OVERVIEW

REVIEW OF ANATOMY AND PHYSIOLOGY

Structures and Functions of the Respiratory System

(Figure 7-1: The respiratory system)

A. The upper portion of the respiratory system filters, moistens, and warms air during inspiration
   1. Nose: lining is ciliated mucosa; divided by septum; turbinates (conchae) projected from lateral walls; contains olfactory receptors for smell; aids in phonation
   2. Paranasal sinuses draining into the nose: frontal, maxillary, sphenoidal, ethmoidal; aid in phonation
   3. Pharynx: nasopharynx, oropharynx, and laryngopharynx; composed of muscle with mucous lining; contain tonsils, adenoids, and other lymphoid tissue that help destroy incoming bacteria
   4. Larynx: formed by cartilage including the thyroid cartilage (Adam's apple), epiglottis (the lid cartilage), cricoid (the signet ring cartilage), and vocal cords (fibroelastic bands stretched across the hollow interior of the larynx); the paired vocal cords (folds) and the posterior arytenoid cartilages make up the glottis; voice production—during expiration, air passing through the larynx causes the vocal cords to vibrate; short, tense cords produce a high pitch; long, relaxed cords, a low pitch
   5. Trachea: smooth muscle walls contain C-shaped rings of cartilage that keep the tube open at all times; lined with ciliated mucosa; extends from larynx to bronchi; 10 to 12 cm long; furnishes open passageway for air going to and from lungs
B. The lower portion of the respiratory system consists of the lungs, which enable the exchange of gases between blood and air to regulate arterial Po_2, Pco_2, and pH; the left lung has two lobes and the right lung has three lobes
   1. Bronchi: right and left, formed by branching of the trachea; right bronchus slightly larger and more vertical than left; each primary bronchus branches into segmental bronchi in each lung; primary and segmental bronchi all contain C-shaped cartilage
   2. Bronchioles: small branches off the secondary bronchi, distinguished by lack of C-shaped cartilage and a duct diameter of about 1 mm; bronchi further branch into terminal bronchioles, respiratory bronchioles, and then alveolar ducts
   3. Alveoli: microscopic sacs composed of a single layer of extremely thin squamous epithelial cells (type I cell) enveloped by a network of pulmonary capillaries that allow for rapid gas exchange; type II cells produce surfactant to prevent alveolar collapse, and type III cells are macrophages that protect against bacteria by phagocytosis
   4. Covering of lung: visceral layer of pleura that joins with the parietal pleura lining the thorax and diaphragm; the space between these two linings is the pleural space and contains a small amount of fluid to eliminate friction; negative pressure in the pleural space relative to atmospheric pressure is essential for breathing

Physiology of Respiration

A. Mechanism of breathing
   1. Following phrenic nerve stimulation, the diaphragm and other respiratory muscles contract
   2. Thorax increases in size
   3. Intrathoracic and intrapulmonic pressures decrease
   4. Air rushes from positive pressure in the atmosphere to negative pressure in the alveoli
   5. Inspiration is completed with stimulation of stretch receptors
   6. Expiration occurs passively as a result of recoil of elastic lung tissue
B. Control of respiration
   1. Alveolar stretch receptors respond to inspiration by sending inhibitory impulses to inspiratory neurons in brainstem to prevent lung overdistention (Hering-Breuer reflex)
   2. Central and peripheral chemoreceptors stimulate respirations in response to lowered pH, increased Pco_2, or decreased Po_2
   3. Medulla oblongata and pons control the rate and depth of respirations
C. Amount of air exchanged in breathing: directly related to gas pressure gradient between atmosphere and alveoli and inversely related to resistance that opposes airflow; positions such as orthopneic and Fowler's can lower abdominal organs and reduce pressure against diaphragm; pulmonary function can be evaluated with a spirometer (Figure 7-2: Lung volumes and capacities)

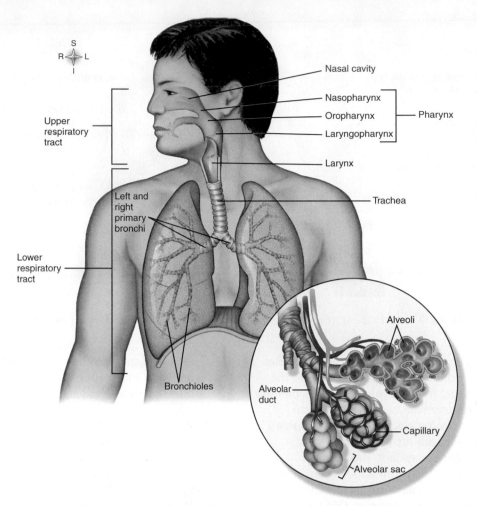

Figure 7-1 The respiratory system. The inset shows the alveolar sacs where the interchange of oxygen and carbon dioxide takes place through the walls of the grapelike alveoli. (From Thibodeau GA, Patton KT: *Anatomy and physiology,* ed 6, St Louis, 2007, Mosby.)

1. Tidal volume: average amount expired after normal inspiration; approximately 500 mL
2. Expiratory reserve volume (ERV): largest additional volume of air that can be forcibly expired after a normal inspiration and expiration; normal ERV is 1000 to 1200 mL
3. Inspiratory reserve volume (IRV): largest additional volume of air that can be forcibly inspired after a normal inspiration; normal IRV is 3000 mL
4. Residual volume: air that cannot be forcibly expired voluntarily from lungs; about 1200 mL; increased in chronic obstructive pulmonary disease (COPD) as lungs lose elasticity and ability to recoil, resulting in air trapping
5. Vital capacity: amount of air that can be forcibly expired after forcible inspiration; varies with size of thoracic cavity, which is determined by various factors (e.g., size of rib cage, posture, volume of blood and interstitial fluid in the lungs, size of the heart); about 4600 mL; decreased with COPD, neuromuscular disease, atelectasis
6. Forced expiratory volume (FEV): volume of air that can be forcibly exhaled within a specific time,

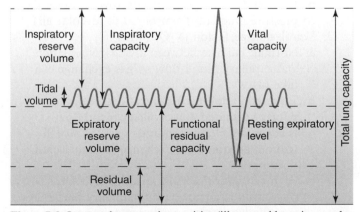

Figure 7-2 Lung volumes and capacities (illustrated by spirography tracing). (From Monahan FD et al: *Phipps' medical-surgical nursing: health and illness perspectives,* ed 8, St Louis, 2007, Mosby.)

   usually 1 to 3 seconds; decreased with increased airway resistance (e.g., bronchospasm, COPD)
7. Inspiratory capacity: largest amount of air that can be inspired after a normal exhalation; about 3500 mL
8. Functional residual capacity: amount of air left in the lungs after a normal exhalation; about 2300 mL; increased with COPD

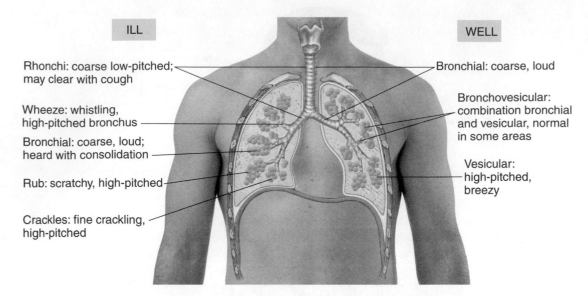

ILL

Rhonchi: coarse low-pitched; may clear with cough

Wheeze: whistling, high-pitched bronchus

Bronchial: coarse, loud; heard with consolidation

Rub: scratchy, high-pitched

Crackles: fine crackling, high-pitched

WELL

Bronchial: coarse, loud

Bronchovesicular: combination bronchial and vesicular, normal in some areas

Vesicular: high-pitched, breezy

Figure 7-3 Breath sounds in the ill and well client. (From Seidel HM, Dains JE, Benedict GW: *Mosby's guide to physical examination*, ed 6, St Louis, 2006, Mosby.)

9. Total lung capacity: amount of air in the lungs after maximum inhalation; about 5800 mL; equal to the sum of tidal volume, residual volume, and inspiratory and expiratory reserve volumes; increased with COPD; decreased with atelectasis and pneumonia

D. Diffusion of gases between air and blood
   1. Occurs across alveolar-capillary membranes (in lungs between air in alveoli and venous blood in lung capillaries); adequate diffusion depends on a balanced ventilation-perfusion (V/Q) ratio
   2. Direction of diffusion
      a. Oxygen: net diffusion toward lower O_2 pressure gradient (from alveolar air to blood)
      b. Carbon dioxide: net diffusion toward lower CO_2 pressure gradient (from blood to alveolar air)
   3. Ventilation-perfusion (V/Q) ratios
      a. Normal: balance between alveolar ventilation and capillary blood flow so gas exchange can take place
      b. Low ventilation-perfusion ratio: alveoli are poorly ventilated, but capillary blood flow is adequate; blood is shunted past the alveoli without adequate gas exchange (e.g., atelectasis, pneumonia)
      c. High ventilation-perfusion ratio: alveolar ventilation is adequate, but capillary blood flow is not; adequate gas exchange does not take place because of dead space (e.g., pulmonary embolism, cardiogenic shock)
      d. Absence of ventilation and perfusion: causes a silent unit; no gas exchange (e.g., pneumothorax)

E. Blood transports O_2 as a solute and primarily as oxyhemoglobin; oxygen saturation of hemoglobin (Sao_2) is normally 95% to 100%

F. Blood transports CO_2
   1. Primarily as a bicarbonate ion (HCO_3^-) formed by ionization of carbonic acid; in the lungs the

molecule splits in the presence of carbonic anhydrase to form CO_2 and H_2O; CO_2 diffuses into the alveoli and the majority of water is retained
   2. As a solute in plasma
   3. In combination with hemoglobin (carboxyhemoglobin)

G. Normal breath sounds (Figure 7-3: Breath sounds in the ill and well client)
   1. Bronchial sounds (over trachea, larynx): result of air passing through larger airways; sounds are loud, harsh, high-pitched; expiration longer than inspiration
   2. Vesicular sounds (over entire lung field except large airways): result of air moving in and out of alveoli; may reflect sound of air in larger passages that is transmitted through lung tissue; sounds are quiet, low-pitched; inspiration longer than expiration
   3. Bronchovesicular sounds (near main stem bronchi); result of air moving through smaller air passages; sounds are moderately pitched, breezy; inspiratory and expiratory phases equal

H. Adventitious breath sounds (Figure 7-3: Breath sounds in the ill and well client)
   1. Fine crackles
      a. Result of sudden opening of small airways and alveoli that contain fluid
      b. Short, high-pitched bubbling sounds; sounds may be simulated by rubbing a few strands of hair between fingers next to the ear
      c. Most common during height of inspiration
      d. Associated with conditions such as pneumonia and pulmonary edema
   2. Coarse crackles
      a. Rush of air passing through airway intermittently occluded by mucus

b. Short, low-pitched bubbling sounds

c. Most common on inspiration and at times expiration

d. Associated with pneumonia, COPD, and pulmonary edema

3. Wheezes

   a. Result of air passing through narrowed small airways

   b. Sounds are high-pitched and musical (sibilant wheezes), or low-pitched and rumbling (sonorous wheezes or rhonchi)

   c. Most common on expiration

   d. Associated with conditions causing narrowing of airways, such as asthma, and with conditions that involve partial obstruction of airway by mucus, foreign body, or tumor

4. Pleural friction rub

   a. Result of roughened pleural surfaces rubbing across each other

   b. Sounds are crackling, grating

   c. Most common during height of inspiration

   d. Associated with conditions that cause inflammation of pleura

REVIEW OF MICROORGANISMS

A. Bacterial pathogens

1. *Bordetella pertussis:* small, gram-negative coccobacillus; causes pertussis or whooping cough

2. *Streptococcus pneumoniae:* gram-positive, encapsulated diplococcus; causes pneumococcal pneumonia (most commonly lobar) and often responsible for sinusitis, otitis media, and meningitis

3. *Haemophilus influenzae:* small, gram-negative, highly pleomorphic bacillus; causes acute meningitis and upper respiratory tract infections

4. *Klebsiella pneumoniae* (Friedländer's bacillus): gram-negative, encapsulated, non–spore-forming bacillus; causes pneumonia and urinary tract infections

5. *Mycobacterium tuberculosis* (tubercle bacillus): acid-fast actinomycete causes tuberculosis

6. *Pseudomonas aeruginosa:* gram-negative, non–spore-forming bacillus; important cause of hospital-acquired infections; respiratory equipment can be source; causes pneumonia, urinary tract infections, and the sepsis that complicates severe burns

B. Rickettsial pathogen: *Coxiella burnetii;* only *Rickettsia* species not associated with a vector; causes Q fever, an infection clinically similar to primary atypical pneumonia

C. Viral pathogens

1. DNA viruses: adenoviruses cause acute respiratory tract disease, adenitis, pharyngitis, and other respiratory tract infections, as well as conjunctivitis

2. RNA viruses

   a. Coronaviruses: frequently associated with a mild upper respiratory tract infection

   b. Picornaviruses: cause poliomyelitis, coxsackie disease, common cold

   c. Retroviruses: invade T lymphocytes and are associated with malignancies, human immunodeficiency virus, and acquired immunodeficiency syndrome (AIDS)

D. Fungal pathogens

1. *Histoplasma capsulatum:* dimorphic fungus producing chlamydospores in infected tissue; causes histoplasmosis

2. *Aspergillus fumigatus:* rapidly proliferating fungus found in soil; inhalation of spores can cause pneumonia

3. *Pneumocystis jiroveci:* a unicellular organism thought to be transmitted by airborne droplets; causes pneumonia

RELATED PHARMACOLOGY

Bronchodilators and Antiasthmatics

A. Description

1. Reverse bronchoconstriction, thus opening air passages in the lungs

2. Act by stimulating beta-adrenergic sympathetic nervous system receptors, relaxing bronchial smooth muscle, or inhibiting inflammation and reducing edema

3. Available in oral, parenteral (IM, Sub-Q, IV), rectal, and inhalation preparations

B. Examples

1. Beta agonists act at beta-adrenergic receptors in bronchi and bronchioles to relax smooth muscle to increase respiratory volume and inhibit histamine release from mast cells to suppress reaction to allergens: albuterol (Proventil); isoproterenol (Isuprel); epinephrine HCl (Adrenalin, Sus-Phrine); metaproterenol sulfate (Alupent); terbutaline sulfate (Brethine); salmeterol (Serevent), which is long-acting

2. Xanthines act directly on bronchial smooth muscle, decreasing spasm and relaxing smooth muscle of the vasculature, but are used less frequently because of side effects and drug interactions: aminophylline; theophylline (Elixophyllin, Theo-Dur), oxtriphylline (Choledyl), dyphylline (Dilor)

3. Anticholinergics inhibit action of acetylcholine at receptor sites on the bronchial smooth muscle and prevent bronchospasm: ipratropium (Atrovent)

4. Inhaled steroids exert antiinflammatory effect on airways: fluticasone (Flovent, Flonase); budesonide (Pulmicort Turbuhaler); beclomethasone (Beclovent, Beconase, Vanceril); triamcinolone (Azmacort); combination product—fluticasone and salmeterol (Advair Diskus)

5. Leukotriene receptor antagonists block action of leukotriene to reduce bronchoconstriction and inflammation associated with asthma: montelukast sodium (Singulair), zafirlukast (Accolate), zileuton (Zyflo)

C. Major side effects: dizziness (decrease in blood pressure); CNS stimulation (sympathetic stimulation); palpitations and hypertension (beta-adrenergic stimulation); gastric irritation (local effect)

D. Nursing care
1. Avoid administration to clients with hypertension, hyperthyroidism, and cardiovascular dysfunction
2. Avoid concurrent administration of CNS stimulants (adrenergics) and bronchoconstricting agents (beta blockers)
3. Administer during waking hours
4. Assess vital signs, breath sounds, Sao_2
5. Assess intake and output
6. Administer with food
7. Teach use of metered-dose inhalers (MDIs), spacers, and peak flow meters; rinse mouth piece, cap, and mouth after each use (oropharyngeal fungal infections are common with inhaled steroids)
8. Explain the need to comply with therapy to decrease the need for short-acting beta agonists
9. Explain the need to avoid stimulants and over-the-counter medications

Mucolytic Agents and Expectorants

A. Description
1. Liquefy secretions in the respiratory tract, promoting a productive cough
2. Mucolytics act directly to break up mucus plugs in tracheobronchial passages
3. Expectorants act indirectly to liquefy mucus by increasing respiratory tract secretions via oral absorption
4. Mucolytic agents are available in inhalation preparations (oral form of acetylcysteine is used to treat acetaminophen toxicity); expectorants are available in oral preparations

B. Examples: mucolytic—acetylcysteine (Mucomyst); expectorants—guaifenesin (Robitussin); potassium iodide (SSKI)

C. Major side effects: GI irritation (local effect); skin rash (hypersensitivity); oropharyngeal irritation and bronchospasm with mucolytics

D. Nursing care
1. Promote adequate fluid intake
2. Encourage coughing and deep breathing
3. Avoid administering fluids immediately after taking liquid expectorants
4. Assess respiratory status
5. Have suction apparatus available

Antitussives

A. Description
1. Suppress the cough reflex
2. Inhibit the cough reflex either by direct action on the medullary cough center or by indirect action peripherally on sensory nerve endings
3. Available in oral preparations

B. Examples: opioid—codeine, hydrocodone bitartrate (Hycodan); nonopioid—dextromethorphan hydrobromide (Robitussin DM), benzonatate (Tessalon); diphenhydramine HCl (Benadryl) is an antihistamine that may be used for coughs

C. Major side effects: drowsiness (CNS depression); nausea (GI irritation); dry mouth (anticholinergic effect of antihistamine in combination products)

D. Nursing care
1. Provide adequate fluid intake
2. Avoid administering fluids immediately after liquid preparations
3. Encourage high-Fowler's position
4. Avoid use postoperatively, and for clients with head injury or asthma
5. Administer opioids cautiously: avoid giving with CNS depressants; caution client to avoid hazardous activity

Opioid Antagonist

A. Description
1. Displace opioids at respiratory receptor sites via competitive antagonism
2. Reverse respiratory depression caused by opioid overdosage
3. Available in parenteral (IV, Sub-Q, IM) preparations

B. Example: naloxone (Narcan)

C. Major side effects: CNS depression (acts on opioid receptors in CNS); nausea, vomiting

D. Nursing care
1. Assess vital signs, especially respirations
2. Have O_2 and emergency resuscitative equipment available
3. Continue to monitor after effects of naloxone wear off because opioids have a longer duration of action

Antihistamines

A. Description
1. Block the action of histamine at H_1 receptor sites via competitive inhibition; also exert antiemetic, anticholinergic, and CNS depressant effects
2. Relieve symptoms of the common cold and allergies that are mediated by the chemical histamine
3. Available in oral and parenteral (IM, IV) preparations

B. Examples: brompheniramine maleate (Dimetane); diphenhydramine HCl (Benadryl); loratadine (Claritin); fexofenadine (Allegra); cetirizine (Zyrtec)

C. Major side effects
1. Drowsiness and dizziness particularly for first-generation antihistamines (CNS depression); GI irritation (local effect); dry mouth (anticholinergic effect)
2. Excitement (paradoxic effect)

D. Nursing care
1. Avoid administration with CNS depressants
2. Caution client to avoid engaging in hazardous activities
3. Administer with food or milk to avoid GI irritation
4. Offer gum or hard candy to promote salivation
5. Avoid using as a hypnotic for older adults

Antituberculars

A. Description
   1. Used to treat tuberculosis; administered in combination (first-line and second-line drugs) over a prolonged time period to reduce the possibility of mycobacterial drug resistance
   2. Available in oral and parenteral (IM) preparations
B. Examples
   1. First-line drugs
      a. Ethambutol (Myambutol): interferes with mycobacterial RNA synthesis
      b. Isoniazid (INH, Nydrazid): interferes with mycobacterial cell-wall synthesis
      c. Pyrazinamide (PMS): bacteriostatic; mechanism unknown
      d. Rifampin (Rifadin), rifabutin (Mycobutin), rifapentine (Priftin): interferes with mycobacterial RNA synthesis
      e. Streptomycin sulfate: inhibits mycobacterial protein synthesis
   2. Second-line drugs inhibit mycobacterial cell metabolism: capreomycin (Capastat) and cycloserine (Seromycin)
C. Major side effects
   1. GI irritation (direct tissue irritation)
   2. Suppressed absorption of fat and B complex vitamins, especially folic acid and B_{12}; depletion of vitamin B_6 by isoniazid
   3. Dizziness (CNS effect)
   4. CNS disturbances (direct CNS toxic effect)
   5. Liver disturbances (direct liver toxic effect)
   6. Blood dyscrasias (decreased RBCs, WBCs, platelet synthesis)
   7. Streptomycin: ototoxicity (direct auditory [eighth cranial] nerve toxic effect); nephrotoxicity
   8. Ethambutol: visual disturbances (direct optic [second cranial] nerve toxic effect)
   9. Rifampin: red discoloration of all body fluids; increases metabolism of corticosteroids, opioids, Coumadin, oral contraceptives, and hypoglycemics
   10. Isoniazid: inhibits phenytoin metabolism; peripheral neuritis
D. Nursing care
   1. Support natural defense mechanisms of client; encourage intake of foods rich in immune-stimulating nutrients such as vitamins A, C, and E, and the minerals selenium and zinc
   2. Obtain sputum specimens for acid-fast bacillus
   3. Monitor blood work during therapy (e.g., liver enzymes)
   4. Instruct the client to take the drugs regularly as prescribed; reinforce need for medical supervision; when compliance is an issue, mandated directly observed therapy ensures treatment is ongoing
   5. Offer client emotional support during long-term therapy
   6. Use safety precautions (supervise ambulation) if CNS effects are manifested
   7. Instruct client regarding nutritional side effects and encourage foods rich in B complex vitamins
   8. Encourage client to avoid use of alcohol during therapy
   9. Ethambutol: encourage frequent visual examinations
   10. Rifampin: instruct client that body fluids may appear orange-red; monitor for drug interactions; decreases effectiveness of oral contraceptives
   11. Streptomycin: encourage frequent auditory examinations
   12. Isoniazid: administer pyridoxine as ordered to prevent neuritis
   13. Instruct client to avoid exposing others to droplets from coughing and to dispose of tissues in a moisture-proof container until no longer contagious (2 to 8 weeks)
   14. Evaluate client's response to medication

✿ RELATED PROCEDURES

Abdominal Thrust (Heimlich Maneuver)

A. Definition: short, abrupt pressure against the abdomen, two fingerbreadths above the umbilicus, to raise intrathoracic pressure; external compression will force out residual lung volume, which will dislodge the obstruction, such as a bolus of food or a foreign body
B. Symptoms of obstruction
   1. Partial: noisy respiration, stridor, dyspnea, light-headedness, dizziness, flushing of face, bulging of eyes, repeated coughing
   2. Total: cessation of breathing, inability to speak or cough, extension of head, facial cyanosis, bulging of eyes, panic, unconsciousness
C. Nursing care
   1. Assess client no longer than 3 to 5 seconds
      a. Ask whether client is choking
      b. Determine whether victim can speak or cough
      c. Observe for universal choking sign (thumb and forefinger encircling throat)
      d. Assess respirations: observe for rise and fall of chest; listen for escape of air from nose and mouth on expiration; feel for flow of air from nose and mouth
   2. Initiate intervention in the presence of a partial obstruction
      a. Allow the individual's expulsive cough to dislodge the obstruction
      b. Assess for signs of total obstruction
      c. Remove foreign bodies coughed up into the mouth
      d. Activate emergency medical service (EMS) system if victim is having difficulty breathing
   3. Initiate intervention in the presence of a total obstruction
      a. Standing behind the conscious victim, encircle the waist and thrust upward and inward against the diaphragm with intertwined clenched fists; repeat thrusts until the object is expelled or the victim becomes unresponsive

    b. If victim becomes unconscious, activate EMS
       system
    c. Begin CPR
    d. Determine patency of airway; remove foreign
       objects from mouth; attempt rescue breathing
    e. If an airway cannot be established, an emergency
       cricothyrotomy may be necessary

Bronchoscopy

A. Definition
  1. Visualization of the tracheobronchial tree via a
    scope advanced through the mouth or nose into the
    bronchi
  2. Performed to remove foreign body, to remove
    secretions, or to obtain specimens of tissue or
    mucus for further study

B. Nursing care
  1. Obtain an informed consent
  2. Keep NPO for 6 to 8 hours before procedure
  3. Administer ordered preprocedure medications to
    produce sedation and decrease anxiety
  4. Inform client to expect some soreness, dysphagia,
    and hemoptysis after the procedure
  5. Advise client to avoid coughing or clearing
    throat
  6. Observe for signs of hemorrhage and/or respiratory
    distress; keep head of bed elevated
  7. Monitor vital signs until stable
  8. Do not allow fluids until the gag reflex
    returns; protect the airway until local anesthetic
    dissipates

Chest Physiotherapy

A. Definition: activities to assist the client to mobilize
  respiratory secretions that could lead to atelectasis
  and/or pneumonia

B. Types of interventions
  1. Incentive spirometer: mechanical device used to
    promote maximum inspiration and loosening of
    secretions; measures air inspired, providing visual
    feedback to client
  2. Percussion (clapping): use of cupped hands to
    repeatedly strike chest wall over congested areas;
    action causes loosening of secretions
  3. Vibration: palmar surface of hands placed on chest
    over congested area and vibrated as client exhales;
    used to loosen secretions
  4. Postural drainage: positioning client to permit
    gravity drainage of congested lung segments

C. Nursing care
  1. Assess baseline breath sounds, Sao_2, and ability of
    client to tolerate procedure
  2. Administer prescribed bronchodilators, mucolytics,
    analgesics
  3. Position client
    a. Fowler's position for incentive spirometry and to
      drain upper lung segments
    b. Side-lying and prone positions with head
      lower than affected segment for postural
      drainage

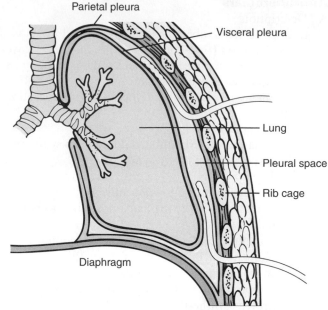

Figure 7-4 Chest tube placement. (From Lewis SL et al: *Phipps' medical-surgical nursing: assessment and management of clinical problems,* ed 7, St Louis, 2007, Mosby.)

  4. Teach use of incentive spirometer
    a. After exhaling, form seal around mouthpiece
      with lips
    b. Take slow, continuous deep breath and hold
      indicator afloat for several seconds before exhaling
    c. Repeat 10 times per hour or as ordered
  5. Perform percussion and vibration for several
    minutes over affected areas being managed with
    postural drainage
  6. Encourage coughing and expectoration of secretions;
    provide tissues and appropriate receptacle
  7. Allow rest periods as needed; avoid scheduling near
    meal times
  8. Evaluate color and amount of secretion, quality of
    breath sounds after procedure
  9. Encourage a 2- to 3-L fluid intake daily to liquefy
    secretions

Chest Tubes

A. Definition
  1. Use of tubes and suction to return negative pressure
    to the intrapleural space, expands lungs by
    removing positive pressure from the pleural space
  2. To drain air from intrapleural space, a chest
    tube is placed in second or third intercostal
    space; to drain blood or fluid, catheter would
    be placed at a lower site, usually eighth or ninth
    intercostal space (Figure 7-4: Chest tube placement)

B. Commercial drainage systems
  1. Water-seal drainage system (e.g., PleurEvac)
    (Figure 7-5: Water seal drainage system)
    a. Calibrated collection chamber for drainage
    b. Water-seal chamber: prevents atmospheric air
      from entering pleural space; fluid level fluctuates

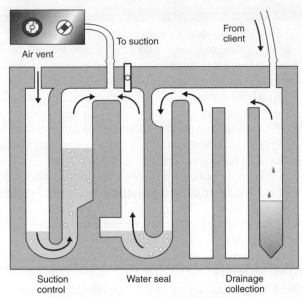

Air vent • **To suction** • **From client**

Suction control • Water seal • Drainage collection

Figure 7-5 Water-seal drainage system. (From Ignatavicius DD, Workman ML: *Medical-surgical nursing: critical thinking for collaborative care,* ed 5, St Louis, 2006, Saunders.)

with respirations until lung is fully expanded; continuous bubbling may indicate air leak; requires instillation of sterile fluid to 2-cm level and then set up for use

   c. Suction control chamber: controls amount of suction, requires instillation of sterile fluid usually to 10 to 20 cm H_2O; when set up for use bubbling indicates suction level is maintained

2. Dry suction water-seal drainage system: has three chambers like water-seal drainage, but does not require fluid in the suction control chamber; quieter than traditional water-seal drainage

3. One-way valve systems (e.g., Heimlich valve): used to remove air from the pleural space; valve prevents air from reentering pleural space

C. Nursing care

1. Ensure that the tubing is not kinked and is positioned on mattress to avoid dependent loops; tape all connections to prevent separation

2. "Milking and stripping" chest tubes is generally not a safe practice because it increases negative intrapleural pressure and does not significantly affect tube patency; consult agency policy

3. Maintain drainage system below level of chest

4. Turn client frequently, making sure chest tubes are not compressed and are free of restrictions to prevent accidental dislodgement

5. Monitor and mark drainage in system; report drainage on dressing immediately since this is not a normal occurrence

6. Observe for fluctuation of fluid in water-seal chamber (tidalling); the level will rise on inhalation and fall on exhalation; if there are no fluctuations, either the lung has expanded fully or the chest tube is clogged; length of time for lung expansion depends on etiology

7. Palpate the area around the chest tube insertion site for subcutaneous emphysema or crepitus, which indicates that air is leaking into subcutaneous tissue; usually a benign finding

8. Situate the drainage system to avoid breakage

9. Place two clamps at the bedside for use when changing systems or if a leak is suspected; clamps are used judiciously and only in emergency situations because they can cause tension pneumothorax

10. Encourage movement, coughing, and deep breathing every 2 hours, splinting the area as needed; assess breath sounds; effective pain management improves compliance

11. Assess for tracheal deviation, a sign of tension pneumothorax

12. Verify that chest radiography has been done before chest tubes are removed

13. If wall suction is stopped, ensure that system is open to atmosphere so air from the pleural space can escape

14. Instruct the client to exhale or strain (Valsalva maneuver) as the tube is withdrawn by physician; apply a gauze dressing immediately and firmly secure to make an airtight dressing

Mechanical Ventilation

A. Definition: use of a mechanical device to maintain ventilation and oxygenation using positive or negative pressure

B. Types of ventilators

1. Negative pressure ventilators create a negative pressure chamber around the chest; operate on the same principle as the iron lung used for polio victims in the past, but are fitted to the individual (e.g., Pneumowrap, Tortoise shell)

2. Positive pressure ventilators

   a. Pressure-cycled: delivers a volume of gas with positive pressure during inspiration; used for short term

   b. Volume-cycled: delivers a preset tidal volume of inspired gas regardless of pressure; most commonly used

   c. Time-cycled: delivers volume of gas for a predetermined inspiratory time; not generally used for adults

C. Modes of ventilation

1. Controlled mandatory ventilation (CMV): client receives a specified volume and rate with no triggering of the machine by the client; the nurse may have to administer drugs such as pancuronium bromide (Pavulon) or morphine to decrease the client's own respiratory response

2. Assist-control ventilation (ACV): client triggers the machine so that the rate may vary; however, if

client has apnea, the machine will initiate respirations at a preset tidal volume

3. Intermittent mandatory ventilation (IMV): client receives a predetermined tidal volume and number of breaths per minute; client controls respirations between mechanical ventilations; rate can be gradually reduced as a client is weaned from the ventilator; rarely used today

4. Synchronized intermittent mandatory ventilation (SIMV): same as IMV but the ventilator breaths are synchronized with the client's own breaths; often used for weaning

5. Pressure support ventilation (PSV): client initiates all breaths, which are then supplemented by positive pressure, improving the tidal volume and reducing respiratory efforts; may be used alone or with IMV/SIMV

6. Positive end-expiratory pressure (PEEP): maintains positive pressure at the end of expiration to keep alveoli open, increasing the functional residual capacity (FRC)

7. Proportional assist ventilation (PAV): synchronizes with and augments client's inspiratory efforts proportionately

8. Continuous positive airway pressure (CPAP): similar to PEEP but exerts positive pressure throughout the respiratory cycle; the client must be breathing spontaneously; used without intubation or mechanical ventilation; used with a tight-fitting face or nose mask; indicated for sleep apnea or heart failure

9. Bi-level positive airway pressure ventilation mode (BiPAP): noninvasive method to deliver air through nose and mouth; inspiratory positive airway pressure (IPAP) and expiratory positive airway pressure (EPAP) are different; will deliver breath if client's rate falls below preset frequency (f)

D. Nursing care
1. Maintain ventilator settings and notify respiratory department and physician if distress occurs

2. Maintain a sealed system between the ventilator and the client so that volume to be delivered is kept constant and air is not lost around the tubing; this is accomplished by inflating the cuff of the endotracheal tube or tracheostomy tube to the minimum occlusive volume

3. Prevent high-pressure alarm: perform suction as needed (humidified oxygen helps liquefy secretions); use bite block if client is biting endotracheal tube; consult with physician about need for sedative or neuromuscular blocking agent if client seems to "fight" or "buck" ventilator

4. Prevent low-pressure alarm: secure connections between tubes and ventilator, maintain endotracheal or tracheostomy tube cuff pressure; may need to ventilate manually if caused by ventilator problem

5. Assess for signs of respiratory insufficiency such as adventitious breath sounds, hypoventilation, tachypnea, cyanosis, and changes in sensorium

6. Check pulse oximetry and blood gases as ordered to determine effectiveness of ventilation

7. Establish a means of communication because client will be unable to speak while on a ventilator

8. Provide oral care, and suction oral cavity as needed

9. Provide tracheostomy care or endotracheal tube care as per agency policy

10. Participate with respiratory therapist to gradually increase spontaneous breathing trials (SBTs) to wean hemodynamically stable client from ventilator; a T-piece can be used to supply supplemental oxygen through the artificial airway during the trials

Oxygen Therapy

A. Definition: administration of supplemental oxygen to prevent or treat tissue hypoxia

B. Methods: depend on client's condition
1. Nasal cannula: 1 to 6 L/min (24% to 43%); least restrictive

2. Simple mask: 5 to 8 L/min (40% to 60%)

3. Partial rebreathing mask: 8 to 11 L/min (50% to 90%)

4. Nonrebreather mask: 12 to 15 L/min (90% to 100%)

5. Venturi mask: delivers precise percentage of oxygen inspired (Figure 7-6: Venturi mask)

C. Nursing care
1. Monitor for signs of hypoxia: agitation, confusion, lethargy, pallor, diaphoresis, tachycardia, cyanosis (late)

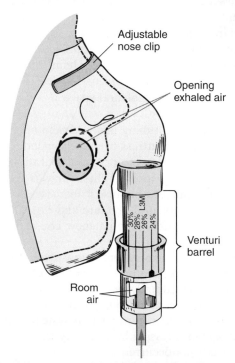

Figure 7-6 Venturi mask. (From Potter PA, Perry AG: *Fundamentals of nursing*, ed 7, St Louis, 2009, Mosby.)

2. Monitor arterial O_2 saturation as ordered with pulse oximeter
   a. Attach sensor, usually to finger or earlobe; avoid extremity with impediment to blood flow
   b. Check preset alarm for O_2 saturation (Sao_2); if less than 85%, adjustment is needed
3. Maintain safety precautions (O_2 supports combustion): place "oxygen in use" sign on door; remind client and visitors not to smoke or use faulty electric devices; be aware of fire extinguishers and O_2 turn-off valve
4. To prevent CO_2 narcosis, verify client does not have COPD before administering high concentration of O_2
5. Provide for humidification of O_2 flow rates greater than 4 L/min to prevent drying of secretions
6. Specific care related to method
   a. Cannula—care for nares with water-soluble lubricant
   b. Rebreather masks—ensure that bag does not deflate completely
   c. Venturi mask—set L/min to deliver specified Fio_2; use appropriate adapter to mix room air with O_2; ensure ports are not obstructed

Suctioning of Airway

A. Definition
   1. Mechanical aspiration of mucous secretions from the tracheobronchial tree by application of negative pressure
   2. Used to maintain a patent airway, obtain a sputum specimen, or stimulate coughing
   3. May be nasotracheal, oropharyngeal, or through an endotracheal or tracheostomy tube
B. Nursing care
   1. Place client in semi-Fowler's position
   2. Obtain vital signs and auscultate breath sounds for presence of secretions
   3. Assess functioning of equipment before and after use
   4. Hyperoxygenate by increasing flow rate; encourage deep breathing or manually ventilate with 100% O_2
   5. Lubricate the sterile suction catheter with sterile saline, water, or water-soluble gel
   6. Insert the catheter: if tracheal suction is being used, insert to the end of the tube (approximately 4 inches); if nasotracheal suction is being used, insert until the cough reflex is induced or resistance is met; when resistance is met, withdraw catheter 2 cm before initiating suction
   7. Apply no suction while the catheter is being inserted
   8. Rotate and withdraw the catheter while suction is applied; do not exceed 10 to 15 seconds
   9. Clear the catheter with sterile solution and encourage the client to breathe deeply
   10. Discontinue suctioning and hyperoxygenate for distress or O_2 desaturation; reassess vital signs and breath sounds

Thoracentesis

A. Definition
   1. Removal of fluid or air from pleural space; done for diagnostic purposes or to alleviate respiratory distress; a needle biopsy of pleura may be done
   2. No more than 1000 mL of fluid should be removed at a time; fluid withdrawn should be sent to the laboratory for culture and sensitivity, analysis of glucose and protein levels, and pH determination
   3. Complications include pneumothorax from trauma to the lung and pulmonary edema resulting from sudden fluid shifts
B. Nursing care
   1. Obtain an informed consent
   2. Ensure that chest x-ray examination is done before and after the procedure
   3. Support the client in the sitting position
   4. Inform the client not to cough during the procedure to prevent trauma to lungs
   5. Assess vital signs before, during, and after the procedure
   6. Note and record the amount, color, and clarity of the fluid withdrawn
   7. Position client on opposite side for 1 hour to promote lung expansion if tolerated; obtain chest x-ray film
   8. Observe the client for coughing, decreased breath sounds, bloody sputum, and rapid pulse rate and report their occurrence immediately
   9. Monitor for subcutaneous emphysema (crepitus)

Tracheostomy Care

A. Definition: removal of dried secretions from the cannula to maintain a patent airway, prevent infection, and prevent irritation
B. Nursing care
   1. Provide tracheostomy care at least every 8 hours
   2. Suction to remove secretions from the lumen of the tube (see Suctioning of Airway under Related Procedures)
   3. If an inner cannula is present
      a. Remove disposable inner cannula and replace with new one using sterile technique
      b. Care for nondisposable inner cannula using surgical aseptic technique; remove and place in peroxide; remove secretions within the cannula with a sterile brush; rinse with normal saline; drain excess saline before reinserting the tube, which is then locked in place
   4. Clean around the stoma with saline, using sterile technique; apply antiseptic ointment if ordered
   5. Change the tracheostomy tape or use commercially available ties, being careful not to dislodge the cannula; request assistance to secure tracheostomy tube; tie with a double knot
   6. Place a tracheostomy dressing or fenestrated 4 × 4 inch (unfilled) dressing below the stoma to absorb expelled secretions
   7. Humidify inhaled air if ordered because air is bypassing normal humidification process in the nasopharynx

MAJOR DISORDERS OF THE RESPIRATORY SYSTEM

✻ PULMONARY EMBOLISM AND INFARCTION

Data Base

A. Etiology and pathophysiology
1. Emboli develop from thrombi in peripheral circulation; associated with venous stasis resulting from immobility, coagulopathy, vascular disease, surgery, aging, oral contraceptives, obesity, and constrictive clothing
2. When an embolus lodges in the pulmonary artery, causing hemorrhage and necrosis of lung tissue, it is called a pulmonary infarction
B. Clinical findings
1. Subjective: sudden onset of severe dyspnea; anxiety; restlessness; sharp pleuritic chest pain
2. Objective: increased temperature, pulse rate, and respirations; violent coughing with hemoptysis; diaphoresis; spiral CTs of the chest, V/Q (ventilation-perfusion) scans, and pulmonary angiography are diagnostic measures to identify nonperfused areas of the lung; D-dimer assay to identify the end products of fibrin clot degradation in venous blood serves as a marker for the presence of venous clots
C. Therapeutic interventions
1. Anticoagulation with heparin IV until therapeutic PTT is attained; sodium warfarin is used for maintenance therapy
2. Thrombolytic therapy if respiratory status is severely compromised
3. Angiography; if the condition is severe, an embolectomy may be indicated
4. Vena caval interruption; a filter (Greenfield or umbrella) may be implanted in inferior vena cava, preventing passage of large thrombi
5. Infusion of dobutamine (Dobutrex) for hypotension

Nursing Care of Clients With Pulmonary Embolism and Infarction

A. Assessment/Analysis
1. Data related to causative factors, especially surgery of the pelvic floor or lower extremities
2. Presence of clinical findings
B. Planning/Implementation
1. Place in the high-Fowler's position, administer oxygen
2. Auscultate breath sounds, monitor Sao$_2$, and ECG
3. Monitor for hypoxemia and right heart failure
4. Administer thrombolytics/anticoagulants as ordered; monitor for bleeding
5. Administer analgesics to reduce pain and decrease anxiety
6. Maintain calm environment to decrease fear
7. Educate client regarding anticoagulants and prevention of thrombophlebitis

C. Evaluation/Outcomes
1. Maintains acceptable breathing patterns
2. Exchanges adequate gases to maintain tissue perfusion
3. Verbalizes feelings of control over situation

✻ PULMONARY EDEMA

Data Base

A. Etiology and pathophysiology
1. An acute emergency condition characterized by a rapid accumulation of fluid in lung tissue and alveolar spaces, resulting from increased pressure within the pulmonary system caused by acute heart failure
2. Possible causes include myocardial infarction, valvular disease, or hypertension leading to left-ventricular failure; circulatory overload, aspiration of gastric contents, drowning, or severe CNS damage
B. Clinical findings
1. Subjective: history of shortness of breath, paroxysmal nocturnal dyspnea, wheezing, and orthopnea; acute anxiety, apprehension, restlessness
2. Objective: rapid, thready pulse and rapid respirations; pink, frothy sputum; wheezing; crackles; pallor or cyanosis; cold, clammy skin; JVD; low PO$_2$; elevated PCWP and CVP
C. Therapeutic interventions
1. O$_2$ in high concentrations may require intubation and mechanical ventilation
2. Fowler's position
3. Morphine to reduce anxiety and peripheral resistance
4. Reduction of preload with diuretics, nitrates for vasodilation, and possible phlebotomy
5. Reduction of afterload with antihypertensive drugs such as nitroprusside
6. Support of cardiac function with inotropic drugs such as dobutamine
7. Hemodynamic monitoring and possible intraaortic balloon pump

Nursing Care of Clients With Pulmonary Edema

A. Assessment/Analysis
1. Presence of clinical findings (e.g., crackles, wheezes, JVD, frothy or blood-tinged sputum, decreased Sao$_2$)
2. Signs of hypoxemia
3. Precipitating factors
B. Planning/Implementation
1. Support client in the orthopneic, high-Fowler's, or semi-Fowler's position with legs dependent
2. Observe and record vital signs, Sao$_2$, ECG, and intake and output
3. Provide a reassuring environment and morphine sulfate to allay anxiety
4. Maintain O$_2$; suction secretions as needed to maintain a patent airway
5. Administer and monitor effects of medications to reduce preload and afterload

6. Prevent complications of bed rest: pressure ulcers, venous stasis, constipation, deconditioning
7. Educate client regarding pharmacology and prevention of heart failure

C. Evaluation/Outcomes
1. Demonstrates activity tolerance within level of cardiac function
2. Maintains adequate gas exchange
3. Verbalizes decreased anxiety

✿ PNEUMONIA
Data Base
A. Etiology and pathophysiology
1. Inflammatory disease of the lung; may cause a collection of pus (empyema) or fluid (pleural effusion) or consolidation within the pleural space
2. May be caused by an infectious agent (bacterial, viral, or fungal) but may also be caused by inhalation of chemicals and aspiration of gastric contents
   a. Community-acquired pneumonia (CAP) is most commonly caused by *Streptococcus pneumoniae* (pneumococcal), *Haemophilus influenzae*, *Legionella pneumophila*, *Mycoplasma pneumoniae*, *Chlamydia* species (*Chlamydia pneumoniae*; more common *psittaci*); viruses
   b. Hospital-acquired pneumonia (HAP) is most commonly caused by *Staphylococcus aureus*, *Pseudomonas aeruginosa*, *Klebsiella pneumoniae*, *Serratia marcescens*, *Streptococcus pneumoniae* (pneumococcal), *Haemophilus influenzae*; misuse of antimicrobial agents led to the emergence of resistant strains such as methicillin-resistant *Staphylococcus aureus* (MRSA)
   c. Aspiration pneumonia occurs when the normal flora of the upper respiratory tract, gastric contents, or chemicals are aspirated into the lung
   d. Pneumonias in immunocompromised hosts include *Pneumocystis* pneumonia (PCP) caused by *Pneumocystis jiroveci* and other fungal pneumonias (e.g., aspergillosis) and *Mycobacterium tuberculosis*
   e. Severe acute respiratory syndrome (SARS): rapidly spreading atypical pneumonia caused by a new coronavirus (SARS-CoV); death rate 10% for people less than 64 years of age and 50% for those more than 64 years of age; health care workers at particular risk because of exposure before implementation of infection control precautions
3. Risk factors include age, COPD, alcoholism, smoking, neutropenia, ineffective cough, immobility, HIV infection, endotracheal intubation
4. Pneumonia is commonly spread by respiratory droplets

B. Clinical findings
1. Subjective: lassitude; dyspnea; chest pain that increases on inspiration

2. Objective
   a. Elevated temperature, increased WBCs
   b. Chest x-ray shows pulmonary infiltration
   c. Cough with sputum production; culture identifies pathogen
      (1) Pneumococcal: purulent, rusty sputum
      (2) Staphylococcal: yellow, blood-streaked sputum
      (3) *Klebsiella* species: red, gelatinous sputum
      (4) Mycoplasmal: nonproductive that advances to mucoid sputum

C. Therapeutic interventions
1. Culture and sensitivity tests on blood and sputum to determine appropriate antibiotic; specimen must be obtained before antimicrobial therapy is started
2. Antimicrobial therapy: antibiotics, antiviral, or antifungal therapy; *Aspergillus* infection is treated with amphotericin B, azole agents such as itraconazole, or the newer antifungal agents, echinocandins such as caspofungin (Cancidas)
3. Respiratory support including O_2, intubation, and ventilation as needed
4. Nutritional supplementation and fluid and electrolyte replacement
5. Bronchodilators
6. Chest physiotherapy and suctioning as needed
7. For SARS: no effective vaccine or treatment identified; supportive care
8. Global surveillance plan to limit influenza and SARS pandemic

Nursing Care of Clients With Pneumonia
A. Assessment/Analysis
1. Vital signs, breathing patterns, Sao_2
2. Color, amount, and consistency of sputum
3. Adventitious sounds on auscultation of lung
4. Mental status changes

B. Planning/Implementation
1. Encourage coughing and deep breathing after chest physiotherapy, splinting the chest as necessary
2. Collect morning sputum specimen for culture and sensitivity tests in sterile container; notify the physician if organism is resistant to the antibiotic being given
3. Increase fluid intake to 3 L daily to thin secretions
4. Maintain semi-Fowler's position
5. Monitor for signs of respiratory distress, such as labored respirations; cool, clammy skin; cyanosis; and change in mental status
6. Balance rest periods to conserve O_2 with activity to mobilize secretions
7. Instruct client to cover nose and mouth when coughing; dispose of tissues properly
8. Administer antibiotics as ordered
9. Teach preventive measures, including the following: role of nutrition and fluids; avoidance of respiratory irritants; vaccination against *Streptococcus pneumoniae* and influenza; balance of activity and rest; cessation of smoking; oral hygiene

10. Follow agency policy regarding transmission-based precautions
11. Nursing care associated with SARS
    a. Use contact precautions (gloves, gowns, and eye protection); airborne precautions (N-95 disposable respirators)
    b. Place client in negative-pressure isolation room
    c. Provide client with surgical mask until infection control precautions can be implemented and during transport in hospital or to home
    d. Isolate client in home for 10 days after resolution of fever and respiratory symptoms
    e. Teach client and family members transmission-based precautions to be followed in home
C. Evaluation/Outcomes
    1. Maintains patent airway and adequate Sao_2
    2. Performs activities of daily living (ADLs) without assistance
    3. Abstains from smoking

PULMONARY TUBERCULOSIS (TB)
Data Base
A. Etiology and pathophysiology
    1. Infection of lungs caused by *Mycobacterium tuberculosis*, an acid-fast bacterium, commonly transmitted by inhalation of droplets
    2. Macrophages surround the bacilli and form a fibrous tissue mass around a Ghon tubercle; necrosis and calcification of the mass within the lungs causes the bacilli to be dormant; future compromised immune responses can cause the Ghon tubercle to ulcerate and activate the bacilli
    3. Predisposing factors include substance abuse, diabetes mellitus, antirejection drugs used in organ transplants, HIV infection, cirrhosis, and other debilitating diseases, as well as inadequate nutrition, crowded living conditions, institutionalization (e.g., prisons, psychiatric institutions), and immigration from countries with high prevalence
    4. The emergence of drug-resistant TB has complicated management of the disease
    5. Chronic; progressive; reinfection phase frequently is encountered in adults and involves progression or reactivation of primary lesions after months or years of latency
    6. Swallowing infected sputum may lead to laryngeal, oropharyngeal, and intestinal TB; TB may also involve bone, kidneys, and meninges
B. Clinical findings
    1. Subjective: malaise; pleuritic pain; easy fatigability
    2. Objective
        a. Fever, night sweats, weight loss; cough that progressively becomes worse; hemoptysis
        b. Chest x-ray film may reveal presence of active or calcified lesions, pleural effusion
        c. Analysis of sputum and gastric contents shows presence of acid-fast bacilli

d. QuantiFERON TB Gold (QFT-G) test detects the release of interferon-gamma when the blood of a client who has been exposed to TB is incubated with synthetic peptides representing protein present in the TB bacillus; results are available in less than 24 hours and more specific than the tuberculin skin test
e. Tuberculin skin test (Mantoux test) involves intradermal injection of purified protein derivative (PPD) from tubercle bacillus extract
    (1) Determines antibody response to TB bacillus; induration of 10 mm or greater 48 to 72 hours later indicates a positive finding; induration of 5 mm may also be significant, particularly for immunocompromised clients
    (2) A positive finding indicates prior infection; may or may not indicate active disease state (a sudden change from negative to positive requires follow-up)
    (3) Immunocompromised clients may not have a positive reaction despite being infected with *M. tuberculosis*
    (4) Clients who have received bacille Calmette-Guérin (BCG) vaccine will also continue to have a positive reaction
C. Therapeutic interventions
    1. Multiple antituberculin drugs for 8 weeks in the initial treatment phase, followed by 4- to 7-month continuation phase during which two drugs are continued (see Antituberculars under Related Pharmacology)
    2. Bed rest until symptoms abate or therapeutic regimen is established
    3. Surgical resection of the involved lobe if symptoms such as hemorrhage develop or chemotherapy is unsatisfactory; rarely done
    4. Isoniazid (INH) preventive therapy (IPT) for 6 to 12 months to immediate contacts (all cases and follow-up of contacts must be reported to public health agency)
    5. High-carbohydrate, high-protein, high-vitamin diet with supplemental vitamin B_6 to counter INH side effects

Nursing Care of Clients With Pulmonary Tuberculosis
A. Assessment/Analysis
    1. Detailed history related to exposure, travel, or BCG inoculation
    2. Fatigue, anorexia, low-grade fever, and night sweats
    3. Sputum for color, amount, and consistency
B. Planning/Implementation
    1. Teach client to provide for scheduled rest periods
    2. Teach which foods to include in the diet and which are nutritious between-meal supplements
    3. Help client plan a realistic schedule for taking the large number of necessary medications

4. Teach the importance of continued follow-up and adherence, without variation, to the drug program that has been established; monitor compliance
5. Instruct client to be alert to the early symptoms of adverse drug reactions (e.g., optic and peripheral neuritis, eighth cranial nerve damage, nephrotoxicity, hepatitis, dermatitis) and to contact the physician immediately if any occur
6. Use standard precautions and airborne precautions with high-efficiency particulate air (HEPA) filter; teach the proper techniques to prevent spread of infection to family members and others: frequent handwashing; covering the mouth when coughing; using and disposing of tissues properly; cleansing of eating utensils and disposal of food wastes
7. Encourage coughing and deep breathing
8. Encourage client to express feelings about disease and the many ramifications (stigma, isolation, fear) it creates

C. Evaluation/Outcomes
   1. Performs ADLs without shortness of breath
   2. Maintains adequate body weight
   3. Complies with treatment regimen
   4. Attains sputum free of *M. tuberculosis*

OBSTRUCTIVE AIRWAY DISEASES

Data Base

A. Etiology and pathophysiology
   1. Asthma: reversible bronchospasms, mucosal edema, and increased secretions that last an hour or more; severity classified as mild intermittent, mild persistent, moderate persistent, or severe persistent; an asthmatic attack that is difficult to control is referred to as status asthmaticus (asthma is no longer grouped together with other diseases that comprise the broad classification of COPD but is included here for review of common clinical findings and care)
   2. Chronic obstructive pulmonary disease (COPD): progressive airflow limitation associated with inflammatory response; four stages classified as mild, moderate, severe, and very severe
      a. Chronic bronchitis: inflammation of the bronchial walls with hypertrophy of the mucous goblet cells; characterized by a chronic cough
      b. Emphysema: characterized by distended, inelastic, or destroyed alveolar walls; these alterations greatly impair the diffusion of gases through the alveolar capillary membrane and increase air trapping, making exhalation difficult
   3. Traditionally it was believed that clients with COPD become accustomed to an elevated residual carbon dioxide level and did not respond to high CO_2 concentrations as the normal respiratory stimulant, responding instead to a drop in O_2 concentration in the blood; newer theories (e.g., Haldane effect) suggest the adverse effects of administering high concentrations of O_2 are caused by the inability of

the O_2-saturated hemoglobin molecules to transport CO_2, leading to increased hypercapnia
   4. May precipitate pulmonary hypertension, cor pulmonale, right ventricular heart failure, or pneumothorax

B. Clinical findings
   1. Subjective: anxiety, restlessness, fatigue, and weakness; dyspnea; headache; impaired sensorium
   2. Objective
      a. Orthopnea, expiratory wheezing, stertorous breathing sounds, cough
      b. Barrel chest, cyanosis, clubbing of fingers, use of accessory muscles; pursed lip breathing (COPD)
      c. Increased P_{CO_2} and decreased P_{O_2} of arterial blood gases; polycythemia (COPD)
      d. Decreased forced expiratory volume; increased residual volume
      e. Distended neck veins, peripheral edema (with right heart failure)

C. Therapeutic interventions
   1. Medications to reduce airway restriction and inflammation (see Bronchodilators and Antiasthmatics under Related Pharmacology in this chapter) Antibiotics and Antivirals under Related Pharmacology in Chapter 3, and Adrenocorticoids under Related Pharmacology in Chapter 9)
   2. Antibiotics to prevent/treat infection
   3. Mucolytics and expectorants to liquefy secretions and to facilitate their removal
   4. Oxygen at 1 to 3 L even if hypoxia is severe
   5. Respiratory therapy program to include nebulizer therapy, postural drainage, and exercise
   6. High-protein soft diet in small, frequent feedings is most easily tolerated
   7. Pneumococcal and influenza vaccines to decrease risk of pneumonia
   8. Surgery for end-stage emphysema: lung volume reduction; lung transplant

Nursing Care of Clients With Obstructive Airway Disease

A. Assessment/Analysis
   1. History of increased symptoms: during early morning, in cold weather, when sleeping, and when smoking
   2. Breathing patterns: abdominal, paradoxical, pursed lip, asynchronous; breath sounds, orthopnea
   3. Frequency of respiratory tract infections
   4. Evidence of chronic and acute hypoxia
   5. Nutritional status

B. Planning/Implementation
   1. Monitor vital signs, SaO_2, breath sounds, and arterial blood gases
   2. Emphasize smoking cessation and avoidance of other external irritants, such as dust and allergens, as much as possible
   3. Supervise client's respiratory exercises, such as pursed-lip or diaphragmatic breathing; orthopneic position aids in exhalation

4. Encourage participation in physical conditioning program
5. Provide fluids to maintain hydration
6. Teach proper use of inhalers and other special equipment (e.g., spacer, peak flow meter)
7. Carefully observe for symptoms of hypoxia and CO_2, intoxication (CO_2 narcosis) such as restlessness, mental confusion
8. Teach client to adjust activities to avoid overexertion and exposure to cold
9. Teach client to avoid crowds and people with respiratory tract infections
10. Teach the client to avoid the use of sedatives or hypnotics, which could compromise respirations
11. Teach client to maintain the highest resistance possible by getting adequate rest, eating nutritious food, dressing properly for weather conditions, maintaining fluid intake, receiving vaccinations against pneumonia and influenza
12. Teach client to be alert for early symptoms of infection, hypoxia, hypercapnia, or adverse response to medications including glucocorticoids
13. Encourage client to continue with close medical supervision
14. Encourage client to express feelings about disease and therapy
15. Assist client to cope effectively with lifelong activity restrictions
16. Encourage client and family to take an active role in planning therapy
17. Prevent complications of bed rest

C. Evaluation/Outcomes
1. Demonstrates pursed-lip breathing and diaphragmatic breathing
2. Describes and complies with treatment regimen
3. States methods for reducing/controlling feelings of anxiety/fear

✤ PNEUMOTHORAX/CHEST INJURY

Data Base

A. Etiology and pathophysiology
1. Collapse of a lung resulting from disruption of the negative pressure that exists within the intrapleural space caused by the presence of atmospheric air in the pleural cavity (should be differentiated from atelectasis, a collapse of alveoli caused by airway obstruction)
2. Reduces the surface area for gaseous exchange and leads to hypoxia and retention of CO_2 (hypercapnia)
3. Types
   a. Spontaneous or simple: thought to occur when a weakened area of the lung (bleb) ruptures; air then moves from the lung to the intrapleural space, causing collapse; highest incidence is in men 20 to 40 years of age
   b. Traumatic: disruption of pleural space by invasive chest procedures, laceration (e.g., a stab wound)

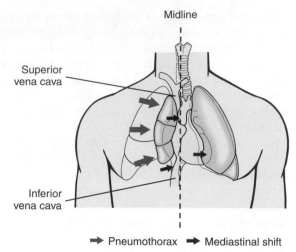

Figure 7-7 Tension pneumothorax. As pleural pressure on the affected side increases, mediastinal displacement ensues, with resultant respiratory and cardiovascular compromise. (From Lewis SL et al: *Medical-surgical nursing: assessment and management of clinical problems,* ed 7, St Louis, 2007, Mosby.)

through the chest wall into the intrapleural space, or penetration by a fractured rib
   c. Hemothorax: collection of blood within the pleural cavity often accompanies traumatic pneumothorax; blood disrupts negative pressure of pleural space
   d. Tension: buildup of pressure as air accumulates within the pleural space; the pressure increase causes the lung to collapse, which results in a mediastinal shift (pressure displaces the trachea, esophagus, heart, and great vessels toward the unaffected side), causing increased thoracic pressure, reduced venous return, and decreased cardiac output (Figure 7-7: Tension pneumothorax)
4. Flail chest: instability of chest wall related to fractures of the ribs or detached sternum; caused by blunt trauma

B. Clinical findings
1. Subjective: sudden unilateral pleuritic chest pain, may be described as mild discomfort or as sharp and increasing on exertion; dyspnea; anxiety, drowsiness
2. Objective
   a. Tachycardia; hypotension; rapid, shallow respirations (nonsymmetric); diaphoresis
   b. Flail chest: loose chest segment moves inward during inspiration and outward during expiration (paradoxical respiration)
   c. Breath sounds on the affected side will be diminished or absent
   d. Chest x-ray examination will reveal extent of the pneumothorax
   e. Increased P_{CO_2}; decreased P_{O_2}

C. Therapeutic interventions
1. Bed rest initially
2. Analgesics and antibiotics
3. Return of negative pressure in the intrapleural space by the insertion of chest tubes attached to suction
4. Restoration of blood volume loss as a result of trauma

Nursing Care of Clients With Pneumothorax

A. Assessment/Analysis
1. Auscultation of lung fields for diminished or absent breath sounds
2. Chest percussion for hyperresonance and palpation for tracheal deviation toward unaffected side in tension pneumothorax
3. Chest motion during inhalation/exhalation
4. Vital signs, Sao_2
5. Skin for changes in color

B. Planning/Implementation
1. Maintain constant supervision until stable
2. Maintain patency of chest tubes (see Chest Tubes under Related Procedures)
3. Place in high-Fowler's position
4. Offer fluids frequently
5. Monitor vital signs, particularly respirations, breath sounds, and Sao_2

C. Evaluation/Outcomes
1. Maintains adequate gas exchange
2. Verifies reduction or absence of chest pain

✾ MALIGNANT LUNG TUMORS

Data Base

A. Etiology and pathophysiology
1. Carcinoma of the lungs may be primary or metastatic
2. Smoking is the most significant risk factor; inhalation of carcinogens responsible for 80% to 90% of cases
3. Leading type of cancer that causes death
4. Incidence highest in men older than 60 years; incidence in women is increasing
5. Symptoms may occur after metastasis to other organs such as the lymph nodes, bone, liver, adrenal glands, mediastinal organs, kidneys, and brain
6. Classification and incidence of lung cancers: adenocarcinoma, 30% to 40%; epidermoid (squamous cell), 30%; small cell (oat cell carcinoma), 20% to 25%; large cell (undifferentiated), 10% to 15%
7. Staging based on tumor size, node involvement, and presence of metastasis

B. Clinical findings
1. Subjective: dyspnea; chills; fatigue; chest pain
2. Objective: persistent cough; change in voice quality; hemoptysis; unilateral wheeze; weight loss; clubbing of fingers; chest x-ray film reveals pleural effusion and "coin" lesions; CT scans and MRI detect metastasis; bronchial washings and brushings from bronchoscopy, CT-guided needle biopsy, and cytologic test of sputum positive for cancer cells

C. Therapeutic interventions
1. Surgical
   a. Lobectomy: removal of one lobe of the lung when the lesion is limited to one area
   b. Wedge resection: removal of a small segment for confined lesion; may also be done for biopsy
   c. Pneumonectomy: removal of an entire lung
   d. Thoracentesis for pleural effusion (see Related Procedures)
2. Radiation therapy may be used as an adjunct therapy or to alleviate symptoms of pain, dyspnea, and hemoptysis
3. Chemotherapy (see Related Pharmacology under Neoplastic Disorders in Chapter 3)

Nursing Care of Clients With Malignant Lung Tumors

A. Assessment/Analysis
1. Sputum quantity and characteristics
2. Lung auscultation for absent breath sounds
3. Chest percussion for dullness over tumors
4. Respirations for shallowness, stridor, and use of accessory muscles
5. Persistent cough

B. Planning/Implementation
1. Monitor vital signs, breath sounds, Sao_2
2. Encourage coughing and deep breathing
3. Change client's position frequently; semi-Fowler's or high-Fowler's position promotes greater lung expansion
4. After pneumonectomy, most commonly positioned on operative side to promote lung expansion; assess position of trachea for mediastinal shift
5. Provide specific care based on therapy being used: care of client with chest tubes (see Related Procedures), radiation therapy, and chemotherapy (see General Nursing Care of Clients With Neoplastic Disorders in Chapter 3)
6. Provide high-protein, high-calorie diet and supplements
7. Use interventions to manage pain: analgesics, distraction, relaxation, imagery

C. Evaluation/Outcomes
1. Verbalizes a reduction of pain
2. Maintains adequate Sao_2
3. States understanding of treatment
4. Breathes with minimal effort

✾ CANCER OF THE LARYNX

Data Base

A. Etiology and pathophysiology
1. Most tumors of the larynx (vocal cords, epiglottis, and laryngeal cartilages) are squamous cell carcinoma
2. Cigarette smoking, secondhand smoke, air pollution, asbestos, chronic respiratory tract infections, heavy alcohol consumption, and voice strain appear to be related to increased incidence
3. More common in men 50 to 70 years of age

B. Clinical findings
1. Subjective: sore throat; dyspnea; dysphagia; weakness
2. Objective: increasing hoarseness; weight loss; enlarged cervical lymph nodes; foul breath; dysphagia

C. Therapeutic interventions
   1. Radiation therapy
   2. Chemotherapy is not curative but is used preoperatively to decrease tumor size; postoperatively, chemotherapy is used to decrease metastasis
   3. Surgical intervention
      a. Partial laryngectomy used in early stages; one vocal cord and part of larynx removed with tumor
      b. Total laryngectomy: removal of total larynx with construction of a permanent tracheal stoma
      c. Radical neck dissection (used when the tumor has metastasized into surrounding tissue and lymph nodes): removal of larynx, surrounding tissue and muscle, lymph nodes, and glands with a permanent tracheal stoma; chest tubes may be needed if thoracic duct leakage occurs; total parenteral nutrition (TPN) if needed
      d. Laser: to eradicate small tumors, vocal cord tumors, or in conjunction with chemotherapy

Nursing Care of Clients With a Total Laryngectomy

A. Assessment/Analysis
   1. Voice for hoarseness
   2. Oropharyngeal inspection for masses
   3. Neck palpation for masses and nodal enlargement
B. Planning/Implementation
   1. Provide time to discuss the diagnosis and the ramifications of surgery
   2. Encourage the client to express feelings
   3. Involve family in preoperative planning
   4. Arrange for individuals with laryngectomies to visit and discuss the rehabilitative process
   5. Establish methods of communication that will be used after surgery (e.g., slate board and chalk, pencil and paper, sign language, electronic voice)
   6. Observe for obstruction of airway by mucous plugs, edema, or blood (e.g., air hunger, dyspnea, cyanosis, gurgling); keep head elevated
   7. Observe for signs of hemorrhage (e.g., increased pulse rate, drop in blood pressure, cold clammy skin, appearance of blood on dressing, frequent swallowing)
   8. Provide, at the bedside, suction apparatus and catheters (additional laryngectomy tube and a surgical instrument set with additional hemostats should be immediately available in case tube becomes dislodged or blocked)
   9. Suction the laryngectomy tube as necessary (see Suctioning of Airway under Related Procedures)
   10. Provide hydration and humidity to compensate for loss of normal humidification of air in the nasopharynx; later the stoma may be covered with a moistened, unfilled gauze pad
   11. Expect and accept a period of mourning, but prevent withdrawal from reality by involving in laryngectomy care; keeping channels of communication open; supporting strengths; encouraging a return to ADLs
   12. Encourage the client to become involved in speech therapy (esophageal, electric larynx, tracheoesophageal puncture)
   13. Teach skills necessary to handle altered body functioning: tracheobronchial suctioning; changing, cleaning, and securing the laryngectomy tube; care of skin around the stoma; providing humidified air for inspiration to prevent drying of secretions (can be achieved by use of moist dressing or cloth bib)
   14. Teach the client to avoid activities that may permit water or irritating substances to enter the trachea; avoid showers (unless wearing a protective cover), swimming, dust, high winds, hair spray, and other volatile substances
   15. Teach the client to avoid wearing clothes with constricting collars or necklines
   16. Teach the client that certain other activities will be impossible (e.g., sipping through a straw, whistling, blowing the nose)
   17. Teach the client to drink fluids and use a humidifier to keep secretions loose
C. Evaluation/Outcomes
   1. States a reduction in feelings of fear
   2. Maintains patent airway
   3. States acceptance of body image

ACUTE RESPIRATORY DISTRESS SYNDROME (ARDS)

Data Base

A. Etiology and pathophysiology
   1. Respiratory failure as a complication of trauma, aspiration, prolonged mechanical ventilation, severe infection, open heart surgery, fat emboli, shock
   2. Involves
      a. Alveolar capillary damage with loss of fluid and pulmonary edema
      b. Impaired alveolar gas exchange causes V/Q mismatch and shunting; tissue hypoxia results
      c. Alteration in surfactant production; decreased lung compliance
      d. Atelectasis, resulting in labored and inefficient respiration
B. Clinical findings
   1. Subjective: restlessness; anxiety; dyspnea
   2. Objective: tachycardia; grunting respirations; intercostal retractions; cyanosis; Pco_2 initially decreased and later increased and decreased Po_2; chest x-ray examination shows pulmonary edema
C. Therapeutic interventions
   1. Relieve the underlying cause
   2. Mechanical ventilation with positive end-expiratory pressure (PEEP): this setting on

a mechanical ventilator maintains positive pressure within the lungs at the end of expiration, which increases the residual capacity, reducing hypoxia

3. Interleukin-1 receptor antagonists, surfactant replacement therapy, antioxidants, and corticosteroids may be used
4. Maintenance of fluid volume and nutrition

Nursing Care of Clients With Acute Respiratory Distress Syndrome

A. Assessment/Analysis
   1. Vital signs, especially characteristics of respirations
   2. Breath sounds, Sao_2, ECG
   3. Pain that increases on inspiration
B. Planning/Implementation
   1. Allow frequent rest periods between therapeutic interventions
   2. Provide tranquil, supportive environment; sedation is contraindicated because of its depressant effect on respirations unless mechanically ventilated
   3. Observe behavioral changes and vital signs because confusion and hypertension may indicate cerebral hypoxia
   4. Auscultate breath sounds to observe for signs of pneumothorax when the client is on PEEP (lung tissue that is frail may not withstand increased intrathoracic pressure, and pneumothorax occurs)
   5. Monitor arterial blood gases, as ordered; use a heparinized syringe
   6. Maintain a patent airway
   7. Care for the client on mechanical ventilation (see Mechanical Ventilation under Related Procedures)
   8. Establish system for communication when client is intubated
   9. Measure central venous and pulmonary artery pressures
   10. Change client's position frequently
C. Evaluation/Outcomes
   1. Maintains adequate gas exchange
   2. Communicates reduction in anxiety
   3. Performs activities without respiratory distress or fatigue

CARBON MONOXIDE POISONING

Data Base
A. Etiology and pathophysiology: carbon monoxide combines with hemoglobin more readily than does O_2, resulting in tissue anoxia; caused by inadequately vented combustion devices
B. Clinical findings
   1. Subjective: headache; dizziness; confusion; palpitations; weakness
   2. Objective: color normal, cyanotic, or flushed, but usually cherry pink; paralysis; loss of consciousness; ECG changes; elevated carboxyhemoglobin levels
C. Therapeutic interventions
   1. Mechanical ventilation with 100% O_2 until carboxyhemoglobin is reduced to less than 5% and respirations are normal
   2. Hyperbaric pressure chamber to increase O_2 concentration and accelerate formation of CO_2, which can be exhaled

Nursing Care of Clients With Carbon Monoxide Poisoning

A. Assessment/Analysis
   1. History to determine extent of exposure
   2. Color of skin
   3. Level of consciousness
B. Planning/Implementation
   1. Remove the individual from the immediate area of poisoning
   2. Monitor cardiopulmonary and neurologic function
   3. Institute cardiopulmonary resuscitation if necessary and maintain until additional help arrives
   4. Administer O_2 as prescribed
   5. Maintain respirations with assistance if needed
   6. Maintain body temperature
   7. Monitor vital signs, with special concern for respirations and breath sounds
   8. Determine whether accidental or intentional; obtain a psychiatric referral if cause was intentional
C. Evaluation/Outcomes
   1. Maintains adequate O_2 levels
   2. Remains conscious and alert

Nursing Care of Clients With Gastrointestinal System Disorders

OVERVIEW

REVIEW OF ANATOMY AND PHYSIOLOGY

Functions of the Gastrointestinal System

Digestion

A. All changes to food in the alimentary canal occur so it can be absorbed and metabolized

B. Types
1. Mechanical digestion: movements of the alimentary tract that
   a. Change physical state of foods
   b. Propel food along the alimentary tract
      (1) Deglutition: swallowing
      (2) Peristalsis: wavelike movements that squeeze food downward in the tract
      (3) Sequential contractions: movements that mix gastric and intestinal contents with digestive juices
2. Chemical digestion: series of hydrolytic processes dependent on specific enzymes and chemicals; an additional substance may be necessary to act as a catalyst to facilitate the process

Absorption

A. Passage of small molecules from food sources through the intestinal mucosa into the blood or lymph

B. Accomplished mainly through the movement of molecules against a concentration gradient because of energy (adenosine triphosphate [ATP]) expenditure (active transport) by the intestinal cells; makes it possible for water and solutes to move through the intestinal mucosa in a direction opposite that expected in osmosis and diffusion

C. Majority occurs in the small intestine; most water is absorbed from large intestine

Metabolism

A. Definition: sum of all chemical reactions in body engaged in energy production and expenditure

B. Anabolism: synthesis of various compounds from simpler compounds

C. Catabolism: metabolic process in which complex substances are broken down into simple compounds; energy is liberated for use in movement, energy storage, and heat production

D. Metabolism of carbohydrates
1. Glucose transport through cell membranes and phosphorylation
   a. Insulin promotes transport of glucose and amino acids through cell membranes
   b. Glucose phosphorylation: conversion of glucose to glucose 6-phosphate; insulin increases the activity of glucokinase and promotes glucose phosphorylation, which is essential before both glycogenesis and glucose catabolism
2. Glycogenesis: conversion of glucose to glycogen for storage in liver and muscle cells
3. Glycogenolysis
   a. In muscle cells glycogen is catabolized to glucose 6-phosphate
   b. In liver cells glycogen is converted to glucose; glucagon and epinephrine accelerate liver glycogenolysis
4. Glucose catabolism
   a. Glycolysis: breakdown of one glucose molecule into two pyruvic acid molecules, with conversion of about 5% of energy stored in glucose to heat and ATP molecules
   b. Krebs citric acid cycle with the electron transport chain: breakdown of two pyruvic acid molecules into six carbon dioxide and six water molecules; Krebs cycle releases about 95% of the energy stored in glucose
5. Gluconeogenesis: chemical reaction that converts protein or fat compounds into glucose; occurs in liver cells
6. Principles of carbohydrate metabolism
   a. Principle of preferred energy fuel: most cells catabolize glucose first, sparing fats and proteins; when the glucose supply becomes inadequate, most cells catabolize fats next; nerve cells require glucose, thus causing proteins to be sacrificed to provide the amino acids needed to produce more glucose (gluconeogenesis); small amounts of glucose can be made from the glycerol portion of fats
   b. Principle of glycogenesis: glucose in excess of about 120 to 140 mg per 100 mL of blood brought to liver cells undergoes glycogenesis and is stored as glycogen
   c. Principle of glycogenolysis: when blood glucose concentration decreases below the midpoint of expected level, liver glycogenolysis accelerates and tends to raise the blood glucose concentration back toward the midpoint of expected level
   d. Principle of gluconeogenesis: when blood glucose concentration decreases below expected level or when the amount of glucose entering the cells is

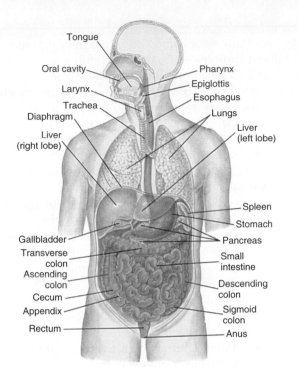

Tongue
Oral cavity
Larynx
Trachea
Diaphragm
Liver
(right lobe)
Pharynx
Epiglottis
Esophagus
Lungs
Liver
(left lobe)
Spleen
Stomach
Pancreas
Gallbladder
Transverse colon
Ascending colon
Cecum
Appendix
Rectum
Small intestine
Descending colon
Sigmoid colon
Anus

Figure 8-1 Structures of the digestive system. (From Thompson et al: *Mosby's clinical nursing*, ed 4, St Louis, 1997, Mosby.)

inadequate, liver gluconeogenesis accelerates and raises blood glucose levels

e. Principle of glucose storage as fat: when the blood insulin content is adequate, glucose in excess of the amount used for catabolism and glycogenesis is converted to fat

Structures of the Gastrointestinal System

(Figure 8-1: Structures of the digestive system)

Mouth (Buccal Cavity)

A. Lips and cheeks
B. Hard palate; soft palate
C. Gums (gingivae); teeth
D. Tongue
   1. Papillae: rough elevations on surface
   2. Taste buds: receptors of cranial nerves VII (facial) and IX (glossopharyngeal); located in papillae
E. Tonsils: lymphatic tissue that produces lymphocytes; defense against infection
F. Salivary glands
   1. Parotid, submandibular, and sublingual
   2. Produce saliva, a mixture of water, mucin, salts, and the enzyme salivary amylase (ptyalin)

Esophagus

A. Posterior to the trachea; anterior to the vertebral column
B. Extends from the pharynx through an opening in the diaphragm (hiatus) to the stomach
C. Collapsible muscular tube; about 25 cm (10 inches) long
D. Secretes mucus; facilitates movement of food

Stomach

A. Size varies in different persons and according to degree of distention

B. Elongated pouch, with greater curve forming the lower left border
C. In epigastric and left hypochondriac portions of the abdominal cavity
D. Divisions
   1. Fundus: the uppermost portion; the bulge adjacent to and extending above the esophageal opening
   2. Body: central portion
   3. Pylorus: constricted lower portion
E. Sphincters
   1. Cardiac: at opening of the esophagus into the stomach
   2. Pyloric: at opening of the pylorus into the duodenum
F. Secretes gastric juice
   1. Stomach wall cells secrete gastrin that stimulates the flow of gastric juices
   2. Chief cells secrete pepsin
   3. Parietal cells secrete hydrochloric acid and intrinsic factor
   4. Goblet cells secrete mucin
G. Functions: food storage and liquefaction (chyme)

Small Intestine

A. Size: approximately 2.5 cm (1 inch) in diameter; 6.1 m (29 feet) in length when relaxed
B. Divisions
   1. Duodenum: joins pylorus of the stomach; C-shaped
   2. Jejunum: middle section
   3. Ileum: lower section; no clear boundary between jejunum and ileum
C. Functions: digestion and absorption; enzymes include sucrase, lactase, and maltase; cholecystokinin stimulates release of bile from the gallbladder
D. Processes: mixing movements; peristalsis; secretion of water, ions, mucus; receives secretions from the liver, gallbladder, and pancreas

Large Intestine

A. Size: approximately 6.3 cm (2.5 inches) in diameter; 1.5 m (5 to 6 feet) long when relaxed
B. Divisions
   1. Cecum: first 2 to 3 inches
   2. Colon: consists of ascending, transverse, descending, and sigmoid colon
   3. Rectum: last 7 to 8 inches
   4. Anus: terminal opening of the alimentary canal
C. Functions: water and sodium ion absorption; temporary storage of fecal matter; defecation
D. Processes: weak mixing movements, mass movements, and peristalsis

Vermiform Appendix

A. Blind-end tube off the cecum just beyond the ileocecal valve
B. Function: part of the immune system

Liver

A. Occupies most of the right hypochondrium and part of the epigastrium
B. Divided into thousands of lobules

C. Ducts
   1. Hepatic duct: from liver
   2. Cystic duct: from gallbladder
   3. Common bile duct: formed by the union of the hepatic and cystic ducts; drains bile into the duodenum at the sphincter of Oddi
D. Functions
   1. Carbohydrate metabolism: converts glucose to glycogen by glycogenesis, converts glycogen to glucose by glycogenolysis, and forms glucose from proteins and fats by gluconeogenesis
   2. Fat metabolism
      a. Ketogenesis: fatty acids are broken down into molecules of acetyl coenzyme A (acetyl-CoA) (beta oxygenation), which then form ketone bodies (acetoacetic acid, acetone, beta-hydroxybutyric acid)
      b. Fat storage
      c. Synthesis of triglycerides, phospholipids, cholesterol, and B complex factor choline
   3. Protein metabolism
      a. Anabolism: synthesis of various blood proteins (e.g., prothrombin, fibrinogen, albumins, alpha and beta globulins, and clotting factors V, VII, IX, and X)
      b. Deamination: chemical reaction by which amino group is split off from amino acid to form ammonia and a keto acid
      c. Urea formation: liver converts most of ammonia formed by deamination to urea
   4. Secretes bile, a substance important for emulsifying fats before digestion and as a vehicle for excretion of cholesterol and bile pigments
   5. Detoxifies various substances (e.g., drugs, hormones)
   6. Vitamin metabolism: stores vitamins A, D, K, and B_{12}; bile salts needed to absorb fat-soluble vitamins A, D, E, and K
   7. Intestinal bacteria produce almost all vitamin K produced in the body

Gallbladder
A. Lies on the undersurface of the liver
B. Sac made of smooth muscle, lined with mucosa arranged in rugae
C. Functions: concentrates and stores bile

Pancreas
A. Structure
   1. Fish-shaped, with body, head, and tail; extends from the duodenal curve to the spleen
   2. A duct and ductless gland
      a. Pancreatic cells: secrete pancreatic juice via a duct to the duodenum; enzymes include trypsin, lipase, and amylase; stimulated by the duodenal hormones secretin and pancreozymin and by parasympathetic impulses
      b. Islets of Langerhans: clusters of cells not connected with pancreatic ducts; composed of alpha and beta cells

B. Functions
   1. Pancreatic juice composed of enzymes that help digest carbohydrates, proteins, and fats
   2. Islet cells constitute the endocrine gland
      a. Alpha cells secrete the hormone glucagon, which accelerates liver glycogenolysis and initiates gluconeogenesis; tends to increase blood glucose level
      b. Beta cells secrete insulin, which exerts a profound influence on the metabolism of carbohydrates, proteins, and fats
         (1) Accelerates the active transport of glucose, along with potassium and phosphate ions, through cell membranes; decreases blood glucose level and increases glucose utilization by the cells for either catabolism or anabolism
         (2) Stimulates the production of liver cell glucokinase; promotes liver glycogenesis, which lowers blood glucose concentration
         (3) Inhibits liver cell phosphatase and therefore inhibits liver glycogenolysis
         (4) Accelerates the rate of amino acid transfer into cells, promoting anabolism of proteins within the cells
         (5) Accelerates the rate of fatty acid transfer into cells, promotes fat anabolism (lipogenesis); inhibits fat catabolism

REVIEW OF NUTRIENTS
Sources of Energy
A. Carbohydrates (4 g per 1 calorie): sugars (simple) and starches (complex); help provide basic fuel for energy (see Metabolism of carbohydrates under Functions of the Gastrointestinal System); food sources: sugars, honey, fruit, milk, syrups, bread, cereal, potatoes, rice, legumes, and flour products such as pasta, crackers, cake, and cookies
B. Proteins (4 g per 1 calorie): basically amino acids and are necessary for body growth, development, and normal functioning; protein is needed to maintain nitrogen balance; food sources: meat, fish, poultry, dry beans, eggs, nuts, milk, and cheese
C. Fats (9 g per 1 calorie): include neutral fats, oils, fatty acids, cholesterol, and phospholipids; contribute to cellular transport; dietary source of fuel and fuel reserve; vitamin absorption and transport; insulation and protection afforded by adipose tissue; food sources: animal fat, coconut and palm oil, dairy products, whole milk, vegetable oils, butter, margarine, mayonnaise, salad dressings, and baked goods and snacks that contain significant fat

Vitamins
A. Organic compounds needed to catalyze metabolic processes; essential for growth, development, and maintenance of body processes

B. Types
1. Vitamin A: fat-soluble vitamin needed for night vision, healthy epithelium, skeletal and tooth development, and energy regulation; sources: carrots, cantaloupe, sweet potatoes, apricots, squash, broccoli, cabbage, spinach and collards, fortified milk products, egg yolk, liver, and kidney; deficiency: slow adaptation to dim light, sinus problems, sore throat, epithelial thickening of tissue over the eye
2. Vitamin D: fat-soluble vitamin that enhances bone mineralization by promoting absorption of calcium, normal muscle contraction; sources: sunlight, cod liver oil, fortified milk; deficiency: rickets (soft, fragile bones, skeletal deformities), osteomalacia (softening of bone causing flexible, brittle bones, skeletal deformities), tetany resulting from low serum calcium level (vitamin D necessary for calcium absorption)
3. Vitamin E: fat-soluble vitamin that is an antioxidant; sources: vegetable oils, whole grains, wheat germ, milk, eggs, meats, fish, and leafy vegetables; deficiency: muscle weakness, anemia; rarely occur
4. Vitamin K: fat-soluble vitamin associated with blood clotting and bone metabolism; 50% produced by intestinal bacteria; sources: liver, green leafy vegetables (lettuce, spinach, cabbage, kale, broccoli, Brussels sprouts), cauliflower, asparagus; deficiency: prolonged antibiotic therapy and fat absorption problems, which contribute to prolonged blood clotting time
5. Vitamin C: water-soluble vitamin associated with wound and fracture healing, antioxidant, adrenal gland function, iron absorption, and folic acid conversion; sources: citrus fruits, tomatoes, green and red peppers, white potatoes, cabbage, broccoli, kale, asparagus, chard, turnip greens, berries, melons, pineapple and guavas; deficiency: (scurvy) tender, sore, bleeding gums; loose teeth; small skin hemorrhages and bleeding around joints, stomach, and heart; ends of long bones soften; delayed wound healing
6. B-complex vitamins: B_1 (thiamine), B_2 (riboflavin), B_3 (niacin), pyridoxine, folic acid, B_{12} (cyanocobalamin), B_6 (pantothenic acid), and biotin; function as coenzymes, each having its own action; sources: each has its own; deficiency: each has its own clinical findings; often seen in clients who drink alcohol, experience weight loss, consume excessive sugar; may turn urine bright yellow

Minerals
A. Inorganic substances that regulate body functions; help build body tissues; most important minerals: calcium, sodium, potassium, iron, iodine, and fluorine (see Table 3-5: Fluid/Electrolyte Imbalances: Etiology, Assessments, and Treatments)

B. Types
1. Calcium: needed for bone and tooth growth, coagulation, nerve conduction, and muscle contraction; sources: milk and dairy products, leafy green vegetables, whole grains, nuts, legumes, and seafood
2. Sodium: major role in fluid balance, transmission of electrochemical impulses along nerve and muscle membranes; sources: table salt, processed foods, milk and milk products (for additional foods, see foods to avoid in Low-sodium diet under Review of Diets)
3. Potassium: regulates fluid balance, conduction of nerve impulses, and muscle contraction, especially the heart; sources: oranges, bananas, dried apricots or peaches, cantaloupe, prune juice, baked potato with skins, pinto beans, winter squash, lima beans, broccoli
4. Iron: essential to hemoglobin and myoglobin formation, constituent of enzyme systems; sources: liver, lean meat, eggs, spinach, fortified cereals, dried beans
5. Iodine: component of thyroid hormones, which help regulate metabolism, cell function and growth; sources: saltwater fish, shellfish and seaweed, table salt fortified with iodine
6. Fluoride (ionized form of fluorine): maintains bone structure and strengthens tooth enamel; sources: added to water, toothpaste, mouthwashes, and provided with supplements

REVIEW OF DIETS

A. MyPyramid diet: recommended by the U.S. Department of Agriculture, Center for Nutrition Policy and Promotion (Figure 8-2: MyPyramid); includes food groups appropriate for a healthy diet; amounts individually calculated based on personal characteristics and needs; recommended number of calories decreases with aging
B. Clear liquid diet: minimizes stimulation of the gastrointestinal tract; examples: clear broth, bouillon, clear juices, plain gelatin, fruit-flavored water, ices, ginger ale, coffee, tea
C. Full liquid diet: for a client with a GI disturbance or inability to tolerate solid or semi-solid food; may follow a clear liquid diet postoperatively; examples: all foods on a clear liquid diet plus milk and items made with milk, such as cream soups, milk drinks, sherbet, ice cream, puddings, custard, yogurt
D. Soft diet: for clients who have difficulty chewing or swallowing; examples: all foods on clear and full liquid diets plus soft, refined cereals, pasta, rice, white bread and crackers, eggs, cheese, shredded or chopped meat, potatoes, cooked vegetables, soft cake, bread pudding, cooked fruits, and a few soft ripe plain fruits without membranes or skins
E. Regular diet: full, well-balanced diet of all foods as desired and tolerated; generally 2000 calories or as ordered by physician

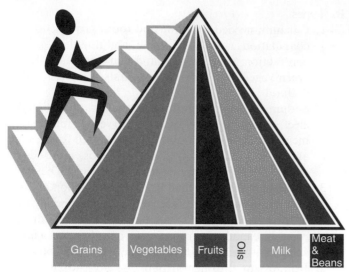

Figure 8-2 MyPyramid. In the MyPyramid, each food group is characterized by varying widths, representative of the proportion of each group that should be eaten. The person climbing the side of the pyramid indicates the need to include daily physical activity in a healthy lifestyle. (Modified from U.S. Department of Agriculture, Center for Nutrition Policy and Promotion; available at www.Mypyramid.gov.)

F. Low-residue diet: minimizes fecal volume and residue; used for severe diarrhea, partial bowel obstruction, and during an acute episode of inflammation of the bowel; can be used in the progression to a regular diet; foods to avoid: milk and milk products, food with seeds, nuts, grains, and raw or dried vegetables and fruits

G. High-fiber diet: foods high in fiber resist digestion, causing a bulky stool that increases peristalsis; increases water content of stool; sources: whole grain foods, bran, root vegetables and their skins, prunes, nuts, fruits, beans

H. Restrictive diets: individually designed to meet specific needs of client
   1. Low-sodium diet: diet may include fresh fish, meat and poultry, fresh or frozen vegetables, pasta, unsalted butter, cooking oil, coffee, tea, lemonade, unflavored gelatin, jam, jelly, honey and maple syrup, unsalted nuts and popcorn; foods to avoid: salt, monosodium glutamate, soy sauce, milk, cheese, processed luncheon meats and bacon, snack foods (chips, pretzels, etc.), bouillon, canned or packaged soup, rice/noodles, pickles, olives, sauerkraut, tomato juice, mustard, most bottled and canned drinks, canned vegetables unless low-sodium type, salad dressings, smoked or salted meat or fish, corned beef, powdered milk drinks, highly processed convenience foods, meat extracts, meat tenderizers, sugar substitutes containing sodium, and sauces such as catsup, tartar, horseradish, Worcestershire, and teriyaki
   2. Low-fat diet: to reduce saturated fat, reduce cholesterol, and prevent coronary heart disease; foods to avoid: candy, ice cream, cake, cookies, and fried foods; strategies to reduce dietary fat: grill, bake, broil, or microwave food; eat less meat; eat leaner cuts of meat; remove fat from meat and poultry before cooking; use skim milk; use less butter or margarine; eat more fish, lima beans, and navy beans for protein
   3. Calorie restriction: calories are restricted to reduce weight
   4. Renal diet: low sodium, potassium, protein, and possibly fluid restriction
   5. Nonallergic diet: food causing the allergic response is eliminated from diet
   6. Diabetic diet: recommended by the American Diabetic Association to control weight and nutritional intake

I. Consistency modifications: foods may be cut up, chopped, or pureed to make them easier for the client to ingest

REVIEW OF PHYSICAL PRINCIPLES

Law of Motion
The greater the force of contraction of the intestinal wall and the more frequent the contractions, the more rapid the propulsion of food and fecal matter through the digestive tract.

Light
A. Refraction: total internal reflection in fiberoptics permits viewing of interior walls of stomach (gastroscopy) and intestines (colonoscopy)
B. X-rays: GI series and barium enemas allow visualization of the soft tissues of the upper and lower gastrointestinal tract; the barium salts coat the inner walls of the tract and absorb the x-rays, outlining organ surfaces

REVIEW OF CHEMICAL PRINCIPLES

Oxidation and Reduction
A. Uniting oxygen with a substance results in oxidation
B. Uniting hydrogen with a substance results in reduction
C. Oxidation of nutrients such as glucose results in the formation of high-energy ATP molecules and heat
D. Some forms of life (anaerobes) can use substances other than oxygen for cellular oxidation (e.g., *Clostridium perfringens* found in gangrenous tissue)

Types of Compounds
Organic Acids
A. Lactic acid: end product of anaerobic muscle metabolism
B. Citric acid: one intermediate in the Krebs citric acid cycle

Amino Acids
A. Able to act as an acid and as a base (amphoteric character)
B. Essential amino acids cannot be synthesized well enough in the body to maintain health and growth and must be supplied in the food

Carbohydrates

A. Include simple sugars, starches, celluloses, gums, and resins; contain carbon, hydrogen, and oxygen
B. Classification
   1. Monosaccharide: a simple sugar (e.g., glucose, fructose)
   2. Disaccharide (e.g., sucrose, lactose, maltose)
   3. Polysaccharide (e.g., starch, glycogen)

Lipids

A. Fatty acids are important constituents of all lipids except sterols
   1. Usually straight-chain carboxylic acids; 3 fatty acids and 1 glycerol molecule form a triglyceride
   2. Saturated fatty acids: have no double bonds between their carbon atoms; solid at room temperature; mainly animal fats
   3. Unsaturated fatty acids: have one or more double bonds between their carbon atoms; liquid at room temperature
   4. Essential fatty acids: cannot be synthesized by the body; must be taken in by diet
B. Cholesterol: a sterol found in human and animal tissue; important component of cellular membranes; found in blood at normal levels of 150 to 200 mg/mL; high cholesterol associated with increased intake of saturated fats and arterial atherosclerosis

Proteins

A. Simple proteins
   1. Albumins: necessary for plasma colloid osmotic pressure (oncotic pressure), which helps control (through osmosis) the flow of water between the plasma and interstitial fluid; with starvation, a decreased serum albumin level causes a fall in the plasma colloid osmotic pressure; this results in edema as less fluid is drawn by osmosis into the capillaries from the interstitial spaces
   2. Globulins: necessary to form antibodies (e.g., serum gamma globulin)
B. Compound proteins
   1. Lipoproteins: simple proteins combined with lipid substances
      a. Low-density lipoprotein cholesterol (LDL)
         (1) Chief carriers of cholesterol; low in triglycerides
         (2) Contribute to atherosclerotic plaque formation
      b. High-density lipoprotein cholesterol (HDL)
         (1) Consist of 50% protein and 20% cholesterol
         (2) Inversely associated with coronary heart disease
   2. Nucleoproteins: proteins complexed with nucleic acids; chromosomes are sometimes referred to as nucleoprotein structures
      a. Ribonucleic acid (RNA) and deoxyribonucleic acid (DNA) are nucleic acids
      b. RNA and DNA store and transmit genetic information from one generation to another
   3. Metalloproteins: proteins containing metal ions (e.g., ferritin, the iron-transporting compound of plasma)

REVIEW OF PATHOGENS

A. Bacterial pathogens
   1. *Brucella:* small, gram-negative bacilli cause brucellosis, an infection that can be acquired by drinking infected milk
   2. *Escherichia coli:* small, gram-negative bacilli that is part of the normal flora of the large intestine; certain strains cause urinary tract infections and diarrhea
   3. *Clostridium difficile:* anaerobic, spore-forming bacterial pathogen; produces toxins that affect bowel mucosa; major cause of nosocomial diarrhea
   4. *Salmonella:* genus of gram-negative, rod-shaped bacteria; origin: raw foods of animal origin (poultry, eggs, dairy products, beef; also vegetables and fruit when irrigated or washed with contaminated water or packed with contaminated ice for transport)
   5. *Shigella:* gram-negative bacilli, similar to *Salmonella; Shigella dysenteriae* causes bacillary dysentery or shigellosis
B. Protozoal pathogens
   1. *Balantidium coli:* ciliated protozoan; causes enteritis
   2. *Entamoeba histolytica:* an amoeba; causes amebiasis (amoebic dysentery)
   3. *Giardia lamblia:* flagellated protozoan; causes enteritis
C. Parasitic pathogens
   1. Nematodes (roundworms): include *Necator americanus* (hookworm), *Ascaris lumbricoides, Enterobius vermicularis* (pinworm), *Trichuris trichiura* (whipworm), all of which may be found in the intestine
   2. Cestodes (tapeworm): may be found in adult form in the intestine; the larval stage (hydatid) of some forms may develop and form cysts in the liver, lungs, and kidneys
   3. Trematodes (flukes): may be found in the lungs, liver, and abdominal cavity

RELATED PHARMACOLOGY

Antiemetics

A. Description
   1. Diminish the sensitivity of the chemoreceptor trigger zone (CTZ) to irritants or decrease labyrinthine excitability
   2. Alleviate nausea and vomiting
   3. Prevent and control emesis and motion sickness
   4. Available in oral, parenteral (IM, IV), rectal, and transdermal preparations
B. Examples
   1. Centrally acting agents: ondansetron HCl (Zofran); prochlorperazine (Compazine); trimethobenzamide HCl (Tigan)
   2. Agents for motion sickness control: dimenhydrinate (Dramamine); meclizine HCl (Antivert, Bonine); promethazine HCl (Phenergan)
   3. Agents that promote gastric emptying: metoclopramide (Reglan)

C. Major side effects: drowsiness (CNS depression); hypotension (vasodilation via central mechanism); dry mouth (decreased salivation from anticholinergic effect); blurred vision (pupillary dilation from anticholinergic effect); incoordination (an extrapyramidal symptom resulting from dopamine antagonism)

D. Nursing care
1. Observe incidences and characteristics of vomitus, provide oral hygiene
2. Eliminate noxious substances from the diet and environment
3. Administer before chemotherapy to limit nausea and vomiting
4. Caution client to avoid engaging in hazardous activities
5. Offer sugar-free chewing gum or hard candy to promote salivation
6. Instruct client to change positions slowly
7. Offer soothing fluids or ice chips in small amounts

Anorexiants
A. Description
1. Suppress the desire for food at the hypothalamic appetite centers; generally produce CNS stimulation
2. Available in oral preparations
B. Examples: amphetamine sulfate (Benzedrine); dextroamphetamine sulfate (Dexedrine)
C. Major side effects: nausea, vomiting (irritation of gastric mucosa); constipation (delayed passage of stool in GI tract); tachycardia (sympathetic stimulation); CNS stimulation (sympathetic activation)
D. Nursing care
1. Educate client regarding
   a. Drug misuse (controlled substances)
   b. Concurrent exercise and diet therapy
   c. Need for medical supervision during therapy
   d. Possibility of affecting ability to engage in hazardous activities
2. Monitor weight

Antacids
A. Description
1. Provide a protective coating on the stomach lining and lower the gastric acid pH; allow more rapid movement of stomach contents into the duodenum
2. Neutralize gastric acid; effective in the treatment of ulcers
3. Available in oral preparations
B. Examples: aluminum hydroxide gel (Amphojel); aluminum and magnesium hydroxides (Maalox); sodium bicarbonate, a systemic antacid, may cause alkalosis
C. Major side effects
1. Constipation (aluminum compounds: aluminum delays passage of stool in GI tract)
2. Diarrhea (magnesium compounds: magnesium stimulates peristalsis in GI tract)
3. Alkalosis (systemic antacids: absorption of alkaline compound into the circulation)

4. Reduced absorption of calcium, iron, and most medications (increase in gastric pH)
D. Nursing care
1. Instruct the client regarding
   a. Prevention of overuse of antacids, which can result in rebound hyperacidity
   b. Need for continued supervision
   c. Dietary restrictions related to gastric distress
   d. Foods high in calcium and iron
   e. Need to take 1 hour before or 2 hours after other oral medications
2. Caution client on a sodium-restricted diet because many antacids contain sodium
3. Shake oral suspensions well before administration
4. Administer with small amount of water to ensure passage to stomach

Anticholinergics
A. Description
1. Inhibit smooth muscle contraction in the GI tract
2. Alleviate pain associated with peptic ulcer
3. Available in oral and parenteral (IM, IV) preparations
B. Examples: atropine sulfate; dicyclomine HCl (Bentyl); glycopyrrolate (Robinul); propantheline bromide (Pro-Banthine)
C. Major side effects (all related to decreased parasympathetic stimulation)
1. Abdominal distention and constipation (decreased peristalsis)
2. Dry mouth (decreased salivation)
3. Urinary retention (decreased parasympathetic stimulation)
4. CNS disturbances (direct CNS toxic effect) (e.g., blurred vision, dizziness)
D. Nursing care
1. Provide dietary counseling with emphasis on bland foods
2. Provide oral hygiene

Antisecretory Agents
A. Description
1. Inhibit gastric acid secretion
2. Act at the H_2 receptors of the stomach's parietal cells to limit gastric secretion (H_2 antagonists)
3. Inhibit hydrogen/potassium ATPase enzyme system to block acid production (proton pump inhibitors)
4. Available in oral and parenteral (IM, IV) preparations
B. Examples
1. H_2 antagonists: famotidine (Pepcid); ranitidine (Zantac)
2. Proton pump inhibitors: omeprazole (Prilosec); lansoprazole (Prevacid); esomeprazole magnesium (Nexium)
C. Major side effects
1. CNS disturbances (decreased metabolism of drug because of liver or kidney impairment)
2. Blood dyscrasias (decreased RBCs, WBCs, platelet synthesis)

3. Skin rash (hypersensitivity)
4. Decrease in bone density with long-term use of acid suppression medications esomeprazole (Nexium), lansoprazole (Prevacid), and omeprazole (Prilosec); similar but less risk with cimetidine (Tagamet) and famotidine (Pepcid)

D. Nursing care
1. Do not administer at same time as antacids; allow 1 hour before or 2 hours after other oral drugs
2. Administer oral preparations with meals
3. Assess for potentiation of oral anticoagulant effect
4. Instruct client to follow prescription exactly
5. Administration should not exceed 8 weeks without medical supervision

Antidiarrheals

A. Description
1. Slow passage of stool through intestines
2. Promote formation of formed stools; alleviate diarrhea
3. Available in oral and parenteral (IM) preparations

B. Examples
1. Fluid adsorbents: decrease the fluid content of stool: bismuth subcarbonate; kaolin and pectin (Kaopectate)
2. Enteric bacteria replacements: enhance production of lactic acid from carbohydrates in intestinal lumen; acidity suppresses pathogenic bacterial overgrowth; examples include *Lactobacillus acidophilus* (Bacid) and *Lactobacillus bulgaricus* (Lactinex)
3. Motility suppressants: decrease GI tract motility so that more water is absorbed from the large intestine: diphenoxylate HCl (Lomotil); loperamide HCl (Imodium)

C. Major side effects
1. Fluid adsorbents: GI disturbances (local effect); CNS disturbances (direct CNS toxic effect)
2. Enteric bacteria replacements: excessive flatulence (increased microbial gas production); abdominal cramps (increased microbial gas production)
3. Motility suppressants: urinary retention (decreased parasympathetic stimulation); tachycardia (vagolytic effect on cardiac conduction); dry mouth (decreased salivation from anticholinergic effect); sedation (CNS depression); paralytic ileus (decreased peristalsis); respiratory depression (depression of medullary respiratory center); constipation

D. Nursing care
1. Monitor bowel movements for color, characteristics, and frequency
2. Assess for fluid/electrolyte imbalance
3. Assess and eliminate cause of diarrhea
4. Motility suppressants
   a. Warn client of interference with ability to perform hazardous activities and risk of physical dependence with long-term use
   b. Offer sugar-free chewing gum and hard candy to promote salivation

Cathartics/Laxatives

A. Description
1. Alleviate or prevent constipation and promote evacuation of stool
2. Available in oral and rectal preparations

B. Examples
1. Intestinal lubricants: decrease dehydration of feces; lubricate intestinal tract; examples—mineral oil, olive oil
2. Fecal softeners: lower surface tension of feces, allowing water and fats to penetrate; examples—docusate calcium (Surfak), docusate sodium (Colace)
3. Bulk-forming laxatives: increase bulk in intestinal lumen, which stimulates propulsive movements by pressure on mucosal lining; examples—methylcellulose (Cellothyl), psyllium hydrophilic mucilloid (Metamucil)
4. Colon irritants: stimulate peristalsis by reflexive response to irritation of intestinal lumen; examples—bisacodyl (Dulcolax), senna (Senokot)
5. Saline cathartics: increase osmotic pressure within intestine, drawing fluid from blood and bowel wall, thus increasing bulk and stimulating peristalsis; examples—effervescent sodium phosphate (Fleet Phospho-Soda), magnesium citrate, Milk of Magnesia

C. Major side effects
1. Laxative dependence with long-term use (loss of normal defecation mechanism)
2. GI disturbances (local effect)
3. Intestinal lubricants: inhibit absorption of fat-soluble vitamins A, D, E, K; can cause anal leaking of oil (accumulation of lubricant near rectal sphincter)
4. Saline cathartics: dehydration (fluid volume depletion resulting from hypertonic state in GI tract); hypernatremia (increased sodium absorption into circulation; shift of fluid from vasculature to intestinal lumen)

D. Nursing care
1. Instruct client regarding overuse of cathartics and intestinal lubricants; increasing intake of fluids and dietary fiber; increasing activity level; compliance with bowel-retraining program
2. Monitor bowel movements for consistency and frequency of stool
3. Intestinal lubricants: use peripad to protect clothing
4. Bulk-forming laxatives: mix thoroughly in 8 oz of fluid and follow with another 8 oz of fluid to prevent obstruction
5. Administer at bedtime to promote defecation in the morning
6. Encourage to develop healthy bowel habits

Intestinal Antibiotics

See Aminoglycosides under Antibiotics in Related Pharmacology under Infection in Chapter 3

Pancreatic Enzymes

A. Description
1. Replace natural endogenous pancreatic enzymes (protease, lipase, amylase); promote digestion of proteins, fats, and carbohydrates
2. Available in oral preparations

B. Examples: pancrelipase (Viokase), Cotazym
C. Major side effects: nausea and diarrhea (GI irritation)
D. Nursing care
   1. Administer with meals or snacks
   2. Avoid crushing enteric-coated preparations
   3. Provide a balanced diet to prevent indigestion

RELATED PROCEDURES

Colostomy Irrigation

A. Definition
   1. Instillation of fluid into the lower colon via a stoma on the abdominal wall to stimulate peristalsis and facilitate the expulsion of feces
   2. Cleansing the colostomy stoma and collection of feces (stool consistency will depend on location of the ostomy; a colostomy of the sigmoid colon will tend to produce formed stools; a transverse or ascending colostomy will produce less-formed stools)
B. Nursing care
   1. Irrigate the stoma at the same time each day to approximate usual bowel habits; provide for uninterrupted bathroom use
   2. Insert a well-lubricated catheter tip (use a cone) into the stoma approximately 7 to 8 cm in the direction of the remaining bowel
   3. Hold the irrigating container 12 to 18 inches above the colostomy; temperature of irrigating solution should be 105° F (40.5° C)
   4. Stop the flow of fluid temporarily if cramping occurs
   5. Provide privacy while waiting for fecal returns or permit the client to ambulate with the collection bag in place to further stimulate peristalsis
   6. Cleanse the peristomal area with soap and water; apply a protective skin barrier
   7. Apply a colostomy bag with the opening ⅛ inch away from the stoma; use a gauze dressing if the colostomy is well regulated
   8. Teach the client to control odor when necessary by placing commercially available deodorizer in the colostomy bag

Endoscopy

A. Definition: visualization of internal organs of the body using a hollow tube with a lighted end: gastroscopy, stomach; esophagoscopy, esophagus; colonoscopy, large colon; proctoscopy, rectum; endoscopic retrograde cholangiopancreatography (ERCP), common bile and pancreatic ducts; capsule endoscopy, swallowed; virtual colonoscopy, series of computed tomography images of the intestine
B. Nursing care
   1. Obtain an informed consent for the procedure
   2. Ensure bilirubin level is greater than 3 to 5 mg/dL before a cholangiopancreatography (ERCP) because cannulization may cause edema, increasing obstruction
   3. If rectal examination is indicated, administer cleansing enemas before the test
   4. Restrict diet (NPO) before procedure
   5. After the procedure, observe for bleeding, changes in vital signs, or nausea
   6. If the throat is anesthetized (as for a gastroscopy or esophagoscopy), check for the return of gag reflex before offering oral fluids
   7. Assess for bleeding or clinical findings of pancreatitis
   8. Place in knee-chest position for sigmoidoscopy
   9. Provide nursing care before capsule endoscopy: instruct client to fast for 12 hours before test; apply antenna patch and belt holding battery and data recorder; instruct client to hold capsule under tongue for 1 minute as unit verifies that light source is functioning and then swallow capsule with 8 ounces of water
   10. Provide nursing care after ingestion of capsule endoscopic device: teach client to notify physician immediately if experiencing dysphagia, abdominal or chest pain, nausea/vomiting, or fever (risk for obstruction); avoid strong electromagnetic field source until capsule is defecated; avoid strenuous activity, bending, or stooping during test; check that recorder is working every 15 minutes; return the device after capsule is excreted

Enemas

A. Definitions
   1. Tap-water: introduction of water into the colon to stimulate evacuation
   2. Soapsuds: introduction of soapy water into the colon to stimulate peristalsis by bowel irritation; contraindicated as a preparation for an endoscopic procedure because it may alter the appearance of the mucosa
   3. Hypertonic: commercially prepared small-volume enema that works on the principle of osmosis
   4. Harris flush or drip: repeated alternate introduction of water into the colon and drainage of that water from the colon through the same tubing to facilitate exit of flatus
   5. Instillation/retention: introduction of a liquid (usually mineral oil) into the colon to facilitate fecal activity through lubricating effect
B. Nursing care
   1. Provide privacy, place client in the left side-lying or Sims' position
   2. Obtain the correct solution
   3. Lubricate the tip of a rectal catheter with water-soluble jelly
   4. Insert the catheter 3 to 4 inches into the rectum
   5. Allow the solution to enter slowly; keep it no more than 12 inches above the rectum; solution may be raised 15 to 18 inches for a high cleansing enema; temporarily interrupt flow if cramping occurs

6. Allow ample time for the client to expel the enema; encourage prolonged retention of an instillation/retention enema
7. Observe and record the amount and consistency of returns

Gastrointestinal Series

A. Definition: introduction of barium, an opaque medium, into the upper GI tract via the mouth (upper GI series) or into the lower GI tract via the rectum for the purpose of x-ray visualization for pathologic changes
B. Nursing care
1. Prepare the client for the procedure by
   a. Maintain the client NPO for 8 to 10 hours before the test
   b. Administering cathartics and/or enemas as ordered to evacuate the bowel
2. Inspect stool after the procedure for the presence of barium
3. Administer enemas and/or cathartics as ordered if the stool does not return as expected
4. Encourage fluid intake after the procedure

Gavage (Tube Feeding)

A. Definitions
1. Nasogastric tube (NGT): placement of a tube through the nose into the stomach (has the highest risk of aspiration of all types of feeding tubes)
2. Intestinal tube: placement of a tube through the nose into the small intestine
3. Surgically placed feeding tubes
   a. Cervical esophagostomy: tube is sutured directly into the esophagus for clients who have had head and neck surgery
   b. Gastrostomy (GT): tube is placed directly into stomach through the abdominal wall and sutured in place; used for clients who require tube feeding on a long-term basis
   c. Jejunostomy: tube is inserted directly into the jejunum for clients with pathologic conditions of the upper GI tract
4. Percutaneous endoscopic gastrostomy (PEG) and low-profile gastrostomy device (G-Button)
   a. Stomach is punctured during endoscopy procedure
   b. Associated with reduced risks, but accidental removal may occur; low risk with button
   c. Dressing should be changed daily; clean with sterile saline if exudate is present
B. Nursing care
1. Verify placement of tube before feeding
   a. Confirm by radiography before initiating tube feedings; test aspirate for acid pH (pH of 1 to 4 confirms gastric placement although can be as high as 6 if client is receiving drugs to reduce gastric acid); inject a small amount of air into the tube and, with a stethoscope placed over the epigastric area, listen for the passage of air into the stomach (less reliable than testing for gastric pH)
   b. Small-bore tube placement must be verified by x-ray examination
2. Aspirate contents of stomach before feeding to determine residual; follow physician's orders or agency policy regarding holding a feeding based on residual amounts; general guidelines: reinstill 300 mL to avoid electrolyte imbalance and call physician for orders; if residual is greater than half of last feeding call physician for orders or follow agency policy; some agencies delay tube feedings for 1 hour if residual amount specified is aspirated when volume is assessed
3. Intermittent feeding
   a. Position the client so that the head is elevated during the feeding
   b. Verify placement of tube
   c. Introduce 30 mL of water to verify the patency of the tube; the tube should not be allowed to empty during feeding
   d. Slowly administer the feeding to prevent regurgitation; administer at room or body temperature; observe and question the client to determine tolerance
   e. Administer 30 mL of water to clear the tube at the completion of the feeding
   f. Clamp the tubing and clean the equipment
   g. Place client in sitting position for 1 hour after feeding; place infant in right side-lying position
4. Continuous feeding
   a. Place prescribed feeding in gavage bag and prime tubing to prevent excess air from entering stomach
   b. Check for residual as per agency policy to verify peristalsis
   c. Set rate of flow; rate of flow can be manually regulated by setting drops per minute or mechanically regulated by using an infusion pump
   d. Position the client to keep the head elevated throughout the feeding
   e. Verify placement of tube every 4 hours; generally done when adding additional fluid to a continuous feeding
   f. Flush tube intermittently with water to prevent occlusion of tube with feeding; change tubing per protocol
   g. Monitor for gastric distention and aspiration; because smaller amounts of feeding are generally administered within a given period, gastric distention and subsequent aspiration are less frequent
   h. Discard unused fluid that has been in gavage administration bag at room temperature for longer than 4 hours
5. Care common for all clients receiving tube feedings
   a. Elevate head of bed: helps to prevent aspiration; facilitates gastric emptying and peristalsis
   b. Monitor for abdominal distention; changes in bowel sounds; assess for diarrhea caused by high osmolarity of feeding

c. Stop tube feeding if nausea and/or vomiting occur or if bowel sounds are not audible
d. Provide oral hygiene
e. When appropriate, encourage the client to chew foods that will stimulate gastric secretions while providing psychologic comfort; chewed food may or may not be swallowed
f. Provide special skin care; if the client has a gastrostomy tube sutured in place, the skin may become irritated from gastrointestinal enzymes; if the client has a nasogastric tube, the skin may become excoriated at point of entry because of irritation
g. Provide supplemental water to balance hypertonic formula if ordered by physician

Parenteral Replacement Therapy

A. Definitions
  1. Peripheral parenteral nutrition (PPN): short-term use
    a. Administration of isotonic lipid and amino acid solutions through a peripheral vein
    b. Amino acid content should not exceed 4%; dextrose content should not be greater than 10%; helps maintain a positive nitrogen balance
    c. Therapy usually limited to 2 weeks
  2. Total parenteral nutrition (TPN): long-term use
    a. Administration of carbohydrates, amino acids, vitamins, and minerals via a central vein because of high osmolality of the solution
    b. High-osmolality solutions (25% dextrose) are administered in conjunction with 5% to 10% amino acids, electrolytes, minerals, and vitamins; helps maintain a positive nitrogen balance
    c. Long-term home nutritional therapy may be delivered by atrial catheters (Hickman/Broviac or Groshong) that are surgically inserted
  3. Intralipid therapy
    a. Infusion of 10% to 20% fat emulsion that provides essential fatty acids
    b. Provides increased caloric intake to maintain positive nitrogen balance
  4. Total nutrient admixture (TNA or "3 in 1")
    a. Combination of dextrose, amino acids, and lipids in one container; vitamins and minerals may be used
    b. Administered through a central line over 24 hours
B. Nursing care
  1. Ensure proper placement of the tube by chest x-ray examination after insertion; accidental pneumothorax can occur during insertion
  2. Precisely regulate the fluid infusion rate; an intravenous pump should be used
    a. Rapid infusion may result in movement of the fluid into the intravascular compartment, causing dehydration, circulatory overload, and hyperglycemia
    b. Slow infusion may result in hypoglycemia because the body adapts to the high osmolality

of this fluid by secreting more insulin; for this reason, therapy is never terminated abruptly but is gradually discontinued
  3. Use aseptic technique when handling the infusion or removing soiled dressing
  4. Use a filter for TPN; filters not used for lipids
  5. Use surgical aseptic technique when changing tubing and applying a new dressing
  6. Record daily weights and monitor urinary glucose and acetone or blood glucose levels frequently
  7. Check laboratory reports daily, especially glucose, creatinine, BUN, and electrolytes; check serum lipids and liver function studies if lipids are administered
  8. Monitor temperature every 4 hours because infection is the most common complication of TPN; if the client has a temperature elevation, order cultures of blood, urine, and sputum to rule out other sources of infection

Paracentesis

A. Definition: removal of fluid from the peritoneum to reduce intraabdominal tension or obtain fluid for culture
B. Nursing care
  1. Obtain informed consent
  2. Have client void before procedure
  3. Position upright at edge of bed
  4. Assess vital signs after procedure; assess for clinical findings of hypovolemia, including pallor, oliguria, dyspnea, tachycardia; maintain pressure to dressing over needle insertion site

MAJOR DISORDERS OF THE GASTROINTESTINAL SYSTEM

OBESITY

Data Base

A. Etiology and pathophysiology
  1. Caloric intake exceeds metabolic needs
  2. Complex illness involving metabolic, genetic, and psychologic factors; one in three African-American and Hispanic-American adults is obese; one in four European-American adults is obese
  3. Research indicates that a stomach hormone, ghrelin, triggers hunger and may be a significant factor in managing weight for a small number of obese clients
  4. Major risk factor in coronary heart disease (CHD), brain attack, hypertension, diabetes, arthritis, asthma, bronchitis, and decreased respiratory function; also may increase the risk of endometrial, breast, colon, kidney, and gallbladder cancer, and degenerative joint disease
  5. Research shows that obese individuals are leptin resistant; leptin is thought to communicate to the brain when stored fat is sufficient and food intake should cease

B. Clinical findings
   1. Subjective: undesirable eating patterns; feelings of low self-esteem, depression, and disturbed body image; fatigue
   2. Objective
      a. Obesity—20% or more over ideal body weight
      b. Morbid obesity—100 lb or more over ideal body weight
      c. Triceps skinfold greater than 15 mm in men and greater than 25 mm in women
      d. Observed dysfunctional eating habits
      e. Behaviors that indicate low self-esteem, depression, and/or disturbed body image
C. Therapeutic interventions
   1. Weight reduction diet; exercise program; behavior modification
   2. Pharmacologic management: appetite suppressants (sibutramine [Meridia]); multivitamins; antidepressants; lipase inhibitors: orlistat (Xenical, 120-mg capsules; and Alli, 60-mg capsules)
   3. Bariatric surgery—surgery for morbid obesity
      a. Gastric bypass: stomach capacity reduced to less than 50 mL; proximal jejunum is transected and the distal end anastomosed to the newly created stomach; the proximal segment is anastomosed to the jejunum
      b. Vertical banded gastroplasty: a pouch is created with a band on the lower end of the stomach, providing a stoma that will not stretch
      c. Gastroplasty with circumgastric banding: an inflatable band placed around the fundus of the stomach limits stomach size; adjusted externally; reversible
      d. Body contouring surgery after weight loss: lipoplasty to remove fat deposits; panniculectomy to remove excess abdominal skinfolds
      e. Women of childbearing age should not become pregnant before surgery and for at least 1 to 2 years postoperatively

Nursing Care of Clients With Obesity

A. Assessment/Analysis
   1. Diet (24-hour recall, food frequency, and food diary), weight, and exercise history
   2. Family history of obesity
   3. Emotions just before eating
   4. Concurrent health problems and complications of obesity (Figure 8-3: Health risks associated with obesity)
   5. Adherence to weight reduction program
   6. Medication history for contributing factors; e.g., steroids contribute to weight gain
B. Planning/Implementation
   1. Review with client diet and eating patterns to increase awareness of amount and type of foods consumed, and emotions that affect intake

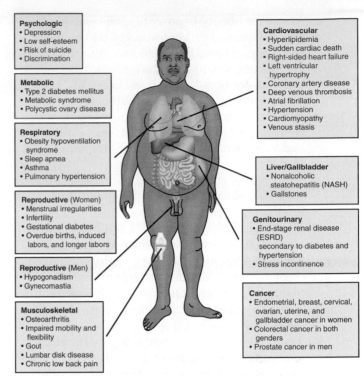

Figure 8-3 Health risks associated with obesity. (From Lewis SL et al: *Medical-surgical nursing: assessment and management of clinical problems*, ed 7, St Louis, 2007, Mosby.)

   2. Review high- and low-calorie foods, snacks, and beverages; determine how to achieve daily caloric intake
   3. Teach behavior modification techniques
   4. Encourage small plates, preparation of small portions, eating slowly, and chewing thoroughly
   5. Encourage a daily walking program and supervised exercise program
   6. Suggest every opportunity to increase activity in daily life
   7. Support emotional needs
   8. Encourage counseling and participation in a self-help group
   9. Teach client about modifiable risk factors for CHD and diabetes mellitus and strategies to minimize complications of diabetes
   10. Teach about medications (e.g., with lipase inhibitors can experience flatus with discharge, fecal urgency, oily evacuation)
   11. Provide postoperative care after bariatric surgery (see General Nursing Care of Clients During the Postoperative Period in Chapter 3; also see postoperative care after gastric resection under Nursing Care of Clients With Peptic Ulcer Disease)
      a. Assess for wound dehiscence and slow wound healing associated with insufficient blood supply to adipose tissue and excessive skinfolds
      b. Provide instruction regarding use of an abdominal binder; be able to slip one finger beneath the binder easily; remove binder every 4 hours to assess skin for irritation

c. Assess for obesity hypoventilation syndrome
d. Use devices to provide for safety and comfort (e.g., large gowns; large bed that converts to a chair; extra wide, heavy-duty wheelchair, walker, and transfer board); ensure accuracy of assessments (e.g., correct size BP cuff)
e. Position in semi-Fowler's position; use continuous positive airway pressure ventilation at night if experiencing obstructive sleep apnea
f. Provide medication in liquid form
g. Once eating, encourage six small feedings (usually 600 to 800 calories daily) and fluid intake to prevent dehydration
h. Encourage high-protein foods and avoidance of alcohol, sugar, fat, and sweetened beverages
i. Teach the clinical findings of infection, deep venous thrombosis (DVT), and dehydration and the need to immediately report these to the physician
j. Encourage client to seek help with psychologic issues
k. Teach the client with bypass surgery the risk for anemia and calcium and vitamin B_{12} deficiencies; these deficiencies may require lifelong nutritional supplementation

C. Evaluation/Outcomes
1. Achieves and maintains an ideal body weight
2. Verbalizes acceptance of self
3. Remains free of injury
4. Maintains skin integrity
5. Demonstrates adequate depth of respirations

FRACTURE OF THE JAW
Data Base
A. Etiology and pathophysiology
1. Generally the result of trauma such as automobile collisions or physical combat
2. Blowout fractures of the orbit may accompany fractured jaw; these are stabilized surgically with wires, plates, and screws
B. Clinical findings
1. Subjective: history of trauma to the face; pain in the face and jaw; double vision
2. Objective: bloody discharge from the mouth; swelling of face on the affected side; difficulty opening or closing the mouth; malocclusion
C. Therapeutic interventions
1. Separated fragments of the broken bone are reunited and immobilized by wires and rubber bands; usually placed without surgical incision
2. Open reduction of the jaw is indicated for severely fractured or displaced bones; interosseous wiring is done

Nursing Care of Clients With Fracture of the Jaw
A. Assessment/Analysis
1. Respiratory status for presence of distress
2. Presence of nausea and potential for vomiting

3. Structures of the face and neck for clinical findings of edema
4. Assessment of drainage from nose or ears for presence of cerebrospinal fluid (CSF); CSF dries in concentric rings
B. Planning/Implementation
1. Postoperatively control vomiting and reduce the chance for aspiration pneumonia by positioning client on side
2. Keep wire cutters at the bedside to release the wires and rubber bands if emesis occurs and aspiration cannot be prevented by suctioning
3. Establish an alternate means of communication
4. Explain diet to the client and family; no solid foods are permitted; encourage high-protein liquids or soft foods pureed in a blender
5. Stress the importance of regular oral hygiene and institute it in the postoperative period
C. Evaluation/Outcomes
1. Adheres to nutritionally balanced safe diet
2. Demonstrates oral hygiene techniques
3. Describes technique for releasing wires and rubber bands if emesis occurs

CANCER OF THE ORAL CAVITY
Data Base
A. Etiology and pathophysiology
1. Primarily in clients who smoke or drink alcohol in large quantities; usually discovered by the dentist
2. Cancer of the lip easily diagnosed; prognosis is good; incidence highest in pipe smokers
3. Cancer of the tongue usually occurs with cancer of the floor of the mouth; metastasis to the neck is common
4. Cancer of the submaxillary glands; highly malignant and grows rapidly
B. Clinical findings
1. Subjective: pain (not an early symptom); alterations of taste
2. Objective: leukoplakia (white patches on mucosa), which is considered precancerous; ulcerated, bleeding areas in the involved structure; lymphadenopathy
C. Therapeutic interventions
1. Reconstructive surgery if indicated
2. Radiation or implantation of radioactive material may arrest growth of tumor
3. TPN, enteral tube feedings
4. Tracheostomy and tube feedings/TPN with extensive head and neck surgery

Nursing Care of Clients With Cancer of the Oral Cavity
A. Assessment/Analysis
1. History of hemoptysis and pain
2. Baseline nutritional data including weight, dietary intake, and ability to chew
3. Characteristics of lesions in oral cavity

B. Planning/Implementation
1. Maintain a patent airway; keep a tracheostomy set at the bedside
2. Maintain fluid, electrolyte, and nutritional balance; administer TPN, enteral tube feedings as ordered
3. Relieve dryness of the mouth by frequent saline mouthwashes and ample fluids if client is receiving radiation therapy
4. Consider time and distance in relation to the radioactive implants when giving nursing care

C. Evaluation/Outcomes
1. Maintains airway patency
2. Maintains nutritional status

GASTROESOPHAGEAL REFLUX DISEASE (GERD)

Data Base

A. Etiology and pathophysiology
1. Backflow of gastric contents into the esophagus, gradually breaking down esophageal mucosa
2. Etiology includes inadequate lower esophageal sphincter (LES) tone, corrosive effects of gastric acid on the esophagus, and delayed esophageal and gastric emptying; may be associated with hiatal hernia, obesity, pregnancy, and caffeine, chocolate, and high-fat food ingestion
3. May lead to Barrett's esophagus, a pathologic condition that can progress to esophageal cancer

B. Clinical findings
1. Subjective: dyspepsia, dysphagia, heartburn (pyrosis), oral release of salty secretions (water brash)
2. Objective: eructation, regurgitation, hoarseness, chronic cough, wheezing, recurrent pneumonia if severe; esophageal pH reveals acid reflux; endoscopy reveals tissue damage

C. Therapeutic interventions
1. Medical management with histamine receptor agonists, antacids, proton pump inhibitors, cholinergics
2. Small, frequent feedings; avoid spices, fats, and alcohol; avoid eating 2 to 3 hours before lying down or remain upright for 2 hours after meals
3. Weight reduction if indicated
4. Surgical intervention if medical management is unsuccessful
   a. Nissen fundoplication: suturing to tighten the fundus around the esophagus
   b. Hill procedure: narrows esophageal opening
5. Endoscopic therapy (Stretta procedure): use of radiofrequency energy at high temperatures via an endoscopic catheter, causing tiny lesions in the lower esophageal sphincter (LES) while client is under conscious sedation; causes tissue tightening, establishing a barrier to reflux, and reducing LES relaxation

Nursing Care of Clients With Gastroesophageal Reflux Disease

A. Assessment/Analysis
1. History of heartburn, regurgitation, dysphagia
2. Establishment of baseline weight to determine need for weight loss
3. Dietary and medication history to determine contributing factors

B. Planning/Implementation
1. Teach client dietary guidelines
   a. Eat small, frequent meals to avoid gastric distention
   b. Limit fatty foods, which delay gastric emptying
   c. Avoid foods that decrease LES pressure, such as alcohol, peppermints, caffeine, and chocolate
   d. Avoid eating or drinking 2 to 3 hours before bedtime
2. Teach client to maintain desirable body weight and avoid tight-fitting clothing and activities that increase intraabdominal pressure
3. Support smoking cessation efforts
4. Elevate the head of the bed on blocks; use extra pillows; advise client to avoid exercising or lying down after meals
5. Provide care after endoscopic therapy (Stretta procedure): ensure patent airway; elevate head of bed 45 degrees; monitor vital signs for complications; assess oxygen saturation; suction client's secretions gently if necessary; report pain higher than 5 (on a scale of 0 to 10) because this may indicate perforation; provide discharge instructions: avoid nonsteroidal antiinflammatory drugs (NSAIDs) for 10 days, consume a soft diet for 2 weeks, crush all pills, and report fever, nausea and vomiting, dysphagia, abdominal discomfort, chest pain, bleeding, and shortness of breath

C. Evaluation/Outcomes
1. Reports incidence of heartburn is greatly reduced
2. Maintains desirable body weight

CANCER OF THE ESOPHAGUS

Data Base

A. Etiology and pathophysiology
1. Occurs predominantly in persons with a history of alcohol abuse; ingestion of hot, spicy foods; smoking; or GERD
2. Tumor most commonly occurs in the middle and lower third of esophagus

B. Clinical findings
1. Subjective: dysphagia; substernal burning pain, particularly after hot fluids
2. Objective: regurgitation; esophagogastroduodenoscopy (EGD) with biopsy and brushings that show malignant cells

C. Therapeutic interventions
 1. Surgical removal of the esophagus is the treatment of choice
  a. Esophagogastrostomy: resection of a portion of the esophagus in which the stomach may be brought up to the remaining end of the esophagus (gastric pull through)
  b. Esophagectomy: removal of part or all of the esophagus, which is replaced by a Dacron graft or portion of the colon (colon interposition)
  c. Gastrostomy: opening directly into the stomach in which a feeding tube is usually inserted to bypass the esophagus
 2. Radiation and/or chemotherapy may be used before or instead of surgery as a palliative measure
 3. Total parenteral nutrition, enteral tube feedings
 4. Photodynamic therapy is used for palliative treatment; Photofrin is injected and several days later a fiberoptic probe in the esophagus activates the absorbed drug in cancer cells, shrinking them

Nursing Care of Clients With Cancer of the Esophagus

A. Assessment/Analysis
 1. History of nutritional status and weight loss
 2. Presence of pain and dysphagia
 3. History of foul breath, eructation, nausea, and vomiting
B. Planning/Implementation
 1. Observe for respiratory distress caused by pressure of tumor on the trachea; place in a semi-Fowler's or high-Fowler's position to facilitate respirations
 2. Monitor vital signs, especially respirations
 3. Provide oral care because dysphagia may result in accumulation of saliva in mouth
 4. Maintain nutritional status by providing TPN, tube feedings, high-protein liquids, and vitamin and mineral replacements as ordered
 5. Suction oral secretions if necessary
C. Evaluation/Outcomes
 1. Maintains airway
 2. Maintains nutritional status

❋ HIATAL HERNIA
Data Base
A. Etiology and pathophysiology
 1. Portion of the stomach protruding through a hiatus (opening) in the diaphragm into the thoracic cavity
 2. Caused by congenital weakness of the diaphragm or from injury, pregnancy, or obesity
 3. Function of the cardiac sphincter is lost; gastric juices enter the esophagus, causing inflammation

B. Clinical findings
 1. Subjective: substernal burning pain or fullness after eating; dyspepsia in the recumbent position; nocturnal dyspnea
 2. Objective: barium swallow, upper GI series, and endoscopy show protrusion of the stomach through the diaphragm; regurgitation
C. Therapeutic interventions
 1. Small, frequent, bland feedings
 2. Pharmacologic therapy (see Therapeutic interventions under GERD) and dietary management
 3. Surgical repair (done infrequently)

Nursing Care of Clients With Hiatal Hernia
See Nursing Care of Clients With Gastroesophageal Reflux Disease

❋ PEPTIC ULCER DISEASE (PUD)
Data Base
A. Etiology and pathophysiology
 1. Ulcerations of the GI mucosa and underlying tissues caused by gastric secretions that have a low pH (acid)
 2. Causes include conditions that increase the secretion of hydrochloric acid by the gastric mucosa or conditions that decrease that tissue's resistance to the acid
  a. Infection of the gastric and/or duodenal mucosa by *Campylobacter pylori* or *Helicobacter pylori*
  b. Zollinger-Ellison syndrome: tumors secreting gastrin, which will stimulate the production of excessive hydrochloric acid
  c. Certain drugs—such as aspirin, steroids, NSAIDs, and indomethacin—will decrease tissue resistance
  d. Smoking
 3. Peptic ulcers may be present in the esophagus, stomach (pyloric portion most common site), or duodenum
 4. Complications include pyloric or duodenal obstruction, hemorrhage, iron depletion and perforation
B. Clinical findings
 1. Subjective: gnawing or burning epigastric pain that occurs 1 to 2 hours after eating (gastric) or 2 to 4 hours after eating (duodenal); nausea; heartburn (pyrosis); relieved by food or antacids (duodenal)
 2. Objective
  a. History of gastritis
  b. If bleeding occurs: clinical findings of anemia; passage of tarry stools (melena); vomitus that is the color of coffee grounds or port wine; low hemoglobin and hematocrit levels
  c. Presence of *Helicobacter pylori* serum antibodies via urea breath test or via biopsy during esophagogastroduodenoscopy
C. Therapeutic interventions
 1. Bland foods and restriction of irritating substances such as nicotine, caffeine, alcohol, spices, and gas-producing foods

2. Antibiotic therapy if microorganism is identified; tetracycline, metronidazole, and bismuth
3. Histamine H$_2$ receptor antagonists or proton pump inhibitors to limit gastric acid secretion; antacids to reduce acidity
4. Sedatives, tranquilizers, anticholinergics, and analgesics for pain and restlessness
5. Antiemetics for nausea and vomiting
6. Vasoconstrictor to control bleeding
7. Type and cross-match so blood will be available if gastric hemorrhage occurs
8. A nasogastric tube for decompression, instillation of vasoconstrictors, and/or saline lavages when hemorrhage occurs
9. Surgical intervention
   a. Esophagogastroduodenoscopy to treat area with electrocoagulation or heater probe therapy
   b. Vagotomy: cutting the vagus nerve, which innervates the stomach, to decrease the secretion of hydrochloric acid
   c. Billroth I: removal of the lower portion of the stomach and attachment of the remaining portion to the duodenum; treatment for carcinoma
   d. Billroth II: removal of the antrum and distal portion of the stomach and subsequent anastomosis of remaining section to the jejunum; treatment for carcinoma
   e. Antrectomy: removal of the antral portion of the stomach
   f. Gastrectomy: removal of 60% to 80% of the stomach
   g. Common complications of partial or total gastric resection
      (1) Dumping syndrome: involves rapid passage of food from stomach to jejunum; food, being hypertonic (especially if high in carbohydrates), will draw fluid from circulating blood into jejunum, causing diaphoresis, faintness, and palpitations
      (2) Hemorrhage
      (3) Pneumonia
      (4) Pernicious anemia

Nursing Care of Clients With Peptic Ulcer Disease
A. Assessment/Analysis
   1. Characteristics of pain and relationship to types of food ingested and time food is consumed; gnawing sensation relieved by food
   2. Abdomen for epigastric tenderness, guarding, and bowel sounds
   3. History of dietary patterns, foods ingested, and alcohol consumption
B. Planning/Implementation
   1. Allow time to express concerns
   2. Administer and assess effects of sedatives, antacids, anticholinergics, H$_2$ receptor antagonists, antibiotics, and dietary modifications

3. Encourage hydration to reduce anticholinergic side effects and dilute hydrochloric acid in stomach
4. Instruct client to
   a. Eat small- to medium-sized meals because this helps prevent gastric distention; encourage between-meal snacks to achieve adequate calories when necessary
   b. Avoid foods that increase gastric acid secretion or irritate gastric mucosa, such as alcohol, caffeine-containing foods and beverages, decaffeinated coffee, red or black pepper; replace with decaffeinated soft drinks and teas; use seasonings such as thyme, basil, sage, etc. to replace pepper
   c. Avoid foods that cause distress; varies for individuals but common offenders are the gas producers (legumes, carbonated beverages, the cruciferous vegetables)
   d. Eat meals in pleasant, relaxing surroundings to reduce acid secretion
   e. Take calcium and iron supplements as ordered if client's medication increases gastric pH
5. Refrain from administering drugs such as salicylates, NSAIDs, steroids, and adrenocorticotropic hormone (ACTH)
6. Observe for complications such as gastric hemorrhage, perforation, and drug toxicity
7. Provide postoperative care after gastric resection
   a. Monitor vital signs; assess the dressing for drainage
   b. Maintain a patent nasogastric tube to suction secretions; this will help prevent stress on the suture line; instill or irrigate as ordered; monitor electrolytes
   c. Observe the color and amount of nasogastric drainage; excessive bleeding or the presence of bright red blood after 12 hours should be reported immediately
   d. Have the client cough, deep breathe, and change position frequently to prevent the occurrence of pulmonary complications
   e. Monitor intake and output
   f. Apply antiembolism stockings; ambulate client early to prevent vascular complications
   g. To prevent dumping syndrome, instruct the client to
      (1) Eat smaller meals at more frequent intervals
      (2) Avoid high-carbohydrate intake and concentrated sweets
      (3) Consume liquids only between meals
      (4) Remain sitting for 1 hour after eating
   h. Time antacids 1 hour before or 2 hours after other medications
C. Evaluation/Outcomes
   1. States pain is reduced or relieved
   2. Identifies clinical findings of complications and the need for immediate medical care
   3. Follows a nutritionally sound diet

CANCER OF THE STOMACH

Data Base
A. Etiology and pathophysiology
1. Risk factors include *H. pylori* in the stomach; ingestion of smoked meats, salted fish, nitrates; and smoking
2. Often not diagnosed until metastasis occurs; the stomach is able to accommodate the growth of a tumor, and pain occurs late in the disease
3. May metastasize by direct extension, lymphatics, or blood to the esophagus, spleen, pancreas, liver, or bone
4. Heredity apparently a factor in the development of carcinoma of the stomach, as is the presence of precursors such as ulcerative disease and pernicious anemia
5. Incidence higher in men more than 40 years of age; the Japanese have a greater rate of cancer of the stomach than do Americans
B. Clinical findings
1. Subjective: anorexia (lack of interest in food); nausea; belching (eructation); heartburn
2. Objective: weight loss; stools positive for occult blood; anemia; achlorhydria (absence of hydrochloric acid); pale skin and acanthosis nigricans (a hyperpigmented, velvety thickening of the skin in the neck, axilla, and groin)
C. Therapeutic interventions
1. Surgical resection
2. Radiation
3. Chemotherapy
4. Combination of radiation and chemotherapy after surgery

Nursing Care of Clients With Cancer of the Stomach
A. Assessment/Analysis
1. History of causative factors, presence of pain, and weight loss
2. Axillary lymph nodes and left supraclavicular nodes for hardness indicative of metastasis
3. Skin for color and presence of lesions associated with cancer of the GI tract
B. Planning/Implementation
1. Encourage verbalization of fears (e.g., cancer, death, family problems, self-image)
2. Provide care after a gastric resection (see Peptic Ulcer Disease earlier in this chapter for nursing care); in addition, if a total gastrectomy is performed, the chest cavity is usually entered, so the client will have chest tubes (see Chest Tubes in Chapter 7 for nursing care)
3. Modify diet to include smaller, more frequent meals (see Peptic Ulcer Disease for more dietary information)
4. If total gastrectomy has been performed, the client will have a vitamin B_{12} deficiency (see Pernicious Anemia under Anemias and Blood Disorders in Chapter 6)

5. Client may require gavage feedings (see Gavage under Related Procedures)
C. Evaluation/Outcomes
1. States relief from discomfort and pain
2. Maintains adequate nutritional status
3. Verbalizes feelings

CHOLELITHIASIS/CHOLECYSTITIS

Data Base
A. Etiology and pathophysiology
1. Inflammation of the gallbladder; usually caused by infection or the presence of stones (cholelithiasis), which are composed of cholesterol, bile pigments, and calcium; may be related to hepatic *Helicobacter* bacteria
2. Diseased gallbladder is unable to contract in response to fatty foods entering the duodenum because of obstruction by calculi or edema
3. When the common bile duct is completely obstructed, the bile is unable to pass into the duodenum and is absorbed into the blood, leading to hyperbilirubinemia and jaundice
4. Incidence is highest in obese women in the fourth decade
B. Clinical findings
1. Subjective: indigestion after eating fatty or fried foods; pain, usually in the right upper quadrant of the abdomen, which may radiate to the back; nausea; itchy skin
2. Objective
   a. Vomiting; elevated temperature and WBC count; clay-colored stool, dark urine, and jaundice may be present
   b. Abdomen has rebound tenderness increasing on inspiration, indicating peritoneal inflammation
   c. Diagnostic tests
      (1) Levels of serum bilirubin and alkaline phosphatase are elevated
      (2) Ultrasonography determines the presence of gallstones
      (3) Endoscopic retrograde cholangiopancreatography (ERCP) reveals presence of gallstones
C. Therapeutic interventions
1. Medical management
   a. Nasogastric suctioning to reduce nausea and eliminate vomiting
   b. Opioids to decrease pain
   c. Antispasmodics and anticholinergics to reduce spasms and contractions of the gallbladder
   d. Antibiotic therapy if infection is suspected
   e. When clients are poor surgical risks or radiolucent cholesterol stones are small, oral chenodiol (Chenix) or ursodiol (Actigall) for 6 to 12 months to dissolve the stones
   f. Dissolution of stones by infusing a solvent such as methyl tertiary terbutyl ether (MTBE) into the gallbladder through ERCP

g. Endoscopic papillotomy via ERCP to retrieve stones in the common bile duct

h. Lithotripsy: fragmentation of stones by ultrasonic sound waves enable their passage without surgical intervention

i. Low-fat diet to avoid stimulating the gallbladder, which contracts to excrete bile with subsequent pain; calories principally from carbohydrate foods in acute phases; if weight loss is indicated, calories may be reduced to 1000 to 1200; postoperatively clients may follow fat-restricted diets initially but progress to regular diets

2. Surgical intervention

a. Abdominal cholecystectomy: removal of the gallbladder through an abdominal incision

b. Laparoscopic cholecystectomy: removal of the gallbladder through an endoscope inserted through the abdominal wall; also called endoscopic laser cholecystectomy (not used if infection is present)

c. Choledochotomy: incision into the common bile duct for removal of stones

Nursing Care of Clients With Cholelithiasis/Cholecystitis

A. Assessment/Analysis

1. Characteristics of pain

2. Presence of pain in relation to ingestion of foods high in fat

3. Abdomen for rebound tenderness that increases on inspiration (peritoneal inflammation)

4. Stools for color (clay-colored) and fat (steatorrhea); urine for color (dark)

5. Laboratory values for abnormal liver function tests

B. Planning/Implementation

1. Teach dietary modification to achieve a low-fat intake initially because reduced bile flow will reduce fat absorption; supplementation with water-miscible forms of vitamins A and E may be prescribed

2. Relieve pain both preoperatively and postoperatively; opioids are drugs of choice because of ability to relax smooth muscle

3. Observe for clinical findings of bleeding (vitamin K is fat-soluble and is not absorbed in the absence of bile); administer vitamin K preparations as ordered

4. Provide care after a cholecystectomy

a. Monitor nasogastric tube attached to suction to prevent distention

(1) Maintain patency of the tube

(2) Assess and measure drainage

b. Provide fluids and electrolytes via intravenous route

(1) Monitor intake and output

(2) Check IV site for redness, swelling, heat, or pain

c. Maintain a low-Fowler's position

d. Encourage coughing and deep breathing; splint the incision (incision is high and midline, making coughing extremely uncomfortable)

e. Provide care for the client with a T-tube (if the common bile duct has been explored, a T-tube is inserted to maintain patency)

(1) Secure the drainage bag; avoid kinking of the tube

(2) Measure drainage at least every shift; drainage during the first day may reach 500 to 1000 mL and then gradually decline

(3) Apply ordered protective ointments around tube to prevent excoriation

(4) When the tube is removed, usually in 7 days, observe stool for normal brown color, which indicates bile is again entering the duodenum

C. Evaluation/Outcomes

1. Verbalizes a decrease in pain

2. Maintains nutritional status

ACUTE PANCREATITIS

Data Base

A. Etiology and pathophysiology

1. Inflammation of pancreas caused by autodigestion by pancreatic enzymes, primarily trypsin

2. May result from gallstones, alcoholism, carcinoma, acute trauma to the pancreas or abdomen, or hyperlipidemia

3. Inflammation with or without edema of pancreatic tissues, suppuration, abscess formation, hemorrhage, necrosis, or duct obstruction

B. Clinical findings

1. Subjective

a. Abrupt onset of aching, burning, stabbing, or pressing central epigastric pain that may radiate to shoulder, chest, and back

b. Abdominal tenderness

c. Nausea

d. Pruritus associated with jaundice

2. Objective

a. Elevated temperature

b. Shallow respirations

c. Vomiting, weight loss

d. Change in character of stools

e. Shock, tachycardia, hypotension

f. Jaundice

g. Grossly elevated serum amylase and lipase levels

h. Decreased serum calcium level

i. Boardlike abdomen with peritonitis

j. Abnormal pancreatic findings on CT scan

3. Severity of clinical findings depends on the cause of the problem, the amount of fibrous replacement of normal duct tissue, the degree of autodigestion of the organ, the type of associated biliary disease if present, and the amount of interference in blood supply to the pancreas

4. Clinical findings may be exaggerated by the development of complications such as pseudocysts (dilated space containing blood, necrotic tissue, and enzymes), abscesses, and pancreatic fistulas

C. Therapeutic interventions
1. Antacids to neutralize gastric secretions
2. Opioids to control pain
3. Bed rest to decrease metabolic demands and promote healing
4. Nothing by mouth and nasogastric decompression to control nausea, reduce stimulation of the pancreas to secrete enzymes, and remove gastric hydrochloric acid
5. Anticholinergics to suppress vagal stimulation and decrease gastric motility and duodenal spasm
6. Antibiotics to prevent secondary infections and abscess formation
7. Diet regulated according to the client's condition: nothing by mouth; parenteral administration of fluids and electrolytes, total or peripheral parenteral nutrition; diet low in fats and proteins, with restriction of stimulants such as caffeine and alcohol; pancreatic rest until largely free of pain and bowel sounds return
8. Pancreatic enzymes and bile salts if necessary
9. Surgical intervention if the client fails to respond to medical management, exhibits persistent jaundice, develops a pseudocyst or bleeds; type of surgery is determined by the cause (e.g., biliary tract surgery, removal of gallstones, drainage of cysts, temporary stent placement)
10. Monitor for hyperglycemia and replace insulin as necessary (beta cells of pancreas may be affected by disease process)

Nursing Care of Clients With Acute Pancreatitis

A. Assessment/Analysis
1. History of causative factors, pain, and recent weight loss
2. Presence of jaundice
3. Abdomen for rigidity and guarding
4. Presence of hyperglycemia
B. Planning/Implementation
1. Provide care for a client with a nasogastric tube
   a. Observe for electrolyte imbalances (manifested by clinical findings such as tetany, irritability, jerking, muscular twitching, mental changes, and psychotic behavior)
   b. Observe for clinical findings of adynamic ileus (e.g., nausea and vomiting, abdominal distention)
   c. Maintain tube patency
2. Monitor for hyperglycemia
3. Monitor vital signs and oxygen saturation
4. Administer prescribed analgesics
5. Maintain NPO during the acute stage of illness; monitor intake and output
6. Place in semi-Fowler's position and encourage deep breathing and coughing to promote deeper respirations and prevent respiratory problems
7. Closely monitor parenteral therapy until oral feedings can be tolerated

8. Teach dietary modifications as required by the client's condition, usually starting with small feedings of low-fat, non–gas-producing liquids and progressing to a more liberalized diet that is low in fat but high in protein and carbohydrates; if fat malabsorption is severe, supplemental vitamins A and E may be necessary; daily supplements of calcium and zinc may also be needed; if insulin secretion is impaired, an American Diabetes Association (ADA) diet is indicated
9. Teach the client and family the importance of dietary discretion, especially the avoidance of alcohol, coffee, spicy foods, and heavy meals
10. Teach importance of taking medication containing pancreatic enzymes (amylase, lipase, trypsin) with each meal to improve digestion of food if the disease becomes chronic
C. Evaluation/Outcomes
1. Reports decrease in pain
2. Maintains nutritional status
3. Demonstrates adequate depth of respirations
4. Maintains fluid and electrolyte balance
5. Avoids the complication of hyperglycemia

CANCER OF THE PANCREAS

Data Base

A. Etiology and pathophysiology
1. Malignant growth from the epithelium of the ductal system, producing cells that block the ducts of the pancreas
2. Fibrosis, pancreatitis, and obstruction of the pancreatic duct
3. Lesion tends to metastasize by direct extension to the duodenal wall, splenic flexure of the colon, posterior stomach wall, and common bile duct
4. Heredity, environmental toxins, alcohol, a high-fat diet, and smoking are associated with increased incidence
5. History of chronic pancreatitis, diabetes mellitus, and alcoholism is common
6. More common in middle-aged men than women
B. Clinical findings
1. Subjective: anxiety; depression; anorexia; nausea; dull, achy pain progressing to severe pain; pruritus associated with jaundice
2. Objective
   a. Jaundice; weight loss; diarrhea and steatorrhea; clay-colored stools; dark urine; ascites
   b. Decreased serum amylase and lipase levels because of decreased secretion of enzymes
   c. Increased serum bilirubin and alkaline phosphatase levels when biliary ducts are obstructed
C. Therapeutic interventions
1. Preparation for surgical intervention: RBC and blood volume replacement; medications to correct coagulation problems and nutritional deficiencies

2. Chemotherapy with gemcitabine (Gemzar) is useful in inhibiting movement of cells from G1 to S phase of cell cycle
3. Chemotherapy and radiation when surgery is not possible or desired to provide comfort, or in conjunction with surgery to limit metastasis
4. Glucose monitoring and insulin replacement to control hyperglycemia
5. Drug therapy such as pancreatic enzymes, bile salts, and vitamin K to correct deficiencies
6. Analgesics and tranquilizers for pain
7. A biliary stent may be used to relieve jaundice
8. Surgery is treatment of choice, although postsurgical prognosis is grim: Whipple's procedure (removal of head of pancreas, duodenum, portion of stomach, and common bile duct) or a cholecystojejunostomy (creation of an opening between gallbladder and jejunum to direct bile flow)

Nursing Care of Clients With Cancer of the Pancreas

A. Assessment/Analysis
1. Presence of jaundice
2. Stool for clay color
3. Urine for dark amber color and frothy appearance
4. Abdomen for enlargement of liver and gallbladder
5. Characteristics of pain
6. History of anorexia, nausea, and weight loss
7. Abdominal dullness on percussion indicating early ascites

B. Planning/Implementation
1. Provide emotional support for the client and family, and set realistic goals when planning care
2. Administer analgesics as ordered and as soon as needed to promote rest and comfort
3. Use soapless bathing and antipruritic agents to relieve pruritus
4. Observe for complications such as peritonitis, gastrointestinal obstruction, jaundice, hyperglycemia, and hypotension
5. Observe the stools for undigested fat
6. Frequently monitor the vital signs, observing for wound hemorrhage caused by coagulation deficiency
7. Administer vitamin K parenterally as ordered
8. Monitor for respiratory tract infection caused by limited chest expansion because of pain at the site of the incision; encourage coughing, turning, and deep breathing
9. Monitor I&O; measure abdominal girth
10. Observe for chemotherapeutic and radiation side effects (e.g., skin irritation, anorexia, nausea, vomiting)
11. Maintain skin markings for radiation therapy
12. Support natural defense mechanisms of the client by encouraging frequent and supplemental feedings of high nutrient density foods as tolerated; stress the immune-stimulating nutrients, especially vitamins A, C, and E, and the mineral selenium
13. Control nausea and vomiting before feedings, if possible
14. Administer vitamin supplements, bile salts, and pancreatic enzymes, as ordered
15. Provide oral hygiene and maintain a pleasant environment, especially at mealtime
16. Provide care after pancreatic surgery (see General Nursing Care of Clients During the Postoperative Period in Chapter 3; also see postoperative care after gastric resection under Nursing Care of Clients With Peptic Ulcer Disease)
    a. Monitor and maintain mechanical ventilation (see Mechanical Ventilation under Related Procedures in Chapter 7)
    b. Ensure patency and maintain multiple drainage tubes and venous and arterial lines
    c. Assess for hyperglycemia and malabsorption syndrome
    d. Assess for delayed wound healing; may be at risk because of hyperglycemia
    e. Assess for hemorrhage, vascular collapse, and hepatorenal failure
    f. Meet emotional needs during this critical and stressful postoperative period
    g. Prevent infection: maintain skin integrity, protect integrity of surgical incision, use sterile technique when changing dressing

C. Evaluation/Outcomes
1. States that pain is controlled
2. Maintains nutritional status
3. Maintains fluid and electrolyte balance
4. Discusses feelings and concerns
5. Avoids hyperglycemia and its complications
6. Avoids infection

HEPATITIS

Data Base

A. Etiology and pathophysiology
1. Hepatitis is an acute or chronic inflammation of the liver caused by bacterial or viral infection, parasitic infestation (usually by contaminated water or food), or chemical agents
2. Hepatic involvement may impair clotting mechanisms
3. Hepatitis A (formerly known as infectious hepatitis)
   a. Caused by hepatitis A virus (HAV)
   b. Transmitted via fecal-oral route, contamination associated with flood waters, or contaminated food (e.g., shellfish)
   c. Excreted in large quantities in feces 2 weeks before and 1 week after the onset of clinical findings
   d. Incubation period is 15 to 50 days
   e. Confers immunity on individual
   f. Carrier state is possible

g. Serum studies
  (1) Anti-HAV: antibody usually apparent once clinical findings appear and lasts up to 12 months
  (2) IgM anti-HAV: antibody indicates recent infection
h. Vaccine: hepatitis A vaccine provides long-term protection

4. Hepatitis B (formerly known as serum hepatitis)
  a. Caused by hepatitis B virus (HBV)
  b. Transmitted by
    (1) Contaminated blood products or articles (e.g., toothbrush, razor, needle)
    (2) Other body secretions (e.g., saliva, semen, urine)
    (3) Introduction of infectious material into eye, oral cavity, lacerations, or vagina
    (4) Shared contaminated needles
  c. Incubation period is 28 to 160 days
  d. Serum studies
    (1) HBsAg—hepatitis B surface antigen: indicates infectious state
    (2) Anti-HBs: antibody to surface antigen indicates immune response
    (3) HBeAg—hepatitis Be antigen: indicates highly infectious state and possible progression to chronic hepatitis
    (4) Anti-HBe: antibody found in recovery
    (5) HBcAg: core antigen of hepatitis B; found in liver cells
    (6) Anti-HBc: antibody most sensitive indicator of prior HBV infection
  e. Vaccine: three doses of hepatitis B vaccine provides immunity in 90% of healthy adults

5. Hepatitis C
  a. Caused by hepatitis C virus (HCV)
  b. Transmitted through blood and blood products
  c. Incubation period is 15 to 160 days following exposure (average 50 days)
  d. Serum studies
    (1) Hepatitis C virus antibodies
    (2) Hepatitis C virus RNA
    (3) Hepatitis C genotyping
  e. Chronic carrier state possible; associated with hepatic cancer

6. Hepatitis D
  a. Caused by hepatitis D virus (HDV)
  b. Transmitted through blood and blood products and close personal contact
  c. Incubation period is unknown
  d. Chronic carrier state possible
  e. Serum studies
    (1) HDAg—hepatitis D antigen: can be detected early
    (2) Anti-HDV antibody: indicates past or present infection

7. Hepatitis E
  a. Caused by hepatitis E virus (HEV)
  b. Transmitted through fecal-oral route
  c. Incubation period is 15 to 65 days
  d. Onset of clinical findings is similar to that of other types of hepatitis; clinical findings are severe in pregnant women

8. Hepatitis G
  a. Caused by hepatitis G virus (HGV)
  b. Transmitted percutaneously through blood, needles, body fluids
  c. Incubation period unknown
  d. It is a bloodborne RNA virus frequently found in clients with HIV

9. Nonviral, toxic, or drug-induced hepatitis: may be caused by drug therapy or other chemicals (e.g., carbon tetrachloride, chloroform, gold compounds, isoniazid [INH], halothene, acetaminophen)

10. Phases of disease: prodromal (preicteric), icteric, and recovery

11. Progression to cirrhosis, hepatic coma, and death may occur

B. Clinical findings
  1. Prodromal (preicteric) phase: malaise, anorexia, nausea, vomiting, and weight loss; clinical findings of upper respiratory tract infection; intolerance for cigarette smoke
  2. Icteric phase: jaundice, bile-colored urine that foams when shaken; acholic (clay-colored) stools
  3. Recovery phase: easy fatigability

C. Therapeutic interventions
  1. Rest
  2. Diet therapy
    a. Moderate to high protein to heal liver tissue; total protein intake should approximate 75 to 100 g daily; alcohol should be avoided
    b. High carbohydrate to meet energy needs and restore glycogen reserves; total carbohydrate intake should be 300 to 400 g
    c. Low fat
    d. High calorie to meet increased energy needs for disease process and tissue regeneration and to spare protein for healing; total should be 2500 to 3000 calories daily
    e. Vitamins A and E when steatorrhea is present; mineral supplements of calcium and zinc
  3. Bile acid sequestrants such as cholestyramine (Questran) to reduce pruritus
  4. Avoidance of hepatotoxic drugs such as acetaminophen, aminoglycoside antibiotics, sedatives
  5. Antiviral agents such as interferon; chronic hepatitis B: telbivudine (Tyzeka), lamivudine (Epivir, Epivir HBV); hepatitis C: interferon (Intron A) and ribavirin (Rebetol)

Nursing Care of Clients With Hepatitis

A. Assessment/Analysis
  1. History of exposure to virus; foreign travel
  2. History of exposure to environmental factors over previous 6 months

3. Right upper quadrant for liver tenderness, firmness
4. Presence of jaundice in skin, sclera, and mucous membranes
5. Temperature to determine presence of fever (associated with type A) or low-grade fever (associated with types B and C); fatigue
6. Presence of bleeding tendencies

B. Planning/Implementation
1. Encourage rest and quiet activities; protect from injury to prevent bleeding
2. Attempt to stimulate the appetite
   a. Provide oral hygiene
   b. Select foods based on the client's preferences
   c. Provide a pleasant, unhurried atmosphere
   d. Provide small, frequent feedings because they are usually tolerated better than large meals
3. Use standard precautions to prevent the spread to others; for hepatitis A or E, use contact precautions when exposed to client's feces
4. Teach prevention
   a. Thorough handwashing
   b. Contact precautions for exposure to feces, blood, or body secretions
   c. Careful handling of needles (dispose of needles without recapping to prevent self-injury and contamination, dispose of needles in hard-sided container)
   d. Administration of immune serum globulin (ISG) after exposure to HAV and administration of hepatitis B immune serum globulin after exposure to HBV to provide passive immunity
   e. Vaccinations against HAV (Havrix, Vaqta) and against HBV (Recombivax HB)
   f. When client has hepatitis that can be transmitted sexually, instruct to use condoms

C. Evaluation/Outcomes
1. States a decrease in fatigue
2. Adheres to prescribed diet
3. Remains free from injury
4. Follows precautions to prevent transmission

HEPATIC CIRRHOSIS
Data Base
A. Etiology and pathophysiology
1. Irreversible fibrosis and degeneration of the liver
2. Types of cirrhosis
   a. Alcoholic (Laënnec's) cirrhosis: related to alcohol abuse
   b. Postnecrotic or macronodular: most common form worldwide; related to viral hepatitis B and C and industrial chemical exposure
   c. Biliary: related to biliary stasis in hepatic ducts; may be an autoimmune response
   d. Cardiac: results from long-term right-sided heart failure; least common form
3. Pressure rises in the portal system (which drains blood from the digestive organs), causing stasis and backup of fluids in digestive organs and lower extremities (portal hypertension)
4. There is a buildup of protein metabolic wastes and increased ammonia levels
5. As liver failure progresses, there is increased secretion of aldosterone, decreased absorption and utilization of the fat-soluble vitamins (A, D, E, K), and ineffective detoxification of protein wastes
6. GI bleeding results from esophageal varices
7. Hepatic coma (hepatic encephalopathy) may result from high blood ammonia levels when the liver is unable to convert the ammonia to urea
8. Fat accumulation in liver tissue

B. Clinical findings
1. Subjective: anorexia; nausea; weakness; fatigue; abdominal discomfort; pruritus
2. Objective
   a. Loss of muscle mass with weight gain caused by fluid retention; ascites; esophageal varices resulting from portal hypertension; hemorrhoids; varicose veins; edema of extremities; hematemesis; jaundice (icterus); delirium caused by rising blood ammonia levels; fetor hepaticus (sweet odor to breath)
   b. Elevated liver enzymes (aspartate aminotransferase [AST], alanine aminotransferase [ALT], alkaline phosphatase [ALP], gamma-glutamyl transferase [GGT])
   c. Decreased serum albumin level; elevated serum bilirubin level; prolonged prothrombin time; hemorrhage resulting from decreased formation of prothrombin

C. Therapeutic interventions
1. Rest for energy conservation
2. Restriction of alcohol intake
3. Vitamin therapy: especially the fat-soluble vitamins A, D, E, and K and vitamin B (thiamine chloride and nicotinic acid); zinc and calcium supplements
4. Diuretics to control ascites and edema
5. Neomycin and lactulose may be prescribed for elevated blood ammonia levels
6. Colchicine, an antiinflammatory agent, may increase survival in moderate cirrhosis
7. Maintenance of respiratory function and adequate oxygen saturation; paracentesis if respiratory distress occurs as a result of ascites
8. Surgical intervention to decrease portal hypertension: a portal caval shunt, in which the circulation from the portal vein bypasses the liver and enters the vena cava; a peritoneovenous shunt (LeVeen or Denver) to move fluid from abdominal cavity to superior vena cava
9. Balloon tamponade with Sengstaken-Blakemore tube for bleeding esophageal varices to apply direct pressure to the varices; vasopressin may be administered IV to control GI bleeding

10. Endoscopic sclerotherapy: via an endoscope a sclerosing agent is injected endoscopically into the varices, causing thrombosis and hemostasis; first-line treatment for active variceal bleeding
11. Dietary modification
    a. Cirrhosis
       (1) Protein as tolerated (80 to 100 g); with increasing liver damage, protein metabolism is hindered
       (2) High carbohydrate, moderate fat; provides for energy; vitamin, mineral, and electrolyte supplements
       (3) Low sodium (500 to 1000 mg daily); helps control increasing ascites
       (4) Soft foods if esophageal varices are present; prevents danger of rupture and bleeding
       (5) Supplementation with B vitamins and fat-soluble vitamins A, D, E, and K
       (6) Alcohol and hepatotoxic agents contraindicated; avoids irritation and malnutrition
    b. Hepatic coma
       (1) Protein is reduced to 15 to 30 g when blood ammonia level rises to above 200 mcg/dL
       (2) High-calorie diet (1500 to 2000 g) to prevent catabolism and liberation of nitrogen
       (3) Fluid carefully controlled according to output and presence of ascites and edema

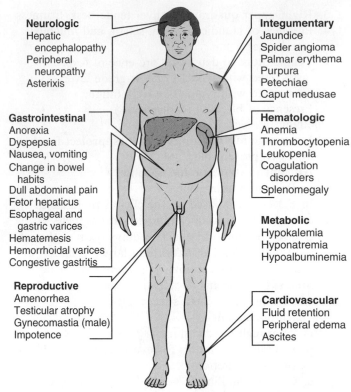

Neurologic
Hepatic encephalopathy
Peripheral neuropathy
Asterixis

Gastrointestinal
Anorexia
Dyspepsia
Nausea, vomiting
Change in bowel habits
Dull abdominal pain
Fetor hepaticus
Esophageal and gastric varices
Hematemesis
Hemorrhoidal varices
Congestive gastritis

Reproductive
Amenorrhea
Testicular atrophy
Gynecomastia (male)
Impotence

Integumentary
Jaundice
Spider angioma
Palmar erythema
Purpura
Petechiae
Caput medusae

Hematologic
Anemia
Thrombocytopenia
Leukopenia
Coagulation disorders
Splenomegaly

Metabolic
Hypokalemia
Hyponatremia
Hypoalbuminemia

Cardiovascular
Fluid retention
Peripheral edema
Ascites

Figure 8-4 Systemic clinical manifestations of liver cirrhosis. (From Lewis SL et al: *Medical-surgical nursing: assessment and management of clinical problems*, ed 7, St Louis, 2007, Mosby.)

Nursing Care of Clients With Hepatic Cirrhosis

A. Assessment/Analysis
(Figure 8-4: Systemic clinical manifestations of liver cirrhosis)
1. History of anorexia, dyspepsia, alcohol abuse or exposure to hepatotoxic agent; loss of muscle mass with weight gain caused by fluid retention
2. Abdomen for pain and liver tenderness; dullness when percussing enlarged liver
3. Abdominal girth measurements for baseline data relative to ascites; weight gain
4. Skin for presence of jaundice, dryness, petechiae, ecchymoses, spider angiomas, and palmar erythema
5. Clinical findings of hepatic coma such as confusion, flapping of extremities

B. Planning/Implementation
1. Observe for bleeding
2. Monitor liver function studies, CBC, and renal function studies
3. Provide high-calorie, protein-restricted diet
4. Provide special skin care and keep client's nails trimmed because pruritus is associated with jaundice
5. Maintain the client in a semi-Fowler's position to prevent ascites from causing dyspnea
6. Monitor intake and output, abdominal girth, and daily weight to assess fluid balance
7. Assist with paracentesis (see Paracentesis under Related Procedures)

8. Provide care when a Sengstaken-Blakemore tube is in place
   a. Maintain traction once the tube is passed and the gastric balloon is inflated to ensure proper placement
   b. Maintain the esophageal balloon at inflated level (30 to 35 mm Hg)
   c. Deflate the balloon for a few minutes at specific intervals if ordered to prevent necrosis
   d. Irrigate with saline if ordered
   e. Maintain a patent airway; suction orally as necessary because the client is unable to swallow saliva
9. Provide care after endoscopic sclerotherapy: monitor for complications of perforated esophagus (pain), aspiration pneumonia, pleural effusion, and increasing ascites; support respiratory status
10. Repeat instructions; ability of client to understand and remember is often impaired because of hepatic encephalopathy; include family in instructions
11. Monitor for clinical findings of impending hepatic coma

C. Evaluation/Outcomes
1. Follows dietary regimen
2. Maintains fluid balance
3. Remains free from injury

❋ CANCER OF THE LIVER
Data Base
A. Etiology and pathophysiology
   1. May be primary or metastatic carcinoma; primary carcinoma (hepatocellular cancer, hepatoma) of the liver is rare
   2. Contributing factors include hepatitis B and C, cirrhosis, alcoholism, and anabolic steroid use
   3. Lack of bile causes inadequate vitamin K absorption, resulting in deficient prothrombin synthesis and subsequent bleeding
   4. Poor prognosis
B. Clinical findings
   1. Subjective: anorexia; ache in epigastric area, weakness, malaise
   2. Objective: weight loss; bleeding; fever; anemia; jaundice; ascites; increased serum bilirubin level; increased alkaline phosphatase level; confusion, lethargy, lower-extremity edema
C. Therapeutic interventions
   1. Generally palliative
   2. Hepatic lobectomy if the tumor is confined
   3. Percutaneous infusions with cytotoxic agents (ethanol, yttrium 90)
   4. Radiofrequency ablation, cryosurgery, embolization of blood vessels supplying the tumor
   5. External radiation therapy

Nursing Care of Clients With Cancer of the Liver
A. Assessment/Analysis
   1. Weight to assess ascites and nutritional status
   2. Skin for jaundice, bleeding, and pallor
   3. Presence of dullness when percussing over liver; ascites
   4. Detailed history including exposure to any known causative agents
B. Planning/Implementation
   1. Provide for comfort and pain relief; help to combat fatigue and conserve energy
   2. Be available to both the client and family members to discuss their feelings
   3. Maintain fluid and electrolyte balance; monitor intake and output
   4. Observe for clinical findings of bleeding, esophageal varices, hypoglycemia, and other metabolic dysfunctions resulting from impaired liver function
   5. Have client cough, deep breathe, and change position frequently to prevent pulmonary and circulatory complications
   6. Because the thoracic cavity may be entered during hepatic surgery, be aware of the care of a client with chest tubes
C. Evaluation/Outcomes
   1. Verbalizes feelings about diagnosis and prognosis
   2. Maintains fluid balance
   3. States relief from discomfort
   4. Remains free from injury-related altered coagulation

❋ APPENDICITIS
Data Base
A. Etiology and pathophysiology
   1. Compromised circulation and inflammation of the vermiform appendix; inflammation may be followed by edema, necrosis, and rupture
   2. Causes include obstruction by a fecalith, foreign body, or kinking
B. Clinical findings
   1. Subjective: anorexia; nausea; right lower quadrant pain (McBurney's point); rebound tenderness
   2. Objective: vomiting; fever; leukocytosis; abdominal distention and paralytic ileus if appendix has ruptured
C. Therapeutic interventions
   1. Surgical removal of the appendix without delay to decrease the chance of rupture and the risk for peritonitis
   2. Prophylactic use of antibiotics
   3. Fluid and electrolyte maintenance
   4. Analgesics for pain

Nursing Care of Clients with Appendicitis
A. Assessment/Analysis
   1. History of characteristics of pain and presence of nausea and vomiting
   2. Presence of anorexia or the urge to pass flatus
   3. Presence of rebound tenderness when palpating abdomen
   4. Presence of tenderness/rigidity when palpating McBurney's point (Rovsing sign)
   5. Temperature for baseline data
   6. Presence and extent of bowel sounds
B. Planning/Implementation
   1. Provide emotional support because this condition is unanticipated and the individual needs to ventilate any fear of surgery
   2. Monitor fluid and electrolyte balance
   3. Assess for clinical findings of infection; maintain a semi-Fowler's position to help localize infection if the appendix ruptures
   4. Assess for return of bowel function (bowel sounds, flatus, bowel movement); encourage ambulation
C. Evaluation/Outcomes
   1. States pain is alleviated
   2. Remains free from infection

❋ IRRITABLE BOWEL SYNDROME (IBS)
Data Base
A. Etiology and pathophysiology
   1. Functional motility disorder of the intestines of unknown cause
   2. Possibly related to serotonin associated with neurologic hormonal regulation; vascular or metabolic disturbance; infection; irritation; heredity; psychologic stress; depression and anxiety; high-fat diet; irritating foods; alcohol
   3. Affects approximately 25% of the population; affects more women than men

B. Clinical findings
   1. Subjective: pain; pain precipitated by eating, bloating, abdominal cramps, dyspepsia
   2. Objective: constipation, diarrhea, or a combination of both; abdominal distention; barium enema and colonoscopy may indicate spasm or mucus accumulation in the intestines
C. Therapeutic interventions
   1. Hydrophilic colloids (bulk) and antidiarrheal agents to control diarrhea; anticholinergics and calcium channel blockers minimize smooth muscle spasm
   2. NPO initially and gradual reintroduction of foods to a healthy high-fiber diet
   3. Antidepressants; stress reduction and/or behavior modification program
   4. Broad-spectrum antibiotic: rifaximin (Xifaxan) shown to reduce overall clinical findings

Nursing Care of Clients With Irritable Bowel Syndrome

A. Assessment/Analysis
   1. Presence of pain, bloating, and abdominal cramps; emotional factors precipitating an event; dietary habits
   2. History of pattern and characteristics of bowel elimination
   3. Presence and extent of bowel sounds
B. Planning/Implementation
   1. Instruct client to
      a. Eliminate irritating and gas-producing substances
      b. Add fiber to diet
      c. Schedule meals regularly
      d. Chew thoroughly and eat slowly
      e. Minimize beverages with meals to avoid distention
      f. Avoid smoking and alcohol
   2. Administer antidiarrheal, bulk-forming laxatives, and/or antispasmodics as ordered
   3. Instruct client to maintain hydration
   4. Encourage the use of stress management strategies; provide emotional reassurance
   5. Provide or teach the importance of meticulous perianal skin care
C. Evaluation/Outcomes
   1. Reports a reduction in pain
   2. Reports a decrease in diarrhea/constipation
   3. Maintains nutritional status
   4. Maintains fluid and electrolyte balance
   5. Implements strategies to reduce emotional stress
   6. Maintains skin integrity

MALABSORPTION SYNDROME

Data Base
A. Etiology and pathophysiology
   1. Failure to absorb one or more of the necessary ingested nutrients; can occur anywhere along the digestive process
   2. May be a primary disorder (celiac sprue or lactase deficiency) or secondary to gastric or intestinal

surgery (e.g., short-bowel syndrome), inflammatory disease, infection, radiation, or drug side effects
B. Clinical findings
   1. Subjective: weakness, fatigue, anorexia, and decreased feeling of well-being
   2. Objective: weight loss, flatulence, borborygmus (loud bowel sounds), abdominal distention, may experience diarrhea or bulky stool, steatorrhea (greasy, bulky, mushy stool with foul odor), clinical findings of protein deficiency, clinical findings related to deficiency in fat-soluble vitamins, dehydration, low serum values (albumin, transferrin, total lymphocyte count, hemoglobin, and hematocrit), positive results of lactose tolerance tests, biopsy of mucosa; and various deficiency specific absorption tests
C. Therapeutic interventions
   1. Resolve precipitating event
   2. Dietary therapy: avoid aggravating substances, supplement needed nutrients, reduce gluten intake with celiac sprue, restrict milk and/or enzyme supplementation in lactose intolerance; tube feedings, PPN or TPN during exacerbations
   3. Administration of antidiarrheals, antispasmodics, antibiotics, and vitamins as indicated

Nursing Care of Clients With Malabsorption Syndrome

A. Assessment/Analysis
   1. Weight, dietary habits, fluid and electrolyte status
   2. Stool for frequency, color, consistency, and steatorrhea
   3. Extent of bowel sounds, abdominal distention, flatulence
   4. Clinical findings associated with specific deficiencies (e.g., protein, vitamins)
   5. Presence of fatigue, weakness, and anorexia
   6. Laboratory data reflective of nutritional status
B. Planning/Implementation
   1. Monitor weight, fluid and electrolyte balance; look for clinical findings associated with the cause of the client's malabsorption
   2. Instruct client regarding dietary restrictions/ modifications
   3. Provide supplements or assist with PPN or TPN
C. Evaluations/Outcomes
   1. Maintains or regains weight
   2. Adheres to dietary regimen
   3. Maintains fluid and electrolyte balance
   4. Verbalizes a decrease in fatigue
   5. Reports a decrease in frequency of diarrhea

INFLAMMATORY BOWEL DISEASE, REGIONAL ENTERITIS (CROHN'S DISEASE)

Data Base
A. Etiology and pathophysiology
   1. Various theories exist, involving genetic predisposition, autoimmune reaction, or environmental causes

2. Cobblestone ulcerations along the mucosal wall of the terminal ileum, cecum, and ascending colon form scar tissue that inhibits food and water absorption
3. Ulceration of the intestinal submucosa accompanied by congestion, thickening of the small bowel, and fissure formations; fistulas and abscesses may form

B. Clinical findings
1. Subjective: nausea; severe abdominal pain, cramping, and spasms; exacerbations related to emotional upsets or dietary indiscretions with milk, milk products, and fried foods
2. Objective
   a. Weight loss; fever; elevated WBC count; diarrhea with mucus; electrolyte disturbances; presence of blood and fat in feces; enlargement of regional lymph nodes
   b. Barium study of upper GI tract shows stricture of the ileum (string sign)
   c. Endoscopy and biopsy to confirm diagnosis
   d. Fecal fat test determines fat content, an abnormal amount of which is significant in malabsorptive disorders or hypermotility
   e. Erythema nodosum, conjunctivitis, and arthritis
   f. D-Xylose tolerance test determines absorptive ability of upper intestinal tract
   g. CT scan shows bowel wall thickening and fistulas

C. Therapeutic interventions
1. NPO and TPN when inflammatory episodes are severe
2. Clear fluid diet progressing to bland, low-residue, low-fat diet, but increased calories, carbohydrates, proteins, and vitamins, especially K and B_{12} (when a large portion of the ileum is involved)
3. Pharmacologic management: antidiarrheals such as loperamide (Imodium, Kaopectate II, Pepto-Bismol); antispasmodics such as propantheline bromide (Pro-Banthine); immunosuppressives such as infliximab (Remicade); anticholinergics; antiinfectives such as metronidazole (Flagyl) and ciprofloxacin (Cipro); antiinflammatory therapy with steroids and adalimumab (Humira); vitamins
4. Surgery when complications such as fistulas or intestinal obstruction occur; anastomosis or temporary or permanent ostomy
5. Maintain fluid and electrolyte balance

Nursing Care of Clients With Crohn's Disease
A. Assessment/Analysis
1. Weight, temperature, and intake and output
2. Feces for color, consistency, and steatorrhea
3. Tenderness and guarding of abdomen, especially right lower quadrant
4. Presence and extent of bowel sounds

B. Planning/Implementation
1. Encourage verbalization of feelings; encourage client and family to participate in the Crohn's and Colitis Foundation of America

2. Observe for clinical findings of fluid and electrolyte imbalances; monitor intake and output
3. Observe for clinical findings of complications such as elevated temperature, increasing nausea and vomiting, abdominal rigidity
4. Assist with TPN if ordered (see Parenteral Replacement Therapy under Related Procedures)
5. Teach the client
   a. Dietary restrictions and modifications (see Inflammatory Bowel Disease, Ulcerative Colitis)
   b. To avoid taking laxatives and salicylates that irritate the intestinal mucosa
   c. How to take antidiarrheals and mucilloid drugs effectively
   d. Skin care if the perianal area is irritated
   e. The importance of seeking help early when exacerbations occur
6. Provide preoperative and postoperative care for intestinal surgery (see Preoperative and Postoperative Care in Inflammatory Bowel Disease, Ulcerative Colitis)

C. Evaluation/Outcomes
1. Reports a reduction in pain
2. Has a decrease in the number of bowel movements
3. Maintains nutritional status
4. Maintains fluid and electrolyte balance
5. Implements strategies to reduce emotional stress

INFLAMMATORY BOWEL DISEASE, ULCERATIVE COLITIS
Data Base
A. Etiology and pathophysiology
1. May be caused by emotional stress, autoimmune response, genetic predisposition, or bacterial infection before onset
2. Edema of mucous membrane of colon leads to bleeding and shallow ulcerations
3. Abscess formation occurs; the bowel wall shortens and becomes thin and fragile
4. Associated with increased risk for colon cancer

B. Clinical findings
1. Subjective: weakness; debilitation; anorexia; nausea; abdominal cramps
2. Objective: dehydration with tenting of skin; frequent passage of bloody, purulent, mucoid, watery stools; anemia; hypocalcemia; low-grade fever

C. Therapeutic interventions
1. Dietary management
   a. During acute episode, low-residue diet progressing to a regular diet; raw bran may be effective in controlling bouts of diarrhea and constipation
   b. Unrestricted fluid intake if tolerated; high-protein, high-calorie diet; avoidance of food allergens, especially milk
2. Pharmacologic management: antiemetics, anticholinergics, corticosteroids, antibiotics, sedatives, analgesics, tranquilizers, and

antidiarrheals; antiinflammatory agents: mesalamine (Lialda), Asacol, a once daily oral treatment for mild to moderate ulcerative colitis

3. Replacement of fluids and electrolytes that are lost because of diarrhea; TPN may be instituted
4. Surgical intervention: indicated when medical management is unsuccessful
   a. Segmental or partial colectomy with anastomosis
   b. Total colectomy with ileostomy
   c. Total colectomy with incontinent or continent ileostomy
   d. Total colectomy with ileoanal anastomosis (creation of an ileal pouch that maintains anal sphincter function)

Nursing Care of Clients With Ulcerative Colitis

A. Assessment/Analysis
   1. Localized areas of tenderness found over diseased bowel on palpation
   2. History of patterns and characteristics of bowel elimination
   3. Feces for color, consistency, and characteristics
   4. Temperature and weight for baseline data
   5. Presence and extent of bowel sounds
   6. Nutritional status

B. Planning/Implementation
   1. Instruct client to adhere to the following dietary program:
      a. Eat small, frequent meals of high-protein, high-calorie foods; low-fat diet helps decrease steatorrhea; if steatorrhea is present, vitamins A and E may be required as supplements
      b. Avoid irritating foods and spices
      c. Replace iron, calcium, and zinc losses with supplements; if there is ileal involvement, intramuscular injections of vitamin B_{12} may be prescribed monthly to reduce anemia
      d. Avoid all food allergens, especially milk; milk may be reintroduced when client is relatively asymptomatic; however, lactose intolerance is common and dairy restrictions may be permanent; lactase enzymes can be added to milk products to hydrolyze lactose
   2. Involve client in dietary selection; recognize preferences as much as possible
   3. Initiate administration and recording of fluid, electrolyte, or blood replacements
   4. Provide gentle, thorough perineal care
   5. Observe for complications such as rectal hemorrhage, fever, dehydration
   6. Allow the client and family time to verbalize feelings and participate in care; encourage participation in the Crohn's and Colitis Foundation of America
   7. Provide preoperative care: a nurse specialist should assist in preoperative stoma site assessment and marking; poorly placed stoma will prevent a tight seal of pouch, contributing to leakage, skin

excoriation, incompatibility with clothing, and decreased quality of life

8. Provide postoperative care
   a. Maintain nasogastric suction during the immediate postoperative period
   b. Provide colostomy care (see Related Procedures) monitor fecal drainage and fluid balance (Figure 8-5: Consistency of feces depending on intestinal location)
   c. Assess for clinical findings of peritonitis
   d. Assess viability of stoma: expected—brick red; inadequate perfusion—gray, pale pink, dark purple
   e. Teach client ileostomy care
      (1) Ileostomy: skin care, continuous use of appliance because the stoma drains continuously
      (2) Continent ileostomy (Kock pouch): pouch will stretch over time to hold over 500 mL; must be catheterized to drain effluent every 4 to 6 hours; external appliance unnecessary; a small dressing covers the stoma
   f. Teach dietary guidelines
      (1) Initial low-residue diet to promote healing
      (2) Avoidance of kernels or seeds that can cause obstruction

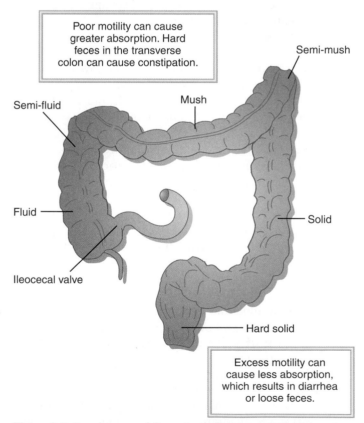

Poor motility can cause greater absorption. Hard feces in the transverse colon can cause constipation.

Semi-mush

Mush

Semi-fluid

Fluid

Solid

Ileocecal valve

Hard solid

Excess motility can cause less absorption, which results in diarrhea or loose feces.

Figure 8-5 Consistency of feces depending on intestinal location. As the feces move from the ileocecal valve to the anus, water is absorbed and the feces become more solid. The characteristics of the output from a colostomy depend on its location in the colon. (From Mahan LK, Escott-Stump S: *Krause's food and nutrition therapy*, ed 12, St Louis, 2008, Saunders.)

(3) Increased fluid intake to compensate for losses

g. Provide emotional support; involve enterostomal therapy nurse; refer to local ostomy organizations

9. Anticipate that stress can precipitate peristalsis

C. Evaluation/Outcomes

1. Maintains or regains weight
2. Adheres to dietary regimen
3. Establishes an acceptable pattern of soft, formed bowel movements
4. Client or family member demonstrates ability to perform ostomy care
5. Implements strategies to reduce emotional stress

✸ INTESTINAL OBSTRUCTION

Data Base

A. Etiology and pathophysiology

1. Interference with normal peristaltic movement of intestinal contents because of neurologic or mechanical impairments
2. Causes (Figure 8-6: Bowel obstructions)
   a. Carcinoma of the bowel
   b. Hernias
   c. Fecal impaction
   d. Adhesions (scar tissue that forms abnormal connections after surgery or inflammation)
   e. Intussusception (telescoping of the bowel on itself)
   f. Volvulus (twisting of the intestines)
   g. Paralytic ileus (interference with neural innervation of the intestines, resulting in a decrease in or absence of peristalsis; may be caused by surgical manipulation, electrolyte imbalance, or infection)
   h. Mesenteric infarction (occlusion of arterial blood supply to bowel, leading to necrosis of bowel)

B. Clinical findings

1. Subjective: colicky abdominal pain; constipation that may be accompanied by urge to defecate without results and seepage of fecal liquid
2. Objective: abdominal distention; vomiting that may contain fecal matter; decreased or absent bowel sounds; clinical findings of dehydration and electrolyte imbalance; obstipation; flat plate of the abdomen shows the bowel distended with air

C. Therapeutic interventions

1. Restriction of oral intake; administration of parenteral fluid and electrolytes
2. Surgical intervention: correction of cause (e.g., hernias, adhesions); colostomy, cecostomy, or ileostomy
3. Decompression of GI tract by means of a nasogastric or intestinal tube

Nursing Care of Clients With Intestinal Obstruction

A. Assessment/Analysis

1. Detailed history to determine risk and causative factors

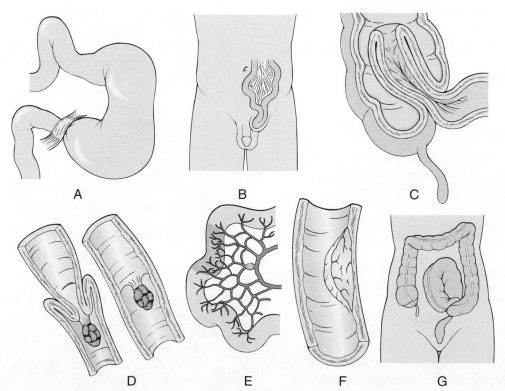

Figure 8-6 Bowel obstructions. **A,** Adhesions. **B,** Strangulated inguinal hernia. **C,** Ileocecal intussusception. **D,** Intussusception from polyps. **E,** Mesenteric occlusion. **F,** Neoplasm. **G,** Volvulus of the sigmoid colon. (From Lewis SL et al: *Medical-surgical nursing: assessment and management of clinical problems,* ed 7, St Louis, 2007, Mosby.)

2. Abdomen for peristaltic waves, distention
3. Presence and characteristics of bowel sounds
4. Previous pattern and characteristics of bowel elimination

B. Planning/Implementation
1. Assess for dehydration and electrolyte imbalance; monitor intake and output
2. Auscultate for bowel sounds; note the passage of flatus
3. Administer oral hygiene frequently
4. Provide special care for the client with an intestinal tube
   a. Once the tube reaches the stomach, position the client on the right side to facilitate passage of tube through the pylorus; then in a semi-Fowler's position to continue the gradual advance into the intestines
   b. Coil and loosely attach extra tubing to the client's gown to avoid tension against peristaltic action
   c. Instill or irrigate with sterile saline every 6 to 8 hours or as ordered to maintain patency
   d. Assess placement of the tube; record the level of advancement; advance (usually 2 to 3 inches every hour) as ordered
   e. When the tube is discontinued, remove gradually because it is being pulled against peristalsis
5. Encourage fluids and foods high in fiber if constipated

C. Evaluation/Outcomes
1. Establishes a regular pattern of bowel elimination
2. Maintains fluid and electrolyte balance

DIVERTICULAR DISEASE

Data Base
A. Etiology and pathophysiology
1. Diverticulosis: multiple pouchlike herniations of intestinal mucosa, as a result of weakness and increased intraabdominal pressure; may be asymptomatic
2. Diverticulitis: inflammation caused by food or feces trapped in a diverticulum; may lead to bleeding, perforation, peritonitis, and bowel obstruction
3. Most commonly occurs in the sigmoid colon, but could occur anywhere along the GI tract
4. Incidence increases with age; inadequate dietary fiber, history of constipation with straining at stool, and genetic predisposition are risk factors

B. Clinical findings
1. Subjective: cramping, colicky pain in left lower quadrant; nausea; malaise
2. Objective
   a. Diarrhea or constipation; frank blood in stool; abdominal distention; fever; leukocytosis
   b. Diagnostic tests: CT scan, abdominal x-ray, and colonoscopy provide direct evidence of the disease

C. Therapeutic interventions
1. Prevention through high-fiber diet; may be encouraged to avoid nuts and foods with small seeds (e.g., berries, caraway seeds, sesame seeds, popcorn)
2. NPO or clear liquids during acute diverticulitis
3. Pharmacologic management: analgesics (morphine sulfate is avoided because it can increase intracolonic pressure), antibiotics, antispasmodics, and bulk-forming laxatives and stool softeners
4. Fluid and electrolyte replacement
5. Surgery: hemicolectomy, temporary loop colostomy, and removal of involved bowel

Nursing Care of Clients With Diverticular Disease
A. Assessment/Analysis
1. History of constipation and/or diarrhea with progression of clinical findings
2. Foods that may precipitate acute diverticulitis
3. Stool for consistency and presence of blood
4. Abdomen for distention
5. Presence and extent of bowel sounds

B. Planning/Implementation
1. Teach client: importance of high-fiber and high-fluid intake; foods to avoid to prevent diverticulitis
2. Prevent constipation with dietary bran and bulk laxatives as ordered
3. Maintain NPO and gastric decompression if ordered during acute episode
4. Monitor for clinical findings of peritonitis: pain, hypotension, abdominal rigidity, abdominal distention, and leukocytosis
5. Administer fluid and electrolyte replacement
6. Teach the importance of completing antibiotic regimen
7. Provide care related to bowel surgery (see Nursing Care of Clients With Cancer of the Small Intestine, Colon, or Rectum)

C. Evaluation/Outcomes
1. Exhibits normal pattern of soft, formed bowel movements
2. Increases intake of high-fiber foods
3. Avoids foods that should be eliminated from diet
4. Reports relief from pain
5. Maintains fluid and electrolyte balance

CANCER OF THE SMALL INTESTINE, COLON, OR RECTUM

Data Base
A. Etiology and pathophysiology
1. Tumor causes narrowing of lumen of bowel, ulcerations, necrosis, or perforation
2. Predisposing factors: familial polyps, aging, chronic ulcerative colitis, bowel stasis, ingestion of food additives, and a high-fat, low-fiber diet

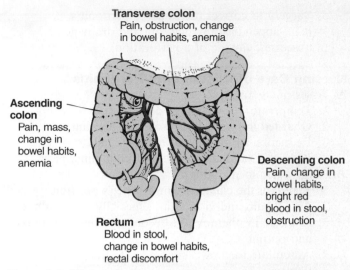

Transverse colon
Pain, obstruction, change
in bowel habits, anemia

Ascending colon
Pain, mass,
change in
bowel habits,
anemia

Descending colon
Pain, change in
bowel habits,
bright red
blood in stool,
obstruction

Rectum
Blood in stool,
change in bowel habits,
rectal discomfort

Figure 8-7 Clinical findings of colorectal cancer by location of primary lesion. (McCance KL, Heuther SE: *Pathophysiology: the biological basis for disease in adults and children*, ed 5, St. Louis, 2006, Mosby.)

3. Cancer of the colon is more common in males, and incidence increases after 50 years of age
4. Cancer of the small intestine is rare; adenocarcinoma of the large intestine is relatively common

B. Clinical findings (Figure 8-7: Clinical findings of colorectal cancer by location of primary lesion)
  1. Subjective: abdominal discomfort or pain; weakness and fatigue
  2. Objective
    a. Alterations in usual bowel function (constipation or diarrhea or alternating constipation and diarrhea); pencil-shaped or ribbon-shaped stool
    b. Abdominal distention
    c. Weight loss
    d. Frank or occult blood in stool; secondary anemia
    e. Digital examination detects any palpable masses
    f. Proctosigmoidoscopy or colonoscopy to visualize the bowel directly and determine the presence of abnormalities; permit biopsy
    g. Cytologic examination of tissue from GI tract detects malignant cells
    h. Elevated alkaline phosphatase and aspartate aminotransferase (AST) levels detect metastasis to the liver
    i. Elevated serum carcinoembryonic antigen (CEA) level may indicate carcinoma of the colon

C. Therapeutic interventions
  1. Surgical intervention to remove the mass and restore bowel function (e.g., colostomy, hemicolectomy, abdominal perineal resection)
  2. Radiation in nonsurgical situations may be used to limit clinical findings; may be used preoperatively to reduce size of tumor or postoperatively to limit metastases
  3. Chemotherapy to reduce the lesion and limit metastases

4. Preparation for surgery
  a. Antibiotics (e.g., neomycin or sulfonamides) to reduce bacteria in the bowel
  b. Type and cross-match of blood for transfusions to correct anemia
  c. Vitamin supplements to improve nutritional status
  d. Gastric or intestinal decompression
  e. Bowel preparation
  f. Postoperative care of the stoma

Nursing Care of Clients With Cancer of the Small Intestine, Colon, or Rectum

A. Assessment/Analysis
  1. Detailed history of clinical findings and risk factors
  2. Stool for frequency, color, consistency, shape
  3. Weight for baseline data
  4. Areas of abdominal discomfort on palpation
  5. Presence and extent of bowel sounds

B. Planning/Implementation
  1. Observe vital signs, increasing abdominal pain, nausea, and vomiting to detect early clinical findings of complications
  2. Monitor patency of gastric or intestinal tube; instill or irrigate with normal saline as ordered; note the amount and character of drainage
  3. Implement preoperative bowel preparation and intestinal antisepsis
  4. Administer chemotherapeutic drugs if ordered; observe for significant side effects such as stomatitis, dehydration, nausea and vomiting, diarrhea, leukopenia
  5. Administer electrolyte and parenteral fluid replacement as ordered in situations of bleeding, vomiting, and/or obstruction
  6. Administer progressive diet as ordered; assess tolerance; teach dietary modifications to client and family, including non–gas-forming foods, avoidance of stimulants, adequate fluid intake; diet should be as close to the client's usual diet as possible
  7. Teach the importance of diet in supporting the body's natural defenses; emphasize high nutrient dense foods from the fruit, vegetable, cereal grain, and legume groups with some lean meat, fish, and poultry; encourage client to eat as great a variety of foods as can be tolerated; vitamin and mineral supplements can be encouraged, especially the immune-stimulating factors
  8. Provide preoperative and postoperative care for colon surgery (see Preoperative and Postoperative Care in Inflammatory Bowel Disease, Ulcerative Colitis)
  9. Assess the client's reaction to the colostomy, recognizing that it will depend on how the client views the colostomy as affecting lifestyle, physical and emotional status, social and cultural background, and place and role in the family; client may demonstrate the stages of grieving

10. Provide colostomy care (see Colostomy Irrigation under Related Procedures); encourage involvement in colostomy care as soon as physical and emotional status permits
11. Recognize that the client with a cecostomy or colostomy is especially sensitive to odors, gestures, and facial expressions
12. Teach the client and family the following: care of the colostomy; measures to facilitate acceptance and adjustment; resumption of activities including sexual activities; avoidance of contact sports; and the need for regular medical supervision
13. Teach the client that colostomy drainage begins in 3 to 4 days; it can be controlled by following a regular irrigation schedule and dietary modifications for colostomy in distal colon; adequate uninterrupted time for colostomy care is necessary
14. Arrange for follow-up care with community agencies as required (e.g., public health, home care programs, American Cancer Society, ostomy resource person)
15. Teach the need to periodically dilate the stoma to prevent strictures
16. Instruct client and family to prevent postoperative infection through vigorous handwashing, avoidance of sick individuals and people with pneumonia or influenza vaccinations if possible
C. Evaluation/Outcomes
    1. Maintains adequate fluid and electrolyte balance
    2. Resumes a regular pattern of bowel elimination
    3. Client or family member demonstrates ability to perform ostomy care
    4. Discusses feelings concerning diagnosis, prognosis, and ostomy
    5. Maintains nutritional status

PERITONITIS
Data Base
A. Etiology and pathophysiology
    1. Inflammation of the peritoneum (most commonly caused by *Escherichia coli*)
    2. Generally caused by infection from perforation of GI tract, chemical stress, or trauma
B. Clinical findings
    1. Subjective: abdominal pain, rebound tenderness; malaise; nausea
    2. Objective: abdominal muscle rigidity; vomiting; elevated temperature, WBCs, and neutrophil count
C. Therapeutic interventions
    1. Bed rest in a semi-Fowler's position to localize drainage to the dependent portion of the abdominal cavity
    2. Nasogastric decompression until the client passes flatus
    3. Parenteral replacement of fluids and electrolytes; TPN
    4. Antibiotic therapy

5. Surgery to correct the cause of peritonitis (e.g., appendectomy, incision and drainage of abscesses, closure of a perforation)

Nursing Care of Clients With Peritonitis
A. Assessment/Analysis
    1. Temperature for baseline data
    2. Guarded movements and/or self-splinting
    3. Reduction or absence of bowel sounds
    4. Presence and characteristics of abdominal pain
B. Planning/Implementation
    1. Maintain the client in semi-Fowler's position
    2. Assess pain and vital signs, especially temperature
    3. Monitor IV therapy, GI decompression, and intake and output
    4. Auscultate for bowel sounds; note the passage of flatus
    5. Administer IV antibiotics
    6. Provide pain management with opioid analgesics
C. Evaluation/Outcomes
    1. Reports absence of pain
    2. Maintains fluid and electrolyte balance
    3. Reestablishes regular pattern of bowel elimination

HEMORRHOIDS
Data Base
A. Etiology and pathophysiology
    1. Varicosities of the rectum that can be internal or external
    2. Precipitated by constipation, prolonged sitting or standing, straining at defecation, obesity, and pregnancy
B. Clinical findings
    1. Subjective: anal pain; pruritus
    2. Objective: protrusion of varicosities around the anus; rectal bleeding and mucus discharge
C. Therapeutic interventions
    1. Low-roughage diet (elimination of raw fruits and vegetables) during acute exacerbations
    2. High-fiber diet during remissions to prevent constipation
    3. Stool softeners to facilitate passage of stool
    4. Analgesic suppositories and ointments; sitz baths or ice compresses for discomfort
    5. Surgical intervention: ligation (internal hemorrhoids may be ligated with rubber bands); cryosurgery; laser; sclerotherapy; hemorrhoidectomy

Nursing Care of Clients With Hemorrhoids
A. Assessment/Analysis
    1. History of causative factors
    2. Presence and characteristics of pain/bleeding
    3. Presence of hemorrhoids in perianal area
B. Planning/Implementation
    1. Help relieve pain by sitz baths, ice compresses, local analgesics
    2. Provide privacy and sufficient time for defecation, especially after meals

3. Encourage intake of high-fiber foods; promote intake of at least 8 glasses of fluid per day
4. Discourage routine use of laxatives, which results in dependency; bulking agents such as Metamucil or stool softeners such as Colace may be prescribed
5. Instruct client to implement regular bowel habits
6. Provide care for the client having a hemorrhoidectomy
   a. Administer cleansing enemas preoperatively
   b. Observe for rectal hemorrhage and urinary retention postoperatively; explain that some bleeding with a bowel movement is expected
   c. Teach how to administer a retention enema on the second or third postoperative day, if ordered, to stimulate defecation and soften the stool
C. Evaluation/Outcomes
   1. Reports increased comfort, particularly on defecation
   2. Adheres to treatment regimen
   3. Establishes a pattern of regular bowel movements without straining or use of laxatives

HERNIAS

Data Base
A. Etiology and pathophysiology
   1. Protrusion of an organ or structure through a weakening in the abdominal wall; may result from a congenital or acquired defect
   2. If the protruding structure can be manipulated back in place, the hernia is said to be reducible; if it cannot, it is considered incarcerated
   3. Strangulation occurs when blood supply to the tissues within the hernia is disrupted; this is an emergency situation, since gangrene occurs
   4. Hernias are named by location: incisional, umbilical, femoral, inguinal
B. Clinical findings
   1. Subjective: history of appearance of swelling after lifting, coughing, or exercise; pain caused by incarceration or strangulation; nausea can accompany strangulation
   2. Objective: swelling (lump) in the groin or umbilicus, or near an old surgical incision that may subside when the client is in a recumbent position; vomiting and abdominal distention when strangulation occurs

C. Therapeutic interventions
   1. Manual reduction by gently pushing the mass back into the abdominal cavity
   2. When the client is a poor surgical risk, a truss (pad worn next to skin held in place under pressure by a belt) may be ordered
   3. Herniorrhaphy: repair of the defect in the abdominal musculature or fascia
   4. Hernioplasty: insertion of wire, mesh, or plastic to strengthen abdominal wall

Nursing Care of Clients With Hernias
A. Assessment/Analysis
   1. History of potential causative factors
   2. Presence or absence of bowel sounds on auscultation
   3. Abdomen with client in standing and lying positions to determine if hernia reduces with positional change
B. Planning/Implementation
   1. Avoid abdominal palpation if hernia is strangulated
   2. Provide care after surgery
      a. Instruct to avoid coughing if possible; use deep breathing and incentive spirometry to prevent respiratory complications; encourage self-splinting
      b. Administer mild cathartics as ordered to prevent straining and increased intraabdominal pressure
      c. Apply an ice bag and scrotal support if the scrotum is edematous postoperatively to reduce edema and pain
      d. Administer medication for pain as ordered
      e. Instruct to avoid lifting or strenuous exercise on discharge until permitted by the surgeon
C. Evaluation/Outcomes
   1. Reports decreased pain
   2. Restates discharge instructions
   3. Avoids straining on defecation

EATING DISORDERS

For anorexia nervosa and bulimia nervosa, see Eating Disorders and General Nursing Care of Clients With Eating Disorders in Chapter 20. See Obesity in this chapter.

Nursing Care of Clients With Endocrine System Disorders

OVERVIEW
REVIEW OF ANATOMY AND PHYSIOLOGY

Function of the Endocrine System

Endocrine glands continuously secrete products called hormones, which are chemical messengers that deliver stimulatory or inhibitory signals to target cells as a result of a feedback mechanism; once secreted, hormones usually remain present in the body for 4 to 6 hours

Structures of the Endocrine System

(See Figure 9-1: Principal endocrine glands)

Thyroid Gland

A. Overlies thyroid cartilage below the larynx
B. Thyroid hormones: accelerate cellular reactions in most body cells
  1. Thyroxine: stimulates metabolic rate; essential for normal physical and mental development
  2. Triiodothyronine: inhibits anterior pituitary secretion of thyroid-stimulating hormone
  3. Calcitonin (thyrocalcitonin): decreases loss of calcium from bone; promotes hypocalcemia; action opposite that of parathormone

Parathyroid Gland

A. Small glands (2 to 12) embedded in the posterior part of the thyroid
B. Parathyroid hormone (parathormone)
  1. Increases blood calcium concentration
    a. Breakdown of bone with release of calcium into blood (requires the active form of vitamin D)
    b. Calcium absorption from intestine into blood
    c. Kidney tubule reabsorption of calcium
  2. Decreases blood phosphate concentration by slowing its reabsorption from the kidneys, thereby decreasing calcium loss in urine

Testes and Ovaries

See Structures of the Male Reproductive System in Chapter 12 and Structures of the Female Reproductive System in Chapter 23

Adrenal Glands

A. Two closely associated structures, adrenal medulla and adrenal cortex, positioned at each kidney's superior border

B. Adrenal hormones
  1. Adrenal medulla: produces two catecholamines, epinephrine and norepinephrine
    a. Stimulate liver and skeletal muscle to break down glycogen to produce glucose
    b. Increase oxygen use and carbon dioxide production
    c. Increase blood concentration of free fatty acids through stimulation of lipolysis in adipose tissue
    d. Cause constriction of nearly all blood vessels of body, thus increasing total peripheral resistance and arterial pressure to shunt blood to vital organs
    e. Increase heart rate and force of contraction and thus raise cardiac output
    f. Inhibit contractions of gastrointestinal and uterine smooth muscle
    g. Epinephrine significantly dilates bronchial smooth muscle
  2. Adrenal cortex: secretes the mineralocorticoid aldosterone and the glucocorticoids cortisol and corticosterone
    a. Aldosterone
      (1) Markedly accelerates sodium and water reabsorption by kidney tubules
      (2) Markedly accelerates potassium excretion by kidney tubules
      (3) Aldosterone secretion increases as sodium ions decrease or potassium ions increase
    b. Cortisol and corticosterone
      (1) Accelerate mobilization and catabolism of tissue protein and fats
      (2) Accelerate liver gluconeogenesis (a hyperglycemic effect)
      (3) Decrease antibody formation (immunosuppressive, antiallergic effect)
      (4) Slow the proliferation of fibroblasts characteristic of inflammation (antiinflammatory effect)
      (5) Decrease adrenocorticotropic hormone (ACTH) secretion
      (6) Mildly accelerate sodium and water reabsorption and potassium excretion by kidney tubules
      (7) Increase release of coagulation factors

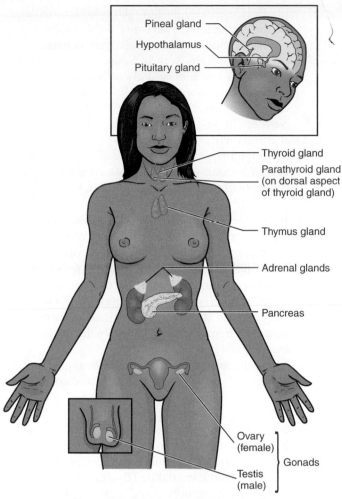

Figure 9-1 Principal endocrine glands.

Labels in figure:
Pineal gland
Hypothalamus
Pituitary gland
Thyroid gland
Parathyroid gland (on dorsal aspect of thyroid gland)
Thymus gland
Adrenal glands
Pancreas
Ovary (female)
Testis (male)
Gonads

Thymus Gland
A. Located at root of neck and anterior thorax
B. Thymic hormone (thymosin)
  1. Regulates immunologic processes
  2. Just after birth produces T lymphocytes that migrate to the lymph nodes and spleen to provide cell-mediated immunity
  3. Synthesizes hormones that regulate the rate of development of lymphoid cells, particularly T cells

Pineal Gland
A. Located in midbrain attached to third ventricle
B. Pineal hormone (melatonin)
  1. May regulate diurnal fluctuations of hypothalamic-hypophyseal hormones
  2. Inhibits numerous endocrine functions, particularly gonadotropic hormones

Pituitary Gland
A. Located in cranial cavity in sella turcica of sphenoid bone; near optic chiasm
B. Composed of an anterior lobe (adenohypophysis) and a posterior lobe (neurohypophysis)
C. Pituitary hormones
  1. Hormones secreted by the anterior lobe
    a. Growth hormone (GH)
      (1) Promotes protein anabolism
      (2) Promotes fat mobilization and catabolism
      (3) Slows carbohydrate metabolism
    b. Thyroid-stimulating hormone (TSH): stimulates synthesis and secretion of thyroid hormones
    c. Adrenocorticotropic hormone (ACTH)
      (1) Stimulates growth of adrenal cortex
      (2) Stimulates the secretion of glucocorticoids; slightly stimulates mineralocorticoid secretion
    d. Follicle-stimulating hormone (FSH)
      (1) Stimulates primary graafian follicle to grow and develop
      (2) Stimulates follicle cells to secrete estrogen
      (3) Stimulates development of seminiferous tubules and spermatogenesis
    e. Luteinizing hormone (LH)
      (1) Stimulates maturation of follicle and ovum; required for ovulation
      (2) Forms corpus luteum in ruptured follicle following ovulation; stimulates corpus luteum to secrete progesterone
      (3) In males, LH is called interstitial cell–stimulating hormone (ICSH); stimulates testes to secrete testosterone
    f. Prolactin (PRL)
      (1) Promotes breast development during pregnancy
      (2) Initiates milk production after delivery
      (3) Stimulates progesterone secretion by corpus luteum

Pancreas
A. Retroperitoneal in abdominal cavity
B. Pancreatic hormones: regulate glucose and protein homeostasis through the action of insulin and glucagon
  1. Insulin: secreted by beta cells of islets of Langerhans
    a. Promotes the cellular uptake of glucose
    b. Stimulates intracellular macromolecular synthesis, such as glycogen synthesis (glyconeogenesis), fat synthesis (lipogenesis), and protein synthesis
    c. Stimulates cellular uptake of sodium and potassium (latter is significant in the treatment of diabetic coma with insulin)
  2. Glucagon: secreted by alpha cells of islets of Langerhans
    a. Induces liver glycogenolysis; antagonizes the glycogen synthesis stimulated by insulin
    b. Inhibits hepatic protein synthesis; this makes amino acids available for gluconeogenesis and also increases urea production
    c. Stimulates hepatic ketogenesis and release of glycerol and fatty acids from adipose tissue when cellular glucose level falls

2. Hormones secreted by the posterior lobe
   a. Antidiuretic hormone (ADH, vasopressin)
      (1) Increases water reabsorption by distal and collecting tubules of kidneys
      (2) Stimulates vasoconstriction, raising blood pressure
   b. Oxytocin
      (1) Stimulates contractions by pregnant uterus
      (2) Stimulates milk ejection from alveoli of lactating breasts into ducts
   c. Melanocyte-stimulating hormone (MSH): stimulates synthesis and dispersion of melanin in skin, causing darkening

RELATED PHARMACOLOGY

Antidiabetic Agents

A. Description
   1. Used to treat diabetes mellitus
   2. Classified into two types: insulin for parenteral use and oral antidiabetics
   3. Insulin
      a. Acts to facilitate the transport of glucose and amino acids across the cell membrane; promotes glycogenesis and protein synthesis
      b. Available in three forms: human, beef, and pork; human insulin is the least antigenic; administered parenterally; brands or forms should not be substituted without medical supervision; nonhuman insulin rarely used since recombinant forms became available
      c. Available in rapid-acting, intermediate-acting, and long-acting forms; rapid-acting and intermediate-acting forms are available in mixed preparations (e.g., Humulin 70/30, which contains 70% NPH and 30% regular insulin)
   4. Oral antidiabetics
      a. Require some functioning beta cells
      b. Lower serum glucose level in a variety of ways depending on the drug

B. Examples
   1. Insulin
      a. Rapid-acting
         (1) Lispro (Humalog), aspart (Novolog), glulisine (Apidra); onset: 10 to 15 minutes; peak: 1 hour; duration: 3 hours
         (2) Exubera: short-acting inhalation insulin; used in conjunction with a long-acting insulin; taken 10 minutes before meals
      b. Short-acting: regular (Humulin R, Novolin R); onset: 0.5 to 1 hour; peak: 2 to 3 hours; duration: 4 to 6 hours
      c. Intermediate-acting: NPH (Humulin N) and Lente; onset: 3 to 4 hours; peak: 4 to 12 hours; duration: 16 to 20 hours
      d. Long-acting
         (1) Ultralente: onset: 6 to 8 hours; peak: 12 to 16 hours; duration: 20 to 30 hours

(2) Peakless basal insulin: glargine (Lantus) and insulin detemir (Levemir): slow, prolonged absorption leads to a relatively constant concentration over 24 hours without peaks; usually taken once daily at bedtime
      e. Combination: isophane insulin suspesion (NPH) and regular insulin (Humulin 70/30 or 50/50; Novolin 70/30)
   2. Oral antidiabetics (hypoglycemics)
      a. Sulfonylureas: stimulate beta cells to produce insulin; second-generation sulfonylureas: glipizide (Glucotrol), glyburide (Micronase), glimepiride (Amaryl)
      b. Biguanides: reduce the rate of endogenous glucose production by liver; increase the use of glucose by muscle and fat cells; metformin (Glucophage)
      c. Thiazolidinediones: improve insulin sensitivity, thus improving peripheral glucose uptake; rosiglitazone (Avandia), pioglitazone (Actos)
      d. Meglitinides: stimulate quick release of insulin by beta cells; repaglinide (Prandin), nateglinide (Starlix)
      e. Alpha-glucosidase inhibitors: block digestion of ingested carbohydrates and slow absorption of glucose; acarbose (Precose), miglitol (Glyset)
      f. DPP4 inhibitor: sitagliptin (Januvia)
      g. Synthetic analog of human amylin: decreases gastric emptying; pramlintide acetate (Symlin)
      h. Incretin mimetic: stimulates insulin production in type 2 diabetes; exenatide (Byetta)
      i. Combination: glyburide and metformin (Glucovance); sitagliptin and metformin hydrochloride (Janumet); pioglitazone HCl and metformin (Actoplus Met)

C. Major side effects
   1. Insulin: hypoglycemia—irritability, tachycardia, hunger, moist skin, tremor, headache, confusion, seizures; lipodystrophy (incidence decreased dramatically since advent of human recombinant insulin); inhalation insulin—cough, dry mouth, chest discomfort
   2. Oral antidiabetics: hypoglycemia; skin rash, allergic reactions, pruritus (hypersensitivity); jaundice (hepatic alterations); thrombocytopenia, lactic acidosis, vitamin B_{12} deficiency; not recommended for clients diagnosed with heart failure (Glucophage); bloating, gas pains, and diarrhea (Precose, Glyset); hepatotoxicity, increased fracture risk (Avandia)

D. Nursing care
   1. Assess clients for clinical findings of hypoglycemia and side effects of medications
   2. Instruct client to
      a. Use proper medication administration procedure
      b. Comply with dietary program, including snacks
      c. Avoid alcohol, especially when taking Glucophage
      d. Perform self-monitoring of blood glucose (SMBG) levels
      e. Carry medical alert card

f. Be prepared for hypoglycemic incidents; administer rapid-acting glucose (e.g., glucose solution or tablets) followed by complex carbohydrate and protein (e.g., cheese and crackers) to stabilize blood glucose level

g. Comply with regular laboratory testing such as measurements of blood glucose, glycosylated hemoglobin (glycohemoglobin, Hgb A_{1c}), liver enzymes

3. Administer insulin

a. Administer all but inhalation forms of insulin subcutaneous because insulin is destroyed by gastric juices if taken by mouth; regular or rapid-acting insulins can be used in continuous Sub-Q insulin infusion devices

b. Use only regular insulin for IV administration

c. If premixed insulin is not prescribed and two forms are to be mixed, draw up regular insulin first so as not to accidentally dilute the regular insulin vial with NPH; peakless basal insulin cannot be mixed with other insulins because it results in precipitation

d. Rotation of sites not necessary with recombinant insulin; abdomen is preferred site because absorption is not influenced by exercise

e. Dosage adjustment will be necessary for NPO status and when ill

4. Offer emotional support to client; therapy is lifelong

5. Metformin: withhold drug before diagnostic studies requiring iodinated contrast media; increased risk of hypoglycemia when given concurrently with allopurinol (Zyloprim)

6. Instruct to prevent complications of hyperglycemia with frequent glucose monitoring and multiple daily injections of insulin as needed

Thyroid Enhancers

A. Description
   1. Regulate the metabolic rate of body cells; aid in growth and development of bones and teeth; and affect protein, fat, and carbohydrate metabolism
   2. Replace thyroid hormone in clients experiencing a reduction in or absence of thyroid gland function
   3. Available in oral and parenteral (IV) preparations

B. Examples: levothyroxine sodium (Synthroid) is drug of choice; liothyronine sodium (Cytomel); liotrix (Thyrolar)

C. Major side effects: increased metabolism (increased serum T_3, T_4); hyperactivity (increased metabolic rate); cardiac stimulation (increased cardiac metabolism)

D. Nursing care
   1. Instruct client to
      a. Report the occurrence of any side effects to the physician immediately
      b. Take medication as scheduled at the same time daily; do not stop abruptly
      c. Take radial pulse rate; notify physician if greater than 100 beats/min
      d. Carry medical alert card
      e. Keep all scheduled appointments with physician; medical supervision is necessary

2. Assess for potentiation of anticoagulant effect
3. Offer emotional support to client; therapy usually is lifelong
4. Assess client for clinical findings of hyperthyroidism

Thyroid Inhibitors

A. Description
   1. Interfere with the synthesis and release of thyroid hormone; inhibit oxidation of iodides to prevent their combination with tyrosine in formation of thyroxine
   2. Treat hyperthyroidism
   3. Available in oral and parenteral (IV) preparations

B. Examples: iodine (potassium iodide); methimazole (Tapazole); propylthiouracil (PTU)

C. Major side effects: agranulocytosis (decreased WBCs); skin disturbances (hypersensitivity); nausea, vomiting (irritation of gastric mucosa); decreased metabolism (decreased production of serum T_3, T_4); iodine: bitter taste, stains teeth (local oral effect on mucosa and teeth)

D. Nursing care
   1. Instruct client to
      a. Report the occurrence of any side effects to physician, especially sore throat, jaundice, and fever
      b. Avoid crowded places and potentially infectious situations
   2. Administer liquid iodine preparations diluted in beverage of choice; use a straw to avoid staining teeth
   3. Assess for clinical findings of hypothyroidism

Adrenocorticoids

A. Description
   1. Interfere with the release of factors important in producing the normal inflammatory and immune responses (immunosuppression)
   2. Remove fluid accumulation from brain, thereby decreasing cerebral edema
   3. Increase glucose and fat formation and promote protein breakdown
   4. Used for hormonal replacement therapy
   5. Available in oral, parenteral (IM, IV), inhalation, intraarticular, and topical (including ophthalmic) preparations

B. Examples
   1. Glucocorticoids
      a. Long-acting: dexamethasone (Decadron)
      b. Intermediate-acting: methylprednisolone (Medrol, Solu-Medrol)
      c. Short-acting: hydrocortisone (Solu-Cortef)
   2. Mineralocorticoids: fludrocortisone (Florinef)

C. Major side effects
   1. Cushingoid clinical findings (increased glucocorticoid activity; causing facial edema, fluid retention, etc.)
   2. Hypertension (sodium and water retention)
   3. Hyperglycemia (increased carbohydrate catabolism; gluconeogenesis)
   4. Mood changes (CNS effect)
   5. GI irritation and ulcer formation (local GI effect)
   6. Cataracts (hyperglycemia)
   7. Hypokalemia (potassium excretion)
   8. Decreased wound healing; leukopenia

9. Osteoporosis
10. Derivatives with 17-ketosteroid properties: masculinization in females

D. Nursing care
1. Administer oral preparations with food, milk, or antacid
2. Monitor weight, BP, and serum electrolytes during therapy
3. Avoid placing client in potentially infectious situations
4. Assess for GI bleeding; monitor blood glucose level in people with diabetes
5. In addition to carrying a medical alert card, instruct client to
   a. Avoid exposure to infections; notify physician if fever or sore throat occurs; avoid immunizations during therapy
   b. Avoid using salt; encourage foods high in potassium
   c. Avoid missing, changing, or withdrawing drug suddenly
   d. Avoid NSAIDs and OTC medications
6. Withdraw drug therapy gradually to permit adrenal recovery; teach to take medications only as directed, and explain why

Antidiuretic Hormone

A. Description
1. Promotes water reabsorption by the distal renal tubules and causes vasoconstriction and increased muscle tone of the bladder, GI tract, uterus, and blood vessels
2. Treatment for diabetes insipidus
3. Available in parenteral (IM, Sub-Q) or nasal preparation

B. Examples
1. Lypressin (Diapid) for intranasal administration; vasopressin (Pitressin)

C. Major side effects
1. Increased intestinal activity (direct peristaltic stimulant)
2. Hyponatremia (water reabsorption)
3. Pallor (hemodilution)
4. Water intoxication (water reabsorption)
5. Cardiac disturbances (fluid/electrolyte imbalance)
6. Nasal irritation (lypressin has local effect on nasal mucosa)

D. Nursing care
1. Assess for clinical findings of water intoxication during therapy, monitor intake and output and urine specific gravity
2. Assess vital signs, especially blood pressure
3. If drug is administered to improve bladder or bowel tone, assess for passage of flatus and urine output

MAJOR DISORDERS OF THE ENDOCRINE SYSTEM

HYPERPITUITARISM

Data Base
A. Etiology and pathophysiology
1. May result from overactivity of gland or from an adenoma

2. Characterized by an excessive concentration of pituitary hormones (e.g., growth hormone [GH], adrenocorticotrpon [ACTH], prolactin [PRL]) in the blood, overactivity, and changes in the anterior lobe of the pituitary gland
3. Two classifications of GH overproduction
   a. Gigantism: generalized increase in size, especially in children; involves the long bones
   b. Acromegaly: occurs after epiphyseal closing, with subsequent enlargement of cartilage, bone, and soft tissues of body
4. ACTH overproduction leads to Cushing's syndrome

B. Clinical findings
1. Subjective: headaches; depression; weakness
2. Objective
   a. Increased soft tissue and bone thickness
   b. Facial features become coarse and heavy, with enlargement of lower jaw, lips, and tongue
   c. Enlarged hands and feet
   d. Increased GH, ACTH, or PRL
   e. X-ray examination of long bones, skull (sella turcica area), and jaw demonstrates change in structure
   f. Amenorrhea
   g. Clinical findings of increased intracranial pressure such as vomiting, papilledema, focal neurologic deficits
   h. Diabetes and hyperthyroidism may also occur

C. Therapeutic interventions
1. Medications
   a. Somatostatin analog octreotide (Sandostatin)
   b. Dopamine agonist bromocriptine (Parlodel)
   c. Medications to relieve clinical findings of other endocrine imbalances resulting from pituitary hyperfunctioning
2. Surgical intervention (hypophysectomy) or irradiation of the pituitary

Nursing Care of Clients With Hyperpituitarism
A. Assessment/Analysis
1. Changes in energy level, sexual function, and menstrual patterns; signs of increased intracranial pressure
2. Face, hands, and feet for thickening, enlargement; changes in the size of hat, gloves, rings, or shoes
3. Presence of dysphagia or voice changes
4. Presence of hypogonadism as a result of hyperprolactinemia
5. Reaction to changes in physical appearance and sexual function

B. Planning/Implementation
1. Help to accept the altered body image that is irreversible
2. Assist family to understand what the client is experiencing
3. Help to recognize that medical supervision will be lifelong

4. Help to understand the basis for the change in sexual functioning
5. Encourage to express feelings
6. Care after a hypophysectomy
   a. Encourage following the established medical regimen
   b. Protect from stressful situations
   c. Protect from infection
   d. Follow and maintain an established schedule for hormone replacement
7. Care for the client undergoing intracranial surgery
   a. Perform neurologic assessments; monitor for increased intracranial pressure
   b. Monitor I&O, and check daily weight to identify complication of diabetes insipidus
   c. Check clear nasal drainage for glucose to determine presence of CSF
   d. Encourage deep breathing, but not coughing
   e. Institute measures to prevent constipation because straining increases intracranial pressure
   f. Maintain client in a position no lower than semi-Fowler's
C. Evaluation/Outcomes
   1. Verbalizes an improved body image
   2. Reports satisfying sexual relationship
   3. Continues medical regimen and supervision

HYPOPITUITARISM
Data Base
A. Etiology and pathophysiology
   1. Deficiency of one or more anterior pituitary hormones
   2. Total absence of pituitary hormones referred to as panhypopituitarism (Simmonds' disease)
   3. Occurs when there is destruction of the anterior lobe of the gland by trauma, tumor, or hemorrhage
   4. Clinical findings vary with target organs affected
B. Clinical findings
   1. Subjective: lethargy; loss of strength and libido; decreased tolerance for cold
   2. Objective
      a. Decreased temperature
      b. Postural hypotension
      c. Hypoglycemia
      d. Decreased levels of GH, ACTH, TSH, FSH, and LH
      e. Sterility; loss of secondary sexual characteristics
      f. Visual disturbances if tumor impinges on optic nerve
C. Therapeutic interventions: replace hormones; intervene surgically if tumor is present

Nursing Care of Clients With Hypopituitarism
A. Assessment/Analysis
   1. Baseline vital signs
   2. Sexual patterns: loss of libido; painful intercourse; inability to maintain an erection
   3. Past and present menstrual patterns

4. Visual acuity
5. Loss of secondary sexual characteristics
6. Activity tolerance
B. Planning/Implementation
   1. Monitor effects of hormone replacement therapy
   2. Discuss the importance of adhering to medical regimen on a long-term basis
   3. Allow ample time to verbalize feelings regarding the long-term nature of the disease and impact on quality of daily life
   4. Provide adequate rest periods
C. Evaluation/Outcomes
   1. Adheres to medical regimen
   2. Expresses positive feelings of body image
   3. Establishes satisfying sexual relationship

DIABETES INSIPIDUS
Data Base
A. Etiology and pathophysiology
   1. Deficient production or secretion of antidiuretic hormone (ADH) by the posterior pituitary gland, decreasing reabsorption of water in nephron tubules; may be familial, idiopathic, or secondary to trauma, surgery, tumors, infections, or autoimmune disorders
   2. Neurogenic diabetes insipidus: renal tubular defect resulting in decreased water absorption; may be familial or result from renal disorders, primary aldosteronism, or excessive water intake (primary polydipsia); results in impaired renal concentrating ability
B. Clinical findings
   1. Subjective: polydipsia; craving for cold water
   2. Objective
      a. Polyuria (5 to 25 L/24 hr)
      b. Dilute urine; specific gravity 1.001 to 1.005; osmolality 50 to 200 mOsm/kg
      c. Increased serum sodium level and plasma osmolality
      d. Clinical findings of dehydration (poor skin turgor, dry mucous membranes, elevated temperature)
C. Therapeutic interventions
   1. Antidiuretic hormone replacement: vasopressin (Pitressin), lypressin (Diapid), desmopressin (DDAVP), vasopressin tannate (Pitressin tannate)
   2. Treatment of underlying cause
   3. Hypophysectomy

Nursing Care of Clients With Diabetes Insipidus
A. Assessment/Analysis
   1. Intake and output, weight, and specific gravity of urine to establish baseline data
   2. Results of serum electrolyte evaluation
   3. Dryness of skin and mucous membranes
B. Planning/Implementation
   1. Monitor fluid and electrolyte status: intake and output, daily weight, skin turgor, electrolyte levels
   2. Replace fluids
   3. Monitor response to ADH replacement

4. Teach client about long-term vasopressin therapy and the need for daily weight records, recognition of polyuria, and wearing a medical alert bracelet; overdosage may cause syndrome of inappropriate antidiuretic hormone (SIADH), leading to water retention and hyponatremia
5. Advise to avoid alcohol because it suppresses ADH secretion

C. Evaluation/Outcomes
1. Maintains fluid balance
2. States clinical findings of overmedication and undermedication with ADH replacement

SYNDROME OF INAPPROPRIATE ANTIDIURETIC HORMONE SECRETION

Data Base

A. Etiology and pathophysiology
1. Excessive ADH secretion leads to fluid retention and dilutional hyponatremia
2. May be caused by head trauma, tumors, or infection; malignant tumor cells may produce ADH

B. Clinical findings
1. Subjective: anorexia; nausea; fatigue; headache
2. Objective
   a. Reduced urine output; hyponatremia
   b. Decreased deep tendon reflexes
   c. Change in mental status, seizures, coma
   d. Clinical findings of fluid retention such as weight gain, crackles, jugular vein distention
   e. Decreased serum sodium level and osmolality

C. Therapeutic interventions: fluid restriction; hypertonic parenteral fluids

Nursing Care of Clients With Syndrome of Inappropriate Antidiuretic Hormone Secretion

A. Assessment/Analysis
1. History of malignancy, infection, or increased intracranial pressure
2. I&O, daily weight, vital signs
3. Serum and urine for sodium concentration and osmolality
4. Neurologic evaluations

B. Planning/Implementation
1. Monitor fluid and electrolyte status
2. Restrict fluid intake; administer hypertonic intravenous solutions as ordered
3. Institute seizure precautions and protect from injury
4. Provide supportive measures for related disorders

C. Evaluation/Outcomes
1. Maintains fluid balance
2. Remains seizure-free

HYPERTHYROIDISM (GRAVES' DISEASE, THYROTOXICOSIS)

Data Base

A. Etiology and pathophysiology
1. Excessive concentration of thyroid hormones in the blood as a result of thyroid disease or increased levels of TSH; leads to a hypermetabolic state
2. Etiology of Graves' disease is mediated by immunoglobulin G (IgG) antibody that activates TSH receptors on the surface of thyroid cells
3. Etiology of Graves' disease is believed to be involved with an autoimmune process of impaired regulation; associated with other autoimmune disorders
4. The gland may also enlarge (goiter) as a result of decreased iodine intake; there may or may not be an increase in the secretion of thyroid hormones
5. Therapy for hypothyroidism: thyroid medication such as levothyroxine (Synthroid, Levothroid)

B. Clinical findings
1. Subjective: polyphagia; emotional lability; apprehension; heat intolerance
2. Objective
   a. Weight loss; loose stools; tremors, hyperactive reflexes; restlessness; diaphoresis; insomnia; exophthalmos, corneal ulceration; increased systolic BP, temperature, pulse rate, and respiration
   b. Decreased TSH levels if thyroid disorder; increased TSH levels if secondary to a pituitary disorder
   c. Graves' disease generally involves hyperthyroidism, goiter, and exophthalmos
   d. Increased triiodothyronine (T_3), thyroxine (T_4), radioactive iodine uptake test (RAI), long-acting thyroid stimulator (LATS)
   e. Thyrotoxic crisis (thyroid storm): a state of hypermetabolism that may lead to heart failure; usually precipitated by a period of severe physiologic or psychologic stress, thyroid surgery, or radioactive iodine therapy

C. Therapeutic interventions
1. Antithyroid medications such as propylthiouracil (PTU) and methimazole (Tapazole) to block the synthesis of thyroid hormone
2. Antithyroid medications such as iodine (potassium iodide, SSKI) to reduce the vascularity of the thyroid gland
3. Radioactive iodine, ^{131}I (atomic cocktail), to destroy thyroid gland cells, thereby decreasing the production of thyroid hormone
4. Medications to relieve the clinical findings related to the increased metabolic rate such as adrenergic blocking agents
5. Well-balanced, high-calorie diet with vitamin and mineral supplements
6. Surgical intervention involves a subtotal or total thyroidectomy

Nursing Care of Clients With Hyperthyroidism

A. Assessment/Analysis
1. History of weight loss, diarrhea, insomnia, emotional lability, palpitations, and heat intolerance
2. Eyes for exophthalmos, tearing, and sensitivity to light (photophobia)

3. Neck palpation for enlarged thyroid gland
4. Weight and vital signs to establish baseline
B. Planning/Implementation
  1. Use measures such as decreased stimulation, medications, and back rub to establish a climate for uninterrupted rest; provide relaxing and calm environment
  2. Protect from stress-producing situations
  3. Keep the room cool
  4. Provide diet high in calories, proteins, and carbohydrates with supplemental feedings between meals and at bedtime; vitamin and mineral supplements as ordered
  5. Understand that client is upset by lability of mood and exaggerated response to environmental stimuli; explain disease processes involved; avoid rushing and surprises; prepare client for procedures
  6. Protect the eyes (eye drops, patches, tinted eyeglasses, elevation of head of bed)
  7. Care for the client before a thyroidectomy
    a. Teach importance of taking prescribed antithyroid medications to achieve euthyroid state
    b. Teach deep-breathing exercises and use of hands to support neck to avoid strain on suture line after surgery
  8. Care for the client after a thyroidectomy
    a. Observe for clinical findings of respiratory distress and laryngeal stridor caused by tracheal edema (keep tracheotomy set available); a sore throat when swallowing is expected
    b. Maintain semi-Fowler's position to reduce edema
    c. Observe dressings at operative site and back of neck and shoulders for clinical findings of hemorrhage
    d. Observe for clinical findings of thyrotoxicosis such as high temperature, tachycardia, irritability, delirium, coma; may result from manipulation of the gland during surgery, which releases thyroid hormone into bloodstream
    e. Notify the physician immediately if clinical findings of thyrotoxicosis occur; administer propranolol (Inderal), iodides, propylthiouracil, and steroids as ordered
    f. Observe for clinical findings of tetany such as numbness or twitching of extremities, spasm of the glottis; hypocalcemia can occur after accidental trauma or removal of the parathyroid glands; if tetany occurs, give calcium gluconate or calcium chloride (IV) as prescribed
    g. Assess for hoarseness; may result from endotracheal intubation or laryngeal nerve damage
  9. Provide client teaching regarding radioactive iodine therapy
    a. Client is mildly radioactive and should follow radiation precautions for 7 days (avoid close prolonged contact with children or sleeping with another person; flush toilet twice after use; thorough handwashing)
    b. Hospitalization in isolation may be required for several days if larger dose is used
    c. Clinical findings of hyperthyroidism may take 3 to 4 weeks to subside
  10. Teach client clinical findings of
    a. Hypothyroidism as a result of treatment
    b. Hyperthyroidism as a result of thyrotoxicosis or overmedication with thyroid hormone replacement therapy
  11. Teach the importance of taking antithyroid medications regularly and to observe for adverse effects
  12. Instruct client to comply with periodic serum studies to monitor hormone levels
C. Evaluation/Outcomes
  1. Maintains ideal body weight
  2. Establishes regular routine of activity and rest

✿ HYPOTHYROIDISM

Data Base

A. Etiology and pathophysiology
  1. Congenital thyroid defects
  2. Defective hormone synthesis
  3. Prenatal and postnatal iodine deficiency
  4. Autoimmune diseases such as Hashimoto's disease and sarcoidosis
  5. Classified according to the time of life in which it occurs
    a. Cretinism: hypothyroidism found at birth
    b. Lymphocytic thyroiditis most frequently appears after 6 years of age and peaks during adolescence; generally self-limiting
    c. Hypothyroidism without myxedema: mild degree of thyroid failure in older children and adults
    d. Hypothyroidism with myxedema: severe degree of thyroid failure in older individuals
  6. Decreased levels of thyroid hormones (T_3 and T_4) slow the basal metabolic rate (BMR); the decreased BMR affects lipid metabolism, increases cholesterol and triglyceride levels, and affects RBC production, leading to anemia and folate deficiency
  7. Myxedema coma is the most severe degree of hypothyroidism, representing a potentially fatal endocrine emergency; precipitated by a severe physiologic stress, myxedema coma involves hypothermia, bradycardia, hypoventilation, and progressive loss of consciousness
B. Clinical findings
  1. Subjective: dull mental processes; apathy; lethargy; loss of libido; intolerance to cold; anorexia
  2. Objective
    a. Lack of facial expression; weight gain; constipation; subnormal temperature and pulse rate; dry, brittle hair and nails; pale, dry, coarse skin; enlarged tongue; drooling; hoarseness;

thinning of lateral eyebrows; scalp, axilla, and pubic hair loss; diminished hearing; anemia; periorbital edema
   b. Decreased BMR
   c. Decreased thyroxine (T_4) and triiodothyronine (T_3) levels, decreased radioactive iodine uptake; delayed or poor response to TSH stimulation test in secondary hypothyroidism, increased TSH in primary hypothyroidism
C. Therapeutic interventions: thyroid hormones; maintenance of vital functions; prevention: screening every 5 years after age 35 for status of hypothyroidism

Nursing Care of Clients With Hypothyroidism

A. Assessment/Analysis
   1. History that may have contributed to condition
   2. Activity tolerance, bowel elimination, sleeping patterns, sexual function, and intolerance to cold
   3. Skin and hair for characteristic changes
   4. Weight and vital signs to establish baseline
   5. Clinical findings of anemia, atherosclerosis, or arthritis
B. Planning/Implementation
   1. Have patience with a lethargic client; activity tolerance and mental functioning will improve with therapy
   2. Teach the client and family to be alert for clinical findings of complications
      a. Angina pectoris: chest pain, indigestion
      b. Cardiac failure: dyspnea, palpitations
      c. Myxedema coma: weakness, syncope, slow pulse rate, subnormal temperature, slow respirations, lethargy
   3. Teach to seek medical supervision regularly and when clinical findings of illness develop
   4. Explain the importance of continued hormone replacement throughout life
   5. Review the clinical findings of hypothyroidism and hyperthyroidism to help client recognize clinical findings of undermedication or overmedication
   6. Explain that increased sensitivity to opioid analgesics and tranquilizers necessitates dosage adjustment; OTC drugs should be avoided unless approved by physician
   7. Help the client and family recognize that client's inability to adapt to cold temperature requires additional protection and modification of outdoor activity in cold weather
   8. Teach to avoid constipation: increase fluid intake and fiber in the diet
   9. Apply moisturizers to skin
   10. Teach the need to restrict calories, cholesterol, and fat in the diet
C. Evaluation/Outcomes
   1. Completes activities of daily living (ADLs) without fatigue

   2. Adheres to dietary, exercise, and medication regimen
   3. Establishes regular pattern of bowel elimination

HYPERPARATHYROIDISM

Data Base
A. Etiology and pathophysiology
   1. Hyperfunction of the parathyroid glands; usually caused by adenoma; hypertrophy and hyperplasia of the glands may also be responsible
   2. As a result of hyperparathyroidism, the reabsorption of calcium and the excretion of phosphorus by the kidneys are increased
   3. If dietary intake is not enough to meet calcium levels demanded by high levels of parathormone, demineralization of bone occurs
B. Clinical findings
   1. Subjective: apathy, fatigue; muscular weakness; anorexia; nausea; emotional irritability; deep bone pain (if demineralization occurs); backache
   2. Objective
      a. Bone cysts, pathologic fractures
      b. Renal calculi composed of calcium; pyelonephritis; renal damage; polyuria
      c. Vomiting; constipation
      d. Elevated serum calcium and parathormone levels
      e. Decreased serum phosphorus level
      f. Cardiac dysrhythmias
C. Therapeutic interventions
   1. Surgical excision of a parathyroid tumor
   2. Calcium intake restricted
   3. Administration of furosemide (Lasix) to increase renal excretion of calcium
   4. Administration of gallium nitrate, calcitonin, or plicamycin with glucocorticoid to lower calcium level

Nursing Care of Clients With Hyperparathyroidism

A. Assessment/Analysis
   1. Presence of GI disturbance or bone pain
   2. History of renal calculi or fractures
   3. Clinical findings of renal calculi such as hematuria or flank pain
   4. Use of thiazide diuretics or vitamin D, which can increase serum calcium level
   5. Serum calcium and phosphorus levels
   6. Baseline vital signs, particularly heart rate and rhythm
B. Planning/Implementation
   1. Strain the urine, observing for calculi
   2. Encourage fluid intake
   3. Assist with ambulation, which helps prevent demineralization; instruct client to avoid high-impact activities
   4. Monitor I&O
   5. Encourage foods with fiber to limit constipation
   6. Instruct to limit intake of foods high in calcium, especially milk products

7. Provide cardiac monitoring if hypercalcemia is severe
8. If surgery is performed, provide the same postoperative care as for clients undergoing thyroidectomy (see Hyperthyroidism)

C. Evaluation/Outcomes
1. Maintains skeletal integrity
2. Remains free of urinary complications

❁ HYPOPARATHYROIDISM

Data Base
A. Etiology and pathophysiology
1. Parathyroid glands may not secrete a sufficient amount of parathormone after thyroid surgery, parathyroid surgery, or radiation therapy of the neck; idiopathic hypoparathyroidism is rare
2. As levels of parathormone drop, the serum calcium level also drops, causing clinical findings of tetany; a concomitant rise in serum phosphate level occurs

B. Clinical findings
1. Subjective: photophobia; muscle cramps; irritability; dyspnea; tingling of extremities
2. Objective
   a. Trousseau's sign (carpopedal spasm)
   b. Chvostek's sign (contraction of the facial muscle in response to tapping near the angle of the jaw)
   c. Decreased serum calcium and parathormone levels; elevated serum phosphate level
   d. Stridor, wheezing from laryngeal spasm; tremors; seizures
   e. X-ray examination reveals increased bone density
   f. Cardiac dysrhythmias; alkalosis; cataracts if the disease is chronic

C. Therapeutic interventions
1. Calcium chloride or calcium gluconate given IV for emergency treatment of overt tetany
2. Calcium salts administered orally (calcium carbonate, calcium gluconate)
3. Vitamin D (dihydrotachysterol, ergocalciferol) to increase absorption of calcium from the GI tract
4. Parathormone injections
5. High-calcium, low-phosphate diet
6. Aluminum hydroxide to decrease absorption of phosphorus from the GI tract

Nursing Care of Clients With Hypoparathyroidism
A. Assessment/Analysis
1. History of muscle spasms, numbness or tingling of extremities, visual disturbances, or seizures
2. Presence of neuromuscular irritability
3. Status of respiratory functioning
4. Heart rate and rhythm
5. Serum calcium and phosphate levels

B. Planning/Implementation
1. Observe for respiratory distress and have emergency equipment available for tracheostomy and mechanical ventilation
2. Maintain seizure precautions
3. Reduce environmental stimuli
4. Provide drug and dietary instruction including elimination of milk, cheese, and egg yolks because of high phosphorus content; encourage to include dietary sources of calcium that are low in phosphorus content
5. Teach clinical findings of hypocalcemia and hypercalcemia; instruct client to contact physician immediately if either should occur

C. Evaluation/Outcomes
1. Remains free from neuromuscular irritability
2. Maintains respiratory functioning within acceptable limits

❁ DIABETES MELLITUS

Data Base
A. Etiology and pathophysiology
1. Hyperglycemia occurs when there is insufficient secretion of insulin, peripheral cells become insulin-resistant, and/or hepatic glucose production is increased
2. Body attempts to rid itself of excess glucose by excreting some via kidneys; an osmotic force is created within the kidneys because of this glucose excretion and body fluid is lost
3. If the body is unable to use carbohydrates for cellular function fat is oxidized as an energy source; oxidation of fats produces ketone bodies
4. Risk factors
   a. Type 1: genetic predisposition; environmental factors such as toxins or viruses; age less than 30 years
   b. Type 2: family history, obesity, usually age 45 years or older, history of gestational diabetes, increasing incidence in childhood and adolescence
5. Classification
   a. Type 1: formerly known as insulin-dependent diabetes mellitus (IDDM); destruction of beta cells leads to an inability to produce insulin; requires exogenous insulin
   b. Type 2: formerly known as non–insulin-dependent diabetes mellitus (NIDDM); has a gradual onset and the pancreas produces some insulin so that ketoacidosis is not likely; may be controlled with adherence to a diet and exercise program that promotes maintenance of a desirable weight; accounts for 90% of diabetes
   c. Gestational: detected during 24 to 28 weeks' gestation; glucose levels are generally normal 6 weeks postpartum; more likely to develop type 2 diabetes 5 to 10 years after delivery; neonate exhibits macrosomia, hypoglycemia, hypocalcemia, and hyperbilirubinemia
   d. Diabetes mellitus associated with other conditions or syndromes (formerly known as secondary diabetes); associated with

glucocorticoid medication and conditions such as Cushing's syndrome and pancreatic disease

  e. Impaired glucose tolerance; high glucose levels but not sufficiently high to be diagnostic for diabetes; prediabetes—fasting serum glucose level of 100 to 125 mg/dL

6. Acute increases in serum glucose levels: diabetic ketoacidosis (DKA) and hyperglycemic hyperosmolar nonketotic syndrome (HHNS) constitute medical emergencies

  a. Causes: insufficient insulin, major stresses (e.g., infection, surgery, trauma, pregnancy, emotional turmoil, nausea and vomiting); drugs (steroids); glucose load

  b. Pathophysiology

    (1) DKA is associated with type 1; with inadequate insulin to support basal needs, proteins and fats are used for energy; ketones are excreted via urine and breathing; dehydration and electrolyte imbalances occur; serum glucose level 300 to 600 mg/dL

    (2) HHNS is associated with type 2; hyperglycemia increases intravascular osmotic pressure, leading to polyuria and cellular dehydration; serum glucose level 500 to 900 mg/dL

7. Acute decrease in serum glucose level: hypoglycemia

  a. Causes: excess insulin or oral antidiabetic medications; too little food or too much exercise when receiving antidiabetic medications

  b. Pathophysiology: excessive insulin lowers serum glucose level as glucose is carried into cells; decreased food intake in relation to prescribed antidiabetic medications results in hypoglycemia; excessive exercise uses glucose for metabolism, decreasing serum glucose level

8. Long-term complications of diabetes: all types of diabetes subject to the same complications and include microangiopathy (retinopathy, nephropathy), macroangiopathy (peripheral vascular diseases, arteriosclerosis, coronary heart disease, cerebral vascular disease), neuropathy, skin problems (cellulitis, fungal infections, boils), periodontal disease (Figure 9-2: Long-term complications of diabetes mellitus)

B. Clinical findings

  1. Subjective: polydipsia; polyphagia; fatigue; blurred vision (retinopathy; osmotic changes); peripheral neuropathy

  2. Objective

    a. Polyuria; weight loss; glycosuria; peripheral vascular changes; ulcers; delayed wound healing; infection; gangrene

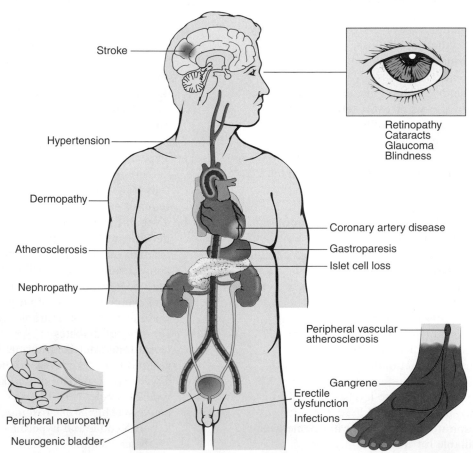

Figure 9-2 Long-term complications of diabetes mellitus. (From Kumar V, Abbas AK: *Robbins and Cotran pathologic basis of disease,* ed 7, Philadelphia, 2005, Saunders.)

b. Hyperglycemia: detected by casual plasma glucose measurement of 200 mg/dL or higher, fasting plasma glucose level of 126 mg/dL or higher, and 2-hour postload glucose level of 200 mg/dL or higher; monitored by hemoglobin A_{1c} (glycosylated hemoglobin) measurement, which reflects average glucose level over preceding 2 to 3 months and should not exceed 7%

3. DKA and HHNS
   a. Hyperglycemia, glycosuria, polyuria
   b. Dehydration: flushed, hot, dry skin; decreased skin turgor (tenting); hyperosmolar blood; hypotension; tachycardia; thirst; headache; confusion; drowsiness
   c. Metabolic acidosis (DKA only): Kussmaul respirations as body attempts to blow off carbon dioxide; ketonuria, sweet breath odor, anorexia, nausea, vomiting, decreased serum pH, decreased PCO_2, decreased HCO_3^- level

4. Hypoglycemia (insulin shock or reaction because of excessive insulin, deficient glucose, or excessive exercise)
   a. Clinical findings occur as a result of sympathetic nervous system (SNS) stimulation or reduced cerebral glucose supply
   b. CNS effects: mental confusion, blurred vision, diplopia, slurred speech, fatigue, seizures
   c. SNS (adrenergic) effects: nervousness, weakness, pallor, diaphoresis, tremor, tachycardia, hunger

C. Therapeutic interventions
1. Lifestyle changes
   a. Weight control: obesity leads to insulin resistance; this can be reversed by weight loss
   b. Exercise: increases insulin sensitivity but must be regular; brisk walking, swimming, and bicycling are recommended
   c. Diet: current recommendations
      (1) Caloric control to maintain ideal body weight
      (2) 50% to 60% of caloric intake should be from carbohydrates with emphasis on complex carbohydrates, high-fiber foods rich in water-soluble fiber (oat bran, peas, all forms of beans, pectin-rich fruits and vegetables); foods with a high glycemic index should be avoided; glycemic index refers to effect of particular foods on blood glucose level
      (3) Protein: intake should be consistent with the U.S. Dietary Guidelines, usually between 60 and 85 g; should be 12% to 20% of daily calories
      (4) Fat intake not to exceed 30% of daily calories (70 to 90 g/day); keep saturated fat intake low; emphasize monounsaturated and polyunsaturated fats
      (5) Dietary ratio: carbohydrate to protein to fat ratio usually about 5:1:2

(6) Distribute food evenly throughout the day in three or four meals, with snacks added between meals and at bedtime as needed in accordance with total food allowance and therapy (insulin or oral hypoglycemics)
(7) Consistent and regulated food intake is basic to disease control along with consistent exercise, medication, and glucose monitoring
(8) Basic tools for planning diet: food composition tables showing nutrient content and glycemic index of commonly used foods

d. Self-monitoring of blood glucose (SMBG) level
   (1) Blood glucose monitoring: finger stick—a drop of blood from the fingertip is put on a special reagent strip, which is read by a glucose monitor
   (2) Interstitial glucose monitoring: continuous interstitial testing (via biosensor inserted subcutaneously) or intermittent transdermal testing (via interstitial fluid drawn through the skin and tested with an electrochemical sensor)

e. Alternate site testing: forearm, upper arm, abdomen, thigh, base of thumb; gives fingertips a rest; alternate sites have less capillary blood flow than fingertips and may not reflect glucose levels that rapidly rise and fall; use one site consistently unless otherwise instructed by the physician because results at various sites differ
   (1) Use fingertip if hypoglycemia is expected or if client is experiencing rapid change in glucose level
   (2) Rub forearm vigorously until warm before testing
   (3) Use monitor designed for alternate site testing
   (4) Avoid use in arm on side of mastectomy; results likely to be low; reduce risk of infection and lymphedema

2. Insulin administration
   a. Adjusted after considering the client's physical and emotional stresses; a specific type of insulin and schedule are prescribed; aggressive insulin therapy regimens are the gold standard of care
   b. Somogyi effect: insulin-induced hypoglycemia rebounds to hyperglycemia
      (1) Epinephrine and glucagon are released in response to hypoglycemia
      (2) These reactions cause mobilization of the liver's stored glucose and induce hyperglycemia
      (3) Somogyi phenomenon is treated by gradually lowering insulin dosage while monitoring blood glucose level, particularly during the night (when hypoglycemia is most likely to occur)

c. Dawn phenomenon: early morning hyperglycemia attributed to increased secretion of growth hormone; this requires delaying administration of PM insulin or increased dosage

d. Insulin pump

(1) External battery-operated device that delivers insulin through a needle inserted into subcutaneous tissue

(2) Small (basal) doses of regular insulin are programmed into computer to be delivered every few minutes; bolus doses (extra preset amounts) are delivered before meals

(3) Improves glucose control for clients with wide variations in insulin need as a result of irregular schedules, pregnancy, or growth requirements

(4) A prescribed amount of insulin for 24 hours plus priming is drawn into syringe

(5) The administration set is primed and needle inserted aseptically, usually into subcutaneous tissue of abdomen

e. Jet injectors: deliver medication through skin under pressure

3. Oral antidiabetics for certain clients with type 2 diabetes who cannot be managed with lifestyle changes alone; must have some functioning beta cells in the islets of Langerhans

4. Other therapies include pancreatic islet cell grafts, pancreas transplants, implantable insulin pumps that continually monitor blood glucose level and release insulin accordingly, cyclosporin therapy to prevent beta cell destruction in type 1 diabetes

5. Management of DKA and HHNS

a. IV to provide fluid replacement and direct access to the circulatory system, and an indwelling urinary catheter to monitor urine output

b. Titration of IV regular insulin according to serum glucose levels

c. Replacement of lost electrolytes, particularly sodium and potassium, using blood studies to determine dosage; when insulin is administered potassium reenters the cell, resulting in hypokalemia

d. Cardiac monitoring if circulatory collapse is imminent or dysrhythmias associated with electrolyte imbalance occur

e. Acidosis treated according to cause

f. Monitoring for hypoglycemia as a result of treatment

6. Management of hypoglycemia (insulin shock or reaction)

a. 10 to 15 g of simple sugar (e.g., glucose tablets, 4 to 6 ounces of juice or soda, hard candy) followed by complex carbohydrate and protein (e.g., cheese and crackers)

b. Insertion of an intravenous line for circulatory access if hemodynamically unstable

c. Administration of 50% dextrose solution for profound hypoglycemia

d. If unconscious, glucagon injection to stimulate glycogenolysis

7. Acetylcysteine therapy when contrast radiologic studies are performed to prevent contrast medium nephrotoxicity

Nursing Care of Clients With Diabetes Mellitus

A. Assessment/Analysis

1. Familial history of diabetes mellitus
2. Cardinal signs of polyuria, polydipsia, and polyphagia
3. History of fatigue, visual changes, impaired wound healing, urinary tract infections, fungal infections, and altered sensation
4. Blood glucose levels, hemoglobin A_{1c} measurement
5. Visual acuity and retinal changes
6. Vital signs and weight for baseline data
7. Urine for acetone levels, microalbumin levels
8. Renal function
9. Dietary and exercise patterns

B. Planning/Implementation

1. Assist the client and family to understand the disease process
2. Encourage to express feelings about illness and the necessary changes in lifestyle and self-image
3. Help with the administration of medication until self-administration is both physically and psychologically possible
4. Assist in recognizing the need for activities and diet that promote and maintain ideal body weight
5. Monitor serum glucose level with routine finger sticks
6. Test urine for ketones if glucose level is high; obtain double-voided specimen or specimen from port of retention catheter using sterile technique
7. Teach client and family to

a. Use blood glucose monitoring system to test blood glucose level; finger sticks are the most reliable; continuous glucose monitoring systems supplement but should not replace finger stick; test blood glucose monitor for accuracy

b. Test urine for ketones when blood glucose level is high

c. Avoid infection

d. Seek professional foot care to cut toenails, provide foot care daily: wash, dry, and lubricate feet but not between toes; inspect feet for irritation etc.; use mirror for soles and heels; protect feet (wear socks and well-fitting, closed shoes; avoid OTC corn medications etc.; do not apply heating pads, ice, or tape to the feet); report any problems immediately to the physician

e. Administer insulin by using sterile technique, rotating injection sites (abdomen preferred) within an anatomic location if using nonhuman form of insulin (prevents lipodystrophy), measuring dosage, and noting types, strengths of insulin, and peak action periods; teach use of insulin pump if ordered (teach how to change subcutaneous needle and tubing every 3 days)

  f. Use food tables when planning dietary intake

  g. Avoid tight shoes and smoking, which will constrict circulation

  h. Recognize clinical findings of impending hypoglycemia (insulin shock, reaction); carry a carbohydrate source

  i. Recognize clinical findings of impending hyperglycemia (DKA, HHNS); carry insulin supplies and glucose monitoring equipment

  8. Encourage to continue medical supervision, including visits to an eye care specialist and podiatrist

  9. Encourage follow-up nutritional counseling

  10. Instruct to maintain regular medical care and to prevent hyperglycemia and complications of diabetes

  11. Screen client regularly for microalbuminuria (assesses kidney function)

C. Evaluation/Outcomes

  1. Adheres to medical regimen of diet, exercise, and medications

  2. Maintains blood glucose and hemoglobin A_{1c} levels within an expected range

  3. Verbalizes diabetes survival skills

  4. Remains free of complications

✳ PRIMARY ALDOSTERONISM (CONN'S SYNDROME)

Data Base

A. Etiology and pathophysiology

  1. Excessive secretion of aldosterone, a mineralocorticoid secreted in response to the renin-angiotensin system and ACTH, causes the kidneys to retain sodium and excrete potassium and hydrogen

  2. Usually caused by an adenoma of the adrenal cortex, but may also be caused by hyperplasia or carcinoma

B. Clinical findings

  1. Subjective: muscle weakness and cramping; polydipsia; polyuria; paresthesia

  2. Objective: hypertension; hypokalemia; hypernatremia; alkalosis; elevated urinary aldosterone levels; renal damage: proteinuria, decreased urine specific gravity

C. Therapeutic interventions

  1. Surgical removal of the tumor

  2. Temporary management with spironolactone

  3. Bilateral adrenalectomy involving lifelong corticosteroid therapy is necessary

Nursing Care of Clients With Primary Aldosteronism

A. Assessment/Analysis

  1. Vital signs

  2. Electrolyte levels

  3. Intake and output, urine specific gravity

  4. Motor and sensory functions for alterations

  5. Cardiac dysrhythmias as a result of hypokalemia

B. Planning/Implementation

  1. Regulate fluid intake

  2. Encourage continued medical supervision

  3. Provide care after a bilateral adrenalectomy

    a. Monitor vital signs, hemodynamic state, and blood glucose level

    b. Administer steroids with antacid, proton pump inhibitor (PPI), or H_2-blocker to prevent GI erosion

    c. Protect from infection and stressful situations

    d. Explain drug and side effects to client

    e. Instruct to carry medical alert identification card

    f. Monitor fluid balance; BP for hypotension

    g. Monitor for emotional upset, which may require an increase in steroid medications

  4. Provide dietary instruction; encourage intake of foods high in potassium and avoidance of foods that contain sodium

C. Evaluation/Outcomes

  1. Maintains BP at an expected level

  2. Selects foods low in sodium and high in potassium

  3. Performs routine ADLs without fatigue

✳ CUSHING'S SYNDROME

Data Base

A. Etiology and pathophysiology

  1. Results from excess secretion of adrenocortical hormones

  2. Caused by hyperplasia or by a tumor of the adrenal cortex; however, the primary lesion may occur in the pituitary gland, causing excess production of ACTH

  3. Administration of excess glucocorticoids or ACTH will also cause Cushing's syndrome

B. Clinical findings

  1. Subjective: weakness; decreased libido; mood swings; steroid psychosis

  2. Objective

    a. Obese trunk, thin arms and legs; moon face; buffalo hump; acne; hirsutism; ecchymotic areas; purple striae on breast and abdomen; amenorrhea; increased susceptibility to infections

    b. Hypertension

    c. Hyperglycemia; hypokalemia; elevated plasma cortisol level

    d. Elevated levels of 17-hydroxycorticosteroids and 17-ketosteroids in urine

    e. Osteoporosis; fractures; kyphosis

    f. Protein wasting, which causes muscle wasting and weakness

    g. Hypernatremia caused by sodium and water retention, resulting in edema and hypertension

C. Therapeutic interventions

  1. Reduce dosage of externally administered corticoids

  2. If lesion on pituitary is causing hypersecretion of ACTH, a hypophysectomy or irradiation of the pituitary may be done; stereotatic irradiation is under study

  3. Surgical excision of adrenal tumors (adrenalectomy)

  4. Adrenal enzyme inhibitors

  5. Potassium supplements

  6. High-protein diet with sodium restriction

Nursing Care of Clients With Cushing's Syndrome

A. Assessment/Analysis

  1. Baseline vital signs, weight, blood glucose level, and electrolytes

  2. Urine specimens for diagnostic purposes

  3. Physical appearance (Figure 9-3: Common characteristics of Cushing's syndrome)

  4. Changes in coping and sexuality from history

B. Planning/Implementation

  1. Monitor vital signs, daily weight, intake and output, blood glucose level, and electrolyte level

  2. Protect from exposure to infections

  3. Encourage ventilation of feelings by the client and spouse because changes in body image and sex drive can alter spousal support

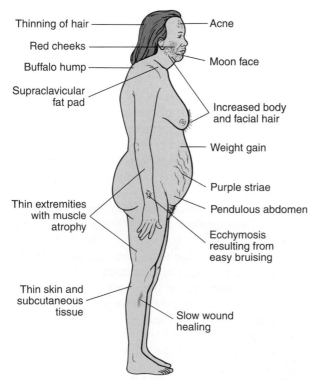

Figure 9-3 Common characteristics of Cushing's syndrome. (From Lewis SL et al: *Medical-surgical nursing: assessment and management of clinical problems*, ed 7, St Louis, 2007, Mosby.)

Labels: Thinning of hair; Red cheeks; Buffalo hump; Supraclavicular fat pad; Thin extremities with muscle atrophy; Thin skin and subcutaneous tissue; Acne; Moon face; Increased body and facial hair; Weight gain; Purple striae; Pendulous abdomen; Ecchymosis resulting from easy bruising; Slow wound healing

  4. Attempt to minimize stress in the environment by measures such as limiting visitors and explaining procedures carefully

  5. Instruct client regarding diet and supplementation; encourage diet rich in nutrient-dense foods such as fruits, vegetables, whole grains, and legumes to improve and maintain nutritional status and prevent any possible drug-induced nutrient deficiencies

  6. Care for the client after a bilateral adrenalectomy (see Primary Aldosteronism)

  7. Care for the client after a hypophysectomy (see Hyperpituitarism)

C. Evaluation/Outcomes

  1. Maintains fluid balance

  2. Remains free of infection

  3. Discusses feelings regarding physical changes

ADDISON'S DISEASE (PRIMARY ADRENAL INSUFFICIENCY)

Data Base

A. Etiology and pathophysiology

  1. Hyposecretion of adrenocortical hormones

  2. Generally caused by autoimmune destruction of the cortex or by idiopathic atrophy; may be seen in clients with AIDS and TB

  3. Addisonian crisis (acute adrenal insufficiency) can be precipitated by stresses such as pregnancy, surgery, infection, dehydration, emotional turmoil; fatal if not treated

  4. Risk factors include endocrine disorders, sudden cessation of glucocorticoids, adrenalectomy, tuberculosis

B. Clinical findings

  1. Subjective: weakness; fatigue; anorexia; nausea

  2. Objective

    a. Increased bronze pigmentation of skin

    b. Vomiting; diarrhea

    c. Impaired protein anabolism resulting in emaciation and fatigue

    d. Hypotension

    e. Decreased levels of serum cortisol, 17-ketosteroids, and 17-hydroxysteroids; increased plasma ACTH level; hyponatremia; hypoglycemia; hyperkalemia

C. Therapeutic interventions

  1. Replacement of hormones: glucocorticoids to correct metabolic imbalance and mineralocorticoids to correct electrolyte imbalance and hypotension; additional hormone replacement during illness or stress to prevent addisonian crisis

  2. Correction of fluid, electrolyte, and glucose imbalances

  3. High-carbohydrate, high-protein diet

  4. Prevention of osteoporosis, which may develop with the use of steroid therapy that breaks down protein matrix in the bones

Nursing Care of Clients With Addison's Disease

A. Assessment/Analysis
1. Baseline vital signs, weight, electrolytes, and serum glucose
2. 24-hour urine specimens for diagnostic purposes (17-hydroxycorticosteroids and 17-ketosteroids)
3. Appearance of skin
4. Changes in energy or activity from history

B. Planning/Implementation
1. Monitor vital signs four times a day; be alert for elevation in temperature (infection, dehydration), alterations in pulse rate and rhythm (hyperkalemia), and alterations in blood pressure
2. Observe for clinical findings of sodium and potassium imbalance
3. Monitor intake and output and weigh daily
4. Collect 24-hour urine specimen
   a. Teach client about foods and medications to be avoided before the test
   b. Have client void at the beginning of the 24-hour time period and discard the urine
   c. Place urine from every voiding into collection container; ensure that appropriate preservative is used and container is kept refrigerated, if necessary
   d. Have client void at the end of the 24-hour time period and place the urine in the container
5. Administer steroids as ordered; give with antacid, PPI, or H_2-blocker to limit ulcerogenic factor of the drug
6. Assign a private room to prevent contact with clients with infectious diseases
7. Limit the number of visitors to reduce stress and risk of infection
8. Advise to avoid physical and emotional stress
9. Teach need for lifelong hormone replacement therapy with increased dosage during stress
10. Review clinical findings of adrenal hypofunction and hyperfunction so client can recognize need for adjustment of steroid dose
11. Instruct to wear medical alert band
12. Encourage diet consistent with the U.S. Dietary Goals with emphasis on diet high in nutrient-dense foods and adequate sodium
13. Administer antiemetics to prevent fluid and electrolyte loss by vomiting

C. Evaluation/Outcomes
1. Maintains fluid balance
2. Maintains electrolyte balance

PHEOCHROMOCYTOMA

Data Base

A. Etiology and pathophysiology
1. Catecholamine-secreting tumor of the adrenal medulla; usually benign
2. Causes increased secretion of epinephrine and norepinephrine (catecholamines)
3. Familial tendency; peak incidence 25 to 50 years of age

B. Clinical findings
1. Subjective: headache; visual disturbances; palpitations; anxiety; psychoneurosis
2. Objective
   a. Hypertension, postural hypotension; tachycardia; diaphoresis; tremors; hyperglycemia; brain attack or blindness may occur
   b. Increased levels of plasma and urinary catecholamines and vanillylmandelic acid (VMA), a product of catecholamine breakdown

C. Therapeutic interventions
1. Surgical removal of the tumor
2. Antihypertensive and antidysrhythmic drugs such as nitroprusside (Nipride), propranolol (Inderal), phentolamine (Regitine)

Nursing Care of Clients With Pheochromocytoma

A. Assessment/Analysis
1. Blood pressures with client in upright and horizontal positions
2. Clinical findings associated with hypertension
3. 24-hour urine specimens for VMA and catecholamine studies

B. Planning/Implementation
1. Instruct to avoid coffee, chocolate, beer, wine, citrus fruit, bananas, and vanilla before the test for VMA
2. Administer parenteral fluids and blood as ordered before and after surgery to maintain blood volume
3. Decrease environmental stimulation
4. If bilateral adrenalectomy is performed
   a. Instruct the client regarding maintenance doses of steroids (see Care for the Client After a Bilateral Adrenalectomy under Primary Aldosteronism)
   b. Postoperatively: instruct client about need to take antihypertensives and to monitor BP until it returns to expected range
5. Emphasize the importance of continued medical supervision and screening for other family members

C. Evaluation/Outcomes
1. Maintains BP at an expected level
2. Remains free of complications of hypertension

Nursing Care of Clients With Integumentary System Disorders

OVERVIEW

REVIEW OF ANATOMY AND PHYSIOLOGY

Functions of the Integumentary System
A. Prevents loss of body fluids
B. Protects deeper tissues from pathogenic organisms, noxious chemicals, and short-wavelength ultraviolet radiation
C. Helps regulate body temperature
D. Provides location for sensory reception of touch, pressure, temperature, pain, wetness, tickle, etc.
E. Assists in vitamin D synthesis
F. Plays excretory role

Structures of the Integumentary System
A. Epidermis (outer layer)
   1. Contains no blood or lymphatic vessels; nourished by diffusion from underlying dermal papillae
   2. Melanocytes produce melanin, which colors skin
   3. Exceptional epidermal regions
      a. Conjunctiva: epidermis so thin it is transparent
      b. Lips: epidermis very thin and highly vascular
B. Dermis
   1. Vascular fabric of collagen and elastic fibers woven for strength and flexibility
   2. Contains abundant touch receptors
   3. Provides fingerprint pattern as unique arrangement of ridges projected to epidermal surface
   4. Skin stretched beyond certain limits (e.g., during pregnancy) may rupture dermal collagen and elastic fibers; consequent scar tissue repair produces striae gravidarum
C. Glands
   1. Eccrine: sweat glands opening in pores that secrete clear fluid
   2. Apocrine: scent glands found in the axillary, mammary, and genital areas
   3. Ceruminous: wax glands in external auditory canal
   4. Sebaceous: small, saclike glands lacking innervation, usually forming close to hairs and opening into upper portion of hair follicle
   5. Mammary: milk-secreting, alveolar glands developing to full extent only during pregnancy
D. Hair
   1. About the same number of follicles in males and females; hormones stimulate differential growth
   2. Arrector pili (smooth muscle) attached at one end to connective sheath in middle of the hair

follicle and at other end to the papillary region of the dermis; on contraction produces "goosebumps"

Tissue Repair
A. Inflammation
   1. Vascular changes: initial vasoconstriction for hemostasis; vessel walls become lined with leukocytes (margination); then vasodilation and increased vessel permeability (effects of histamine from mast cells, kinins, and prostaglandins); platelets clump and lymphatics become plugged with fibrin to wall off damaged area
   2. Leukocytes leave the vessels (diapedesis) and phagocytize foreign substances
   3. Chronic inflammation: macrophages predominate and fibroblasts deposit collagen around each group of macrophages and foreign substances; stage of granuloma formation
B. Fibroplasia
   1. Epithelialization: epithelial cells of the epidermis begin to cover tissue defect
   2. Deep in the wound, fibroblasts synthesize collagen and ground substance; process begins about fourth or fifth day and continues for 2 to 4 weeks
   3. Capillaries regenerate and tissue becomes red (granulation tissue)
   4. Fibrin plugs are lysed
C. Scar maturation
   1. Collagen fibers rearranged into a stronger, more organized pattern
   2. Scar remodels, gradually softens, and fades; if collagen synthesis exceeds breakdown, a hypertrophic scar or keloid forms
   3. Contraction of wound margins begins about 5 days after injury; fibroblasts migrate into the wound and assist in closing the defect; may result in contractures that can be debilitating

REVIEW OF PHYSICAL PRINCIPLES: HEAT

A. Conduction: transfer of heat from one object to another by direct contact
B. Evaporation: water vapor released by the skin (perspiration) cools the body surface, which decreases body temperature

C. Radiation: transfer of heat from one object to another without actual contact

D. Convection: transfer of heat away from the body by air movement

RELATED PHARMACOLOGY

Pediculicides/Scabicides

A. Description
1. Act at the parasite's nerve cell membrane to produce death of the organism
2. Destroy parasitic arthropods
3. Available in topical preparations

B. Examples: permethrin (Nix), pyrethrin with piperonyl (RID), lindane (Kwell)

C. Major side effects: skin irritation (hypersensitivity); contact dermatitis (local irritation); hepatotoxic and nephrotoxic

D. Nursing care
1. Inspect skin, particularly the scalp, for scabies and pediculosis before and after treatment; assess for skin irritation
2. Use gown, gloves, and cap to prevent spread of parasitic arthropods because scabies and pediculosis are highly contagious
3. Keep linen of an infected client separate to prevent reinfection of client or family
4. Avoid drug contact with the eyes and mucous membranes
5. Follow manufacturer's directions on length of direct exposure to agent and frequency of use, especially with children; avoid use during pregnancy

Antiinfectives

A. Description
1. Have bactericidal effect on the bacterial cell wall or alter cellular function
2. Available in topical preparations

B. Examples: mafenide acetate (Sulfamylon); silver nitrate 0.5% solution; silver sulfadiazine (Silvadene)

C. Major side effects
1. Silver sulfadiazine: skin irritation; hemolysis in clients with glucose-6-phosphate dehydrogenase (G-6-PD) deficiency
2. Mafenide acetate: metabolic acidosis; burning sensation when first applied
3. Silver nitrate: electrolyte imbalance; brownish black discoloration of skin

D. Nursing care
1. Adhere to strict surgical asepsis, cleanse and ensure débridement before application
2. Apply prescribed medications
   a. Silver sulfadiazine: apply thin layer; monitor G-6-PD level before treatment
   b. Mafenide acetate: assess for clinical findings of acidosis during therapy
   c. Silver nitrate: apply dressings soaked in silver nitrate; protect self from contact with drug; assess for electrolyte imbalances during therapy

d. Prevent contamination of topical medication container

Antipruritics

A. Description
1. Inhibit sensory nerve impulse conduction at the local site and exert a local anesthetic effect
2. Relieve itching and promote comfort
3. Available in topical preparations

B. Examples: benzocaine (Anbesol, Solarcaine), tetracaine HCl (Pontocaine)

C. Major side effects: skin irritation (hypersensitivity); contact dermatitis (local irritation)

D. Nursing care
1. Assess lesion for location, size, and irritation
2. Discourage scratching; keep client's nails well trimmed; avoid contact with open wounds
3. Advise medical follow-up because these medications provide only temporary relief of clinical findings
4. Prevent contamination of topical agent container

Antiinflammatory Agents

A. Description
1. Reduce clinical findings of inflammation
2. Produce vasoconstriction, which decreases swelling and pruritus
3. Available in topical preparations

B. Examples: dexamethasone (Decaderm; Hexadrol); hydrocortisone (Acticort); triamcinolone (Aristocort, Kenalog, Trimolone)

C. Major side effects: skin irritation (hypersensitivity); contact dermatitis (local irritation); skin atrophy; adrenal insufficiency if absorbed systemically (suppression of hypothalamic-pituitary-adrenal axis); fungal overgrowth

D. Nursing care
1. Assess lesions for color, location, and size
2. Protect skin from scratching or rubbing
3. Avoid contact with eyes
4. Cleanse skin before application and reapplication
5. Assess client for clinical findings of sensitivity
6. Avoid occlusive dressings unless directed otherwise
7. Prevent contamination of topical agent container

Dermal Agents

A. Description
1. Inhibit keratinization and sebaceous gland function to improve cystic acne and reduce sebum excretion
2. Available preparations: oral and topical

B. Examples: isotretinoin (Accutane), vitamin A acid (Retin-A)

C. Major side effects: visual disturbances: corneal opacities, decreased night vision (vitamin A toxicity—effect on visual rods); papilledema, headache (pseudotumor cerebri); hepatic dysfunction (hepatotoxicity); cheilitis (vitamin A toxicity); pruritus, skin fragility (dryness); hypertriglyceridemia (increased plasma triglycerides)

D. Nursing care
1. Assess visual and hepatic status before administration
2. Monitor levels of blood lipids before and during therapy

Table 10-1 Primary Skin Lesions

Lesion		Description
Macule	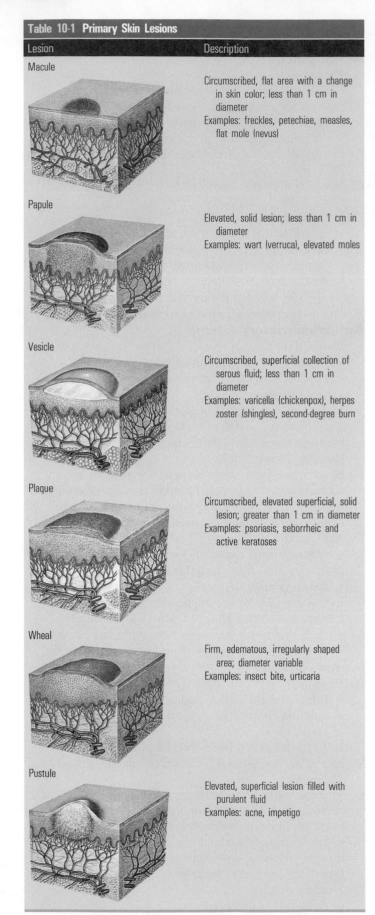	Circumscribed, flat area with a change in skin color; less than 1 cm in diameter Examples: freckles, petechiae, measles, flat mole (nevus)
Papule		Elevated, solid lesion; less than 1 cm in diameter Examples: wart (verruca), elevated moles
Vesicle		Circumscribed, superficial collection of serous fluid; less than 1 cm in diameter Examples: varicella (chickenpox), herpes zoster (shingles), second-degree burn
Plaque		Circumscribed, elevated superficial, solid lesion; greater than 1 cm in diameter Examples: psoriasis, seborrheic and active keratoses
Wheal		Firm, edematous, irregularly shaped area; diameter variable Examples: insect bite, urticaria
Pustule		Elevated, superficial lesion filled with purulent fluid Examples: acne, impetigo

From Lewis SL et al: *Medical-surgical nursing: assessment and management of clinical problems*, ed 7, St Louis, 2007, Mosby.

3. Instruct client to
   a. Avoid pregnancy during and for 1 month after therapy; use contraception if sexually active
   b. Avoid vitamin A supplements
   c. Side effects are reversible when therapy is discontinued
4. Assess for depression or suicidal ideation

MAJOR DISORDERS OF THE INTEGUMENTARY SYSTEM

SKIN LESIONS

Primary Lesions
(Table 10-1: Primary Skin Lesions)
Secondary Lesions
(Table 10-2: Secondary Skin Lesions)

PRESSURE ULCERS (DECUBITUS ULCERS)

Data Base
A. Etiology and pathophysiology
   1. Caused by interruption of circulation when pressure on the skin exceeds capillary pressure of 32 mm Hg for prolonged periods
   2. Pressure compresses capillaries and microthrombi form to occlude blood flow; tissue becomes damaged as a result of tissue hypoxia
   3. Most ulcers commonly occur over bony prominences: sacrum, greater trochanter, heels, scapulae, elbows, malleoli, occiput, ears, and ischial tuberosities (Figure 10-1: Common sites for pressure ulcers and frequency of ulceration per site)
   4. Contributing factors
      a. Immobility—results in prolonged pressure
      b. Aging—decreased epidermal thickness, elasticity, and secretion by sebaceous glands
      c. Moisture—causes skin maceration
      d. Imbalanced nutrition—loss of subcutaneous tissue reduces padding; inadequate protein intake leads to negative nitrogen balance, decreased muscle mass, and impaired wound healing
      e. Pyrexia—causes increased cellular demand for oxygen
      f. Inadequate tissue oxygenation—edema, anemia, and circulatory disturbances result in less oxygen delivered to tissues
      g. Incontinence—substances in urine and feces irritate the skin
      h. Dryness—skin less supple
      i. Shearing force or friction—exerts excessive tension on skin
      j. Cognitive impairments—client unaware of discomfort and does not self-protect
      k. Equipment—causes pressure, tension, or shearing forces on skin

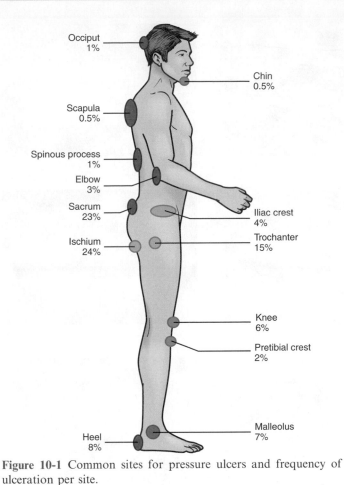

Figure 10-1 Common sites for pressure ulcers and frequency of ulceration per site.

5. Staging determined by depth and color (Figure 10-2: Staging of pressure ulcers)
   a. Depth of tissue damage
      (1) Suspected deep tissue injury: purple or maroon localized area of intact skin or blood-filled blister; area may be firm, boggy, warmer, cooler, or painful in comparison with nearby tissue
      (2) Stage I: nonblanchable area of erythema; skin is intact; usually over bony prominence
      (3) Stage II: partial-thickness ulceration of epidermis and/or dermis; presents as an abrasion, blister, or shallow crater; red/pink wound bed; without tissue sloughing; may be intact/open serum-filled blister
      (4) Stage III: full-thickness ulceration involving the epidermis, dermis, and subcutaneous tissue; sloughing may be present; presents as a deep crater with or without undermining; bone, tendon, or muscle is not exposed
      (5) Stage IV: extensive tissue damage involving full-thickness skin loss and damage to muscle, bone, and/or tendon; sloughing or eschar may be present on parts of

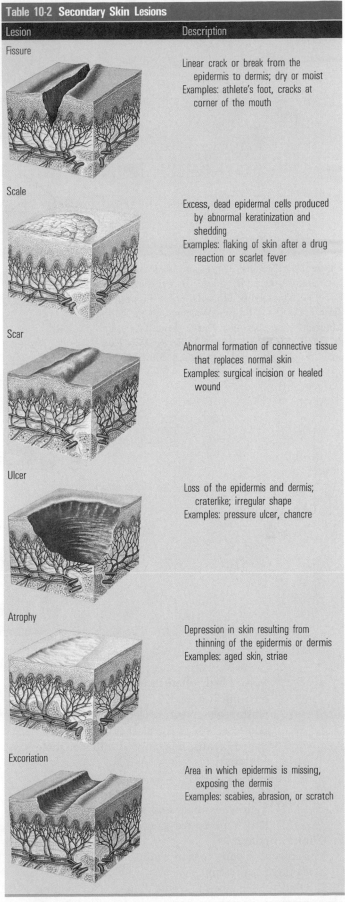

Table 10-2 Secondary Skin Lesions

Lesion	Description
Fissure	Linear crack or break from the epidermis to dermis; dry or moist Examples: athlete's foot, cracks at corner of the mouth
Scale	Excess, dead epidermal cells produced by abnormal keratinization and shedding Examples: flaking of skin after a drug reaction or scarlet fever
Scar	Abnormal formation of connective tissue that replaces normal skin Examples: surgical incision or healed wound
Ulcer	Loss of the epidermis and dermis; craterlike; irregular shape Examples: pressure ulcer, chancre
Atrophy	Depression in skin resulting from thinning of the epidermis or dermis Examples: aged skin, striae
Excoriation	Area in which epidermis is missing, exposing the dermis Examples: scabies, abrasion, or scratch

From Lewis SL et al: *Medical-surgical nursing: assessment and management of clinical problems*, ed 7, St Louis, 2007, Mosby.

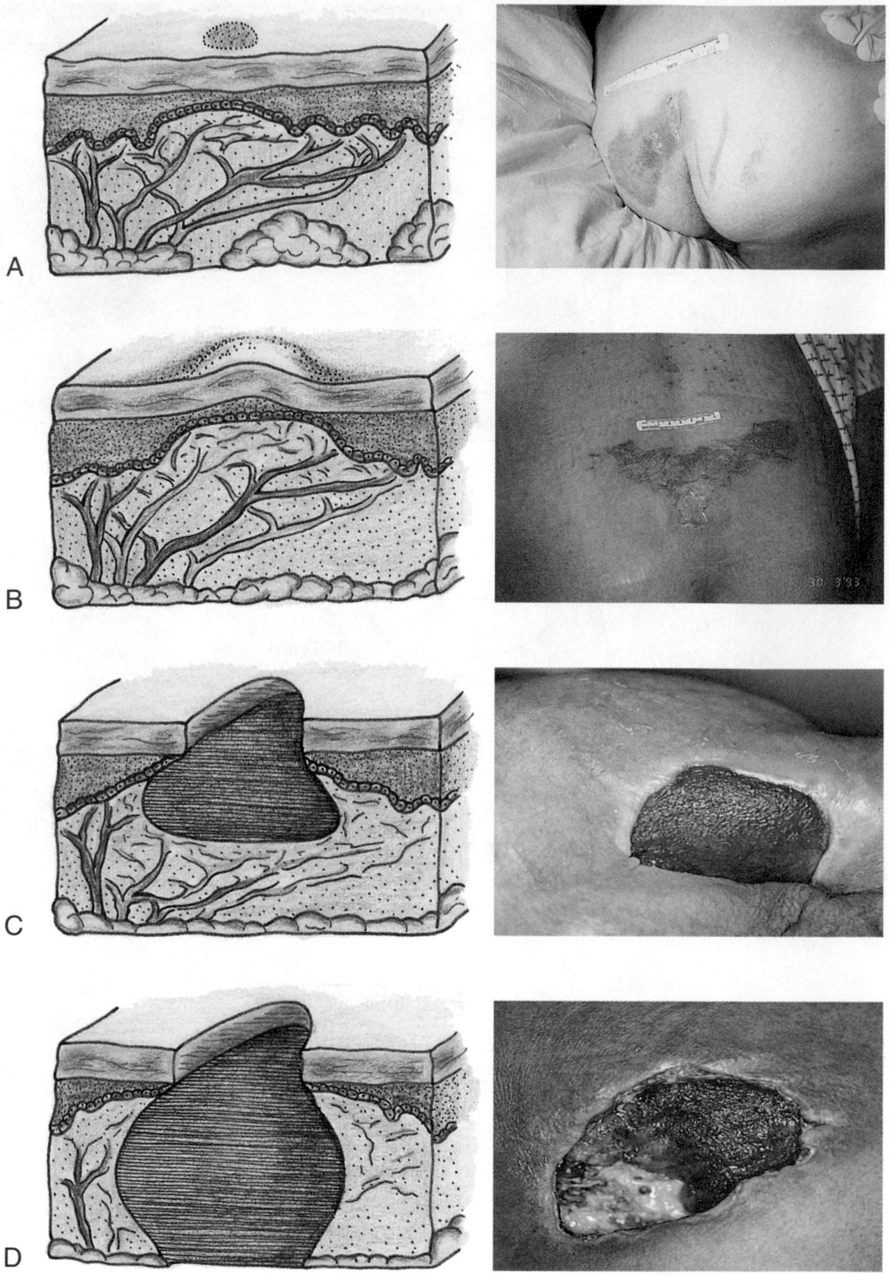

Figure 10-2 Staging of pressure ulcers. **A,** Stage I pressure ulcer. **B,** Stage II pressure ulcer. **C,** Stage III pressure ulcer. **D,** Stage IV pressure ulcer. (Courtesy Laurel Wiersma, RN, MSN, Clinical Nurse Specialist, Barnes-Jewish Hospital, St Louis, MO. In Potter PA, Perry AG: *Fundamentals of nursing,* ed 7, St Louis, 2009, Mosby.)

wound bed; often includes undermining or tunneling
      (6) Unstageable pressure ulcer: full-thickness skin loss; base of the ulcer is unable to be staged because it is covered with sloughing or eschar
   b. Color of wound
      (1) Black: necrotic
      (2) Yellow: exudate and yellow fibrous debris
      (3) Red: pink to red granulation
B. Clinical findings
   1. Subjective: pain; loss of sensation if sensory nerve damage is present
   2. Objective: erythema; tissue damage (see staging of pressure ulcers); exudate; pyrexia and leukocytosis if systemic infection is present

C. Therapeutic interventions
   1. Elimination/minimization of pressure on the ulcer through frequent repositioning and use of supportive devices (e.g., air-fluidized beds, low–air-loss beds, or kinetic beds)
   2. Administration of protein supplements or total parenteral nutrition (TPN) to prevent negative nitrogen balance if client has serum albumin level less than 3.5 g, is anorexic, or is less than 80% of ideal body weight
   3. Administration of vitamin and mineral supplements (particularly vitamin C and zinc) to promote wound healing
   4. Débridement of necrotic tissue, which interferes with healing and promotes bacterial growth: mechanical irrigation; chemical débridement with enzyme

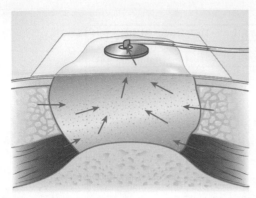

Figure 10-3 Wound V.A.C. system using negative pressure to remove fluid from area surrounding the wound, reducing edema and improving circulation to the area.

preparations; surgical débridement; wet-to-damp dressings

5. Application of dressings to promote healing
   a. Moist gauze: maintains wound humidity, which promotes epithelial cell growth
   b. Polyurethane film: provides barrier to bacteria and external fluid; promotes moist environment; permits view of wound
   c. Hydrocolloid dressing: maintains wound humidity, liquefies necrotic debris, and provides a protective cushion
   d. Absorptive dressing: absorbs drainage
   e. Vacuum-assisted wound closure: negative pressure applied to wound bed to remove exudate and facilitate angiogenesis (Figure 10-3: Wound V.A.C. system)
6. Antibiotic therapy
7. Skin grafts
8. Growth hormone therapy

Nursing Care of Clients With Pressure Ulcers

A. Assessment/Analysis
   1. Stage, size, and location
   2. Type and amount of exudate
   3. Risk factors: immobility, incontinence, malnutrition
B. Planning/Implementation
   1. Emphasize preventive care as soon as contributing factors are identified
   2. Change client's position at least every 1 to 2 hours
   3. Use supportive devices (e.g., pillows, heel and elbow pads, cushions, special mattresses or bed) to reduce pressure on bony prominences
   4. Encourage activity to enhance circulation
   5. Teach client to change position every hour; teach how to shift weight to minimize pressure
   6. Keep skin clean (bathing removes irritants and stimulates circulation), dry, and lubricated
   7. Massage around bony prominences, but avoid massaging reddened areas that are already damaged
   8. Ensure adequate fluid intake

9. Provide well-balanced diet; emphasize importance of protein, zinc, and vitamins C, A, and B
10. Avoid shearing force by lifting, not dragging, the client during position changes
11. Assess skin of high-risk clients daily

C. Evaluation/Outcomes
   1. Maintains intact skin
   2. Consumes diet high in protein, zinc, and vitamins C, A, and B
   3. Changes position every hour

BURNS

Data Base

A. Etiology and pathophysiology
   1. Thermal, radiation, electrical, and chemical (acids, bases) burns; cause cell destruction and result in depletion of fluid and electrolytes
   2. Extent of the fluid and electrolyte loss directly related to extent and degree of the burn (Figure 10-4: Classification of burn injury)
      a. Partial thickness
         (1) Superficial partial-thickness (first-degree) burn affects epidermis, causing erythema, edema, and pain; fluid loss slight, especially if less than 15% of body surface is involved (e.g., sunburn)
         (2) Deep partial-thickness (second-degree) burn affects epidermis and dermis, causing erythema, pain, vesicles with oozing; fluid loss slight to moderate, especially if less than 15% of body surface is involved (e.g., scalding)
      b. Full-thickness (third-degree) burn affects entire dermis and at times the subcutaneous tissue, resulting in charred or pearly white, dry skin and absence of pain; fluid loss usually severe, especially if more than 2% of body surface is involved (e.g., flame, electric, chemical)
      c. Full-thickness (fourth-degree) burn involves skin, fat, muscle, and bone; areas are charred or burned away (e.g., flame, electrical, chemical)
   3. Classification of burns
      a. Minor burns: no involvement of hands, face, or genitalia; total partial-thickness burn area does not exceed 15%
      b. Moderate burns: partial-thickness involvement of 15% to 25% of body; but full-thickness burns do not exceed 10% of body area
      c. Major burns: involvement exceeds 25% (if partial-thickness) or 10% (if full-thickness) of body surface; involvement of hands, face, genitalia, or feet; this classification is also used if the client has a preexisting chronic health problem, is younger than 18 months or more than 50 years of age, or has additional injuries

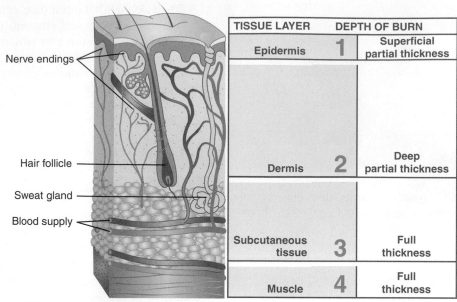

TISSUE LAYER		DEPTH OF BURN
Epidermis	1	Superficial partial thickness
Dermis	2	Deep partial thickness
Subcutaneous tissue	3	Full thickness
Muscle	4	Full thickness

Nerve endings

Hair follicle

Sweat gland

Blood supply

Figure 10-4 Classification of burn injury. (From Mahan LK, Escott-Stump S: *Krause's food and nutrition therapy*, ed 12, St Louis, 2008, Saunders.)

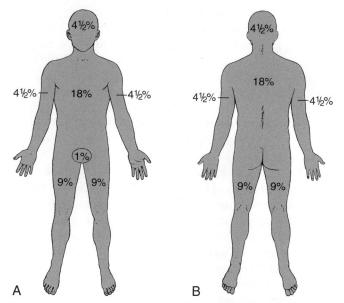

Figure 10-5 Rule of Nines. A commonly used assessment tool with estimates of the percentages (in multiples of 9) of the total body surface area burned. **A,** Adults (anterior view). **B,** Adults (posterior view). (From Thompson JM et al: *Mosby's clinical nursing*, ed 5, St Louis, 2002, Mosby.)

4. Pulmonary injury should be suspected if two of the following factors are present, and expected if three or all four are present
   a. Hair in nostrils singed; soot around mouth or nostrils
   b. Client was trapped in a closed space
   c. Face, nose, and lips burned
   d. Initial blood sample contains carboxyhemoglobin
5. Percentage of body surface area involved is determined; estimated by Lund-Browder chart or Rule of Nines (Figure 10-5: Rule of Nines)

6. Phases of burn injury
   a. Emergent: initial life-threatening stage; usually 24 to 48 hours; major concerns are respiratory status because of smoke inhalation, hypovolemia because of fluid shifts out of cells, and hyperkalemia because of cellular destruction
   b. Acute: begins with mobilization of fluids and electrolytes back into cells and ends when burns are healed or covered by skin grafts; may take days, weeks, or months; major concerns are hypervolemia and hypokalemia as a result of fluid and electrolyte shifts back into the intravascular and intracellular compartments, and infection
   c. Rehabilitation: begins when wounds are healed and client is able to resume self-care; may take weeks to months; major concern is resuming functional roles and coping with body image disturbances
7. Curling's ulcer may occur after a burn
   a. The client may complain of gastric discomfort, or there may be profuse bleeding; usually occurs by end of the first week after burn injury
   b. Treatment essentially the same as for a gastric ulcer; however, mortality after surgical repair is high because of the client's debilitated state
8. Suppressed immune system involving lymphocytes, immunoglobulin production, and changes in neutrophil and macrophage functioning
B. Clinical findings
   1. Subjective: extreme anxiety; restlessness (may indicate cerebral hypoxia); pain (depends on severity of burn); paresthesia; disorientation

2. Objective
   a. Changes in appearance of skin indicate degree of burn
   b. Hematuria; blood hemolysis with subsequent rise in plasma hemoglobin level may occur with full-thickness burns
   c. Elevated hematocrit level as a result of fluid loss or deceptively normal values because of protein losses from weeping wounds
   d. Electrolyte imbalance: cellular destruction results initially in hyperkalemia, hyponatremia, and hyperuricemia
   e. Presence of clinical findings of hypovolemic shock caused by circulatory failure, resulting from seepage of water, plasma, proteins, and electrolytes from burned area
   f. Presence of clinical findings of neurogenic shock (clinical findings similar to hypovolemic shock) caused by the fright, terror, hysteria, and pain involved in the situation
   g. Evidence of renal impairment (e.g., increased BUN and creatinine levels) if acute tubular necrosis occurs as a result of circulatory collapse

C. Therapeutic interventions
   1. Establishment of airway and administration of oxygen; mechanical ventilation as needed
   2. IV replacement (electrolyte solutions and colloids such as blood and plasma) to maintain circulation
      a. Volume of fluid replacement is based on percentage of body surface area involved and client's weight (e.g., Parkland/Baxter and Brooke Army formulas)
      b. Half of fluid is administered in first 8 hours; second half is administered over next 16 hours
   3. Reduction of total IV solutions during second 24 hours depends on the urinary output, blood work, and hemodynamic pressures
   4. Insertion of urinary retention catheter; hourly urinary output to monitor kidney function and influence fluid replacement
   5. Insertion of central line to monitor hemodynamic pressures (e.g., central venous pressure [CVP], pulmonary capillary wedge pressure [PCWP])
   6. Vital signs monitored every 15 minutes
   7. Serum electrolytes and blood gases to observe for levels and assist in deciding replacement therapy
   8. Tetanus toxoid booster administration; tetanus human immune globulin for passive immunity if not previously immunized
   9. Nothing by mouth except mineral water for first 24 to 48 hours; clear liquids as tolerated after 2 days; then high-protein, high-carbohydrate, high-fat, high-vitamin diet as tolerated
   10. Maintenance of surgical asepsis
   11. Daily hydrotherapy; water temperature should be tepid (98° to 100° F)
   12. Skin grafting to close wounds, limit fluid loss, promote healing, and limit contractures
      a. Heterograft (xenograft): skin from animals, usually pigs (porcine xenograft)
      b. Homograft (allograft): skin from another person or cadaver
      c. Autograft: skin from another part of the client's body
         (1) Mesh graft: machine used to mesh skin obtained from a donor site so it can be stretched to cover a larger area of burn
         (2) Postage stamp graft: earlier method of accomplishing the same goal as a mesh graft; a small amount of skin is used to cover a larger area; the donor skin is cut into small pieces and applied to the burn
         (3) Sheet grafting: large strips of skin placed over the burn as close together as possible
         (4) Cultured epithelial autografting is used for massive burn treatment
      d. Synthetic coverings
   13. Surgical, mechanical, or enzymatic débridement to promote healing and decrease infection
   14. IV antibiotics (based on wound culture and sensitivity [C&S]) and topical antibiotics (mafenide acetate ointment, silver nitrate solution, silver sulfadiazine, neomycin sulfate, bacitracin, polymyxin B) to limit infection
   15. Opioids to reduce pain and sedatives to decrease anxiety; given IV or orally because of decreased muscle absorption

Nursing Care of Clients With Burns

A. Assessment/Analysis
   1. Clinical findings of airway involvement: burns of face, neck, or chest; sooty sputum; or hoarseness
   2. Vital signs, arterial blood gases, and breath sounds to establish a baseline for respiratory function
   3. CVP or PCWP, and urine output, to establish baseline for assessment of circulation
   4. Estimated body surface area involvement and severity of burns

B. Planning/Implementation
   1. Apply cool, moist dressing at site of injury; neutralize the burn if caused by a chemical (acid, base); flush with water and apply the opposite chemical in a weak form as ordered
   2. Monitor vital signs, CVP or PCWP, and I&O (hourly urine output) as ordered; notify physician if output falls below 30 mL/hr or rises above 50 mL/hr
   3. Observe for clinical findings of electrolyte imbalance (calcium, potassium, and sodium) and metabolic acidosis

4. Administer fluid and electrolytes as ordered
5. Monitor respiratory function: characteristics of respirations, breath sounds, arterial blood gases, and pulse oximetry
6. Administer oxygen as ordered
7. Elevate head of the bed
8. Encourage coughing, deep breathing, and incentive spirometer use
9. Prevent infection
   a. Monitor for clinical findings of infection (rising temperature and WBC count, odor); promptly culture exudate if infection is suspected
   b. Follow principles of protective precautions (gown, gloves, mask, hair covering) during contact because of the client's compromised ability to resist infection
   c. Administer tetanus toxoid as ordered
   d. Administer IV and topical antibiotics as ordered
   e. Use sterile technique for wound care
10. Apply pressure dressings as ordered to reduce contractures and scarring
11. Support joints and extremities in functional position and perform range-of-motion (ROM) exercises; use beds or mattresses designed to avoid pressure
12. Provide care related to skin graft
   a. Keep donor sites (which are covered with a nonadherent dressing and wrapped in an absorbent gauze) dry; remove absorbent gauze as nonadherent dressing will separate as healing occurs
   b. Monitor the grafts, which are generally left with a light pressure dressing for approximately 3 days; after the graft has "taken," roll cotton-tipped applicators gently over the graft to remove underlying exudate; exudate allowed to remain could promote infection and prevent the graft from adhering; instruct client to restrict mobility of the affected part
   c. Monitor for foul-smelling drainage, temperature elevation, and other clinical findings of infection; promptly culture exudate if infection is suspected
   d. Instruct the client to avoid exposure of the graft and donor sites to the sun
13. Support the client physically and emotionally while turning
14. Keep room temperature warm and humidity high
15. Prevent GI erosion
   a. Observe for clinical findings of stress ulcer
   b. Give ordered drugs to decrease or neutralize hydrochloric acid
   c. Provide small, frequent feedings; diet high in protein, carbohydrates, vitamins, and minerals; moderate in fat, with adequate calories for protein sparing

16. Give medication for pain as ordered and particularly before dressing change
17. Provide emotional support
   a. Expect client to express negative feelings; accept negative feelings
   b. Explain need for staff wearing gowns and masks
   c. Assist client to cope with change in body image
   d. Give realistic reassurance; convey a positive attitude
   e. Encourage participation in self-care
   f. Refer client and family to support groups and rehabilitative services
C. Evaluation/Outcomes
   1. Maintains respiratory function
   2. Maintains fluid balance
   3. Remains free of infection
   4. Expresses feelings about altered body image

CELLULITIS

Data Base
A. Etiology and pathophysiology
   1. Infection of deep layers of the dermis; spreads along connective tissue planes
   2. Usually caused by streptococcal or staphylococcal organisms
   3. Organism enters tissue through abrasion, bite, trauma, or wound
   4. Erysipelas is an acute infection of superficial dermis and lymphatics caused by beta-hemolytic group A streptococci
   5. Necrotizing fasciitis is cellulitis that extends to the fascia, causing thrombosis of subcutaneous vessels and gangrene of tissue
B. Clinical findings
   1. Subjective: pain; itching
   2. Objective: swelling; redness; warmth; leukocytosis
C. Therapeutic interventions
   1. IV, IM, or oral antibiotic therapy following cultures of the area
   2. Rest with elevation of extremity
   3. Warm compresses

Nursing Care of Clients With Cellulitis
A. Assessment/Analysis
   1. Progression of clinical findings
   2. Clinical findings of inflammation
   3. Evidence of trauma
   4. Evidence of impaired immune response from history
   5. Vital signs and WBC count for data base
B. Planning/Implementation
   1. Monitor vital signs and WBC count for evidence of systemic involvement; assess peripheral tissue perfusion
   2. Use contact precautions and surgical asepsis as indicated
   3. Administer analgesics and antibiotics as ordered
   4. Elevate extremity
   5. Apply warm compresses as ordered; protect from thermal trauma

C. Evaluation/Outcomes
1. Experiences resolution of inflammatory process
2. Reports relief of pain

CANCER OF THE SKIN
Data Base
A. Etiology and pathophysiology
1. Most common cancer; slow progression and high cure rate if detected early for some types
2. Exposure to the sun, irritating chemicals, and chronic friction implicated; more common in persons with fair complexions
3. Types (Figure 10-6: Cancer of the skin)
   a. Basal cell carcinoma: generally located on the face and appears as a waxy nodule that may have telangiectasia visible; the most common type of skin cancer, but metastasis is rare

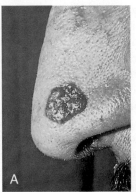
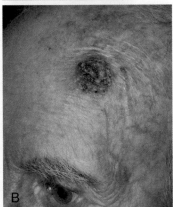
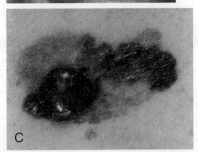

Figure 10-6 Cancer of the skin. **A,** Basal cell carcinoma. **B,** Squamous cell carcinoma. **C,** Melanoma. (**A,** from Belcher AE: *Cancer nursing*, St Louis, 1992, Mosby. **B,** from Habif TP: *Clinical dermatology: a color guide to diagnosis and therapy*, ed 3, St Louis, 1996, Mosby. **C,** from Zitelli BJ, Davis HW: *Atlas of pediatric physical diagnosis*, ed 5, St Louis, 2007, Mosby.)

b. Squamous cell carcinoma: found most frequently on upper extremities and face, which are exposed to the sun; appears as a small, red, nodular lesion; may develop secondarily to precancerous lesions such as keratosis and leukoplakia; develops rapidly and may metastasize through local lymph nodes
c. Malignant melanoma: arises from the pigment-producing melanocytes; the color of the lesion may vary greatly (white, flesh, gray, brown, blue, black); suspected with changes in size, color, sensation, or characteristics of a mole; most serious type of skin cancer; metastasis via blood can be extensive

B. Clinical findings
1. Subjective: pruritus may or may not be present; localized soreness
2. Objective: change in color, size, or shape of preexisting lesion; oozing, bleeding, or crusting; biopsy of tumor reveals type of cancer; lymphadenopathy if metastasis has occurred

C. Therapeutic interventions
1. Surgical excision of the lesion and surrounding tissue
2. Chemosurgery, which involves the use of zinc chloride to fix the cells before they are dissected by layers
3. Cryosurgery—using liquid nitrogen to destroy the tumor cells by freezing
4. Radiation (malignant melanoma does not respond well to this mode of treatment)
5. Electrodesiccation and curettage—mechanical disruption of cells by heat; cells are then cut away with curet
6. Laser light is used to vaporize lesions
7. Chemotherapy
8. Nonspecific immunostimulants such as bacille Calmette-Guérin (BCG) vaccine

Nursing Care of Clients With Cancer of the Skin
A. Assessment/Analysis
1. History of changes in size, color, shape, sensation, or unusual bleeding of lesions
2. Risk factors from history
3. Skin for presence of suspicious lesions, documenting objective and subjective characteristics

B. Planning/Implementation
1. Instruct to examine moles for changes and have those subject to chronic irritation (bra or belt line) removed
2. Encourage to avoid sun exposure; use sunscreens with a rating higher than 15 SPF (solar protection factor); wear protective clothing (long sleeves, pants, and hat)
3. Emphasize continued medical supervision
4. Encourage verbalization; maintain a therapeutic environment
5. Provide care to the client receiving radiation: observe skin for local reaction; avoid use of ointments, or powders containing metals

6. Provide care related to specific chemotherapeutic agents (see Related Pharmacology under Neoplastic Disorders in Chapter 3)
7. Support natural defense mechanisms of client; encourage intake of nutrient-dense foods with emphasis on fruits, vegetables, whole grains, and legumes, especially those high in the immune-stimulating nutrients selenium and vitamins A, C, and E; beta-carotene has been associated with prevention of skin cancer
8. Encourage client to verbalize fears

C. Evaluation/Outcomes
1. Avoids exposure to the sun and known irritants
2. Examines skin lesions regularly and reports changes to physician
3. Verbalizes acceptance of physical appearance after surgical excision of lesions

✿ HERPES ZOSTER (SHINGLES)

Data Base

A. Etiology and pathophysiology
1. Acute viral infection of structures along the pathway of peripheral nerves caused by reactivation of latent varicella-zoster virus
2. Occurs in clients who have had chickenpox and are exposed to an affected individual
3. Commonly occurs in immunosuppressed clients (e.g., leukemia, lymphoma) who have previously had chickenpox
4. May involve the eye, leading to keratitis, uveitis, and blindness

B. Clinical findings
1. Subjective: pain; paresthesias; pruritus
2. Objective: vesicles along the involved nerves; stains made from lesion exudate isolate the organism

C. Therapeutic interventions
1. Administration of acyclovir (Zovirax) or valacyclovir (Valtrex)
2. Medications for pain, relaxation, itching, and prevention of secondary infection
3. Pain control by blocking the nerve through injection of drugs such as lidocaine or applying medication such as triamcinolone (Kenalog)
4. Antiinflammatory drugs such as systemic or topical steroids
5. Prevention: Vaccine available (Zostavax) for people 60 years or older; reduces development of and chronic pain associated with shingles, which is common in older adults

Nursing Care of Clients With Herpes Zoster

A. Assessment/Analysis
1. Progression of clinical findings from history, includes factors that compromise the immune response (e.g., age, disease, chemotherapy)
2. Presence of characteristic lesion

B. Planning/Implementation
1. Administer analgesics and other medications as ordered
2. Reduce itching and protect lesions from air by the application of salves, ointments, lotions, and sterile dressings as ordered
3. Protect from pressure by use of air mattress, bed cradle, and light, loose clothing (avoid synthetic and woolen materials and use cotton fabrics)
4. Use airborne and/or contact precautions as indicated
5. Administer antibiotics as ordered
6. Encourage client to avoid scratching and to use gloves at night to limit trauma from accidental scratching; explain basis for the rash and pruritus
7. Allay fears about shingles by providing objective information
8. Encourage the client to express feelings
9. Encourage diet rich in nutrient-dense foods such as fruits, vegetables, whole grains, and legumes to improve and maintain nutritional status and prevent possible drug-induced nutrient deficiencies; encourage intake of vitamin C because it has been reported to stimulate the immune response to viral infection by increasing interferon, which limits viral reproduction in early stages
10. Teach handwashing to help prevent spread of the virus; individuals who have not had chickenpox should not be assigned to provide care
11. Emotionally support client dealing with severe pain and social isolation

C. Evaluation/Outcomes
1. Experiences an improvement in skin integrity
2. Reports that pain and pruritus have subsided

✿ SYSTEMIC LUPUS ERYTHEMATOSUS (SLE)

Data Base

A. Etiology and pathophysiology
1. Origin unknown; affects the connective tissue and is thought to result from a defect in the body's immunologic mechanisms, genetic predisposition, or environmental stimuli
2. Immune complex deposits in blood vessels, among collagen fibers, and on organs
3. Necrosis of the glomerular capillaries, inflammation of cerebral and ocular blood vessels, necrosis of lymph nodes, vasculitis of the GI tract and pleura, and degeneration of the basal layer of skin
4. More common in females, ages 15 to 40

B. Clinical findings
1. Subjective: malaise; photosensitivity; joint pain
2. Objective: fever; butterfly erythema on the face; erythema of palms; positive lupus erythematosus preparation (LE prep); increased antinuclear antibodies (ANAs) in blood; Raynaud's phenomenon; weight loss; evidence of impaired renal, gastrointestinal, cardiac, respiratory, and neurologic functions

C. Therapeutic interventions
   1. Corticosteroids and analgesics to reduce inflammation and pain
   2. Supportive therapy as major organs become affected
   3. Plasmapheresis to remove autoantibodies and immune complexes from the blood
   4. Life-threatening SLE may be treated with stem cell transplants

Nursing Care of Clients With Systemic Lupus Erythematosus

A. Assessment/Analysis
   1. Progression of clinical findings from the history
   2. Presence of skin lesions
   3. Sensitivity to light (photosensitivity)
   4. Vital signs for baseline data
   5. Heart and lung sounds
   6. Abdomen for enlargement of liver and spleen
   7. Neurologic status
   8. Renal function (review BUN and creatinine analysis results)
B. Planning/Implementation
   1. Administer corticosteroids and observe for side effects, teaching client to do the same (see Antiinflammatory Agents under Related Pharmacology in this chapter)
   2. Help client and family cope with severity of the disease and its poor prognosis
   3. Explain the importance of protecting skin: use of mild soap; avoidance of exposure to sunlight; use of sun-blocking agents
   4. Help to establish program of exercise balanced by rest periods to avoid fatigue
   5. Instruct to alter consistency and frequency of meals if dysphagia and anorexia exist
   6. Encourage diet rich in nutrient-dense foods such as fruits, vegetables, whole grains, and legumes to improve and maintain nutritional status and compensate for nutrient interactions of corticosteroid and other therapeutic medications; emphasize vitamin C because it is essential in the biosynthesis of collagen, and large doses have been found to increase total collagen synthesis
   7. Teach to prevent infection (e.g., handwashing and avoidance of individuals with infections)
   8. Emphasize the need for continued medical supervision
C. Evaluation/Outcomes
   1. Demonstrates a reduction in skin lesions
   2. States that pain is reduced
   3. Verbalizes fears with family and health care providers

PROGRESSIVE SYSTEMIC SCLEROSIS (SCLERODERMA)

Data Base

A. Etiology and pathophysiology
   1. Thought to be caused by an autoimmune defect; occurs in women more frequently than in men
   2. Systemic disease that causes fibrotic changes in connective tissue throughout the body
   3. May involve the skin, blood vessels, synovial membranes, esophagus, heart, lungs, kidneys, or GI tract
   4. CREST syndrome refers to a group of clinical findings associated with a poor prognosis: Calcium deposits in organs; Raynaud's phenomenon; Esophageal dysfunction; Sclerodactyly (scleroderma of the digits); Telangiectasia (vascular lesions formed by dilation of a group of small blood vessels)
B. Clinical findings
   1. Subjective: articular pain; muscle weakness
   2. Objective
      a. Hard skin that eventually adheres to underlying structures; face becomes masklike; body motion restricted
      b. Telangiectases on the lips, fingers, face, and tongue
      c. Dysphagia
      d. Raynaud's phenomenon
      e. Positive LE preparation, elevated gamma-globulin levels, presence of antinuclear antibodies
C. Therapeutic interventions
   1. Immunosuppressants: cyclosporine and methotrexate; corticosteroids are rarely prescribed because they can cause a sudden decrease in renal function
   2. Salicylates or analgesics for joint pain
   3. Vasodilators for clinical findings of Raynaud's phenomenon; angiotensin-converting enzyme inhibitors; calcium channel blockers; alpha blockers; nitroglycerin topical ointment to digits
   4. Physical therapy

Nursing Care of Clients With Scleroderma

A. Assessment/Analysis
   1. Onset and progression of clinical findings from history
   2. Skin, particularly of the hands and face
   3. Joints for inflammation
B. Planning/Implementation
   1. Support the client and family emotionally; there is no cure at present
   2. Use mild soaps and lotions for skin care
   3. Instruct to avoid smoking and exposure to cold
   4. Encourage deep-breathing exercises
   5. Teach the importance of observing for side effects of corticosteroids or other immunosuppressive drugs (e.g., infection)
   6. Monitor function of all vital organs (e.g., cardiac, respiratory, and renal status)
C. Evaluation/Outcomes
   1. Maintains skin integrity
   2. Verbalizes acceptance of changes in appearance and disease
   3. Reports clinical findings of vital organ involvement

Nursing Care of Clients With Neuromusculoskeletal System Disorders

OVERVIEW

REVIEW OF ANATOMY AND PHYSIOLOGY

Structures and Functions of the Nervous System

Overview

A. Central nervous system (CNS)
1. Brain
2. Spinal cord
B. Peripheral nervous system (PNS)
1. Cranial nerves
2. Spinal nerves
3. Autonomic nervous system (ANS)
   a. Sympathetic nervous system: mediated by neurotransmitter norepinephrine
   b. Parasympathetic nervous system: mediated by neurotransmitter acetylcholine

Neurons

Nerve cells: basic structural and functional units
A. Types
1. Sensory (afferent) neurons: transmit impulses to spinal cord or brain
2. Motoneurons (efferent): transmit impulses away from brain or spinal cord to muscles or glands
   a. Upper motor neurons: located in CNS; destruction causes loss of voluntary control, muscle spasticity, and hyperactive reflexes
   b. Lower motor neurons: extend to myoneural junction; destruction causes loss of voluntary control, muscle flaccidity, and loss of reflexes
B. Impulse transmission
1. Dendrites: carry impulses toward cell body
2. Cell body: contains a nucleus and other cytoplasmic matter
3. Axon: carries impulse away from cell body
4. Myelin: multiple, dense layers of membrane around an axon or dendrite; myelinated nerve fibers transmit nerve impulses more rapidly than nonmyelinated fibers
5. Synapse
   a. Point of contact between axon of one cell and dendrite of another
   b. Axons enlarge here to form synaptic terminals that secrete neurotransmitters
   c. Some synapses are excitatory and others inhibitory

Brain

A. General considerations
1. Has large blood supply and high O_2 consumption
2. Can use only glucose for energy metabolism; therefore hypoglycemia can seriously alter brain function
3. Protected by the blood-brain barrier, a selective filtration system that isolates the brain from certain substances in the general circulation
4. Basic tissue types: neuron cell aggregations (gray matter) and tracts of myelinated fibers (white matter)
B. Brainstem
1. Consists of medulla, pons, and midbrain
2. Conducts impulses between the cord and brain; most motor and sensory fibers decussate (cross over) in medulla
3. Contains reflex centers for heart, blood vessel diameter, respiratory reflexes, vomiting, coughing, and swallowing
4. Cranial nerves III through XII originate in brainstem
C. Cerebellum: exerts synergic control over skeletal muscles, producing smooth, precise movements; coordinates skeletal muscle contractions; promotes posture, equilibrium, and balance
D. Diencephalon
1. Thalamus
   a. Crudely translates sensory impulses into sensations but does not localize them
   b. Processes motor information from the cerebral cortex and cerebellum and projects back to the motor cortex
   c. Contributes to emotional component of sensations (pleasant or unpleasant)
2. Hypothalamus
   a. Part of the neural path by which emotions and other cerebral functions can alter vital, automatic functions such as the heartbeat, BP, peristalsis, and secretion by glands
   b. Secretes neuropeptides that influence secretion of various anterior pituitary hormones
   c. Makes antidiuretic hormone (ADH) and oxytocin, which are secreted by the posterior pituitary
   d. Contains appetite center and satiety center

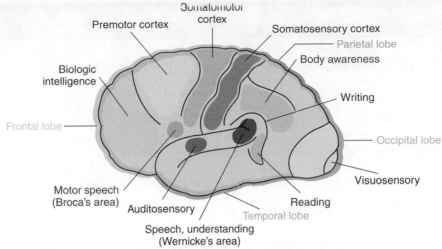

Figure 11-1 Cerebral cortex. (Modified from Monahan FD et al: *Phipps' medical-surgical nursing: health and illness perspectives*, ed 8, St Louis, 2007, Mosby.)

e. Serves as a heat-regulating center by relaying impulses to lower autonomic centers for vasoconstriction, vasodilation, and sweating, and to somatic centers for shivering

f. Maintains waking state; part of arousal or alerting neural pathway

3. Optic chiasm: the point of crossing over (decussation) of optic nerve fibers

E. Cerebral cortex: consists of multiple lobes divided into two hemispheres covered by gray matter forming folds (convolutions) composed of hills (gyri) and valleys (sulci) (Figure 11-1: Cerebral cortex)

1. Frontal lobe
   a. Influences abstract thinking, sense of humor, and uniqueness of personality
   b. Controls contraction of skeletal muscles and synchronization of muscular movements
   c. Exerts control over hypothalamus; influences basic biorhythms
   d. Controls muscular movements necessary for speech (Broca's area)

2. Parietal lobes
   a. Translate nerve impulses into sensations (e.g., touch, temperature)
   b. Interpret sensations; provide appreciation of size, shape, texture, and weight
   c. Interpret sense of taste

3. Temporal lobes
   a. Translate nerve impulses into sensations of sound and interpret sounds (Wernicke's area; usually in dominant hemisphere)
   b. Interpret sense of smell
   c. Control behavior patterns

4. Occipital lobe
   a. Interprets sense of vision
   b. Provides appreciation of size, shape, and color

F. Brain and spinal cord protection
   1. Vertebrae around the cord; cranial bones around the brain

2. Meninges
   a. Dura mater: white fibrous tissue, outer layer
   b. Arachnoid: "cobwebby" middle layer
   c. Pia mater: innermost layer; adheres to outer surface of the cord and brain; contains blood vessels

3. Spaces
   a. Subarachnoid space around the brain and cord between arachnoid and pia mater, contains cerebral spinal fluid
   b. Subdural space between dura mater and arachnoid
   c. Epidural space between the dura mater and cranial bones

4. Ventricles and cerebral aqueduct inside the brain; four cavities known as first, second, third, and fourth ventricles
   a. Cerebrospinal fluid (CFS) formed by plasma filtering from network of capillaries (choroid plexus) in each ventricle
   b. CFS circulates throughout ventricles, brain, and subarachnoid space and returns to blood via venous sinuses of brain

Cranial Nerves

Are 12 pairs. (Table 11-1: Distribution and Function of Cranial Nerve Pairs and Figure 11-2: Cranial nerves)

Spinal Cord

A. Structure
   1. Inner core of gray matter shaped like a three-dimensional H
   2. Long columns of white matter surround the cord's inner core of gray matter; namely, right and left anterior, lateral, and posterior columns; composed of numerous sensory and motor tracts

B. Functions
   1. Sensory tracts conduct impulses up cord to brain (e.g., spinothalamic tracts, two of the six ascending tracts, conduct sensations of pain, temperature, vibration, and proprioception)

Table 11-1 Distribution and Function of Cranial Nerve Pairs*

Name and Number	Distribution	Function
Olfactory (I)	Nasal mucosa, high up along the septum especially	Sense of smell (sensory only)
Optic (II)	Retina of eyeball	Vision (sensory only)
Oculomotor (III)	Extrinsic muscles of eyeball, except superior oblique and external rectus; also intrinsic eye muscles (iris and ciliary)	Eye movements; constriction of pupil and bulging of lens, which together produce accommodation for near vision
Trochlear (IV), smallest cranial nerve	Superior oblique muscle of eye	Eye movements
Trigeminal (V) (or trifacial), largest cranial nerve	Sensory fibers to skin and mucosa of head and to teeth; muscles of mastication (sensory and motor fibers)	Sensation in head and face; chewing movements
Abducent (VI)	External rectus muscle of eye	Abduction of eye
Facial (VII)	Muscles of facial expression; taste buds of anterior two thirds of tongue; motor fibers to submaxillary and sublingual salivary glands	Facial expressions; taste; secretion of saliva
Acoustic (VIII) (vestibulocochlear)	Inner ear	Hearing and equilibrium (sensory only)
Glossopharyngeal (IX)	Posterior third of tongue; mucosa and muscles of pharynx; parotid gland; carotid sinus and body	Taste and other sensations of tongue; secretion of saliva; swallowing movements; function in reflex arcs for control of blood pressure and respiration
Vagus (X) (or pneumogastric)	Mucosa and muscles of pharynx, larynx, trachea, bronchi, esophagus; thoracic and abdominal viscera	Sensations and movements of organs supplied; for example, slows heart, increases peristalsis and gastric and pancreatic secretion; voice production
Spinal accessory (XI)	Certain neck and shoulder muscles (muscles of larynx, sternocleidomastoid, trapezius)	Shoulder movements; turns head; voice production; muscle sense
Hypoglossal (XII)	Tongue muscles	Tongue movements, as in talking; muscle sense

*Note: The first letters of the words in the following sentence are the first letters of the cranial nerves, and many generations of anatomy students have used it as an aid to memorizing the names: "On Old Olympus' Towering Tops, A Finn and German Viewed Some Hops." (There are several slightly different versions of the mnemonic.)

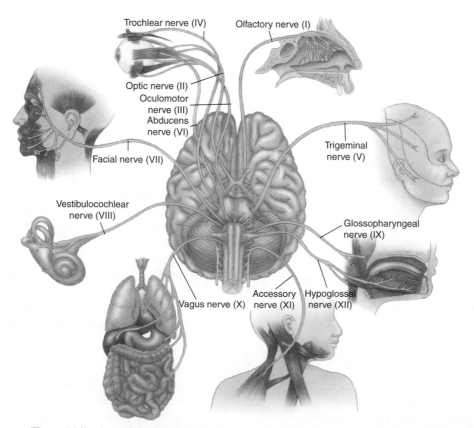

Figure 11-2 Cranial nerves. (From Thibodeau GA, Patton KT: *Anatomy and physiology,* ed 6, St Louis, 2007, Mosby.)

2. Motor tracts (pyramidal and extrapyramidal tracts) conduct impulses down cord from brain (e.g., the two corticospinal tracts decussate, controlling voluntary movement on the side of the body opposite the cerebral cortex from which the impulse initiated; three vestibulospinal tracts are involved with some autonomic functions)
3. Gray matter of cord contains reflex centers for all spinal cord reflexes

Spinal Nerves

A. Are 31 pairs, each containing a dorsal root and a ventral root
B. Branches of the spinal nerves form intricate networks of fibers (e.g., brachial plexus), from which nerves emerge to supply various parts of the skin, mucosa, and skeletal muscles
C. All spinal nerves are composed of both sensory dendrites (dorsal root) and motor axons (ventral root)

Autonomic Nervous System

A. Conducts impulses from the brainstem or cord out to visceral effectors: cardiac muscle, smooth muscle, and glands
B. Consists of two divisions
1. Sympathetic (adrenergic fibers) secretes norepinephrine: influences heart, smooth muscle of blood vessels and bronchioles, and glandular secretion
2. Parasympathetic (cholinergic fibers) secretes acetylcholine: influences digestive tract and smooth muscle to promote digestive gland secretion, peristalsis, and defecation; influences the heart to decrease rate and contractility
C. Autonomic antagonism and summation: sympathetic and parasympathetic impulses tend to produce opposite effects (Table 11-2: Autonomic Functions)
D. Under conditions of stress, sympathetic impulses to the visceral effectors dominate over parasympathetic impulses; however, in some individuals under stress,

Table 11-2 Autonomic Functions

Autonomic Effector	Effect of Sympathetic Stimulation (Neurotransmitter: Norepinephrine Unless Otherwise Stated)	Effect of Parasympathetic Stimulation (Neurotransmitter: Acetylcholine)
Cardiac Muscle	Increased rate and strength of contraction (beta receptors)	Decreased rate and strength of contraction
Smooth Muscle of Blood Vessels		
Skin blood vessels	Constriction (alpha receptors)	No effect
Skeletal muscle blood vessels	Dilation (beta receptors)	No effect
Coronary blood vessels	Constriction (alpha receptors) Dilation (beta receptors)	Dilation
Abdominal blood vessels	Constriction (alpha receptors)	No effect
Blood vessels of external genitals	Constriction (alpha receptors)	Dilation of blood vessels causing erection
Smooth Muscle of Hollow Organs and Sphincters		
Bronchioles	Dilation (beta receptors)	Constriction
Digestive tract, except sphincters	Decreased peristalsis (beta receptors)	Increased peristalsis
Sphincters of digestive tract	Constriction (alpha receptors)	Relaxation
Urinary bladder	Relaxation (beta receptors)	Contraction
Urinary sphincters	Constriction (alpha receptors)	Relaxation
Reproductive ducts	Contraction (alpha receptors)	Relaxation
Eye		
Iris	Contraction of radial muscle; dilated pupil	Contraction of circular muscle; constricted pupil
Ciliary	Relaxation; accommodates for far vision	Contraction; accommodates for near vision
Hairs (pilomotor muscles)	Contraction produces goose pimples, or piloerection (alpha receptors)	No effect
Glands		
Sweat	Increased sweat (neurotransmitter: acetylcholine)	No effect
Lacrimal	No effect	Increased secretion of tears
Digestive (salivary, gastric, etc.)	Decreased secretion of saliva; not known for others	Increased secretion of saliva
Pancreas, including islets	Decreased secretion	Increased secretion of pancreatic juice and insulin
Liver	Increased glycogenolysis (beta receptors); increased blood glucose level	No effect
Adrenal medulla*	Increased epinephrine secretion	No effect

From Thibodeau GA, Patton KT: *Anatomy and physiology*, ed 6, St Louis, 2007, Mosby.
*Sympathetic preganglionic axons terminate in contact with secreting cells of the adrenal medulla. Thus the adrenal medulla functions, to quote someone's descriptive phrase, as a "giant sympathetic postganglionic neuron."

parasympathetic impulses via the vagus nerve increase to glands and smooth muscle of the stomach, stimulating hydrochloric acid secretion and gastric motility

Nerve Impulse Conduction

A. Sodium-potassium pump: transports sodium out and potassium into the cell; requires adenosine triphosphate (ATP) to work

B. Resting potential: exists when cells are in an unstimulated or resting state

C. Action potential: composed of depolarization and repolarization; known as the nerve impulse

D. Reflex arc: pathway to spinal cord and back to effector organ that elicits a single, specific response; primitive nerve activity

E. Types of neurotransmitters (there are at least 30 types)
1. Monoamines (norepinephrine, dopamine, serotonin, acetylcholine); axons that release acetylcholine are called cholinergic; those that release norepinephrine are called adrenergic
2. Amino acids (gamma-aminobutyric acid [GABA], glutamic acid, glycine, taurine); GABA is the most common inhibitory transmitter in the brain
3. Neuropeptides (e.g., vasopressin, enkephalins, and endorphins); some influence hormone levels and others affect perception and integration of pain and emotional experience
4. Prostaglandins: some inhibit and some excite; may moderate the action of other transmitters by influencing the neuronal membrane

Sense Organs

A. Taste
1. Taste buds consist of groups of receptors connected to cranial nerves VII and IX
2. Responds to sweet at tongue tip; sour and salt at tip and sides; bitter at back
3. Olfaction involved in sense of taste

B. Olfaction
1. Receptors in epithelium of the nasal mucosa; odors sensed as chemicals interact with receptors on sensory hairs of olfactory cells
2. Olfactory pathways utilize cranial nerve I

C. Sight
1. Sclera and cornea (outer coat); choroid; ciliary body; suspensory ligament holding lens; iris (middle coat); retina (inner coat)
2. Anterior cavity contains aqueous humor; posterior cavity contains vitreous humor
3. Extrinsic muscles move eyeball in various directions; intrinsic muscles (e.g., ciliary muscles) control size of pupil and shape of lens, accomplishing accommodation
4. Accessory structures (provide protection): eyebrows, eyelashes, lacrimal apparatus, and eyelids; lined with mucous membrane (conjunctiva) that continues over surface of eyeball; inner and outer canthi at junction of eyelids

5. Physiology of vision
a. Refraction, accommodation, and constriction of pupils are necessary to focus image on the retina
b. Binocular vision: visual fields of two eyes overlap; although each eye sees some areas of the environment that the other eye cannot, both eyes also see large areas in common; the human brain interprets these overlapping fields in terms of depth; optic chiasm is the site of the crossover of fibers of the optic nerves, permitting binocular vision
c. Stimulation of the retina: rods considered receptors for night vision; cones are receptors for daylight and color vision; macula lutea, center of the retina, receives and analyzes light only from the center of the visual field and contains the fovea centralis where cones are concentrated
d. Conduction to visual area in occipital lobe of cerebral cortex by fibers of cranial nerve II and optic tract

6. Errors of refraction
a. Myopia (nearsightedness): focuses rays anterior to the retina
b. Hyperopia (farsightedness): focuses rays posterior to the retina
c. Astigmatism: irregular curvature of the surface of the cornea that focuses rays unevenly on the retina

D. Hearing
1. External ear: consists of the auricle (or pinna), external acoustic meatus (ear opening), and external auditory canal
2. Middle ear: separated from the external ear by the tympanic membrane; middle ear contains auditory ossicles (malleus, incus, stapes) and openings from the eustachian tubes, mastoid cells, external ear, and internal ear
3. Inner ear (or labyrinth)
a. Vestibule contains maculae acusticae; vestibular nerve (branch of eighth cranial [acoustic or vestibulocochlear] nerve); provides information about equilibrium, position of the head, and acceleration and deceleration
b. Semicircular canals contain crista ampullaris, the sense organ for sensations of equilibrium and head movements
c. Cochlea contains membranous cochlear duct in which is located the organ of Corti, the hearing sense organ; cochlear nerve (branch of eighth cranial nerve) supplies organ of Corti
4. Physiology of hearing
a. Sound waves strike tympanic membrane, causing it to vibrate; the vibrations sequentially move the malleus, incus, and stapes
b. Movement of the stapes against the oval window starts a ripple in the perilymph, which is transmitted to the endolymph inside the cochlear duct; this stimulates the organ of Corti

c. Cochlear nerve conducts impulses from the organ of Corti to the brain; hearing occurs when impulses reach the auditory area in the temporal lobe of the cerebral cortex

Structures and Functions of the Muscular System

A. Purpose: movement, posture, and heat production
B. Types of muscles and neural control
   1. Striated: controlled by voluntary nervous system via somatic motoneurons in spinal and some cranial nerves
   2. Smooth: controlled by autonomic nervous system via autonomic motoneurons in autonomic, spinal, and some cranial nerves; not under voluntary control
   3. Cardiac: control is identical to that of smooth muscle
C. Bursa: synovial fluid–filled sac situated in places where friction occurs; facilitates movement of tendons over bone, relieving pressure between moving parts
D. Tendons: bands of fibrous tissue connecting muscle to bone
E. Ligaments: bands of fibrous tissue connecting bone to cartilage; support and strengthen joints

Skeletal Muscles

A. Anatomy
   1. Muscle fibers coated with fibrous connective tissue (fascia) that binds muscle to surrounding tissues
   2. Attach to at least two bones; bone that moves is called insertion bone, and that which remains stationary is called the origin bone
   3. Muscle fibers contain myofibrils specialized for contraction; composed of protein myofilaments, containing actin and myosin
B. Physiology of muscle contraction
   1. Basic principles of muscle contraction
      a. Contract only if stimulated; anything that prevents impulse conduction paralyzes the muscle
      b. Skeletal muscles almost always act in groups; classified as prime movers, synergists, or antagonists
      c. Contraction of a skeletal muscle either shortens the muscle (producing movement) or increases muscle tension (tone)
         (1) Tonic contractions: produce muscle tone; do not shorten the muscle to produce movements
         (2) Isometric contractions: increase the degree of muscle tone; do not shorten the muscle to produce movements; daily isometric contractions gradually increase muscle strength
         (3) Isotonic contractions: the muscle shortens, thereby producing movement
      d. Treppe (staircase phenomenon): when a muscle contracts a few times, subsequent contractions are more powerful
      e. Shivering: rapid, repetitive, involuntary muscle contractions caused by hypothalamic temperature regulating center; most of the energy of ATP is converted to heat but a small part goes to muscle contraction; consumes large amounts of O_2
   2. Energy of muscle contraction
      a. Electrical energy flows along transverse intracellular tubules associated with sarcoplasmic reticulum
      b. Calcium ions released by electrical energy inactivate troponin, which normally blocks the interaction between actin and myosin
      c. Myosin releases and uses energy from ATP to cause contraction
      d. Creatine phosphate replenishes the supply of ATP as needed; the source of energy is glucose and fatty acids oxidized aerobically to CO_2 and water
      e. Anaerobic breakdown of glucose during prolonged and vigorous muscle contraction results in lactic acid buildup associated with fatigue and an aching feeling; this O_2 debt is reversed during rest or increased O_2 saturation to reverse the anaerobic state
   3. Neuromuscular junction
      a. Axon terminal, containing synaptic vesicles, forms a junction with the sarcolemma of muscle fiber; tiny synaptic cleft separates the presynaptic membrane (axon) from postsynaptic membrane (sarcolemma)
      b. When a nerve impulse reaches the axon terminal, acetylcholine is released from synaptic vesicles into the synaptic cleft; when acetylcholine binds to receptor sites on the sarcolemma, a channel opens and sodium and potassium ions flow down their concentration gradients; the sarcolemma is depolarized, and electrical energy flows into the muscle fiber; cholinesterase inactivates acetylcholine to prevent static contraction
   4. Changes in muscle mass
      a. Hypertrophy is physical enlargement of a muscle resulting from an increase in cellular components. Muscle fibers do not divide to produce more fibers
      b. Atrophy is a wasting of a muscle resulting from a variety of factors (e.g., diminished cellular proliferation, death of cells, decreased activity, hormonal changes)
      c. Hyperplasia is a proliferation of normal cells, increasing the volume of the tissue

Structures and Functions of the Skeletal System

A. Purpose
   1. Provides supporting framework; protects viscera and brain
   2. Bones serve as levers and joints as fulcrums
   3. Hemopoiesis by red bone marrow: formation of all kinds of blood cells; some lymphocytes and monocytes are formed in lymphatic tissue
   4. Mineral storage: calcium, phosphorus, and sodium

B. Skeleton: contains 206 bones
C. Joint: junction of two or more bones
  1. Synarthrotic (fibrous): generally nonmovable; no joint cavity or capsule; bones held together by fibrous tissue (e.g., sutures)
  2. Amphiarthrotic (cartilaginous): slightly movable; no joint cavity or capsule; bones held together by cartilage and ligaments (e.g., symphysis pubis)
  3. Diarthrotic: freely movable; lined by a layer of hyaline cartilage covering the articular surfaces of the joining bones; held together by a fibrous capsule lined with synovial membrane and ligaments
    a. May be ball and socket (e.g., hip), hinge (e.g., elbow), condyloid (e.g., wrist), pivot, gliding, or saddle
    b. Movement depends on type of joint
      (1) Flexion: bending one bone on another, decreasing the angle between adjacent bones
      (2) Extension: stretching one bone away from another, increasing the angle between adjacent bones
      (3) Abduction: moving bone away from body's midline
      (4) Adduction: moving bone toward the body's midline
      (5) Rotation: pivoting bone on its axis
      (6) Internal rotation: turning of a limb toward the midline of the body
      (7) External rotation: turning of a limb away from the midline of the body
      (8) Circumduction: circular movement of a limb
      (9) Supination: forearm movement turning the palm forward or upward
      (10) Pronation: forearm movement turning the palm backward or downward
      (11) Inversion: ankle movement turning the sole of the foot inward
      (12) Eversion: ankle movement turning the sole of the foot outward
      (13) Protraction: moving a part, such as the lower jaw, forward
      (14) Retraction: pulling a part back; opposite of protraction
      (15) Plantar flexion: pointing toes downward away from the body
      (16) Dorsiflexion: pointing toes upward toward the body
D. Variations in skeletons
  1. Male skeleton larger and heavier than female skeleton
  2. Male pelvis deep and funnel shaped with narrow, pubic arch; female pelvis shallow, broad, and flaring with wider pubic arch
  3. From infancy to adulthood, bones grow and their relative sizes change due in part to stimulation of somatotrophic hormone (e.g., the torso becomes proportionately larger to the head, the pelvis relatively larger, and the legs proportionately longer)

  4. From young adulthood to old age, bone margins and projections change gradually; marginal lipping and spurs occur, thereby restricting movement
  5. Demineralization results in a reduction in the mass of bone per unit of volume (osteoporosis); mostly occurs in postmenopausal women; related to decreased hormone production, lack of exercise that stresses skeleton, and inadequate intake of calcium, magnesium, and vitamins A, C, and D

Bone Formation
A. Ossification process
  1. Types of bone: cancellous (spongy) and compact (dense)
  2. Formation of bone matrix (the intercellular substance of bone): made up of collagen fibers and a cementlike ground substance; the osteoblasts (bone-forming cells) synthesize collagen and cement substance from proteins provided by the diet; exercise and estrogens act to stimulate osteoblasts to form bone matrix
  3. Calcification of bone matrix: calcium salts deposit in the bone matrix
  4. Balance of osteoblastic (bone building) and osteoclastic (bone resorption) activity continuously turn over bone tissue; osteopenia and osteoporosis occur when osteoclastic activity is greater than osteoblastic activity
B. Nutrients required for growth, maintenance, and remodeling of bone
  1. Vitamin A: promotes chondrocyte function and synthesis of lysosomal enzymes for osteoclast activity
  2. Vitamin C: promotes synthesis of collagen and bone matrix
  3. Vitamin D: promotes calcium and phosphorus absorption
  4. Calcium: needed to form calcium phosphate and hydroxyapatite
  5. Magnesium: important enzyme activator in the mineralization process
  6. Phosphorus: needed to form calcium phosphate and hydroxyapatite
C. Repair of bone
  1. When bone is fractured, connective tissue called a callus grows into and around fracture
  2. Macrophages reabsorb damaged/dead cells
  3. Osteoclasts dissolve bone fragments
  4. Osteoblasts produce new bone substance and fuse bone together
  5. Final bone shape slowly remodeled; complete process takes several months; slower than epithelial tissue, which has a higher metabolic rate and richer blood supply

REVIEW OF PHYSICAL PRINCIPLES
A. Lever: rigid bar that moves about a fixed point known as the fulcrum; a small force is applied through a large

distance and the other end of the lever exerts a large force over a small distance; related to effective body mechanics

B. Pulleys: can multiply force at the expense of distance; used in traction

C. Center of gravity
1. Area of a body where the majority of weight is located; in a human the center of gravity is in the pelvic cavity; should be over the base of support for stability and balance
2. When bending over, the body's center of gravity shifts from a stable position between the legs to an unstable position outside the legs; keeping the legs apart widens the base of support

D. Buoyancy of water: reduces the energy to move muscles or objects against the force of gravity

E. Pascal's principle: when pressure is applied to a fluid in a closed, nonflexible container, it is transmitted undiminished throughout all parts of the fluid and acts in all directions (e.g., brain tumor and hydrocephalus); increasing pressure causes pain

F. Electromagnetic fields: use of a strong magnetic field (MRI) or high-energy electromagnetic radiation (x-ray, CT) to diagnose abnormalities

G. Sound
1. Mechanical vibration progresses better through solids and liquids than through gases (e.g., bowel sounds, breath sounds)
2. Ultrasonic vibrational frequencies exceeding the upper level of human hearing
   a. Low-intensity ultrasonic waves are used to treat arthritis and bursitis, to break kidney stones, and to help dissolve scars
   b. Sonograms are pictures of the body derived through differential reflection or transmission of sound waves
3. Hearing aids: electronic devices that amplify sounds and assist persons with impaired hearing to hear
   a. Air-conduction type sends an amplified sound wave into the ear, thus using the person's own middle ear
   b. Bone-conduction type bypasses the middle ear and transmits amplified vibrations to the skull bones, which in turn produce vibrations in the inner ear

REVIEW OF MICROORGANISMS

A. Bacterial pathogens
1. *Clostridium tetani:* large, gram-positive, motile bacillus forming large terminal spores; an obligate anaerobe; causes tetanus (lockjaw)
2. *Neisseria meningitidis:* gram-negative diplococcus; causes epidemic (meningococcic) meningitis
3. *Borrelia burgdorferi:* transmitted by tick bite; causes Lyme disease

B. DNA viruses: varicella (chickenpox), herpes zoster (shingles), infectious mononucleosis, and cytomegalic inclusion disease

C. RNA viruses: mostly borne by mosquitoes and ticks; cause eastern equine encephalomyelitis, western equine encephalomyelitis, and Venezuelan equine encephalomyelitis

D. Nematode: *Trichinella spiralis:* a small parasitic nematode; causes trichinosis

RELATED PHARMACOLOGY
Anticonvulsants (Antiseizure)

A. Description
1. Modify bioelectric activity at subcortical and cortical sites by stabilizing the nerve cell membrane and/or raising the seizure threshold to incoming stimuli
2. Decrease the occurrence, frequency, and/or severity of convulsive episodes
3. Available in oral and parenteral (IM, IV) preparations

B. Examples
1. Hydantoins used for tonic-clonic (formerly called grand mal) and psychomotor seizures: phenytoin (Dilantin), mephenytoin (Mesantoin), fosphenytoin (Cerebyx)
2. Barbiturates used for tonic-clonic and partial seizures: phenobarbital (Luminal), primidone (Mysoline), mephobarbital (Mebaral)
3. Benzodiazepines are both anticonvulsant and antianxiety agents; diazepam (Valium) and lorazepam (Ativan) are used for status epilepticus; clonazepam (Klonopin) is used for absence (formerly called petit mal) seizures
4. Succinimides are used for absence seizures: ethosuximide (Zarontin), methsuximide (Celontin), phensuximide (Milontin)
5. Gabapentin (Neurontin) is used for partial seizures; also used to control pain of herpes zoster (shingles) and other neurologic disorders
6. Carbamazepine (Tegretol) is used for tonic-clonic and psychomotor seizures; also used to control pain of trigeminal neuralgia and other neurologic disorders
7. Valproic acid (Depakene, Depakote) is used for absence seizures

C. Major side effects
1. Dizziness, drowsiness (CNS depression)
2. Nausea, vomiting (irritation of gastric mucosa)
3. Skin rash (hypersensitivity)
4. Blood dyscrasias (decreased RBCs, WBCs, platelet synthesis)
5. Hepatotoxicity
6. Phenytoin: ataxia (neurotoxicity); gingival hyperplasia (gum irritation leading to tissue overgrowth); hirsutism (virilism); hypotension (decreased atrial and ventricular conduction); reddish brown urine; therapeutic serum level is 10 to 20 mcg/mL

D. Nursing care
1. Administer with food to reduce GI irritation
2. Instruct client to
   a. Avoid alcohol and other CNS depressants
   b. Notify physician if fever, sore throat, or skin rash develops

c. Carry medical alert card

d. Report seizure activity, unusual bleeding, or loss of balance

e. Avoid abrupt discontinuation; dose must be tapered

3. Encourage diet rich in nutrient-dense foods such as fruits, vegetables, whole grains, and legumes to improve and maintain nutritional status and prevent possible drug-induced deficiencies of folic acid, calcium, and vitamin D

4. Instruct client to review other medications, supplements, and herbal remedies with physician and pharmacist because of drug interactions (e.g., phenytoin increases metabolism of oral contraceptives and anticoagulants; gingko may decrease phenytoin's effectiveness as an anticonvulsant)

5. Monitor therapeutic blood levels

6. Maintain client safety

7. Care for clients receiving phenytoin (Dilantin)

a. Avoid mixing with other IV infusions; incompatible with 5% dextrose

b. Provide oral hygiene; inspect oral mucosa for infection

c. Assess for initial potentiation of anticoagulant effect followed by inhibition

d. Assess urine; drug may discolor urine pink to red-brown

e. Assess for tissue necrosis because phenytoin is highly irritating to veins

Osmotic Diuretics

A. Description

1. Reduce cerebral edema and intraocular pressure by increasing the osmotic pressure within the vasculature, thus causing fluid to leave the tissues and be excreted in the urine

2. Available in parenteral (IV) preparations

B. Example: mannitol (Osmitrol)

C. Major side effects

1. Headache (dehydration)

2. Nausea (fluid and electrolyte imbalance)

3. Chills (fluid and electrolyte imbalance)

4. Rebound edema when discontinued (fluid and electrolyte imbalance)

5. Fluid/electrolyte imbalances (hyponatremia, hypokalemia resulting from promotion of sodium and potassium excretion)

D. Nursing care

1. Monitor I&O, daily weight, and levels of serum electrolytes

2. Question administration to clients with heart failure or impaired renal function

3. Elevate head of bed during therapy

4. Assess client for signs of increased intracranial pressure (decreasing pulse rate, widening pulse pressure, increasing systolic pressure, unequal pupils, change in level of consciousness, vomiting)

Calcium Enhancers

A. Description

1. Calcium ion replacement directly increases serum calcium concentration

2. Vitamin D replacement improves absorption of calcium from intestines

3. Bisphosphonates absorb calcium phosphate crystals in bone and may directly block dissolution of hydroxyapatite crystals of bone; inhibit resorption of bone by osteoclast

4. Parathyroid agents decrease bone resorption

5. Hormone replacement therapy (see Osteoporosis in Chapter 24 and Estrogens under Related Pharmacology in Chapter 23)

B. Examples

1. Calcium ion replacement: calcium carbonate (OsCal); calcium chloride; calcium gluconate

2. Vitamin D replacement: calcitriol (Rocaltrol) and cholecalciferol (Calciferol)

3. Bisphosphonates: alendronate (Fosamax), risedronate (Actonel), ibandronate (Boniva) (which is taken once a month), pamidronate (Aredia) (which is given intravenously)

4. Parathyroid agents: calcitonin (Miacalcin) nasal spray or injection, teriparatide (Forteo) subcutaneous injection

C. Major side effects

1. Nausea, vomiting, renal calculi, muscle flaccidity (hypercalcemia)

2. Constipation (increased serum calcium level delays passage of stool in GI tract)

3. Calcium preparations: cardiac disturbances (stimulation of cardiac conduction)

4. Vitamin D: dry mouth; metallic taste (early vitamin D toxicity associated with hypercalcemia)

5. Bisphosphonates: bone pain, headache, abdominal pain, nausea

6. Parathyroid agents: diarrhea, urinary frequency, headache, chest pressure, and dyspnea

D. Nursing care

1. Assess for signs of hypercalcemia and tetany

2. Monitor levels of serum electrolytes during course of therapy

3. Encourage increased fluid intake and acid-ash diet to reduce potential of renal calculi and constipation; stress vitamin D and calcium-rich foods such as eggs, cheese, whole-grain cereals, and cranberries; limit milk, fruits, and vegetables

4. Calcium preparations: assess for potentiation of digitalis effect

5. Oral bisphosphonates: instruct client to take on empty stomach with a full glass of water and to remain upright for 30 to 60 minutes; can cause esophageal ulcers

Antiparkinson Agents

A. Description

1. Anticholinergic drugs act at central sites to inhibit cerebral motor impulses and to block efferent impulses that cause rigidity of the musculature

2. Dopaminergic agents supply or cause the release of dopamine required for norepinephrine synthesis and maintenance of the neurohormonal balance at subcortical, cortical, and reticular sites that control motor function
3. Catechol *O*-methyltransferase (COMT) inhibitors deter enzymes involved in the breakdown of levodopa, thereby prolonging the duration of action of levodopa in the CNS
4. Monoamine oxidase B (MAO-B) inhibitor exerts a neuroprotective effect
5. Antiviral agent may cause release of dopamine from storage site

B. Examples
   1. Anticholinergic drugs: benztropine mesylate (Cogentin) and trihexyphenidyl HCl (Aparkane, Apo-Trihex)
   2. Dopaminergic agents: levodopa (Dopar, Larodopa), carbidopa-levodopa (Sinemet); bromocriptine (Parlodel), pergolide (Permax), ropinirole (Requip), pramipexole (Mirapex) are dopaminergic receptor agonists
   3. COMT inhibitors: entacapone (Comtan), tolcapone (Tasmar)
   4. MAO-B inhibitor: selegiline (Eldepryl)
   5. Antiviral agent: amantadine (Symmetrel)

C. Major side effects
   1. Anticholinergic drugs (decrease parasympathetic stimulation)
      a. Dry mouth (decreased salivation)
      b. Blurred vision (pupillary dilation)
      c. Constipation (decreased peristalsis)
      d. Urinary retention (decreased muscle tone)
   2. Other drugs
      a. Orthostatic hypotension (loss of compensatory vasoconstriction with position change)
      b. Ataxia, involuntary movements, blepharospasm (neurotoxicity)
      c. CNS disturbances and emotional disturbances including suicidal ideation (CNS effect)
      d. Nausea, vomiting (irritation of gastric mucosa)
      e. Bone marrow depression
      f. Neuroleptic malignant syndrome (muscle rigidity, fever, mental status changes, unstable BP) is associated with dopaminergics

D. Nursing care
   1. Instruct client to
      a. Avoid discontinuing drug suddenly
      b. Understand that treatment controls symptoms but is not a cure
      c. Continue health supervision
      d. Take COMT inhibitors in conjunction with dopaminergic agents or no benefit will be derived
   2. Offer emotional support; therapy is usually for life
   3. Encourage diet rich in nutrient-dense foods such as fruits, vegetables, whole grains, and legumes to improve and maintain nutritional status and prevent possible drug-induced nutrient deficiencies

4. Care for the client receiving anticholinergic drugs
   a. Offer sugar-free chewing gum and hard candy to increase salivation
   b. Explain that ability to perform potentially hazardous activities may be impaired
   c. Increase fluids, roughage, and activity to prevent constipation
   d. Monitor for urinary retention
5. Care for the client receiving levodopa
   a. Limit or eliminate vitamin B_6 from diet (e.g., pork, veal, lamb, potatoes, legumes, oatmeal, wheat germ)
   b. Inform client regarding dosage and "holiday" periods
   c. Instruct client and family to monitor for extrapyramidal effects (unsteady gait, involuntary movements)
   d. Instruct client and family to report muscle rigidity and fever, which may be signs of neuroleptic malignant syndrome
   e. Monitor CBC, BP
6. Care for the client receiving selegiline
   a. Inform families that selegiline may be started early in the course of the disease because neuroprotective actions are expected
   b. Use safety precautions because drug can cause orthostatic hypotension
   c. Avoid foods containing tyramine such as wine, cheese, and chocolate because this drug is an MAOI; ingestion of these foods can cause a severe hypertensive crisis

Cholinesterase Inhibitors

A. Description
   1. Prevent enzymatic breakdown of acetylcholine at nerve endings, thus allowing accumulation of the neurotransmitter
   2. Improve the strength of contraction in all muscles, including those involved with the process of respiration
   3. Used to diagnose and treat myasthenia gravis
   4. Available in oral and parenteral (IM, IV) preparations

B. Examples: edrophonium (Tensilon) (used for diagnostic purposes), neostigmine bromide (Prostigmin), pyridostigmine (Mestinon), ambenonium (Mytelase)

C. Major side effects
   1. Nausea, vomiting (irritation of gastric mucosa)
   2. Diarrhea (increased peristalsis)
   3. Hypersalivation (increased parasympathetic stimulation)
   4. Muscle cramps (increased skeletal muscle contraction)
   5. CNS disturbances (CNS effect)
   6. Acute toxicity (cholinergic crisis): profound muscle weakness, pulmonary edema, and respiratory failure (bronchial constriction); must be differentiated from myasthenic crisis with edrophonium test

D. Nursing care
 1. Administer medications on time exactly as prescribed; monitor client; dosage is adjusted according to needs
 2. Have atropine sulfate available for treatment of overdosage
 3. Administer with food to reduce GI irritation
 4. Instruct client to
  a. Carry a medical alert card
  b. Take medication before meals to improve chewing and swallowing
  c. Encourage diet rich in nutrient-dense foods such as fruits, vegetables, whole grains, and legumes to improve and maintain nutritional status and prevent possible drug-induced nutrient deficiencies
  d. Report respiratory distress immediately

Skeletal Muscle Relaxants
A. Description
 1. Central agents act by CNS depression to bring about relaxation of voluntary muscles
 2. Peripheral agents block nerve impulse conduction at the myoneural junction
 3. Relieve muscle spasms
 4. Available in oral and parenteral (IM, IV) preparations
B. Examples
 1. Carisoprodol (Soma)
 2. Cyclobenzaprine (Flexeril)
 3. Diazepam (Valium)
 4. Methocarbamol (Robaxin)
 5. Baclofen (Lioresal)
C. Major side effects
 1. Dizziness, drowsiness (CNS depression)
 2. Nausea (irritation of gastric mucosa)
 3. Headache (central antimuscarinic effect)
 4. Tachycardia (brainstem stimulation)
D. Nursing care
 1. Encourage diet rich in nutrient-dense foods such as fruits, vegetables, whole grains, and legumes to improve and maintain nutritional status and prevent possible drug-induced nutrient deficiencies
 2. Teach client receiving central agents to use safety precautions during initial therapy and to avoid engaging in potentially hazardous activities or using alcohol and other CNS depressants

Nonsteroidal Antiinflammatory Drugs (NSAIDs)
A. Description
 1. Interfere with prostaglandin synthesis
 2. Alleviate inflammation and subsequent discomfort of rheumatoid conditions
 3. Available in oral and parenteral (IM) preparations
B. Examples
 1. Diclofenac (Voltaren)
 2. Etodolac (Lodine)
 3. Ibuprofen (Motrin)
 4. Naproxen (Naprosyn)
 5. Salicylates (ASA)
 6. Ketorolac (Toradol)
 7. COX-2 inhibitors: newer NSAIDs with less GI irritation: celecoxib (Celebrex), nabumetone (Relafan)
C. Major side effects
 1. GI ulceration, tarry stools (melena)
 2. Skin rash (hypersensitivity)
 3. Blood dyscrasias (decreased RBCs, WBCs, platelet synthesis)
 4. CNS and genitourinary (GU) disturbances
 5. Increased liver enzymes
D. Nursing care
 1. Administer with meals to reduce GI irritation; instruct client to avoid other gastric irritants such as alcohol and smoking
 2. Monitor coagulation and liver profiles
 3. Assess vital signs; may increase BP
 4. Instruct client to report the occurrence of any side effects to the physician such as bleeding or hearing disturbance; aspirin toxicity causes tinnitus
 5. Encourage diet rich in nutrient-dense foods such as fruits, vegetables, whole grains, and legumes to improve and maintain nutritional status and prevent possible drug-induced nutrient deficiencies; restrict sodium intake because fluid retention may occur

Antigout Agents
A. Description
 1. Act by decreasing uric acid formation and increasing its excretion
 2. Prevent and arrest gout attacks that are caused by high levels of uric acid in the blood
 3. Available in oral and parenteral (IV) preparations
B. Examples
 1. Allopurinol (Zyloprim): blocks formation of uric acid within the body
 2. Colchicine: decreases uric acid crystal deposits by inhibiting lactic acid production by leukocytes; used for acute attacks
 3. Probenecid (Benemid): prevents formation of tophi by inhibiting the reabsorption of uric acid by the kidneys
C. Major side effects
 1. Nausea, vomiting, diarrhea (irritation of gastric mucosa)
 2. Blood dyscrasias (decreased RBCs, WBCs, and platelet synthesis)
 3. Liver damage (hepatotoxicity)
 4. Skin rash (hypersensitivity)
D. Nursing care
 1. Administer antiinflammatory drugs (prednisone, indomethacin (Indocin)) in addition to drugs that will lower serum uric acid level during the acute phase
 2. Increase fluids to discourage the formation of renal calculi
 3. Encourage weight reduction if overweight
 4. Monitor serum urate levels to determine effectiveness of treatment

5. Administer with meals to reduce GI irritation
6. Instruct client to avoid high-purine foods such as organ meats, anchovies, sardines, and shellfish; encourage diet rich in nutrient-dense foods such as fruits, vegetables, and whole grains, as well as milk, cheese, and eggs; teach the importance of preventing drug-induced nutrient deficiencies

Ophthalmic Agents

A. Description
   1. Produce a variety of actions (e.g., constriction, dilation, antiinflammatory, antiinfective)
   2. Diagnose and treat conditions affecting the eyes
   3. Available in a variety of topical preparations; drugs having a systemic action are available in oral and parenteral (IM, IV) preparations
B. Examples
   1. Miotics: constrict the pupil, pulling the iris away from the filtration angle and improving outflow of aqueous humor; used to treat chronic open-angle glaucoma
      a. Beta-blocker miotics: betaxolol (Betoptic), timolol (Timoptic)
      b. Anticholinesterase miotics: demecarium (Humorsol)
      c. Cholinergic miotics: carbachol (Isopto-carbachol)
   2. Mydriatics: dilate pupil (mydriasis) by causing contraction of the dilator muscle of the iris with minimal effect on the ciliary muscle, which lessens the effect on accommodation; include anticholinergics (which relax the ciliary muscle) and cycloplegic agents (which paralyze accommodation); used to facilitate eye examinations and surgery
      a. Atropine
      b. Tropicamide (Mydriacyl, Tropicacyl)
      c. Cyclopentolate (Cyclogyl)
      d. Dipivefrin (Propine)
   3. Carbonic anhydrase inhibitors: decrease production of aqueous humor to control intraocular pressure
      a. Acetazolamide (Diamox)
      b. Brinzolamide (Azopt)
      c. Dorzolamide (Trusopt)
   4. Osmotic agents: administered systemically to increase blood osmolality, which mobilizes fluid from the eye to reduce volume of intraocular fluid; used to decrease intraocular pressure in glaucoma and corneal edema
      a. Glycerin (glycerol, Osmoglyn, Ophthalgan)
      b. Mannitol (Osmitrol)
      c. Urea (Ureaphil)
      d. Isosorbide (Isomotic)
   5. Corticosteroids: administered topically to decrease the inflammatory response
      a. Dexamethasone (Decadron, AK-Dex)
      b. Prednisolone (Econopred, Inflamase)
C. Major side effects
   1. Miotics
      a. Twitching of eyelids and brow ache (increased cholinergic stimulation)
      b. Headache (vasodilation)
      c. Conjunctival pain (irritation of conjunctiva)
      d. Contact dermatitis (local irritation)
   2. Mydriatics (decreased parasympathetic stimulation)
      a. Dry mouth (decreased salivation)
      b. Flushing, fever, and ataxia (CNS effect)
      c. Blurred vision, photophobia (pupillary dilation)
      d. Skin rash (hypersensitivity)
      e. Tachycardia (decreased vagal stimulation)
   3. Carbonic anhydrase inhibitors
      a. Diuresis (increased excretion of sodium and water in renal tubule); metabolic acidosis
      b. Paresthesia (fluid/electrolytc imbalance)
      c. Bone marrow depression
      d. CNS disturbances (CNS effect)
   4. Osmotic agents
      a. Headache (cerebral dehydration)
      b. Nausea, vomiting (fluid/electrolyte imbalance)
   5. Corticosteroids
      a. Blurred vision
      b. Increased intraocular pressure
D. Nursing care
   1. Instruct client regarding proper method of application and need for medical supervision during therapy; emphasize need for handwashing before instilling drops and to apply pressure on the lacrimal duct during instillation to prevent systemic absorption
   2. Assess for occurrence of side effects and/or worsening of condition
   3. Encourage diet rich in nutrient-dense foods such as fruits, vegetables, whole grains, and legumes to improve and maintain nutritional status and prevent possible drug-induced nutrient deficiencies
   4. Provide care for the client receiving mydriatics: caution that vision will be blurred temporarily; advise that sunglasses will relieve photophobia; caution about engaging in hazardous activities

RELATED PROCEDURES

Computerized Tomography (CT)

A. Definition
   1. Cross-sectional visualization of the head or other body cavity determined by computer analysis of relative tissue density as an x-ray beam passes through the body
   2. Provides three-dimensional information about location and extent of tumors, infarcted areas, atrophy, and vascular lesions
   3. May be done with IV injection of contrast agent for enhanced visualization
B. Nursing care
   1. Explain procedure; inform the client that it will be necessary to lie still and that the equipment is complex but will cause no discomfort; infants and cognitively impaired or anxious clients may need to be sedated
   2. Obtain informed consent
   3. If contrast is planned, assess for allergy to iodine, a component of the contrast material

4. Withhold food for approximately 2 hours before contrast testing; dye may cause nausea in sensitive clients
5. Remove wigs, clips, and pins before CT of head
6. Encourage fluids after the procedure if contrast agent is used
7. Critically ill clients may need continuous monitoring and nursing care during the procedure

Magnetic Resonance Imaging (MRI)
A. Definition
   1. Uses magnetic fields and radio waves to produce cross-sectional images
   2. Produces accurate images of blood vessels, bone marrow, gray and white brain matter, spinal cord, globe of the eye, heart, abdominal structures, and breast tissue; can monitor blood velocity; particularly useful in diagnosis of multiple sclerosis
B. Nursing care
   1. Explain procedure; obtain informed consent
   2. Screen for claustrophobia; assess ability to withstand confining surroundings because client must remain in the tunnel-like machine for up to 90 minutes; sedation may be required; open MRI may be an option for clients who cannot tolerate closed spaces
   3. Instruct client to lie still, expect a series of intermittent thumping sounds, and communicate via a microphone located in the scanner
   4. Have client remove jewelry, clothing with metal fasteners, dentures, hearing aids, glasses, and any transdermal patches with foil layers before entering scanner
   5. Review history for contraindications: orthopedic hardware; pacemaker; artificial heart valves; or other implants that may be dislodged or malfunction as a result of the magnetic field; keep area free of metal objects; arrange for supplemental oxygen beforehand because oxygen tanks cannot enter the room

Lumbar Puncture
A. Definition: involves the introduction of a needle into the subarachnoid space below the spinal cord, usually between L3 and L4 or between L4 and L5
B. Purposes
   1. Withdrawal of CSF for diagnostic purposes or to reduce spinal pressure (usually is 70 to 200 cm H_2O)
   2. Measurement of spinal pressure (Queckenstedt's test involves compression of the jugular veins; pressure should rise; but if blockage exists, pressure will not rise)
   3. Injection of medication such as anesthetics
C. Nursing care
   1. Explain procedure; obtain informed consent
   2. Assist the client into a position that will enlarge opening between vertebrae
      a. Lying on side with feet drawn up and head lowered to chest; back near edge of mattress
      b. Sitting on side of bed, leaning on overbed table, feet supported on a flat surface

3. After procedure: maintain client in prone position for 2 hours; flat side-lying for 2 to 3 hours; and then avoid elevating the head for 6 more hours to prevent post–lumbar puncture headache
4. Label specimens and send to laboratory; note color and amount of fluid
5. Assess immediate response for signs of shock and complications such as CSF leakage, infection, and brain herniation if space-occupying lesion is present; prolonged headaches may indicate leakage of CSF
6. Administer fluids unless contraindicated

Positron Emission Tomography (PET)
A. Definition
   1. Client is given strong radioactive tracers that emit signals; computer analysis of the emitted gamma rays forms images
   2. Determines blood flow, glucose metabolism, and oxygen extraction
   3. Effective in diagnosis of brain attack, brain tumors, epilepsy; can evaluate progress of Alzheimer's disease, Parkinson's disease, bipolar disorders, and head injuries
B. Nursing care
   1. Explain procedure; obtain informed consent
   2. Maintain NPO 4 hours before test
   3. Explain that client must lie still for about 45 minutes; sedation may be needed

Neurologic Assessment (Including Glasgow Coma Scale)
A. Definition: systematic evaluation of the cranial nerves, motor and sensory functioning, and mental status to detect neurologic abnormalities
   1. Critical aspects of a complete neurologic assessment are generally extracted and compose a "neuro checklist," which is used when the nature of the situation does not warrant complete evaluation
   2. Glasgow Coma Scale (Table 11-3: Glasgow Coma Scale and Figure 11-3: Types of posturing)
B. Nursing care
   1. Cranial nerves (see Table 11-1 and Figure 11-2)
      a. Olfactory (I): ability to identify familiar odors such as mint or alcohol with eyes closed and one nostril occluded at a time
      b. Optic (II): visual acuity measured by use of Snellen chart or by gross estimation with reading material; gross comparison of visual fields with those of examiner; color perception
      c. Oculomotor (III), trochlear (IV), and abducent (VI): ability of the pupils to react equally to light and to accommodate to varying distances; range of extraocular movement (EOM) evaluated by asking the client to follow a finger or object with the eyes; also assess for nystagmus (jerking motion of eyes), particularly when eyes are directed laterally
      d. Trigeminal (V): sensations of the face evaluated by lightly stroking cotton across forehead, chin,

Table 11-3 Glasgow Coma Scale

Assessed Behavior	Adult Criteria	Infant and Young Child Criteria	Score*
Eye opening	Spontaneous opening	Spontaneous opening	4
	To verbal stimuli	To loud noise	3
	To pain	To pain	2
	No response	No response	1
Verbal response	Oriented to appropriate stimulation	Smiles, coos, cries	5
	Confused	Irritable, cries	4
	Inappropriate words	Inappropriate crying	3
	Incoherent	Grunts, moans	2
	None	No response	1
Motor response	Obeys commands	Spontaneous movement	6
	Localizes pain	Withdraws to touch	5
	Withdraws from pain	Withdraws to pain	4
	Flexion to pain (decorticate)	Abnormal flexion (decorticate)	3
	Extension to pain (decerebrate)	Abnormal extension (decerebrate)	2
	None	No response	1

Modified from Teasdale G, Jennett B: Assessment of coma and impaired consciousness: a practical scale, *Lancet* 2:81-84, 1974; James HE: Neurologic evaluation and support of the child with acute brain insult, *Pediatr Ann* 15:17, 1986.
*Add the numbers from each category. Maximum score = 15. Minimum score = 3.

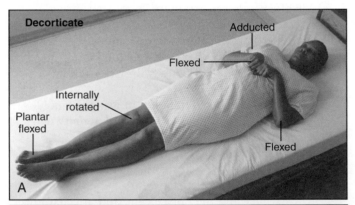

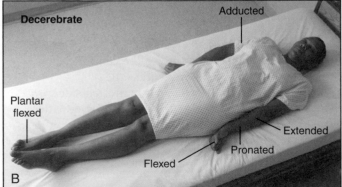

Figure 11-3 Types of posturing. **A,** Decorticate. **B,** Decerebrate. (From Monahan FD et al: *Phipps' medical-surgical nursing: health and illness perspectives,* ed 8, St Louis, 2007, Mosby.)

and cheeks while the client's eyes are closed; ability to clench the teeth (jaw closure)

e. Facial (VII): symmetry of the facial muscles as the client speaks or is asked to make faces

f. Acoustic or vestibulocochlear (VIII): hearing acuity determined by a watch tick or whispered numbers;

Weber's test may be performed by holding the stem of a vibrating tuning fork at midline of the skull (should be heard equally in both ears)

g. Glossopharyngeal (IX) and vagus (X): uvula should hang in midline; swallow and gag reflexes should be intact

h. Spinal accessory (XI): symmetric ability to turn the head or shrug the shoulders against counterforce of the examiner's hands

i. Hypoglossal (XII): ability to protrude the tongue without deviation, to left or right, and without tremors

2. Motor function (including cerebellar function)

a. Balance
   (1) Observation of gait
   (2) Romberg's test: positive if the client fails to maintain an upright position with feet together when the eyes are closed

b. Coordination: ability to touch the finger to the nose when arms are extended or to perform similar tasks smoothly

c. Muscle strength: evaluated by having the client move symmetrical muscle groups against opposition supplied by the examiner

3. Sensory function: bilateral testing of the response to light touch with cotton, sharp versus dull stimuli, vibration of a tuning fork

4. Mental status (cerebral functioning)

a. Level of consciousness: determined by the response to stimuli (verbal, tactile, or painful)

b. Orientation to person, place, and time: determined by general conversation and direct questioning

c. Judgment, memory, and ability to perform simple calculations

d. Appropriateness of behavior and mood

5. Reflexes
   a. Deep tendon reflexes (biceps, triceps, patellar, Achilles) with a reflex hammer; classification from 0 (absent) to 4+ (hyperactive); 2+ is expected
   b. Plantar: plantar flexion of the foot when the sole is stroked firmly with a hard object such as a tongue blade; abnormal adult response (dorsiflexion of the foot and fanning of the toes) is described as a positive Babinski's reflex and is indicative of corticospinal tract disease
   c. Oculocephalic (doll's eyes movements): when head of comatose client is turned to side, eyes should move in opposite direction; absence of reflex suggests brainstem injury; contraindicated with a neck injury
   d. Oculovestibular (caloric test): when warm or ice water is instilled into the ear of a comatose client, nystagmus occurs; eyes should deviate toward the stimulated ear if ice water is used and away with warm water; absence of reflex suggests brainstem damage; contraindicated if eardrum is perforated
6. Accurately record findings; report any deviations
7. Explain to and reassure the client and family when the examination must be repeated frequently
8. Coordinate other care with frequent neurologic assessments to promote rest between assessments

Continuous Passive Motion (CPM) Device
A. Definition: a machine that provides for passive range of motion, most commonly for the knee
B. Purposes
   1. Move joint without weight bearing or straining muscles after orthopedic surgery
   2. Stimulate regeneration of articular tissues or maintain/increase range of motion
C. Nursing care
   1. Align extremity in padded CPM device
   2. Set foot cradle at the angle ordered by the physician
   3. Adjust device according to length of client's extremity
   4. Set flexion, extension, and speed dials as ordered by the physician; these are generally increased gradually as tolerated to maximize mobility
   5. Demonstrate use of control cord to client
   6. Ensure pain control measures are implemented before procedure

Braces or Splints
A. Purposes
   1. Support and protect weakened muscles
   2. Prevent and correct anatomic deformities
   3. Aid in controlling involuntary muscle movements
   4. Immobilize and protect a diseased or injured joint
   5. Aid in ambulating with physical impairments
B. Nursing care
   1. Keep equipment in good repair (e.g., oil joints, replace straps when worn)
   2. Ensure adequate shoes (e.g., heels low and wide, high top to hold heel in shoe)

3. Examine skin daily for evidence of breakdown at pressure points
4. Check alignment of braces (e.g., leg brace: joints should coincide with body joints; back brace: upright bars in center of back, brace should grip pelvis and trochanter firmly, lacing should begin from bottom)
5. Coordinate the use of assistive devices appropriate for braces and splints with the physical therapist

Mobility: Assistive Devices
A. Purposes
   1. Improve or maintain stability of client with a lower limb disability to prevent injury
   2. Provide security while developing confidence in ambulating
   3. Relieve pressure on weight-bearing joints
   4. Assist in increasing speed of ambulation with less fatigue
   5. Provide for greater mobility and independence
B. Nursing care: use of a cane
   1. Ascertain ability to bear weight on the affected extremity
   2. Ensure ability to use the upper extremity opposite the affected lower extremity
   3. Measure to determine length of cane required: highest point should be approximately level with greater trochanter; hand piece should allow 30 degrees of flexion at elbow with wrist held in extension
   4. Explain the proper techniques in using a cane
      a. Hold in hand opposite affected extremity and close to body
      b. Advance cane and affected extremity simultaneously, and then unaffected leg
      c. When climbing, step up with unaffected extremity and then place cane and affected lower extremity on step; when descending, reverse procedure
   5. Walk on client's affected side
   6. Observe for incorrect use of the cane
      a. Leaning the body over the cane
      b. Shortening the stride on unaffected side
      c. Inability to develop the usual walking pattern
      d. Persistence of an abnormal gait pattern after cane is no longer needed
C. Nursing care: crutch walking
   1. Teach exercises to strengthen triceps, finger flexors, and wrist and elbow extensors
   2. Ensure proper fit of crutches
      a. Measure distance from anterior fold of axilla to 15 cm (6 inches) out from heel
      b. Axillary bars must be 5 cm (2 inches) below axillae and should be padded
      c. Hand bars should allow almost complete extension of arm with elbows flexed about 30 degrees when client places weight on hands
   3. Ensure that rubber crutch tips are in good condition

4. Assist in use of proper technique, depending on ability to bear weight and to take steps with either one or both of the lower extremities
   a. Four-point alternate crutch gait
      (1) Right crutch, left foot, left crutch, right foot; always three points of support on floor
      (2) Equal but partial weight bearing on each limb; slow, stable gait
      (3) Client must be able to bear weight on and manipulate both extremities, and get one foot ahead of the other
   b. Two-point alternate crutch gait
      (1) Right crutch and left foot simultaneously; always two points of support on floor
      (2) More rapid version of four-point gait and requires more balance and strength
   c. Three-point gait
      (1) Advance both crutches and the weaker lower extremity simultaneously, then the stronger lower extremity
      (2) Fairly rapid gait, but requires more balance and strength in the arms and the unaffected lower extremity
      (3) Used when one leg can support the whole body weight and the other cannot take full weight bearing
   d. Swing crutch gaits: used when client has bilateral paralysis of legs and hips
      (1) Swing-to gait: place both crutches forward, lift and swing body up to crutches, then place crutches in front of body and continue; always two points of support on floor; needs power in upper arms
      (2) Swing-through gait: place both crutches forward, lift and swing body through crutches, then place crutches in front of body and continue; a difficult gait that necessitates rolling pelvis forward and arching back to get center of gravity in front of hips; needs power in trunk and upper extremities, excellent balance, and self-confidence
   e. Ascending stairs: transfer weight to crutches and move unaffected leg up to next step; transfer weight to unaffected leg; bring crutches and affected leg up to the step
   f. Descending stairs: transfer weight to unaffected leg; move crutches and affected leg down a step; transfer weight to crutches; bring unaffected leg down to the step
5. Observe for incorrect use of crutches
   a. Hiking hips with abduction gait (common in amputees)
   b. Lifting crutches while still bearing down on them
   c. Walking on ball of foot with foot turned outward and flexion at hip or knee level
   d. Hunching shoulders (crutches usually too long) or stooping shoulders (crutches usually too short)

   e. Looking downward while ambulating
   f. Bearing weight under arms should be avoided to prevent injury to the nerves in the brachial plexus; damage to these nerves can cause paralysis and is known as crutch palsy
D. Nursing care: use of a walker
   1. Assist in selecting a walker
      a. Device should be used when the client is not able to ambulate with a cane; partial weight bearing required
      b. Measurements are same as those for a cane
      c. Requires strong elbow extensors and shoulder depressors and partial strength in hands and wrist muscles to lift a standard walker; two- and four-wheeled walkers available
      d. Device cannot be used on steps
   2. Assist in ambulating with the walker
      a. Lift device off floor and place forward a short distance, then advance between walker
      b. Two-wheeled walkers: raise back legs of the device off the floor, roll walker forward, then advance to it
      c. Four-wheeled walkers: push device forward on floor and then walk to it
   3. Observe for incorrect use of the walker
      a. Keeping arms rigid and swinging through to counterbalance position of lower extremity
      b. Tending to lean forward with abnormal flexion at hips
      c. Tending to step forward with unaffected leg and shuffle affected leg up to walker

Mobility: Wheelchair

A. Purpose
   1. Support and move a client on a special chair that has wheels; the client is propelled or propels self
   2. Provide mobility for those who cannot ambulate or those who can ambulate but whose ambulation is unsteady, unsafe, or too strenuous
   3. Decrease oxygen demands and cardiac workload
   4. Promote independence and stimulate activities
B. Nursing care
   1. Instruct the client that prolonged sitting in one position can cause flexion contractures of the hips and knees and ischial pressure ulcers (encourage the client to change body positions and to use padded cushions and exercises such as push-ups every hour to relieve pressure)
   2. Ensure that device is in operating condition (e.g., wheel brakes, arm locks, seat belts, swing foot rests); inform client about accessories (e.g., removable arms, lap boards, extra-long leg panels, battery or motor propulsion)
   3. Assist client with transfer; keep wheelchair in close proximity to bed or chair when transferring; position wheelchair on the unaffected side if client has unilateral weakness (except clients on total hip precautions who often transfer toward the affected side to avoid adduction)

Instillation of Eye Medications

A. Purpose: to provide therapeutic effect of medication ordered
B. Nursing care
   1. Position the client with the head slightly backward
   2. Pull lower eyelid down and instill solution in center of conjunctival sac; ointment applied from inner canthus outward
   3. Have client close the eyes gently and instruct that they should not be rubbed
   4. Apply pressure to the nasolacrimal duct if liquid instillation to reduce systemic effects

Irrigations of the Ear

A. Definition
   1. Introduction of fluid into the external auditory canal
   2. Usually done for cleansing but can be used to apply antiseptic solutions
B. Nursing care
   1. Verify if tympanic membrane is intact
   2. Assist the client to a sitting position with the head tilted to affected side for an irrigation to facilitate drainage; for instillations, the client should lie on the unaffected side
   3. Straighten canal to promote flow of fluid: gently pull on the external ear up and back for an adult and pull down and back for a child less than 3 years of age
   4. Direct solution into the canal without exerting excessive force; collect returns in a basin
   5. Dry the outer ear
   6. Record the procedure, type of drainage, etc.

MAJOR DISORDERS OF THE NEUROMUSCULOSKELETAL SYSTEM

❋ TRAUMATIC BRAIN INJURIES

Data Base

A. Etiology and pathophysiology
   1. Motor vehicle accidents are the most common cause; can result from assaults, falls, and sport-related accidents
   2. Caused by a sudden force to the head
      a. Acceleration injury: immobile head struck by moving object
      b. Deceleration injury: head hits stationary object
      c. Deformation injury: force disrupts the integrity of the skull
   3. Fractures
      a. Linear: simple break in the bone
      b. Depressed: break that results in fragments of bone penetrating brain tissue
      c. Basilar: occurs over the base of frontal and temporal lobes; ecchymosis is common over areas involved
   4. Hemorrhages (secondary brain injury)
      a. Epidural: hematoma forms between the dura and the skull; may result from a laceration of the middle meningeal artery

      b. Subdural: hematoma forms between the dura and arachnoid layers; generally follows venous damage
      c. Intracerebral hematoma
   5. Concussion: temporary disruption of synaptic activity; brief loss of consciousness (less than 5 minutes)
   6. Contusions: bruising of brain tissue, with slight bleeding of small cerebral vessels into surrounding tissues at site of impact (coup) or opposite to site (contrecoup) as a result of rebound reaction
      a. Cerebral contusions manifest depending on areas involved
      b. Brainstem contusions result in unresponsiveness
   7. Complications include cerebral edema, increased intracranial pressure, brain abscess, meningitis, diabetes insipidus, hydrocephalus (from blocked absorption of CSF), death
B. Clinical findings
   1. Subjective: lethargy; indifference to surroundings; altered sensory function (e.g., visual or auditory)
   2. Objective
      a. Signs of increased intracranial pressure (see Brain Tumors)
      b. Lack of orientation to time and place
      c. Positive Babinski's reflex
      d. Seepage of CSF from nose or ears; usually indicative of basilar skull fracture
C. Therapeutic interventions
   1. Control seizures with anticonvulsants
   2. Mechanical ventilation; hyperventilation constricts cerebral vessels, lowering intracranial pressure
   3. Monitor intracranial pressure with external catheter such as ventricular catheter or subarachnoid screw
   4. Reduce cerebral edema with glucocorticoids and loop diuretics; there is disagreement regarding their efficacy
   5. Maintain adequate fluid and electrolyte balance
   6. Surgical intervention in cases of depressed skull fractures or hematomas

Nursing Care of Clients With Traumatic Brain Injuries

A. Assessment/Analysis
   1. Airway and breathing pattern
   2. Neurologic status (see Neurologic Assessment [Including Glasgow Coma Scale] under Related Procedures)
   3. Signs of increased intracranial pressure (see Brain Tumors)
   4. Circumstances of injury
   5. Presence of glucose in clear drainage from nose or ears, which indicates CSF
B. Planning/Implementation
   1. Institute neurologic assessments including Glasgow Coma Scale every 15 minutes for several hours, progressing to every hour and then every 4 hours as client's condition stabilizes
   2. Maintain airway by suctioning as necessary (coughing increases intracranial pressure); use an airway or endotracheal tube

3. Keep client's head elevated 30 degrees to reduce venous pressure within cranial cavity; maintain straight alignment of head and neck
4. Administer glucocorticoids and/or diuretics if ordered
5. Institute seizure precautions; administer anticonvulsants if ordered; protect from injury
6. Monitor for fluid or electrolyte imbalances; diabetes insipidus or syndrome of inappropriate antidiuretic hormone may occur
7. If the client's eyes remain open, protect the corneas with artificial tears, or ointment as ordered
8. Support client's nutritional needs; administer tube feedings or assist with small, frequent meals
9. Position the client to prevent pressure ulcers
10. Provide range-of-motion exercises and splints to prevent contractures
11. Provide auditory and tactile stimulation
12. Assist client to avoid activities that increase intracranial pressure such as the Valsalva maneuver, lifting, sneezing, and neck flexion; administer stool softeners
13. Recognize that confusion after return of consciousness may be a defense against stress or indication of a neurologic deficit
14. Utilize hypothermia as ordered to reduce temperature and metabolic demands
15. Encourage client and family to participate in planning and care
16. Provide opportunity for expression of feelings

C. Evaluation/Outcomes
1. Maintains a patent airway
2. Improves level of consciousness
3. Remains free from complications of immobility
4. Participates in decisions about administration of care

✿ BRAIN TUMORS

Data Base

A. Etiology and pathophysiology
1. Either benign or malignant; intervention required, because of the rise in intracranial pressure since the skull cannot accommodate the increasing size of the tumor
2. Classified according to tissue of origin
   a. Meningioma: occurs outside brain from covering meninges; usually benign
   b. Acoustic neuroma: tumor of the eighth cranial nerve
   c. Gliomas: most common; originate in neural tissue; usually malignant and include astrocytoma, glioblastoma, oligodendroglioma
   d. Angiomas: occur from within blood vessels
   e. Metastatic tumors: originate elsewhere in the body, most commonly the lung, breast, kidney, and site of malignant melanoma

B. Clinical findings
1. Subjective: headache that increases when supine or stooping; lethargy; nausea

2. Objective: signs of increased intracranial pressure; abnormal CT scan, MRI, EEG; vomiting; papilledema
3. Symptoms may vary depending on location
   a. Frontal lobe: personality changes, focal seizures, blurred vision, hemiparesis, altered thought processes
   b. Temporal lobe: seizures, headache, papilledema, receptive aphasia, tinnitus
   c. Parietal lobe: visual loss, motor and sensory focal seizures
   d. Occipital region: focal seizures, visual hallucinations, homonymous hemianopsia
   e. Cerebellar region: loss of coordination, tremors, nystagmus

C. Therapeutic interventions
1. Radiation therapy and/or chemotherapy
2. Brachytherapy: radioactive source is implanted surgically
3. Surgery for partial or complete removal of the lesion
   a. Craniotomy with removal of lesion and invaded tissue
   b. Stereotactic radiosurgery; employs computer-directed radiation to eradicate tissue
4. Steroids, anticonvulsives, osmotic diuretics, and antiemetics to control symptoms

Nursing Care of Clients With Brain Tumors

A. Assessment/Analysis
1. History from client and family to identify behavioral changes, coping skills, and neurologic deficits
2. Neurologic status (see Neurologic Assessment [Including Glasgow Coma Scale] under Related Procedures)
3. Signs of increased intracranial pressure
   a. Decreased level of consciousness
   b. Unilateral nonreactive and/or dilated pupil progressing to bilateral
   c. Rapid rise in body temperature; decreased pulse rate; changes in respiratory pattern
   d. Increased systolic pressure; widening pulse pressure
   e. Restlessness
   f. Headache most common in the morning after the body has been horizontal for several hours; intensified by coughing, sneezing, or straining, which increase intracranial pressure
   g. Weakness or paralysis
   h. Visual and other sensory disturbances; papilledema
   i. Vomiting
   j. Seizures
4. Nutritional status

B. Planning/Implementation
1. Monitor neurologic status
2. Provide emotional support for client and family; refer to support groups and hospice if indicated

3. Administer corticosteroids and antiemetics as ordered
4. Provide small, frequent feedings, supplements, and oral hygiene
5. Provide care for the client requiring brain surgery
   a. Obtain consent for surgery and removal of hair
   b. After surgery keep the client's head elevated 30 degrees
   c. Support respiratory function by encouraging deep breathing, appropriate positioning, and suctioning to maintain the airway
   d. Use strict aseptic technique with intracranial pressure monitoring
   e. Observe dressings for CSF leakage or hemorrhage
   f. Monitor intake and output
   g. Use hypothermia as ordered if the client is febrile; fever increases metabolic needs of the brain
6. Help focus on abilities rather than disabilities
7. Emphasize need for continued health care
C. Evaluation/Outcomes
1. Maintains adequate respiratory function
2. Performs ADLs with assistance
3. Establishes effective communication

BRAIN ATTACK/CEREBRAL VASCULAR ACCIDENT (CVA)

Data Base
A. Etiology and pathophysiology
1. Destruction (infarction) of brain cells caused by effects of a reduction in O_2 supply
   a. Ischemic attack results when brain tissues are blocked from O_2 supply by thrombus or embolus; 83% of attacks are this type
   b. Hemorrhagic attack results from bleeding into brain tissue or subarachnoid space
2. Effects depend on the area of the brain involved and extent of damage; may be masked or delayed because of compensatory collateral circulation through the circle of Willis
3. Risk factors include hypertension, hyperlipidemia, obesity, smoking, cerebral arteriosclerosis, cerebral aneurysm, atrial fibrillation, diabetes mellitus, advanced age, African-American ancestry
4. Transient ischemic attacks (TIAs) may also occur without causing permanent damage; these last a few minutes to 24 hours; highly predictive of impending brain attack
B. Clinical findings
1. Subjective: syncope; headache; changes in level of consciousness; unilateral paresthesias; mood swings
2. Objective
   a. Hemiparesis (weakness on one side of the body) or hemiplegia (paralysis on one side of the body) on side opposite the lesion (initially flaccid, then spastic)

b. Aphasia: brain unable to fulfill its communicative functions because of damage to input, integrative, or output centers
   (1) Expressive (motor or Broca's) aphasia: difficulty making thoughts known to others; speaking and writing are most affected
   (2) Receptive (sensory or Wernicke's) aphasia: difficulty understanding what others are trying to communicate; interpretation of speech and reading is most affected
   (3) Global aphasia: affects both expression and reception
   (4) Dysarthria: difficulty speaking because of paralysis of muscles needed for articulation
c. Dysphagia: difficulty swallowing
d. Visual changes
   (1) Homonymous hemianopsia: loss of vision in half of the same visual field in both eyes
   (2) Agnosia: disturbance in ability to recognize objects and attach meaning to them
   (3) Ptosis and paralysis of ocular muscles (Horner's syndrome)
e. Alterations in reflexes
f. Altered bladder and bowel function (e.g., incontinence, retention)
g. CSF is bloody if cerebral or subarachnoid hemorrhage is present
h. Abnormal EEG, CT scan, MRI
i. Cerebral angiography may reveal vascular abnormalities such as aneurysms, narrowing, or occlusions
j. Signs of increased intracranial pressure (see Brain Tumors)
C. Therapeutic interventions
1. Modify risk factors for prevention (e.g., weight loss, antiplatelet therapy for atrial fibrillation, low-fat diet and statins for hyperlipidemia, smoking cessation)
2. Complete bed rest with sedation as needed if brain attack occurs
3. Maintenance of oxygenation by O_2 therapy or mechanical ventilation
4. If ischemic type, thrombolytic therapy with recombinant tissue plasminogen activator (t-PA) within 3 hours of onset
5. Maintenance of nutrition by the parenteral route or nasogastric feedings if the client is unable to swallow
6. Anticoagulant therapy if thrombus or embolus is present; antiplatelet therapy
7. Antihypertensives and anticonvulsants if indicated
8. Antiinflammatory or osmotic diuretics may be used to reduce cerebral edema and intracranial pressure
9. Surgical intervention
   a. Carotid endarterectomy or stent placement (may be done prophylactically) to improve cerebral blood flow when carotid arteries are narrowed by arteriosclerotic plaques
   b. Performed to relieve pressure and control bleeding if hemorrhage is present

Nursing Care of Clients With Brain Attacks

A. Assessment/Analysis
   1. Adequacy of airway and respiratory function
   2. Neurologic status (see Neurologic Assessment [Including Glasgow Coma Scale] under Related Procedures)
   3. Presence of signs of increased intracranial pressure (see Brain Tumors)

B. Planning/Implementation
   1. Perform neurologic assessments; note signs of increased intracranial pressure
   2. Monitor vital signs; avoid using affected extremity for BP measurement because reading may be falsely lowered
   3. Maintain patency of the airway by positioning, suctioning, and inserting an artificial airway
   4. Place client in low semi-Fowler's position to decrease intracranial pressure; turn to side to drain oral secretions and prevent aspiration; provide O_2 as necessary
   5. Encourage deep breathing; use mechanical ventilation if ordered
   6. Involve all health care team members to plan care
   7. Assist client and family to set realistic goals; provide encouragement
   8. Accept and explore feelings of fear, anger, and depression; accept mood swings
   9. Provide frequent oral hygiene; use artificial tears if blink reflex is absent
   10. Institute seizure precautions
   11. Provide elastic or pneumatic stockings
   12. Prevent pressure ulcers (see Pressure Ulcers in Chapter 10)
   13. Prevent contractures: prevent muscle atrophy and contractures
       a. Provide passive range-of-motion exercises; active range-of-motion and other exercises may be instituted later
       b. Maintain functional alignment: use devices to prevent footdrop, flexion of fingers, external rotation of hips, adduction of shoulders and arms; turn every 1 to 2 hours; raise side rails for safety and to facilitate self-turning
       c. Collaborate with physical therapist about rehabilitation plan
   14. Provide tube feedings if swallowing and gag reflexes are depressed or absent
   15. Provide food in a suitable form based on the degree of dysphagia (mechanical soft, pureed, thickening products); encourage intake of nutrient-dense foods; when client is capable of chewing, introduce dietary fiber to promote bowel function
   16. Assist with feeding (e.g., use a padded spoon handle; feed on the unaffected side of mouth; feed in as close to a sitting position as possible); allow sufficient time for adequate chewing and swallowing
   17. Encourage the client with dysarthria or aphasia to communicate
       a. Be aware of own reactions to the speech difficulty
       b. Evaluate extent of the client's ability to understand and express self
       c. Reinforce exercises learned in speech therapy; provide positive feedback
       d. Convey that there is a problem with communication, not with intelligence; try to reduce anxiety related to communication
       e. Avoid pushing to point of frustration
       f. Minimize distractions that interfere with message reception and interpretation
       g. Face client directly when communicating; speak slowly, clearly, and in short sentences; do not raise your voice; connect words with objects
       h. Use alternative means of communication; develop a system of cues
       i. Involve the client in social interactions
       j. Be alert for clues and gestures when speech is garbled
   18. Make a definite transition between tasks to prevent or reduce confusion
   19. Attempt to prevent fecal impaction and/or urinary tract problems
       a. Assess for signs of urinary retention: abdominal distention, frequency
       b. Provide adequate fluid intake
       c. Provide a diet with enough roughage of sufficient quantity for bowel content and proper consistency for evacuation (a full rectum puts pressure on the bladder, which promotes urinary incontinence); avoid straining at stool because it can raise intracranial; administer stool softeners as ordered
       d. Avoid preoccupation with elimination; avoid encouragement of incontinence
       e. Stimulate elimination by exercise
       f. Help develop regular bowel and bladder patterns
       g. Respect the individual; provide for privacy and individuality of routine
       h. Utilize physical and psychologic techniques to stimulate elimination
   20. Create environment that keeps sensory monotony to a minimum; orient to time and place; increase social contacts; provide visual stimuli
   21. Promote self-esteem; encourage wearing own clothes, self-care activities, decision making
   22. Instruct client to report further neurologic deficits immediately so treatment can be initiated to prevent a brain attack

C. Evaluation/Outcomes
   1. Maintains respiratory function
   2. Remains alert and oriented
   3. Communicates effectively
   4. Remains free of complications of immobility
   5. Family and client participate in decisions and care

✤ EPILEPSY (SEIZURE DISORDERS)

Data Base

A. Etiology and pathophysiology
1. Abnormal discharge of electric impulses by nerve cells in brain from idiopathic or secondary causes, resulting in loss of consciousness; seizures; motor, sensory, behavioral changes
2. Onset of idiopathic epilepsy generally before age 30; seizures can be associated with brain tumor, brain attack, Alzheimer's disease, hypoglycemia, head trauma, fluid shifts in the brain
3. Types of seizures
   a. Partial seizures (seizures beginning locally)
      (1) Simple: focal motor or sensory effect; no loss of consciousness
      (2) Complex: cognitive, psychosensory, psychomotor, or affective effect; brief loss of consciousness
   b. Generalized seizures (bilaterally symmetric and without local onset)
      (1) Absence (petit mal): brief transient loss of consciousness with or without minor motor movements of eyes, head, or extremities; most common in childhood and adolescence
      (2) Myoclonic: brief, transient rigidity or jerking of extremities, singly or in groups
      (3) Tonic-clonic (grand mal): aura, loss of consciousness, rigidity followed by tonic-clonic movements, interruption of respirations, loss of bladder and bowel control; may last 2 to 5 minutes
      (4) Atonic: loss of muscle control; loss of consciousness may be brief
   c. Status epilepticus: prolonged repetitive seizures without recovery between attacks; may result in complete exhaustion, cerebral injury, or death
B. Clinical findings (tonic-clonic seizures)
1. Subjective: seizure often preceded by an aura or warning sensation such as seeing spots or feeling dizzy; lethargy following return to consciousness (postictal phase)
2. Objective
   a. Shrill cry as seizure begins and air is forcefully exhaled
   b. Loss of consciousness during seizure
   c. Tonic-clonic movement of the muscles
   d. Incontinence
   e. Abnormal EEG
C. Therapeutic interventions
1. Anticonvulsant therapy usually continued throughout life; diazepam (Valium) or lorazepam (Ativan) given IV to treat status epilepticus (see Antianxiety/Anxiolytic Medications under Related Pharmacology—Psychotropic Medications in Chapter 16)
2. Sedatives used to reduce emotional stress
3. Neurosurgery is sometimes indicated if seizures are caused by tumors or vascular problems

Nursing Care of Clients With Epilepsy

A. Assessment/Analysis
1. History of type, frequency, and duration of seizures; precipitating factors
2. Sensations associated with the seizure that may constitute an aura
B. Planning/Implementation
1. Provide protection from injury during and after the seizure; nothing should be forced into the mouth because this may cause tongue to occlude airway; position on side if possible to facilitate drainage of oral secretions
2. Help the client with an aura to plan for self-protection before seizure develops
3. Encourage use of a medical alert tag
4. Help plan a schedule that provides adequate rest and reduction of stress
5. Teach the client and family to determine the presence of an aura and monitor the initial point of seizure, type of seizure, level of consciousness, progression of seizure, incontinence, and postictal condition
6. Encourage expression of feelings about illness and necessary changes in lifestyle
7. Assist client and family to accept the diagnosis and develop understanding of the disease
8. Refer for job counseling as necessary
9. Encourage client and family to attend local epilepsy association meetings
10. Refer client to state laws regarding driving
11. Teach about anticonvulsants (see Anticonvulsants [Antiseizure] under Related Pharmacology) and need for continued medical supervision
C. Evaluation/Outcomes
1. Remains free from injury
2. Verbalizes willingness to follow lifelong medication regimen

✤ BELL'S PALSY (FACIAL PARALYSIS)

Data Base

A. Etiology and pathophysiology
1. Paralysis that occurs on one side of the face as a result of an inflamed seventh cranial (facial) nerve; generally lasts only 2 to 8 weeks but may last longer in older clients
2. Cause unknown; possibly viral, ischemic, or autoimmune link
3. Most common between ages 20 and 50 years
B. Clinical findings
1. Subjective: facial pain; altered taste; impaired ability to chew and swallow
2. Objective: distortion of face; drooping of mouth on affected side; difficulty with articulation; diminished blink reflex; upward movement of eyeball when closing eye; increased lacrimation
C. Therapeutic interventions
1. Diagnostic evaluation to rule out (eliminate) brain attack as the cause
2. Prednisone therapy

3. Heat, massage, and electric stimulation to maintain circulation and muscle tone
4. Prevention of corneal irritation with eye drops and use of protective eye shield

Nursing Care of Clients With Bell's Palsy
A. Assessment/Analysis
1. Presence or absence of blink reflex and ability to close the eye
2. Facial pain; extent of facial paralysis and altered sensation
3. Nutritional intake; ability to chew and swallow
B. Planning/Implementation
1. Teach prevention of corneal irritation by using artificial tears, manually closing the eye, and applying an eye shield; use of wrap around sunglasses
2. Teach importance of keeping face warm
3. Teach gentle massage of face; simple exercises such as blowing when acute phase is over
4. Encourage ventilation of feelings
5. Support nutritional status by providing privacy and small, frequent feedings; encourage favoring the unaffected side while eating
C. Evaluation/Outcomes
1. Maintains corneal integrity
2. Expresses a positive body image
3. States pain is reduced

TRIGEMINAL NEURALGIA (TIC DOULOUREUX)
Data Base
A. Etiology and pathophysiology
1. Disorder of the fifth cranial (trigeminal) nerve characterized by intense knifelike pain along the branches of the nerve
2. May result from abnormalities of ganglion, tumors, vascular anomalies, or dental infection
3. Incidence higher in clients with multiple sclerosis, particularly men
B. Clinical findings
1. Subjective: unilateral burning or knifelike pain lasting 1 to 15 minutes, usually in lip, chin, or teeth; pain precipitated by brushing hair, eating, cold drafts; exhaustion from prolonged pain
2. Objective: sudden closure of an eye; twitching of mouth and cheek
C. Therapeutic interventions
1. Anticonvulsants such as carbamazepine (Tegretol) to relieve and prevent acute attacks
2. Skeletal muscle relaxants such as baclofen (Lioresal) may help control symptoms
3. Surgical intervention
a. Microscopic relocation of arterial loop that may cause vascular compression of trigeminal nerve; preserves facial sensation, but pain relief lasts about 2 years

b. Percutaneous radio frequency trigeminal gangliolysis: destroys nerve, providing permanent relief for most clients; alters facial sensation and corneal reflex

Nursing Care of Clients With Trigeminal Neuralgia
A. Assessment/Analysis
1. Description of pain and factors that precipitate attacks
2. Effect on activities (e.g., eating, shaving, washing the face, brushing the teeth) because of fear of precipitating an attack
B. Planning/Implementation
1. Teach factors to limit triggering an attack, which can result in exhaustion
a. Avoid foods that are too cold or too hot
b. Chew soft foods on unaffected side
c. Use cotton pads to gently wash face and for oral hygiene
d. Keep the room free of drafts; avoid jarring
e. Instruct client to use scarves and hats to protect face from cold temperatures
2. Provide teaching to clients who have sensory loss as a result of treatment
a. Inspection of the eye for irritation and foreign bodies
b. Warm normal saline irrigation of the affected eye two or three times a day is helpful in preventing a corneal infection
c. Dental checkups every 6 months, because caries will not produce pain
3. Teach about anticonvulsants (see Anticonvulsants [Antiseizure] under Related Pharmacology) and the need for continued medical supervision
C. Evaluation/Outcomes
1. Reports decreased severity of pain and number of attacks
2. Consumes nutritionally balanced diet
3. Develops mechanisms to cope with fear

PARKINSON'S DISEASE (PARALYSIS AGITANS)
Data Base
A. Etiology and pathophysiology
1. Progressive disorder in which there is a destruction of nerve cells in the basal ganglia and substantia nigra of the brain, which results in dopamine deficiency and subsequent generalized degeneration of muscular function
2. Risk factors: advanced age; family history
B. Clinical findings (Figure 11-4: Parkinson's disease: clinical findings)
1. Subjective: fatigue; mild, diffuse, muscular pain; stiffness and rigidity, particularly of large joints; depression
2. Objective
a. Diminished voluntary motion: increased difficulty in performing usual activities, such as

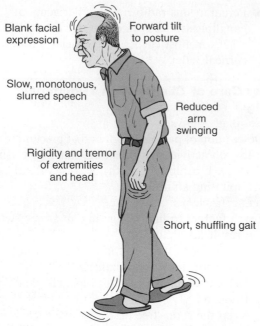

Blank facial expression

Forward tilt to posture

Slow, monotonous, slurred speech

Reduced arm swinging

Rigidity and tremor of extremities and head

Short, shuffling gait

Figure 11-4 Parkinson's disease: clinical findings. (Modified from Lewis SL et al: *Medical-surgical nursing: assessment and management of clinical problems*, ed 7, St Louis, 2007, Mosby.)

writing, dressing, eating, swallowing, and walking (e.g., reduced arm swing, bent posture, difficulty rising from a sitting position, shuffling propulsive gait)

(1) Bradykinesia: slowness of voluntary movement
(2) Hypokinesia: decreased movement
(3) Akinesia: inability to move

b. Generalized tremor commonly accompanied by "pill-rolling" movements of the thumb against the fingers; non-intention tremors usually reduced by purposeful movements
c. Masklike facial expression, unblinking eyes
d. Low-pitched, slow, poorly modulated, poorly articulated speech
e. Drooling; difficulty in swallowing saliva
f. Various autonomic symptoms (e.g., lacrimation, constipation, incontinence, decreased sexual capacity, excessive perspiration)
g. Dementia and confusion in approximately 60% of individuals, especially older adults

C. Therapeutic interventions
1. Medical regimen is palliative rather than curative
2. Pharmacologic intervention (see Antiparkinson Agents under Related Pharmacology)
3. Physiotherapy to reduce rigidity of muscles and prevent contractures
4. The role of surgical intervention is limited
   a. Deep brain stimulation by implanted electrode attached to pulse generator (similar to a pacemaker)
   b. Destruction of thalamus or globus pallidus for intractable tremor and rigidity using stereotactic nerve stimulation
   c. Neural transplant and gene transfer technique are being studied

Nursing Care of Clients With Parkinson's Disease

A. Assessment/Analysis
1. History of onset and progression of symptoms, and use of antiparkinson medications
2. Observations of tremors, posture, gait, facial expression
3. Nutritional status
4. Elimination status
5. Horizontal and vertical blood pressures to identify postural hypotension

B. Planning/Implementation
1. Provide a safe environment
2. Teach client or family to cut food into small bite-sized pieces or alter the consistency to prevent choking; encourage diet rich in nutrient-dense foods such as fruits, vegetables, whole grains, and legumes to improve and maintain nutritional status and prevent possible drug-induced nutrient deficiencies
3. Suction client's secretions as needed to maintain an adequate airway (usually advanced stages)
4. Encourage an adequate intake of roughage and fluids to avoid constipation
5. Teach activities to limit postural deformities (e.g., use firm mattress without a pillow, periodically lie prone, keep head and neck as erect as possible, avoid leaning forward when walking)
6. Teach activities to maintain appropriate gait; use cane or walker as necessary
7. Teach and encourage daily physical therapy to limit rigidity and prevent contractures (e.g., warm baths, passive and active exercises)
8. Avoid rushing as stress intensifies symptoms
9. Encourage continuation of medications even though results may be minimal
10. Teach client and family about antiparkinson agents (see Antiparkinson Agents under Related Pharmacology)
11. Assist in setting achievable goals to improve self-esteem

C. Evaluation/Outcomes
1. Maintains patent airway
2. Participates in daily exercise program
3. Complies with prescribed medical therapy
4. Remains free from injuries

MULTIPLE SCLEROSIS (DISSEMINATED SCLEROSIS)

Data Base
A. Etiology and pathophysiology
1. Randomly scattered plaques of sclerotic tissue on demyelinated axons; frequently affected areas include optic nerves, cerebrum, brainstem, cerebellum, and spinal cord
2. Chronic, debilitating, progressive disease with periods of remission and exacerbation

3. Cause unknown; viral, environmental, and immunologic causes have been implicated
4. Onset in early adult life (20 to 40 years); higher incidence in females, Caucasians, and those living in temperate climates
5. Fatigue, stress, and heat tend to increase symptoms

B. Clinical findings
1. Subjective
   a. Numbness; altered position sense; increased incidence of trigeminal neuralgia
   b. Dysphagia
   c. Weakness; fatigue
   d. Blurred vision; diplopia
   e. Altered emotional affect (depression, apathy, or euphoria)
2. Objective
   a. Charcot's triad: intention tremor; nystagmus; scanning (clipped) speech
   b. Ataxia; shuffling gait; increased deep tendon reflexes; spastic paralysis
   c. Impaired bowel and bladder function
   d. Impotence
   e. Cognitive loss (advanced stage)
   f. Pallor of optic discs; blindness
   g. Increased immunoglobulin G (IgG) levels in the CSF
   h. MRI indicates demyelination and presence of multiple sclerosis plaques

C. Therapeutic interventions
1. Generally palliative
2. Disease-modifying therapy
   a. Interferon beta-1a (Avonex) given IM and (Rebif) given Sub-Q
   b. Interferon beta-1b (Betaseron) given Sub-Q
   c. Glatiramer acetate (Copaxone) given Sub-Q
   d. Mitoxantrone HCl (Novantrone) given IV every 3 months
3. Additional drugs: corticosteroids to shorten duration of relapses, baclofen (Lioresal) for spasticity, carbamazepine (Tegretol) for trigeminal neuralgia, ascorbic acid to acidify urine, immunosuppressive agents
4. Physical therapy and psychotherapy

Nursing Care of Clients With Multiple Sclerosis

A. Assessment/Analysis
1. History of onset and progression of motor and sensory loss
2. Factors that intensify symptoms
3. Neurologic status (see Neurologic Assessment [Including Glasgow Coma Scale] under Related Procedures)

B. Planning/Implementation
1. Incorporate frequent rest periods
2. Avoid hot baths, which can increase symptoms
3. Teach client and family about medications; reinforce injection technique; explain Avonex may cause flulike symptoms
4. Assist family to understand why client should be encouraged to be active; teach use of assistive devices for ADLs
5. Assist client and family to plan and implement a bowel and bladder regimen; teach urinary self-catheterization if appropriate
6. Explain the disease process to both client and family in understandable terms
7. Do not encourage false hopes during periods of remission
8. Spend time listening to both client and family; encourage ventilation of feelings
9. Encourage counseling and rehabilitation
10. Explain to client and family that mood swings and emotional alterations are part of the disease
11. Help client maintain self-esteem
12. Teach how to compensate for problems with gait: walk with feet farther apart to broaden base of support; use low-heeled shoes; use assistive devices when necessary (tripod cane, walker, wheelchair)
13. Teach how to compensate for loss of sensation: use a thermometer to test water temperature; avoid constricting stockings; use protective clothing in cold weather; change position frequently
14. Teach how to compensate for difficulty in swallowing: take small bites; chew well; use a straw with liquids; eat foods of more solid consistency
15. Provide a diet rich in nutrient-dense foods such as fruits, vegetables, whole grains, and legumes to improve and maintain nutritional status and compensate for nutrient interactions of corticosteroid medications; some practitioners advise avoidance of "night shade" foods (e.g., tomatoes, peppers, eggplant) and adherence to a low-fat diet
16. Provide skin care to prevent formation of pressure ulcers; turn frequently
17. Prevent dysfunctional contractures; provide range-of-motion exercises; splints
18. Refer client and family to the local chapter of the National Multiple Sclerosis Society

C. Evaluation/Outcomes
1. Maintains a patent airway
2. Remains free from injury
3. Establishes exercise/activity and rest/sleep routine that avoids fatigue
4. Maintains bowel and bladder function
5. Remains free from urinary tract infection
6. Copes with changes in physical abilities and lifestyle changes

MYASTHENIA GRAVIS

Data Base

A. Etiology and pathophysiology
1. Chronic, progressive, neuromuscular disorder with remissions and exacerbations; a disturbance in the transmission of impulses at the myoneural junction, resulting in profound weakness

2. Dysfunction caused by reduced acetylcholine receptors (AChR) and altered postsynaptic membrane of muscle end plates
3. Autoimmune theory: antibodies to AChR cause accelerated destruction and blockage of AChR
4. Highest incidence in young adult women ages 20 to 40; peak incidence in men is 60 to 70 years old
5. Myasthenic crisis refers to sudden inability to swallow or maintain respirations because of the weakness of the muscles of respiration

B. Clinical findings
1. Subjective: extreme muscle weakness; becomes progressively worse with use, but improves with rest; dyspnea; transient respiratory insufficiency, dysphagia (difficulty chewing and swallowing); dysarthria (difficulty speaking); diplopia
2. Objective
   a. Physical: ptosis; strabismus; weak voice (dysphonia); myasthenic smile (snarling, nasal smile); ineffective cough; enlarged thymus
   b. Diagnostic measures: spontaneous relief of symptoms with IV administration of edrophonium (Tensilon); edrophonium also used to distinguish myasthenic crisis from cholinergic crisis (toxic effects of excessive neostigmine)

C. Therapeutic interventions
1. Medications that block the action of cholinesterase at the myoneural junction (see Cholinesterase Inhibitors under Related Pharmacology)
2. Radiation therapy or surgical removal of the thymus may cause partial remission by producing antigen-specific immunosuppression
3. Corticosteroids to suppress antibody production
4. Tracheostomy with mechanical ventilation as necessary in myasthenic crisis
5. Plasmapheresis and immunosuppressives to reduce circulating antibody titer
6. Tube feedings if experiencing difficulty swallowing

Nursing Care of Clients With Myasthenia Gravis

A. Assessment/Analysis
1. History of onset and progression of motor and sensory loss
2. Neurologic status (see Neurologic Assessment [Including Glasgow Coma Scale] under Related Procedures)
3. Respiratory status: vital signs, depth of respirations, breath sounds, Sao$_2$, arterial blood gases

B. Planning/Implementation
1. Administer medications on strict time schedule to prevent onset of symptoms; medication may need to be administered during night
2. Monitor for signs of dyspnea, dysphagia, and dysarthria; may be caused by worsening of myasthenia (myasthenic crisis) or overdose of anticholinergic drugs (cholinergic crisis); drooping eyelids is often first sign of impending muscle weakness

3. Keep head of bed elevated; keep a tracheostomy set at bedside
4. Plan activity to avoid fatigue based on the individual's tolerance; collaborate with client to develop individualized energy-saving strategies
5. Teach client and family to avoid people with upper respiratory tract infections (pneumonia may develop as a result of respiratory impairment) and to wash hands correctly
6. Encourage carrying medical alert information
7. Avoid administering morphine to clients receiving cholinesterase inhibitors; these drugs potentiate effects of morphine and may cause respiratory depression
8. Provide emotional support and close client contact to allay anxiety
9. Schedule meals to coincide with peak drug action; administer tube feedings as ordered
10. Administer artificial tears to keep cornea moist if client has difficulty closing eyes
11. Encourage client and family to participate in planning care
12. Ensure that client understands the signs and symptoms of myasthenic and cholinergic crises
13. Refer client and family to Myasthenia Gravis Foundation and local self-help groups
14. In severe instances anticipate all needs, because the client is too weak to turn, drink, or even request assistance
15. Maintain a patent airway; suction client's secretions as necessary; provide tracheostomy care; maintain mechanical ventilation as ordered

C. Evaluation/Outcomes
1. Maintains a balance between activity and rest
2. Maintains effective respiratory function
3. Identifies signs and symptoms of crises

GUILLAIN-BARRÉ SYNDROME (POLYRADICULONEURITIS)

Data Base

A. Etiology and pathophysiology
1. Autoimmune response that destroys peripheral nerve myelin
2. May follow respiratory or gastrointestinal viral infection, vaccination, pregnancy, or surgery
3. After initial and plateau periods, recovery may take 2 years; although most fully recover, some experience residual deficits or die of complications

B. Clinical findings
1. Subjective: ascending weakness that begins in the lower extremities; paresthesia; dysphagia; diplopia
2. Objective
   a. Paralysis begins in lower extremities; ascends within the body; maximal deficit usually by 4 weeks
   b. Respiratory paralysis

  c. Autonomic neuropathy (e.g., hypertension, bradycardia, tachycardia, diaphoresis)
  d. Abnormal CSF and electrophysiologic studies
C. Therapeutic interventions
  1. IV therapy with IgG
  2. Plasmapheresis
  3. Support of vital functions

Nursing Care of Clients With Guillain-Barré Syndrome

A. Assessment/Analysis
  1. Respiratory function including airway, respiratory rate, breath sounds, Sao$_2$, and arterial blood gases
  2. Neurologic status (see Neurologic Assessment [Including Glasgow Coma Scale] under Related Procedures); does not affect level of consciousness or cognitive function
  3. History of any recent illness (particularly viral infections)
  4. Onset and progression of symptoms
B. Planning/Implementation
  1. Monitor vital signs, breath sounds, and Sao$_2$
  2. Maintain airway; keep tracheostomy set at bedside; mechanical ventilation may be needed
  3. Monitor gag and swallow reflexes; maintain gastrostomy tube feedings as necessary; monitor bowel sounds (paralytic ileus may occur); monitor urinary output
  4. Provide emotional support for the client and family because of the severity of adaptations and lengthy convalescent period
  5. Prevent complications of immobility: skin care; range-of-motion exercises; position changes; coughing and deep breathing; antiembolism stockings
  6. Refer client and family to Guillain-Barré Foundation for additional information and community resources
C. Evaluation/Outcomes
  1. Maintains effective respiratory function
  2. Remains free from complications of immobility
  3. Discusses feelings with family and other health care team members

✳ AMYOTROPHIC LATERAL SCLEROSIS (ALS)

Data Base
A. Etiology and pathophysiology
  1. Progressive, degenerative process involving the motor neurons of the spinal cord, medulla, and cortex; both upper and lower motor neurons are affected
  2. Occurs more frequently in men than women in the fifth and sixth decades
  3. Cause unknown; autoimmune diseases and genetic causes are implicated
  4. Death from respiratory complications frequently occurs within 3 to 5 years
  5. Often called Lou Gehrig's disease

B. Clinical findings
  1. Subjective: muscular weakness; malaise; fatigue
  2. Objective
    a. Fasciculations (irregular spasmodic twitching of small muscle groups); spasticity; atrophy
    b. Overactive deep tendon reflexes
    c. Difficulty in breathing, chewing, swallowing, speaking
    d. Outbursts of laughter or crying
    e. Abnormal electromyography
C. Therapeutic interventions
  1. Physiotherapy and skeletal muscle relaxants to relieve spasticity
  2. Respiratory function support with mechanical ventilation
  3. Riluzole (Rilutek) to inhibit glutamate accumulation, possibly preventing injury or death of neurons

Nursing Care of Clients With Amyotrophic Lateral Sclerosis

A. Assessment/Analysis
  1. History of onset and progression of symptoms
  2. Neurologic status (see Neurologic Assessment [Including Glasgow Coma Scale] under Related Procedures)
  3. Respiratory status (vital signs, respiratory depth, Sao$_2$, spirometry)
B. Planning/Implementation
  1. Encourage client to remain active as long as possible, employing supportive devices
  2. Encourage range-of-motion exercises
  3. Monitor swallowing ability; positioning and consistency of diet to prevent aspiration; provide enteral feedings via percutaneous endoscopic gastrostomy (PEG) tube as vital capacity drops
  4. Provide alternate means of communication as speech declines
  5. Encourage client and family to discuss feelings; explore advance directives while client is still able to speak
  6. Maintain respiratory function: increased fluids, positioning, chest physiotherapy, coughing and deep-breathing exercises, suctioning, and mechanical ventilation as needed
  7. Support natural defense mechanisms; encourage a diet consisting of nutrient-dense foods, especially those rich in the immune-stimulating nutrients selenium and vitamins A, C, and E
  8. Teach the avoidance of situations that may contribute to infection
  9. Refer client and family to ALS Association
C. Evaluation/Outcomes
  1. Maintains effective respiratory function
  2. Discusses feelings with family and other health care team members

✳ ARTHRITIS

Data Base

A. Etiology and pathophysiology
  1. Rheumatoid arthritis (RA)
     a. Altered immune response, in which enzymes destroy collagen; the synovial membrane proliferates, forming pannus, which destroys cartilage and bone; HLA-DR4 antibody usually present
     b. Other effects include fever, weight loss, anemia, Raynaud's phenomenon, arteritis, neuropathy, pericarditis, ankylosis, and Sjögren's syndrome
     c. Etiology unclear; apparent genetic predisposition; incidence higher in women
  2. Osteoarthritis (OA) (degenerative arthritis)
     a. Characterized by degeneration of articular cartilage
     b. Considered a noninflammatory joint disease with no systemic effects
     c. Risk factors include age; obesity; injury; repetitive trauma from sports, occupation, or other activity; presence of *ank* gene
  3. Gouty arthritis (GA)
     a. Disorder in purine metabolism, leading to increased uric acid in blood and deposition of uric acid crystals (tophi) in tissues, especially joints; followed by an inflammatory response
     b. Incidence highest in males; familial tendency
     c. Renal urate lithiasis (kidney stones) may result from precipitation of uric acid in the presence of a low urinary pH
B. Clinical findings
  1. Subjective
     a. Joint pain
        (1) OA: insidious onset of asymmetric pain in hips, knees, fingers, or spine that increases with weight-bearing activity and is relieved by rest
        (2) RA: symmetrical pain in small joints of hands and feet; knees, shoulders, hips, elbows, and ankles affected as disease progresses; not relieved by rest
        (3) GA: sudden onset of asymmetric joint pain usually in metatarsophalangeal joint of the great toe
     b. Morning stiffness: less than 1 hour with OA; more than 1 hour with RA
     c. Anorexia, fatigue, and malaise (RA, GA)
  2. Objective
     a. Decreased range of motion
     b. Inflammation (swelling, heat, redness) of involved joints (RA, GA)
     c. Deformities (Figure 11-5: Arthritic hand deformities)
        (1) Ulnar drift, Boutonnière deformity, swan neck deformity, rheumatoid nodules (RA), bony ankylosis
        (2) Heberden's and Bouchard's nodes (bony hypertrophy) symmetrically occurring on fingers (OA)

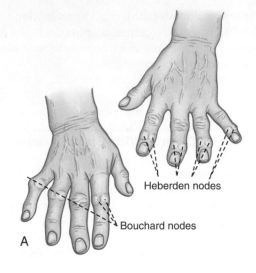

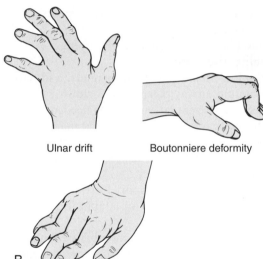

Figure 11-5 Arthritic hand deformities. **A,** Characteristics of osteoarthritis. **B,** Characteristics of rheumatoid arthritis. (**A** from Mourad L: *Orthopedic disorders*, St Louis, 1991, Mosby. **B** from Lewis SL et al: *Medical-surgical nursing: assessment and management of clinical problems*, ed 7, St Louis, 2007, Mosby.)

        (3) Tophi in outer ear, hands, feet, elbows, or knees (GA)
     d. Crepitus when joint is moved (OA)
     e. Fever (RA, GA)
     f. Laboratory findings
        (1) RA: presence of rheumatoid factor (RF), elevated erythrocyte sedimentation rate (ESR), decreased RBC count, and positive C-reactive protein and antinuclear antibody (ANA) tests; joint fluid analysis demonstrates inflammation
        (2) GA: elevated serum uric acid
C. Therapeutic interventions
  1. Pharmacologic management
     a. Acetaminophen (OA)
     b. Nonsteroidal antiinflammatory drugs (RA, OA, GA) (see Nonsteroidal Antiinflammatory Drugs [NSAIDs] under Related Pharmacology)

c. Tumor necrosis factor inhibitors: etanercept (Enbrel), infliximab (Remicade), adalimumab (Humira)

d. Disease-modifying antirheumatic drugs (DMARDs) such as anakinera (Kineret), azathioprine (Imuran), cyclosporine (Sandimmune), hydroxychloroquine (Plaquenil), gold compounds, leflunomide (Arava), methotrexate (Rheumatrex), sulfasalazine (Azulfidine) (RA)

e. Hyaluronic acid (Orthovisc) joint injections to lubricate knee joints (OA)

f. Antigout Agents (see Related Pharmacology)

g. Corticosteroids (RA and resistant GA) to reduce inflammation

h. While research has not supported the efficacy of glucosamine and chondroitin, some clients report reduced pain with supplements (OA); glucosamine has a glucose base that interferes with antidiabetic medications

2. Weight loss if indicated

3. Physical therapy to preserve joint function; application of heat/cold

4. Use of splints and assistive devices

5. Surgical intervention (RA, OA); often done in a laminar air flow room

a. Synovectomy: removal of the enlarged synovial membrane before bone and cartilage destruction occurs

b. Arthrodesis: fusion of a joint when the joint surfaces are severely damaged; this leaves client with no range of motion of affected joint

c. Arthroplasty: surgical repair of joint or replacement with a prosthetic device (see Fracture of the Hip)

6. Apheresis treatment with protein A immunoadsorption column (Prosorba), which binds RA antibodies before blood is returned to client (RA)

Nursing Care of Clients With Arthritis

A. Assessment/Analysis
1. Extent of range of motion of involved joints; presence of bony deformities
2. History of onset and progression of symptoms, noting degree to which pain interferes with daily activities
3. Presence of risk factors such as obesity

B. Planning/Implementation
1. Assist with activities that require using affected joints; allow for rest periods
2. Maintain functional alignment of joints
3. Provide range-of-motion exercises up to point of pain, recognizing that some discomfort is always present; apply heat or cold before exercises if ordered
4. Relieve discomfort and edema by medications or application of heat/cold (warm compresses should be between 98.6° and 105° F)

5. Allow ample time to verbalize feelings regarding limited motion and changes in lifestyle; help set realistic goals, focusing on strengths
6. Support client through weight loss program if indicated
7. Encourage client to follow physical therapist's instruction regarding regular exercise and use of supportive devices to maintain independence; encourage muscle strengthening and stretching to increase joint stability
8. Administer and teach about prescribed pharmacologic therapy (e.g., gold compounds can cause nephrotoxicity and blood dyscrasias; Plaquenil can cause visual disturbances)
9. Provide dietary instructions
   a. Encourage diet rich in nutrient-dense foods such as fruits, vegetables, whole grains, and legumes to improve and maintain nutritional status and vitamin and mineral intake, and compensate for nutrient interactions of corticosteroid and other treatment medications (RA, GA); avoid high-purine foods such as organ meats, anchovies, sardines, and shellfish (GA)
   b. Increase fluid intake to 2000 to 3000 mL daily to prevent formation of calculi; alkaline-ash diet to increase the pH of urine to discourage precipitation of uric acid and enhance the action of drugs such as probenecid (GA)
10. Provide care for the client with RA or OA requiring joint replacement (see Nursing Care of Clients With Fractures of the Extremities or Hip)
11. Refer client and family to the Arthritis Foundation

C. Evaluation/Outcomes
1. Reports reduction in pain
2. Completes activities of daily living using supportive devices as needed
3. Accepts and adjusts to deformities

OSTEOMYELITIS

Data Base

A. Etiology and pathophysiology: infection of bone by direct or indirect invasion, usually by *Staphylococcus aureus;* may be acute or chronic
1. Indirect entry: via blood from another site; usually in young males; most often occurs in growing long bones; associated with local trauma
2. Direct entry: extends from open wound to bone via arterial blood; ischemia results in formation of sequestrum (dead bone tissue), leading to chronic osteomyelitis; not age related

B. Clinical findings
1. Subjective: pain and tenderness of bone; malaise; headache
2. Objective: signs of sepsis or tissue infection such as fever; edema and erythema over bone; drainage if chronic; positive culture from bone biopsy and positive radionuclide bone scan; MRI useful in confirmation of diagnosis

C. Therapeutic interventions
1. Intravenous antibiotic therapy for 4 to 6 weeks followed by oral antibiotics for 2 to 3 months; antibiotic-impregnated beads may be placed in the wound
2. Incision and drainage of a bone abscess
3. Sequestrectomy: surgical removal of the dead, infected bone and cartilage; muscle or bone grafts may be needed
4. A closed suction irrigation system can be applied to the wound to eliminate debris
5. Preventive measures include prophylactic antibiotics before surgery; early removal of invasive lines

Nursing Care of Clients With Osteomyelitis

A. Assessment/Analysis
1. History of trauma, infections, or surgery
2. Involved tissue for signs of inflammation
3. Onset and characteristics of pain
B. Planning/Implementation
1. Monitor neurovascular status of extremity
2. Administer analgesics, antibiotics, and warm soaks as ordered
3. Use surgical asepsis for wound care
4. Maintain functional body alignment and promote comfort
5. Use room deodorizer if a foul odor is apparent
6. Allow expression of feelings about length of recovery
7. Encourage nutrient-dense diet to compensate for impact of long-term antibiotic therapy on nutritional status
C. Evaluation/Outcomes
1. Reports reduction in pain
2. Resolves infectious process

OSTEOGENIC SARCOMA

Data Base
A. Etiology and pathophysiology
1. Malignant bone tumor that usually begins in long bones, especially around knee
2. Metastasis to the lungs common and occurs early; prognosis is poor
3. Highest incidence between 10 and 30 years
B. Clinical findings
1. Subjective: bone pain; malaise
2. Objective: local swelling; weight loss; anemia; elevated serum calcium alkaline phosphatase level; neoplastic cells
C. Therapeutic interventions
1. Surgery: wide excision of tumor, reconstructive surgery, bone grafts, amputation of limb
2. Chemotherapy
3. Radiation

Nursing Care of Clients With Osteogenic Sarcoma

A. Assessment/Analysis
1. Description of onset and progression of symptoms
2. Extent of support system and home environment

B. Planning/Implementation
1. Maintain safe environment to decrease risk for pathologic fractures
2. Help client control pain by relaxation, imagery, distraction, and medication
3. Be available for the client and family to discuss fears, concerns, and treatment
4. Encourage diet of nutrient-dense foods, especially those rich in the immune-stimulating nutrients selenium and vitamins A, C, and E, as well as protein; increase fluid intake
5. Administer care based on therapeutic interventions (see General Nursing Care of Clients With Neoplastic Disorders in Chapter 3, and Amputation)
6. Refer client and family to cancer support groups
7. Collaborate with physical therapist about the need for and safe use of assistive devices
C. Evaluation/Outcomes
1. Reports reduction in pain
2. Remains free from injury

MULTIPLE MYELOMA

Data Base
A. Etiology and pathophysiology
1. Malignant overgrowth of plasma cells in bone and bone marrow produce a specific nonfunctional immunoglobulin (monoclonal protein); osteoclast activating factor produced by the plasma cells and other substances cause bone breakdown
2. Cause unknown; risk factors include exposure to ionizing radiation and occupational chemicals; genetic and viral factors are being studied
3. Occurs primarily in older men
B. Clinical findings
1. Subjective: bone pain (back and ribs); progressive weakness
2. Objective
a. Anemia; platelet deficiency; weight loss
b. Idiopathic bone fractures; punched-out appearance of the bones on radiograph
c. Serum electrophoresis for monoclonal protein level to monitor extent of disease
d. Presence of Bence Jones protein in urine
e. Hypercalcemia and hyperuricemia, which may result in renal damage
f. Diagnosis confirmed by bone marrow biopsy
C. Therapeutic interventions
1. Chemotherapeutic agents, especially dexamethasone (Decadron) or prednisone; melphalan (Alkeran), cyclophosphamide (Cytoxan), doxorubicin (Adriamycin)
2. Radiation therapy
3. Bone marrow transplantation or peripheral blood stem-cell transplantation
4. Analgesics and opioids for pain
5. Supportive therapy such as transfusions, vertebroplasty with orthopedic cement,

bisphosphonates such as pamidronate (Aredia) to strengthen bone

6. Thalidomide (Thalomid) has been effective against multiple myeloma; clients must be counseled about use of contraception because this drug is associated with severe birth defects

Nursing Care of Clients With Multiple Myeloma

A. Assessment/Analysis
   1. Description of onset and progression of symptoms
   2. Signs of myelosuppression
   3. Renal function; precipitation of protein, calcium, and uric acid in urine

B. Planning/Implementation
   1. Allow time to express feelings about the disease and related therapies
   2. Help control pain by relaxation, imagery, distraction, and use of analgesics
   3. Assist with movement to prevent pathologic fractures; back braces may be used for support
   4. Increase fluid intake to prevent renal damage
   5. Provide care for the client receiving radiation or chemotherapy (see General Nursing Care of Clients With Neoplastic Disorders in Chapter 3)
   6. Encourage diet high in nutrient-dense foods, especially those rich in the immune-stimulating nutrients selenium and vitamins A, C, and E, as well as protein

C. Evaluation/Outcomes
   1. Reports decrease in pain
   2. Remains free from injury (fractures, renal damage)

❋ DEGENERATIVE DISK DISEASE

Data Base

A. Etiology and pathophysiology
   1. Herniation and protrusion of the nucleus pulposus into the spinal canal with subsequent compression of the cord or nerve roots; usually occurs as a result of aging or trauma
   2. Most common site is lumbosacral area (between L4 and L5), but herniation can also occur in the cervical region (between C5 and C6 or between C6 and C7)

B. Clinical findings
   1. Subjective
      a. Lumbosacral disk
         (1) Acute pain or paresthesias in lower back, radiating across buttock and down leg (sciatic pain); pain increases with activities that raise intraspinal pressure
         (2) Pain on affected side when raising extended leg
         (3) Weakness of the foot
      b. Cervical disk
         (1) Neck pain that may radiate to hand
         (2) Paresthesias and weakness of the affected upper extremity
   2. Objective
      a. Straightening of lumbar curve scoliosis away from affected side (lumbosacral disk) is associated with scoliosis

b. Atrophy of biceps and triceps (cervical disk)
      c. Spinal defect on MRI; myelogram or CT scan also may be used

C. Therapeutic interventions
   1. Bed rest initially during acute phase; physical therapy for muscle strengthening and flexibility
   2. Back brace or support; cervical collar or traction
   3. Local application of heat or cold
   4. NSAIDs, muscle relaxants, analgesics
   5. Surgical intervention (for progressive deficit)
      a. Laminectomy: excision of the ruptured portion of the nucleus pulposus through an opening created by removal of part of the vertebra
      b. Diskectomy: removal of herniated disk; cervical diskectomy may be done through an anterior or posterior incision; bone grafts and hardware may be used
      c. Microdiskectomy: uses a magnifying lens to facilitate removal of pieces of disk that press on nerve; incision is generally 1 inch
      d. Laminotomy: incision into the lamina
      e. Spinal fusion: if two or more disks are involved, the affected vertebrae are permanently fused to stabilize the spine with bone graft
      f. Percutaneous diskectomy: disk material is removed through a trocar; laser may be used to destroy damaged disk

Nursing Care of Clients With Degenerative Disk Disease

A. Assessment/Analysis
   1. Characteristics and radiation of pain
   2. Contributing factors such as trauma, obesity, degenerative joint disease, scoliosis
   3. Posture and gait alterations
   4. Extent of muscle strength and sensory function of involved extremities

B. Planning/Implementation
   1. Administer skeletal muscle relaxants, analgesics, and other medications as ordered
   2. Use a firm mattress and bed board
   3. Make certain that traction and/or braces are correctly applied and maintained and that weights hang freely
   4. Use a fracture bedpan to avoid lifting of hips
   5. Provide frequent back care to relax muscles and promote circulation
   6. Support body alignment at all times
   7. Use log-rolling to turn (instruct client to fold arms across chest, bend knee on side opposite direction of turn, and then roll over)
   8. Teach the importance of weight loss, low-heeled shoes, and body mechanics, avoiding activities that increase intraspinal pressure (e.g., coughing, lifting, straining on defecation)
   9. Increase fluid intake and encourage diet rich in nutrient-dense foods such as fruits, vegetables, whole grains, and legumes to improve and maintain

nutritional status and prevent constipation; use stool softeners to prevent straining

10. Provide care for client undergoing disk surgery
    a. Explain that pain may persist postoperatively because of edema
    b. Protect client's airway, particularly after cervical spine surgery
    c. Place bedside table, phone, and call bell within reach to prevent twisting
    d. Observe the dressing for hemorrhage and leakage of spinal fluid
    e. Observe for adequate ventilation in clients who have undergone a cervical laminectomy, diskectomy, or fusion
    f. Assess for changes in neurologic function (e.g., sensory changes in extremities)
    g. Assist with back brace or cervical collar if ordered; instruct client to wear cervical brace as directed to prevent spinal cord injury
    h. Instruct client that pain and muscle spasm will improve gradually
11. Foster independence
12. Encourage prescribed exercises
13. Encourage the client to express feelings

C. Evaluation/Outcomes
    1. Reports reduction in pain
    2. Remains free from injury
    3. Increases mobility

✳ FRACTURES OF THE EXTREMITIES

Data Base

A. Etiology and pathophysiology
    1. Break in bone continuity, accompanied by localized tissue response and muscle spasm
    2. Caused by trauma or pathologic fractures as a result of osteoporosis, multiple myeloma, or bone tumors
    3. Types
        a. Complete fracture: bone completely separated into two parts; transverse or spiral
        b. Incomplete fracture: only part of width of bone broken
        c. Comminuted fracture: bone broken into several fragments
        d. Greenstick fracture: splintering on one side of bone, with bending of other side; occurs only in pliable bones, usually in children
        e. Simple (closed) fracture: bone broken but skin is intact
        f. Compound (open) fracture: break in skin at the time of fracture with or without protrusion of bone
    4. Stages of healing include formation of a hematoma; fibrocartilage formation; callus formation; ossification; consolidation and remodeling of the callus
B. Clinical findings
    1. Subjective: pain aggravated by motion; tenderness; neurovascular changes and numbness

2. Objective
    a. Loss of motion; crepitus (grating sound) heard when affected limb is moved
    b. Edema; ecchymosis
    c. X-ray examination reveals break in continuity of bone
    d. Shortening of extremity caused by change in bone alignment
    e. Muscle spasm
    f. Loss of function
    g. Impaired local circulation (cool, dusky color, diminished pulses) if arteries are damaged
    h. Shock when accompanied by blood loss
C. Therapeutic interventions
    1. Traction may be used to reduce the fracture or to maintain alignment of bone fragments until surgery or healing occurs
        a. Skin traction: weights pull on device (e.g., foam boot) applied to an extremity to exert a straight pull on a limb (e.g., Buck's extension/traction; often used temporarily to immobilize the leg while awaiting surgery for a fractured hip)
        b. Skeletal traction: weights pull on pins surgically attached to bone (e.g., Steinmann pin, Kirschner's wire, skeletal tongs, halo traction for cervical fractures)
    2. Surgical intervention to align the bone (open reduction), often with plates, screws, nails (e.g., intramedullary nails) to hold fracture in alignment (internal fixation)
    3. Manipulation to reduce fracture (closed reduction)
    4. Application of cast to maintain alignment and immobilize limb; may be plaster or fiberglass
    5. Use of external fixation device when fractures accompany soft tissue injury

Nursing Care of Clients With Fractures of the Extremities

A. Assessment/Analysis
    1. Ability of client to move extremity
    2. Altered appearance of involved body part
    3. Factors precipitating injury
    4. Neurovascular assessment; soft tissue injury or edema may compromise circulatory or neurologic functioning; 5 Ps—pain, pulselessness, pallor, paresthesias, paralysis
B. Planning/Implementation
    1. Provide emergency care
        a. Evaluate the client's general physical condition; treat for shock
        b. Splint extremity in position found before moving client; consider all suspected fractures as fractures until radiography is performed
        c. Cover open wound with sterile dressing if available
    2. Observe for signs of emboli (fat or blood): severe chest pain, dyspnea, pallor, diaphoresis, petechiae (fat)

3. Observe for signs of gas gangrene, which develop. 2 to 5 days after deep wound injury
   a. Culture shows *Clostridium perfringens, C. welchii, C. novyi*
   b. Bronzed or blackened wound tissue; necrosis
   c. Crepitus; pallor
4. Provide care for a client with a cast
   a. Observe for signs of circulatory impairment: change in skin temperature or color, numbness or tingling, decrease in peripheral pulse, inability to move toes/fingers, prolonged blanching of toes/fingers after compression, increasing unrelieved pain; excessive tissue pressure within the fascial compartment can compromise circulation to the area, causing ischemia and leading to edema, which further compromises circulation (compartment syndrome)
   b. Protect the cast from damage until dry: elevate on pillow; handle with palms of hands only
   c. Promote drying of the cast by leaving it uncovered
   d. Maintain bed rest until the cast is dry and ambulation is permitted
   e. Observe for signs of hemorrhage and measure extent of drainage on cast
   f. Observe for irritation caused by rough cast edges, and pad as necessary for comfort and to prevent soiling
   g. Observe for swelling and notify the physician if necessary
   h. Administer analgesics judiciously and report unrelieved pain
   i. Observe for signs of infection (e.g., elevated temperature, odor from cast, swelling)
   j. Teach isometric exercises to prevent muscle atrophy
5. Provide care for a client in traction
   a. Check that weights are hanging freely and that the affected limb is not resting against anything that will impede the pull of the traction; never interrupt skeletal traction
   b. Maintain affected extremity in functional alignment; encourage use of trapeze or side rails to facilitate movement; teach client how to use the trapeze to lift body during linen change to avoid shearing force, which contributes to skin breakdown
   c. Observe for footdrop with Buck's extension/traction, because this may indicate nerve damage
   d. Observe site of insertion of skeletal traction for irritation or infection; use surgical asepsis when cleansing site of insertion of skeletal traction (an antiseptic ointment may be ordered)
6. Observe for signs of thromboembolytic complications such as deep venous thrombosis (DVT) and pulmonary embolus (PE); prevent clots by administering ordered anticoagulants, antiembolism devices (e.g., sequential compression device)
7. Encourage high-protein, high-vitamin diet to promote healing; high-calcium diet is not recommended for clients on prolonged bed rest, because decalcification of bone will continue until activity is restored, and a high calcium intake could lead to formation of renal calculi
8. Encourage fluids to help prevent constipation, renal calculi, urinary tract infection, and maintain hydration
9. Reposition every 1 to 2 hours, use pressure-relieving devices, and provide skin care to prevent pressure ulcers
10. Teach isometric exercises to promote muscle strength and tone for crutch walking
11. Teach appropriate crutch-walking technique; non–weight bearing (three-point swing-through); weight bearing (four point) progressing to use of cane (see Mobility: Assistive Devices under Related Procedures)

C. Evaluation/Outcomes
1. Remains free from infection
2. Maintains neurovascular functioning
3. Remains free from complications
4. Regains mobility and function after healing

FRACTURE OF THE HIP
Data Base
A. Etiology and pathophysiology
1. Fractures of head or neck of femur (intracapsular) or trochanteric area (extracapsular); loss of blood supply to head of femur will result in aseptic necrosis
2. Incidence highest may be used for older females because osteoporosis and degenerative joint disease increase likelihood of sustaining a fracture from a fall
B. Clinical findings
1. Subjective: pain; changes in sensation
2. Objective: affected leg appears shorter; external rotation of the affected limb; x-ray examination reveals lack of continuity of bone
C. Therapeutic interventions
1. Buck's extension/traction as a temporary measure to limit soft tissue injury and relieve pain of muscle spasm; leg is kept extended with slight internal rotation and the client's body weight is used as counter-traction
2. Closed reduction with hip spica cast may be used for fractures of the intertrochanteric region
3. Open reduction and internal fixation (ORIF)
4. Total hip replacement (THR) when fracture site or joint degeneration will not permit internal fixation

Nursing Care of Clients With Fracture of the Hip
A. Assessment/Analysis
1. Shortening and external rotation of leg
2. Degree and nature of pain
3. Neurovascular assessment; 5 Ps—pain, pulselessness, pallor, paresthesias, paralysis
4. Other health problems that may affect recovery

B. Planning/Implementation
1. See Nursing Care of Clients With Fractures of the Extremities
2. Encourage the use of a trapeze to facilitate movement and prevent shearing force on skin; lift pelvis by using trapeze and unaffected leg
3. Use a fracture pan for elimination or elevated commode (clients with total hip replacements must avoid flexing the hip >90 degrees)
4. Provide postoperative care for THR
   a. Monitor neurovascular status
   b. Maintain portable wound suction drainage device (e.g., Hemovac); anticipate up to 500 mL in the first 24 hours; usually removed by second postoperative day when daily drainage decreases to approximately 30 mL
   c. Administer analgesics; patient-controlled analgesia (PCA) and/or continuous regional analgesia (e.g., ropivacaine [Naropin])
   d. Determine if surgeon wants client to turn from side to side or must avoid turning on the operative side; place pillow between legs when turning on unaffected side; use pillow to maintain abduction after hip replacement and instruct client to avoid crossing legs to prevent dislodging the prosthesis
   e. Encourage quadriceps setting exercises
   f. Assist client to ambulate; first use a walker and progress to a cane; support on unaffected side; follow orders for extent of weight bearing permitted on affected extremity because this will depend on type of surgery performed and type of device inserted
   g. Avoid activities that may dislocate the prosthesis (see Figure 11-6: Total hip replacement: do's and do not's related to body mechanics)
   h. Prevent complication of thromboembolism: administer anticoagulants; apply antiembolism stockings; encourage dorsiflexion of feet; monitor coagulation profile; observe dressing and under client for bleeding
   i. Prevent pulmonary complications: encourage coughing and deep breathing; explain use of incentive spirometer; assist with frequent position changes; assess for adaptations related to pulmonary embolus (e.g., chest pain, shortness of breath)
   j. Encourage weight reduction if needed
   k. Collaborate with other health professionals for physical therapy and rehabilitation
C. Evaluation/Outcomes
1. Maintains alignment of affected leg
2. Demonstrates improved mobility
3. Avoids complications of immobility

❀ SPINAL CORD INJURY

Data Base
A. Etiology and pathophysiology
1. Sudden impingements on the spinal cord as a result of trauma

2. Fractures of vertebrae can cut, compress, or completely sever the spinal cord; signs and symptoms depend on location (lumbar, thoracic, cervical) and extent of damage (complete transection, partial transection, compression) and may be temporary or permanent; sensation and mobility of areas supplied by nerves below the level of the lesion are affected
3. Highest incidence ages 16 to 30
B. Clinical findings
1. Subjective: paresthesias or loss of sensation below the level of the injury
2. Objective
   a. Inability to move body below level of injury
   b. Early symptoms of spinal shock
      (1) Sudden loss of reflexes below the level of the injury; particularly bowel and bladder, which may lead to paralytic ileus and urinary retention
      (2) Flaccid paralysis (immobility accompanied by weak, soft, flabby muscles) below level of injury
      (3) Neurogenic shock: absence of sympathetic innervation leads to peripheral vasodilation and venous pooling, hypotension, bradycardia, and inability to perspire
   c. Later symptoms of spinal cord injury
      (1) Reflex hyperexcitability (spastic paralysis): muscles below site of injury become spastic and hyperreflexic
      (2) State of diminished reflex excitability (flaccid paralysis) below site of injury follows the state of reflex hyperexcitability in all instances of total cord damage and may occur in some instances of partial cord damage
      (3) In total cord damage both upper and lower motoneurons are destroyed; signs and symptoms depend totally on location of injury; loss of motor and sensory function present at this time is usually permanent
         (a) Sacral region: paralysis (usually flaccid) of lower extremities (paraplegia) accompanied by atonic (autonomous) bladder and bowel with impairment of sphincter control
         (b) Lumbar region: paralysis of lower extremities that may extend to pelvic region (usually flaccid) accompanied by a spastic (automatic) bladder and loss of bladder and anal sphincter control
         (c) Thoracic region: same signs and symptoms as those for lumbar region except paralysis extends to trunk below level of diaphragm
         (d) Cervical region: same signs and symptoms as those for thoracic region except paralysis extends from neck down and includes paralysis of all extremities (quadriplegia); if injury is above C4, there is an absence of independent respirations
      (4) In partial cord damage either the upper or the lower motoneurons, or both, may be destroyed; therefore symptoms depend not only

Do   **Do Not**

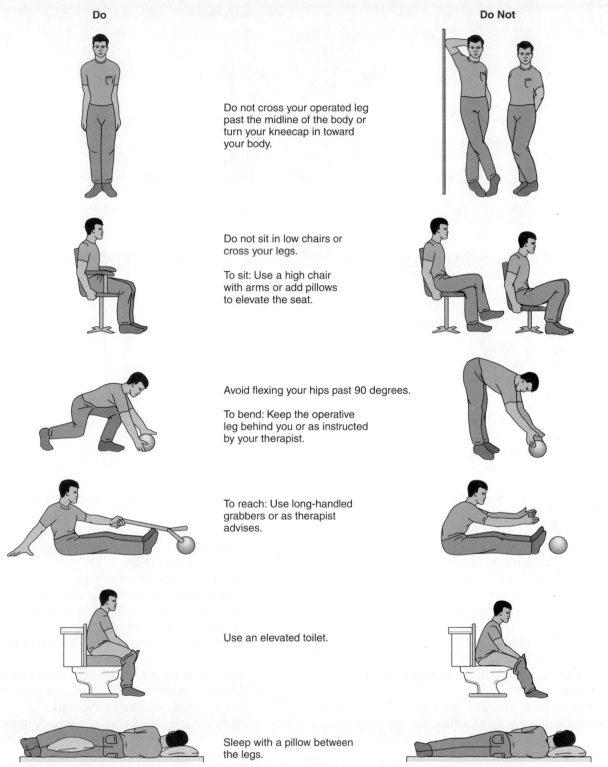

Do not cross your operated leg
past the midline of the body or
turn your kneecap in toward
your body.

Do not sit in low chairs or
cross your legs.

To sit: Use a high chair
with arms or add pillows
to elevate the seat.

Avoid flexing your hips past 90 degrees.

To bend: Keep the operative
leg behind you or as instructed
by your therapist.

To reach: Use long-handled
grabbers or as therapist
advises.

Use an elevated toilet.

Sleep with a pillow between
the legs.

Figure 11-6 Total hip replacement: do's and do not's related to body mechanics. Home-going instructions illustrating do's and do not's for clients with a total hip replacement. Clients are to avoid extreme flexion (past 90 degrees), adduction, and internal rotation of operated hip—any of which may cause dislocation of the prosthesis. (From Monahan FD et al: *Phipps' medical-surgical nursing: health and illness perspectives,* ed 8, St Louis, 2007, Mosby.)

on location but also on type of neurons involved; destruction of lower motoneurons will result in atrophy and flaccid paralysis of involved muscles, whereas destruction of upper motoneurons causes spasticity

(5) Autonomic dysreflexia (hyperreflexia): exaggerated autonomic response to factors such as a distended bowel or bladder; leads to bradycardia, hypertension, headache, piloerection (goose bumps), diaphoresis, and

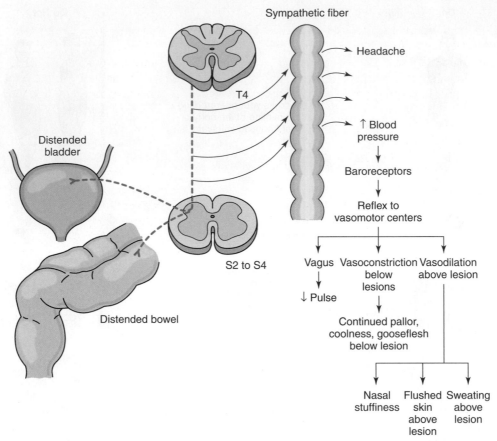

Figure 11-7 Autonomic dysreflexia (hyperreflexia): causes and clinical findings. (From Monahan FD et al: *Phipps' medical-surgical nursing: health and illness perspectives*, ed 8, St Louis, 2007, Mosby.)

nasal congestion (Figure 11-7: Autonomic dysreflexia: causes and clinical findings)

C. Therapeutic interventions
1. Maintenance of vertebral alignment
   a. At site of injury, maintain client in position found until transportation with a head and back stabilizer in place can occur
   b. Bed rest with supportive devices or with total immobilization
   c. Skeletal traction (Crutchfield or Vinke tongs; halo device)
   d. Corsets, braces, and other devices when mobility is permitted
2. Surgery to reduce pain or pressure and/or stabilize spine (e.g., laminectomy, spinal fusion)
3. Respiratory therapy, mechanical ventilation as needed
4. Temperature control via hypothermia
5. High doses of steroids to reduce inflammatory process at site of injury
6. Extensive rehabilitation therapy

Nursing Care of Clients With Spinal Cord Injuries

A. Assessment/Analysis
1. Respiratory status
2. Neurologic status (see Neurologic Assessment [Including Glasgow Coma Scale] under Related Procedures)
3. Abdomen for bladder or bowel distention
4. Skin integrity
5. Health problems that impact recovery
6. Client's coping skills and support systems

B. Planning/Implementation
1. Maintain frequent monitoring of cardiovascular, respiratory, and neurologic functioning
2. Maintain spinal alignment at all times; use the log-rolling method to turn
3. Maintain surgical asepsis with skeletal traction or spinal surgery
4. Institute measures to prevent thrombophlebitis
5. Maintain body parts in a functional position; prevent dysfunctional contractures
6. Institute active and passive range-of-motion exercises as soon as approved; exercises may be performed in water
7. Encourage verbalization and accept feelings
8. Include client in decision-making process; encourage independence when possible
9. Involve client, family, and entire health team in developing a plan of care
10. Help with adjustment to altered body image, lifestyle, and self-concept
11. Set realistic short-term goals so success can be achieved, promoting motivation
12. Examine skin for signs of pressure from positioning, braces, or splints; use techniques to prevent

pressure; provide skin care; use pressure-relieving devices or beds; reposition every 1 to 2 hours

13. Provide an opportunity to touch, grasp, and manipulate objects of different sizes, weights, and textures to stimulate tactile sensation

14. Protect affected limbs by proper positioning during transfer

15. Teach use of unaffected extremities to manipulate, move, and stabilize affected parts

16. Attempt to establish a scheduled pattern of bowel function

 a. Compare client's bowel habits before illness to current pattern; establish a specific time for bowel movement; schedule evacuation after a meal to utilize the gastrocolic reflex (peristaltic wave in the colon induced by entrance of food into a fasting stomach)

 b. Determine if client senses the need to defecate (e.g., feeling of fullness or pressure in the rectum, flatus, borborygmus)

 c. Encourage assumption of a position most near the physiologic position for defecation

 d. Utilize the following assistive measures to induce defecation

 (1) Teach bearing down and contracting abdominal muscles (Valsalva maneuver should be avoided by people with cardiac problems)

 (2) Teach leaning forward to increase intraabdominal pressure by compressing abdomen against thighs

 (3) Digital stimulation

 (4) Use suppository if necessary

 (5) Use enemas only as a last resort

 e. Provide a diet with bowel-stimulating properties, with emphasis on fruits, vegetables, cereal grains, and legumes, because these are rich sources of dietary fiber; fiber absorbs water, swells, and stretches the bowel, promoting peristalsis

 f. Encourage sufficient fluid intake: 2000 to 3000 mL per day

 g. Encourage activities to develop tone and strength of muscles that can be used

 h. Provide for adaptation of equipment as necessary (e.g., elevated toilet seat, grab bars, padded backrest)

 i. Teach the family the bowel training program

17. Attempt to establish bladder function

 a. Determine the type of bladder problem

 (1) Neurogenic bladder: any disturbance in bladder functioning caused by a lesion of the nervous system

 (2) Spastic bladder (reflex or automatic): disorder caused by a lesion of spinal cord above bladder reflex center, in the conus medullaris; there is a loss of conscious sensation and cerebral motor control; the bladder empties automatically when the detrusor muscle is sufficiently stretched (about 500 mL) to prevent overdistention

 (3) Flaccid bladder (atonic, nonreflex, or autonomous): disorder caused by a lesion of the spinal cord at the level of the sacral conus or below; the bladder continues to fill, becomes distended, and periodically overflows; the bladder muscle does not contract forcefully and therefore does not empty except with a conscious effort

 b. Review the client's bladder habits before illness as well as the current pattern of elimination; record output, voiding times, and times of incontinence

 c. Encourage activity

 d. Encourage sufficient fluid intake: 3000 to 4000 mL per 24-hour period; a glass of water with each attempt to void

 e. Restrict fluid after 6 PM to limit amount of urine in bladder during night

 f. Encourage assumption of as normal a position as possible for voiding

 g. Establish a voiding schedule

 (1) Begin trial voiding at the time the client is most often incontinent

 (2) Attempt voiding every 2 hours all day and 2 to 3 times during the night

 (3) Time intervals between voiding should be shorter in morning than later in day

 (4) As ability to maintain control improves, lengthen the time between attempts

 (5) Time of intervals is not as important as regularity

 h. Determine whether there is an awareness of need or act of urination (e.g., fullness or pressure, flushing, chilling, goose pimples, cold sweats)

 i. Utilize assistive measures to induce urination by teaching the client to

 (1) Use Credé maneuver: manual expression of the urine from the bladder with moderate external pressure, downward and backward, from the umbilicus to over the suprapubic area

 (2) Bend forward to increase intraabdominal pressure

 (3) Stimulate "trigger points"—areas that, for the particular individual, will instigate urination (e.g., stroke the thigh, pull pubic hair, touch meatus)

 j. Provide for adaptive equipment as necessary (e.g., elevated toilet seats, commode, urinals, drainage systems)

18. Discuss need for sexual expression and options available; include discussion of penile implants

19. Care for the client experiencing autonomic dysreflexia

 a. Place in a high-Fowler's position

 b. Ensure patency of urinary drainage system

     c. Assess for fecal impaction

     d. Eliminate other stimuli such as drafts

     e. Notify physician; administer prescribed antihypertensives

  20. When permitted, encourage and support use of tilt table to imitate weight bearing and reduce loss of calcium from bones caused by immobility

  21. Refer client to National Spinal Cord Injury Association

C. Evaluation/Outcomes

  1. Maintains respiratory functioning

  2. Avoids complications of immobility

  3. Establishes program to maintain bowel function

  4. Establishes program to maintain bladder function

  5. Adjusts to changes in lifestyle

  6. Functions satisfactorily sexually

❀ AMPUTATION

Data Base

A. Etiology and pathophysiology

  1. Removal of a body part as a result of trauma or surgical intervention

  2. Necessitated by malignant tumor, trauma, arterial insufficiency

B. Clinical findings

See Osteogenic Sarcoma (this chapter) and Vascular Disease: Thrombophlebitis, Varicose Veins, and Peripheral Vascular Disease (Chapter 6)

C. Therapeutic interventions

  1. Below-the-knee amputation (BKA) common in peripheral vascular disease; facilitates successful adaptation to prosthesis because of retained knee function

  2. Above-the-knee amputation (AKA) necessitated by trauma or extensive disease

  3. Upper extremity amputation usually necessitated by severe trauma, malignant tumors, or congenital malformation

Nursing Care of Clients With Amputations

A. Assessment/Analysis

  1. Neurovascular status of involved extremity

  2. History to determine causative factors and health problems that can compromise recovery

  3. Understanding of the surgery

  4. Coping skills and support system

B. Planning/Implementation

  1. Provide care preoperatively

     a. Initiation of exercises to strengthen muscles of extremities in preparation for crutch walking

     b. Coughing and deep-breathing exercises

     c. Emotional support for anticipated alteration in body image

  2. Monitor vital signs and dressing for signs of hemorrhage or infection

  3. Elevate the foot of the bed briefly if ordered by the surgeon to decrease edema; avoid elevation of the residual limb on a pillow in order to prevent hip flexion contractures

  4. Provide residual limb care

     a. Maintain elastic bandage to reduce edema and subcutaneous fat and shape residual limb in preparation for prosthesis

     b. When wound is healed, wash daily, avoiding the use of oils, which may cause maceration

     c. Apply pressure to end of residual limb with progressively firmer surfaces to toughen

     d. Encourage client to move the affected limb; keep extended in functional alignment

     e. Place the client with a lower extremity amputation in a prone position twice daily to stretch the flexor muscles and prevent hip flexion contractures

  5. Teach client about phantom limb pain/sensation caused by severed nerves

     a. Characteristics: pain/sensation may be constant or intermittent; varies from numbness and tingling to severe pain; may be burning, squeezing, shooting; gradually decreases over 2 years

     b. Institute care that may help provide relief: have client look at the residual limb or close eyes and put the limb through range-of-motion as if the extremity were still there

     c. If severe pain continues for long duration, medical therapy may include

       (1) Transcutaneous electric nerve stimulation (TENS), local anesthetic agents, ultrasound, antidepressants

       (2) Surgical revision of the residual limb

  6. Consider the special needs related to an upper extremity amputation

     a. Mastery of an upper extremity prosthesis is more complex than that of a lower extremity prosthesis

     b. Bilateral shoulder exercises must be done to prepare for fitting the prosthesis

     c. Artificial arms cannot be used above head or behind back because of harnessing

     d. No artificial hand can duplicate all the fine movements of the fingers and thumb of the hand, although the development of electronic limbs does not negate this future possibility

     e. There is a loss of sensory feedback; therefore visual control must be used at all times (a blind person could not adequately use a functional prosthesis)

  7. Support client through fitting, application, utilization, and care of prosthesis

  8. Allow expression of emotions; encourage family to participate in care

C. Evaluation/Outcomes

  1. Remains safe from injury

  2. Verbalizes acceptance of altered body image

  3. Maximizes independence

  4. Copes with phantom limb sensation/pain

✤ CATARACT

Data Base

A. Etiology and pathophysiology
   1. Opacity of the crystalline lens or its capsule
   2. Results from aging, injury, infection, cigarette smoking, obesity, diabetes mellitus, exposure to sun, corticosteroids

B. Clinical findings
   1. Subjective: distortion of vision (e.g., haziness, cloudiness, diplopia); photophobia
   2. Objective: progressive loss of vision; black pupil appears clouded, progressing to milky white appearance

C. Therapeutic interventions
   1. Corrective lenses as eyes become more myopic
   2. Surgical intervention to remove the opaque lens
      a. Surgery most frequently performed in an ambulatory surgery setting
      b. Extracapsular extraction involves removing the anterior capsule and lens through a small incision after the lens has been fragmented through a phacoemulsification technique; most common procedure
      c. Intracapsular extraction involves removal of the entire lens as a unit
      d. Intraocular lens implantation usually done at the time of cataract extraction
      e. Corrective lenses after cataract surgery
      f. Antiemetics, analgesics, and stool softeners postoperatively

Nursing Care of Clients With Cataracts

A. Assessment/Analysis
   1. Description of onset and progression of symptoms
   2. Visual acuity
   3. Characteristics of lens

B. Planning/Implementation
   1. Provide thorough orientation to environment
   2. Place call bell, phone, and other items on unaffected side
   3. Avoid glaring lights; provide eye protection from lights
   4. Provide auditory stimulation such as television, radio, and talking books
   5. Remove environmental hazards
   6. Provide care after cataract removal
      a. Instruct the client to prevent pressure on eye by avoiding the following: touching, rubbing, tightly closing the eyes, sneezing, bending from the waist, coughing, rapid head movements, straining at stool, lifting, lying on the affected side
      b. Instruct the client about prescribed analgesics, antiemetics, and stool softeners as required
      c. Reduce the amount of light and encourage the use of sunglasses when the eye patch is removed
      d. Teach signs of increased intraocular pressure (e.g., pain, restlessness, increased pulse rate) and infection (e.g., pain, changes in vital signs)

e. Explain that vision may be altered but will clear and glasses will help to compensate for distortion

C. Evaluation/Outcomes
   1. Remains free from injury
   2. Demonstrates increased visual acuity

✤ GLAUCOMA

Data Base

A. Etiology and pathophysiology
   1. The pressure within the eyeball is higher than the expected range of 10 to 21 mm Hg causing optic nerve damage; increased incidence in older adults
   2. Open-angle glaucoma
      a. Occurs when aqueous fluid does not drain properly from the eye; related to pathologic changes in the trabecular meshwork or Schlemm's canal
      b. The intraocular pressure increases and destroys retinal nerve fibers, causing progressive vision loss in affected areas
      c. Most common type of glaucoma
   3. Angle-closure glaucoma
      a. Occurs when iris lies close to drainage channels, creating a mechanical blockage of trabecular meshwork that interferes with exit of aqueous humor from anterior chamber
      b. Trapped aqueous humor causes the intraocular pressure to rise suddenly
      c. Occurs more commonly in African Americans and people older than 60

B. Clinical findings
   1. Open-angle glaucoma
      a. Subjective: halos around lights
      b. Objective: gradual loss of peripheral vision; increased intraocular pressure (24 to 32 mm Hg) as measured by a tonometer
   2. Angle-closure glaucome
      a. Subjective: nausea; halos around lights; severe frontal headache
      b. Objective: loss of peripheral vision; steamy cornea; redness and swelling of the conjunctiva; increased intraocular pressure (50 to 70 mm Hg) as measured with a tonometer

C. Therapeutic interventions
   1. Lowering the intraocular pressure with topical alpha-adrenergics, prostaglandins, beta blockers, and cholinergics; oral carbonic anhydrase inhibitors
   2. Surgical intervention to facilitate drainage of the aqueous humor: laser iridotomy or trabeculectomy; laser trabeculoplasty; filtering procedures

Nursing Care of Clients With Glaucoma

A. Assessment/Analysis
   1. Description of onset and progression of symptoms
   2. Visual acuity; peripheral vision
   3. Characteristics of sclera, pupil, and anterior chamber

B. Planning/Implementation
  1. Teach the importance of thorough eye examinations including visual field mapping to identify forms of glaucoma
  2. Explain the importance of continued use of eye medications as ordered to prevent further visual loss
  3. Explain the need for continued medical supervision for measurement of intraocular pressure to ensure control of the disorder
  4. Teach avoidance of exertion, stooping, straining for a bowel movement, coughing, or heavy lifting, and use of atropine because these increase intraocular pressure
  5. Instruct to report severe eye or brow pain and nausea to the physician
C. Evaluation/Outcomes
  1. Maintains present level of visual acuity
  2. Remains free from injury

❖ DETACHED RETINA

Data Base
A. Etiology and pathophysiology
  1. Retina separates from the choroid and vitreous humor seeps behind the retina
  2. May result from trauma, the aging process, or cataract surgery; also seen in clients with myopia greater than −6 or diabetes mellitus
B. Clinical findings
  1. Subjective: flashes of light; floaters; sensation of a veil in the line of sight
  2. Objective: loss of vision; retinal separation noted on ophthalmoscopy
C. Therapeutic interventions
  1. Bed rest, with area of detachment in a dependent position to promote healing
  2. Tranquilizers for rest and to reduce anxiety
  3. Surgical intervention
    a. Cryosurgery: supercooled probe causes retinal scarring to reattach retina
    b. Photocoagulation: laser beam through the pupil produces a retinal burn, which causes scarring of the involved area
    c. Scleral buckling: depressing the sclera to force choroid closer to retina
    d. Pneumatic retinopexy: injection of a gas bubble or other substance into the vitreous cavity to apply pressure on the detached portion of the sensory retina, keeping it in contact with the retinal pigment epithelium; used with cryosurgery or photocoagulation
    e. Vitrectomy: a small incision is made in the sclera to allow for specialized instruments; the vitreous gel is suctioned from inside the eye and replaced with gas to reposition the retinal layers; the body naturally replaces the fluid over time as the gas is absorbed; may be combined with scleral buckling

Nursing Care of Clients With Detached Retina
A. Assessment/Analysis
  1. Description of onset and progression of symptoms; history to identify contributing factors such as trauma or recent surgery of the eye
  2. Visual acuity
  3. Status of retina via ophthalmoscopic examination
B. Planning/Implementation
  1. Provide accurate information in a calm voice; client's anxiety is high as a result of the sudden, unexpected vision loss
  2. Keep on bed rest in position as ordered
  3. Provide a call bell and answer promptly
  4. Maintain protective eye patch
  5. Instruct client to avoid activities that increase intraocular pressure such as coughing, straining, and stooping
  6. Observe for signs and symptoms of hemorrhage postoperatively (e.g., severe pain, restlessness)
  7. Diminish lights in the room
  8. Position clients who have had pneumatic retinoplasty so that gas bubble is in the best location to seal the detachment
C. Evaluation/Outcomes
  1. Reports improved vision
  2. Remains free from injury

❖ OTOSCLEROSIS

Data Base
A. Etiology and pathophysiology
  1. Fixation of the stapes caused by the growth of bone, preventing transmission of vibrations and resulting in a progressive conductive hearing loss
  2. Cause unknown, but incidence higher in females; autosomal dominant trait
B. Clinical findings
  1. Subjective: hearing loss; possible tinnitus
  2. Objective: use of a tuning fork shows bone conduction better than air conduction (Rinne test); presence of spongy bone in the labyrinth
C. Therapeutic interventions
  1. Hearing aids to amplify sound
  2. Stapedectomy: removal of the diseased portion of the stapes and replacement with a prosthetic implant to conduct vibrations from the middle to inner ear

Nursing Care of Clients With Otosclerosis
A. Assessment/Analysis
  1. History of onset and progression of symptoms
  2. Extent of hearing loss via audiometry
  3. Rinne test to evaluate loss of air conduction
B. Planning/Implementation
  1. Position postoperatively according to orders: lying on the operated side facilitates drainage; lying on the nonoperated side helps prevent displacement of graft
  2. Instruct client to alter position gradually to prevent vertigo

3. Question about pain, headache, vertigo, or unusual sensations in ear
4. Instruct avoidance of sneezing, blowing nose, swimming, showering, and flying until permitted by physician; if the client must sneeze, instruct to keep mouth open to equalize pressure in ear
5. Explain that because of edema from surgery and the presence of packing, hearing will be diminished but will improve

C. Evaluation/Outcomes
1. Reports improved hearing ability
2. Remains free from injury
3. Establishes effective communication

MÉNIÈRE'S DISEASE (ENDOLYMPHATIC HYDROPS)

Data Base
A. Etiology and pathophysiology
1. Chronic, inner ear disease that incapacitates because of sudden, severe attacks of vertigo
2. Caused by endolymph in the vestibular and semicircular canals
3. Incidence highest in males between 20 and 60 years of age
B. Clinical findings
1. Subjective: vertigo; nausea; headache; tinnitus; sensitivity to loud sounds; sensory hearing loss, usually unilateral; aural fullness
2. Objective: vomiting; diaphoresis; nystagmus during attacks; Weber test and auditory testing document unilateral hearing loss
C. Therapeutic interventions
1. Pharmacologic therapy: meclizine (Antivert); diuretics; antihistamines; diazepam (Valium)

2. Destruction of vestibular nerve, which can cause deafness depending on the approach
3. Insertion of endolymphatic drainage shunt may relieve symptoms without loss of hearing
4. Low-sodium diet

Nursing Care of Clients With Ménière's Disease
A. Assessment/Analysis
1. Description of onset and progression of symptoms; situations that precipitate an attack
2. History of allergies or infections that may complicate the disorder
3. Extent of hearing loss via audiometry
4. Weber test to determine auditory loss
B. Planning/Implementation
1. Support emotionally
2. Encourage avoidance of rapid movements to limit the onset of symptoms
3. Teach self-protection from injury during attack (e.g., pull off the road if driving, lie down); maintain bed rest in the presence of severe vertigo
4. Ensure client understands that surgical options are considered for management of vertigo, and hearing loss may continue
5. Teach avoidance of foods high in salt, such as salted meats and fish, cheese, condensed milk, carrots, and spinach
C. Evaluation/Outcomes
1. Reports a reduction in frequency and intensity of vertigo
2. Remains free from injury
3. Establishes effective communication

Nursing Care of Clients With Urinary/Reproductive System Disorders

OVERVIEW

REVIEW OF ANATOMY AND PHYSIOLOGY OF THE URINARY SYSTEM

Functions of the Urinary System

A. Secrete urine
B. Eliminate urine from body
  1. Excrete normal and abnormal metabolic wastes
  2. Regulate BP and the composition and volume of blood; maintain fluid, electrolyte, and acid-base balance

Structures of the Urinary System

(Figure 12-1: Structures of the male and female urinary systems)

Kidneys

A. Gross anatomy
  1. Shaped like lima beans; lie against posterior abdominal wall, behind peritoneum at level of last thoracic and first three lumbar vertebrae; right kidney slightly lower than left
  2. External structures: hilum, renal capsule
  3. Internal structures: cortex, medulla, pyramids, columns, papillae, calyces, pelvis
B. Blood flow in the kidney
  1. Kidneys receive 20% of cardiac output during rest; reduced to 2% to 4% during physical or emotional stress
  2. Abdominal aorta gives rise to renal arteries, which enter the hilum of each kidney; eventually branch into afferent arterioles, which enter glomerular capillary beds
  3. Efferent arterioles leave the glomerular capillary bed; eventually converge into progressively larger veins until leaving the kidney
C. Nephron
  1. Anatomic and functional unit of the kidney; approximately 1 million per kidney
  2. Functions via principles of filtration, reabsorption, and secretion (Figure 12-2: Glomerular filtration, tubular reabsorption, and tubular secretion)
    a. Glomerulus: urine formation starts with filtration; water and solutes (except cellular elements of blood, albumins, fibrinogen, and other blood proteins) filter out of capillaries through glomerular-capsular membrane and into Bowman's capsule
    b. Bowman's capsule: filtrate collects here before flow to the tubules
    c. Tubular reabsorption and secretion
      (1) Proximal tubule
        (a) Reabsorption of glucose and other nutrients mainly by active transport
        (b) Reabsorption of electrolytes from the tubule filtrate to blood in the peritubular capillaries; forms network of capillaries around tubules; cations (notably sodium) reabsorbed by active transport, stimulated by aldosterone; anions (notably chloride and bicarbonate) are reabsorbed by diffusion following cation transport
        (c) Reabsorption of about 80% of the water from the tubular filtrate to the blood by osmosis
      (2) Loop of Henle: establishes osmotic conditions that promote water reabsorption and actively transport chloride ions from the filtrate, thus passively removing sodium ions with the chloride
      (3) Distal tubule
        (a) Reabsorption of electrolytes, particularly sodium; influenced by the mineralocorticoid aldosterone
        (b) Reabsorption of water into the blood by osmosis; controlled by antidiuretic hormone
        (c) Secretion of hydrogen, potassium, and ammonia from blood in the peritubular capillaries to the tubular filtrate, via active transport
D. Collecting tubules: final osmotic reabsorption of most of the remaining water in urine occurs; under antidiuretic hormone influence
E. Urine description/composition
  1. Amount: 1.5 L/day average (30 mL/hr)
  2. Color: light yellow to dark amber
  3. Odor: aromatic; food and drugs alter odor and color
  4. Specific gravity: 1.005 to 1.030 is average; varies greatly depending on fluid intake and the quantity of solutes; lower specific gravity—more dilute the urine; higher specific gravity—more concentrated the urine
  5. Urine pH: usually acidic (4.5 to 7.5 is average)

F. Urine volume control

1. Glomerular filtration rate (GFR): usually constant (about 125 mL/min); in certain pathologic conditions the GFR may change markedly and alter urine volume (e.g., in shock the GFR decreases, causing oliguria; a decrease in plasma proteins lowers the colloid oncotic pressure, increasing the GFR)
2. Solutes in tubular filtrate: an increase in tubular solutes causes decreased osmosis of water from proximal tubule back into blood and therefore an increase in urine volume (e.g., in diabetes, excess glucose in the tubular filtrate leads to increased urine volume [polyuria, diuresis])
3. Aldosterone mechanism: stimulates kidney tubules to reabsorb sodium, and water follows the sodium
4. Antidiuretic hormone (ADH): produced in hypothalamus and secreted into blood by posterior pituitary gland; secretion stimulated by an increase in the osmotic pressure of extracellular fluid or a decrease in the volume of extracellular fluid; ADH acts on distal and collecting tubules, causing water to osmose from the tubular filtrate back into the blood; this increased water reabsorption tends to increase the total volume of body fluid by decreasing the urine volume

G. Control of amount of blood flow through kidneys

1. Reduced renal blood flow results in renal excretion of the hormone renin
2. Renin interacts with blood proteins, producing angiotensin II
3. Angiotensin II causes vasoconstriction and aldosterone secretion, resulting in an increase in blood pressure and renal blood flow

6. Urea: waste product of protein and amino acid metabolism
7. Uric acid: end product of purine metabolism or oxidation in the body
8. Creatinine: waste product of muscle metabolism
9. Electrolytes: potassium, sodium, calcium, chloride
10. Hormones and their breakdown products
11. Abnormal constituents: glucose, protein, RBCs, ketone bodies, bilirubin, calculi, WBCs

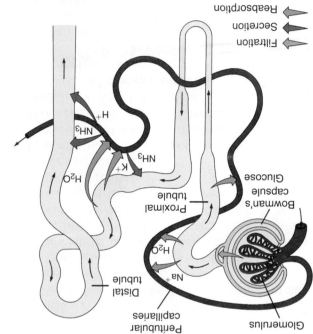

Figure 12-2 Mechanism of urine formation—filtration, reabsorption, and secretion—and where they occur in the nephron. (From Thibodeau GA, Patton KT: *Anatomy and physiology*, ed 4, St. Louis, 2007, Mosby.)

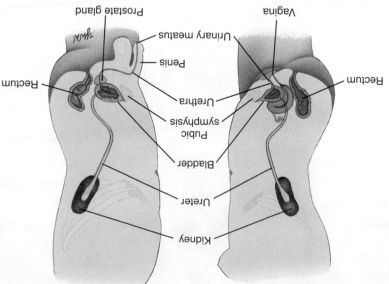

Figure 12-1 Structures of the male and female urinary systems. Sagittal section of the female urinary system (*left*) and male urinary system (*right*), each showing a partially distended bladder. (From Thibodeau GA, Patton KT: *Anatomy and physiology*, ed 6, St Louis, 2007, Mosby.)

Ureters

A. Location: behind the parietal peritoneum
B. Structure: ureter expands as it enters the kidney to form the renal pelvis; subdivided into calyces, each of which contains renal papillae
C. Function: collect urine secreted by the kidney cells and propel it to the bladder by peristaltic waves

Urinary Bladder

A. Location: behind symphysis pubis, below parietal peritoneum
B. Structure: collapsible bag of smooth muscle lined with mucosa arranged in rugae, three openings—two from ureters and one into the urethra
C. Functions: reservoir for urine until sufficient amount accumulated for elimination and expulsion of urine from body by way of urethra

Urethra

A. Location
 1. Female: behind the symphysis pubis, anterior to the vagina
 2. Male: extends through the prostate gland, fibrous sheet, and penis
B. Structure: musculomembranous tube lined with mucosa; opening to exterior called urinary meatus
C. Functions
 1. Female: passageway for expulsion of urine
 2. Male: passageway for expulsion of both urine and semen

REVIEW OF ANATOMY AND PHYSIOLOGY OF THE REPRODUCTIVE SYSTEM

Structures of the Male Reproductive System
(Figure 12-3: External and internal male sex organs)

Glands

A. Main male sex glands (gonads) are the testes
 1. Location: in the scrotum, one testis in each compartment (two compartments)
 2. Structure: composed of tiny tubules called seminiferous tubules, embedded in connective tissue containing interstitial cells; ducts emerge to enter head of epididymis
 3. Functions
  a. Seminiferous tubules form spermatozoa (male sex cells or gametes); process called spermatogenesis (occurs at puberty)
  b. Interstitial cells secrete testosterone, the main androgen, or male hormone; increases protein synthesis, induces growth of secondary sexual characteristics, and promotes development of brain in fetus
B. Accessory glands
 1. Seminal vesicles: secrete nutrient-rich fluid estimated to constitute about 30% of semen
 2. Prostate gland: secretes estimated 60% of semen; prostatic secretion is alkaline, which increases sperm motility, and contains abundance of the enzyme acid phosphatase; therefore blood level of this enzyme increases in metastasizing cancer of prostate
 3. Bulbourethral glands (Cowper's glands): secrete alkaline fluid that lubricates urethra before ejaculation

Ducts

A. Epididymis: conducts seminal fluid (semen) from testes to vas deferens; sperm mature while semen is stored before ejaculation
B. Vas deferens (seminal ducts): conduct sperm and small amount of fluid from each epididymis to an ejaculatory duct
C. Ejaculatory ducts: ejaculate semen into urethra
D. Urethra: see description under Structures of the Urinary System

Supporting Structures

A. External: scrotum and penis
 1. Scrotum: contains testes, epididymis, and first part of seminal duct; allows sperm to develop

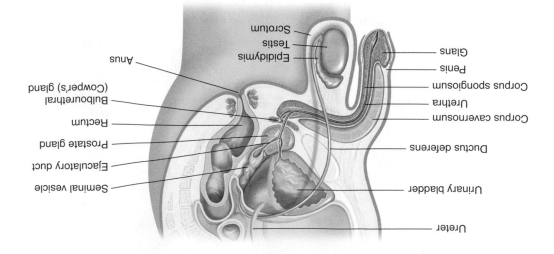

Figure 12-3 External and internal male sex organs. (From Thibodeau GA, Patton KT: *The human body in health and disease*, ed 4, St. Louis, 2005, Mosby.)

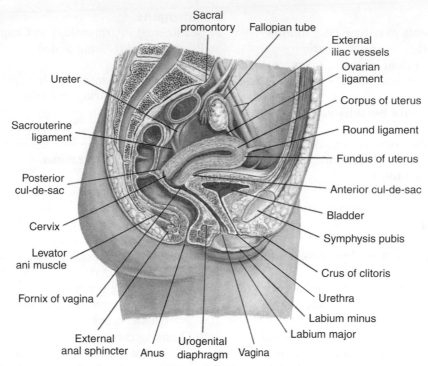

Figure 12-4 Female reproductive tract and related organs. (From Seidel HM et al: *Mosby's guide to physical examination*, ed 6, St Louis, 2006, Mosby.)

at 2 to 3 degrees below body temperature, which is ideal for sperm development

2. Penis: contains large vascular spaces that when filled with blood cause erection of penis; contains the urethra

B. Internal: spermatic cords are fibrous tubes located in each inguinal canal; torsion of testes twists the cords, destroys sperm, interrupts blood supply, and can result in cell death and gangrene

Structures of the Female Reproductive System

(Figure 12-4: Female reproductive tract and related organs) See Female Reproductive System

REVIEW OF MICROORGANISMS

Bacterial Pathogens

A. *Enterobacter aerogenes:* gram-negative bacillus; causes urinary tract infections

B. *Haemophilus ducreyi:* gram-negative bacillus; causes the venereal ulcer called chancroid (soft chancre)

C. *Neisseria gonorrhoeae:* gram-negative diplococcus; causes gonorrhea; transmitted sexually

D. *Pseudomonas aeruginosa:* gram-negative bacillus; infection characterized by blue-green pus; a common secondary invader of wounds, burns, outer ear, and urinary tract; transmitted by catheters and other hospital instruments if contaminated

E. *Treponema pallidum:* highly motile spirochete; causes syphilis; transmitted sexually

F. *Chlamydia trachomatis:* intracellular parasite characterized as a bacteria because of cell wall composition and process of reproduction; they

reproduce only within cells; causes a variety of diseases including genital infections in men and women

Protozoal Pathogen

A. *Trichomonas vaginalis:* a flagellated protozoan; causes trichomonas vaginitis; transmitted sexually

Viral Pathogens

A. Human immunodeficiency virus (HIV): causes acquired immunodeficiency syndrome (AIDS); primarily transmitted sexually and by blood

B. Herpesvirus hominis: causes herpes genitalis; transmitted via genital or oral-genital routes

C. Human papillomavirus (genital or venereal warts [condylomata acuminata]): characterized by papillary or cauliflower-like masses in or on the genitourinary structures; may be a precursor to cancer of the cervix; vaccine available

RELATED PHARMACOLOGY

Kidney-Specific Antiinfectives

A. Description

1. Exert an antibacterial effect on renal tissue and the ureters and bladder

2. Used to treat local urinary tract infections

3. Available in oral and parenteral (IV) preparations

B. Examples: nalidixic acid (NegGram), nitrofurantoin (Macrobid, Macrodantin)

C. Major side effects: nausea, vomiting (irritation of gastric mucosa); skin rash (hypersensitivity); CNS disturbances (neurotoxicity); blood dyscrasias (decreased RBCs, WBCs, and platelet synthesis); hepatotoxicity; exfoliative dermatitis; interstitial pneumonitis

D. Nursing care
1. Administer with meals to reduce GI irritation
2. Monitor blood work, cultures, and urinary output
3. Encourage increased fluid intake to promote drug excretion and prevent toxicity and crystal formation
4. Nalidixic acid: assess for potentiation of anticoagulant effect
5. Nitrofurantoins: dilute oral suspensions in milk or juice to prevent staining of teeth; instruct client that the urine will appear brown

Sulfonamides
See Sulfonamides under Related Pharmacology in Chapter 3

Urinary Spasmolytics
A. Description
1. Directly affect the smooth muscle of the urinary tract
2. Used for symptomatic relief of incontinence
B. Examples: flavoxate HCl (Urispas), oxybutynin Cl (Ditropan), tolterodine (Detrol)
C. Major side effects related to anticholinergic effect: tachycardia, palpitations, dry mouth, constipation, drowsiness, blurred vision, urinary retention, allergic reaction
D. Nursing care
1. Do not administer if GI obstruction is present
2. Administer cautiously to clients with glaucoma
3. Advise client to avoid driving and other hazardous activities; avoid hot environments
4. Monitor urinary output

Androgens
A. Description
1. Hormones that promote secondary sex characteristics in men and have anabolic properties; stimulate building and repair of body tissue
2. Used in debilitating conditions, for inoperable breast cancer, and to restore hormone levels in males; treatment of fibrocystic breast disease, dysmenorrhea, and severe postpartum breast engorgement in nonnursing mothers
3. Available in oral, parenteral (IM, Sub-Q), and buccal preparations
B. Examples: fluoxymesterone (Halotestin); danazol (Danocrine)
C. Major side effects: weight gain, edema (sodium and water retention); acne, changes in libido (androgen effect); hoarseness, deep voice (virilism—androgen effect); nausea, vomiting (irritation of gastric mucosa; hypercalcemia), emotional lability
D. Nursing care
1. Assess for clinical findings of virilization in females
2. Encourage a diet high in calories and proteins to aid in building body tissues and low in sodium to limit edema
3. Administer with meals to reduce GI irritation
4. Monitor BP during course of therapy
5. Assess for potentiation of anticoagulant effect

Estrogens
See Related Pharmacology in Chapter 23, Nursing Care to Promote Childbearing and Women's Health
Progestins
See Related Pharmacology in Chapter 23, Nursing Care to Promote Childbearing and Women's Health

RELATED PROCEDURES

Urinary Catheterization
A. Definitions
1. Sterile introduction of a catheter through the urethra into the bladder
2. Intermittent (straight) catheterization: to drain urine, obtain a urine specimen, or determine a residual volume (amount of urine left in the bladder after voiding)
3. Indwelling (retention) catheterization: inflated balloon holds catheter in place; attached to a collecting bag; bladder is continually emptied by gravity
B. Nursing care
1. Explain procedure to client; provide privacy
2. Position the female client supine with the knees flexed and abducted and the male client supine with the knees slightly abducted
3. Use sterile technique; test balloon by inflating and deflating before insertion
4. Place a sterile fenestrated drape over the external genitalia, exposing meatus
5. Cleanse the urinary meatus using cotton balls saturated with suitable solution
   a. For female clients separate the labia minora with thumb and forefinger and cleanse from anterior to posterior using one pledget for each stroke (keep labia separated once cleansing begins)
   b. For male clients hold the penis between thumb and forefinger and cleanse from meatus to shaft using one pledget for each stroke (retract foreskin during this procedure and replace after procedure)
6. Insert lubricated catheter into the bladder
   a. For female clients insert approximately 7.5 cm or slightly past the point at which urine returns
   b. For male clients, hold the penis perpendicular to the body and insert catheter 17 to 25 cm or well past the point at which urine returns
   c. Attempt balloon inflation; if any resistance is met, deflate balloon, insert catheter further, and reattempt inflation
7. Drain urine slowly by gravity
   a. Intermittent catheterization: remove catheter when bladder is empty
   b. Retention catheterization: inflate balloon with sterile solution and place closed collection system below level of bladder; hang bag from bed frame, not siderails
8. Assist the client to a comfortable position and record data on appropriate records

9. Ensure patency of catheter: eliminate kinks, dependent loops, and clogs; secure catheter to client's leg to prevent telescoping action in urethra
10. Wash genital area with soap and water daily and as necessary
11. Keep system closed at all times; collect urine specimen from port along tubing using sterile technique
12. Monitor output hourly if client is critically ill
13. Prepare for removal of indwelling catheter by intermittently clamping tubing to restore muscle tone; flaccidity of urinary sphincter may occur after catheter is removed; situational incontinence and dribbling may occur temporarily; monitor for urinary output of sufficient quantity (200 mL or more) within 6 to 8 hours after removal of indwelling catheter

Continuous Bladder Irrigation (CBI)

A. Definition
1. Instillation of sterile isotonic solution into the bladder through a triple-lumen catheter: one for instillation of fluid into balloon tip, one for instillation of fluid into bladder, and one for return of fluid and urine from the bladder (Figure 12-5: Continuous bladder irrigation)
2. Used to prevent occlusion of catheter by clots or to administer local antibiotic treatment

B. Nursing care
1. Connect catheter port to irrigant via intravenous tubing using sterile technique
2. Set rate of infusion as ordered; order may state that flow should be sufficient to keep the drainage pink; if red, bloody drainage or clots occur, CBI should be increased to achieve pink drainage
3. Maintain infusion continuously, observing color, clarity, and amount of drainage
4. Assess for clinical findings of dilutional hyponatremia
5. Deduct irrigant from total urinary output to calculate actual urine output

MAJOR DISORDERS OF URINARY/ REPRODUCTIVE SYSTEMS

See Chapter 24, Nursing Care Related to Major Disorders Affecting Women's Health for additional disorders

URINARY TRACT INFECTIONS (UTIs)

Data Base

A. Etiology and pathophysiology
1. Cystitis is inflammation of the bladder wall usually caused by an ascending bacterial infection (*Escherichia coli* is most common)
   a. Common in females: shorter urethra, childbirth, anatomic proximity of the urethra to rectum
   b. Occurs in men secondary to epididymitis, prostatitis, renal calculi

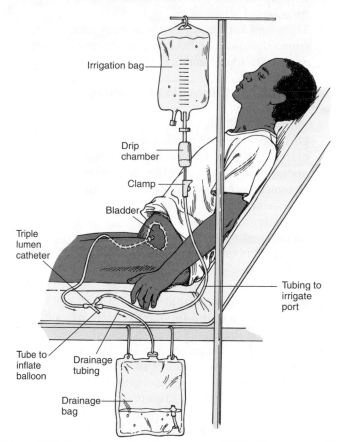

Figure 12-5 Continuous bladder irrigation (CBI). (From Potter PA, Perry AG: *Fundamentals of nursing*, ed 6, St Louis, 2005, Mosby.)

2. Urethritis is inflammation of the urethra caused by staphylococci, *Escherichia coli, Pseudomonas* species, and streptococci
   a. Although inflammatory clinical findings are similar to gonorrheal urethritis, sexual contact is not the cause
   b. May cause prostatitis and epididymitis
3. Urosepsis is caused by gram-negative bacteria
   a. May result from an indwelling urinary catheter or an untreated urinary tract infection
   b. Can lead to septic shock and death

B. Clinical findings
1. Subjective: urgency; frequency; pain when bearing down during urination
2. Objective: nocturia; hematuria; pyuria; cloudy urine; positive urine culture

C. Therapeutic interventions
1. Identification of causative organism through urine culture
2. Pharmacologic therapy with antibiotics, urinary antiseptics, antispasmodics
3. Diet directed toward altering the properties of urine (e.g., cranberry juice—contributes to hostile environment for bacterial growth; eliminate caffeine because it contributes to bladder irritability)
4. Additional fluids to dilute the urine
5. Warm sitz baths to provide comfort

6. Urinary dilation and instillation of antiseptic solutions
7. Treatment for urosepsis: IV therapy with aminoglycosides or beta-lactam antibiotics such as aztreonam (Azactam)

Nursing Care of Clients With Urinary Tract Infections

A. Assessment/Analysis
   1. Urine for color, clarity, odor, blood, or mucus; presence of dysuria, burning, discharge
   2. Suprapubic area for bladder distention
   3. In males, rectal examination for prostate tenderness or enlargement
B. Planning/Implementation
   1. Obtain urine specimen for culture and sensitivity before administering ordered antibiotics; refrigerate specimen if it cannot be sent to the laboratory immediately
   2. Teach to seek medical attention at first sign of clinical findings and to take medications as directed
   3. Encourage the intake of additional fluids
   4. Promote physical comfort
   5. Teach preventive measures such as performing perineal care, avoiding tub baths, voiding after intercourse, wearing cotton underwear
   6. Teach clients at risk for recurrent UTIs that frequent follow-up care with culture and sensitivity testing of the urine is indicated
C. Evaluation/Outcomes
   1. Expresses relief of pain on urination
   2. Resumes expected urinary patterns
   3. Describes methods to prevent recurrence of infection

✿ UROLITHIASIS AND NEPHROLITHIASIS

Data Base

A. Etiology and pathophysiology: formation of stones in the urinary tract; stones may be composed of calcium phosphate, uric acid, or oxalate; they tend to recur and may cause obstruction, infection, and/or hydronephrosis
B. Clinical findings
   1. Subjective: severe pain in kidney area radiating down flank to pubic area (renal colic), frequency, urgency, nausea; history of associated health problems (e.g., gout, hyperparathyroidism, immobility, dehydration, UTIs)
   2. Objective: diaphoresis, pallor, grimacing, vomiting, hematuria, and pyuria if infection is present
C. Therapeutic interventions
   1. Opioids and NSAIDs for pain
   2. Antispasmodics to reduce renal colic
   3. Allopurinol (Zyloprim) or sulfinpyrazone (Anturane) to reduce uric acid excretion
   4. Antibiotics to reduce infection
   5. Intake and output; strain urine
   6. Diet therapy
      a. Large fluid intake to produce dilute urine
      b. Diet altered according to type of stone

(1) Calcium stones: low-calcium diet (400 mg daily), achieved by eliminating dairy products; if phosphate involvement, limit high-phosphorus foods (e.g., dairy products, meat); if oxalate involvement, avoid oxalate-rich foods (e.g., tea, almonds, cashews, chocolate, cocoa, beans, spinach, rhubarb); because calcium stones have an alkaline chemistry, an acid-ash diet can be used to create an acidic urinary tract, which is less conducive to their formation; encourage whole grains, eggs, cranberry juice; limit milk, vegetables, fruit; provide riboflavin, vitamins A and C, and folic acid supplements

(2) Uric acid stones: uric acid is a metabolic product of purines; limit purine foods (e.g., meat [especially organ meats], meat extracts, and to a lesser extent whole grains and legumes); alkaline-ash diet because the stone composition is acid

(3) Cystine stones (rare): low methionine intake because methionine is the essential amino acid from which the nonessential amino acid cystine is formed; limit protein foods (meat, milk, eggs, cheese); alkaline-ash diet, because the stone is an acid composition

7. Surgical intervention if stone is not passed or complications are present (e.g., nephrolithotomy, ureterolithotomy, cystolithectomy)
8. Percutaneous ultrasonic lithotripsy (PUL)
   a. Less traumatic alternative to surgery
   b. Nephroscope is inserted through skin into kidney
   c. Ultrasonic waves disintegrate stones that are then removed by suction and irrigation
9. Laser lithotripsy: utilizes lasers with ureteroscope
10. Extracorporeal shock-wave lithotripsy (ESWL): client is exposed to shock waves that disintegrate stones so that they can be passed with urine

Nursing Care of Clients With Urolithiasis and Nephrolithiasis

A. Assessment/Analysis
   1. Vital signs, particularly temperature, for baseline data
   2. Urine for color, clarity, pH, odor
   3. Urine for presence of stones (strain all urine); intake and output
B. Planning/Implementation
   1. Administer analgesics as ordered
   2. Encourage to set own pattern of activity; provide periods for undisturbed rest
   3. Encourage fluid intake of 3000 to 4000 mL daily
   4. Administer antibiotics as ordered to prevent infection
   5. Encourage to remain on diet; teach to read labels on food for presence of contraindicated additives such as calcium or phosphate

6. Encourage daily weight-bearing exercise, when not contraindicated, to prevent hypercalciuria caused by release of calcium from the bones
7. Provide care after a nephrolithotomy or percutaneous ultrasonic lithotripsy
   a. Change dressings frequently during the first 24 hours after a nephrolithotomy
   b. Maintain patency of urethral catheter to prevent hydronephrosis; call physician if urine output is less than 50 mL/hr
   c. Encourage use of incentive spirometry and coughing and deep breathing to prevent atelectasis

C. Evaluation/Outcomes
   1. States relief of pain
   2. Establishes expected urine flow
   3. Describes strategies for prevention of stone formation

ACUTE KIDNEY FAILURE

Data Base

A. Etiology and pathophysiology
   1. Usually follows trauma to the kidneys or overwhelming physiologic stress (e.g., burns, septicemia, nephrotoxic drugs and chemicals, hemolytic blood transfusion reaction, severe shock, renal vascular occlusion) that decreases blood flow to the glomeruli or to the nephrons
   2. Sudden and almost complete loss of glomerular and/or tubular function
   3. May cause death from acidosis, potassium intoxication, pulmonary edema, or infection
   4. May progress from anuric or oliguric phase through diuretic phase to convalescent phase (which can take 6 to 12 months) to return of function or may progress to chronic renal failure

B. Clinical findings
   1. Subjective: irritability; headache; anorexia; circumoral numbness; tingling of extremities (hypocalcemia); lethargy and drowsiness that can progress from stupor to coma
   2. Objective
      a. Sudden drop in urinary output appearing a few hours after the causative event; oliguria—output less than 400 mL but more than 100 mL/24 hours; anuria—output less than 100 mL/24 hours
      b. Restlessness, twitching, seizures
      c. Nausea and vomiting
      d. Skin pallor, anemia, and increased bleeding time, which can progress to epistaxis and internal hemorrhage
      e. Ammonia (urine) odor to breath and perspiration, which can progress to uremic frost on skin and pruritus
      f. Generalized edema, hypervolemia, hypertension, and increased venous pressure; can progress to pulmonary edema and heart failure
      g. Deep, rapid respirations to compensate for metabolic acidosis
      h. Elevated serum levels of BUN, creatinine, potassium; decreased pH, carbon dioxide combining power, and serum levels of calcium and sodium
      i. Albumin in urine, decreased urine specific gravity

C. Therapeutic interventions
   1. Correct the underlying cause of acute renal failure (e.g., treat shock, eliminate drugs and toxins, treat transfusion reactions, restore integrity of urinary tract)
   2. Complete bed rest
   3. Diet therapy
      a. Calories and protein adequate for maintenance and to prevent tissue breakdown: 2000 to 2500 daily; protein low to moderate according to tolerance: 30 to 50 g; carbohydrate relatively high for energy: 300 to 400 g; fat relatively moderate: 70 to 90 g
      b. Sodium controlled according to serum levels and excretion tolerance: varying from 400 to 2000 mg; potassium controlled according to serum levels and excretion capacities: varying from 1300 to 1900 mg
      c. Water controlled according to excretion: about 800 to 1000 mL
      d. Calcium intake of 1000 mg/day to prevent or delay progression of renal osteodystrophy or demineralization of bone, which results from chronic acidosis and altered vitamin A metabolism; vitamin supplements because of dietary restrictions; calcium supplements only when serum phosphate is under control because of risk for precipitation of calcium phosphate in the kidney; phosphorus intake of less than 600 mg/day to delay progression of renal insufficiency; restriction of milk (1 cup or less per day), meats, poultry, fish, eggs, and cereal grain products; avoid soft drinks and beer
      e. Renal diet low in water-soluble vitamins, iron, and zinc, necessitating daily supplements; dialyzed clients need daily supplements of vitamin B_6 (5 to 10 mg), vitamin C (70 to 100 mg), and folic acid (1 mg)
      f. Total parenteral nutrition (TPN) and parenteral intralipid therapy
   4. Packed RBCs, electrolytes, and glucose IV as necessary
   5. Exchange resins to decrease serum potassium level
   6. Antibiotics to reduce possibility of infection
   7. Peritoneal dialysis, hemodialysis, or hemofiltration

Nursing Care of Clients With Acute Kidney Failure

A. Assessment/Analysis
   1. Daily weight, fluid balance, electrolytes, BUN, and creatinine levels
   2. Clinical findings of hyperkalemia and hyponatremia
   3. History of clinical findings and potential causative factors

B. Planning/Implementation
1. Monitor I&O and hourly urine/output; assess for clinical findings of overhydration (e.g., pitting, dependent, sacral, or periorbital edema; crackles or dyspnea; headache, distended neck veins, and hypertension)
2. Provide for fluid and electrolyte balance by monitoring, replacing, or limiting fluids and electrolytes as ordered
3. Provide periods of undisturbed rest to conserve energy and oxygen
4. Protect client from injury caused by bleeding tendency, the possibility of seizures, and a clouded sensorium
5. Observe for early clinical findings of complications (e.g., hemorrhage, seizures, cardiac problems, pulmonary edema, infection)
6. Provide special skin care to prevent breakdown and remove uremic frost
7. Encourage intake of ordered diet; allow choices in the selection of food while recognizing that little variation is possible
8. Support client receiving peritoneal dialysis, hemodialysis, or hemofiltration
C. Evaluation/Outcomes
1. Maintains fluid and electrolyte balance within acceptable limits
2. Adheres to treatment protocols
3. Maintains nutritional status
4. Remains free from injury

CHRONIC KIDNEY FAILURE/ END-STAGE RENAL DISEASE

Data Base
A. Etiology and pathophysiology
1. Occurs as the result of chronic kidney infections, developmental abnormalities, vascular disorders, and destruction of kidney tubules
2. Ongoing deterioration in renal function results in uremia
B. Clinical findings
1. Subjective: lethargy; drowsiness; headache; nausea; pruritus
2. Objective
a. Oliguria; anuria; vomiting; anemia; hypertension; anasarca; uremic frost; urochromatic pigmentation (bronze pigmentation)
b. Decreased serum calcium level (causing tetany) and pH (metabolic acidosis); increased serum phosphate and potassium levels; azotemia; radiograph reveals renal osteodystrophy
c. Kussmaul respirations, mental clouding, seizures, coma, death
C. Therapeutic interventions
1. Fluid and sodium restriction
2. Antihypertensive medications
3. Recombinant human erythropoietin (Epogen) to manage anemia

4. Dietary management
a. Very low protein (20 g); minimal essential amino acids makes body use own excess urea nitrogen to synthesize nonessential amino acids needed for tissue protein production
b. Controlled electrolytes, especially potassium (1500 mg)
c. See Acute Kidney Failure for additional diet therapy information
5. Continuous arteriovenous hemofiltration (CAVH); hemofiltration is based on the principle of convection, which is that some elements in plasma fluid are conveyed across a semipermeable membrane as a result of differences in hydrostatic pressure in the system; can use previously established fistulas or externally placed access points without the need for external pumps or dialysis machines; the client's BP is the driving force
6. Peritoneal dialysis: dialyzing solution is introduced via a catheter inserted in the peritoneal cavity; the peritoneal membrane is used as a dialyzing membrane to remove toxic substances, metabolic wastes, and excess fluid
a. Intermittent: involves 6 to 48 hours several times a week
b. Continuous ambulatory peritoneal dialysis (CAPD): involves approximately three or four exchanges a day, 7 days a week, and can be administered at home
7. Hemodialysis: the client is attached (via a surgically created arteriovenous fistula or loop graft; see Figure 12-6: Types of access for hemodialysis) to a machine that pumps the blood along a semipermeable membrane; dialyzing solution is on the other side of the membrane, and osmosis and/or diffusion of wastes, toxins, and fluid from the client occurs
8. Kidney transplant from compatible donor
a. Human leukocyte antigen (HLA) tests and tissue and blood typing are done to decrease risk for rejection; least risk for rejection occurs if donor and recipient are identical twins
b. Client's own kidney is not removed unless it is infected or enlarged; new kidney is placed generally in the iliac fossa retroperitoneally and the donor's ureter is attached to the bladder to prevent reflux of urine
9. Steroids and immunosuppressives (e.g., cyclosporine [Sandimmune] if a kidney transplant is performed)

Nursing Care of Clients With Chronic Kidney Failure/End-Stage Renal Disease
A. Assessment/Analysis
1. Data related to urinary elimination patterns; hourly output; urine for color, consistency, odor, and amount; electrolyte status; vital signs and BP

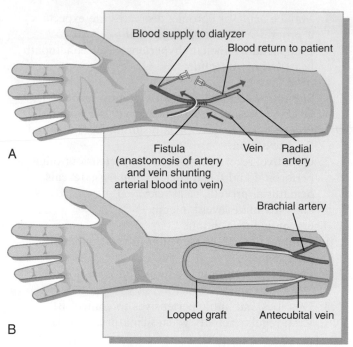

Figure 12-6 Types of access for hemodialysis. **A,** Arteriovenous fistula. **B,** Artificial loop graft. (From Mahan LK, Escott-Stump S: *Krause's food and nutrition therapy*, ed 12, St Louis, 2008, Saunders.)

2. Neurologic status including attention span, weakness, and neuropathies
3. Breath for an ammonia odor
4. Skin for color and the presence of uremic frost
5. Clinical findings of infection associated with dialysis: particularly for pneumonia and of vascular access site
6. Clinical findings of bleeding because of impaired platelet function
7. Emotional status of client and significant others

B. Planning/Implementation
1. Monitor vital signs and intake and output
2. Provide skin care
3. Provide care for the client undergoing dialysis
   a. Explain the procedure and answer questions; assure that a staff member will be available
   b. Weigh before and after procedure
   c. Take vital signs before and after and every 15 minutes during the procedure; assess for hypotension and hemorrhage
   d. Use surgical asepsis in preparation of the site (abdomen or area of fistula); if an abdominal catheter is not in place for peritoneal dialysis, have the client void before inserting catheter
   e. During peritoneal dialysis keep an accurate flow chart and monitor for clinical findings of respiratory distress and peritonitis; reposition to promote drainage from abdomen; drain abdomen if respiratory distress occurs; wash catheter site with soap and water during daily shower; protect site with gauze dressing; monitor serum glucose level
   f. During hemodialysis, watch the site for clotting; check clotting time and administer heparin as

prescribed by the physician; monitor for patency of internal fistula between treatments by palpating for a thrill and auscultating for a bruit; ensure cannulas and tubing are intact; exsanguination can occur in minutes if dislodged; protect access device from trauma or manipulation
   g. Check tubes for patency during both procedures
   h. Provide back care to promote comfort and diversional activities to help pass the time because both procedures are long
   i. Refer for nutritional counseling; stress importance of lifelong dietary modifications
   j. Avoid taking BP or phlebotomy in arm with arteriovenous fistula or graft
   k. Monitor for electrolyte imbalances particularly those associated with potassium and sodium
4. Provide care for the client undergoing kidney transplantation
   a. Prepare client and family emotionally for possible outcomes of surgery
   b. Maintain patency of drainage tubes, including the retention catheter; urine is expected; gross hematuria or clots are not expected postoperatively
   c. Monitor fluid and electrolyte balance; initial output is increased because of sodium diuresis; sharp decrease may signal rejection; monitor serum electrolytes, BUN, and creatinine
   d. Monitor weight and vital signs, particularly temperature; isolation may be necessary to prevent infection
   e. Observe for clinical findings of opportunistic infections such as candidiasis, cytomegalovirus infection, and *Pneumocystis jiroveci* pneumonia; teach need to prevent infection by avoiding crowds and using aseptic techniques, especially thorough handwashing
   f. Administer steroids and immunosuppressives as ordered to prevent rejection; explain need for lifelong immunosuppressive therapy
   g. Observe for and teach clinical findings of rejection: malaise, fever, flank pain or tenderness, decreasing urinary output; serum creatinine level will increase

C. Evaluation/Outcomes
1. Maintains fluid and electrolyte balance within expected limits
2. Remains free from infection
3. Adheres to dietary and fluid restrictions
4. Verbalizes feelings
5. Describes clinical findings of transplant rejection

ADENOCARCINOMA OF THE KIDNEY
Data Base
A. Etiology and pathophysiology
1. Most common cancer affecting the kidneys; incidence higher in males
2. Common sites of metastasis include lungs, liver, and long bones

B. Clinical findings
   1. Subjective: may be absent until metastasis occurs; dull back pain; weakness
   2. Objective: weight loss; anemia; elevated temperature; painless hematuria; and enlarged kidney palpable during physical examination
C. Therapeutic interventions
   1. Radical nephrectomy
   2. Partial nephrectomy (heminephrectomy) when neoplasm is bilateral or when only one kidney is functioning
   3. Radiation therapy if tumor is sensitive
   4. Chemotherapy; hormonal therapy with medroxyprogesterone (Provera); drugs for primary renal cell carcinoma: multikinase inhibitor—sorafenib (Nexavar) decreases renal cell tumor growth and angiogenesis; sunitinib (Sutent) inhibits renal cell tumor growth because it interferes with the tumor receiving the blood and nutrients it needs to grow; temsirolimus (Torisel) enzyme inhibitor
   5. Palliative care if condition is terminal

Nursing Care of Clients With Adenocarcinoma of the Kidney

A. Assessment/Analysis
   1. Presence of hematuria, pain
   2. Flank regions for asymmetry
B. Planning/Implementation
   1. Monitor I&O; increase fluids
   2. Administer analgesics as ordered
   3. Observe urine for color, amount, and any abnormal components
   4. Support natural defenses; encourage intake of foods rich in the immune-stimulating nutrients, especially vitamins A, C, and E, and the mineral selenium
   5. Care for the client after a nephrectomy
      a. Encourage coughing and deep breathing while splinting the incision
      b. Examine dressing and linen under the client; more serosanguineous drainage is expected after a partial nephrectomy than a total nephrectomy
      c. Maintain integrity of the urinary drainage system; avoid kinking of tubes; output should exceed 30 mL/hr
C. Evaluation/Outcomes
   1. States reduction in pain
   2. Discusses feelings related to prognosis
   3. Maintains expected urine output

❧ GLOMERULONEPHRITIS

Data Base
A. Etiology and pathophysiology
   1. Damage to both kidneys resulting from filtration and trapping of antigen-antibody complexes within the glomeruli; inflammatory and degenerative changes affect all renal tissue
   2. Often follows a streptococcal infection such as tonsillitis

3. May be acute or chronic; decreases life expectancy if progressive renal damage occurs
4. Complications include hypertensive encephalopathy, heart failure, infection
B. Clinical findings
   1. Subjective: flank pain; costovertebral tenderness; headache; visual disturbances; malaise; weakness; fatigue; anorexia; dyspnea resulting from salt and fluid retention
   2. Objective: fever; tachycardia; hypertension; oliguria; periorbital and facial edema; urinalysis reveals hematuria, protein, casts; elevated plasma, BUN, and creatinine levels; anemia
C. Therapeutic interventions
   1. Antibiotics such as penicillin to treat underlying infection
   2. Dietary restriction of sodium, fluids, and protein based on clinical status
   3. Diuretics and antihypertensives to control BP
   4. Rest; regular activity when hematuria and proteinuria resolve

Nursing Care of Clients With Glomerulonephritis

A. Assessment/Analysis
   1. History of recent upper respiratory tract or skin infections, or invasive procedures
   2. BP for baseline data
   3. Urine for blood, protein
   4. Presence of dyspnea, edema, neck vein engorgement
B. Planning/Implementation
   1. Monitor I&O, daily weight, urine specific gravity
   2. Monitor vital signs, particularly temperature; protect from infection
   3. Provide special prophylactic skin care to prevent skin breakdown because of edema
   4. Observe for complications such as renal failure, heart failure, and hypertensive encephalopathy
   5. Monitor urinalysis, serum electrolytes, BUN, and creatinine levels
   6. Encourage continued medical supervision
   7. Refer for case management as needed; the long-term nature of the illness may create economic and familial problems
C. Evaluation/Outcomes
   1. Maintains fluid balance within acceptable limits
   2. Maintains nutritional status
   3. Describes clinical findings of complications

❧ BLADDER TUMORS

Data Base
A. Etiology and pathophysiology
   1. Most frequent in men more than 50 years of age
   2. Risk factors include smoking, radiation, exposure to certain chemicals over prolonged time, and schistosomiasis
   3. Common sites of metastasis include lymph nodes, bone, liver, and lungs

B. Clinical findings
1. Subjective: frequency and urgency of urination; dysuria
2. Objective: painless hematuria, direct visualization by cystoscopic examination with bladder washings

C. Therapeutic interventions
1. Surgical intervention
   a. Resection of tumor
   b. Cystectomy may be partial (resulting in a decreased capacity) or radical (which requires a urinary diversion)
      (1) Ileal conduit: section of ileum is resected and attached to ureters; one end of ileal segment is sutured closed and other is brought to skin as an ileostomy to drain urine; technique most widely used to divert urine; appliance needed because urine flow is continuous
      (2) Continent ileal urinary reservoir (Indiana, Florida, Koch, or Charleston pouch): similar to an ileal conduit, but involves creation of a nipplelike valve that can be drained by insertion of a catheter
      (3) Nephrostomy: catheter inserted in kidney through an incision
      (4) Ureterostomy: ureters implanted in abdominal wall to drain urine
      (5) Neobladder: the urethra and external anatomy are unchanged, and a new bladder is created internally
2. Radiation therapy
3. Chemotherapy

Nursing Care of Clients With Bladder Tumors

A. Assessment/Analysis
1. Abdomen for bladder distention
2. Urine for hematuria

B. Planning/Implementation
1. Allow time to verbalize fears of surgery, cancer, death, and body-image alterations
2. Prepare bowel preoperatively with laxatives, antibiotics, and enemas as ordered
3. Assess color and amount of urine (at least 50 mL/hr); maintain patency of drainage system; turn and position to promote urine flow
4. Care for the client with an ileal conduit
   a. Cleanse the skin around the stoma and under the drainage bag with soap and water; inspect for excoriation
   b. Dry skin, apply skin adhesive to the area around the stoma, and apply collection device
   c. Maintain the urinary drainage bag, which is fitted snugly around but not touching the stoma, to collect the continuous flow of urine
   d. Encourage self-care; teach the client to change the appliance
5. Care for the client with a continent ileal urinary reservoir: teach client to insert catheter through

nipple valve to drain urine at prescribed times, thus preventing absorption of metabolic wastes from the urine as well as urine reflux into the ureters
6. Expect a variety of psychologic manifestations (e.g., denial, anger or depression)
7. Arrange visit from member of an ostomy club
8. Support natural defenses of client; encourage intake of foods rich in the immune-stimulating nutrients, especially vitamins A, C, and E, and the mineral selenium

C. Evaluation/Outcomes
1. Discusses feelings
2. Demonstrates correct care of stoma and appliance

BENIGN PROSTATIC HYPERPLASIA (BPH)

Data Base

A. Etiology and pathophysiology
1. Slow enlargement of the prostate gland common in men more than 40 years of age
2. Constriction of urethra and subsequent interference in urination; predisposition to hydronephrosis

B. Clinical findings
1. Subjective: frequency, urgency, difficulty initiating stream (hesitancy), feeling of incomplete emptying of bladder after urination
2. Objective: nocturia, hematuria, decreased force of stream, urinary retention; enlarged prostate on digital rectal examination or transurethral ultrasound; biopsy reveals hyperplasia rather than malignancy

C. Therapeutic interventions
1. Relief of acute obstruction by insertion of indwelling or suprapubic cystostomy catheter
2. Pharmacologic management
   a. 5-α-Reductase inhibitors: block the uptake and utilization of androgens by the prostate, reducing glandular hyperplasia; examples include finasteride (Proscar) and dutasteride (Avodart)
   b. α_1-Adrenergic receptor blocking agents, such as terazosin (Hytrin)
   c. Urinary antiseptics and antibiotics to prevent infection from stasis of urine
3. Surgery of the prostate
   a. Transurethral: instruments are inserted through urethra; transurethral ultrasound-guided laser incision of prostate (TULIP), transurethral incision of the prostate (TUIP), and transurethral resection of the prostate (TURP)
   b. Suprapubic: requires incision of abdomen and bladder
   c. Retropubic: requires abdominal incision
   d. Perineal: requires perineal incision; highest risk for incontinence, impotence, and wound contamination

4. Continuous bladder irrigation (CBI) after surgery to promote hemostasis and limit clots that block the catheter
5. Transurethral dilatation of prostate: reduction of prostatic obstruction of urethra via balloon catheter, stent, or coils

Nursing Care of Clients With Benign Prostatic Hyperplasia

A. Assessment/Analysis
1. Urinary function for frequency, urgency, hesitancy; size and force of stream
2. Abdomen for bladder distention
3. Clinical findings indicating impaired urinary function as a result of prolonged obstruction

B. Planning/Implementation
1. Encourage increased fluid intake (2400 to 3000 mL/day)
2. Administer antiseptics and antibiotics as ordered to prevent or treat urinary tract infections after urine for culture is obtained
3. Instruct to avoid anticholinergics and antihistamines because they can cause urinary retention
4. Assist the hospitalized client to a standing position to void; moist heat or a warm shower may relax the urinary sphincter
5. Care for the client after prostate surgery
   a. Observe for clinical findings of hemorrhage (e.g., change in vital signs, pain, clinical findings of shock, frank bleeding)
   b. Maintain patency of the catheter: unobstructed gravity flow, adequate fluid intake, CBI, sterile irrigation as ordered; bladder distention and pain may indicate tube obstruction
   c. Monitor output; volume of irrigant must be subtracted from drainage for clients with CBI (see Continuous Bladder Irrigation under Related Procedures)
   d. Administer prescribed stool softeners to prevent straining and pressure on the operative site, and advise to avoid prolonged sitting, both of which can precipitate hemorrhage
   e. Maintain suprapubic and cystotomy catheters after suprapubic prostatectomy; change dressings frequently after removal of catheter because of urine leakage
   f. Encourage to express concerns about sexual functioning
   g. Provide as much privacy as possible
   h. Instruct to perform perineal exercises to regain urinary control; initially dribbling is common after surgery; notify physician if stream decreases as it may indicate urethral stricture

C. Evaluation/Outcomes
1. Verbalizes concerns about urinary and sexual functioning
2. Achieves expected pattern of urinary elimination

CANCER OF THE PROSTATE

Data Base
A. Etiology and pathophysiology
1. Slow, malignant change in prostate gland that spreads by direct invasion of surrounding tissues and metastasizes to bony pelvis and spine
2. Incidence increases with age; family history is an important risk factor

B. Clinical findings
1. Subjective: frequency; urgency; difficulty initiating stream; back, groin, or lower abdominal pain
2. Objective
   a. Decreased force of stream, urinary retention
   b. Elevated serum acid phosphatase and carcinoembryonic antigen (CEA) levels; increased prostate-specific antigen (PSA) value; alkaline phosphatase level rises with bone metastasis
   c. Digital rectal examination (DRE) reveals enlarged hardened prostate; transurethral ultrasound (TRUS) reveals mass, detects nonpalpable masses; biopsy demonstrates malignancy
   d. Radiolabeled monoclonal antibody capromab pendetide with indium-111 (ProstaScint): an antibody attracted to prostate-specific membrane antigen on prostate cancer cells; the radioactive element is then visualized on scanning; detects metastasis before or after treatment

C. Therapeutic interventions
1. Type of surgical intervention depends on extent of lesion, client's physical condition, and client's acceptance of outcome (impotence follows radical prostatectomy)
2. Radical prostatectomy, done by perineal or retropubic approach, removing the seminal vesicles and a portion of the bladder neck
3. Radiation therapy alone or in conjunction with surgery preoperatively or postoperatively to reduce lesion and limit metastases; high doses of external-beam radiotherapy and/or seed therapy
4. Diethylstilbestrol (estrogen) may be necessary to reduce the size of an inoperable lesion or postoperatively to limit metastases
5. Orchiectomy may be necessary to limit production of testosterone and thus slow the spread of the disease

Nursing Care of Clients With Cancer of the Prostate

A. Assessment/Analysis
1. Progression of urinary clinical findings; presence and location of pain
2. Alterations in urinary functioning
3. Presence of metastasis to bone, lungs, liver, or kidneys

B. Planning/Implementation
1. Provide care similar to that for the client who has undergone prostate surgery for benign prostatic hyperplasia (see Benign Prostatic Hyperplasia)
2. Explain that development of secondary female characteristics will occur as a result of estrogen therapy and not the surgery
3. Allow time and opportunity to express concerns about diagnosis of cancer and impotence; support the client's male image
4. Monitor for evidence of metastasis
5. Provide care for the client receiving radiation (see Radiation and General Nursing Care of Clients With Neoplastic Disorders in Chapter 3)

C. Evaluation/Outcomes
1. Verbalizes concerns regarding sexuality and prognosis
2. Maintains expected pattern of urinary elimination
3. Maintains satisfying sexual expression

CANCER OF THE TESTES

Data Base

A. Etiology and pathophysiology
1. Etiology unknown; contributing factors include infection, cryptorchidism, genetics, and hormone levels
2. Leading cause of death from cancer in men 20 to 35 years old
3. Most are germ cell tumors (seminomas, embryonal carcinomas, teratomas, and choriosarcomas)
4. Metastasizes to the retroperitoneal nodes, lungs, and CNS

B. Clinical findings
1. Subjective: heaviness or dull ache in scrotal area; backache or abdominal pain
2. Objective
   a. Weight loss; enlarged testes; palpable mass; hydrocele

b. Elevated tumor markers: alpha-fetoprotein, beta–human chorionic gonadotropin
c. CT scan of chest and abdomen may show metastasis

C. Therapeutic interventions
1. Orchiectomy (removal of the testis)
2. Retroperitoneal lymph node dissection (RPLND)
3. Radiation
4. Chemotherapy: cisplatin, dactinomycin, vinblastine sulfate

Nursing Care of Clients With Cancer of the Testes

A. Assessment/Analysis
1. Palpation of the testes for enlargement
2. Evidence of metastasis: back pain, dyspnea, cough, dysphagia, altered mental state, and visual changes

B. Planning/Implementation
1. Discuss the possibility of banking sperm before treatment because of risk for sterility
2. Encourage discussion of feelings
3. Provide care for the client receiving either chemotherapy or radiation (see Radiation and General Nursing Care of Clients With Neoplastic Disorders in Chapter 3)

C. Evaluation/Outcomes
1. Verbalizes feelings about sexuality, treatment, and prognosis
2. Maintains satisfying sexual expression

Nursing Care of Clients With Infectious Diseases

OVERVIEW

See Infection in Chapter 3, Integral Aspects of Nursing Care, p. 24, for additional information

MAJOR INFECTIOUS DISEASES

✿ GAS GANGRENE

Data Base

A. Etiology and pathophysiology
   1. Caused by an anaerobic gram-positive clostridium *(Clostridium perfringens, C. welchii, C. novyi)* that enters through a deep wound
   2. Bacilli colonize in muscle tissue around wound; occurs 2 to 5 days after injury
B. Clinical findings
   1. Subjective: pain; apprehension; anorexia; chills
   2. Objective
      a. Bronzed or blackened wound tissue; crepitus; sweetish, foul-smelling watery exudate; necrosis of muscle tissues
      b. Pallor; diarrhea; vomiting; temperature elevation (may be slight)
      c. Presence of *Clostridia* on culture, low hemoglobin (Hgb) value
C. Therapeutic interventions
   1. Multiple incisions for decompression and drainage
   2. Complete removal (extirpation) and debridement of involved tissue followed by copious irrigations
   3. Penicillin G, tetracycline, chloramphenicol, or erythromycin, depending on culture and sensitivity (C&S)
   4. Amputation
   5. Hyperbaric oxygenation
   6. Whole blood, packed RBCs, or plasma transfusions to combat hemolysis and profound anemia
   7. Antitoxin therapy may be started

Nursing Care of Clients With Gas Gangrene

A. Assessment/Analysis
   1. Monitor for specific clinical findings
B. Planning/Implementation
   1. Refer to Chapter 3, Integral Aspects of Nursing Care: Infection, (General Nursing Care of Clients at Risk for Infection)
   2. Prevent further infection from fecal contamination (organism is found in feces)

   3. Use standard and contact precautions
   4. Monitor fluid, electrolyte, and cardiovascular status
C. Evaluation/Outcomes
   1. Adapts to complications
   2. Remains free from infection

✿ TOXOPLASMOSIS

Data Base

A. Etiology and pathophysiology
   1. Caused by protozoan *(Toxoplasma gondii)*, a parasite
   2. Contracted by eating raw meat containing cysts or exposure to contaminated cat feces
   3. Most common opportunistic CNS infection of those with AIDS
   4. During pregnancy can cause congenital anomalies or death of fetus even though mother may be asymptomatic
   5. Leading cause of encephalitis in immunosuppressed clients
B. Clinical findings
   1. Subjective: malaise; fatigue; headache
   2. Objective: fever; seizures; cognitive and motor impairment; lymphadenopathy; positive cultures; brain abscesses
C. Therapeutic interventions
   1. Pregnant women and immunosuppressed clients may be treated with pyrimethamine (Daraprim), azithromycin (Zithromax), sulfadiazine (Microsulfon), clindamycin (Cleocin), and leucovorin (Wellcovorin)
   2. Usually no treatment required for otherwise healthy adults

Nursing Care of Clients With Toxoplasmosis

A. Assessment/Analysis
   1. Monitor for specific clinical findings
B. Planning/Implementation
   1. Refer to Chapter 3, Integral Aspects of Nursing Care: Infection (General Nursing Care of Clients at Risk for Infection)
   2. Use standard precautions
   3. Encourage a diet rich in nutrient-dense foods
   4. Caution pregnant clients to avoid cleaning cat litter pans or gardening where they may be exposed to cat feces

5. Teach about proper handling, preparation, and storage of meat, washing fruits and vegetables, and care of cat litter

C. Evaluation/Outcomes

1. Remains free from infection
2. Continues with follow-up supervision as necessary

✿ MALARIA

Data Base

A. Etiology and pathophysiology

1. Caused by a protozoan *(Plasmodium falciparum, P. vivax, P. ovale, P. malariae)* from a bite by an infected *Anopheles* mosquito, through the use of dirty needles, or by a transfusion from an infected donor
2. Parasite enters the bloodstream and invades RBCs; destruction of RBCs, blockage of capillaries, and irreversible damage to the spleen and liver may follow
3. "Blackwater fever," which causes intravascular hemolysis and hemoglobinuria, is a rare complication
4. Sickle cell trait provides natural resistance

B. Clinical findings

1. Subjective: malaise; headache; muscle aches; chills; thirst
2. Objective: high fever; anemia; enlarged spleen; dehydration; renal failure

C. Therapeutic interventions

1. Antimalarial drugs (pyrimethamine, chloroquine phosphate): for treatment and chemoprophylaxis 1 week before visiting endemic areas and regularly while in the area
2. Aspirin
3. Prevention: avoidance of stagnant pools; insect repellants and protective clothing to prevent mosquito bites

Nursing Care of Clients With Malaria

A. Assessment/Analysis

1. Monitor for specific clinical findings

B. Planning/Implementation

1. Refer to Chapter 3: Integral Aspects of Nursing Care: Infection (General Nursing Care of Clients at Risk for Infection)
2. Monitor fluid and electrolyte balance; maintain hydration
3. Use therapeutic measures to decrease fever
4. Maintain bed rest until the fever and other clinical findings have ceased
5. Support natural defense mechanisms; encourage intake of nutrient-dense foods with emphasis on fruits, vegetables, whole grains, and legumes, especially those high in the immune-stimulating nutrients selenium and vitamins A, C, and E
6. If client is receiving quinine, teach to observe for clinical findings of cinchonism (e.g., tinnitus, vertigo, and deafness) and to take medication with meals to reduce GI irritation

C. Evaluation/Outcomes

1. Continues prophylaxis as necessary
2. Recognizes that organism is always present in blood

✿ RABIES (HYDROPHOBIA)

Data Base

A. Etiology and pathophysiology

1. Caused by a virus (rhabdovirus) spread by bite of an infected animal; the animal can be a carrier and not be ill with the disease
2. Incubation period is 10 to 50 days with bites in the upper parts of the body, 4 months with bites in the lower parts
3. Bites are usually unprovoked; suspected animals are observed for 10 days
4. Virus spreads from the soft tissue surrounding the wound to the peripheral nerves and ultimately affects the CNS; may cause punctate hemorrhages and neuronal destruction
5. Early treatment with vaccine is necessary as once disease develops it is usually fatal

B. Clinical findings

1. Subjective
   a. Anxiety; depression; malaise; lethargy; irritability; headaches; stiff neck; photophobia; dyspnea
   b. Thirst; anorexia; nausea
   c. Paresthesia or pain near the bite or in the bitten extremity
2. Objective
   a. Respiratory difficulty such as wheezing, hyperventilation, and spasms
   b. Hydrophobia: sight, sound, or thought of water triggers painful pharyngeal muscle contractions that expel fluid from mouth
   c. Excessive salivation, frothy drooling, severe difficulty swallowing, choking
   d. Nuchal rigidity, seizures
   e. Apnea, cardiac dysrhythmias
   f. Paralysis, coma

C. Therapeutic interventions

1. Cleansing of the wound with soap and water
2. Tracheostomy if severe respiratory impairment develops
3. Sedatives or anesthetics as necessary; phenytoin (Dilantin) used for seizures
4. Human rabies immune globulin for passive immunity; dose given in the buttock; wound is bathed with the drug
5. Human diploid cell vaccine is used to induce active immunity; treatment consists of five doses over 4 weeks followed by a sixth dose after 2 months

Nursing Care of Clients With Rabies

A. Assessment/Analysis

1. Monitor for specific clinical findings

B. Planning/Implementation

1. Refer to Chapter 3, Integral Aspects of Nursing Care: Infection (General Nursing Care of Clients at Risk for Infection)

2. Avoid contact with the saliva of an infected client
3. Monitor blood gases, fluid and electrolyte balance, and ECGs
4. Keep room dark and quiet to limit agitation
5. Monitor tracheostomy and suction secretions as needed
6. Prevent drafts, which may result in spasms
7. Encourage the client/family to verbalize feelings

C. Evaluation/Outcomes
1. Recovers after vaccine is administered
2. Avoids contact with potential sources of infection
3. Function returns to body part affected by bite

ROCKY MOUNTAIN SPOTTED FEVER

Data Base

A. Etiology and pathophysiology
1. Transmitted by a tick infected with *Rickettsia rickettsii;* there may or may not be a history of a tick bite
2. Sudden onset, with an incubation period of 3 to 17 days
3. Organism attacks endothelial cells and extends into the vessel walls, causing thrombi, inflammation, and necrosis

B. Clinical findings
1. Subjective: malaise; insomnia; headache; anorexia; photophobia; joint and muscle discomfort; hearing loss
2. Objective
   a. Fever; enlarged spleen; hypotension; circulatory collapse; renal collapse
   b. Rash (rose-colored macules); edema; subcutaneous hemorrhage; necrosis

C. Therapeutic interventions
1. Prompt recognition and treatment vital
2. Tetracycline or chloramphenicol therapy continued until the client is afebrile for 3 to 5 days
3. Treatment of clinical findings and complications as they develop

Nursing Care of Clients With Rocky Mountain Spotted Fever

A. Assessment/Analysis
1. Monitor for specific clinical findings

B. Planning/Implementation
1. Refer to Chapter 3, Integral Aspects of Nursing Care: Infection (General Nursing Care of Clients at Risk for Infection)
2. Assure family that client's disturbed emotional responses are associated with the disease
3. Monitor clinical findings to determine progression of the disease
4. Assess the cardiovascular status to determine developing circulatory collapse
5. Reassure that hearing loss will last only several weeks
6. Teach prevention such as wearing tick repellents, checking pants and animals for the presence of ticks, and removing ticks

7. Teach individuals to remove ticks with tweezers to prevent contamination of fingers

C. Evaluation/Outcomes
1. Continues with follow-up supervision as necessary
2. Avoids contact with potential sources of infection

LYME DISEASE

Data Base

A. Etiology and pathophysiology
1. Caused by spirochete bacteria *(Borrelia burgdorferi)* transmitted by carrier tick that acquired bacterium from infected host; disease is most often carried by mice, deer, or raccoons; cats, dogs, and horses may also be carriers
2. Tick injects spirochete-laden saliva into bloodstream, incubates 3 to 32 days, and then migrates outward, causing a rash
3. Initial rash and flulike clinical findings; later neuromusculoskeletal and cardiac clinical findings
4. Most common vector-borne illness in the United States
5. Infectious organism can survive in host 10 years or more

B. Clinical findings
1. Subjective: chills; muscle aches; joint pain; headache; dizziness; stiff neck; nausea
2. Objective
   a. Fever; red-ringed, circular rash (erythema chronicum migrans); swollen joints; lack of coordination; facial palsy; paralysis; dementia
   b. Blood tests include antibody titers, enzyme-linked immunosorbent assay, Western blot assay; a positive result may indicate past or current infection

C. Therapeutic interventions
1. Antibiotics such as penicillin, doxycycline, ceftriaxone sodium (Rocephin)
2. Symptomatic treatment

Nursing Care of Clients With Lyme Disease

A. Assessment/Analysis
1. Monitor for specific clinical findings

B. Planning/Implementation
1. Refer to Chapter 3, Integral Aspects of Nursing Care: Infection (General Nursing Care of Clients at Risk for Infection)
2. Assure family that client's disturbed emotional responses are associated with the disease
3. Monitor clinical findings to determine progression of the disease
4. Question clients with arthritic clinical findings about possible exposure
5. Teach clients to
   a. Avoid tall grass and wooded areas; use chemical repellents; wear light colors to enhance tick identification; wear long sleeves and pants tucked in high boots when walking in areas with tick infestation
   b. Shower and inspect skin

c. Remove ticks with tweezers, grasping close to skin to avoid breaking mouth parts
6. Advise clients who are at risk to receive vaccine
7. Administer antibiotics as ordered
   a. Early Lyme disease: doxycycline, amoxicillin
   b. Severe Lyme disease: ceftriaxone (Rocephin), cefotaxime (Claforan), penicillin G
C. Evaluation/Outcomes
   1. Continues follow-up supervision as necessary
   2. Avoids contact with potential sources of tick

❁ TETANUS (LOCKJAW)

Data Base
A. Etiology and pathophysiology
   1. Caused by an anaerobic bacillus, *Clostridium tetani,* that is transmitted through an open wound; clinical findings from 2 days to 3 weeks after exposure
   2. Toxins from the bacillus invade the nervous tissue, and the motor and sensory nerves become hypersensitive, resulting in prolonged contractions and respiratory failure
B. Clinical findings
   1. Subjective: irritability; restlessness; pain from muscle spasms
   2. Objective: muscle rigidity; spastic contractions of voluntary muscles; spasm of masticatory muscles (trismus); spasms of respiratory tract; grotesque grinning expression (risus sardonicus) caused by spasms of facial muscles
C. Therapeutic interventions
   1. Prompt recognition of potential contamination and treatment vital; tetanus immune globulin (TIG) used to provide temporary passive immunity; tetanus toxoid may also be given in a different site
   2. Once clinical findings develop, specific therapy is ineffective; therefore institution of supportive therapy is necessary until toxins are reduced by time
   3. Maintenance of adequate pulmonary ventilation
   4. Debridement of wound to allow exposure to air
   5. Control of muscle spasms; sedation to limit spasms
   6. Antibiotics to limit secondary infection
   7. Maintenance of fluid balance and nutrition via enteral feedings

Nursing Care of Clients With Tetanus
A. Assessment/Analysis
   1. Monitor for specific clinical findings
B. Planning/Implementation
   1. Refer to Chapter 3, Integral Aspects of Nursing Care: Infection (General Nursing Care of Clients at Risk for Infection)
   2. Prevent the disease through immunization with tetanus toxoid to provide active immunity; prophylaxis in suspect injuries
   3. Initiate seizure precautions; maintain a quiet environment to decrease excessive stimuli, which may result in seizures

4. Frequently assess respiratory status; administer oxygen as needed; mechanical ventilation may be required
5. Suction airway as necessary to maintain patency and promote ventilation; keep an endotracheal tube and tracheostomy set at the bedside
6. Encourage the client/family to verbalize feelings
7. Need to boost immunity with "booster shot" every 10 years
C. Evaluation/Outcomes
   1. Maintains active immunity
   2. Seeks medical assistance with potentially infectious injuries

❁ TYPHOID FEVER

Data Base
A. Etiology and pathophysiology
   1. Caused by the bacterium *Salmonella typhi,* which is carried in human feces and transmitted through sewage, flies, and shellfish; incubation period 3 to 20 days
   2. Bacterium invades the GI tract and localizes in lymph tissue of the intestinal wall (Peyer's patches); these areas may become thrombosed and tissue sloughs off
   3. Hemorrhage, peritonitis, perforation, and hepatitis are serious complications
B. Clinical findings
   1. Subjective: headache; drowsiness
   2. Objective: fever; bradycardia; rose-colored papules on the abdomen; enlarged spleen and liver; delirium; constipation during the early stage; diarrhea during the late stage
C. Therapeutic interventions
   1. Amoxicillin (Amoxil), sulfamethoxazole and trimethoprim (Bactrim), ciprofloxacin (Cipro)
   2. Corticosteroids the first 4 to 5 days of treatment
   3. Maintenance of fluid balance and nutrition
   4. Symptomatic treatment

Nursing Care of Clients With Typhoid Fever
A. Assessment/Analysis
   1. Monitor for specific clinical findings
B. Planning/Implementation
   1. Refer to Chapter 3, Integral Aspects of Nursing Care: Infection (General Nursing Care of Clients at Risk for Infection)
   2. Maintain safety if delirium is present
   3. Encourage a soft diet rich in high-nutrient density and high-calorie foods
   4. Employ methods to decrease the fever
   5. Monitor fluid and electrolytes to prevent imbalance
   6. In addition to standard precautions, use contact precautions if the client is incontinent of feces
   7. Encourage client and family to verbalize concerns precipitated by the illness
   8. Educate the public to prevent disease through proper sewage treatment

9. Encourage vaccination programs with booster injections every 3 years in endemic areas
C. Evaluation/Outcomes
1. Maintains active immunity
2. Practices proper personal hygiene

VIRAL AND BACTERIAL INFECTIOUS GASTROENTERITIS

Data Base

A. Etiology and pathophysiology
1. Gastroenteritis involves inflammation of the stomach and intestines; usually related to contaminated water and food
2. *Staphylococcus aureus:* caused by a strain that clots plasma (coagulase positive); most virulent type; causes a variety of infections
   a. Found in unrefrigerated creams, mayonnaise, stuffing, meats, and fish
   b. Usually transmitted to food on the hands of food handlers
   c. Incubation period is 1 to 6 hours after ingestion of contaminated food, with symptoms lasting 24 to 48 hours
3. *Clostridium botulinum* (botulism): a serious, often fatal form; its exotoxin is the most powerful biologic toxin known
   a. Found in improperly processed foods, mostly canned foods
   b. Blocks neuromuscular transmission in cholinergic nerve fibers by possibly binding with acetylcholine
   c. Incubation period usually 12 to 72 hours after ingestion of contaminated food, but may be as long as 4 to 8 days
4. *Salmonella* (salmonellosis): causes a local GI infection in which organisms multiply in the intestines but do not enter blood
   a. Found in inadequately cooked meats
   b. Incubation period usually 10 to 24 hours after ingestion of contaminated food, and symptoms usually last 2 to 3 days
5. *Clostridium difficile:* spore-forming gram-positive bacteria
   a. Frequent cause of nosocomial infection in clients receiving antibiotic therapy
   b. Toxin can cause pseudomembranous colitis and sepsis
6. Vancomycin-resistant enterococcus (VRE): gram-positive bacteria normally residing in the GI tract
   a. Frequent cause of nosocomial infection
   b. May resist all antimicrobial agents
B. Clinical findings
1. Subjective
   a. Nausea, abdominal cramps and pain, malaise
   b. Botulism: diplopia, muscle weakness, dysphasia
2. Objective
   a. Diarrhea 1 to 8 hours after ingestion

   b. Vomiting, fever, chills
   c. Botulism: diminished visual acuity and gag reflex, loss of pupillary light reflex
C. Therapeutic interventions
1. Elimination of chemical, mechanical, and/or thermal irritation
2. Adequate fluid and electrolytes orally or parenterally
3. Bed rest
4. For botulism
   a. Darkened room
   b. Parenteral feedings to prevent aspiration
   c. Tracheostomy and other supportive measures
   d. Cathartics and cleansing enemas to remove toxins from the body
   e. Trivalent antitoxins as necessary
   f. Gastric lavage
5. For *C. difficile*
   a. Discontinuation of antibiotic therapy if implicated as the cause
   b. Administration of metronidazole (Flagyl) or oral vancomycin for moderate to severe symptoms
   c. Surgical intervention for pseudomembranous colitis may be necessary

Nursing Care of Clients With Infectious Gastroenteritis

A. Assessment/Analysis
1. History of ingestion of contaminated foods
2. Frequency and characteristics of stool
3. Temperature for baseline data
4. Presence of nausea and vomiting
5. For botulism establish neurologic baseline data, especially gag reflex
6. Clinical findings of fluid and electrolyte imbalance
B. Planning/Implementation
1. Obtain stool specimen for culture
2. Offer small amounts of fluids as tolerated; maintain IV fluids
3. Maintain contact precautions; engage in meticulous handwashing
4. Monitor clients who are immunocompromised or receiving antimicrobial therapy for profuse watery diarrhea indicative of *C. difficile*
5. Teach the importance of properly storing and cooking foods
6. For botulism
   a. Prevent aspiration pneumonia by elevating the head of the bed; keep suction equipment available at the bedside
   b. Observe neurologic status to determine progression of the disease
   c. Prevent contractures and emboli by the use of range-of-motion exercises
C. Evaluation/Outcomes
1. Reports decreased bowel activity
2. Maintains fluid and electrolyte balance
3. Maintains nutritional status

✺ SYPHILIS

Data Base

A. Etiology and pathophysiology
  1. Caused by the spirochete *Treponema pallidum*
  2. Transmitted primarily during the primary or secondary stages; usually sexually transmitted; may be congenital
  3. Stages
     a. Primary: occurs 10 to 90 days after contact; adaptations generally localized
     b. Secondary: occurs up to 6 months after exposure; a systemic response
     c. Latent: begins after the secondary stage and may last several months to years; client is asymptomatic
     d. Tertiary: may occur 18 to 20 years later
        (1) Gummas (granulomas) attack any organ and cause cardiovascular syphilis (aortitis and thoracic aortic aneurysms) and neurosyphilis
        (2) Rare for an individual to infect another; however, a fetus can be infected

B. Clinical findings
  1. Primary syphilis
     a. Chancre on genitalia, mouth, or anus; serous drainage from chancre
     b. Enlarged lymph nodes
     c. Positive test for syphilis: Venereal Disease Research Laboratory (VDRL), rapid plasma reagin circle card test (RPR-CT), automated reagin test (ART), fluorescent treponemal antibody absorption test (FTA-ABS)
  2. Secondary syphilis
     a. Skin rash on palms and soles of feet, alopecia
     b. Erosions of oral mucous membrane
     c. Fever, enlarged lymph nodes
  3. Latent syphilis: asymptomatic
  4. Tertiary syphilis
     a. Cardiovascular changes: aortitis, aortic aneurysm, stroke
     b. Neurologic changes: personality changes, ataxia, blindness

C. Therapeutic interventions
  1. Penicillin; probenecid to delay excretion of penicillin
  2. Tetracycline or erythromycin if client is allergic to penicillin

Nursing Care of Clients With Syphilis

A. Assessment/Analysis
  1. Progression of clinical findings
  2. Genitalia, rectum, and oropharynx for inflammation, lesions, or drainage
  3. Regional lymph nodes for enlargement
  4. History of allergy to penicillin

B. Planning/Implementation
  1. Provide a supportive, nonjudgmental environment
  2. Encourage early screening and educational programs such as STI clinics, hot lines, and workshops
  3. Teach about the disease and its transmission; cleansing of the genitals and condoms help prevent transmission of most STIs
  4. Encourage identification of prior contacts so they can be treated
  5. Inform client that the disease must be reported to the health department, but that confidentiality will be maintained
  6. Explain need to complete course of antibiotic therapy
  7. Instruct to avoid any sexual activity until tests are negative; encourage monogamous relationship
  8. Implement contact precautions
  9. Teach meticulous handwashing to prevent autoinoculation

C. Evaluation/Outcomes
  1. Avoids sexual contact until follow-up testing indicates transmission will not occur
  2. Identifies "safer sex" practices to reduce risk for reinfection

✺ GONORRHEA

Data Base

A. Etiology and pathophysiology
  1. Caused by *Neisseria gonorrhoeae,* a gram-negative diplococcus; penicillinase-producing *N. gonorrhoeae* is a newer strain resistant to penicillin
  2. Clinical findings depend on nature of sexual contact and may appear within a few days after exposure; may remain asymptomatic
  3. When untreated, inflammation subsides in 2 to 4 weeks, but client may become a carrier

B. Clinical findings
  1. Subjective: dysuria, urgency, anal pruritus, lower abdominal discomfort, joint pain, painful defecation
  2. Objective
     a. Purulent penile or vaginal discharge
     b. Fever
     c. Urethral or endocervical smear positive for gonococcus; cultures should be obtained from the urethra, endocervix, anal canal, and pharynx
     d. If untreated, clinical findings of complications such as salpingitis, infertility, urethral stricture, prostatitis, epididymitis, inflammation of the rectum (proctitis), and pharyngitis can occur

C. Therapeutic intervention: CDC recommends a cephalosporin (e.g., Rocephin)

Nursing Care of Clients With Gonorrhea

A. Assessment/Analysis
  1. See Assessment/Analysis under Nursing Care of Clients With Syphilis

B. Planning/Implementation
  1. Instruct to wash hands to prevent conjunctivitis
  2. Make arrangements for follow-up culture 2 weeks after therapy is initiated
  3. Monitor urinary and bowel elimination
  4. Allow time to verbalize concerns about potential infertility

5. Identify sexual contacts; encourage use of condoms to prevent future infections
6. See Nursing Care of Clients With Syphilis for additional information

C. Evaluation/Outcomes
   1. Maintains reproductive functions
   2. Identifies "safer sex" practices to reduce risk for reinfection

HERPES GENITALIS

Data Base

A. Etiology and pathophysiology
   1. Most commonly caused by herpes simplex type 2 (herpesvirus hominis type 2); may also be caused by type 1, which is most often associated with lesions (cold sores) of the mouth

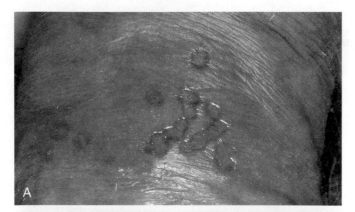

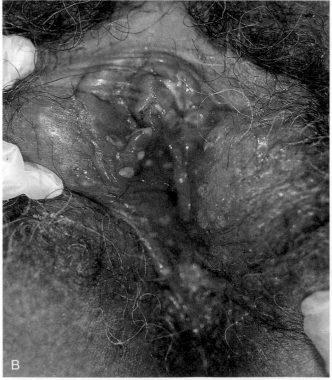

Figure 13-1 Herpes simplex virus type 2, in male **(A)** and female **(B)** clients. (From Habif TP: *Clinical dermatology: a color guide to diagnosis and therapy,* ed 4, St. Louis, 2004, Mosby.)

2. Lesions occur 3 to 7 days after infection and may last several weeks
3. When clinical findings resolve, virus lies dormant in spinal root ganglia and is capable of repeatedly causing lesions
4. Transmitted through sexual contact when active lesions are present; newborn may be infected during vaginal birth
5. May cause aseptic meningitis, proctitis, and prostatitis; associated with higher rate of cervical cancer

B. Clinical findings
   1. Subjective: dysuria; flulike clinical findings; tingling sensation before vesicles appear; genital itching and pain
   2. Objective: leukorrhea; vaginal bleeding; vesicles and papules on genitalia (Figure 13-1: Herpes simplex virus type 2); urinary retention; culture reveals herpesvirus type 2

C. Therapeutic interventions
   1. No cure; acyclovir sodium (Zovirax), valacyclovir (Valtrex), or famciclovir (Famvir) reduce healing time and severity of clinical findings
   2. Sedation for severe pain
   3. Alcohol (topical) may be used to dry lesions

Nursing Care of Clients With Herpes Genitalis

A. Assessment/Analysis
   1. See Assessment/Analysis under Nursing Care of Clients With Syphilis

B. Planning/Implementation
   1. Provide emotional support to deal with incurable, contagious nature of disease
   2. Help to develop stress-reducing strategies; stress precipitates recurrences
   3. Encourage increased fluid intake
   4. Relieve local discomfort as ordered: analgesics, topical anesthetic agents, sitz baths, application of heat or cold
   5. Stress the need to avoid sexual contact when lesions exist; avoid intercourse during the last 6 weeks of pregnancy; teach safer sex practices
   6. Advise to have annual Papanicolaou smears
   7. Implement contact precautions
   8. Teach to avoid touching area unnecessarily and meticulous handwashing to prevent autoinoculation
   9. Keep area clean and dry; encourage use of cotton underwear and loose-fitting clothing
   10. See Planning/Implementation under Nursing Care of Clients With Syphilis for additional information

C. Evaluation/Outcomes
   1. Reports relief of dysuria and pain
   2. Exhibits intact skin without lesions
   3. Abstains from sexual contact when lesions are present

ACQUIRED IMMUNODEFICIENCY SYNDROME (AIDS)

Data Base
A. Etiology and pathophysiology
1. Caused by the human immunodeficiency virus (HIV); a retrovirus; most commonly caused by HIV-1; other strains include HIV-2 and HIV-3
2. HIV infects helper T lymphocytes (T4/CD4 cells), B lymphocytes, macrophages, promyelocytes, fibroblasts, and epidermal Langerhans cells
3. When the T4/CD4 cell count falls below 200/µL opportunistic infections are greatest because the immune system is severely depressed
4. Opportunistic infections and disorders associated with AIDS: protozoal (*Pneumocystis jiroveci* pneumonia, toxoplasmosis, cryptosporidiosis); fungal (candidiasis, cryptococcosis, histoplasmosis, tinea); bacterial *(Mycobacterium avium-intracellulare* complex, *Mycobacterium tuberculosis* [MTB]); viral (herpes simplex, varicella-zoster, cytomegalovirus, molluscum contagiosum, human papillomavirus, and Epstein-Barr); and malignancies (Kaposi's sarcoma, B-cell lymphomas, non-Hodgkin's lymphoma)
5. Classification system for HIV infection according to Centers for Disease Control and Prevention
   a. T4/CD4 categories
      (1) Category 1: 500 cells/µL or more
      (2) Category 2: 200 to 499 cells/µL
      (3) Category 3: Less than 200 cells/µL
   b. Clinical categories
      (1) Category A: categories B and C have not occurred; asymptomatic HIV infection; persistent generalized lymphadenopathy; acute (primary) HIV infection
      (2) Category B: category C has not occurred; presence of conditions attributed to HIV infection; conditions that are considered to have a clinical course or that require management that is complicated by HIV infection
      (3) Category C: includes all clinical conditions listed as advanced HIV disease or AIDS; once a person is in category C, the person remains in this category
6. The HIV is present in blood, semen, vaginal secretions, blood-tinged saliva, tears, breast milk, and CSF; transmission occurs through contact with infected blood, semen, and vaginal secretions; the virus is not viable outside the body
7. The adult is considered HIV positive when blood tests reveal the presence of HIV or antibodies to the HIV
8. Once individuals are infected with HIV, they are capable of transmitting the virus
9. Incubation period estimates range from 6 months to 10 years and may be longer; the antibodies produced by the body can generally first be detected in the blood in 2 weeks to 3 months or longer after infection; a test that detects the presence of virus within 24 hours of exposure is available

B. Clinical findings
1. Subjective: anorexia, fatigue, dyspnea, chills, sore throat
2. Objective
   a. Positive test for HIV antibody: clients are screened using ELISA (enzyme-linked immunosorbent assay); clients with a positive ELISA have results confirmed using the Western blot
   b. Positive test for presence of HIV itself; polymerase chain reaction (PCR); HIV RNA provides evidence of viral load
   c. Decreased T4/CD4 cells to less than 200/µL
   d. Decreased ratio of T4 cell (helper cell) to T8 cell (suppressor cell)
   e. Night sweats
   f. Enlarged lymph nodes
   g. Wasting syndrome: weight loss exceeding 10% baseline weight, chronic diarrhea for more than 30 days, chronic weakness or constant fever
   h. HIV encephalopathy: memory loss, lack of coordination, partial paralysis, mental deterioration
   i. Presence of associated opportunistic infections and malignancies
3. Women with AIDS may have gynecologic manifestations (see AIDS in Nursing Care Related to Major Disorders Affecting Women's Health in Chapter 24)

C. Therapeutic interventions
1. There is no cure; prevention is the key to control
2. Pharmacologic therapy: highly active antiretroviral therapy (HAART) involves drug combinations; combinations and the order in which they are given influence effectiveness
   a. Nucleoside analogue reverse transcriptase inhibitors (NRTIs)
      (1) Interfere with DNA chain
      (2) Examples: zidovudine (AZT, Retrovir), emtricitabine (Emtriva), lamivudine (Epivir), abacavir sulfate (Ziagen)
      (3) Side effects: lactic acidosis, hepatomegaly, peripheral neuropathy, rash
   b. Protease inhibitors (PIs)
      (1) Block virus' ability to break down larger protein molecules into smaller functional units
      (2) Examples: ritonavir (Norvir), lopinavir/ritonavir (Kaletra); darunavir (Prezista); tipranavir (Aptivus)
      (3) Side effects: nausea, vomiting, diarrhea, abdominal pain, and anorexia (GI irritation); hyperglycemia (diabetes); peripheral paresthesias (neuropathy); headache (dehydration); renal calculi (calcium precipitation); increased liver enzymes (hepatotoxicity)

   c. Nonnucleoside reverse transcriptase inhibitors (NNRTIs)
     (1) Bind to reverse transcriptase and block RNA and DNA replication
     (2) Examples: efavirenz (Sustiva), tenofovir (Viread)
     (3) Side effects: transient rash, nausea, diarrhea; hepatotoxicity, nephrotoxicity
   d. Fusion inhibitor
     (1) Stops HIV from entering the CD4 cells by inhibiting the fusion of viral and cellular membranes
     (2) Example: enfuvirtide (Fuzeon); Sub-Q injection twice a day
     (3) Side effects: painful skin reactions at local injection site, headache, peripheral neuropathy, hypersensitivity reactions, and pneumonia
   e. Antiviral: valacyclovir (Valtrex) used for herpes zoster and genital herpes but also found to lower HIV levels in blood and genital secretions
   f. Combinations (more effective): **Atripla** (tenofovir [Viread], emtricitabine [Emtriva], efavirenz [Sustiva]); **Combivir** (zidovudine [AZT], lamivudine [Epivir]); **Epzicom** (abacavir [Ziagen], lamivudine [Epivir])
3. Specific treatment of opportunistic infections
   a. *Pneumocystis jiroveci:* trimethoprim-sulfamethoxazole (Bactrim), pentamidine
   b. Tuberculosis: isoniazid (INH), rifampin (Rifadin), ethambutal (Myambutol)
   c. Fungal infections: nystatin (Mycostatin), amphotericin B (Fungizone), ketoconazole (Nizoral)
   d. Viral infections: acyclovir (Zovirax)
4. Management of clinical findings
5. Research to control the disease involves genetic manipulation and vaccines to prevent HIV infection in uninfected individuals
6. Postexposure prophylaxis (PEP) for accidental needle sticks involves treatment with reverse transcriptase inhibitors

Nursing Care of Clients With Acquired Immunodeficiency Syndrome

A. Assessment/Analysis
1. CDC recommends HIV screening for all people 13 to 64 years of age regardless of risk
2. Weight and vital signs for baseline
3. Progression of clinical findings
4. Presence of lymphadenopathy
5. Skin and mucous membranes for evidence of Kaposi's sarcoma (lesions in epidermis that extend into dermis or extracutaneous lesions) or opportunistic infections
6. Respiratory function (e.g., characteristics of respiration, arterial blood gases, breath sounds)

B. Planning/Implementation
1. Use standard precautions for all clients, regardless of diagnosis, because the virus can be transmitted before the client shows clinical findings of disease
2. Encourage verbalization of feelings; provide emotional support
3. Refer client and significant others to counselor or support group because client and family must cope with social rejection and death
4. Protect from secondary infection; assess for clinical findings of opportunistic infections
5. Monitor client receiving zidovudine for blood dyscrasias
6. Teach client taking a protease inhibitor to avoid drinking alcohol (hepatotoxicity) and to drink 8 to 10 glasses of water per day to avoid dehydration
7. Provide frequent rest periods
8. Teach the importance of
   a. Complying with prescribed medication dosage regimen; nonadherence has led to emergence of resistant strains
   b. Informing sexual contacts of diagnosis
   c. Avoiding sexual intercourse/activity unless using a condom; avoiding the use of petroleum jelly because it breaks down condom integrity
   d. Not sharing needles with other individuals
   e. Continuing medical supervision
   f. Preventing opportunistic infections
   g. Avoiding breast-feeding
9. Provide high-calorie, high-protein diet to prevent weight loss; encourage intake of foods rich in the immune-stimulating nutrients, especially vitamins A, C, and E, and the mineral selenium to support natural defense mechanisms; ritonavir (Norvir) and saquinavir (Fortovase) should be taken with a high-fat, high-protein meal, indinavir (Crixivan) should be taken on an empty stomach

C. Evaluation/Outcomes
1. Avoids opportunistic infections
2. Maintains body weight
3. Completes self-care activities without fatigue
4. Maintains skin integrity
5. Experiences decreased frequency of loose stools
6. Shares feelings with family and health care providers
7. Is aware of community support groups

✿ WEST NILE VIRUS (WNV)

Data Base

A. Etiology and pathophysiology
1. Caused by a mosquito-borne *Flavivirus* contracted from infected birds (main host); also by infected blood products and organs
2. Most people do not seek treatment; 20% experience a mild episode resulting in West Nile fever; some experience a severe episode, with 1 in 150 developing encephalitis or meningitis; older adults, infants, and immunocompromised individuals are at greatest risk
3. Incubation period is 3 to 14 days; clinical findings generally last 3 to 6 days

B. Clinical findings
   1. Subjective: mild episode—anorexia, eye pain, headache, malaise, myalgia, nausea; severe episode—clinical findings of mild episode plus weakness and fatigue
   2. Objective: mild episode—vomiting, lymphadenopathy, rash on neck, trunk, arms, or legs, IgM antibody to WNV in serum or cerebrospinal fluid; severe episode—clinical findings of mild episode plus change mental status, flaccid paralysis, and confusion; 1 in 150 develop neurologic clinical findings of encephalitis or meningitis, and some develop coma and death
C. Therapeutic interventions
   1. Supportive care: mild episode—increase fluid intake and rest; severe episode—IV fluids, respiratory support if necessary, treatment to prevent secondary infection, medication for fever, discomfort, and treatment of encephalitis or meningitis if present

Nursing Care of Clients With West Nile Virus
A. Assessment/Analysis
   1. Monitor for specific clinical findings
B. Planning/Implementation
   1. Provide supportive care; encourage rest and an increase in fluid intake
   2. Administer ordered medication for fever, discomfort, and encephalitis or meningitis
   3. Teach how to prevent mosquito bites: use repellents, avoid outdoors during dusk and dawn, wear light long sleeve shirts, pants and socks; secure screens; cover infants with netting when outdoors; prevent or clean up areas that contain stagnant water
C. Evaluation/Outcomes
   1. Maintains normal fluid and electrolyte status
   2. Reports relief of fatigue and fever
   3. Implements strategies to prevent mosquito bites

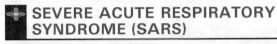

SEVERE ACUTE RESPIRATORY SYNDROME (SARS)

See Chapter 7, Major Disorders of the Respiratory System, Pneumonia

Medical-Surgical Nursing Review Questions With Answers and Rationales

QUESTIONS

GROWTH AND DEVELOPMENT

1. When planning discharge teaching for a young adult, the nurse should include the potential health problems common in this age-group. What should the nurse include in this teaching plan?
   1. Kidney dysfunction
   2. Cardiovascular diseases
   3. Eye problems, such as glaucoma
   4. Accidents, including their prevention

2. When meeting the unique teaching needs of an older adult recently diagnosed with diabetes mellitus, the nurse plans a teaching program based on the principle that learning:
   1. Reduces general anxiety
   2. Is negatively affected by age
   3. Requires continued reinforcement
   4. Necessitates readiness of the learner

3. A 76-year-old male client asks the nurse about the chances of getting osteoporosis like his wife. Which is the best response by the nurse?
   1. "This is only a problem for women."
   2. "Exercise is a good way to prevent this problem."
   3. "You are not at risk because of your small frame."
   4. "You might think about having a bone density test."

4. The nurse is managing acute pain experienced by the older adult client during the first 24 hours after admission to the hospital. The nurse should ensure that:
   1. Pain medication is ordered via the intramuscular route
   2. An order for meperidine (Demerol) is secured for pain relief
   3. Patient-controlled analgesia is avoided in this population
   4. Ordered PRN analgesics are administered on a scheduled basis

5. An older adult is admitted to the hospital after sustaining a hip fracture. When caring for this client the nurse understands that older adults have a high incidence of hip fractures because of:
   1. Carelessness
   2. Fragility of bone
   3. Sedentary existence
   4. Rheumatoid diseases

6. When formulating nursing care plans for older adults, the nurse should include special measures to accommodate for age-related sensory losses such as:
   1. Difficulty in swallowing
   2. Increased sensitivity to heat
   3. Diminished sensation of pain
   4. Heightened response to stimuli

7. The nurse is caring for an older adult with a hearing loss secondary to aging. What can the nurse expect to identify when assessing this client?
   1. Copious, moist cerumen
   2. Tears in the tympanic membrane
   3. Difficulty hearing women's voices
   4. Overgrowth of the epithelial auditory lining

8. A 93-year-old client in a nursing home has been eating less food during meal times. The best intervention for this client would be to:
   1. Substitute a supplemental drink for the meal
   2. Spoon-feed the client until the food is completely eaten
   3. Allow the client a longer period of time to complete the meal
   4. Arrange for a consultation for the placement of a gastrostomy tube

CIRCULATORY SYSTEM (CARDIOVASCULAR, BLOOD, AND LYMPHATIC SYSTEMS)

9. When taking a client's apical pulse, where should the nurse place the stethoscope?
   1. Just to the left of the median point of the sternum
   2. In the fifth intercostal space at the left midclavicular line
   3. Between the sixth and seventh ribs at the left mid-axillary line
   4. Between the third and fourth ribs and to the left of the sternum

10. A client with episodes of a cardiac dysrhythmia is to wear a Holter monitor for 24 hours. When planning teaching for this client, what information should the nurse include about the monitor? The monitor:
    1. Can be taken off while bathing
    2. Can record activities and manifestations of responses

3. Will assist in determining the size and contour of the heart
4. Will record tracings of abnormal cardiac rhythms during activities of daily living

11. A client with angina pectoris is scheduled for an exercise electrocardiogram (stress test). What information should the nurse include when explaining the value of this test? Exercise stress testing is a:
    1. Definitive method to diagnose the cause of chest pain
    2. Diagnostic modality of minimal value in planning treatment for angina
    3. Noninvasive means of assessing cardiovascular conduction and function
    4. Minimally invasive manner of assessing a body's reaction to increases in exercise

12. A client is admitted with chest pain unrelieved by nitroglycerin, an elevated temperature, decreased blood pressure, and diaphoresis. A myocardial infarction is diagnosed. Which is the most accurate explanation for one of these clinical indicators based on the nurse's understanding of the disease process?
    1. Parasympathetic reflexes from the infarcted myocardium cause diaphoresis.
    2. Inflammation in the myocardium causes a rise in the systemic body temperature.
    3. Catecholamines released at the site of the infarction cause intermittent localized pain.
    4. Constriction of central and peripheral blood vessels causes a decrease in blood pressure.

13. The nurse documents that a client's pulse pressure is decreasing. To determine the accuracy of this statement, what must the nurse calculate?
    1. Force exerted against an arterial wall
    2. Difference between the apical and radial rates
    3. Difference between systolic and diastolic readings
    4. Extent of ventricular contraction in relation to output

14. After open-heart surgery a client develops a temperature of 102° F (38.8° C). The nurse notifies the physician because elevated temperatures:
    1. Increase the cardiac output
    2. May indicate cerebral edema
    3. Are likely to lead to diaphoresis
    4. May be a forerunner of hemorrhage

15. The nurse is teaching a group of clients with peripheral vascular disease to stop smoking. Which physiologic effect of nicotine should the nurse explain to the group?
    1. Constriction of the superficial vessels, dilating the deep vessels
    2. Constriction of the peripheral vessels, increasing the force of flow
    3. Dilation of the superficial vessels with constriction of the collateral circulation
    4. Dilation of the peripheral vessels, causing a reflex constriction of visceral vessels

16. During an interview, the nurse discovers that the spouse of a debilitated client regularly digitally removes stool from the client's rectum. The nurse explores other strategies to regulate the client's bowel movements because disimpaction could stimulate the vagus nerve and result in:
    1. Tachycardia
    2. Slowing of the heart
    3. Dilation of the bronchioles
    4. Coronary artery vasodilation

17. The nurse is assessing the skin of a client with a history of chronic venous insufficiency. The nurse understands that the darkening of tissue results from the breakdown of hemoglobin with subsequent formation of:
    1. Heme
    2. Ferric chloride
    3. Ferrous sulfide
    4. Insoluble amino acids

18. When caring for a client with chronic occlusive arterial disease, what precipitating cause is the nurse most likely to identify for development of ulceration and gangrenous lesions?
    1. Emotional stress, which is short-lived
    2. Poor hygiene and limited protein intake
    3. Stimulants such as coffee, tea, or cola drinks
    4. Trauma from mechanical, chemical, or thermal sources

19. A client is prescribed prolonged bed rest after surgery. Which complication does the nurse expect to prevent by teaching the client to avoid pressure on the popliteal space?
    1. Cerebral embolism
    2. Pulmonary embolism
    3. Dry gangrene of a limb
    4. Coronary vessel occlusion

20. The nurse in the postanesthesia care unit is caring for a client who has received a general anesthetic. The nurse should notify the physician if the:
    1. Client pushes the airway out
    2. Client has snoring respirations
    3. Respirations of 16 breaths/min are shallow
    4. Systolic blood pressure drops from 130 to 90 mm Hg

21. After abdominal surgery a client suddenly complains of numbness in the right leg and a "funny feeling" in the toes. What should the nurse do first?
    1. Elevate the legs and tell the client to drink more fluids
    2. Instruct the client to remain in bed and notify the physician
    3. Rub the client's legs to stimulate circulation and cover the client with a blanket
    4. Tell the client about the dangers of prolonged bed rest and encourage ambulation

22. After a bilateral lumbar sympathectomy a client has a sudden drop in blood pressure but there is no evidence of bleeding. What should the nurse recognize as the most likely cause of the change in pressure?
    1. Inadequate fluid intake
    2. Aftereffects of anesthesia
    3. Increased level of epinephrine
    4. Reallocation of the blood supply

23. While convalescing from abdominal surgery a client develops thrombophlebitis. Which clinical indicator

of this complication should the nurse expect to identify when assessing the client?
1. Pitting edema of the lower leg
2. Ecchymotic areas of the extremity
3. Intermittent claudication of the leg
4. Localized warmth of the lower extremity

24. A client is being instructed on the use of antiembolism stockings. The nurse should teach the client that the stockings should be:
1. Alternately kept on 2 hours and off 2 hours
2. Worn only at night when activity is lessened
3. Put on before getting out of bed in the morning
4. Left in place until the physician advises otherwise

25. What should the nurse teach a client to do to minimize orthostatic hypotension?
1. Wear support hose continuously
2. Lie down for 30 minutes after taking medication
3. Avoid tasks that require high energy expenditures
4. Sit on the edge of the bed a short time before arising

26. A client being treated for hypertension reports having a persistent hacking cough. The nurse explains that this may be a side effect associated with:
1. ACE inhibitors
2. Thiazide diuretics
3. Calcium channel blockers
4. Angiotensin receptor blockers

27. To assess the effectiveness of a vasodilator administered to a client, what should the nurse assess?
1. Pulse rate
2. Breath sounds
3. Cardiac output
4. Blood pressure

28. What should the nurse assess to determine if a client is experiencing the therapeutic effect of valsartan (Diovan), an angiotensin II receptor blocking agent?
1. Lipid profile
2. Apical pulse
3. Urinary output
4. Blood pressure

29. When teaching a client with heart disease about risk factors, what should the nurse tell the client about cholesterol? Cholesterol:
1. Causes an increase in serum HDL
2. Can be found in both plant and animal sources
3. Should be eliminated because it causes the disease process
4. Decreases when unsaturated fats are substituted for saturated fats

30. The physician prescribes cholestyramine (Questran) for a client with hyperlipidemia. Which instructions should the nurse include in the client's teaching plan?
1. "Increase your intake of fiber and fluid."
2. "Take the medication before you go to bed."
3. "Check your pulse before taking the medication."
4. "Contact your doctor if your skin or sclera turn yellow."

31. When cardiovascular disease is a concern, reduction of saturated fat in the diet may be desired and substitutes

of polyunsaturated fat may be recommended. What should the nurse instruct the client with cardiovascular disease to avoid?
1. Olive oil
2. Tuna fish
3. Whole milk
4. Soluble fiber

32. When teaching a client with a cardiac problem who must limit saturated fats in the diet, the nurse should stress the importance of increasing the intake of:
1. Enriched whole milk
2. Red meats, such as beef
3. Vegetables and whole grains
4. Liver and other glandular organ meats

33. Which instructions should the nurse include in the teaching plan for a client who will be taking simvastatin (Zocor) when discharged? Check all that apply
1. ☐ Increase dietary intake of potassium
2. ☐ Avoid prolonged exposure to the sun
3. ☐ Schedule regular ophthalmic examinations
4. ☐ Take the medication at least ½ hour before meals
5. ☐ Contact the physician if skin becomes gray-bronze

34. When anticipating the possible health problems encountered in a health clinic in an African-American community, the nurse particularly needs to focus on assessing for signs and symptoms of:
1. Osteoporosis
2. Hypertension
3. Uterine cancer
4. Thyroid disorders

35. Nifedipine (Procardia XL) 90 mg is prescribed for a client with hypertension. The nurse should instruct the client to notify the physician if the client experiences:
1. Blurred vision
2. Dizziness on rising
3. Excessive urination
4. Difficulty breathing

36. A client asks what the coronary arteries have to do with angina. When determining the answer, the nurse should take into consideration that the coronary arteries carry blood:
1. To the lungs
2. To the endocardium
3. From the aorta to the myocardium
4. From the pulmonary system to the heart

37. What should the nurse identify as the primary cause of the pain experienced by a client with a coronary occlusion?
1. Arterial spasm
2. Ischemia of the heart muscle
3. Blocking of the coronary veins
4. Irritation of nerve endings in the cardiac plexus

38. When teaching a client with angina how to use nitroglycerin, what should the nurse instruct the client to do?
1. Place 2 tablets under the tongue when pain occurs
2. Place 1 tablet under the tongue and swallow another when pain is intense

3. Place 1 tablet under the tongue 3 minutes before activity and repeat the dose in 5 minutes if pain occurs
4. Place 1 tablet under the tongue when pain occurs and use an additional tablet after the attack to prevent recurrence

39. When caring for a client after cardiac catheterization, which nursing action is most important?
   1. Administer O_2
   2. Provide for rest
   3. Check the ECG every 5 to 15 minutes
   4. Check a pulse distal to the insertion site

40. During a cardiac catheterization, blood samples from the client's right atrium, right ventricle, and pulmonary artery are analyzed for their O_2 content. Which does the nurse identify as the expected finding?
   1. All samples contain more O_2 than does pulmonary vein blood
   2. The samples of blood all contain about the same amount of O_2
   3. Pulmonary artery blood contains more O_2 than the other samples
   4. Blood from the right atrium has less O_2 than the right ventricle blood

41. Which is one of the more common complications of myocardial infarction identified by the nurse in the coronary care unit?
   1. Dysrhythmia
   2. Hypokalemia
   3. Anaphylactic shock
   4. Cardiac enlargement

42. The nurse prepares a client for insertion of a pulmonary artery catheter (e.g., Swan-Ganz catheter). The nurse explains to the client that the catheter will be inserted to provide information about:
   1. Stroke volume
   2. Venous pressure
   3. Coronary artery patency
   4. Left ventricular functioning

43. A client is admitted with severe chest pain. What laboratory test should the nurse expect the physician to order to confirm a diagnosis of myocardial infarction?
   1. ALT
   2. APTT
   3. Troponin
   4. Potassium

44. A 72-year-old client is admitted with cerebral arteriosclerosis complicated by polycythemia vera. Heparin q6h is prescribed. What clinical finding enables the nurse to conclude the anticoagulant therapy has been effective?
   1. A reduction of confusion
   2. An absence of ecchymotic areas
   3. An APPT twice the usual value
   4. A decreased viscosity of the blood

45. What specifically should the nurse monitor when a client is receiving a platelet aggregation inhibitor such as clopidogrel (Plavix)?
   1. Nausea
   2. Epistaxis

3. Chest pain
4. Elevated temperature

46. A client is receiving warfarin sodium (Coumadin). The nurse should review the results of which test that is specific for calculating the daily dosage of this anticoagulant?
   1. INR
   2. APTT
   3. Bleeding time
   4. Sedimentation rate

47. When preparing a client for discharge after surgery for a coronary artery bypass graft, what should the nurse teach the client to expect?
   1. Mild fever and extreme fatigue for several weeks after surgery
   2. No further drainage from the incisions after hospitalization
   3. Mild incisional pain and tenderness up to 3 to 4 weeks after surgery
   4. Some increase in edema in the leg used for the donor graft when activity increases

48. The nurse assesses a client with heart failure who is receiving bumetanide (Bumex) and digoxin (Lanoxin) for symptoms of electrolyte depletion. What does the nurse understand is the cause of the depletion?
   1. Diuretic therapy
   2. Sodium restriction
   3. Continuous dyspnea
   4. Inadequate oral intake

49. The nurse suspects a client is in cardiogenic shock. What should the nurse understand about this type of shock? Cardiogenic shock is:
   1. An irreversible phenomenon
   2. A failure of the circulatory pump
   3. Usually a fleeting reaction to tissue injury
   4. Generally caused by decreased blood volume

50. The nurse finds an injured person sitting in a chair, obviously in shock. What should the nurse do?
   1. Keep the head elevated; give a stimulant in small sips
   2. Apply tourniquets to three extremities, rotating one every 15 minutes
   3. Surround the body with a warm blanket or chemical heating pads if available
   4. Place the person in the supine position, prevent chilling, and give fluids if possible

51. What clinical indicator is the nurse most likely to identify when completing a history and physical of a client with complete heart block?
   1. Syncope
   2. Cephalalgia
   3. Tachycardia
   4. Hemiparesis

52. The nurse in the emergency department is assigned to care for four clients with serious health problems. Which health problem does the nurse identify as the priority?
   1. Head injury
   2. A fractured femur
   3. Ventricular fibrillation
   4. A penetrating abdominal wound

53. While a pacemaker catheter is being inserted, the client's heart rate drops to 38 beats/min. What medication does the nurse expect the physician to order?
1. Atropine sulfate
2. Digoxin (Lanoxin)
3. Lidocaine (Xylocaine)
4. Procainamide (Pronestyl)

54. A client with a bundle branch block is on a cardiac monitor. What ECG change should the nurse identify on the client's cardiac monitor?
1. Sagging ST segments
2. Absence of P wave configurations
3. Inverted T waves following each QRS complex
4. Widening of QRS complexes to 0.12 second or greater

55. The nurse understands that a pacemaker is used in some clients to serve the function performed by the:
1. SA node
2. AV node
3. Bundle of His
4. Accelerator nerves to the heart

56. The nurse observes the following dysrhythmia on a client's cardiac monitor. What rhythm does the nurse identify?

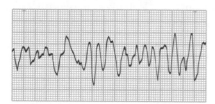

1. Atrial flutter
2. Atrial fibrillation
3. Ventricular fibrillation
4. Ventricular tachycardia

57. A client is admitted with atrial fibrillation and asks the nurse about cardioversion. The nurse explains that cardioversion is a procedure used to convert certain dysrhythmias to normal sinus rhythm. In addition to atrial fibrillation, for which ventricular dysrhythmia is cardioversion most effective?
1. Standstill
2. Fibrillation
3. Tachycardia
4. Premature complexes

58. The physician has inserted a permanent fixed (asynchronous) pacemaker in a client. When teaching, the nurse should:
1. Instruct the client to sleep on two pillows
2. Teach the client to keep daily accurate records of the pulse
3. Encourage the client to reduce the former level of activity
4. Inform the client that the pacemaker functions when the heart rate drops below a preset rate

59. To evaluate the effectiveness of a client's pacemaker that provides on-demand pacing, the nurse ensures that the pulse remains:
1. In a regular rhythm
2. Above the demand rate

3. Equal to the pacemaker
4. Palpable at all pulse sites

60. When a client develops ventricular fibrillation in a coronary care unit, what is the responsibility of the first person reaching the client?
1. Administer O_2
2. Defibrillate the client
3. Initiate cardiopulmonary resuscitation
4. Administer sodium bicarbonate intravenously

61. A client who has a myocardial infarction is in the coronary unit on a cardiac monitor. The nurse observes ventricular irritability on the screen. What medication should the nurse prepare to administer?
1. Digoxin (Lanoxin)
2. Furosemide (Lasix)
3. Amiodarone (Cardarone)
4. Norepinephrine (Levophed)

62. A client is admitted to the coronary care unit with atrial fibrillation and a rapid ventricular response. The nurse prepares for cardioversion. To avoid the potential danger of inducing ventricular fibrillation during cardioversion, the nurse should ensure that the:
1. Energy level is set at its maximum level
2. Synchronizer switch is in the "on" position
3. Skin electrodes are applied after the T wave
4. Alarm system of the cardiac monitor is functioning simultaneously

63. The nurse understands that a physician's order for digoxin (Lanoxin) is appropriate for which client?
1. Client A

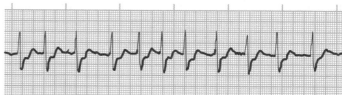

2. Client B

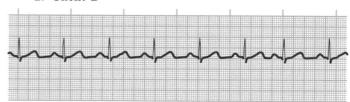

3. Client C

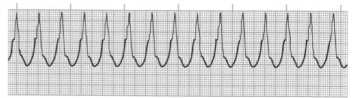

4. Client D

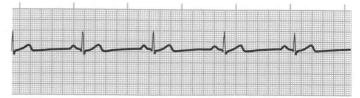

64. What is the most important information the nurse and the rapid response team must keep in mind when caring for a client who has had a cardiac arrest?
    1. Age of the client
    2. Time the client was anoxic
    3. Heart rate of the client before the arrest
    4. Emergency medications available for the client

65. A client is found unconscious and unresponsive. What should the nurse do first?
    1. Initiate a code
    2. Check for a radial pulse
    3. Compress the lower sternum
    4. Give four full lung inflations

66. When performing cardiac compression on an adult client, how far must the nurse depress the lower sternum to maintain circulation until a defibrillator is available?
    1. 1.3 to 2 cm (½ to ¾ inch)
    2. 2 to 2.5 cm (¾ to 1 inch)
    3. 4 to 5 cm (1½ to 2 inches)
    4. 2.5 to 4 cm (1 to 1½ inch)

67. When performing external cardiac compression, how should the nurse exert downward vertical pressure?
    1. Extending the fingers over the sternum and chest with the heels of each hand side by side
    2. Placing the fingers of one hand on the sternum and the fingers of the other hand on top of them
    3. Clenching the hand into a fist and placing the fleshy part of a clenched fist on the lower sternum
    4. Interlocking the fingers with the heel of one hand on the sternum and the heel of the other on top of it

68. A client has edema in the lower extremities during the day, which disappears at night. The nurse understands that this is consistent with which medical problem?
    1. Pulmonary edema
    2. Myocardial infarction
    3. Right ventricular heart failure
    4. Chronic obstructive lung disease

69. A client is admitted to the hospital and has edematous ankles. What should the nurse do to best reduce edema of the lower extremities?
    1. Restrict fluids
    2. Elevate the legs
    3. Apply elastic bandages
    4. Do range-of-motion exercises

70. When taking an admission history of a client with right ventricular heart failure, what clinical indicators will the nurse most likely identify from the client's complaints?
    1. Dyspnea, edema, fatigue
    2. Fatigue, vertigo, headache
    3. Weakness, palpitations, nausea
    4. Syncope, oliguria, increased thirst

71. When assessing the lower extremities of a client with right ventricular heart failure, the nurse expects to identify pitting edema because of what pressure change?
    1. Decrease in the tissue hydrostatic pressure
    2. Increase in tissue colloid osmotic pressure
    3. Increase in the plasma hydrostatic pressure
    4. Decrease in the plasma colloid osmotic pressure

72. The nurse understands that the client with right ventricular heart failure may develop ascites. What is the physiologic change underlying this development?
    1. Loss of cellular constituents in blood
    2. Rapid osmosis from tissue spaces to cells
    3. Increased pressure within the circulatory system
    4. Rapid diffusion of solutes and solvents into plasma

73. Spironolactone (Aldactone) is prescribed for a client. When teaching the client about this medication, what does the nurse instruct the client to avoid when making dietary choices?
    1. Red meats
    2. Citrus juice
    3. Whole grains
    4. Dairy products

74. The nurse is advising a client about the risks associated with failing to seek treatment for acute pharyngitis caused by beta-hemolytic streptococcus. For what health problem is the client at risk?
    1. COPD
    2. Anemia
    3. Endocarditis
    4. Reye's syndrome

75. What effect does anxiety produce that makes it particularly important for the nurse to allay the anxiety of a client with heart failure?
    1. Increases the cardiac workload
    2. Interferes with usual respirations
    3. Decreases the amount of O_2 used
    4. Produces an elevation in temperature

76. What should the nurse do to help alleviate the distress of a client with heart failure and pulmonary edema?
    1. Elevate the lower extremities
    2. Encourage frequent coughing
    3. Prepare for modified postural drainage
    4. Place the client in the orthopneic position

77. During a teaching session with a client who has experienced an anterior septal myocardial infarction, what statement by the client indicates to the nurse that there is a need for further discussion?
    1. "I want to stay as pain-free as possible."
    2. "I am not good at remembering to take medications."
    3. "I should not have any problems in reducing my salt intake."
    4. "I wrote down my medication information for future reference."

78. Two hours after a cardiac catheterization that was accessed via the right femoral route, an adult client complains of numbness and pain in the right foot. What action should the nurse take first?
    1. Call the physician
    2. Check the client's pedal pulses
    3. Take the client's blood pressure
    4. Recognize that this is an expected response

79. A client is returned to the surgical unit immediately after placement of a coronary artery stent that was

accomplished via access through the femoral artery. The nurse understands that the priority nursing assessment should be for:
1. Acute pain
2. Impaired mobility
3. Impaired swallowing
4. Hematoma formation

80. A 55-year-old client is admitted with the diagnosis of possible myocardial infarction. The physician orders enzyme studies for the client. While reviewing the results, which enzyme does the nurse identify as the first enzyme to change in the presence of a myocardial infarction?
1. ALT
2. AST
3. Total LDH
4. Troponin T

81. When a 70-year-old client with heart failure is transferred from the emergency department to the medical service, what should the nurse on the unit do first?
1. Interview the client for a health history
2. Assess the client's heart and lung sounds
3. Monitor the client's pulse and temperature
4. Obtain a blood specimen for measurement of serum electrolytes

82. A client has contrast medium injected into the brachial artery so that a cerebral angiogram can be performed. Immediately after the procedure what nursing assessment of the client is most essential?
1. Stability of gait
2. Presence of a gag reflex
3. Blood pressure in both arms
4. Symmetry of the radial pulses

83. The nurse is leading a discussion in a senior citizen center. What should the nurse respond when asked to identify the most significant risk factor for developing or dying from coronary heart disease (CHD) for women versus men?
1. Obesity
2. Diabetes
3. Elevated CRP levels
4. High levels of HDL-C

84. The nurse is teaching a group of clients about risk factors for heart disease. Which factors increase a client's risk for a myocardial infarction? Check all that apply.
1. ☐ Obesity
2. ☐ Hypertension
3. ☐ Increased HDL
4. ☐ Diabetes insipidus
5. ☐ Asian-American ancestry

85. What is the most important nursing action when measuring a client's pulmonary capillary wedge pressure (PCWP)?
1. Have the client bear down when measuring the PCWP
2. Deflate the balloon as soon as the PCWP is measured
3. Place the client in a supine position before measuring the PCWP
4. Flush the catheter with a heparin solution after the PCWP is determined

86. What criteria should the nurse use to determine normal sinus rhythm for a client on a cardiac monitor? Check all that apply.
1. ☐ The RR intervals are relatively consistent
2. ☐ One P wave precedes each QRS complex
3. ☐ The ST segment is higher than the PR interval
4. ☐ Four to eight complexes occur in a 6-second strip
5. ☐ The QRS complex ranges from 0.12 to 0.2 seconds

87. What is the most important assessment for the nurse to make after a client has had a femoropopliteal bypass for peripheral vascular disease?
1. Incisional pain
2. Pedal pulse rate
3. Degree of hair growth
4. Lower extremity color

88. Which signs cause the nurse to suspect cardiac tamponade after a client has cardiac surgery? Check all that apply.
1. ☐ Tachycardia
2. ☐ Hypertension
3. ☐ Increased CVP
4. ☐ Increased urine output
5. ☐ Jugular vein distention

89. A client with upper GI bleeding develops a mild anemia. What should the nurse expect the physician to order for this client?
1. Epogen
2. Dextran
3. Iron salts
4. Vitamin B_{12}

90. The emergency department nurse is admitting a client after an automobile collision. The physician estimates that the client has lost about 15% to 20% of blood volume. Which assessment finding should the nurse expect this client to exhibit?
1. A urine output of 50 mL/hr
2. A blood pressure of 150/90 mm Hg
3. A respiratory rate of 16 breaths/min
4. An apical heart rate of 142 beats/min

91. The nurse is to administer a unit of blood to a client admitted with esophageal varices. What nursing actions should be taken?
1. Since vital signs were recently recorded, hang the blood and monitor the client's vital signs every 15 minutes until the transfusion is absorbed
2. Hang the blood quickly because the client is pale and moaning and is in critical condition; return in 15 minutes to monitor vital signs
3. Record vital signs in accordance with facility policy and check the blood product against the client's ID bracelet in the presence of the nursing supervisor
4. Take and record baseline vital signs, verify the blood product with another nurse against the client's ID bracelet, and monitor the vital signs according to the facility's policies

92. The physician orders 1 unit of whole blood for a client after gastrointestinal surgery. When administering blood,

the nurse first verifies the type and cross-match and then the next nursing action is to:
1. Use an infusion pump to ensure the accuracy of the infusion
2. Warm the blood to body temperature to prevent chilling the client
3. Draw a blood sample from the client before each unit is transfused
4. Run the blood at a slower rate during the first few minutes of the transfusion

93. During a blood transfusion a client develops chills and a headache. What is the priority nursing action?
1. Cover the client
2. Stop the transfusion at once
3. Notify the physician immediately
4. Decrease the rate of the blood infusion

94. The nurse administers 2 units of packed RBCs (250 mL each) followed by 500 mL of 0.9% sodium chloride. How much total solution (blood and sodium chloride) has infused?
Answer: _____ mL

95. When caring for a client with disseminated intravascular coagulation, what is the priority nursing action?
1. Monitor for Homans' sign
2. Avoid giving intramuscular injections
3. Take temperatures via the rectal route
4. Apply sequential compression stockings

96. A client has a low hemoglobin level, which is attributed to a nutritional deficiency. Which foods should the nurse teach the client to add to the diet? Select all that apply.
1. ☐ Raisins
2. ☐ Squash
3. ☐ Carrots
4. ☐ Spinach
5. ☐ Apricots

97. A client is admitted with a higher than expected red blood cell count. The nurse understands that, in general, the higher the red blood cell count, the:
1. Higher the blood pH
2. Lower the hematocrit
3. Greater the blood viscosity
4. Less it contributes to immunity

98. The nurse understands that the only molecules that do not readily pass through the capillary endothelium are:
1. Blood gases
2. Plasma proteins
3. Glucose and ions
4. Amino acids and water

99. The nurse is caring for a client with an infection caused by group A beta-hemolytic streptococci. The nurse understands that this infection is associated with:
1. Hepatitis A
2. Rheumatic fever
3. Spinal meningitis
4. Rheumatoid arthritis

100. The nurse is caring for a client who is a victim of trauma. When the client expresses fear that AIDS may develop as a result of a blood transfusion, how should the nurse respond?
1. "The blood is treated with radiation to kill the virus."
2. "Screening for the HIV antibodies has minimized this risk."
3. "The ability to directly identify HIV has eliminated this concern."
4. "Consideration should be given to donating your own blood for transfusion."

101. A client has a bone marrow aspiration performed. After the procedure, what is the first nursing action?
1. Position the client on the affected side
2. Cleanse the site with an antiseptic solution
3. Briefly apply pressure over the aspiration site
4. Begin frequent monitoring of the client's vital signs

102. A client is diagnosed with Hodgkin's disease. Which lymph nodes does the nurse expect to be affected first?
1. Axillary
2. Inguinal
3. Cervical
4. Mediastinal

103. The nurse understands that the highest incidence of Hodgkin's disease is in:
1. Children
2. Older adults
3. Young adults
4. Middle-aged persons

104. A client is to have whole-body radiation for Hodgkin's disease. The nurse's teaching plan should center around the likely occurrence of increased:
1. Blood viscosity
2. Susceptibility to infection
3. Red blood cell production
4. Tendency for pathologic fractures

105. A client is admitted to the hospital with a diagnosis of a deep vein thrombosis of the right lower extremity. When caring for this client the nurse understands that fragments of cells in the bloodstream that break down on exposure to injured tissue and begin the chain reaction leading to a blood clot are known as:
1. Platelets
2. Leukocytes
3. Erythrocytes
4. Red blood cells

106. The nurse understands that thromboplastin, which initiates the clotting process, is found in:
1. Bile
2. Plasma
3. Platelets
4. Erythrocytes

107. The nurse is caring for a client with a wound that exhibits signs of blood coagulation and healing. When assessing this wound, the nurse understands that the soluble substance that becomes an insoluble gel is:
1. Fibrin
2. Thrombin

3. Fibrinogen
4. Prothrombin

108. The nurse is caring for a client who sustained a lacerating injury. When caring for this client, the nurse understands that blood clotting requires the presence of the catalyst:
1. F^-
2. Cl^-
3. Ca^{++}
4. Fe^{+++}

109. The nurse is teaching a client about the importance of vitamin K in the diet for blood clotting. The essential information that the nurse should include in this teaching is the fact that vitamin K promotes:
1. Platelet aggregation
2. Ionization of blood calcium
3. Fibrinogen formation by the liver
4. Prothrombin formation by the liver

110. The nurse is caring for a client with a diagnosis of polycythemia vera. The client asks, "Why do I have an increased tendency toward coronary and cerebral thromboses?" The nurse's best response is, "This increased tendency is attributable to:
1. Elevated blood pressure."
2. Increased blood viscosity."
3. Fragility of the blood cells."
4. Immaturity of red blood cells."

111. A serum bilirubin measurement is performed on a client who is weak, dyspneic, and jaundiced. The nurse understands that a bilirubin level greater than 2 mg/100 mL blood volume may indicate:
1. Hemolytic anemia
2. Pernicious anemia
3. Decreased rate of red blood cell destruction
4. Low oxygen-carrying capacity of erythrocytes

112. As a result of a serious automobile collision, a client is admitted with multiple trauma including a ruptured spleen. The nurse understands that a splenectomy is performed because the spleen is:
1. A highly vascular organ
2. The cause of liver disease after rupture
3. The largest lymphoid organ in the body
4. Anatomically adjacent to the diaphragm

113. The nurse is caring for a client who had a splenectomy. In the immediate postoperative period, for which complication should the nurse specifically assess in this client?
1. Infection
2. Peritonitis
3. Intestinal obstruction
4. Abdominal distention

114. A client has a splenectomy after a motor vehicle collision. What is a postoperative nursing concern specific for this type of surgery?
1. Pulmonary embolism
2. Prolonged immobility
3. Adequate lung aeration
4. Decreased blood volume

115. What Respiratory System should the nurse expect when assessing a client who has had a splenectomy?
1. Lung crackles
2. Pain on inspiration
3. Shortness of breath
4. Excessive secretions

116. The client is returned to the surgical unit from the postanesthesia care unit (PACU) after a having a splenectomy. In the immediate postoperative period, the nurse specifically should observe for potential complications. Select all that apply.
1. ☐ Shock
2. ☐ Infection
3. ☐ Intestinal obstruction
4. ☐ Abdominal distention
5. ☐ Pulmonary complications

117. A female client has a low hemoglobin level, which is attributed to a nutritional deficiency. Which food should the nurse recommend the client increase in the diet?
1. Beef
2. Liver
3. Prunes
4. Broccoli

118. While being prepared for surgery for a ruptured spleen, a client complains of feeling lightheaded. The client's color is pale and the pulse is very rapid. The nurse concludes that the client may be:
1. Hyperventilating
2. Going into shock
3. Extremely anxious
4. Developing an infection

RESPIRATORY SYSTEM

119. The nurse understands that in the absence of pathology, a client's respiratory center is stimulated by:
1. Oxygen
2. Lactic acid
3. Calcium ions
4. Carbon dioxide

120. The nurse uses abdominal-thoracic thrusts (Heimlich maneuver) when an older adult in a senior center chokes on a piece of meat. Which volume of air is the basis for the efficacy of the abdominal thrusts (Heimlich maneuver) to expel a foreign object in the larynx?
1. Tidal
2. Residual
3. Vital capacity
4. Inspiratory reserve

121. A client states that the physician said the tidal volume is slightly diminished and asks the nurse what this means. What explanation should the nurse give the client? Tidal volume is the amount of air:
1. Exhaled forcibly after a normal expiration
2. Exhaled after there is a normal inspiration
3. Inspired forcibly above a normal inspiration
4. Trapped in the alveoli that cannot be exhaled

122. The nurse is teaching the client deep-breathing exercises. The nurse understands that air rushes into the alveoli as a result of which change in pressure?
    1. Increasing alveolar pressure
    2. Elevated diaphragmatic pressure
    3. Rising pressure in the pleural space
    4. Lowered pressure within the chest cavity

123. A client is scheduled for a pulmonary function test. The nurse explains that during the test one of the instructions the respiratory therapist will give the client is to breathe normally. What is being measuring when the client follows these directions?
    1. Tidal volume
    2. Vital capacity
    3. Expiratory reserve
    4. Inspiratory reserve

124. The nurse notes that a client's hemoglobin level is decreasing and is concerned about tissue hypoxia. An increase in what diagnostic test result indicates an acceleration in O_2 dissociation from hemoglobin?
    1. pH
    2. po_2
    3. pco_2
    4. HCO_3^-

125. What nursing action will limit hypoxia when suctioning a client's airway?
    1. Lubricate the catheter with saline
    2. Use a sterile suction catheter each time
    3. Apply suction only after catheter is inserted
    4. Limit suctioning with catheter to 30 seconds

126. The nurse repositions a client who is diagnosed with emphysema to facilitate breathing. Which position facilitates maximum air exchange?
    1. Supine
    2. Orthopneic
    3. Low-Fowler's
    4. Semi-Fowler's

127. A client is admitted with suspected atelectasis. Which clinical indicator does the nurse expect to identify when assessing the client?
    1. Slow, deep respirations
    2. Diminished breath sounds
    3. A dry, unproductive cough
    4. A normal oral temperature

128. A client is admitted to the emergency department with carbon monoxide poisoning. The nurse understands that the poisonous nature of carbon monoxide results from:
    1. Its tendency to block CO_2 transport
    2. The inhibitory effect it has on vasodilation
    3. The bubbles it tends to form in blood plasma
    4. Its preferential combination with hemoglobin

129. A client is shot in the chest during a holdup and is transported to the hospital via ambulance. In the emergency department chest tubes are inserted, one in the second intercostal space and one at the base of the lung. What is the purpose of the tube in the second intercostal space?
    1. Remove the air that is present in the intrapleural space

2. Drain serosanguineous fluid from the intrapleural compartment
    3. Provide access for the instillation of medication into the pleural space
    4. Permit the development of positive pressure between the layers of the pleura

130. How should the nurse monitor for the complication of subcutaneous emphysema after the insertion of chest tubes?
    1. Assess for the presence of a barrel-shaped chest
    2. Auscultate the breath sounds for crackles and rhonchi
    3. Palpate around the chest tube insertion sites for crepitus
    4. Compare the length of inspiration with the length of expiration

131. During the first 36 hours after the insertion of chest tubes, when assessing the function of a three-chamber, closed-chest drainage system, the nurse notes that the water in the underwater seal tube is not fluctuating. What initial action should the nurse take?
    1. Inform the physician
    2. Take the client's vital signs
    3. Check whether the tube is kinked
    4. Turn the client to the unaffected side

132. After a laryngectomy a client is concerned about improving the ability to communicate. What topic should the nurse include in a teaching plan for the client?
    1. Sign language
    2. Body language
    3. Esophageal speech
    4. Computer-generated speech

133. After a client has a laryngectomy, what statement by the client indicates to the nurse that the teaching about activities and the stoma was understood? "I should avoid:
    1. Strenuous exercises."
    2. Sleeping with pillows."
    3. All types of water sports."
    4. High-humidity environments."

134. A client is admitted for an exacerbation of emphysema. The client has a fever, chills, and difficulty breathing on exertion. Based on the client's history and present status, what is a priority nursing action?
    1. Checking for capillary refill
    2. Encouraging increased fluid intake
    3. Suctioning secretions from the airway
    4. Administering high concentration of O_2

135. The common factor of scarlet fever, otitis media, bacterial endocarditis, rheumatic fever, and glomerulonephritis that the nurse should understand is that all of these diseases:
    1. Are self-limiting infections caused by spirilla
    2. Can be easily controlled through childhood vaccination
    3. Are caused by parasitic bacteria that normally live outside the body
    4. Result from streptococcal infections that enter via the upper respiratory tract

136. A client is admitted to the intensive care unit with acute pulmonary edema. Which rapidly acting diuretic that can be administered intravenously should the nurse anticipate that the physician will order?
1. Furosemide (Lasix)
2. Chlorothiazide (Diuril)
3. Chlorthalidone (Hygroton)
4. Spironolactone (Aldactone)

137. What nursing action will most help a client obtain maximum benefits after postural drainage?
1. Administer PRN oxygen
2. Place the client in a sitting position
3. Encourage the client to cough deeply
4. Encourage the client to rest for 30 minutes

138. A client with emphysema experiences a sudden episode of shortness of breath and is diagnosed with a spontaneous pneumothorax. What likely cause of the spontaneous pneumothorax should the nurse's response take into consideration?
1. Pleural friction rub
2. Tracheoesophageal fistula
3. Rupture of a subpleural bleb
4. Puncture wound of the chest wall

139. The nurse must be alert for signs of respiratory acidosis in the client with emphysema. In addition to a long-term problem with O_2 maintenance, what problem does this client have?
1. CO_2 retention
2. Localized tissue necrosis
3. Increased respiratory rate
4. Saturated hemoglobin molecules

140. A spontaneous pneumothorax is suspected in a client with a history of emphysema. In addition to calling the physician, what action should the nurse take?
1. Administer 60% O_2 via Venturi mask
2. Place the client on the unaffected side
3. Give O_2 2 L per minute via nasal cannula
4. Prepare for IV administration of electrolytes

141. A client is diagnosed with a spontaneous pneumothorax. Which physiologic effect of a spontaneous pneumothorax should the nurse include in a teaching plan for the client?
1. The heart and great vessels shift to the affected side
2. There is greater negative pressure within the chest cavity
3. Inspired air will move from the lung into the pleural space
4. The other lung will collapse if not treated immediately

142. What clinical indicator should the nurse expect to identify when assessing an individual with a spontaneous pneumothorax?
1. Hematemesis
2. Unilateral chest pain
3. Increased thoracic motion
4. Mediastinal shift toward the involved side

143. A client has a pneumothorax, and a closed-chest drainage system is inserted to reinflate the lung.

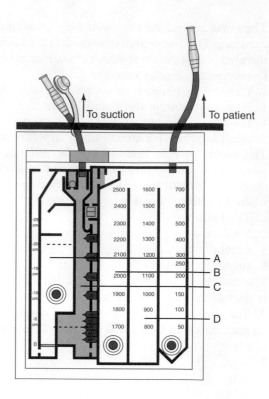

Identify the chamber (by number in the above figure) that provides the water seal.
1. A
2. B
3. C
4. D

144. What is the underlying reason the nurse must assess a client with emphysema for clinical indicators of hypoxia?
1. Pleural effusion
2. Infectious obstructions
3. Loss of aerating surface
4. Respiratory muscle paralysis

145. The nurse administers oxygen at 2 L/min via nasal cannula to a client with emphysema. For which clinical indicators should the nurse closely observe the client?
1. Cyanosis and lethargy
2. Anxiety and tachycardia
3. Hyperemia and increased respirations
4. Drowsiness and decreased respirations

146. When the alveoli lose their normal elasticity as a result of emphysema, why is it important that the nurse teach the client exercises that lead to effective use of the diaphragm?
1. The residual capacity of the lungs has been increased
2. Inspiration has been markedly prolonged and difficult
3. The client has an increase in the vital capacity of the lungs
4. Abdominal breathing is an effective compensatory mechanism that is spontaneously initiated

147. While receiving an adrenergic beta₂ agonist drug for asthma, the client complains of palpitation, chest pain, and a throbbing headache. What is the most appropriate nursing action?

1. Tell the client not to worry; these are expected side effects from the medicine.
2. Withhold the drug until additional orders are obtained from the physician.
3. Ask the client to relax; then give instructions to breathe slowly and deeply for several minutes.
4. Reassure the client that these effects are temporary and will subside as the body becomes accustomed to the drug.

148. What would be the priority goal established for a client with asthma who is being discharged from the hospital? The client:
1. Is able to obtain pulse oximeter readings
2. Demonstrates use of a metered-dose inhaler
3. Knows the primary care provider's office hours
4. Can identify the foods that may cause wheezing

149. A client with a long history of asthma is scheduled for surgery. What information should be included in pre-operative teaching? The client:
1. Will be prone to respiratory tract infections
2. Can use relaxation techniques to consciously limit the severity of asthmatic attacks
3. Needs to avoid coughing forcibly because this increases the intrathoracic pressure
4. Should consider having local anesthesia because it has fewer side effects than general anesthesia

150. A client with asthma is being taught how to use a peak flow meter to monitor how well the asthma is being controlled. What should the nurse instruct the client to do?
1. Perform the procedure once in the morning and once at night.
2. Move the trunk from an upright to a bending position while exhaling.
3. Inhale completely and then blow out as hard and as fast as possible through the mouthpiece.
4. Place the mouthpiece between the lips and in front of the teeth before starting the procedure.

151. When a client suffers a complete pneumothorax, there is danger of a mediastinal shift. If such a shift occurs, what potential effect should cause the nurse be concerned?
1. Rupture of the pericardium
2. Infection of the subpleural lining
3. Decreased filling of the right heart
4. Increased volume of the unaffected lung

152. The physician inserts a chest tube in a client who has been stabbed in the chest and attaches it to a closed-drainage system. Which is an important nursing intervention when caring for the client?
1. Apply a thoracic binder to prevent tension on the tube.
2. Observe for fluid fluctuations in the water-seal chamber.
3. Administer morphine sulfate, because the client will be agitated.
4. Clamp the tubing securely to prevent a rapid decline in pressure.

153. A client has chest tubes attached to a chest tube drainage system. When caring for this client, what should the nurse do?
1. Clamp the chest tubes when suctioning.
2. Palpate the surrounding area for crepitus.
3. Change the dressing daily using aseptic technique.
4. Empty the drainage chamber at the end of the shift.

154. The nurse is caring for a variety of clients. The nurse should implement measures to prevent pulmonary embolism in the client who:
1. Had dental surgery
2. Has thrombocytopenia
3. Had a knee replacement
4. Has bacterial pneumonia

155. The graduate nurse reminds a client who has just had a laryngoscopy not to take anything by mouth until instructed to do so. What conclusion would be made about this intervention by the nurse preceptor who is evaluating the performance of the graduate nurse?
1. Inappropriate, because the client is conscious and may be thirsty after being NPO
2. Appropriate, because such clients usually experience painful swallowing for several days
3. Appropriate, because early eating or drinking after such a procedure may result in aspiration
4. Inappropriate, because the client is likely to be anxious and it is easier to remove the water pitcher

156. A client has a bronchoscopy in ambulatory surgery. What action should the nurse take to prevent laryngeal edema?
1. Place ice chips in the client's mouth
2. Offer the client liberal amounts of fluid
3. Keep the client in the semi-Fowler's position
4. Tell the client to suck on medicated lozenges

157. After a bronchoscopy because of suspected cancer of the lung, a client develops pleural effusion. What should the nurse recognize as the most likely cause of the pleural effusion?
1. Excessive fluid intake
2. Inadequate chest expansion
3. Extension of cancerous lesions
4. Irritation from the bronchoscopy

158. A client who is to be admitted for minor surgery has a chest radiograph as part of the presurgical physical. The nurse is notified that the radiograph reveals that the client has pulmonary tuberculosis. What evidence of tuberculosis is provided by the radiograph?
1. Sensitized T cells
2. Presence of acid-fast bacilli
3. Cavities caused by caseation
4. Microscopic primary infection

159. A tuberculosis (TB) infection is suspected by the nurse when a client demonstrates several adaptations associated with TB. Indicate those findings that would be expected. Select all that apply.
1. ❑ Fatigue
2. ❑ Polyphagia
3. ❑ Hemoptysis

4. ☐ Night sweats

5. ☐ Black tongue

160. A client who is taking rifampin (Rifadin) tells the nurse, "My urine looks orange." What action should the nurse take?

1. Explain this is expected

2. Check the liver enzymes

3. Strain the urine for stones

4. Ask what foods were eaten

161. What must the nurse determine before discontinuing airborne precautions for a client with pulmonary tuberculosis?

1. Tuberculin skin test is negative.

2. Client no longer has the disease.

3. Sputum is free of acid-fast bacteria.

4. Client's temperature has returned to normal.

162. A client has a right pneumonectomy. During surgery the phrenic nerve is accidentally severed. What effect on the client does the nurse understand that this accident will have?

1. Produce a partially atonic diaphragm

2. Limit postoperative pain considerably

3. Allow the diaphragm to partially descend

4. Permit greater excursion of the thoracic cavity

163. The nurse expects that the initial treatment for a client who has a leak of the thoracic duct following radical neck surgery should include insertion of:

1. Gastrostomy tube to drain the fluid, a high-fat diet, and bed rest

2. Chest tube to drain the fluid, total parenteral nutrition, and bed rest

3. Rectal tube to prevent distention, a low-fat diet, and increased activity

4. Nasogastric tube to drain the fluid, a moderate-fat diet, and increased activity

164. After a radical neck dissection a client has two tubes from the area of the incision connected to portable wound drainage. Inspection of the neck reveals moderate edema even though the drainage systems are functioning. For which clinical indicator(s) should the nurse assess the client?

1. Loss of the gag reflex

2. Cloudy wound drainage

3. Restlessness and dyspnea

4. Crackles and abdominal distention

165. What should the nurse include in the plan of care for a client who has just had a total laryngectomy?

1. Instructing the client to whisper

2. Placing the client in the orthopneic position

3. Removing the outer tracheostomy tube PRN

4. Suctioning the tracheostomy tube whenever necessary

166. Which nursing action is important when suctioning the secretions of a client with a tracheostomy?

1. Use a new sterile catheter with each insertion

2. Initiate suction as the catheter is being withdrawn

3. Insert the catheter until the cough reflex is stimulated

4. Remove the inner cannula before inserting the suction catheter

167. A thoracentesis is performed. Following the procedure, it is most important for the nurse to observe the client for:

1. Periods of confusion

2. Expectoration of blood

3. Increased breath sounds

4. Decreased respiratory rate

168. A client with a pulmonary embolus is intubated and placed on mechanical ventilation. What nursing action is important when suctioning the endotracheal tube?

1. Apply negative pressure while inserting the suction catheter

2. Hyperoxygenate with 100% O_2 before and after suctioning

3. Use quick, short movements of the suction catheter to loosen secretions.

4. Suction two to three times in succession to effectively clear the airway.

169. In the first 2½ hours after a radical neck dissection, 40 mL of medium red, bloody fluid is obtained from the drainage system. What should the nurse do? Check all that apply.

1. ☐ Take vital signs

2. ☐ Notify the surgeon

3. ☐ Change the dressing

4. ☐ Apply pressure over the site

5. ☐ Elevate the lower extremities

170. The nurse should refer a client to the pulmonary clinic for suspected tuberculosis based on which clinical indicators reported during the initial client interview?

1. Hemoptysis and night sweats

2. Chest pain and increased cough

3. Weight gain and bilateral crackles

4. Unexplained weight loss and vomiting

171. Which nursing intervention will help prevent atelectasis in a client with fractured ribs as a result of chest trauma?

1. Apply a thoracic binder for support

2. Encourage coughing and deep breathing

3. Defer pain medication the first day after injury

4. Position the client face down on a soft mattress

172. The arterial blood gases of a client with COPD deteriorate, and respiratory failure is impending. For which clinical indicator should the nurse first assess?

1. Cyanosis

2. Bradycardia

3. Mental confusion

4. Distended neck veins

173. The nurse is caring for a client with a Venturi mask who is receiving 40% O_2. What nursing actions are indicated? Select all that apply.

1. ☐ Keep the oxygen source higher than the client's airway.

2. ☐ Adjust the liter flow according to the O_2 saturation.

3. ☐ Prevent the client's blanket from covering the adaptor's orifices

4. ❒ Ensure that the bag does not deflate completely during inspiration
5. ❒ Check that the appropriate adaptor to deliver the prescribed FIO_2 is attached to the mask

174. The nurse is administering O_2 to a client with chest pain who is restless. What is the method of O_2 administration that is least likely to increase apprehension in the client?
1. Cannula
2. Catheter
3. Venturi mask
4. Rebreather mask

175. A client who has acquired immunodeficiency syndrome develops bacterial pneumonia. On admission to the emergency department, the client's Pao_2 is 80 mm Hg. When the arterial blood gases are drawn again, the level is determined to be 65 mm Hg. What should the nurse do?
1. Notify the physician
2. Increase the O_2 flow rate
3. Decrease the tension of O_2 in the plasma
4. Have arterial blood gases performed again to check for accuracy

176. In addition to treatment of the underlying cause, the nurse understands that management of a client with acute respiratory distress syndrome (ARDS) will include which medical intervention?
1. Chest tube insertion
2. Aggressive diuretic therapy
3. Administration of beta blockers
4. Positive end-expiratory pressure

177. When caring for an intubated client receiving mechanical ventilation, the nurse hears the high-pressure alarm. Which action is most appropriate?
1. Obtain arterial blood gases
2. Lower the tidal volume setting
3. Remove secretions by suctioning
4. Check that tubing connections are secure

178. A nurse on a respiratory care unit is orienting a graduate nurse who has experience with clients who have cardiac problems. To build on the graduate's knowledge, the nurse explains that the relationship between two ventilator modes parallels the relationship between a fixed and a demand pacemaker. The two ventilator modes are:
1. IMV and SIMV
2. EPAP and IPAP
3. CMV and MMV
4. CPAP and PEEP

179. A client has an endotracheal tube and is receiving mechanical ventilation. The nurse identifies that periodic suctioning may be necessary. The nurse follows a specific protocol when performing this procedure. After obtaining the client's vital signs the nurse's next intervention should be to:
1. Auscultate the lung sounds
2. Hyperoxygenate for 30 seconds
3. Suction for approximately 10 seconds
4. Rotate the catheter during its withdrawal

180. The nurse is involved in an international committee to address global health problems. What suggestion is most appropriate for the nurse to make to best meet the challenge associated with a potential emerging influenza pandemic? Countries should:
1. Stockpile antibiotics
2. Establish a global surveillance plan
3. Limit vaccination programs to children under the age of 12
4. Initiate vaccination programs during the months of August and September

181. The nurse works with a large population of immigrant clients and is concerned about the debilitating effects of influenza. The nurse understands which action is the first line of defense against an emerging influenza pandemic?
1. Complying with quarantine measures
2. Instituting strict international travel restrictions
3. Seeking aid from the international public health community
4. Reporting surveillance findings to appropriate public health officials

GASTROINTESTINAL SYSTEM

182. The nurse is planning a community health program about screening for cancer. Which information recommended by the American Cancer Society (ACS) should the nurse include?
1. Mammography should be performed annually after age 35 years for women
2. Fecal occult blood testing should be performed yearly beginning at age 50 years
3. Digital rectal exams and PSA testing should be done yearly after age 40 for men
4. Breast self-examination should be performed monthly beginning at age 30 years

183. The nurse is teaching an athletic teenager about nutrients that provide the quickest source of energy. The nurse concludes that understanding has taken place when the adolescent makes which selection from a menu?
1. Glass of milk
2. Slice of bread
3. Chocolate candy bar
4. Glass of orange juice

184. The nurse is planning to teach a client who is newly diagnosed with diabetes about the important role of glucose in the body. The nurse should include the fact that glucose is an important molecule in a cell because primarily it is used for:
1. Production of energy
2. Synthesis of proteins
3. Building of genetic material
4. Formation of cell membranes

185. The nurse is teaching a client about protein digestion. The nurse identifies that learning has taken place when

the client says, "The end products of protein digestion, amino acids, are absorbed from the small intestine by:
1. Simple diffusion because of their small size."
2. Filtration according to the osmotic pressure direction."
3. Active transport with the aid of vitamin B_6 (pyridoxine)."
4. Osmosis caused by their greater concentration in the intestinal lumen."

186. The nurse is teaching a group of senior citizens about nutrition. The nurse should include the information that a complete protein, a food protein of high biologic value, is one that contains:
1. All of the amino acids in sufficient quantity to meet human requirements
2. All of the essential amino acids in correct proportion to meet human needs
3. The essential amino acids in any proportion because the body can always fill in the difference needed
4. Most of the amino acids from which the body will make additional amounts of the essential amino acids needed

187. The nurse identifies that the client understands information about vitamin K when the client states, "Vitamin K is:
1. Found in a wide variety of foods, so there is no danger of deficiency."
2. Produced in sufficient amounts for metabolic needs by intestinal bacterial."
3. Easily absorbed without assistance, so all that is consumed is absorbed."
4. Rarely found in dietary food sources, so a natural deficiency can easily occur."

188. Before the nurse can assess the responses of a client to a deficiency in vitamin C, the nurse needs to understand that vitamin C is related to tissue integrity and hemorrhagic disease. The nurse needs to know that vitamin C controls such disorders by:
1. Preventing tissue hemorrhage by providing essential blood-clotting materials
2. Preserving the structural integrity of tissue by protecting the lipid matrix of cell walls from peroxidation
3. Facilitating adequate absorption of calcium and phosphorus for bone formation to prevent bleeding in the joints
4. Strengthening capillary walls and structural tissue by depositing cementing material to build collagen from ground substance and thus prevent tissue hemorrhage

189. A client describes abdominal discomfort following ingestion of milk. The nurse recognizes that this may be the result of a genetic deficiency of which enzyme?
1. Lactase
2. Maltase
3. Sucrase
4. Amylase

190. To better understand the adaptations presented by a client who is cachectic, it is important for the nurse to understand that the main function of adipose tissue in fat metabolism is synthesizing and:
1. Releasing glucose for energy
2. Regulating cholesterol production
3. Using lipoproteins for fat transport
4. Storing triglycerides for energy reserves

191. The nurse is teaching a client about the differences between the terms saturated and unsaturated, when used in reference to fats. The nurse should include in the teaching that when these terms are used in reference to fats, they relate to which factor?
1. Taste
2. Color
3. Density
4. Digestibility

192. A client has unexpected high levels of fat compounds in the blood. The physician orders a therapeutic diet to limit these compounds. What foods should the nurse expect to be limited in this client's diet?
1. Fruits
2. Grains
3. Animal fats
4. Vegetable oils

193. The nurse is caring for a client who has a high triglyceride level. Which substance is produced by the breakdown of triglyceride molecules?
1. Fatty acids
2. Amino acids
3. Urea nitrogen
4. Simple sugars

194. A client with a high cholesterol level says to the nurse, "Why can't the doctor just give me a medication to eliminate all the cholesterol in my body so it isn't a problem?" The nurse needs to teach the client that cholesterol is important in the human body for:
1. Blood clotting
2. Bone formation
3. Muscle contraction
4. Cellular membrane structure

195. Many vitamins and minerals regulate the chemical changes of cell metabolism by acting in a coenzyme role. The nurse identifies that the client understands the role of a coenzyme when the client states, "A coenzyme role means that the vitamin or mineral:
1. Forms a new compound by a series of complex changes."
2. Is not part of the enzyme controlling a particular reaction."
3. May be necessary for the cellular metabolism to proceed."
4. Prevents unnecessary reactions by neutralizing the controlling enzyme."

196. Because fat is insoluble in water, it cannot travel freely in the blood. Therefore the nurse understands that the main compounds formed to serve as a vehicle of transport are:
1. Lipoproteins
2. Triglycerides

3. Phospholipids

4. Plasma proteins

197. The nurse teaches the client that amino acids are involved in total body metabolism, building and rebuilding various tissues. The nurse identifies that the client understands information about essential amino acids when the client says, "Amino acids:
    1. Can be made by the body because they are essential to life."
    2. Are essential in body processes and the remaining amino acids are not."
    3. Come from the diet because they cannot be synthesized by the human body."
    4. Are used in key processes essential for growth once they are synthesized by the body."

198. A client with hypertension is prescribed a low-sodium diet. The nurse concludes that the client understands the teaching about the diet when the food lowest in natural sodium is identified as:
    1. Milk
    2. Meat
    3. Fruits
    4. Vegetables

199. Megadoses of vitamin A are taken by a client. Why should the nurse question this practice?
    1. This vitamin is highly toxic even in small amounts
    2. The liver has a great storage capacity for the vitamin, even to toxic amounts
    3. This vitamin cannot be stored, and the excess amount would saturate the general body tissues
    4. Although the body's requirement for the vitamin is very great, the cells can synthesize more as needed

200. The nurse is teaching a client about the work of changing raw fuel forms of carbohydrates to the refined usable fuel glucose. The nurse should include the fact that this primarily is accomplished by enzymes located in which body structure?
    1. Oral mucosa
    2. Small intestine
    3. Large intestine
    4. Stomach mucosa

201. A client is deficient in vitamin A (a fat-soluble vitamin) produced from provitamin A, its precursor carotene. To help correct this deficiency, the nurse should teach the client that the main source of this vitamin is:
    1. Oranges
    2. Tomatoes
    3. Skim milk
    4. Leafy greens

202. A client who recently immigrated has a chronic vitamin A deficiency. When assessing the client for clinical indicators of the deficiency, the nurse understands that vitamin A serves as:
    1. An integral part of the retina's pigment called melanin
    2. A component of the rods and cones, which control color blindness
    3. The material in the cornea that prevents the formation of cataracts
    4. The necessary component of rhodopsin (visual purple), which controls light-dark adaptations

203. A client is to have gastric gavage. In which position should the nurse place the client when the gavage tube is being inserted?
    1. Supine position
    2. Mid-Fowler's position
    3. High-Fowler's position
    4. Trendelenburg position

204. A client with the diagnosis of cancer of the stomach expresses aversion to meals and eats only small amounts. What should the nurse provide?
    1. Nourishment between meals
    2. Small portions more frequently
    3. Only foods the client likes in small portions
    4. Supplementary vitamins to stimulate the client's appetite

205. The physician orders a paracentesis. How should the nurse instruct the client to prepare for the radiograph?
    1. Void before the procedure
    2. A laxative the evening before the procedure
    3. Nothing by mouth for 8 hours before the procedure
    4. A low soapsuds enema the morning of the procedure

206. A client asks, "Why do I have to have barium salts for the GI series and barium enema?" Which is the best response by the nurse? "Barium salts:
    1. Give off visible light and illuminate the alimentary tract."
    2. Dye the alimentary tract and thus provide for color contrast."
    3. Provide fluorescence and thus illuminate the alimentary tract."
    4. Absorb x-rays and thus give contrast to the soft tissues of the alimentary tract."

207. A client is scheduled for a sigmoidoscopy. As part of the preparation for this diagnostic procedure, what should the nurse do?
    1. Administer an enema the morning of the test
    2. Withhold fluids and foods for 24 hours before the examination
    3. Explain to the client that a chalklike substance will have to be swallowed
    4. Provide the client with a container for the collection of a stool specimen

208. The physician orders a sigmoidoscopy for one client and a barium enema for another client. Which is a nursing responsibility common to preparing both of these clients for these procedures?
    1. Giving castor oil the afternoon before
    2. Withholding food and fluid for 8 hours
    3. Administering soapsuds enemas until clear
    4. Ensuring the understanding of the procedure

209. The physician orders a high-cleansing enema for a client. What is the maximum height at which the

container of fluid should be held by the nurse when administering this enema?
1. 30 cm (12 inches)
2. 37 cm (15 inches)
3. 45 cm (20 inches)
4. 66 cm (26 inches)

210. During administration of an enema, a client complains of intestinal cramps. What should the nurse do?
1. Give it at a slower rate
2. Discontinue the procedure
3. Stop until cramps are gone
4. Lower the height of the container

211. The nurse explains to a client who is scheduled for a barium enema that visualization of the GI tract is made possible by the:
1. High x-ray absorbing properties of barium
2. Coloring of the intestinal wall with barium
3. High x-ray transmitting properties of barium
4. Chemical interaction between electrolytes and barium

212. A client is receiving a percutaneous endoscopic gastrostomy (PEG) tube feeding. When the nurse assesses the client, which response indicates that the client is unable to tolerate a continuation of the feeding?
1. A passage of flatus
2. Epigastric tenderness
3. A rise of formula in the tube
4. The rapid flow of the feeding

213. Three days after admission for a brain attack (CVA), a client has a nasogastric tube inserted and is receiving continuous tube feedings. What should the nurse do to best evaluate whether the feeding is being absorbed?
1. Aspirate for a residual volume
2. Evaluate the intake in relation to the output
3. Instill air into the client's stomach while auscultating
4. Compare the client's body weight with the baseline data

214. A client is receiving hypertonic tube feedings. The nurse understands that the main reason why this client may experience diarrhea is:
1. Increased fiber intake
2. Bacterial contamination
3. Inappropriate positioning
4. High osmolarity of the feedings

215. The physician orders intermittent nasogastric tube feeding to supplement a client's oral nutritional intake. Which hazard associated with a nasogastric tube feeding will be reduced if the nurse administers this feeding over 30 to 60 minutes?
1. Distention
2. Flatulence
3. Indigestion
4. Regurgitation

216. A client has a fractured mandible that is immobilized with wires. Which is the life-threatening postoperative problem for which the nurse must monitor?
1. Infection
2. Vomiting

3. Osteomyelitis
4. Bronchospasm

217. A client who had an incision and drainage of an oral abscess is to be discharged. The nurse should instruct the client to notify the physician if there is:
1. A foul odor to the breath
2. Pain with swelling after 1 week
3. Pain associated with swallowing
4. A tenderness in the mouth when chewing

218. A client has cancer of the tongue. When conducting a physical assessment of this client, which specific adaptation should the nurse expect to find?
1. Halitosis
2. Leukoplakia
3. Bleeding gums
4. Substernal pain

219. The nurse is collecting a health history from a client who has a diagnosis of cancer of the tongue. For which risk factor commonly associated with cancer of the tongue should the nurse assess when collecting the client's history?
1. Nail biting
2. Poor dental habits
3. Frequent gum chewing
4. Heavy consumption of alcohol

220. A client with gastroesophageal reflux disease complains about having difficulty sleeping at night. What should the nurse instruct the client to do?
1. Sleep on several pillows
2. Eliminate carbohydrates from the diet
3. Suggest a glass of milk before retiring
4. Take antacids such as sodium bicarbonate

221. The nurse is providing discharge instructions for a client with a diagnosis of gastroesophageal reflux disease (GERD). To limit symptoms of GERD, what should the nurse advise the client to do?
1. Avoid heavy lifting
2. Lie down after eating
3. Increase fluid intake with meals
4. Wear an abdominal binder or girdle

222. A client with gastric ulcer disease asks the nurse the reason for antibiotic therapy that includes metronidazole (Flagyl). The nurse explains that antibiotics are prescribed to:
1. Augment the immune response
2. Potentiate the effect of antacids
3. Treat *Helicobacter pylori* infection
4. Reduce hydrochloric acid secretion

223. A client with gastroesophageal reflux disease (GERD) should make diet and lifestyle changes. What instructions should the nurse include in the client's discharge teaching? Check all that apply.
1. ❑ Avoid alcohol
2. ❑ Add milk to coffee or tea
3. ❑ Elevate the foot of the bed 6 inches
4. ❑ Eat three evenly spaced meals daily
5. ❑ Eat slowly while chewing thoroughly
6. ❑ Restrict the diet to small, frequent meals

224. A client with esophageal cancer is to receive total parenteral nutrition. A right subclavian catheter is inserted by the physician. The nurse knows that the primary reason for using a central line is that:
 1. It prevents the development of infection
 2. There is less chance of this infusion infiltrating
 3. It is more convenient so clients can use their hands
 4. The large amount of blood helps to dilute the concentrated solution

225. A client with inflammatory bowel disease is receiving total parenteral nutrition (TPN) via an infusion pump. When administering TPN it is essential that the nurse:
 1. Monitor the client's blood glucose level q2h at the bedside with a glucometer
 2. Change the TPN solution bag every 24 hours even if there is solution left in the bag
 3. Instruct the client to breathe shallowly when changing the TPN tubing using sterile technique
 4. Speed up the rate of the TPN infusion if the amount delivered has fallen behind the prescribed hourly rate

226. A client with a suspected peptic ulcer in the duodenum is admitted to the hospital for diagnostic testing and treatment. When assessing this client's pain, the nurse expects that the client will probably describe the associated pain as:
 1. An ache radiating to the left side
 2. An intermittent colicky flank pain
 3. A gnawing sensation relieved by food
 4. A generalized abdominal pain intensified by moving

227. A client is scheduled for a pyloroplasty and vagotomy because of strictures caused by ulcers unresponsive to medical therapy. The nurse reinforces the client's understanding by stating that the vagotomy serves to:
 1. Increase the heart rate
 2. Hasten gastric emptying
 3. Eliminate pain sensations
 4. Decrease secretions in the stomach

228. Which medical diagnosis can the nurse expect when collecting a health history from a client who is scheduled for an antrectomy?
 1. Cataracts
 2. Otosclerosis
 3. Gastric ulcers
 4. Trigeminal neuralgia

229. After a subtotal gastrectomy for cancer of the stomach, a client develops dumping syndrome. When caring for this client, the nurse understands that dumping syndrome refers to:
 1. Nausea resulting from a full stomach
 2. Reflux of intestinal contents into the esophagus
 3. Rapid passage of osmotic fluid into the jejunum
 4. Buildup of feces and gas within the large intestine

230. Two hours after a subtotal gastrectomy the nurse notes that the drainage from the client's nasogastric tube is bright red. What should the nurse do?
 1. Notify the physician immediately
 2. Clamp the nasogastric tube for 1 hour
 3. Recognize that this is an expected finding
 4. Irrigate the nasogastric tube with iced saline

231. A client is admitted to the surgical unit from the postanesthesia care unit with a Salem sump nasogastric tube that is to be attached to wall suction. Which nursing action should the nurse implement when caring for this client?
 1. Irrigate the client's tube with normal saline
 2. Use sterile technique when irrigating the tube
 3. Withdraw the tube quickly when decompression is terminated
 4. Allow the client to have small sips of ice water unless nauseated

232. After a partial gastrectomy is performed, a client is returned from the postanesthesia care unit to the surgical unit with an IV solution infusing and a nasogastric tube in place. The nurse identifies that there is no nasogastric drainage for 30 minutes. There is an order to instill the nasogastric tube PRN. What should the nurse do? Instill:
 1. 30 mL of normal saline and continue the suction
 2. 20 mL of air and clamp off the suction for 1 hour
 3. 50 mL of saline and increase the pressure of the suction
 4. 15 mL of distilled water and disconnect the suction for 30 minutes

233. A client is admitted to the hospital with a diagnosis of intestinal obstruction. The physician orders intestinal suction via a nasoenteric decompression tube. A serious danger associated with intestinal suctioning is an excessive loss of:
 1. Protein enzymes
 2. Energy carbohydrates
 3. Vitamins and minerals
 4. Water and electrolytes

234. When an intestinal obstruction is suspected, a client has a nasogastric tube inserted and attached to suction. The nurse should critically assess this client for:
 1. Edema
 2. Belching
 3. Dehydration
 4. Excessive salivation

235. The nurse designs a health teaching program specifically for a client who has had a gastrectomy. What should this plan include?
 1. A list of gas-forming foods and how to avoid them
 2. An explanation of the therapeutic effect of a high-roughage diet
 3. Encouragement to resume previous eating habits as soon as possible
 4. Information about dumping syndrome and how to limit it or prevent it

236. The nurse understands that a client may develop pernicious anemia following a gastrectomy because:
 1. Vitamin B_{12} is only absorbed in the stomach
 2. Hemopoietic factor is secreted in the stomach

3. Parietal cells of the stomach secrete the intrinsic factor
4. Chief cells in the stomach promote the secretion of the extrinsic factor

237. After a subtotal gastrectomy a client is returned to the surgical unit. Which is the best nursing action employed by the nurse to prevent pulmonary complications?
1. Ambulating the client to increase respiratory exchange
2. Maintaining a consistent O_2 flow rate to increase oxygen saturation
3. Promoting frequent turning and deep breathing to mobilize secretions
4. Keeping a plastic airway in place to ensure patency of the client's airway

238. An older adult is returned to the surgical unit after having a subtotal gastrectomy. The nurse understands that the most prudent dietary guideline for this client is to:
1. Increase intake of dietary roughage slowly
2. Avoid oral feedings for a prolonged period
3. Resume small, easily digested feedings gradually
4. Allow self-selection of personally preferred foods

239. To help prevent long-term complications associated with gastric bypass surgery, the nurse needs to educate the client. Identify the factors that should be included in the nurse's plan for this client. Check all that apply.
1. ☐ Eat foods rich in calcium
2. ☐ Ingest 3 small feedings daily
3. ☐ Limit fluids to 1500 mL daily
4. ☐ Consume a diet high in protein
5. ☐ Routinely receive vitamin B_{12} injections.

240. Six weeks after discharge, a client with a jejunoiliac bypass for morbid obesity returns to the out-patient clinic complaining of palpitations, abdominal cramps, diarrhea, and dizziness 30 minutes after meals. The inference the nurse should make from the stated complaints is that the client is experiencing:
1. Gastric reflux
2. Reflux gastritis
3. Dumping syndrome
4. Abdominal peritonitis

241. Which statement by a client who is scheduled for bariatric surgery indicates to the nurse that further preoperative teaching is necessary?
1. "I need to eat more high-protein foods."
2. "I'm going to have a figure like a model in about a year."
3. "I'm going to be out of bed and sitting in a chair the first day after surgery."
4. "I will be limiting my intake to 600 to 800 calories a day once I start eating again."

242. When preparing a morbidly obese male for bariatric surgery, the nurse informs the client that he should:
1. Receive medications in liquid form
2. Lie on the right side for 1 hour after meals
3. Ingest a high-carbohydrate diet once he resumes eating
4. Receive patient-controlled analgesia for 6 days after surgery

243. Which clinical indicator should the nurse identify before scheduling a client for endoscopic retrograde cholangiopancreatography (ERCP)?
1. Urine output
2. Bilirubin level
3. Blood pressure
4. Serum glucose level

244. A client has an interference in bile utilization caused by cholecystitis. The nurse understands that the ejection of bile into the alimentary tract is controlled by:
1. Gastrin
2. Secretin
3. Enterocrinin
4. Cholecystokinin

245. The nurse is preparing a teaching plan for a client with a history of cholelithiasis. The nurse should include in this plan that the client will experience discomfort after ingesting fatty foods because:
1. Fatty foods are hard to digest
2. Bile flow into the intestine is obstructed
3. The liver is manufacturing inadequate bile
4. There is inadequate closure of the ampulla of Vater

246. The nurse is caring for a client with cholelithiasis and obstructive jaundice. When assessing this client, the nurse should be alert for which common clinical indicators associated with these conditions? Select all that apply.
1. ☐ Ecchymosis
2. ☐ Yellow sclera
3. ☐ Dark brown stool
4. ☐ Straw-colored urine
5. ☐ Pain in right upper quadrant

247. For which clinical indicator should the nurse monitor when caring for a client with cholelithiasis and obstructive jaundice?
1. Yellow sclera
2. Pain on urination
3. Dark brown stool
4. Coffee-ground vomitus

248. Before a cholecystectomy the physician orders vitamin K. The nurse understands that this is administered because it is used in the formation of:
1. Bilirubin
2. Prothrombin
3. Thromboplastin
4. Cholecystokinin

249. A client is returned to the surgical unit after an abdominal cholecystectomy. What is the main reason why the nurse should assess for clinical indicators of respiratory complications?
1. Length of time required for surgery is prolonged
2. Client's resistance is lowered because of bile in the blood
3. Incision is in close proximity to the client's diaphragm
4. Bloodstream is invaded by microorganisms from the biliary tract

250. A client is admitted to the hospital with a medical diagnosis of acute pancreatitis. When caring for this client, the nurse understands that the hormone stimulating the flow of pancreatic enzymes is:
   1. Enterocrinin
   2. Pancreozymin
   3. Enterogastrone
   4. Cholecystokinin

251. The major digestive changes in fat are accomplished in the small intestine by lipase from the pancreas. When caring for a client with pancreatitis, the nurse understands that the enzymatic activity of lipase:
   1. Synthesizes new triglycerides from the dietary fat consumed
   2. Emulsifies the fat globules and reduces their surface tension
   3. Easily breaks down all the dietary fat to fatty acids and glycerol
   4. Splits off all the fatty acids in about 30% of the total dietary fat consumed

252. A client with a history of pancreatitis is scheduled for surgery to excise a pseudocyst of the pancreas. A pseudocyst of the pancreas is a:
   1. Malignant growth
   2. Sack filled with pancreatic enzymes
   3. Pocket of undigested food particles
   4. Dilated space of necrotic tissue and blood

253. The nurse is caring for a client with a diagnosis of acute pancreatitis and alcoholism. The nurse understands that an acute attack of pancreatitis can be precipitated by heavy drinking because:
   1. Alcohol promotes the formation of calculi in the cystic duct
   2. The pancreas is stimulated to secrete more insulin than it can immediately produce
   3. The alcohol alters the composition of enzymes so they are capable of damaging the pancreas
   4. Alcohol increases enzyme secretion and pancreatic duct pressure and causes backflow of enzymes into the pancreas

254. A client is diagnosed with cancer of the pancreas and is apprehensive and restless. Which nursing action should be included in the plan of care?
   1. Teaching the importance of rest
   2. Administering antibiotics as ordered
   3. Encouraging the expression of concerns
   4. Explaining that everything will be all right

255. The nurse understands that the main reason why the risk for developing respiratory tract infections increases after pancreatic surgery is the:
   1. Length of time required for surgery
   2. Proximity of the incision to the diaphragm
   3. Lowered resistance caused by bile in the blood
   4. Transfer of bacteria from the pancreas to the blood

256. The nurse understands that the main role of the liver in relation to fat metabolism is:
   1. Storing fat for energy reserves
   2. Producing phospholipids to regulate metabolism
   3. Oxidizing fatty acids to produce energy needed for activity
   4. Converting fat to lipoproteins for rapid utilization in metabolic processes

257. A client is recovering from an acute episode of alcoholism that included esophageal involvement. What are the components of a therapeutic diet that are most appropriate for the nurse to include in the teaching plan for this client? Select all that apply.
   1. ☐ Soft diet
   2. ☐ Regular diet
   3. ☐ Low-protein diet
   4. ☐ High-protein diet
   5. ☐ Low-carbohydrate diet
   6. ☐ High-carbohydrate diet

258. The physician orders thiamine chloride and nicotinic acid for a client with alcoholism. The nurse should teach the client that these vitamins are needed to maintain which body function?
   1. Neuronal activity
   2. Bowel elimination
   3. Efficient circulation
   4. Prothrombin formation

259. A client is admitted to the hospital with a diagnosis of alcohol withdrawal syndrome. The nurse understands that the detoxification of alcohol damages tissues. What body organ will be protected by the nurse's encouragement of a high-calorie diet fortified with vitamins?
   1. Liver
   2. Heart
   3. Adrenals
   4. Pancreas

260. When collecting an admission history, the nurse identifies that the client prefers fish and crustaceans over other sources of protein. When planning discharge teaching for this client, the nurse should include the fact that the cooked food most likely to remain contaminated by the virus that causes hepatitis A is:
   1. Canned tuna
   2. Broiled shrimp
   3. Baked haddock
   4. Steamed lobster

261. The nurse understands that prophylaxis for hepatitis B includes:
   1. Preventing constipation
   2. Screening of blood donors
   3. Avoiding shellfish in the diet
   4. Limiting hepatotoxic drug therapy

262. The nurse is caring for a client who is positive for hepatitis A. What should the nurse do?
   1. Use caution when bringing food to the client
   2. Wear a gown when entering the client's room
   3. Use gloves when removing the client's bedpan
   4. Wear a protective mask when entering the client's room

263. A client who is about to have a blood transfusion asks the nurse, "Which type of hepatitis is most frequently transmitted by transfusions?" The nurse should respond, "Although the risk is minimal, the type of hepatitis associated with blood transfusion is hepatitis:
1. A."
2. B."
3. C."
4. D."

264. The nurse educator of a college health course is discussing tattoos with the class. During the discussion, the nurse warns the students that tattoos are associated with which type of hepatitis?
1. A
2. C
3. D
4. E

265. A client in a debilitated state is admitted for palliative treatment of cancer of the liver. On admission, which objective information collected by the nurse is most helpful for future monitoring of the client's condition?
1. Diet history
2. Bowel sounds
3. Present weight
4. Pain description

266. The nurse can expect a client with liver cancer to complain of fatigue. The nurse understands that this is a common complaint because a readily available form of energy, although limited in amount, is stored in the liver by conversion of glycogen to:
1. Glucose
2. Glycerol
3. Tissue fat
4. Amino acids

267. A client is admitted to the hospital with a diagnosis of cirrhosis of the liver. The client has a history of long-standing inadequate nutrition, including a protein deficiency. The nurse understands that this deficiency will contribute to:
1. Tissue anabolism
2. Decreased bile in the blood
3. Fat accumulation in liver tissue
4. Coagulation of blood in microcirculation

268. A client with chronic hepatic failure is soon to be discharged from the hospital. When planning discharge teaching for this client, which diet should the nurse encourage the client to follow?
1. High-fat
2. Low-calorie
3. Low-protein
4. High-sodium

269. A client is admitted to the hospital with a diagnosis of cirrhosis of the liver and ascites. When caring for this client, the nurse understands that the portal vein:
1. Brings blood away from the liver
2. Enters the superior vena cava from the cranium

3. Brings venous blood from the intestinal wall to the liver
4. Is located superficially on the anteromedial surface of the thigh

270. When assessing a client with portal hypertension, the nurse should be alert for clinical indications of which complication?
1. Liver abscess
2. Intestinal obstruction
3. Perforation of the duodenum
4. Hemorrhage from esophageal varices

271. The nurse understands that the clinical indicators identified in clients with cirrhosis are chiefly the result of:
1. Infection of the esophagus
2. Obstruction of the hepatic duct
3. Fatty degeneration of Kupffer cells
4. Obstruction of the portal circulation

272. The nurse is caring for a client with a diagnosis of cirrhosis of the liver. The nurse understands that ascites seen in cirrhosis results in part from:
1. The escape of lymph into the abdominal cavity directly from the inflamed liver sinusoid
2. Increased plasma colloid osmotic pressure caused by excessive liver growth and metabolism
3. The decreased levels of ADH and aldosterone caused by increasing metabolic activity in the liver
4. Compression of the portal veins, with resultant increased back-pressure in the portal venous system

273. The physician orders a gastrointestinal endoscopy with a capsule endoscopic device. The nurse should instruct the client to:
1. Check the recorder every hour
2. Avoid eating food and fluid during the test
3. Avoid stooping and bending during the test
4. Swallow the capsule as soon as it is placed in the mouth

274. A client is diagnosed with cirrhosis of the liver. When assessing this client the nurse should be alert for clinical indicators of varicose veins as a result of which pathologic process?
1. Increased plasma hydrostatic pressure in veins of the lower extremities
2. Toxic and irritating products released into the blood from the diseased organs
3. Ballooning of vein walls from decreased venous pressure and incompetent valves
4. Decreased plasma protein concentration, resulting in the pooling of blood in the venous system

275. A client is a candidate for intubation as a result of bleeding esophageal varices. Which type of tube should the nurse anticipate will most likely be used by the physician to meet the needs of this client?
1. Levin tube
2. Salem sump
3. Miller-Abbott tube
4. Blakemore-Sengstaken tube

276. A client with hepatic cirrhosis begins to develop slurred speech, confusion, drowsiness, and a flapping tremor.

With this evidence of impending hepatic coma, which diet can the nurse expect the physician to order for this client?

1. 20 g of protein, 2000 calories
2. 70 g of protein, 1200 calories
3. 80 g of protein, 2500 calories
4. 100 g of protein, 1500 calories

277. A client eats a meal that contains 13 g of fat, 31 g of carbohydrates, and 5 g of protein. What is this client's total caloric intake for this meal?

1. 196 calories
2. 261 calories
3. 286 calories
4. 351 calories

278. A client is admitted to the hospital with a diagnosis of cirrhosis of the liver. For which classic sign of hepatic coma should the nurse assess this client?

1. Bile-colored stools
2. Elevated cholesterol
3. Flapping hand tremors
4. Depressed muscle reflexes

279. The nurse is concerned that a client with a diagnosis of cirrhosis of the liver may experience the complication of hepatic coma. Which sign is present if the client is experiencing hepatic coma?

1. Icterus
2. Urticaria
3. Uremic frost
4. Hemangioma

280. The nurse understands that a laboratory test can indicate that the liver of a client with cirrhosis is compromised and neomycin enemas might be helpful. Which laboratory test should the nurse monitor that, when abnormal, might identify a client who could benefit from neomycin enemas?

1. Ammonia level
2. Culture and sensitivity
3. White blood cell count
4. Alanine aminotransferase level

281. A male client with cirrhosis has a prolonged prothrombin time and a low platelet count. The physician orders a regular diet. Considering the client's condition, the nurse should instruct the client to:

1. Avoid foods high in vitamin K
2. Check his pulse several times a day
3. Drink a glass of milk when taking aspirin
4. Report signs of bleeding no matter how slight

282. A client is admitted with anorexia, weight loss, abdominal distention, and abnormal stools. A diagnosis of malabsorption syndrome is made. What nursing action should the nurse implement to best meet this client's needs?

1. Allow the client to eat food preferences
2. Institute IV therapy to improve the client's hydration
3. Maintain NPO status, because food precipitates diarrhea
4. Encourage consumption of meats at mealtime and high-protein snacks

283. A client is diagnosed as having malabsorption syndrome secondary to celiac sprue. Striking clinical improvement should be noted by the nurse when assessing the client after administration of:

1. Folic acid
2. Vitamin B_{12}
3. Corticotropin
4. A gluten-free diet

284. When planning dietary teaching for a client with malabsorption syndrome, which food should the nurse teach the client to avoid?

1. Corn
2. Cheese
3. Rye bread
4. Fruit juice

285. For which classic clinical indicator should the nurse assess the stool of clients with malabsorption syndrome?

1. Melena
2. Frank blood
3. Fat globules
4. Currant jelly consistency

286. The nurse is admitting a client with the diagnosis of malabsorption syndrome to the medical unit at lunchtime. Which foods can be included on the client's ordered diet?

1. Breaded veal cutlet with cheese
2. Roast beef sandwich with pickles
3. Chicken noodle soup with crackers
4. Cheese omelet with chopped spinach

287. Which food selection by a client with malabsorption syndrome indicates that the nurse's dietary teaching has been successful?

1. Baked potato
2. Noodle pudding
3. Postum beverage
4. Turkey sandwich

288. An 18-year-old is admitted with an acute onset of right lower quadrant pain. Appendicitis is suspected. For which clinical indicator should the nurse assess the client to determine if the pain is secondary to appendicitis?

1. Urinary retention
2. Gastric hyperacidity
3. Rebound tenderness
4. Increased lower bowel motility

289. A client has an appendectomy and develops peritonitis. The nurse should assess the client for an elevated temperature and which additional clinical indicator commonly associated with peritonitis?

1. Hyperactivity
2. Extreme hunger
3. Urinary retention
4. Local muscular rigidity

290. A client had surgery for a perforated appendix with localized peritonitis. In which position should the nurse place this client?

1. Sims' position
2. Trendelenburg's position

3. Semi-Fowler's position

4. Dorsal recumbent position

291. The physician orders a Harris flush to reduce a client's flatus after abdominal surgery. How many inches should the nurse insert the rectal catheter?

1. 2

2. 4

3. 6

4. 8

292. A 93-year-old client with a history of diverticulitis is admitted with severe abdominal pain, anorexia, nausea, vomiting for 24 hours, a markedly elevated temperature, and increased white blood cells. The nurse understands the most likely reason for surgical intervention is that:

1. Surgery is usually indicated for a diagnosis of diverticulitis

2. The symptoms exhibited by the client on admission are life-threatening

3. In some instances diverticulitis is difficult to differentiate from carcinoma except surgically

4. The client's age indicates immediate correction of the potentially fatal condition is needed

293. A client is admitted to the hospital with a diagnosis of regional enteritis (Crohn's disease). Which is the most likely reason for the physician to order administration of parenteral vitamins to this client?

1. More rapid action results

2. They are ineffective orally

3. They decrease colon irritability

4. Intestinal absorption may be inadequate

294. After many years of coping with colitis, a client makes the decision to have a colectomy as advised by the physician. The nurse understands that a significant factor in this decision is most likely that the client knows:

1. It is temporary until the colon heals

2. Surgical treatment cures ulcerative colitis

3. Ulcerative colitis can progress to Crohn's disease

4. Without surgery eating table foods is contraindicated

295. A self-help group of clients with irritable bowel syndrome has invited a nurse to present a program on nutrition. Which substance should the nurse teach clients to minimize in the diet to decrease GI irritability?

1. Cola drinks

2. Amino acids

3. Rice products

4. Sugar products

296. A client is admitted to the hospital with a diagnosis of colitis. Which clinical indicator should the nurse expect when assessing this client?

1. Fever

2. Diarrhea

3. Hemoptysis

4. Leukocytosis

297. The physician orders daily stool examinations for a client with chronic bowel inflammation. The nurse understands that these stool examinations are ordered to determine:

1. Fat content

2. Occult blood

3. Ova and parasites

4. Culture and sensitivity

298. When advising a college student about dietary choices, the nurse should be aware of the caloric value of the most commonly ordered fast-foods eaten by active young adults. List the following foods in order from the one with the least number of calories to the one with the most number of calories.

1. _____French fries

2. _____Garden salad

3. _____Whopper with cheese

4. _____Six pieces of chicken tenders

299. The nurse is caring for a client with a diagnosis of Crohn's disease. When evaluating a client's response to health care intervention which expected outcome is most important for this client?

1. Does skin care

2. Takes oral fluids

3. Gains a half pound per week

4. Experiences less abdominal cramping

300. The nurse should teach a client with GI irritability to minimize the intake of dietary irritants. Which should be avoided? Check all that apply.

1. ☐ Table salt

2. ☐ Cola drinks

3. ☐ Amino acids

4. ☐ Rice products

5. ☐ Milk products

301. The nurse is collecting a health history for a client with a diagnosis of colitis. Which is a common adaptation to colitis that the nurse should expect to identify when assessing this client?

1. Hemoptysis

2. Weight loss

3. Polycythemia

4. Decreased white blood cells

302. When teaching a client with an acute exacerbation of colitis about diet, the nurse recognizes that dietary teaching has been effective when the client states, "I can have:

1. Orange juice."

2. Scrambled eggs."

3. Vanilla milkshakes."

4. Creamed potato soup."

303. Which explanation is most accurate when the nurse teaches a client about intussusception of the bowel?

1. Kinking of the bowel onto itself

2. A band of connective tissue compressing the bowel

3. Telescoping of a proximal loop of bowel into a distal loop

4. A protrusion of an organ or part of an organ through the wall that contains it

304. When caring for a client with an ileostomy, the nurse should:

1. Teach the client to eat foods high in residue

2. Explain that drainage can be controlled with daily irrigations

3. Expect the stoma to start draining on the third postoperative day

4. Anticipate that any emotional stress can increase intestinal peristalsis

305. A client had part of the ileum surgically removed. When assessing this client, the nurse should monitor for clinical indicators of anemia because:
1. Folic acid is absorbed in the ileum
2. The hemopoietic factor is absorbed in the ileum
3. Iron absorption is dependent on simultaneous bile salt absorption in the ileum
4. The trace elements copper, cobalt, and nickel, required for hemoglobin synthesis, are absorbed in the ileum

306. An active adolescent is admitted to the hospital for surgery for an ileostomy. When planning a teaching session about self-care, the nurse includes sports that should be avoided by a client with an ileostomy. Which should be included on the list of sports to be avoided?
1. Football
2. Swimming
3. Track events
4. Cross country skiing

307. A client is scheduled for a colonoscopy and the physician orders a tap water enema. In which position should the nurse place the client?
1. Sims' position
2. Back-lying position
3. Knee-chest position
4. Mid-Fowler's position

308. A client is admitted to the hospital for a colon resection, and in preparation for surgery the physician orders neomycin. The nurse understands the main reason why this antibiotic is especially useful before colon surgery is because it:
1. Will not affect the kidneys
2. Acts systemically without delay
3. Has limited absorption from the GI tract
4. Is effective against many different organisms

309. The nurse understands a primary step toward achievement of a long-range goal associated with the rehabilitation of a client with a new colostomy is:
1. Mastery of techniques of colostomy care
2. Readiness to accept an altered body function
3. Awareness of available community resources
4. Knowledge of the necessary dietary modifications

310. Neomycin 1 g is ordered preoperatively for a client with a diagnosis of cancer of the colon. The client asks why neomycin is being given. Which is the best response by the nurse?
1. "It will decrease your kidney function and lessen urine production during surgery."
2. "It will kill the bacteria in your bowel and decrease the risk for infection after surgery."
3. "It is used to alter the body flora, which reduces the spread of the tumor to adjacent organs."
4. "It is used to prevent you from getting an infection, particularly a bladder infection, before surgery."

311. A client who had a colon resection and formation of a colostomy 2 days ago is receiving care by the nurse. When assessing the color of the stoma to determine if it is viable, the nurse expects the stoma to be:
1. Pink
2. Gray
3. Brick red
4. Dark purple

312. A nurse is caring for a client who is receiving total parenteral nutrition (TPN) after extensive colon surgery. The nurse concludes that the client understands teaching about the purpose of TPN when the client states, "TPN:
1. Provides short-term nutrition after surgery."
2. Assists in providing supplemental nutrition."
3. Provides total nutrition when GI function is questionable."
4. Assists people who are unable to eat but have active GI function."

313. A female client with the diagnosis of Crohn's disease tells the nurse that her boyfriend dates other women. She believes that this behavior causes an increase in her symptoms. In an effort to counsel the client, what should the nurse do first?
1. Educate the client's boyfriend about her illness
2. Help the client explore attitudes toward herself
3. Suggest the client should not see her boyfriend for a while
4. Schedule a counseling session for the client and her boyfriend

314. The nurse is caring for two clients. One client has ulcerative colitis and the other client has Crohn's disease (regional enteritis). When caring for these clients, the nurse understands that the manifestation that is more likely to be identified in the client with ulcerative colitis than the client in Crohn's disease (regional enteritis) is:
1. Inclusion of transmural involvement of the small bowel wall
2. Correlation with increased malignancy because of malabsorption syndrome
3. Involvement beginning proximally with intermittent plaques found along the colon
4. Involvement starting distally with rectal bleeding and spreading continuously up the colon

315. A client with ulcerative colitis has experienced frequent severe exacerbations over the last several years. The client is admitted to the hospital with intense pain, severe diarrhea, and cachexia. Which therapeutic course should the nurse expect the physician to explore with this client?
1. Intensive psychotherapy
2. Continued medical therapy
3. Surgical therapy (colectomy)
4. Diet therapy (low-residue, high-protein diet)

316. When teaching a client who goes to work every day to care for a new colostomy, the nurse should recommend that the irrigations be implemented at the

same time every day. Which time should the nurse suggest scheduling the client's colostomy irrigations?
1. Approximately 30 minutes after breakfast
2. When it is most convenient for the client
3. Halfway between the two largest meals of the day
4. At the time the client had bowel movements before surgery

317. The nurse is teaching a client with a permanent colostomy about self-care in preparation for discharge from the hospital. Which should the nurse discuss with the client? The:
1. Need for special clothing
2. Periodic dilation of the stoma
3. Importance of limiting activity
4. Bland, low-residue diet regimen

318. A client with cancer of the colon has surgery for a resection of the tumor and the creation of a colostomy. Postoperatively, the nurse teaches the client about nutrition. The nurse evaluates that learning has taken place when the client states, "I should follow a diet that is:
1. Rich in protein."
2. Low in fiber content."
3. As close to usual as possible."
4. Higher in calories than before."

319. The nurse is caring for a client with a nasointestinal tube. Which solution should the nurse plan to use when instilling this tube to ensure its patency?
1. Sterile water
2. Isotonic saline
3. Hypotonic saline
4. Hypertonic glucose

320. After having a transverse colostomy, the client asks what physical effect the surgery will have on future sexual relationships. Which information should the nurse include in a teaching plan for this client?
1. Sexual relationships must be curtailed for several weeks
2. Surgery will temporarily decrease the client's sexual impulses
3. The client will be able to resume usual sexual relationships
4. The partner should be told about the surgery before any sexual activity

321. A client has a transverse loop colostomy. What should the nurse do when inserting a catheter for the colostomy irrigation?
1. Use an oil-based lubricant
2. Instruct the client to bear down
3. Apply gentle but continuous force
4. Direct it toward the client's right side

322. During a colostomy irrigation, a client complains of abdominal cramps. What action should the nurse employ in response to the client's complaints?
1. Discontinue the irrigation
2. Lower the container of fluid
3. Clamp the catheter for a few minutes
4. Advance the catheter approximately 1 inch

323. How many inches should the nurse insert a catheter into the stoma when performing a colostomy irrigation?
1. 5 cm (2 inches)
2. 8 cm (3 inches)
3. 15 cm (6 inches)
4. 20 cm (8 inches)

324. When teaching irrigation of a colostomy, how many inches above the stoma should the nurse teach the client to place the container?
1. 15 cm (6 inches)
2. 25 cm (10 inches)
3. 30 cm (12 inches)
4. 45 cm (18 inches)

325. The client is diagnosed with cancer of the rectum and has surgery for an abdominoperineal resection and colostomy. Which nursing care should be implemented during the postoperative period?
1. Withholding fluids for 72 hours
2. Limiting fluid intake for several days
3. Having the client change the colostomy bag
4. Keeping the client's skin around the stoma clean

326. Before discharge, a client who had a colostomy for colorectal cancer questions the nurse about resuming activities. Which information should the nurse include in a teaching plan about activity?
1. Activities of daily living should be resumed as quickly as possible by the client to avoid depression
2. Most sports activities, except for swimming, can be resumed based on the client's overall physical condition
3. With counseling and medical guidance, a near-normal lifestyle, including complete sexual function, is possible
4. After surgery, changes in activities must be made to accommodate for the physiologic changes caused by the operation

327. Which statement by an older adult client leads the nurse to suspect that the client has become impacted with stool?
1. "I have a lot of gas pains."
2. "I don't have much of an appetite."
3. "I feel like I have to go and just can't."
4. "I haven't had a bowel movement for 2 days."

328. Which clinical indicator identified by the nurse supports the probable presence of a fecal impaction in a client with limited mobility?
1. Tympany
2. Fecal liquid seepage
3. Bright red blood in the stool
4. Decreased number of bowel movements

329. With the knowledge that a client who is bedbound is accustomed to taking enemas periodically to avoid constipation, which action should be implemented by the nurse?
1. Arrange to have enemas ordered for the client.
2. Have the physician order a daily laxative for the client.
3. Obtain an order for a bedside commode to facilitate defecation.
4. Offer a large glass of prune juice with warm water each morning.

330. A client is experiencing chronic constipation. When teaching this client to include more bulk in the diet, the nurse concludes that learning has occurred when the client states, "Bulk in the diet promotes defecation by:
1. Irritating the bowel wall."
2. Stimulating colonic musculature chemically."
3. Acting on the multiflora of the large intestine."
4. Stretching smooth muscle, causing it to contract."

331. A client is scheduled for ligation of hemorrhoids. Which diet should the nurse expect the physician to encourage the client to ingest in preparation for this surgery?
1. Bland diet
2. Clear liquid diet
3. Low-residue diet
4. High-protein diet

332. A client with hemorrhoids asks what caused this problem to occur. Which primary cause of hemorrhoids should be the nurse's focus in response to this client's question?
1. Constipation
2. Hypertension
3. Eating spicy foods
4. Bowel incontinence

333. A client is scheduled for a hemorrhoidectomy. The nurse should observe the client for the presence of which common clinical indicator associated with hemorrhoids?
1. Pruritus
2. Flatulence
3. Anal stenosis
4. Rectal bleeding

334. Postoperative care for a client who has had a hemorrhoidectomy should include which nursing intervention?
1. Administering enemas
2. Administering stool softeners
3. Encouraging showers as needed
4. Providing occlusive dressings to the area

335. A client is diagnosed as having hepatitis B virus (HBV). After reviewing the client's health history, the nurse, looking for possible situations in which exposure could have occurred, should recognize that the disease was most likely acquired when the client:
1. Had a small tattoo on the arm 3 months ago
2. Assisted in the emergency birth of a baby 2 weeks ago
3. Attended an ecologic conference in a large urban center 2 months ago
4. Worked for 5 weeks in an undeveloped area in Mexico 4 months ago

336. A client who is receiving total parenteral nutrition (TPN) complains of nausea, thirst, and a headache. Which clinical indicator should the nurse monitor initially to further assess the client's status?
1. Blood glucose
2. Urinary output
3. Blood pressure
4. Oral temperature

337. A low-residue diet is ordered for a client. When assisting with the selection of foods from the menu, which foods should the nurse suggest that the client choose?
1. Steamed broccoli
2. Creamed potatoes
3. Raw spinach salad
4. Baked sweet potato

338. A client has severe diarrhea and the physician orders intravenous therapy, sodium bicarbonate, and an antidiarrheal medication. The nurse expects that the physician will probably order which most frequently ordered antidiarrheal drug?
1. Bisacodyl (Dulcolax)
2. Psyllium (Metamucil)
3. Docusate sodium (Colace)
4. Loperamide HCl (Imodium)

339. A client with hepatitis B asks the nurse, "Why don't you give me some medication to help me get rid of this problem?" Which is the best response by the nurse?
1. "Sedatives can be given to help you relax."
2. "We can give you immune serum globulin."
3. "There are drugs to help reduce viral load and liver inflammation."
4. "Vitamin supplements are frequently helpful and hasten recovery."

340. The nurse instructs a client with viral hepatitis about the type of diet that should be ingested. Which lunch selected by the client indicates understanding about dietary principles associated with this medical diagnosis?
1. Turkey salad, French fries, sherbet
2. Cottage cheese, mixed fruit salad, milkshake
3. Salad, sliced chicken sandwich, gelatin dessert
4. Cheeseburger, tortilla chips, chocolate pudding

341. The nurse is reviewing discharge plans with a client who is hospitalized with hepatitis A. The nurse concludes that the client understands preventive measures to reduce the risk for spreading the disease when the client states, "I should:
1. Wash my hands frequently."
2. Launder my clothes separately."
3. Put used tissues in the garbage."
4. Wear a mask when leaving the house."

342. An exploratory laparotomy is performed on a client with melena, and gastric cancer is discovered. A partial gastrectomy is performed, and a jejunostomy tube is surgically implanted. A nasogastric tube to suction is in place. During the first 24 hours after surgery, the nurse would expect the client's drainage to:
1. Be green and viscid
2. Contain some blood and clots
3. Contain large amounts of frank blood
4. Be similar to coffee grounds in color and consistency

ENDOCRINE SYSTEM

343. A client is diagnosed with diabetes insipidus. During assessment, which sign does the nurse identify as the most indicative of diabetes insipidus?
1. Increased blood glucose
2. Decreased serum osmolarity
3. Elevation of blood pressure
4. Low urinary specific gravity

344. A client is admitted with a head injury. The nurse identifies that the client's urinary retention catheter is draining large amounts of clear, colorless urine. What does the nurse identify as the most likely cause?
1. Poor renal perfusion
2. Increased serum glucose
3. Inadequate ADH secretion
4. Excess amounts of IV fluid

345. The nurse is caring for a client with a disorder of the posterior pituitary gland. Before assessing this client, the nurse first needs to understand that antidiuretic hormone (ADH) influences kidney function by stimulating the:
1. Nephron tubules to reabsorb water
2. Nephron tubules to reabsorb glucose
3. Glomerulus to withhold the proteins from the urine
4. Glomerulus to control the quantity of fluid passing through it

346. Corticosteroids can cause infections. Which rationale does not support this concept? Corticosteroids:
1. Prevent the production of leukocytes
2. Stop antibody production in lymphatic tissue
3. Promote the growth and spread of enteric viruses
4. Interfere with the inflammatory response of the body

347. When caring for all clients and especially clients with a problem of endocrine gland secretion, the nurse should know approximately how long hormones are present in the body. How many hours do most hormones present in the body at any given time remain in the body once secreted from endocrine glands?
1. 24 hours
2. 4 to 6 hours
3. 8 to 12 hours
4. More than 72 hours

348. After a head injury a client develops a deficiency of antidiuretic hormone (ADH). To assess this client, the nurse first needs to understand that usually secretion of ADH causes:
1. Serum osmolarity to increase
2. Urine concentration to decrease
3. Glomerular filtration to decrease
4. Tubular reabsorption of water to increase

349. After surgical clipping of a cerebral aneurysm, the client develops the syndrome of inappropriate secretion of antidiuretic hormone. The nurse should assess this client for which manifestations of excessive levels of antidiuretic hormone (ADH)? Select all that apply.
1. ☐ Polyuria
2. ☑ Weight gain
3. ☐ Hypotension
4. ☑ Hyponatremia
5. ☐ Decreased specific gravity

350. A client who has acromegaly and diabetes mellitus undergoes a hypophysectomy. The nurse identifies that further teaching about the hypophysectomy is necessary when the client states, "I know I will:
1. Be sterile for the rest of my life."
2. Require larger doses of insulin than I did preoperatively."
3. Have to take thyroxine or a similar preparation for the rest of my life."
4. Have to take cortisone or a similar preparation for the rest of my life."

351. The nurse is caring for a client who had a hypophysectomy. The nurse specifically should observe this client for an early clinical indicator of:
1. Urinary retention
2. Respiratory distress
3. Bleeding at the suture line
4. Increased intracranial pressure

352. The nurse is caring for a client experiencing a stressful emergency. The nurse understands that the rapid adjustments made by the client's body are associated with increased activity of which gland?
1. Thyroid
2. Adrenal
3. Pituitary
4. Pancreatic

353. Which piece of information from the client's history does the nurse identify as a risk factor for developing osteoporosis? The client:
1. Receives long-term steroid therapy
2. Has a history of hypoparathyroidism
3. Engages in strenuous physical activity
4. Consumes high doses of the hormone estrogen

354. The nurse is caring for two clients newly diagnosed with diabetes mellitus. One client has type 1 diabetes and the other client has type 2 diabetes. The nurse understands that the main difference between newly diagnosed type 1 and type 2 diabetes mellitus is that in type 1 diabetes:
1. Onset of the disease is slow
2. Excessive weight is a contributing factor
3. Treatment involves diet, exercise, and oral agents
4. Complications are not present at time of diagnosis

355. A client is scheduled for an adrenalectomy. Which nursing action should the nurse implement when caring for this client?
1. Provide a high-protein diet
2. Administer steroids IM or IV
3. Collect a 24-hour urine specimen
4. Withhold all medications for 48 hours

356. The nurse is caring for a newly admitted client with a diagnosis of Cushing's syndrome. Why should the nurse monitor this client for clinical indicators of diabetes mellitus?
  1. Cortical hormones stimulate rapid weight loss.
  2. Excessive ACTH secretion damages pancreatic tissue.
  3. Tissue catabolism results in a negative nitrogen balance.
  4. Glucocorticoids accelerate the process of gluconeogenesis.

357. When caring for a client with a diagnosis of Cushing's syndrome, the nurse understands the most common cause of Cushing's syndrome is:
  1. Pituitary hypoplasia
  2. Insufficient ACTH production
  3. Hyperplasia of the adrenal cortex
  4. Deprivation of adrenocortical hormones

358. The nurse is assessing a client with Cushing's syndrome. Which clinical indicator can the nurse expect to identify?
  1. Menorrhagia
  2. Buffalo hump
  3. Dependent edema
  4. Migraine headaches *hypopituitarism*

359. When assessing a client with Cushing's syndrome, which clinical indicator can the nurse expect the client to demonstrate?
  1. Lability of mood
  2. A decrease in the growth of hair
  3. Ectomorphism with a moon face
  4. An increased resistance to bruising

360. When caring for a client with a diagnosis of Cushing's syndrome, the nurse understands that excessive amounts of glucocorticoids and mineralocorticoids will increase the client's:
  1. Urine output ↓
  2. Glucose level
  3. Serum potassium ↓
  4. Immune response ↓

361. When collecting a 24-hour urine specimen, what should the nurse do?
  1. Check if preservatives need to be added
  2. Weigh the client before starting the collection
  3. Discard the last voided specimen of the 24-hour period
  4. Check the client's intake and output for the previous 24-hour period

362. A client is scheduled for a bilateral adrenalectomy. Before surgery, steroids are administered to the client. The nurse understands the reason for this is to:
  1. Foster accumulation of glycogen in the liver
  2. Increase the inflammatory action to promote scar formation
  3. Facilitate urinary excretion of salt and water following surgery
  4. Compensate for sudden lack of these hormones following surgery

363. The nurse is caring for a client who is scheduled for a bilateral adrenalectomy. Which medication can the nurse expect the physician to order for this client on the day of surgery and in the immediate postoperative period?
  1. ACTH
  2. Regular insulin
  3. Pituitary extract (Pituitrin)
  4. Hydrocortisone succinate (Solu-Cortef)

364. The nurse is caring for a client who had an adrenalectomy. The nurse understands that until the client is regulated by steroid therapy, the nurse must monitor for:
  1. Hypotension ↓ *aldosterone*
  2. Hyperglycemia
  3. Sodium retention
  4. Potassium excretion

365. A client who has just had an adrenalectomy is told about a death in the family and becomes very upset. After comforting the client, the nurse notifies the physician because the client:
  1. Will probably require mild sedation to ensure rest
  2. Should have the steroid medication dosage reduced
  3. Has a decreased ability to handle stress despite steroid therapy
  4. Will have feelings of exhaustion and lethargy as a result of stress

366. A client with a tentative diagnosis of Cushing's syndrome has an elevated cortisol level. The nurse should assess this client for:
  1. Hypovolemia
  2. Hyperkalemia
  3. Hypoglycemia
  4. Hypernatremia

367. The physician orders a low-sodium, high-potassium diet for a client with Cushing's syndrome. The nurse understands that this diet was ordered for this client because:
  1. The use of salt probably contributed to the disease
  2. Excess weight will be gained if sodium is not limited
  3. The loss of excess salt in the urine requires less renal stimulation
  4. Excessive secretions of aldosterone and cortisone cause renal retention of sodium and loss of potassium

368. The nurse is caring for a client with a diagnosis of Addison's disease. The nurse understands that hypotension associated with this disease involves a disturbance in the production of:
  1. Estrogens
  2. Androgens
  3. Glucocorticoids
  4. Mineralocorticoids

369. The nurse should monitor a client with Addison's disease closely for signs of infectious complications because there is a disturbance in which body mechanism?
  1. Stress response *fight infection*
  2. Electrolyte balance
  3. Metabolic processes
  4. Respiratory function

370. A client is admitted to a medical unit with a diagnosis of Addison's disease. The nurse understands that emaciation, muscular weakness, and fatigue associated with Addison's disease result from a disturbance in which body process?
    1. Fluid balance
    2. Electrolyte levels
    3. Protein anabolism
    4. Masculinizing hormones

371. The nurse is planning care for a client with a diagnosis of Addison's disease. Which is an important nursing intervention that the nurse should include in the plan that is specific for a client with Addison's disease?
    1. Encouraging the client to exercise
    2. Protecting the client from exertion
    3. Restricting the client's fluid intake
    4. Monitoring the client for hypokalemia

372. The physician writes orders addressing the needs of a client with Addison's disease. The nurse understands that the main focus of treatment for this client is to:
    1. Decrease eosinophils
    2. Increase lymphoid tissue
    3. Restore electrolyte balance
    4. Improve carbohydrate metabolism

373. The nurse is caring for a client with Addison's disease. Which information should the nurse include in a teaching plan as a means of encouraging this client to improve dietary intake?
    1. Increased amounts of potassium are needed to replace renal losses
    2. Increased protein is needed to heal the adrenal tissue and thus cure the disease
    3. Supplemental vitamins are needed to supply energy to assist in regaining the lost weight
    4. Extra salt is needed to replace the amount being lost due to lack of sufficient aldosterone to conserve sodium

374. The physician orders fludrocortisone therapy for a client with adrenal insufficiency. The nurse should teach the client to consult with the physician in the event of:
    1. Rapid weight gain
    2. Fatigue in the afternoon
    3. Unpredictable changes in mood
    4. Increased frequency of urination

375. A client newly diagnosed with diabetes states, "I know that glucose is delivered to the cells for production of energy. However, does any hormone control use of glucose by the cell?" Which hormone should the nurse explore with the client when responding to this question?
    1. Insulin
    2. Thyroxine
    3. Adrenal steroids
    4. Growth hormone

376. After assessing a client, the nurse concludes that the client may be experiencing hyperglycemia. Which clinical indicator commonly associated with hyperglycemia supports the nurse's conclusion?
    1. Polydipsia
    2. Polyphasia
    3. Polygalactia
    4. Polydysplasia

377. The nurse is monitoring a client's laboratory results for a fasting plasma glucose level. The nurse understands that the client is considered to be prediabetic when a fasting plasma glucose level is between:
    1. 40 and 60 mg/dL
    2. 80 and 99 mg/dL
    3. 100 and 125 mg/dL
    4. 126 and 140 mg/dL

378. Which nursing intervention takes priority when a client is first admitted with hyperglycemic hyperosmolar nonketotic syndrome (HHNS)?
    1. Providing oxygen
    2. Encouraging carbohydrates
    3. Administering fluid replacement
    4. Teaching facts about dietary principles

379. A client admitted to the emergency department has ketones in the blood and urine. Which situation associated with this development should be the nurse's focus when collecting additional data about this client?
    1. Starvation
    2. Alcoholism
    3. Bone healing
    4. Positive nitrogen balance

380. A client tells the nurse during the admission history that an oral hypoglycemic agent is a medication that is taken daily. The nurse understands that an oral hypoglycemic agent may be used for clients with:
    1. Ketosis
    2. Obesity
    3. Type 1 diabetes
    4. Some insulin production

381. The nurse is admitting a client to the hospital with a diagnosis of hypoglycemia. Identify the clinical indicators that the nurse should expect. Select all that apply.
    1. ☐ Thirst
    2. ☐ Palpitations
    3. ☐ Diaphoresis
    4. ☐ Slurred speech
    5. ☐ Hyperventilation

382. The nurse is caring for a client with a diagnosis of diabetes. When monitoring this client for hyperglycemia, the nurse understands that the adaptations associated with diabetic coma result from an excess accumulation in the blood of:
    1. Sodium bicarbonate, causing alkalosis
    2. Ketones from rapid fat breakdown, causing acidosis
    3. Nitrogen from protein catabolism, causing ammonia intoxication
    4. Glucose from rapid carbohydrate metabolism, causing drowsiness

383. A male physician who is found in a diabetic coma has omitted information about a history of diabetes

mellitus from his health record. This pertinent information has most likely been omitted for which reason?

1. Individuals with diabetes mellitus often have lapses of memory
2. Physicians with diabetes are not accepted for residency in many hospitals
3. He needs assistance in developing a more favorable adaptation to this stress
4. He is unable to handle the psychologic stress related to alterations in body functioning

384. The nurse is caring for a postoperative client who also has diabetes. When caring for this client, the nurse needs to understand that the most common cause of diabetic ketoacidosis is:
1. Emotional stress
2. Presence of infection
3. Increased insulin dose
4. Inadequate food intake

385. A client is admitted to the hospital with a diagnosis of diabetic acidosis. The nurse understands that the common initial medical intervention associated with this diagnosis will include administration of:
1. IV fluids
2. Potassium
3. NPH insulin
4. Sodium polystyrene sulfonate (Kayexalate)

386. A client is diagnosed with diabetic ketoacidosis. Which insulin should the nurse expect the physician to order?
1. Human NPH insulin
2. Human regular insulin
3. Insulin lispro injection
4. Insulin glargine injection

387. The nurse is caring for several clients who have diabetes. When assessing these clients, the nurse should understand that a difference between diabetic coma and hyperglycemic hyperosmolar nonketotic syndrome (HHNS) is that a response clients in diabetic coma experience is:
1. Fluid loss
2. Glycosuria
3. Kussmaul respirations
4. Increased blood glucose level

388. A client with untreated type 1 diabetes mellitus may lapse into a coma because of acidosis. An increased concentration of which element in the serum is the direct cause of this type of acidosis?
1. Ketones
2. Glucose
3. Lactic acid
4. Glutamic acid

389. A client is learning alternate site testing (AST) for glucose monitoring. Which client statement indicates to the nurse that additional teaching is necessary?
1. "I need to rub my forearm vigorously until warm before testing at this site."
2. "The fingertip is preferred for glucose monitoring if hyperglycemia is suspected."

3. "Alternate site testing is unsafe if I am experiencing a rapid change in glucose levels."
4. "I have to make sure that my current glucose monitor can be used at an alternative site."

390. A client with diabetes asks the nurse whether the new forearm stick glucose monitor gives the same results as a fingerstick. The nurse should base the response on the knowledge that:
1. These monitors are meant for children
2. Faster readings come from a fingerstick
3. There is no difference between the readings
4. Readings are on a different scale for each monitor

391. A urine specimen is needed to test for the presence of ketones in a client who is diabetic. What should the nurse do when collecting this specimen from a urinary retention catheter?
1. Disconnect the catheter and drain the urine into a clean container
2. Clean the drainage valve and remove the urine from the catheter bag
3. Wipe the catheter with alcohol and drain the urine into a sterile test tube
4. Use a sterile syringe to remove the urine from a clamped, cleansed catheter

392. When monitoring a client's fasting plasma glucose (FPG) level, at which FPG level should the nurse identify that the client has prediabetes?
1. 70 mg/dL
2. 100 mg/dL
3. 130 mg/dL
4. 160 mg/dL

393. A client has a hypoglycemic reaction to insulin. When the nurse assesses this client, which adaptation is indicative of this response?
1. Glycosuria
2. Perspiration
3. Dry, hot skin
4. Fruity odor of breath

394. The nurse is planning to teach facts about hyperglycemia to a client with a diagnosis of diabetes. The nurse should include in this lesson that diabetic acidosis is precipitated by:
1. Breakdown of fat stores for energy
2. Excessive secretion of endogenous insulin
3. Ingestion of too many highly acidic foods
4. Increased concentrations of cholesterol in the extracellular compartment

395. The nurse is collecting information about a client who is being admitted because of a diabetic ketoacidotic coma. Which factor most likely predisposed this client to this condition?
1. Taking too much insulin
2. Getting too much exercise
3. Running a fever with the flu
4. Eating fewer calories than prescribed

396. The nurse is reviewing the medical record for data associated with a client's admission to the hospital for an episode of diabetic ketoacidosis. Which information

related to this event should the nurse document on the client's medical record? Select all that apply.
1. ☐ Sweating
2. ☐ Low P_{CO_2}
3. ☐ Retinopathy
4. ☐ Acetone breath
5. ☐ Elevated serum bicarbonate level

397. Laboratory tests are performed on a client with diabetic ketoacidosis. Which should the nurse expect the tests to reveal?
1. Dilute urine
2. Hypoglycemia
3. Normal acidity
4. Low CO_2 level

398. The nurse is caring for a client with diabetes who is scheduled for a radiographic study requiring contrast. Which should the nurse expect the physician to order?
1. Acetylcysteine therapy
2. Renal-friendly contrast medium
3. Forced diuresis with mannitol after the test
4. Hydration with dextrose and water before the test

399. The physician orders glucagon for a client with type 1 diabetes. The nurse understands that the primary reason for the use of glucagon to treat this client is:
1. Diabetic acidosis
2. Hyperinsulin secretion
3. Insulin-induced hypoglycemia
4. Idiosyncratic reactions to insulin

400. A client's blood gases reflect diabetic acidosis. Which clinical indicator should the nurse expect to identify when monitoring this client's laboratory values?
1. Increased pH
2. Decreased P_{O_2}
3. Increased P_{CO_2}
4. Decreased HCO_3^-

401. The nurse is caring for a client with a new diagnosis of type 1 diabetes. When the physician tries to regulate this client's insulin regimen the client experiences episodes of hypoglycemia and hyperglycemia. The nurse understands the reason that glucagon may be given to this client if hypoglycemia occurs is that it:
1. Inhibits glycogenesis
2. Stimulates release of insulin
3. Increases blood glucose levels
4. Provides more storage of glucose

402. The nurse administers regular insulin to a client in diabetic ketoacidosis. In addition, the nurse anticipates that the IV solution prescribed should contain potassium to replenish potassium ions in the extracellular fluid that are being:
1. Rapidly lost from the body by copious diaphoresis present during coma
2. Carried with glucose to the kidneys to be excreted in the urine in increased amounts

3. Quickly used up during the rapid series of catabolic reactions stimulated by insulin and glucose
4. Moved into the intracellular fluid compartment because of the generalized anabolism induced by insulin and glucose

403. A client has a hypoglycemic reaction to insulin. The nurse assesses the client and documents the client's adaptations that are indicative of this response. Select all that apply.
1. ☐ Pallor
2. ☐ Tremors
3. ☐ Glycosuria
4. ☐ Acetonuria
5. ☐ Diaphoresis

404. The nurse is monitoring a client's blood glucose level via a fingerstick measurement. The nurse identifies that the client is experiencing a hypoglycemic reaction. Which nursing intervention should be instituted immediately to relieve the symptoms associated with this reaction?
1. Giving 4 oz of fruit juice
2. Administering 5% dextrose solution IV
3. Withholding a subsequent dose of insulin
4. Providing a snack of cheese and dry crackers

405. The nurse working in the diabetes clinic is evaluating a client's success with managing diabetes. Which is the best indication that a client with diabetes mellitus is successfully managing the disease after discharge?
1. Reduction in excess body weight
2. Stabilization of the serum glucose
3. Demonstrated knowledge of the disease
4. Compliance with orders for insulin administration

406. A client with type 1 diabetes mellitus has a fingerstick glucose level of 258 mg/dL at bedtime. An order for sliding scale insulin exists. What should the nurse do?
1. Call the client's physician.
2. Encourage the intake of fluids.
3. Administer the insulin as ordered.
4. Give the client ½ cup of orange juice.

407. A client with diabetes is given instructions about foot care. Which client statement indicates an understanding of the nurse's instructions? "I will:
1. Soak my feet daily for 1 hour."
2. Cut my toenails before bathing."
3. Examine my feet using a mirror at least once a week."
4. Break in new shoes over the course of several weeks."

408. Which client statement indicates to the nurse that learning about diabetes mellitus and diet is understood? "My diet:
1. Should be rigidly controlled to avoid emergencies."
2. Can be planned around a wide variety of commonly used foods."
3. Is based on nutritional requirements that are the same for all people."
4. Must not include eating any combination dishes and processed foods."

409. The physician orders 36 units of NPH insulin and 12 units of regular insulin. The nurse plans to administer these drugs in one syringe. Identify the steps in this procedure by listing the numbers by each picture next to the step below in priority order. (Start with the number of the picture that represents the first step and end with the number by the picture that represents the last step.)

Step 1_____ Step 2_____ Step 3_____ Step 4_____

1. Inject air equal to NPH dose into NPH vial.

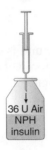

2. Invert regular insulin bottle and withdraw regular insulin dose.

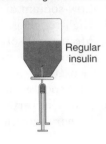

Regular insulin

3. Inject air equal to regular dose into regular vial.

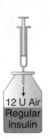

4. Invert NPH vial and withdraw NPH dose.

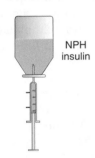

NPH insulin

410. The nurse is caring for a group of clients who have diabetes. In the event that a client experiences hypoglycemia, which insulin has the most rapid onset of action?
1. Lente
2. Lispro
3. Ultralente
4. Humulin N

411. A client with diabetes mellitus states, "I cannot eat big meals; I prefer to snack throughout the day." The nurse should carefully explain that:
1. Regulated food intake is basic to control
2. Salt and sugar restriction is the main concern
3. Small, frequent meals are better for digestion
4. Large meals can contribute to a weight problem

412. The nurse plans an evening snack of milk, crackers, and cheese for an average-sized client who is receiving Humulin N insulin. This snack provides:
1. Encouragement to stay on the diet
2. Added calories to promote weight gain
3. Nourishment to counteract late insulin activity
4. High-carbohydrate nourishment for immediate use

413. When a client has a glycosylated hemoglobin measurement of 6%, the nurse should plan care based on the knowledge that the client:
1. Is experiencing a rebound hyperglycemia

2. Needs the insulin changed to a different type
3. Has followed the treatment plan as prescribed
4. Requires further teaching regarding nutritional guidelines

414. The nurse is formulating a teaching plan for a client recently diagnosed with type 2 diabetes. Identify the interventions that decrease the risk for complications for this client. Check all that apply.
1. ☐ Examining the feet daily
2. ☐ Wearing well-fitting shoes
3. ☐ Performing regular exercise
4. ☐ Visiting the physician weekly
5. ☐ Powdering the feet after showering
6. ☐ Testing bath water with the toes before bathing

415. Which is an independent nursing action that should be included in the plan of care for a client after an episode of ketoacidosis?
1. Monitoring for signs of hypoglycemia as a result of treatment
2. Withholding glucose in any form until the situation is corrected
3. Giving fruit juices, broth, and milk as soon as the client is able to take fluids orally
4. Regulating insulin dosage according to the amount of ketones found in the client's urine

416. A client with diabetes mellitus has an above-the-knee amputation because of severe peripheral vascular disease. Which is the nurse's primary responsibility 2 days following surgery when preparing the client for dinner?
1. Checking the client's serum glucose level
2. Assisting the client out of bed into a chair
3. Placing the client in the high-Fowler's position
4. Ensuring that the client's residual limb is elevated

417. A client with diabetes is being taught to self-administer a subcutaneous injection of insulin. Identify the preferred site for the self-administration of this drug.
1. A
2. B
3. C
4. D

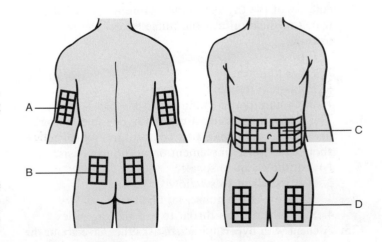

418. The nurse understands that the gland that is the primary regulator of the rate of oxygenation in all the cells in the body is the:
    1. Thyroid gland
    2. Adrenal gland
    3. Pituitary gland
    4. Pancreatic gland

419. The nurse is caring for a client who is experiencing an underproduction of thyroxine. When assessing this client, clinical indicators identified by the nurse are associated with:
    1. Myxedema
    2. Acromegaly
    3. Graves' disease
    4. Cushing's disease

420. The nurse is caring for a client with a congenital defect of the thyroid gland. Which response should the nurse expect the client to exhibit as a result of low levels of T_3 and T_4?
    1. Irritability
    2. Tachycardia
    3. Cold intolerance
    4. Profuse diaphoresis

421. Which adaptations should the nurse expect the client to exhibit when assessing a client with hyperthyroidism?
    1. Listlessness
    2. Weight loss
    3. Bradycardia
    4. Decreased appetite

422. The nurse understands that after radioactive iodine is administered to a client with Graves' disease, the client is:
    1. Not radioactive and can be handled as any other individual
    2. Highly radioactive and should be isolated as much as possible
    3. Mildly radioactive and should be treated with routine safety precautions
    4. Not radioactive but may still transmit some dangerous radiations and must be treated with precautions

423. Understanding the need to decrease the size and vascularity of the thyroid gland before a thyroidectomy, which medication can the nurse expect the physician to order?
    1. Pitressin
    2. Propylthiouracil
    3. Potassium iodide
    4. Potassium permanganate

424. The nurse is assessing a client for possible laryngeal nerve injury following a thyroidectomy. Which action should the nurse implement on an hourly basis?
    1. Ask the client to speak
    2. Ask the client to swallow
    3. Have the client hum a familiar tune
    4. Swab the client's throat to test the gag reflex

425. A client with hyperthyroidism asks the nurse about the tests the physician will be ordering. Which diagnostic tests should the nurse plan to include in a teaching plan for this client?
    1. T_4 and x-ray films
    2. TSH assay and T_3
    3. Thyroglobulin level and Po_2
    4. Protein-bound iodine and SMA

426. The nurse is caring for a newly admitted client with a diagnosis of Graves' disease. Which diet does the nurse anticipate the physician will order for this client?
    1. High-calorie diet
    2. Low-sodium diet
    3. High-roughage diet
    4. Mechanical-soft diet

427. The nurse in the postanesthesia care unit is caring for a client who just had a thyroidectomy. For which client response should the nurse monitor immediately after this surgery?
    1. Urinary retention
    2. Signs of restlessness
    3. Decreased blood pressure
    4. Signs of respiratory obstruction

428. The nurse is caring for a client who just had a thyroidectomy. Because an accidental removal of the parathyroid glands during a thyroidectomy is always a concern, for which client response should the nurse assess?
    1. Tetany
    2. Myxedema
    3. Hypovolemic shock
    4. Adrenocortical stimulation

429. When taking the blood pressure of a client who has had a thyroidectomy, the nurse notices the client is pale and has spasms of the hand. The nurse notifies the physician. While awaiting the physician's orders, the nurse should prepare for replacement of:
    1. Calcium
    2. Magnesium
    3. Bicarbonate
    4. Potassium chloride

430. When a client returns from the postanesthesia care unit following a subtotal thyroidectomy, what should the nurse do immediately?
    1. Inspect the incision
    2. Instruct the client not to speak
    3. Keep the client supine for 24 hours
    4. Place a tracheostomy set at the bedside

431. On the first postoperative day following a thyroidectomy, a client tolerates a full-fluid diet. This is changed to a soft diet on the second postoperative day. The client complains of a sore throat when swallowing. What should the nurse do?
    1. Reorder the full-fluid diet
    2. Notify the physician immediately
    3. Administer analgesics as prescribed before meals
    4. Provide saline gargles to moisten the mucous membranes

432. The nurse is assessing a client with a diagnosis of hypothyroidism. Which adaptation should the nurse expect this client to exhibit?
1. Dry skin
2. Weight loss
3. Resting tremors
4. Heat intolerance

433. The nurse understands that the two interbalanced regulatory agents that control overall calcium balance in the body are:
1. Phosphorus and ACTH
2. Vitamin A and thyroid hormone
3. Ascorbic acid and growth hormone
4. Vitamin D and parathyroid hormone

434. The nurse understands that the hormone that tends to decrease calcium concentration in the blood is:
1. Calcitonin
2. Aldosterone
3. Parathormone
4. Triiodothyronine

435. A client is diagnosed with hyperthyroidism and is experiencing exophthalmia. Which measures should the nurse include when teaching this client how to manage the discomfort associated with exophthalmia? Check all that apply.
1. ☐ Use tinted glasses.
2. ☐ Use warm, moist compresses.
3. ☐ Elevate the head of the bed 45 degrees.
4. ☐ Tape eyelids shut at night if they do not close.
5. ☐ Apply a petroleum-based jelly along the lower eyelid.

436. When assessing for complications of hyperparathyroidism, the nurse should monitor the client for which response?
1. Tetany
2. Seizures
3. Graves' disease
4. Bone destruction

437. The nurse is caring for a client who is admitted to the hospital with the diagnosis of primary hyperparathyroidism. Which action should be included in this client's plan of care?
1. Ensuring a large fluid intake
2. Providing a high-calcium diet
3. Instituting seizure precautions
4. Prescribing bed rest without bathroom privilages

INTEGUMENTARY SYSTEM

438. The nurse is preparing to give a client a tepid bath and uses a bath thermometer to test the water temperature. What is the acceptable temperature range for a tepid bath?
1. 92° to 94° F
2. 95° to 97° F
3. 98° to 100° F
4. 101° to 103° F

439. The physician orders the application of a warm soak to an IV site that has infiltrated. The nurse understands that the application of local heat transfers temperature to the body via the principle of:
1. Radiation
2. Insulation
3. Convection
4. Conduction

440. The nurse is caring for a client who is admitted to the hospital for medical management of heart failure and severe peripheral edema. The nurse understands that if the edema remains unresolved, the client will most likely develop:
1. Proteinemia
2. Contractures
3. Tissue ischemia
4. Thrombus formation

441. The nurse is caring for a client with a diagnosis of psoriasis. When assessing this client, which clinical finding will most likely be present?
1. Scaly lesions
2. Pruritic lesions
3. Multiple petechiae
4. Erythematous macules

442. A client with psoriasis asks the nurse what common treatment can be expected for this condition. Which intervention should the nurse include in a teaching plan for this client?
1. Avoiding exposure to the sun
2. Topical application of steroids
3. Potassium permanganate baths
4. Debridement of necrotic plaques

443. When planning care for a client with scabies, it is important for the nurse to understand that it is:
1. Highly contagious
2. Caused by a fungus
3. Chronic with exacerbations
4. Associated with other allergies

444. The nurse is caring for a client with the diagnosis of pemphigus vulgaris. The nurse needs to plan care to address which resulting problem?
1. Paralysis
2. Infertility
3. Skin lesions
4. Impaired digestion

445. The nurse is caring for a client who is admitted for diagnostic testing to rule out systemic lupus erythematosus (SLE). Which common adaptation to this disease can the nurse expect the client to exhibit?
1. A butterfly rash
2. Firm skin fixed to tissue
3. Muscle mass degeneration
4. An inflammation of small arteries

446. A client newly diagnosed with scleroderma states, "Where did I get this from?" The nurse's best response is, "Although no cause has been determined for scleroderma, it is thought to be the result of:
1. Autoimmunity."
2. Ocular motility."

3. Increased amino acid metabolism."
4. Defective sebaceous gland formation."

447. A client with a spinal cord injury tends to assume the low-Fowler's position excessively. Indicate the area of the body that is most vulnerable to the development of a pressure ulcer in this client.

Answer: _____

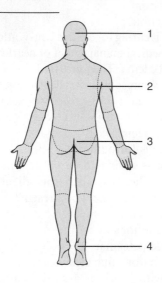

448. The nurse is caring for a client admitted for removal of basal cell carcinoma and reconstruction of the nose. About which contributing factor should the nurse question the client when collecting a health history?
1. Familial tendencies
2. Their dietary patterns
3. Their smoking history
4. Ultraviolet radiation exposure

449. For which adaptation should the nurse assess a client with metastatic melanoma?
1. Oily skin
2. Nikolsky's sign
3. Lymphadenopathy
4. Erythema of the palms

450. A client is admitted for malignant melanoma that was discovered during a routine eye examination. For which preferred treatment does the nurse expect the client to be scheduled?
1. Radiation
2. Enucleation
3. Cryosurgery
4. Chemotherapy

451. When teaching first aid, the nurse explains that the best first-aid treatment for acid burns on the skin is to flush them with water and then apply a solution of which type of sodium?
1. Sulfate
2. Chloride
3. Hydroxide
4. Bicarbonate

452. A nurse educator is teaching a class of nursing students about the best action to employ when providing first-aid treatment for a client who experienced an alkali burn. The students are told that an effective

first-aid treatment for this type of burn is to flush it with water and then with:
1. Weak acid
2. Dilute base
3. Salt solution
4. Antibiotic solution

453. The nurse identifies that learning about skin grafts has occurred when the client says, "A skin graft that is taken from another portion of my own body is known as:
1. An allograft."
2. A xenograft."
3. An autograft."
4. A homograft."

454. A client is scheduled to have a pigskin graft applied to a burned area. The nurse understands that this type of graft is known as:
1. An isograft
2. An allograft
3. A homograft
4. A heterograft

455. The nurse is evaluating a client's fluid loss resulting from extensive burns. Which blood test is most valuable when determining this client's fluid loss?
1. BUN
2. Blood pH
3. Hematocrit
4. Sedimentation rate

456. When evaluating fluid loss in a burned client, the nurse understands that the relationship between body surface area and fluid loss is:
1. Equal
2. Unrelated
3. Inversely related
4. Directly proportional

457. A client is admitted to the emergency department with extensive burns. Which medication should the nurse anticipate the physician ordering for this client as soon after admission as possible?
1. Tetanus toxoid
2. Gamma globulin
3. Isoproterenol (Isuprel)
4. Phytonadione (AquaMEPHYTON)

458. Which is the most difficult problem for the nurse to deal with when meeting the needs of an extensively burned client 3 days after admission?
1. Severe pain
2. Maintenance of sterility
3. Alteration in body image
4. Frequent dressing changes

459. The nurse is caring for a client who has a disturbed body image as a result of a burn injury. Which is an important nursing intervention for this client?
1. Convey a positive attitude toward the client
2. Arrange for the client to meet other clients with burns
3. Remove mirrors until the client's physical appearance has improved
4. Remind family members to refrain from comments about the client's appearance

460. A middle-aged adult is admitted with partial-thickness burns over 42% of the body. The nurse anticipates that the physician will rate this client's condition as:
    1. Fair
    2. Poor
    3. Good
    4. Critical

461. The primary short-term outcome established by the nurse for a client 1 day after sustaining a partial-thickness burn to the lower leg accounting for 5% of the total body surface area is, "The client's:
    1. Airway will remain patent."
    2. Burns will heal free of infection."
    3. Urine output will exceed 30 mL every hour."
    4. Pain will be no higher than 2 on a scale of 0 to 10."

462. A worker is involved in an explosion of a steam pipe and receives a scalding burn to the chest and arms. The burned areas are painful, mottled red, weeping, and edematous. The nurse understands that these burns are classified as:
    1. Eschar
    2. Full-thickness
    3. Deep partial-thickness
    4. Superficial partial-thickness

463. During the first few hours after a client is admitted to the burn unit with partial-thickness burns of the trunk and head, the nurse is least concerned about the development of:
    1. Pain
    2. Leukopenia
    3. Laryngeal edema
    4. Fluid volume deficit

464. In the emergent phase immediately after a severe burn injury, client care is centered on replacement IV fluid therapy. The nurse should question the physician's order if it is designed to provide:
    1. Colloids
    2. Potassium
    3. Hypertonic saline
    4. Lactated Ringer's solution

465. The nurse is caring for a client during the first 24 hours following a burn injury. When assessing this client, which sign indicates adequate fluid replacement therapy?
    1. Falling CVP readings
    2. Urinary output of 15 to 20 mL/hr
    3. Slowing of a previously rapid pulse
    4. Hematocrit level rising from 50% to 55%

466. The nurse places a client with severe burns on a circulating air bed. The primary reason why the nurse implements this action is to:
    1. Increase mobility
    2. Prevent contractures
    3. Limit orthostatic hypotension
    4. Prevent pressure on peripheral blood vessels

467. Which information should the nurse include in a teaching plan for a client whose burns are being treated with the exposure method?
    1. Bathing will not be permitted
    2. Aseptic techniques are required
    3. Dressings will be changed every day
    4. Room temperature must be kept at 72° F

468. A severely burned client has been hospitalized for 2 days. Until now recovery has been uneventful, but the client begins to exhibit extreme restlessness. The nurse concludes that this most likely indicates that the client is developing:
    1. Kidney failure
    2. Fluid overload
    3. Cerebral hypoxia
    4. Metabolic acidosis

469. A female client with 35% of total body surface area burned in a factory fire is now 48 hours post burn. The client's clinical manifestations indicate that she is moving from the emergent to the acute phase of burn management. Which assessment supports this conclusion?
    1. Hypokalemia
    2. Hypoglycemia
    3. Decreased blood pressure
    4. Elevated urine specific gravity

470. The nurse is caring for a client with a diagnosis of necrotizing fasciitis. The nurse understands that the primary concern at this time is:
    1. Fluid volume
    2. Skin integrity
    3. Physical mobility
    4. Urinary elimination

NEUROMUSCULOSKELETAL SYSTEM

471. The student nurse who is administering a beta blocker asks the nurse about its effect on the autonomic nervous system. When formulating a response the nurse should understand which common misconception about the autonomic nervous system?
    1. Both sympathetic and parasympathetic impulses continually affect most visceral effectors
    2. The autonomic nervous system is regulated by impulses from the hypothalamus and other parts of the brain
    3. Sympathetic impulses stimulate while parasympathetic impulses inhibit the functioning of any visceral effector
    4. Visceral effectors (e.g., cardiac muscle, smooth muscle, glandular epithelial tissue) receive impulses only via autonomic neurons

472. The client with a head injury is having problems with several sensory functions. The nurse should understand that the structure that acts as a relay center for sensory impulses is the:
    1. Thalamus
    2. Cerebellum
    3. Hypothalamus
    4. Medulla oblongata

473. The nurse identifies which clinical indicator of parasympathetic dominance in a client under stress?
    1. Constipation
    2. Goose pimples

3. Increased GI secretions

4. Excess epinephrine secretion

474. Which clinical indicator does the nurse identify when assessing a client with hemiplegia?

1. Paresis of both lower extremities

2. Paralysis of one side of the body

3. Paralysis of both lower extremities

4. Paresis of upper and lower extremities

475. The school nurse is attending to a student athlete who is complaining of muscle pain after a practice session. The nurse should explain to the student that an over-exercised muscle that has an insufficient O_2 supply may become sore from a buildup of:

1. Lactic acid

2. Butyric acid

3. Acetoacetic acid

4. Hydrochloric acid

476. The nurse advises a client to participate in an aerobic exercise program to reduce the risk of cardiovascular disease. The nurse expects the O_2 associated with anaerobic activity to produce which effect on muscles?

1. Lower levels of ATP

2. Higher levels of calcium

3. Higher levels of glycogen

4. Lower levels of lactic acid

477. After a head injury, a client reports experiencing changes in emotion. The nurse understands that feelings of pleasantness or unpleasantness, varying in degree from mild to intense, occur when sensory impulses reach the:

1. Thalamus

2. Basal ganglia

3. Hypothalamus

4. Cerebral cortex

478. A client has experienced multiple transient ischemic attacks. The nurse understands an arterial anastomosis present at the base of the brain is important in maintaining the integrity of the cerebral neurons. What is the name of this anastomosis?

1. Volar arch

2. Circle of Willis

3. Brachial plexus

4. Brachiocephalic sinus

479. When caring for a client with a head injury that may have involved the medulla, the nurse bases assessments on the knowledge that the medulla controls a variety of functions. Which ones apply? Select all that apply.

1. ☐ Breathing

2. ☐ Pulse rate

3. ☐ Fat metabolism

4. ☐ Blood vessel diameter

5. ☐ Temperature regulation

480. When performing a neurologic assessment of a client, the nurse identifies that the client has a dilated right pupil. The nurse understands that this suggests a problem with which cranial nerve?

1. Third cranial nerve

2. Second cranial nerve

3. Fourth cranial nerve

4. Seventh cranial nerve

481. The mouth of a client is drawn over to the left. The nurse understands that this suggests injury to which cranial nerve?

1. Left facial nerve

2. Right facial nerve

3. Left abducent nerve

4. Right trigeminal nerve

482. A physician performs a lumbar puncture. The client asks if the needle goes into the spinal cord. The nurse bases a response on the understanding that the physician must insert a needle into the:

1. Pia mater

2. Foramen ovale

3. Subarachnoid space

4. Aqueduct of Sylvius

483. After a brain attack a client remains unresponsive to sensory stimulation. The nurse understands general sensations such as heat, cold, pain, and touch are registered in the:

1. Frontal lobe

2. Parietal lobe

3. Occipital lobe

4. Temporal lobe

484. A client experiences a traumatic brain injury. Which finding identified by the nurse indicates damage to the upper motor neurons?

1. Absent reflexes

2. Flaccid muscles

3. Trousseau's sign

4. Babinski's response

485. When caring for an anxious, fearful client, the nurse would identify which of the following as an indication of sympathetic nervous system control?

1. Dry skin

2. Skin pallor

3. Constriction of pupils

4. Pulse rate of 60 beats/min

486. When transporting a client on a stretcher, the nurse makes certain that the client's arms do not hang down over the edge. To which nerve plexus does the nurse avoid injury by taking this precaution?

1. Solar plexus

2. Celiac plexus

3. Basilar plexus

4. Brachial plexus

487. The nurse assists the physician in performing a lumbar puncture. When pressure is placed on the jugular vein during a lumbar puncture, the spinal fluid pressure is expected to increase. Which sign should the nurse expect the physician to document?

1. Homans' sign

2. Romberg's sign

3. Chvostek's sign

4. Queckenstedt's sign

488. In the postanesthesia care unit, the nurse should assess a client who has had a craniotomy for a meningioma and a ventriculoatrial shunt for:
1. Dehydration
2. Blurred vision
3. Wound infection
4. Narrowing pulse pressure

489. A client is admitted with a tumor near the optic chiasm. The client asks the nurse about the optic chiasm. When formulating a response, what must the nurse understand? The optic chiasm:
1. Forms a cavity in which the eyeball is fixed
2. Receives nerve impulses from the optic tracts
3. Is a crossing of some optic nerves in the cranial cavity
4. Is the space posterior to the lens with the consistency of jelly

490. A client is admitted with paresis of the ciliary muscles of the left eye. The nurse understands contraction of the ciliary muscles:
1. Closes the eyelids
2. Causes the pupils to dilate
3. Focuses the lens on near objects
4. Brings about convergence of both eyes

491. A client develops an inflammatory reaction in the eye. Which drug does the nurse anticipate the physician will probably prescribe?
1. Cortisone
2. Neomycin
3. Nitrofurazone (Furacin)
4. Acetazolamide (Diamox)

492. Which desired effect of therapy should the nurse explain to the client with primary angle-closure glaucoma?
1. Dilating the pupil
2. Resting the eye muscles
3. Controlling intraocular pressure
4. Preventing secondary infections

493. Which clinical indicator is the nurse most likely to identify when exploring the history of a client with open-angle glaucoma?
1. Constant blurred vision
2. Sudden attacks of acute pain
3. Impairment of peripheral vision
4. Sudden, complete loss of vision

494. A client's child asks the nurse what a cataract is. What explanation should the nurse provide? "A cataract is:
1. An opacity of the lens."
2. A thin film over the cornea."
3. A crystallinization of the pupil."
4. An increase in the density of the conjunctiva."

495. After a client has cataract surgery, what should the nurse do?
1. Instruct the client to avoid driving for 2 weeks
2. Teach the client coughing and deep-breathing techniques
3. Encourage eye exercises to strengthen the ocular musculature
4. Advise the client to refrain from vigorous brushing of teeth and hair

496. When a client with a detached retina asks about the condition, the nurse's response should be based on the understanding that retinal detachment is a:
1. Consequence of optic nerve and retinal atrophy
2. Degeneration of the choroid and optic chiasm
3. Division between the photoreceptor and neural layers of the retina
4. Separation between the sensory portion of the retina and the pigment layer

497. A client is scheduled for surgery for a detached retina. Which client statement indicates to the nurse that preoperative teaching is effective? "The goal of surgery is to:
1. Promote growth of new retinal cells."
2. Adhere the sclera to the choroid layer."
3. Graft a healthy piece of retina in place."
4. Create a scar that aids in healing retinal holes."

498. A client in the health clinic reports a hearing loss. The client asks the nurse, "Which part of the car contains the receptors for hearing?" The nurse's response includes an explanation of the function of which part of the ear?
1. Utricle
2. Cochlea
3. Middle ear
4. Tympanic cavity

499. The client has a conductive hearing loss. The nurse explains that the bones that transmit vibrations to the oval window of the cochlea are located in which structure?
1. Earlobe
2. Eardrum
3. Inner ear
4. Middle ear

500. A client with a hearing loss asks the nurse to explain the cause of nerve deafness. The nurse explains that nerve deafness is most likely caused by an injury or infection that damages the:
1. Vagus nerve
2. Cochlear nerve
3. Vestibular nerve
4. Trigeminal nerve

501. A client is scheduled for a labyrinthectomy to treat Ménière's syndrome. The nurse concludes that the client understood preoperative instructions when the client identifies that the surgery results in:
1. Anosmia
2. Absence of pain
3. Decreased cerumen
4. Permanent irreversible deafness

502. The nurse is developing a teaching plan for a client with otosclerosis. What understanding must the nurse have to provide effective instruction?
1. Stapedectomy is the procedure of choice
2. Hearing aids usually restore some hearing
3. The client is usually unable to hear bass tones
4. Air conduction is more effective than bone conduction

503. When considering a client's symptoms, how should the nurse categorize a client's complaint of tinnitus?
    1. Objective
    2. Subjective
    3. Prodromal
    4. Functional

504. The nurse is providing care for a client with otosclerosis. To anticipate the clinical indicators the client will exhibit, the nurse must understand that the three ossicles serve primarily to:
    1. Maintain balance
    2. Translate sound waves into nerve impulses
    3. Amplify the energy of sound waves entering the ear
    4. Communicate with the throat via the eustachian tube

505. The nurse is planning a research study involving nursing care of clients with brain tumors. The nurse is limiting the study to clients with the same diagnosis to control variables. Which diagnosis provides the largest population for the nurse to research?
    1. Glioma
    2. Angioma
    3. Meningioma
    4. Neurofibroma

506. What clinical indicators does the nurse expect to identify when assessing a client with a brain tumor in the occipital lobe?
    1. Hemiparesis
    2. Receptive aphasia
    3. Personality changes
    4. Visual hallucinations

507. A client is to have a parotidectomy to remove a cancerous lesion. For which postoperative complication that may be permanent should the nurse monitor?
    1. A tracheostomy
    2. Frey's syndrome
    3. Facial nerve dysfunction
    4. An increase in salivation

508. A client, who is receiving phenytoin (Dilantin) to control a seizure disorder, questions the nurse regarding this medication after discharge. Which is the nurse's best response? "This medication:
    1. Prevents the occurrence of seizures."
    2. Will probably have to be continued for life."
    3. Needs to be taken during periods of emotional stress."
    4. Can usually be stopped after a year's absence of seizures."

509. A client with a history of seizures is admitted with a partial occlusion of the left common carotid artery. The client has been taking phenytoin (Dilantin) for 10 years. When planning care for this client, what should the nurse do first?
    1. Obtain a history of seizure type and incidence
    2. Place an airway, and restraints at the bedside
    3. Ask the client to remove any dentures and eyeglasses
    4. Observe the client for increased restlessness and agitation

510. What is the primary responsibility of a nurse during a client's generalized motor seizure?
    1. Inserting a plastic airway between the teeth
    2. Determining whether an aura was experienced
    3. Administering the prescribed PRN anticonvulsant
    4. Clearing the immediate environment for client safety

511. A client who has a history of seizures is scheduled for an arteriogram at 10 AM and is to have nothing by mouth before the test. The client is scheduled to receive phenytoin (Dilantin) at 9 AM. What should the nurse do?
    1. Omit the 9 AM dose of the drug
    2. Give the same dosage of the drug rectally
    3. Ask the physician if the drug can be given IV
    4. Administer the drug with 30 mL of water at 9 AM

512. A client is admitted to the emergency department with a brain injury as a result of an automobile collision. The nurse understands that the injury is more likely to cause death if it involves the:
    1. Pons
    2. Medulla
    3. Midbrain
    4. Thalamus

513. After sustaining a head trauma, a client complains of hearing ringing noises. The nurse understands that this clinical indicator suggests injury to the:
    1. Frontal lobe
    2. Occipital lobe
    3. Sixth cranial nerve (abducent)
    4. Eighth cranial nerve (vestibulocochlear)

514. When assessing an unconscious client, which clinical indicator should the nurse expect to identify? An inability to:
    1. Hear voices
    2. Control elimination
    3. Move spontaneously
    4. React to painful stimuli

515. The neurologic assessment of a client who had a craniotomy includes the Glasgow Coma Scale. What does the nurse evaluate to assess the client's score on the Glasgow Coma Scale? Check all that apply.
    1. ☐ Ability of the client's pupils to react to light
    2. ☐ Degree of purposeful movement by the client
    3. ☐ Appropriateness of the client's verbal responses
    4. ☐ Stimulus necessary to cause the client's eyes to open
    5. ☐ Symmetry of muscle strength of the client's extremities

516. A client regains consciousness and has expressive aphasia. What should the nurse include as part of long-range planning for this client?
    1. Provide positive feedback when the client uses a word correctly
    2. Wait for the client to verbally state needs regardless of how long it takes
    3. Suggest that the client get help at home because the disability is permanent
    4. Help the family to accept the fact that the client cannot participate in verbal communication

517. Soon after admission to the hospital with a head injury, a client's temperature rises to 102.2° F (39° C). The nurse understands that this suggests injury to what structure?
    1. Thalamus
    2. Hypothalamus
    3. Temporal lobe
    4. Globus pallidus
518. When caring for a client who has a possible skull fracture as a result of trauma, what action should the nurse take?
    1. Monitor the client for signs of brain injury
    2. Check for hemorrhaging from the oral and nasal cavities
    3. Elevate the foot of the bed if the client develops symptoms of shock
    4. Observe for symptoms of decreased intracranial pressure and temperature
519. A client with a brain tumor is being assessed. Which adaptations would indicate an increase in intracranial pressure? Check all that apply.
    1. ❑ Fever
    2. ❑ Stupor
    3. ❑ Orthopnea
    4. ❑ Rapid pulse
    5. ❑ Hypotension
520. What therapeutic effect does the nurse expect to identify when dexamethasone is administered to a client after a brain attack?
    1. Improved renal blood flow
    2. Reduced intracranial pressure
    3. Maintenance of circulatory volume
    4. Prevention of the development of thrombi
521. When caring for a client who has sustained a head injury, it is important that the nurse assess for which clinical indicator?
    1. Decreased carotid pulses
    2. Bleeding from the oral cavity
    3. Altered level of consciousness
    4. Absence of deep tendon reflexes
522. Two weeks after cranial surgery for a ruptured cerebral aneurysm, a client develops hydrocephalus. The nurse understands that the hydrocephalus is probably related to which physiologic response?
    1. Increased production of CSF
    2. Vasospasm of adjacent cerebral arteries
    3. Ischemic changes in Broca's speech center
    4. Blocked absorption of fluid from the arachnoid space
523. In the immediate postoperative period after a client has had brain surgery, the nurse should assess the client for:
    1. Tachycardia
    2. Constricted pupils
    3. Elevated diastolic pressure
    4. Decreased level of consciousness
524. A client has been receiving dexamethasone (Decadron) during the past 2 weeks for control of cerebral edema.

The nurse understands that the therapeutic response of the client to dexamethasone is based on which action?
    1. Suppressed production of antibodies
    2. Increased elasticity of the ventricle walls
    3. Decreased cerebral capillary permeability
    4. Reduced CSF secretion by the choroid plexus
525. Which health problem does the nurse identify from an older client's history that increases the client's risk factors of a brain attack?
    1. Glaucoma
    2. Hypothyroidism
    3. Continuous nervousness
    4. Transient ischemic attacks
526. Which clinical indicator is the nurse most likely to identify when assessing a client with a ruptured cerebral aneurysm?
    1. Tonic-clonic seizures
    2. Decerebrate posturing
    3. Sudden severe headache
    4. Narrowed pulse pressure
527. A client with a brain attack is comatose on admission. Which clinical indicator is the nurse most likely to identify?
    1. Twitching motions
    2. Purposeful motions
    3. Urinary incontinence
    4. Unresponsiveness to pain
528. When a client experiences a brain attack, in which position should the nurse initially place the client?
    1. Prone position
    2. Supine position
    3. Lateral position
    4. Trendelenburg position
529. The nurse understands that a client with dysphagia has difficulty:
    1. Writing
    2. Focusing
    3. Swallowing
    4. Understanding
530. A client with a brain attack has dysarthria. What should the nurse include in the care plan to address this problem?
    1. Routine hygiene
    2. Liquid formula diet
    3. Prevention of aspiration
    4. Effective communication
531. A client with a brain attack has a right hemiplegia. The nurse understands that blood pressures should not be obtained by using this client's right arm because circulatory impairment may:
    1. Produce inaccurate readings
    2. Hinder restoration of function
    3. Precipitate the formation of a thrombus
    4. Cause excessive pressure on the brachial artery
532. A client is confined to bed rest after a brain attack results in hemiplegia; 24 hours after the brain attack,

which exercises should the nurse incorporate into the client's care plan?
1. Active exercises of the extremities
2. Passive range-of-motion exercises
3. Light weight-lifting exercises of the right side
4. Isotonic exercises that would capitalize on returning muscle function

533. Which clinical indicators does the nurse identify that suggest that a client is experiencing urinary retention and overflow after a brain attack?
1. Frequent voidings
2. Oliguria and edema
3. Continual incontinence
4. Decreased urine production and pH

534. A client has left hemiplegia because of a brain attack. What can the nurse do to contribute to the client's rehabilitation?
1. Begin active exercises
2. Position the client to prevent deformity
3. Make a referral to the physical therapist
4. Avoid moving the affected extremities unless necessary

535. A client has had a brain attack and the practitioner has ordered bed rest. What can the nurse use to best prevent footdrop in this client?
1. Blocks
2. Splints
3. Cradles
4. Sandbags

536. What is the maximum amount of time the nurse should allow an older adult with a brain attack to remain in one position?
1. 1 to 2 hours
2. 3 to 4 hours
3. 15 to 20 minutes
4. 30 to 40 minutes

537. A client with a hemiparesis is reluctant to use a cane. The nurse explains to the client that a cane is needed to:
1. Maintain balance to improve stability
2. Relieve pressure on weight-bearing joints
3. Prevent further injury to weakened muscles
4. Aid in controlling involuntary muscle movements

538. On which principle should the nurse base client teaching when planning to assist a client to reestablish a regular pattern of defecation?
1. Sedentary activities produce muscle atonia
2. Increased fluid promotes ease of evacuation
3. Peristalsis is initiated by the gastrocolic reflex
4. Increased potassium is needed for normal neuromuscular irritability

539. For optimum nutrition, the nurse may find that a client with a brain attack needs assistance with eating. What should the nurse do?
1. Request that the client's food be pureed
2. Feed the client to conserve the client's energy
3. Have a family member assist the client with each meal
4. Encourage the client to participate in the feeding process

540. A client with a brain attack becomes incontinent of feces. When establishing a bowel training program, the nurse understands the action most important to support success is:
1. Using medication to induce elimination
2. Planning a definite time for attempted evacuations
3. Considering previous habits associated with defecation
4. Timing of elimination to take advantage of the gastrocolic reflex

541. The nurse is caring for a client who has urinary incontinence as the result of a brain attack. To limit the occurrence of urinary incontinence the nurse should:
1. Insert a urinary retention catheter
2. Institute measures to prevent constipation
3. Encourage an increase in the intake of caffeine
4. Suggest that a carbonated beverage be ingested daily

542. The spouse of a client who has had a brain attack seems unable to accept the idea that the client must be encouraged to participate in self-care. What is the best response by the nurse?
1. Tell the spouse to let the client do things independently
2. Allow the spouse to assume total responsibility for the client's care
3. Explain that the nursing staff has full responsibility for the client's activities
4. Ask the spouse for assistance in planning those activities most helpful to the client

543. The spouse of a client with a brain attack insists on doing everything for the client during visits. After these visits, the client seems to be depressed. The nurse understands that these visits have what effect on the client?
1. Losing faith in the future
2. Feeling the loss of independence
3. Experiencing guilt about being a burden
4. Recognizing that the wife is now the leader in the relationship

544. A client is diagnosed as having expressive aphasia. What type of impairment does the nurse expect the client to exhibit?
1. Speaking and/or writing
2. Following specific instructions
3. Understanding speech and/or writing
4. Recognizing words for familiar objects

545. What actions should the nurse include when planning for the long-term care of a client with expressive aphasia?
1. Help the client accept this disability as permanent
2. Begin helping the client associate words with physical objects
3. Wait for the client to initiate communication even if it takes a long time
4. Help family members accept the fact that they cannot verbally communicate with the client

546. Which nursing action is specific to the plan of care for a client with trigeminal neuralgia?
1. Apply ice compresses to the affected area.
2. Be alert to prevent dehydration or starvation.

3. Initiate exercises of the jaw and facial muscles.

4. Emphasize the importance of brushing the teeth.

547. Which clinical indicator does the nurse expect to identify when assessing a client with tic douloureux?
   1. Multiple petechiae
   2. Excruciating facial pain
   3. Unilateral muscle weakness
   4. Fine motor tremors of the eyelid

548. What action should the nurse take to prevent precipitating a painful attack in a client with tic douloureux?
   1. Avoid walking swiftly past client
   2. Keep the client in the prone position
   3. Discontinue oral hygiene temporarily
   4. Massage both sides of the face frequently

549. When developing a teaching plan for a client with trigeminal neuralgia, the nurse should include an explanation of the side effects of which medication typically used to treat this disorder?
   1. Ascorbic acid
   2. Morphine sulfate
   3. Allopurinol (Zyloprim)
   4. Carbamazepine (Tegretol)

550. Which clinical indicator does the nurse expect to identify when assessing a client with trigeminal neuralgia (tic douloureux)?
   1. Prolonged periods of sleep because of anxiety
   2. Hyperactivity because of medications received
   3. Exhaustion and fatigue because of the extreme pain
   4. Excessive talkativeness because of anxiety and apprehension

551. What should the nurse instruct the client to do to limit triggering the pain associated with trigeminal neuralgia?
   1. Drink iced liquids
   2. Avoid oral hygiene
   3. Apply warm compresses
   4. Chew on the unaffected side

552. What should the nurse include when planning care for a client with Bell's palsy?
   1. Managing incontinence
   2. Assisting with ambulation
   3. Preventing corneal damage
   4. Maintaining seizure precautions

553. A college freshman comes to the health clinic exhibiting slurring speech, a slight right-sided facial droop, and an inability to close the right eyelid. The client is taken to the emergency department, and Bell's palsy is diagnosed. List the following concerns in priority order for this client.
   1. _____Risk for falls because of altered vision
   2. _____Low self-esteem because of appearance
   3. _____Risk for malnutrition because of facial droop
   4. _____Inability to communicate because of slurred speech

554. Which clinical indicator should the nurse expect a client with an exacerbation of multiple sclerosis to experience?
   1. Double vision
   2. Resting tremors

3. Flaccid paralysis

4. Mental retardation

555. Which statement by a client with multiple sclerosis indicates to the nurse that the client needs further teaching?
   1. "I use a straw to drink liquids."
   2. "I will take a hot bath to help relax my muscles."
   3. "I plan to use an incontinence pad when I go out."
   4. "I may be having a rough time now, but I hope tomorrow will be better."

556. A recently hospitalized client with multiple sclerosis is concerned about generalized weakness and a fluctuating physical status. What is the priority nursing intervention for this client?
   1. Encourage bed rest
   2. Space activities throughout the day
   3. Teach the limitations imposed by the disease
   4. Have one of the client's relatives stay at the bedside

557. What does the nurse understand that clients with myasthenia gravis, Guillain-Barré syndrome, and amyotrophic lateral sclerosis share in common?
   1. Progressive deterioration until death
   2. Deficiencies of essential neurotransmitters
   3. Increased risk for respiratory complications
   4. Involuntary twitching of small muscle groups

558. What nursing intervention is anticipated for a client in the plateau phase of Guillain-Barré syndrome?
   1. Providing a straw to stimulate the facial muscles
   2. Inserting an indwelling catheter to monitor urinary output
   3. Encouraging aerobic exercises to avoid muscle atrophy
   4. Administering antibiotic medication to prevent pneumonia

559. The nurse is leading a support group for clients affected by myasthenia gravis. For what group of individuals does the nurse understand that the incidence of myasthenia gravis is highest?
   1. Males ages 15 to 35
   2. Children ages 5 to 15
   3. Females ages 20 to 30
   4. Both sexes equally before age 40

560. A client with myasthenia gravis asks the nurse why the disease has occurred. What pathology underlies the nurse's reply?
   1. A genetic defect in the production of acetylcholine
   2. An inefficient use of the neurotransmitter acetylcholine
   3. A decreased number of functioning acetylcholine receptor sites
   4. An inhibition of the enzyme AChE, leaving the end-plates folded

561. A client with myasthenia gravis asks the nurse, "What is going to happen to me and to my family?" When formulating a response, the nurse should understand that the prognosis for myasthenia gravis generally is:
   1. Excellent with proper treatment
   2. Slowly progressive without remissions

3. Chronic with exacerbations and remissions
4. Poor, with death occurring in a few months

562. The nursing assistant brings a lunch tray to a client with myasthenia gravis, for whom bed rest has been prescribed. The nurse enters the room and identifies that the client is experiencing increased dysphagia. What should the nurse do first?
1. Call the physician
2. Administer oxygen
3. Suction the trachea
4. Raise the head of the bed

563. To what does the nurse attribute the increased risk of respiratory complications in clients with myasthenia gravis?
1. Narrowed airways
2. Impaired immunity
3. Ineffective coughing
4. Viscosity of secretions

564. A client with myasthenia gravis has been receiving neostigmine (Prostigmin). What understanding of its action should the nurse have before administering this drug?
1. Stimulates the cerebral cortex
2. Blocks the action of cholinesterase
3. Replaces deficient neurotransmitters
4. Accelerates transmission along neural sheaths

565. A client with myasthenia gravis continues to become weaker despite treatment with neostigmine. The nurse understands that edrophonium HCl (Tensilon) is ordered to:
1. Rule out cholinergic crisis
2. Promote a synergistic effect
3. Overcome neostigmine resistance
4. Confirm the diagnosis of myasthenia

566. A client is diagnosed with Parkinson's disease and asks the nurse what causes the disease. On which underlying pathology does the nurse base a response?
1. Disintegration of the myelin sheath
2. Breakdown of the corpora quadrigemina
3. Reduced acetylcholine receptors at synapses
4. Degeneration of the neurons of the basal ganglia

567. When interviewing a client with a tentative diagnosis of Parkinson's disease, the nurse expects the client to report the onset of symptoms occurred:
1. Suddenly
2. Overnight
3. Gradually
4. Irregularly

568. A client with the diagnosis of Parkinson's disease asks the nurse, "Why do I drool so much?" Which is the nurse's best response?
1. "We don't know why this happens."
2. "There is a paralysis of the throat muscles."
3. "You have a loss of involuntary movements."
4. "Muscle rigidity prevents normal swallowing."

569. Which clinical indicator does the nurse expect a client with Parkinson's disease to exhibit?
1. Flattened affect
2. Muscle flaccidity

3. Tonic-clonic seizures
4. A change in pain tolerance

570. When helping a client with Parkinson's disease to ambulate, what instructions should the nurse give the client?
1. Avoid leaning forward
2. Hesitate between steps
3. Rest when tremors are experienced
4. Keep arms close to the center of gravity

571. The nurse administers levodopa (L-dopa) to a client with Parkinson's disease. Which therapeutic effect does the nurse expect the medication to produce?
1. Increase in acetylcholine production
2. Regeneration of injured thalamic cells
3. Improvement in myelination of neurons
4. Replacement of the neurotransmitter in the brain

572. Which clinical indicator does the nurse expect to identify when assessing a client admitted with a herniated lumbar disk?
1. Pain radiating to the hip and leg
2. Bowel and bladder incontinence
3. Paralysis of both lower extremities
4. Overgrowth of tissue on the lower back

573. The nurse expects a client with a herniated intervertebral disk to report that a sudden increase in pain is associated with:
1. Coughing or sneezing
2. Sitting on cold surfaces
3. Standing for extended periods
4. Lying supine or flexing the knees

574. After microdiskectomy for a herniated lumbar disk, for which clinical indicator should the nurse assess the client?
1. Cerebral edema
2. Spasms of the bladder
3. Sensory loss in the legs
4. Pain referred to the flanks

575. After a client has a lumbar laminectomy, what should the nurse do?
1. Encourage the client to cough frequently
2. Log-roll the client by using the draw sheet
3. Assess the client for indications of peritonitis
4. Instruct the client to bend the knees when turning

576. How does the nursing care for a client with a cervical laminectomy differ from the nursing care for a client with a lumbar laminectomy? When caring for a client with a cervical laminectomy, the nurse:
1. Should maintain the client's head in a flexed position
2. Has the added responsibility of removing oral secretions
3. Must keep the client's bed at a 45-degree angle continuously
4. Provides range-of-motion exercise early during the postoperative period

577. A nurse finds a victim under the wreckage of a collapsed building. The individual is conscious, breathing satisfactorily, and lying on the back complaining of

back pain and an inability to move the legs. Which action should the nurse take first?
1. Leave the individual lying on the back with instructions not to move and seek additional help
2. Roll the individual onto the abdomen, place a pad under the head, and cover with any material available
3. Gently raise the individual to a sitting position to see whether the pain either diminishes or increases in intensity
4. Gently lift the individual onto a flat piece of lumber and, using any available transportation, rush to the closest medical institution

578. After a spinal cord injury the physician indicates that a client is a paraplegic. The family asks the nurse what this means. What explanation should the nurse give to the family?
1. Upper extremities are paralyzed
2. Lower extremities are paralyzed
3. One side of the body is paralyzed
4. Both lower and upper extremities are paralyzed

579. A client with a spinal cord injury has paraplegia. The nurse assesses for which major problem the client may experience early in the recovery period?
1. Bladder control
2. Nutritional intake
3. Quadriceps setting
4. Use of aids for ambulation

580. The nurse should expect the client with a spinal cord injury to have some spasticity of the lower extremities. To prevent the development of contractures, what should the nurse include in the care plan for this client?
1. Deep massage
2. Active exercise
3. Use of a tilt board
4. Proper positioning

581. A client has paraplegia as a result of a motorcycle accident. What is the reason the nursing care plan should include turning the client every 1 to 2 hours?
1. Prevent pressure ulcers
2. Keep the client comfortable
3. Prevent flexion contractures of the extremities
4. Improve venous circulation in the lower extremities

582. After a client experiences a spinal cord injury, the nurse encourages the client to drink fluids primarily to prevent:
1. Dehydration
2. Skin breakdown
3. Electrolyte imbalances
4. Urinary tract infections

583. A client has a functional transection of the spinal cord at C7-8, resulting in spinal shock. Which clinical indicator does the nurse expect to identify when assessing the client immediately after the injury?
1. Spasticity
2. Incontinence
3. Flaccid paralysis
4. Respiratory failure

584. After a traumatic spinal severance, a young client is having difficulty accepting the paralysis. One day the client has severe leg spasms and says, "My strength is coming back, and I know I will walk again." The nurse's response should be based on what understanding?
1. The nerves are regenerating and motor function is returning
2. Spinal shock has subsided and client's reflexes are hyperactive
3. The client has developed thrombophlebitis and is experiencing pain
4. Motor function may be returning now that the edema is subsiding

585. When a client with a cervical injury complains of a severe headache and nasal congestion, the nurse should assess for:
1. Suprapubic distention
2. Increased spinal reflexes
3. Adventitious breath sounds
4. Imminent development of shock

586. A client with quadriplegia is placed on a tilt table daily. Each day the angle of the head of the table is gradually increased. When the client asks the reason for the tilt table, what is the nurse's best response? "The tilt table is used to:
1. Facilitate turning."
2. Prevent pressure sores."
3. Promote hyperextension of the spine."
4. Limit loss of calcium from the bones."

587. The nurse in a rehabilitation center teaches clients with quadriplegia to use an adaptive wheelchair. Why is it important that the nurse provide this instruction?
1. It prepares them for bracing and crutch walking
2. They usually are not, and never will be, functional walkers
3. They have the strength in the upper extremities for self-transfer
4. It assists them in overcoming orthostatic hypotension

588. A client with degenerative joint disease asks the nurse, "My doctor mentioned something about synovial fluid and the joint. What is that?" What is the nurse's best response? "The synovial fluid of the joints minimizes:
1. Efficiency."
2. Work output."
3. Friction in the joints."
4. Velocity of movements."

589. The client sustains a hip fracture and asks the nurse why the fall affected that part of the femur. The nurse explains that the shaft and ends of long bones represent two types of bone. Which characteristic does the nurse understand is greater for compact bone than for cancellous bone?
1. Size
2. Weight
3. Volume
4. Density

590. The nurse administers allopurinol (Aloprim) to a client with gout. The nurse explains that the object of this therapy is to:
    1. Increase bone density
    2. Decrease synovial swelling
    3. Decrease uric acid production
    4. Prevent crystallization of uric acid

591. A client is admitted with acute gouty arthritis. Which medication does the nurse anticipate the physician may prescribe to prevent and treat an acute attack of gout?
    1. Colchicine
    2. Hydrocortisone
    3. Ibuprofen (Motrin)
    4. Probenecid (Benemid)

592. To limit painful attacks, which food should the nurse teach a client with gout to avoid?
    1. Eggs
    2. Liver
    3. Cheese
    4. Salmon

593. Two days after a sprain accompanied by edema, the practitioner orders the application of warm compresses. What is the appropriate temperature range for the compresses that the nurse applies?
    1. 65° to 79° F (18.0° to 26.1° C)
    2. 80° to 92° F (26.6° to 33.3° C)
    3. 93° to 97° F (34.0° to 36.1° C)
    4. 98° to 105° F (36.6° to 40.5° C)

594. The nurse suspects the development of compartment syndrome for a client who has sustained blunt trauma to the forearm. For which early sign of compartment syndrome should the nurse assess the client?
    1. Warm skin at site of injury
    2. Escalating pain in the fingers
    3. Rapid capillary refill in affected hand
    4. Bounding radial pulse in the injured arm

595. Which nursing intervention for the client should initially receive the lowest priority immediately after a client experiences a traumatic amputation of a leg in a motor vehicle accident?
    1. Teaching residual limb care
    2. Monitoring hemoglobin levels
    3. Maintaining the compression dressing
    4. Using therapeutic interviewing techniques

596. What instructions should the nurse give the client to prevent a hip flexion contracture following an amputation of a lower limb?
    1. Turn from side to side every 1 to 2 hours
    2. Sit in a chair for 30 minutes three times a day
    3. Lie on the abdomen 30 minutes four times daily
    4. Perform quadriceps muscle setting exercises twice daily

597. What should the nurse do to control edema of the residual limb 1 week after a client has had an above-the-knee amputation?
    1. Administer the prescribed diuretic
    2. Restrict the client's oral fluid intake

    3. Rewrap the elastic bandage as necessary
    4. Keep the residual limb elevated on a pillow

598. Before ambulation is started, what instructions should the nurse provide the client to make walking with crutches easier?
    1. Use of the trapeze to strengthen the biceps muscles
    2. The importance of keeping the affected limb in extension and abduction to prevent contractures
    3. Isometric exercises of the hamstring muscles while sitting in a chair until circulatory status is stable
    4. Exercises with or without weights to strengthen the triceps, finger flexors, wrist extensors, and elbow extensors

599. What should the nurse do to promote early and efficient ambulation after a client has a midthigh amputation?
    1. Keep the head of the bed elevated
    2. Place pillows under the residual limb
    3. Encourage the client to lie on unaffected side
    4. Turn the client to the prone position periodically

600. A client has a total hip replacement. Which clinical indicator of pulmonary embolism indicates that the nursing plan to prevent postoperative thrombus formation has been ineffective?
    1. Flushing of the face
    2. Elevation of temperature
    3. Sudden onset of shortness of breath
    4. Pain rating increase from 2 to 8 in the hip

601. What instructions should the nurse give the client when the client is allowed out of bed after an above-the-knee amputation?
    1. Keep the hip in extension and alignment
    2. Keep the hip raised with the residual limb elevated
    3. Walk with crutches until the residual limb is completely healed
    4. Lift the shoulder and hip of the affected side when taking a step

602. A client has a total knee replacement, and a continuous passive motion device is being used. The nurse understands that preoperative teaching was effective when the client identifies the goal of this treatment as:
    1. Maintaining muscle tone
    2. Improving flexion of joint
    3. Preventing tissue breakdown
    4. Avoiding formation of thrombus

603. When should the nurse engage the client scheduled for an amputation in rehabilitation?
    1. Before the surgery
    2. During the convalescent phase
    3. On discharge from the hospital
    4. When it is time for a prosthesis

604. After an above-the-knee amputation of the leg, a client complains of pain in the foot that is no longer there. The nurse understands the underlying reason for phantom limb sensation is:
    1. Tactile illusions associated with severed blood vessels
    2. An unconscious phenomenon to aid with the grieving over the lost body part

    3. Hallucinations secondary to emotional symptoms associated with the distress of amputation

    4. Sensations in the amputated limb secondary to thalamic localization of stimuli from nerve endings

605. Which crutch gait should the nurse teach the client wearing a prosthesis after a single-leg amputation?
    1. Four-point gait
    2. Three-point gait
    3. Tripod crutch gait
    4. Swing-through crutch gait

606. Which principle should the nurse understand when assisting a client with crutches to learn the four-point gait?
    1. Elbows should be kept in rigid extension
    2. Most of the weight should be supported by axillae
    3. The client must be able to bear weight on both legs
    4. The affected extremity should be kept off the ground

607. A client is in skeletal traction while awaiting surgery for repair of a fractured femur. The client complains of leg discomfort and asks the nurse to release the traction. Which is the nurse's best initial response?
    1. "I will remove half of the weights and notify your physician."
    2. "I'll get your pain medication to help relieve your discomfort."
    3. "I can't do that because the weights are needed to keep your bone in alignment."
    4. "I have to follow the physician's directions, and releasing weights is not ordered."

608. A client's leg is set in a long leg cast. Because of the long leg cast, the nurse should monitor for a clinical indicator of compromised circulation such as:
    1. Foul odor
    2. Swelling of the toes
    3. Drainage on the cast
    4. Increased temperature

609. A client has a long leg cast. What instructions should the nurse give the client in preparation for crutch walking?
    1. Use the trapeze to strengthen the biceps
    2. Keep the affected limb in extension and abduction
    3. Sit up straight in a chair to develop the back muscles
    4. Do exercises in bed to strengthen the upper extremities

610. What intervention should the nurse avoid to prevent contractures of the joints of the lower extremities in a client with paraplegia?
    1. Changing the client's bed position hourly
    2. Using supportive devices to maintain alignment
    3. Providing the client with active exercise instructions
    4. Passively moving the extremities through ROM several times daily

611. The care plan for a client with paraplegia includes nursing actions to prevent the formation of urinary calculi. The nurse explains to the client that the risk for urinary calculi is associated with:
    1. High fluid intake
    2. Inadequate kidney function

    3. Increased intake of calcium
    4. Accelerated bone demineralization

612. A client who has been immobilized for an extended period questions the need for a tilt table. Which is the nurse's best response? "The tilt table is used to help:
    1. Prevent hypertension."
    2. Encourage increased activity."
    3. Encourage circulation to the skin."
    4. Prevent loss of calcium from long bones."

613. A client is placed into a whirlpool tub for range-of-motion exercises. The client asks the nurse about the need to exercise in water. What explanation should the nurse give the client? "Rehabilitating exercises carried out under water utilize the water's:
    1. Vapor."
    2. Pressure."
    3. Buoyancy."
    4. Temperature."

614. When assessing a client with a fracture of the neck of the femur, which clinical indicator should the nurse expect to identify?
    1. Adduction with internal rotation
    2. Abduction with external rotation
    3. Shortening of the affected extremity with external rotation
    4. Lengthening of the affected extremity with internal rotation

615. When placing a client with a fractured hip in traction before surgery, the nurse explains that the purpose of traction is to:
    1. Relieve muscle spasm and pain
    2. Prevent contractures from developing
    3. Keep the client from turning and moving in bed
    4. Maintain the limb in a position of external rotation

616. A client is admitted with a fracture of the neck of the femur. In what position should the nurse maintain the client's affected extremity?
    1. Internal rotation with extension of the knee and hip
    2. Internal rotation with flexion of the knee and hip
    3. External rotation with flexion of the knee and hip
    4. External rotation with extension of the knee and hip

617. The care plan for a client with a fractured hip includes nursing actions to prevent which type of contracture?
    1. Flexion of the hip
    2. Abduction of the hip
    3. Hyperextension of the hip
    4. Internal rotation of the hip

618. A client develops aseptic necrosis after a fracture of the head of the femur. The nurse understands that aseptic necrosis is associated with which risk factor?
    1. Infection at the site of the wound
    2. Weight-bearing before fracture is healed
    3. Immobilization after reduction of the fracture
    4. Loss of blood supply to the head of the femur

619. To reduce a hip fracture, the client is placed in traction before surgery for an open reduction and internal fixation. Because the client keeps slipping down in

bed, increased countertraction is ordered. How does the nurse increase the countertraction?
1. Elevate the head of the bed
2. Add more weight to the traction
3. Use a slight Trendelenburg position
4. Tie a chest restraint around the client

620. The nurse understands that the intramedullary nailing procedure listed on the operating room schedule is for the client with which orthopedic problem?
1. Slipped epiphysis of the femur
2. Fracture of the shaft of the femur
3. Fracture of the neck of the femur
4. Intertrochanteric fracture of the femur

621. After a client has total hip replacement surgery, the nurse should avoid placing the client in which position?
1. Supine position
2. Lateral position
3. Orthopneic position
4. Semi-Fowler's position

622. To prevent thrombus formation after a total hip replacement, the nurse should ensure that the client is:
1. Turned from side to side
2. Encouraged to exercise the ankles
3. Ambulated when the effects of anesthesia are gone
4. Permitted to be up in a chair for as long as tolerated

623. Nursing care of a client with a fractured hip should include the assessment of pedal pulses. The nurse should assess for which important characteristics of the pedal pulses?
1. Contractility and rate
2. Color of skin and rhythm
3. Amplitude and symmetry
4. Local temperature and visible pulsations

624. When the nurse is monitoring a client for hemorrhage following a total hip replacement, which is the priority assessment?
1. Checking vital signs q4h
2. Measuring the girth of the thigh
3. Examining the bedding under the client
4. Observing for ecchymosis at the operative site

625. When a client is in the right side-lying position after the insertion of a left hip prosthesis, the nurse ensures that the client has an abduction pillow placed between the thighs and that the entire length of the upper leg is supported. The most important reason for using the abduction pillow is to prevent:
1. Strain on the operative site
2. Thrombus formation in the leg
3. Flexion contractures of the hip joint
4. Skin surfaces from rubbing together

626. Which is an example of the principles of body mechanics that the nurse uses when caring for immobilized clients?
1. Placing the feet apart to increase the stability of the body
2. Bending at the waist to provide the power for lifting

3. Keeping the body straight when lifting to reduce pressure on the abdomen
4. Relaxing the abdominal muscles while using the extremities to prevent strain

627. After an open reduction and internal fixation of a fractured hip, the nurse should assess the client's affected leg. Select all assessments that apply.
1. ☐ Body temperature
2. ☐ Mobility of the hip
3. ☐ Mobility of the toes
4. ☐ Condition of the pin
5. ☐ Presence of pedal pulse

628. A client with a fractured hip is helped from the bed to a chair after surgery. Why does the nurse instruct the client to bear most of the weight on the unaffected leg before sitting in a chair? Bearing most of the weight on the unaffected leg:
1. Can increase circulation in the lower extremities
2. Will help maintain the strength of the unaffected limb
3. Is the quickest method of getting the client to and from the bed
4. Reduces the amount of help necessary to lift the client from the bed to the chair

629. On the first postoperative day following a hip replacement a client asks for assistance onto the bedpan. What should the nurse instruct the client to do?
1. Use the elbows and hands to lift the pelvis
2. Extend both legs and pull on the trapeze to lift the pelvis
3. Turn gently toward the operative side, lifting the pelvis off the bed
4. Flex the unoperated knee and pull on the trapeze to lift the pelvis off the bed

630. When a client is ready to walk with crutches after knee surgery, which technique will the nurse most likely teach the client?
1. Two-point
2. Four-point
3. Three-point
4. Swing-through

631. When teaching crutch walking to a client following arthroscopic surgery of the knee, on which part of the body should the nurse instruct the client to place weight?
1. The upper arms
2. The axillary region
3. Palms of the hands
4. Both lower extremities

632. The nurse evaluates that a client understands the discharge instructions after a total hip replacement when the client states, "I should avoid:
1. Climbing stairs."
2. Stretching exercises."
3. Sitting in a low chair."
4. Lying prone for 30 minutes."

633. What is the nurse's primary consideration when caring for a client with rheumatoid arthritis?
    1. Surgery
    2. Comfort
    3. Education
    4. Motivation

634. The nurse is caring for a client with rheumatoid arthritis. Based on the client's diagnosis, the nurse should review the result of which laboratory test?
    1. Pancreatic lipase
    2. Bence Jones protein
    3. Antinuclear antibody
    4. Alkaline phosphatase

635. To prevent deformities in a client with rheumatoid arthritis, the nurse plans to alternate rest periods with which intervention?
    1. Active exercise
    2. Passive massage
    3. Bracing of joints
    4. Isometric exercises

636. A regimen of rest, exercise, and physical therapy is ordered for a client with rheumatoid arthritis. What should the nurse explain is the intended purpose of this regimen?
    1. Prevent arthritic pain
    2. Halt the inflammatory process
    3. Help prevent the crippling effects of the disease
    4. Provide for the return of joint motion after prolonged loss

637. The nurse is completing the health history of a client admitted with osteoarthritis. The nurse expects the client to report initial involvement of which joints?
    1. Hips and knees
    2. Ankles and metatarsals
    3. Fingers and metacarpals
    4. Cervical spine and shoulders

638. A client with rheumatoid arthritis asks the nurse why the physician is going to inject hydrocortisone into the knee joint. The nurse explains that the most important reason for the injection is to:
    1. Lubricate the joint
    2. Reduce inflammation
    3. Provide physiotherapy
    4. Prevent ankylosis of the joint

639. When planning nursing care for a client with an acute episode of rheumatoid arthritis, what should the nurse take into consideration?
    1. Inflammation of the synovial membrane will rarely occur
    2. Bony ankylosis of the joint is irreversible and causes immobility
    3. Redness and swelling of a joint signify irreversible damage has occurred
    4. Complete immobility is desired during the acute phase of inflammation

640. When preparing an individualized teaching plan for a client with rheumatoid arthritis, which topic should the nurse omit from the generalized teaching plan for clients with arthritis?
    1. Ulnar drift
    2. Heberden's nodes
    3. Swan neck deformity
    4. Boutonniere deformity

641. The nurse questions a client with rheumatoid arthritis about pain. When should the nurse expect the client to experience increased pain and limited movement of the joints?
    1. After assistive exercise
    2. When the room is cool
    3. In the morning on awakening
    4. When the latex fixation test is positive

642. A client who has intermittently been having painful, swollen knee and wrist joints during the past 3 months is admitted to the hospital for treatment of rheumatoid arthritis. What type of diet should the nurse expect the physician to order?
    1. Salt-free, low-fiber diet
    2. High-calorie, low-cholesterol diet
    3. High-protein diet with minimal calcium
    4. Regular diet with vitamins and minerals

643. Which medication should the nurse anticipate being prescribed to relieve the pain experienced by a client with rheumatoid arthritis?
    1. Xanax, 0.5 mg tid
    2. Aspirin, 0.6 g q4h
    3. Codeine, 30 mg q4h
    4. Meperidine, 30 mg q4h PRN

644. What should the nurse do to prevent deformities of the knee in a client with an exacerbation of arthritis?
    1. Encourage motion of the joint
    2. Maintain a knee brace on the leg
    3. Keep the client on a regimen of bed rest
    4. Immobilize the joint with pillows until pain subsides

645. A client with rheumatoid arthritis has severe pain and swelling of the joints in both hands. Range-of-motion exercises for this client should be:
    1. Passively performed by the nurse
    2. Avoided if the client reports discomfort
    3. Preceded by the application of heat or cold
    4. Gradually increased to improve mobility and independence

646. A client with arthritis reports receiving the following dietary suggestions over the years. Which recommendation for a daily diet should the nurse reinforce?
    1. Wheat germ and yeast
    2. Yogurt and blackstrap molasses
    3. Multiple vitamin supplements in large doses
    4. Adequate foods in a variety of different food groups

647. A client with degenerative arthritis may require a total hip replacement. What should the nurse understand about this surgery? This surgery is done:
    1. In a laminar airflow room
    2. Using three separate stages

3. Early in the disease process
4. With the client in the lithotomy position

URINARY/REPRODUCTIVE SYSTEMS

(For additional questions, see Childbearing and Women's Health Nursing Review Questions with Answers and Rationales, Chapter 28, p. 585.)

648. When caring for a male client who is to receive chemotherapy for a cancerous condition, the nurse understands that spermatogenesis occurs:
1. At the time of puberty
2. At any time after birth
3. Immediately following birth
4. During embryonic development

649. The nurse is caring for a client with an undescended testicle. The nurse understands that the main reason testes are suspended in the scrotum is to:
1. Protect the sperm from the acidity of urine
2. Facilitate the passage of sperm through the urethra
3. Protect the sperm from high abdominal temperatures
4. Facilitate their maturation during embryonic development

650. A client is admitted to the hospital with a diagnosis of condylomata acuminata. When caring for this client it is important that the nurse understands that this term refers to:
1. Scabies
2. Herpes zoster
3. Venereal warts
4. Cancer of the epididymis

651. The nurse is caring for a client with a trichomonal infection. Which organism causes a trichomonal infection?
1. Yeast
2. Fungus
3. Protozoan
4. Spirochete

652. The nurse is caring for a client with a diagnosis of cancer of the prostate. Which serum level should be monitored to follow the course of the disease?
1. Creatinine
2. Blood urea nitrogen
3. Nonprotein nitrogen
4. Prostate-specific antigen

653. When caring for a client with a diagnosis of benign prostatic hyperplasia it is important for the nurse to understand that it:
1. Is a congenital abnormality
2. Usually becomes malignant
3. Predisposes to hydronephrosis
4. Causes an elevated acid phosphatase level

654. The nurse is caring for a client with a fluid and electrolyte imbalance. Which is the most important means of maintaining fluid and electrolyte balance that should be understood by the nurse?
1. Aldosterone
2. The urinary system

3. The respiratory system
4. Antidiuretic hormone

655. The nurse understands which principle is associated with the reabsorption of water from glomerular filtrate in the kidney tubules?
1. Osmosis
2. Diffusion
3. Active dialysis
4. Active transport

656. The nurse is caring for a male client who is scheduled for a dilation of the urethra. Before explaining the procedure, the nurse must understand that the structure surrounding the male urethra is the:
1. Epididymis
2. Prostate gland
3. Seminal vesicle
4. Bulbourethral gland

657. The nurse understands that a female has a higher risk for developing cystitis than a male. Which is the most common contributing factor to this increased risk?
1. Altered urinary pH
2. Hormonal secretions
3. Juxtaposition of the bladder
4. Proximity of the urethra to the anus

658. A routine urinalysis is ordered for a client. What should the nurse do if the specimen cannot be sent immediately to the laboratory?
1. Take no special action.
2. Refrigerate the specimen.
3. Store it in the dirty utility room and send it later.
4. Discard the specimen and collect another specimen later.

659. A client with a urinary retention catheter in place complains of discomfort in the bladder and urethra. What should the nurse do first?
1. Notify the physician
2. Milk the tubing gently
3. Check the patency of the catheter
4. Irrigate the catheter with prescribed solutions

660. A client experiences difficulty in voiding after an indwelling urinary catheter is removed. The nurse concludes that this is most probably related to:
1. Fluid imbalances
2. A sedentary lifestyle
3. Nervous tension following the procedure
4. An interruption in previous voiding habits

661. A client with cancer of the prostate requests the urinal at frequent intervals but either does not void or voids in very small amounts. The nurse concludes that this is most likely caused by which factor?
1. Edema
2. Dysuria
3. Retention
4. Suppression

662. Which nursing action can best prevent infection from urinary retention catheters?
1. Cleansing the perineum
2. Encouraging adequate fluids

3. Irrigating the catheter once daily

4. Cleansing around the meatus periodically

663. The nurse is caring for a client with a continuous bladder irrigation. Which is the most important nursing action?

1. Monitoring urinary specific gravity to determine hydration

2. Subtracting irrigant from output to determine urine volume

3. Recording urinary output every hour to determine kidney function

4. Including irrigating solution in a 24-hour urine specimen to determine urine concentration

664. The nurse is providing client teaching to a woman who has recurrent urinary tract infections. Which information should the nurse include concerning the reason women are more susceptible to urinary tract infections than men?

1. Inadequate fluid intake

2. Poor hygienic practices

3. The length of the urethra

4. The continuity of mucous membranes

665. A client in a nursing home is diagnosed with urethritis. Before initiating treatment orders, what should the nurse plan to do?

1. Start a 24-hour urine collection

2. Prepare for urinary catheterization

3. Teach how to perform perineal care

4. Obtain a urine specimen for culture and sensitivity

666. The nurse is assessing the urine of a client with a urinary tract infection. For which characteristic should the nurse assess each specimen of urine?

1. Clarity

2. Viscosity

3. Specific gravity

4. Glucose and acetone

667. For what should the nurse monitor when caring for a client who has hematuria?

1. Intractable diarrhea

2. Acetone in the urine

3. Symptoms of peritonitis

4. Gross blood in the urine

668. The nurse is caring for a client with glomerulonephritis. What should the nurse instruct the client to do to prevent recurrent attacks?

1. Take showers instead of tub baths

2. Continue the same restrictions on fluid intake

3. Avoid situations that involve physical activity

4. Seek early treatment for respiratory tract infections

669. The immediate objective of nursing care for an overweight, mildly hypertensive client with ureteral colic and hematuria is to decrease which clinical indicator?

1. Pain

2. Weight

3. Hematuria

4. Hypertension

670. The nurse is caring for clients with renal calculi. Which is the most important nursing action?

1. Limit fluid intake at night

2. Strain the urine at each voiding

3. Record the client's blood pressure

4. Administer analgesics every 3 hours

671. The pathology report states that a client's urinary calculus is composed of uric acid. Which should the nurse instruct the client to avoid?

1. Eggs

2. Fruit

3. Meat extracts

4. Raw vegetables

672. A lithotripsy to break up renal calculi is unsuccessful, and a nephrolithotomy is performed. Which postoperative clinical indicator should the nurse report to the physician?

1. Passage of pink-tinged urine

2. Pink drainage on the dressing

3. Intake of 1750 mL in 24 hours

4. Urine output of 20 to 30 mL/hr

673. A client is scheduled to have surgery to remove a calculus in the bladder. The nurse needs to educate the client about which procedure?

1. Cystometry

2. Cystolithiasis

3. Cryoextraction

4. Cystolithectomy

674. The nurse is caring for a client with a diagnosis of renal calculi of calcium phosphate composition. Which type of diet should the nurse explore with the client when providing discharge information?

1. Low purine

2. Low calcium

3. High phosphorus

4. High alkaline ash

675. The pathology report states that a client's urinary calculus is composed of uric acid. Which should the nurse instruct the client to avoid?

1. Milk

2. Cheese

3. Red meats

4. Organ meats

676. The nurse is caring for a client with end-stage renal disease. Which clinical indicator of end-stage renal disease should the nurse expect?

1. Polyuria

2. Jaundice

3. Azotemia

4. Hypotension

677. A client has a heminephrectomy and returns from the postanesthesia care unit with a nephrostomy tube and an indwelling urinary catheter. The client's urinary output is 50 mL/hr. What is the nurse's next action?

1. Record the findings

2. Encourage oral fluids

3. Irrigate the nephrostomy tube

4. Notify the physician immediately

678. A client is diagnosed with bladder cancer, and a cystectomy and an ileal conduit are scheduled. What should the nurse plan to do preoperatively?
    1. Limit fluid intake for 24 hours
    2. Teach range-of-motion and Kegel exercises
    3. Teach the procedure for irrigating the ileal conduit
    4. Administer cleansing enemas and laxatives as ordered

679. The nurse recognizes that the major disadvantage of a conduit diversion is that:
    1. Peristalsis is greatly decreased
    2. Stool continuously oozes from it
    3. Urine continuously drains from it
    4. Absorption of nutrients is diminished

680. After a nephrectomy, a client arrives in the postanesthesia care unit with a plastic airway in place. When observing the client for signs of hemorrhage, which action should be employed by the nurse?
    1. Turn the client to observe the dressings
    2. Press the client's nail beds to note capillary refill
    3. Observe the client for hemoptysis when suctioning
    4. Monitor the client's blood pressure for a rapid increase

681. A client has undergone a suprapubic prostatectomy. The nurse can expect the client to return from the postanesthesia care unit with which type of tube?
    1. Cystostomy
    2. Nasogastric
    3. Nephrostomy
    4. Ureterostomy

682. A client who has just had a suprapubic prostatectomy returns from the postanesthesia care unit and accidentally pulls out the urethral catheter. What is the nurse's next action?
    1. Reinsert a new catheter
    2. Notify the physician immediately
    3. Check for bleeding by irrigating the suprapubic tube
    4. Take no immediate action if the suprapubic tube is draining

683. The nurse is caring for a client with an indwelling urinary catheter. What is the most important action for the nurse to take when planning to irrigate the bladder?
    1. Use sterile equipment
    2. Instill the fluid under high pressure
    3. Warm the solution to body temperature
    4. Aspirate immediately to ensure return flow

684. What should the nurse do to obtain an accurate urine output for a client with a continuous bladder irrigation (CBI)?
    1. Measure the contents of the bedside drainage bag
    2. Stop the irrigation and determine the urine output
    3. Subtract the volume of irrigant from the total drainage
    4. Ensure that urine and irrigant drain into two separate bags

685. The nurse understands that metabolic acidosis develops in kidney failure as a result of:
    1. Inability of the renal tubules to secrete hydrogen ions and conserve bicarbonate
    2. Depressed respiratory rate by metabolic wastes, causing carbon dioxide retention
    3. Inability of the renal tubules to reabsorb water to dilute the acid contents of blood
    4. Impaired glomerular filtration, causing retention of sodium and metabolic waste products

686. A client with acute kidney failure is to receive a very low-protein diet. The nurse understands that this diet is based on the principle that:
    1. A high-protein intake ensures an adequate daily supply of amino acids to compensate for losses
    2. Essential and nonessential amino acids are necessary in the diet to supply materials for tissue protein synthesis
    3. This supplies only essential amino acids, reducing the amount of metabolic waste products, thus decreasing stress on the kidneys
    4. Urea nitrogen cannot be used to synthesize amino acids in the body, so the nitrogen for amino acid synthesis must come from the dietary protein

687. A client with acute kidney failure states, "Why am I twitching and my fingers and toes tingling?" The nurse should respond, "This is caused by:
    1. Acidosis."
    2. Calcium depletion."
    3. Potassium retention."
    4. Sodium chloride depletion."

688. A client with acute kidney failure becomes confused and irritable. The nurse understands that the most likely cause of this behavior is:
    1. Hyperkalemia
    2. Hypernatremia
    3. An elevated BUN
    4. A limited fluid intake

689. The nurse is caring for a client with chronic kidney failure. Which adaptation should the nurse expect?
    1. Polyuria
    2. Hypotension
    3. Muscle twitching
    4. Respiratory acidosis

690. A client with chronic kidney failure is to be treated with continuous ambulatory peritoneal dialysis (CAPD). Which statement indicates to the nurse that the client understands the purpose of this therapy?
    1. "It provides continuous contact of dialyzer and blood to clear toxins by ultrafiltration."
    2. "It exchanges and cleanses blood by correction of electrolytes and excretion of creatinine."
    3. "It decreases the need for immobility because it clears toxins in short and intermittent periods."
    4. "It uses the peritoneum as a semipermeable membrane to clear toxins by osmosis and diffusion."

691. The nurse evaluates that a client scheduled for peritoneal dialysis understands its purpose when the client says, "The purpose of peritoneal dialysis is to:
    1. Reestablish kidney function."
    2. Clean the peritoneal membrane."
    3. Provide fluid for intracellular spaces."
    4. Remove toxins in addition to other metabolic wastes."

692. The nurse is caring for a client with a diagnosis of chronic kidney failure who has just been told by the physician that hemodialysis is necessary. The nurse understands that the reason why hemodialysis is necessary is because the client now has:
    1. Ascites
    2. Acidosis
    3. Hypertension
    4. Hyperkalemia

693. When receiving hemodialysis, the complication of the removal of too much sodium may occur. Therefore the nurse should assess the client for:
    1. Muscle cramps
    2. Chvostek's sign
    3. Cardiac dysrhythmias
    4. Increased temperature

694. The nurse is caring for a client with an external shunt used for hemodialysis. The nurse understands that the most serious complication associated with hemodialysis is:
    1. Septicemia
    2. Clot formation
    3. Exsanguination
    4. Sclerosis of vessels

695. The nurse is caring for a client who just had an arteriovenous shunt inserted for hemodialysis. What should the nurse do?
    1. Cover the cannula with an elastic bandage
    2. Notify the physician if a bruit is heard in the cannula
    3. Use surgical aseptic technique when giving shunt care
    4. Take the blood pressure on the arm with the shunt every 4 hours

696. When assessing a client during peritoneal dialysis, the nurse observes that drainage of the dialysate from the peritoneal cavity has ceased before the required volume has returned. What should the nurse instruct the client to do?
    1. Drink 8 oz of water
    2. Turn from side to side
    3. Deep breathe and cough
    4. Rotate the catheter periodically

697. A client with an invasive carcinoma of the bladder is receiving radiation to the lower abdomen in an attempt to shrink the tumor before surgery. Considering the side effects of radiation, what should the nurse do?
    1. Observe feces for the presence of blood
    2. Monitor the blood pressure for hypertension
    3. Administer enemas to remove sloughing tissue
    4. Provide a high-bulk diet to prevent constipation

698. During the postoperative period after surgery for a kidney transplant, the client's creatinine level is 3.1 mg/dL. Considering this laboratory result, the nurse should first:
    1. Notify the surgeon
    2. Check the intravenous infusions
    3. Assess for decreased urine output
    4. Obtain current blood work reports

INFECTIOUS DISEASES

699. A client is concerned about contracting malaria while visiting relatives in Southeast Asia. To best prevent malaria, what should the nurse teach the client to avoid?
    1. Mosquito bites
    2. Untreated water
    3. Undercooked food
    4. Overpopulated areas

700. The nurse is reviewing the physical examination and laboratory tests of a client with malaria. For which important clinical indicator should the nurse be alert when reviewing data about this client?
    1. Polyuria
    2. Leukocytosis
    3. Splenomegaly
    4. Erythrocytosis

701. Which action should the nurse take when caring for a client with malaria?
    1. Institute seizure precautions
    2. Prepare for blood transfusions
    3. Maintain isolation precautions
    4. Provide nutrition between paroxysms

702. The nurse is teaching a client about drug therapy against *Plasmodium falciparum*. What information should the nurse include in the teaching plan?
    1. The infection can be controlled
    2. Immunity will prevent reinfestation
    3. The infection can generally be eliminated
    4. Immunity from the original infection is temporary

703. Blackwater fever occurs in some clients with malaria. For which adaptation should the nurse assess this client?
    1. Dark-red urine
    2. Low-grade fever
    3. Clay-colored diarrhea
    4. Coffee-ground emesis

704. The nurse is caring for a client who is HIV-positive. It is most important for the nurse to teach the client how to prevent:
    1. Infection
    2. Depression
    3. Social isolation
    4. Kaposi's sarcoma

705. A mother with the diagnosis of AIDS states that she has been caring for her baby even though she has not been feeling well. What important information should the nurse determine?
    1. If she has kissed the baby
    2. If the baby is breastfeeding

3. When the baby last received antibiotics

4. How long she has been caring for the baby

706. The nurse is planning to provide discharge teaching to the family of a client with AIDS. Which statement should the nurse include in the teaching plan?
    1. "Wash the dishes in hot soapy water as you usually do."
    2. "Let the dishes soak in hot water overnight before washing."
    3. "You should boil the client's dishes for 30 minutes after use."
    4. "Have the client eat from paper plates so they can be discarded."

707. During an AIDS education class a client states, "Vaseline works great when I use condoms." Which conclusion about the client's knowledge of condom use can the nurse draw from this statement?
    1. An understanding of safer sex
    2. An ability to assume self-responsibility
    3. Ignorance concerning correct condom use
    4. Ignorance concerning the transmission of HIV

708. A client is diagnosed with gastroenteritis. The nurse understands that the basic intention underlying the unique dietary management for this client is to:
    1. Provide optimal amounts of all important nutrients
    2. Increase the amount of bulk and roughage in the diet
    3. Eliminate chemical, mechanical, and thermal irritation
    4. Promote psychologic support by offering a wide variety of foods

709. The nurse is caring for a client who had *Clostridium welchii (C. perfringens)* cultured from a wound of the lower extremity. Which disease is produced when this organism enters a wound, causing crepitus?
    1. Tetanus
    2. Anthrax
    3. Botulism
    4. Gangrene

710. A client in the emergency department states, "I was bitten by a raccoon while I was fixing a water pipe in the crawl space of my basement." Which is the most effective first-aid treatment for the nurse to use for this client?
    1. Administering an antivenin
    2. Maintaining a pressure dressing
    3. Cleansing the wound with soap and water
    4. Applying a tourniquet proximal to the wound

711. The nurse in the public health clinic is teaching clients how to prevent toxoplasmosis. What should the nurse instruct the clients to avoid?
    1. Contact with cat feces
    2. Working with heavy metals
    3. Ingestion of freshwater fish
    4. Excessive radiation exposure

712. A client is admitted with the diagnosis of tetanus. It is most important for the nurse to observe for which clinical indicator?
    1. Muscular rigidity
    2. Respiratory tract spasms

3. Restlessness and irritability

4. Spastic voluntary muscle contractions

713. A client is suspected of having rabies after being bit by a raccoon. For which clinical indicator should the nurse assess the client?
    1. Diarrhea
    2. Forgetfulness
    3. Urinary stasis
    4. Pharyngeal spasm

714. A client is admitted to the hospital for general paresis as a complication of syphilis. Which therapy should the nurse anticipate will most likely be ordered for this client?
    1. Penicillin
    2. Major tranquilizers
    3. Behavior modification
    4. Electroconvulsive therapy

715. The nurse is counseling a client who has gonorrhea. The nurse should teach this client that gonorrhea is highly infectious and:
    1. Is easily cured
    2. Occurs very rarely
    3. Can produce sterility
    4. Is limited to the external genitalia

716. A client is diagnosed as having gonorrhea. What medication should the nurse expect the physician to order?
    1. Acyclovir (Zovirax)
    2. Colistin (Cortisporin)
    3. Ceftriaxone (Rocephin)
    4. Dactinomycin (actinomycin)

717. A female client is very upset with her diagnosis of gonorrhea and asks the nurse, "What can I do to prevent getting another infection in the future?" The nurse is aware that the teaching has been understood when the client states, "My best protection is to:
    1. Douche after every intercourse."
    2. Avoid engaging in sexual behavior."
    3. Insist that my partner use a condom."
    4. Use a spermicidal cream with intercourse."

718. The nurse is caring for a client with a diagnosis of acute salpingitis. Which condition is most commonly the cause of inflammation of the fallopian tubes?
    1. Syphilis
    2. Abortion
    3. Gonorrhea
    4. Hydatidiform mole

719. A client is diagnosed with herpes genitalis. What should the nurse do to prevent cross-contamination?
    1. Institute droplet precautions
    2. Arrange transfer to a private room
    3. Wear a gown and gloves when giving direct care
    4. Close the door and wear a mask when in the room

720. A client cannot understand how syphilis was contracted because there has been no sexual activity for several days. Which length of time associated with the incubation of syphilis should the nurse include in the teaching plan?
    1. 1 week
    2. 4 months

3. 2 to 6 weeks

4. 48 to 72 hours

721. When preparing a teaching plan for a client with syphilis, the nurse needs to include that syphilis is not considered contagious in the:
1. Primary stage
2. Tertiary stage
3. Incubation stage
4. Secondary stage

722. The nurse is concerned about the public health implications of gonorrhea diagnosed in a 16-year-old adolescent. Which should be of most concern to the nurse?
1. Finding the client's contacts
2. Interviewing the client's parents
3. Determining the reasons for the client's promiscuity
4. Instructing the client about birth control measures

723. The nurse is teaching a client about the drug therapy for gonorrhea. Which fact about drug therapy should the nurse emphasize?
1. It can cure the infection
2. It prevents complications
3. It controls its transmission
4. It can reverse pathologic changes

DRUG-RELATED RESPONSES

724. When assessing the therapeutic action of drugs classified as tumor necrosis factor inhibitors, what client response indicates to the nurse that these drugs are effective? A client with:
1. Ovarian cancer continues in remission
2. Diabetes mellitus develops an increase in insulin production
3. Coronary artery disease experiences vasodilation of the coronary arteries
4. Rheumatoid arthritis sustains a reduction in inflammatory joint pain

725. The nurse uses povidone-iodine (Betadine) on the skin before attempting to obtain a peripheral blood culture because it:
1. Makes the skin more supple
2. Avoids drying the skin as does alcohol
3. Eliminates surface bacteria that would contaminate the culture
4. Provides a cooling agent to diminish the feeling from the puncture wound

726. A client has glaucoma and edema of the lower extremities. The nurse understands that the systemic drug that may be prescribed to produce diuresis and inhibit formation of aqueous humor is:
1. Chlorothiazide (Diuril)
2. Acetazolamide (Diamox)
3. Bendroflumethiazide (Naturetin)
4. Demecarium bromide (Humorsol)

727. A client complains of fatigue and dyspnea and appears pale. The nurse questions the client about medications currently being taken. In light of the symptoms, which medication causes the nurse to be most concerned?
1. Ferrous sulfate (Feosol) 325 mg daily
2. Levothyroxine (Synthroid) 150 mcg daily
3. Famotidine (Pepcid) 20 mg two times a day
4. Methyldopa (Aldomet) 250 mg two times a day

728. The nurse must observe for signs of hyperkalemia when administering:
1. Furosemide (Lasix)
2. Metolazone (Zaroxolyn)
3. Spironolactone (Aldactone)
4. Hydrochlorothiazide (HydroDIURIL)

729. A client is receiving albuterol (Proventil) to relieve severe asthma. For which clinical indicators should the nurse monitor the client?
1. Lethargy
2. Palpitations
3. Visual disturbances
4. Decreased pulse rate

730. The postanesthesia care unit nurse reports the client received intrathecal morphine intraoperatively for postoperative pain control. Because the client has received this medication, what should the nurse include as part of the client's initial 24-hour postoperative care?
1. Assessing the client for tachycardia
2. Monitoring of respiratory rate hourly
3. Observing the client for signs of CNS excitement
4. Administering naloxone (Narcan) every 3 to 4 hours

731. What should the nurse include in a teaching plan aimed at reducing the side effects associated with taking calcium channel blockers such as diltiazem (Cardizem)?
1. Lie down after meals
2. Change positions slowly
3. Avoid dairy products in diet
4. Take the drug with an antacid

732. The nurse is providing discharge instructions for a client with angina. The nurse should teach the client to suspect that nitroglycerin sublingual tablets have lost their potency when:
1. Sublingual tingling is experienced
2. The tablets are more than 3 months old
3. The pain is unrelieved but facial flushing is increased
4. Onset of relief is delayed, but the duration of relief is unchanged

733. If symptoms of warfarin overdose are observed, what should the nurse expect the physician to order?
1. Heparin
2. Vitamin K
3. Protamine sulfate
4. Iron-dextran (Imferon)

734. The nurse should question an order for metoprolol (Lopressor) when it is prescribed for a client with:
1. Hypertension
2. Angina pectoris
3. Sinus bradycardia
4. Myocardial infarction

735. Which of the client's health problems leads the nurse to question an order for a beta blocker?
    1. Heart failure
    2. Hypertension
    3. Sinus tachycardia
    4. Coronary artery disease

736. The nurse evaluates that the simvastatin (Zocor) being administered to a client is effective when there is a reduction in:
    1. INR
    2. Chest pain
    3. Triglycerides
    4. Blood pressure

737. A client with a history of arthritis has an acute episode of right ventricular heart failure and is receiving furosemide (Lasix). The physician lowers the client's usual dosage of aspirin. The client asks the nurse the reason for the lower dose. What is the nurse's best response?
    1. "Aspirin accelerates metabolism of furosemide and decreases the diuretic effect."
    2. "Aspirin in large doses after an acute stress episode increases the bleeding potential."
    3. "Competition for renal excretion sites by the drugs causes increased serum levels of aspirin."
    4. "Use of furosemide and aspirin concomitantly increases formation of uric acid crystals in the nephron."

738. When teaching a client who is to take nitroglycerin tablets, what instructions should the nurse give the client?
    1. Limit the number of tablets to 4 per day
    2. Discontinue the medication if a headache develops
    3. Make certain the medication is stored in a dark container
    4. Increase the number of tablets if dizziness is experienced

739. While taking the health history of a client who is to have surgery in 1 week, the nurse identifies that the client is taking ibuprofen (Advil) for discomfort associated with osteoarthritis. When bringing this to the physician's attention, the nurse would expect that the physician may change the order to:
    1. Naproxen (Aleve)
    2. Ibuprofen (Motrin)
    3. Ketorolac (Toradol)
    4. Acetaminophen (Tylenol)

740. A client who is obtund has a blood pressure of 80/35 mm Hg after a blood transfusion. In an effort to support renal perfusion, the nurse administers dopamine (Intropin) at 2 mcg/kg/min as ordered. What is the most relevant outcome indicating effectiveness of the medication for this client?
    1. A decrease in blood pressure
    2. An increase in urinary output
    3. A decrease in core temperature
    4. An increase in level of consciousness

741. The nurse identifies that a client receiving chemotherapy has lost weight. Which is the best nursing intervention?
    1. Providing low-carbohydrate meals
    2. Explaining effect of chemotherapy
    3. Encouraging the intake of large meals
    4. Administering ordered antiemetics before meals

742. The physician orders ibuprofen (Motrin) and hydroxychloroquine sulfate (Plaquenil) for an older client's arthritis. The nurse teaches the client about hydroxychloroquine toxicity. The nurse determines that the information was understood when the client states, "I will contact the physician immediately if I develop:
    1. Blurred vision."
    2. Urinary retention."
    3. Difficulty swallowing."
    4. Feelings of irritability."

743. One week after being hospitalized for an acute myocardial infarction, a client complains of loss of appetite and a nauseous feeling. Which effect of the prescribed medications does the nurse suspect is the cause of these clinical indications?
    1. Adverse effects of digoxin (Lanoxin)
    2. Therapeutic effects of furosemide (Lasix)
    3. Therapeutic effects of propranolol (Inderal)
    4. Adverse effects of spironolactone (Aldactone)

744. The nurse understands that many of the chemotherapeutic agents used in the treatment of clients with cancer cause:
    1. High leukocyte levels
    2. Bone marrow depression
    3. Lowered sedimentation rate
    4. Increased hemoglobin levels

745. The nurse should teach a client to withhold the prescribed digoxin if the client experiences:
    1. Singultus
    2. Chest pain
    3. Blurred vision
    4. Increased urinary output

746. The nurse is preparing to administer digoxin (Lanoxin) intravenously to a client with atrial fibrillation. In relation to the infusion of the medication, the nurse:
    1. May administer the dose over 1 minute
    2. Should monitor the serum potassium level
    3. May give the drug with other infusing medications
    4. Should withhold the drug if the blood pressure is 115/60 mm Hg

747. The INR of a client receiving Coumadin has been somewhat unstable when checked in the clinic laboratory. The nurse interviews the client to identify factors contributing to the problem. What assessment is most important for the nurse to make? The client's:
    1. Use of analgesics
    2. Serum glucose level
    3. Serum potassium levels
    4. Adherence to the prescribed drug regimen

748. A client is receiving IV heparin sodium and oral warfarin sodium (Coumadin) concurrently for a partial

occlusion of the left common carotid artery. The client expresses concern about why both heparin and Coumadin are needed. What explanation should the nurse provide? "The plan:
1. Allows clot dissolution while prevents new clot formation."
2. Permits the administration of smaller doses of each medication."
3. Immediately provides maximum protection against clot formation."
4. Provides anticoagulant intravenously until the oral drug reaches its therapeutic level."

749. A client with a partial occlusion of the left common carotid artery is to be discharged while still receiving warfarin (Coumadin). The nurse is discussing the adverse effects of warfarin with the client. About which clinical indicator should the nurse tell the client to seek medical consultation?
1. Presence of blood in urine
2. Increased swelling of the ankles
3. Diminished ability to concentrate
4. Occurrence of transient ischemic attacks

750. A client is receiving an anticoagulant for a pulmonary embolism. Which drug should the nurse instruct the client to avoid taking without speaking with the physician?
1. Ferrous sulfate
2. Acetylsalicylic acid
3. Isoxsuprine (Vasodilan)
4. Chlorpromazine (Thorazine)

751. Tissue plasminogen activator (t-PA) is to be administered to a client in the emergency department. Which is the priority nursing assessment?
1. Apical pulse rate
2. Electrolyte levels
3. Signs of bleeding
4. Tissue compatibility

752. A client with tuberculosis asks the nurse why vitamin B$_6$ (pyridoxine) is given with isoniazid (INH). The nurse should explain, "The:
1. Tuberculostatic effect of isoniazid is enhanced."
2. Immunologic defenses of the client are improved."
3. Vitamin is extrinsically needed because with isoniazid natural vitamin synthesis is decreased."
4. Destruction of remaining organisms is accelerated after their reproduction by isoniazid is inhibited."

753. A client receiving morphine is being monitored by the nurse for signs and symptoms of overdose. Check all that apply.
1. ☐ Polyuria
2. ☐ Lethargy
3. ☐ Bradycardia
4. ☐ Dilated pupils
5. ☐ Slow respirations

754. Which medication should the nurse anticipate will be prescribed to relieve anxiety and apprehension in the client with pulmonary edema?
1. Chloral hydrate
2. Morphine sulfate

3. Sodium phenobarbital
4. Hydroxyzine hydrochloride

755. Some clients self-prescribe over-the-counter glucosamine to help relieve joint pain and stiffness. When teaching about glucosamine, the nurse should include that the client needs to reconsider taking this medication if the client has:
1. Osteoarthritis
2. Heart disease
3. Hyperthyroidism
4. Diabetes mellitus

756. Levodopa is prescribed for a client with Parkinson's disease. What should the nurse understand about this drug? Levodopa:
1. Is inadequately absorbed if given with meals
2. Must be monitored by weekly laboratory tests
3. Causes an initial euphoria followed by depression
4. May cause the side effect of orthostatic hypotension

757. The nurse is providing instructions for a client who is receiving phenytoin (Dilantin), but has limited access to health care. The nurse emphasizes meticulous oral hygiene because phenytoin:
1. Causes hyperplasia of the gums
2. Increases alkalinity of the oral secretions
3. Irritates the gingiva and destroys tooth enamel
4. Promotes plaque and bacterial growth at the gum lines

758. The nurse understands that edrophonium HCl (Tensilon) is used for the diagnosis of myasthenia gravis because it will cause an increase in:
1. Symptoms
2. Consciousness
3. Blood pressure
4. Muscle strength

759. A client is receiving phenytoin (Dilantin) for a seizure disorder and heparin for a deep vein thrombosis. Coumadin is added in preparation for discontinuing the heparin. Why must the nurse observe the client closely during the initial days of treatment with Coumadin?
1. Phenytoin increases the clotting potential
2. Coumadin affects the metabolism of phenytoin
3. Coumadin's action is greater in clients with seizure disorders
4. Seizures increase the metabolic degradation rate of Coumadin

760. A client who is receiving phenytoin (Dilantin) asks why folic acid was prescribed. What is the best response by the nurse? Folic acid:
1. Absorption from foods is inhibited
2. Potentiates the action of phenytoin
3. Improves absorption of iron from foods
4. Prevents the neuropathy caused by phenytoin

761. What should the nurse monitor to evaluate the effectiveness of carbamazepine (Tegretol) in the management of a client's trigeminal neuralgia?
1. Pain relief
2. Liver function

3. Cardiac output
4. Seizure activity

762. Ceftriaxone (Rocephin) 2.5 g IVPB every 8 hours is ordered for a client with a severe infection. The pharmacy sends a vial labeled 5 g per 10 mL. What volume of Rocephin should the nurse add to the IVPB solution?
Answer: _____ mL

763. The nurse is caring for a client who had a total knee replacement 2 days ago and who is requesting Darvocet N100 in addition to the patient-controlled analgesia (PCA). The client reports having taken 2 Darvocet tablets every 3 hours for several weeks before surgery. If each tablet contains 650 mg of acetaminophen, how much acetaminophen had the client been ingesting per day?
1. 5200 mg
2. 10,400 mg
3. 15,600 mg
4. 18,800 mg

764. The practitioner orders 500 mg of an antibiotic IVPB every 12 hours. The vial of antibiotic contains 1 g and indicates that the addition of 2.5 mL of sterile water will yield 3 mL of reconstituted solution. How many milliliters of the antibiotic should be added to the 50-mL IVPB bag?
Answer: _____ mL

765. A client is to have mafenide (Sulfamylon) cream applied to burned areas. The nurse understands that a serious side effect of Sulfamylon therapy that the client may experience is:
1. Curling's ulcer
2. Renal shutdown
3. Metabolic acidosis
4. Hemolysis of red blood cells

766. After several days of IV therapy for chloroquine-resistant malaria, the physician replaces the IV medication with oral quinine sulfate, 2 g per day in divided doses. The nurse should administer this medication after meals to:
1. Delay its absorption
2. Minimize gastric irritation
3. Decrease stimulation of appetite
4. Reduce its antidysrhythmic action

767. Preparation of a client for a subtotal thyroidectomy may include the administration of potassium iodide solution. When the client refuses to take the medication, the nurse provides instruction and reinforces which desired effect?
1. Reduction of the total basal metabolic rate
2. Decrease of the thyroid gland's vascularity
3. Maintenance of the parathyroid glands' function
4. Ablation of the cells of the thyroid gland that produce hormones

768. What information should the nurse include when teaching a client about antacid therapy? Antacid tablets:
1. Must be taken 1 hour before meals
2. Are as effective as the liquid forms
3. Should be taken only at 4-hour intervals
4. Interfere with the absorption of other drugs

769. A client who has been diagnosed as having Lyme disease is started on doxycycline, a tetracycline. What should the nurse do when administering this drug?
1. Administer the medication with meals or a snack
2. Provide orange or other citrus fruit juice with the medication
3. Provide medication an hour before milk products are ingested
4. Offer antacids 30 minutes after administration if GI side effects occur

770. An ambulatory female client with relapsing-remitting multiple sclerosis is to receive every-other-day injections of interferon beta-1a (Avonex). When planning to discuss this medication with the client and her husband, what adverse effect should the nurse explain that the client may experience?
1. Anhidrosis
2. Hypercalcemia
3. Flulike symptoms
4. Decreased heart rate

771. Before the discharge of a client with Addison's disease, the physician prescribes hydrocortisone and fludrocortisone. The nurse explains that the medication is being administered to:
1. Control excessive loss of potassium salts
2. Decrease cardiac dysrhythmias and dyspnea
3. Prevent hypoglycemia and permit the client to respond to stress
4. Increase amounts of angiotensin II to raise the client's blood pressure

772. The nurse administers the drug desmopressin acetate (DDAVP) to a client with diabetes insipidus. To evaluate the effectiveness of the drug, the nurse should monitor the client's:
1. Arterial blood pH
2. Intake and output
3. Fasting serum glucose
4. Pulse and respiratory rates

773. A client receiving morphine by patient-controlled analgesia has a respiratory rate of 6 breaths/min. What intervention should the nurse anticipate?
1. Nasotracheal suction
2. Mechanical ventilation
3. Naloxone administration
4. Cardiopulmonary resuscitation

774. A client will be taking nitrofurantoin (Macrobid) 50 mg orally every evening at home to manage recurrent urinary tract infections. What instructions should the nurse give to the client?
1. Increase intake of fluids
2. Strain urine for crystals and stones
3. Stop the drug if the urinary output increases
4. Maintain the exact time schedule for taking the drug

775. A client with rheumatoid arthritis is receiving aspirin. The nurse should teach the client to report symptoms of salicylate intoxication, which include:
1. Polyuria
2. Tinnitus

3. Joint pain

4. Laryngeal spasm

776. What should the nurse include in a teaching plan for a client taking calcium channel blockers such as nifedipine (Procardia)? Check all that apply.
   1. ☐ Reduce calcium intake
   2. ☐ Change positions slowly
   3. ☐ Report peripheral edema
   4. ☐ Expect temporary hair loss
   5. ☐ Avoid drinking grapefruit juice

777. A client with rheumatoid arthritis is receiving aurothioglucose, a gold compound. It is most important that the nurse monitor the client for:
   1. Hypertension
   2. Cutaneous lesions
   3. Thrombocytopenia
   4. Elevated blood glucose

778. The nurse is planning care for a patient with cancer who is receiving the plant alkaloid vincristine (Oncovin). In contrast to the side effects of most chemotherapeutic agents, what is a common side effect of vincristine that the nurse must address in the client's care plan?
   1. Nausea
   2. Alopecia
   3. Constipation
   4. Hyperuricemia

779. The physician orders antibiotic therapy for a client receiving chemotherapy. The nurse understands that that this is a result of the effect of chemotherapy on the client's:
   1. Liver
   2. Blood
   3. Lymph nodes
   4. Bone marrow

780. Why does the nurse expect the client to develop soreness of the mouth and anus during chemotherapy for cancer of the lung?
   1. These tissues are poorly nourished because the client is anorectic
   2. The entire GI tract is involved because of the direct irritating effects of chemotherapy
   3. The tissues that normally divide rapidly are damaged by the chemotherapeutic agent
   4. The side effects of the chemotherapeutic agents used tend to concentrate in these body areas

781. The nurse administers leucovorin calcium to a client before the ordered methotrexate. The client asks the reason for this. The nurse's response is based on the understanding that leucovorin calcium is being given to:
   1. Potentiate the metabolite required for destruction of cancer cells
   2. Supply levels of folic acid required by blood-forming organs
   3. Act synergistically with antineoplastic drugs to destroy cancer cells
   4. Increase production of phagocytic cells required to remove debris liberated by disintegrating cancer cells

782. The physician plans to reduce a client's dexamethasone (Decadron) dosage gradually and to continue a lower maintenance dosage. The nurse explains to the client that the gradual dosage reduction provides which effect?
   1. Production of antibodies by the immune system
   2. Return of cortisone production by the adrenal glands
   3. Building of glycogen and protein stores in liver and muscle
   4. Time to observe for return of increased intracranial pressure

783. A client with rheumatoid arthritis has been taking a steroid medication for the past year. For which complication of the prolonged use of this medication should the nurse assess the client?
   1. Elevated C-reactive protein
   2. Elevated sedimentation rate
   3. Decreased white blood cells
   4. Decreased serum glucose levels

784. Which test result should the nurse review to determine if the antibiotic prescribed for the client will be effective?
   1. Serologic test
   2. Sensitivity test
   3. Serum osmolality
   4. Sedimentation rate

785. After receiving streptomycin sulfate for 2 weeks as part of the medical regimen for tuberculosis, the client states, "I feel like I am walking like a drunken seaman." The nurse withholds the drug and promptly reports the problem to the physician because the symptoms may be a result of the drug's effect on which part of the body?
   1. Pyramidal tracts
   2. Cerebellar tissue
   3. Peripheral motor end-plates
   4. Vestibular branch of the eighth cranial nerve

786. A client says, "I take baking soda in water when I get heartburn." The nurse suggests an antacid containing aluminum and magnesium hydroxide such as Maalox instead of baking soda. What is the advantage these antacids have over baking soda? Aluminum and magnesium hydroxide:
   1. Contain little, if any, sodium
   2. Are readily absorbed by the stomach mucosa
   3. Have no direct effect on the systemic acid-base balance when taken as directed
   4. Cause few side effects such as diarrhea or constipation when they are used properly

787. The physician orders ranitidine (Zantac) for a client with peptic ulcer disease. The client asks the nurse what this medication does. On which action of ranitidine does the nurse base a response?
   1. Increases gastric motility
   2. Neutralizes gastric acidity
   3. Facilitates histamine release
   4. Inhibits gastric acid secretion

788. A terminally ill client has been in the hospice unit for several weeks on a morphine drip. The dose is now above the typical morphine dosage. The client's spouse tells the nurse that the client is again uncomfortable and needs the morphine increased. Medical orders state to titrate morphine to comfort level. What should the nurse do?
    1. Add a placebo to the morphine to appease the spouse
    2. Discuss with the spouse the risk for morphine addiction
    3. Assess the client's pain before increasing the morphine to the next level
    4. Check the client's heart rate before increasing the morphine to the next level

789. Isoniazid (INH) is prescribed as a prophylactic measure for a client whose spouse has active tuberculosis. What statements by the client indicate to the nurse that there is a need for further teaching? Check all that apply.
    1. ❏ "I will still be taking this drug six months from now."
    2. ❏ "I sometimes allow our children to sleep in our bed at night."
    3. ❏ "I plan to start taking pyridoxine supplements with breakfast."
    4. ❏ "I know I also have tuberculosis because the skin test was positive."
    5. ❏ "I'll be skipping the wine, but enjoying the cheese at my neighbor's party."

790. The nurse is reviewing the history and physicals of several clients from the clinic who are taking rifampin (Rifadin) for the treatment of tuberculosis. Which client presents a specific concern for the nurse?
    1. A 45-year-old taking a loop diuretic
    2. A 26-year-old taking oral contraceptives
    3. A 32-year-old taking a proton pump inhibitor
    4. A 72-year-old taking intermediate-acting insulin

791. After surgery a client develops a deep vein thrombosis and a pulmonary embolus. The physician orders heparin via a continuous drip at 1200 units/hr and several hours later orders vancomycin (Vancocin) 500 mg intravenously every 12 hours. The client has one IV site, a peripheral line in the left forearm. The nurse should:
    1. Stop the heparin, flush the line, and administer the vancomycin
    2. Use a piggyback setup to administer the vancomycin into the heparin
    3. Start another IV line for the vancomycin and continue the heparin as ordered
    4. Hold the vancomycin and tell the physician that the drug is incompatible with heparin

792. The practitioner orders valsartan (Diovan), an angiotensin II receptor antagonist, for a client. For which possible side effect should the nurse monitor the client?
    1. Constipation
    2. Hypokalemia
    3. Change in visual acuity
    4. Orthostatic hypotension

793. A female client whose ECG exhibits multiple premature ventricular complexes is to take oral disopyramide (Norpace). When planning to teach the client about this medication, the nurse should discuss signs and symptoms related to the side effect of:
    1. Rhinorrhea
    2. Constipation
    3. Hyperglycemia
    4. Stress incontinence

794. A beta blocker, timolol (Blocadren), has been prescribed for a client with moderate hypertension. After teaching about this medication, the nurse identifies that the client needs further teaching when the client states, "I should:
    1. Change positions slowly."
    2. Take the medication before going to bed."
    3. Expect to feel drowsy when taking this drug"
    4. Count the pulse before taking the medication."

795. A client with type 2 diabetes mellitus develops gout and the physician orders allopurinal (Zyloprim). The client is also taking metformin (Glucophage) and an over-the-counter NSAID. When teaching about the administration of Zyloprim, the nurse should instruct the client to:
    1. Decrease daily dose of NSAIDs
    2. Limit fluid intake to 1 quart a day
    3. Take the medication on an empty stomach
    4. Monitor blood glucose levels more frequently

796. The physician orders a vitamin tablet that contains vitamin B complex. What should the nurse teach the client?
    1. The urine may turn bright yellow
    2. The daily fluid intake should be increased
    3. The vitamin should be taken on an empty stomach
    4. The drug may accumulate in the body if the dose is not followed exactly

797. The nurse is administering 40 mg of furosemide (Lasix) intravenously. The nurse identifies that it is being administered too fast when the client states, "My:
    1. Bladder feels full."
    2. Ears are plugged up."
    3. Heart is beating fast."
    4. Left arm feels numb."

798. The physician orders nesiritide (Natrecor), a vasodilator, for a client with acute heart failure and pulmonary edema. The nurse evaluates that the medication is effective when the client has a decreased occurrence of:
    1. Dyspnea
    2. Hypotension
    3. Unstable angina
    4. Premature heart beats

799. A client is receiving MOPP chemotherapy and asks about its effect on immunity. The nurse identifies that further teaching is necessary when the client states:
    1. "The prednisone I am taking has the side effect of decreasing the immune response."
    2. "I am at increased risk for infection because of decreased white blood cell production."

3. "Being home will place me at greater risk because there are more microorganisms there."

4. "My immune status may decline because nutritional problems I may experience will affect my immunity."

800. The nurse receives a change of shift report for a client who had surgery for a total hip replacement 24 hours ago. After reviewing the client's medical record (shown here) and completing a physical assessment, which complication should the nurse conclude that the client is experiencing?

1. Fat embolism
2. Urinary retention
3. Hypovolemic shock
4. Pulmonary embolism

CLIENT CHART
History
The client is a 43-year-old iron worker who experienced a crushing occupational injury requiring a total hip replacement. He is relatively healthy but is 10% overweight, smokes 2 packs a day, and is borderline for type 2 diabetes.
Vital Signs
T: 101.4° F, P: 100, R: 30, BP: 160/100
Physical Assessment
Dyspnea
Altered mental state
Restlessness and agitation
Petechial rash on the neck and chest
Urine collection bag contains 50 mL output for last hour and the I&O flow sheet indicates 250 mL output over the last 4 hours.

ANSWERS AND RATIONALES

GROWTH AND DEVELOPMENT

1. 4 Accidents are common during young adulthood because of immature judgment and impulsivity associated with this stage of development.

1 Kidney dysfunction is not a problem specific to any one stage of growth. 2 Cardiovascular disease is a common health problem in middle adulthood. 3 Glaucoma is a common health problem in the older adult.

Client Need: Health Promotion and Maintenance; **Cognitive Level:** Application; **Integrated Process:** Teaching/Learning; **Nursing Process:** Planning/Implementation; **Reference:** Ch 5, General Nursing Care of Young Adults

2. 3 Neurologic aging causes forgetfulness and a slower response time; repetition increases learning.

1, 4 This principle is applicable to all learning regardless of the client's age. 2 Learning occurs but it may take longer.

Client Need: Health Promotion and Maintenance; **Cognitive Level:** Application; **Integrated Process:** Teaching/Learning; **Nursing Process:** Planning/Implementation; **Reference:** Ch 5, General Nursing Care of Middle-Older and Old-Older Adults

3. 4 Osteoporosis is not restricted to women; it is a potential major health problem of all older adults; estimates indicate that half of all women have at least one osteoporotic fracture and the risk in men is estimated between 13% and 25%; a bone mineral density (BMD) measurement assesses the mass of bone per unit volume or how tightly the bone is packed.

1 Osteoporosis also can occur in men. 2 Exercise may decrease the occurrence of, but will not prevent, osteoporosis; a regimen including weight-bearing exercises is advised. 3 A small frame is a risk factor for osteoporosis.

Client Need: Health Promotion and Maintenance; **Cognitive Level:** Application; **Integrated Process:** Teaching/Learning; **Nursing Process:** Planning/Implementation; **Reference:** Ch 5, General Nursing Care of Middle-Older and Old-Older Adults

4. 4 Around-the-clock administration of analgesics is recommended for acute pain in the older adult population; this helps to maintain a therapeutic blood level of pain medication.

1 The intramuscular route is not recommended for older adults, who are more likely to experience reduced muscle mass, which can reduce bioavailability of the drug. 2 Meperidine (Demerol) should be avoided because of its potential for toxicity as a result of a decline in physiologic function in the older adult; it should be avoided especially in clients with heart failure or renal impairment, which is often seen in the older adult population. 3 Patient-controlled analgesia should not be avoided in this population; it gives the client control and is an excellent choice for clients who do not have dementia.

Client Need: Pharmacological and Parenteral Therapies; **Cognitive Level:** Application; **Nursing Process:** Planning/Implementation; **Reference:** Ch 5, The Middle-Older and Old-Older Adult, Data Base

5. 2 Bones become more fragile because of loss of bone density associated with the aging process; often associated with lower circulating levels of estrogens or testosterone.

1 Carelessness is a characteristic applicable to certain individuals rather than to people within a developmental level. 3 Although prolonged immobility is associated with bone demineralization, hip fractures also occur in active older adults. 4 Rheumatoid diseases certainly can affect the skeletal system but do not increase the incidence of hip fractures.

Client Need: Health Promotion and Maintenance; **Cognitive Level:** Application; **Nursing Process:** Assessment/Analysis; **Reference:** Ch 5, The Middle-Older and Old-Older Adults, Data Base

6. 3 This may make an older individual unaware of a serious illness, thermal extremes, or excessive pressure.

1 There should be no interference with swallowing in older individuals. 2 Older individuals tend to feel the cold and rarely complain of the heat. 4 There is a decreased response to stimuli in the older individual.

Client Need: Health Promotion and Maintenance; **Cognitive Level:** Application; **Nursing Process:** Planning/Implementation; **Reference:** Ch 5, The Middle-Older and Old-Older Adults, Data Base

7. 3 Generally, female voices have a higher pitch than male voices; older adults with presbycusis (hearing loss caused by the aging process) have more difficulty hearing higher pitched sounds.

1 Cerumen becomes drier and harder as a person ages. 2 There is no greater incidence of tympanic tears caused by the aging process. 4 The epithelium of the lining of the ear becomes thinner and drier.

Client Need: Health Promotion and Maintenance; **Cognitive Level:** Application; **Nursing Process:** Assessment/Analysis, **Reference:** Ch 5, General Nursing Care of Middle-Older and Old-Older Adults

8. 3 Aged clients may display psychomotor retardation and need more time to complete the tasks associated with the activities of daily living; meal times should be relaxing and social.

1 Supplemental drinks should augment meals and be offered between meals, not as a substitute for meals. 2 Clients should be encouraged to feed themselves to remain as independent as possible; spoon feeding may not mirror the pace of eating preferred by the client and forcing the client to eat all of the food may precipitate anxiety, frustration, and agitation. 4 Placement of a gastrostomy tube is premature.

Client Need: Health Promotion and Maintenance; **Cognitive Level:** Application; **Nursing Process:** Planning/Implementation; **Reference:** Ch 5, General Nursing Care of Middle-Older and Old-Older Adults

CIRCULATORY SYSTEM (CARDIOVASCULAR, BLOOD, AND LYMPHATIC SYSTEMS)

9. **2** The heart's apex is between the fifth and sixth ribs at the midclavicular line. It is closest to the chest wall here, so auscultation is easier.
1, 3, 4 Although it may be possible to auscultate the heart in this area, it is usually easier to do so over the apex.
Client Need: Reduction of Risk Potential; **Cognitive Level:** Application; **Nursing Process:** Assessment/Analysis; **Reference:** Ch 6, Review of Anatomy and Physiology, Heart

10. **4** The cardiac rhythm is monitored and rhythm disturbances documented; documented disturbances are stored, printed, and then analyzed in relation to the client's activity/symptom diary.
1 The monitor must remain in place constantly for accurate recordings. **2** The client must keep a record of activities and symptoms while the monitor records cardiac rhythm disturbances, and then an analysis of correlations between the two is made. **3** A chest radiograph, not a Holter monitor, will reveal the size and contour of the heart.
Client Need: Reduction of Risk Potential; **Cognitive Level:** Application; **Integrated Process:** Teaching/Learning; **Nursing Process:** Planning/Implementation; **Reference:** Ch 6, Related Procedures, Cardiac Monitoring

11. **3** This test evaluates the heart's ability to meet the need for additional O_2 in response to the stress of exercising. Changes in the ECG identify dysrhythmias and ST changes indicative of myocardial ischemia.
1 This test assists in the differential diagnosis of chest pain; the diagnosis of heart disease is made via the results of a variety of diagnostic procedures and laboratory tests. **2** This is a valuable test that will influence the diagnosis and treatment of heart disease. **4** This is a noninvasive test.
Client Need: Reduction of Risk Potential; **Cognitive Level:** Application; **Integrated Process:** Teaching/Learning; **Nursing Process:** Planning/Implementation; **Reference:** Ch 6, Related Procedures, Cardiac Monitoring

12. **2** Temperature may increase within the first 24 hours as a result of the inflammatory response to tissue destruction and persist as long as a week.
1 Diaphoresis is caused by activation of the sympathetic, not parasympathetic, nervous system and may indicate cardiogenic shock. **3** Pain is persistent and constant, not intermittent; it is caused by oxygen deprivation and the release of lactic acid. **4** The BP rises initially but then drops because there is a decrease in cardiac output.
Client Need: Physiological Adaptation; **Cognitive Level:** Analysis; **Nursing Process:** Assessment/Analysis; **Reference:** Ch 6, Coronary Artery Disease, Data Base

13. **3** Pulse pressure is obtained by subtracting the diastolic from the systolic reading after the BP has been recorded.
1 This is the definition of BP; it is not the pulse pressure. **2** This is the pulse deficit. **4** This is not pulse pressure.

Client Need: Reduction of Risk Potential; **Cognitive Level:** Application; **Nursing Process:** Assessment/Analysis; **Reference:** Ch 6, Review of Anatomy and Physiology, Blood Vessels

14. **1** Temperatures of 102° F (38° C) or greater lead to an increased metabolism and cardiac workload.
2 An elevated temperature is not an early sign of developing cerebral edema. Open heart surgery is not associated with cerebral edema. **3** Although diaphoresis is related to an elevated temperature, it is not the reason for notifying the physician. **4** Fever is unrelated to hemorrhage; in hemorrhage with shock, the temperature decreases.
Client Need: Physiological Adaptation; **Cognitive Level:** Comprehension; **Integrated Process:** Communication/Documentation; **Nursing Process:** Planning/Implementation; **Reference:** Ch 6, Cardiac Surgery, Nursing Care

15. **2** Constriction of the peripheral blood vessels and the resulting increase in BP impair circulation and limit the amount of O_2 being delivered to body cells, particularly in the extremities.
1 Nicotine constricts all peripheral vessels, not just superficial ones; its primary action is vasoconstriction; it will not dilate deep vessels. **3, 4** Nicotine constricts rather than dilates peripheral vessels.
Client Need: Health Promotion and Maintenance; **Cognitive Level:** Comprehension; **Integrated Process:** Teaching/Learning; **Nursing Process:** Planning/Implementation; **Reference:** Ch 6, Vascular Disease, Nursing Care

16. **2** Vagal stimulation slows the heart. The vagus is the principal nerve of the parasympathetic portion of the autonomic nervous system, and its axon terminals release acetylcholine. The response of the viscera to acetylcholine varies, but in general the organ is in a relaxed state.
1 This is an action of the sympathetic nervous system (accelerator nerve) caused by the release of norepinephrine. **3** Stimulation of the sympathetic nervous system dilates bronchioles in the lungs; the vagus nerve constricts them. **4** There are no parasympathetic fibers to the coronary blood vessels; sympathetic impulses dilate these vessels.
Client Need: Physiological Adaptation; **Cognitive Level:** Application; **Nursing Process:** Planning/Implementation; **Reference:** Ch 6, Review of Anatomy and Physiology, Regulatory Mechanisms Affecting Circulation

17. **3** The release of iron from hemoglobin as erythrocytes disintegrate in tissue results in ferrous sulfide formation, causing darkening of the tissues.
1 Heme constitutes the pigment portion of the hemoglobin molecule, which gives blood its red color; it is not associated with chronic venous insufficiency. **2** Ferric chloride is used as a reagent, topically as an antiseptic, and as an astringent; it is not related to chronic venous insufficiency. **4** All amino acids are soluble.
Client Need: Physiological Adaptation; **Cognitive Level:** Analysis; **Nursing Process:** Assessment/Analysis; **Reference:** Ch 6, Vascular Disease, Data Base

18. 4 Diminished sensation decreases awareness of injury. Injured tissue cannot heal properly because of cellular deprivation of O_2 and nutrients; ulceration and gangrene may result.

1 Emotional stress does not cause tissue injury; however, because of vasoconstriction, it may prolong healing. 2 Inadequate hygiene is only one stress that may cause tissue trauma; protein is not related to this disease. 3 Caffeine stimulates the cerebral cortex; it does not contribute to ulceration or deprivation of oxygen.

Client Need: Physiological Adaptation; Cognitive Level: Application; Nursing Process: Assessment/Analysis; Reference: Ch 6, Vascular Disease, Data Base

19. 2 The pulmonary capillary beds are the first small vessels (capillary beds) that the embolus encounters once it is released from the calf veins.

1, 4 This would not occur because the embolus would enter the pulmonary system first. 3 Dry gangrene occurs when the arterial rather than the venous circulation is compromised.

Client Need: Physiological Adaptation; Cognitive Level: Application; Nursing Process: Planning/Implementation; Reference: Ch 6, Vascular Disease, Nursing Care

20. 4 A drop in BP, rapid pulse rate, cold clammy skin, and oliguria are signs of decreased blood volume and shock, which if not treated promptly can lead to death.

1 This is an expected response; the client will push out the airway as the effects of anesthesia subside. 2 Snoring respirations are common because of the depressant effects of anesthesia. 3 Shallow respirations are common because of the depressant effects of anesthesia.

Client Need: Management of Care; Cognitive Level: Application; Integrated Process: Communication/Documentation; Nursing Process: Planning/Implementation; Reference: Ch 6, Shock, Data Base

21. 2 Localized sensory changes may indicate nerve damage, impaired circulation, or thrombophlebitis. Activity should be limited, and the physician notified.

1 Symptoms may indicate a serious problem, and the physician must be notified. While fluids may be helpful to prevent hemoconcentration and the resulting risk of thrombus formation, fluids should be held in case a surgical procedure or diagnostic test is performed that requires the client to refrain from oral intake. 3 Rubbing or massaging the legs is contraindicated because of possible dislodging of a thrombus if present. 4 Bed rest is indicated to prevent the possibility of further damage or creation of an embolus.

Client Need: Physiological Adaptation; Cognitive Level: Application; Integrated Process: Communication/Documentation; Nursing Process: Planning/Implementation; Reference: Ch 6, Vascular Disease, Data Base

22. 4 A sympathectomy causes dilation of the blood vessels in the lower extremities; the resulting shift in the fixed blood volume lowers systemic BP.

1 Fluid losses associated with surgery may gradually lower BP and are compensated by endocrine and renal mechanisms. 2 Although anesthesia depresses vital signs, generally there is not a sudden drop in BP postoperatively. 3 Epinephrine would increase BP by stimulating cardiac contractility.

Client Need: Physiological Adaptation; Cognitive Level: Comprehension; Nursing Process: Evaluation/Outcomes; Reference: Ch 6, Review of Anatomy and Physiology, Regulating Mechanisms Affecting Circulation

23. 4 Thrombophlebitis is inflammation of a vein that occurs with the formation of a clot. Adaptations include pain, redness, warmth, tenderness, and edema.

1 Pitting edema does not occur in thrombophlebitis. 2 Ecchymosis is a sign of bleeding; thrombophlebitis is caused by a clot. 3 Intermittent claudication (pain when walking, resulting from tissue ischemia) may occur with peripheral arterial disease.

Client Need: Physiological Adaptation; Cognitive Level: Application; Nursing Process: Assessment/Analysis; Reference: Ch 6, Vascular Disease, Data Base

24. 3 Support hose apply external pressure on the veins, preventing the retrograde pressure or flow that may occur in the standing or sitting positions; application before arising prevents the veins from having the opportunity to become engorged.

1 If this schedule is followed, at some point the feet will be dependent before the stockings are put on; venous pooling and edema may occur; application of elastic stockings at this time can cause tissue trauma. 2 Because they promote venous return, they do not need to be worn when the legs are elevated in bed. 4 Stockings must be removed so that the legs can be washed and dried at least daily. They usually need not be worn while in bed with the feet elevated during sleep, because gravity prevents venous pooling.

Client Need: Reduction of Risk Potential; Cognitive Level: Application; Integrated Process: Teaching/Learning; Nursing Process: Planning/Implementation; Reference: Ch 6, Vascular Disease, Nursing Care

25. 4 Sitting on the edge of the bed before getting up gives the body a chance to adjust to the effects of gravity on circulation in the upright position.

1 Support hose may help prevent orthostatic hypotension by increasing venous return. However, they must be applied before getting out of bed and would not be worn continuously. 2 This would not prevent episodes of orthostatic hypotension. 3 Energetic tasks, once standing and acclimated, do not increase hypotension.

Client Need: Safety and Infection Control; Cognitive Level: Application; Integrated Process: Teaching/Learning; Nursing Process: Planning/Implementation; Reference: Ch 6, Hypertension, Nursing Care

26. **1** ACE (angiotensin-converting enzyme) increases the sensitivity of the cough reflex, leading to the common adverse effect sometimes referred to as an ACE cough.

2, 3, 4 A cough is not a side effect of this category of medications.

Client Need: Pharmacological and Parenteral Therapies; **Cognitive Level:** Application; **Integrated Process:** Teaching/Learning; **Nursing Process:** Planning/Implementation; **Reference:** Ch 6, Antihypertensives

27. **4** Vasodilation will lower BP.

1 The peripheral pulse rate is not affected. **2** Breath sounds are not directly affected by vasodilation. **3** The nurse cannot directly assess cardiac output because it involves multiplying the stroke volume by the heart rate.

Client Need: Pharmacological and Parenteral Therapies; **Cognitive Level:** Application; **Nursing Process:** Evaluation/Outcomes; **Reference:** Ch 6, Antihypertensives

28. **4** Angiotensin II receptor blockers lower BP; they block the receptor sites in smooth muscles and the adrenal glands so vasoconstriction is prevented.

1, 2, 3 ARBs do not directly affect this.

Client Need: Pharmacological and Parenteral Therapies; **Cognitive Level:** Application; **Nursing Process:** Evaluation/Outcomes; **Reference:** Ch 6, Antihypertensives

29. **4** Cholesterol is a sterol found in tissue; it is attributed in part to diets high in saturated fats.

1 Exercise, not cholesterol, increases HDL levels and helps decrease the risk of heart disease. **2** Only animal foods furnish dietary cholesterol. **3** Cholesterol is also produced by the body and is needed for the synthesis of bile salts, adrenocortical and steroid sex hormones, and provitamin D.

Client Need: Health Promotion and Maintenance; **Cognitive Level:** Application; **Integrated Process:** Teaching/Learning; **Nursing Process:** Planning/Implementation; **Reference:** Ch 6, Coronary Artery Disease, Nursing Care

30. **1** Fiber and fluids help prevent the most common adverse effect of constipation—fecal impaction.

2 The medication should be taken with meals. **3** The pulse is not affected. **4** Cholestyramine binds bile in the intestine; therefore it reduces the incidence of jaundice.

Client Need: Pharmacological and Parenteral Therapies; **Cognitive Level:** Application; **Integrated Process:** Teaching/Learning; **Nursing Process:** Planning/Implementation; **Reference:** Ch 6, Antilipidemics

31. **3** Whole milk is high in saturated fat.

1 Olive oil contains unsaturated fat. **2** Most fish have a low fat content. **4** Soluble fiber helps to lower cholesterol.

Client Need: Basic Care and Comfort; **Cognitive Level:** Analysis; **Integrated Process:** Teaching/Learning; **Nursing Process:** Planning/Implementation; **Reference:** Ch 6, Coronary Artery Disease, Nursing Care

32. **3** Vegetables and whole grains are low in fat and have soluble fiber, which may reduce the risk for heart disease.

1 Animal-derived products, such as milk, are high in saturated fats. **2** Meats are high in saturated fats. **4** These are high in cholesterol.

Client Need: Basic Care and Comfort; **Cognitive Level:** Application; **Integrated Process:** Teaching/Learning; **Nursing Process:** Planning/Implementation; **Reference:** Ch 6, Coronary Artery Disease, Nursing Care

33. **1** ☐ The medication does not affect levels of potassium.

  2 ☒ The medication increases photosensitivity; client should avoid sun exposure and use sun block.

  3 ☒ The client should be monitored for the adverse effects of glaucoma and cataracts.

  4 ☐ The medication is most effective when taken at bedtime because cholesterol synthesis is highest at night.

  5 ☒ Gray-bronze skin and unexplained muscle pain are signs of rhabdomyolysis.

Client Need: Pharmacological and Parenteral Therapies; **Cognitive Level:** Application; **Nursing Process:** Planning/Implementation; **Reference:** Ch 6, Antilipidemics

34. **2** Hypertension is 78% more prevalent in African Americans than among Caucasian Americans; 1 in 3 African Americans have hypertension.

1 African Americans have approximately 50% less risk for osteoporosis than Caucasian Americans. **3** Caucasian-American women are 30% more likely to be diagnosed with uterine cancer than African-American women. **4** Statistics indicate that African Americans are less likely to develop thyroid disorders than Caucasian Americans.

Client Need: Health Promotion and Maintenance; **Cognitive Level:** Application; **Nursing Process:** Assessment/Analysis; **Reference:** Ch 6, Hypertension, Data Base

35. **4** Dyspnea may indicate development of pulmonary edema, which is a life-threatening condition.

1 This CNS side effect may occur in some people, but it is not life-threatening. **2, 3** This is a common side effect of this medication, which is not life-threatening.

Client Need: Pharmacological and Parenteral Therapies; **Cognitive Level:** Application; **Integrated Process:** Teaching/Learning; **Nursing Process:** Planning/Implementation; **Reference:** Ch 6, Antidysrhythmics

36. **3** The two coronary arteries are the first branches of the aorta and carry blood with a high O_2 content to the myocardium.

1 This is the function of the pulmonary arteries. **2** They carry blood with high O_2 content to the myocardium, not the endocardium. **4** This is a function of the pulmonary veins.

Client Need: Physiological Adaptation; **Cognitive Level:** Knowledge; **Integrated Process:** Teaching/Learning; **Nursing Process:** Planning/Implementation; **Reference:** Ch 6, Review of Anatomy and Physiology, Heart

37. **2** Ischemia causes tissue injury and the release of chemicals, such as bradykinin, that stimulate sensory nerves and produce pain.

1 Arterial spasm, resulting in tissue hypoxia and pain, is associated with angina pectoris. **3** Arteries, not veins, are involved in the etiology of a myocardial infarction. **4** Tissue injury and pain occur in the myocardium.

Client Need: Physiological Adaptation; **Cognitive Level:** Comprehension; **Nursing Process:** Assessment/Analysis; **Reference:** Ch 6, Coronary Artery Disease, Data Base

38. **3** Anginal pain, which can be anticipated during certain activities, may be prevented by dilating the coronary arteries immediately before engaging in the activity.

1 One tablet is generally administered at a time; doubling the dosage may produce severe hypotension and headache. **2** The sublingual form of nitroglycerin is absorbed directly through the mucous membranes and should not be swallowed. **4** When the pain is relieved, rest will generally prevent its recurrence by reducing O_2 consumption of the myocardium.

Client Need: Pharmacological and Parenteral Therapies; **Cognitive Level:** Application; **Integrated Process:** Teaching/Learning; **Nursing Process:** Planning/Implementation; **Reference:** Ch 6, Coronary Vasodilators

39. **4** The pulse should be assessed because the trauma at the insertion site may interfere with blood flow distal to the site. There is also danger of bleeding.

1 This would be determined on an individual basis; it is not routine. **2** Rest is not a priority, although the extremity in which the catheter was inserted usually is immobilized for a period of time to prevent bleeding at the insertion site. **3** The client will be on a cardiac monitor, which will allow for continuous monitoring.

Client Need: Reduction of Risk Potential; **Cognitive Level:** Application; **Nursing Process:** Evaluation/Outcomes; **Reference:** Ch 6, Related Procedures, Cardiac Catheterization

40. **2** Blood samples from the right atrium, right ventricle, and pulmonary artery would all be about the same with regard to O_2 concentration because the lining of the heart consumes very little oxygen from the returning venous blood.

1 These contain less O_2 than does pulmonary vein blood, which carries oxygenated blood back to the heart, where it will be ejected into the circulation. **3, 4** The samples from the right atrium, right ventricle, and pulmonary artery contain the same concentration of O_2.

Client Need: Reduction of Risk Potential; **Cognitive Level:** Comprehension; **Nursing Process:** Assessment/Analysis; **Reference:** Ch 6, Related Procedures, Cardiac Catheterization

41. **1** Myocardial infarction (MI) may cause increased irritability of tissue or interruption of normal transmission of impulses. Dysrhythmias occur in about 90% of clients after MI.

2 Hypokalemia may result when clients are taking cardiac glycosides and diuretics; this is a complication associated with therapy, not a pathologic entity related to the MI itself. **3** Anaphylactic shock is caused by an allergic reaction, not by an MI. **4** Cardiac enlargement is a slow process, so it would not be evident in the coronary care unit.

Client Need: Physiological Adaptation; **Cognitive Level:** Analysis; **Nursing Process:** Assessment/Analysis; **Reference:** Ch 6, Coronary Artery Disease, Data Base

42. **4** The catheter is placed in the pulmonary artery. Information regarding left ventricular function is obtained when the catheter balloon is inflated.

1 Information on stroke volume, the amount of blood ejected by the left ventricle with each contraction, will not be provided by a pulmonary catheter. **2** Although a central venous pressure reading can be obtained with the pulmonary catheter, it is not as specific as a pulmonary wedge pressure, which reflects pressure in the left side of the heart. **3** The patency of the coronary arteries is usually evaluated by cardiac catheterization.

Client Need: Reduction of Risk Potential; **Cognitive Level:** Comprehension; **Integrated Process:** Teaching/Learning; **Nursing Process:** Planning/Implementation; **Reference:** Ch 6, Related Procedures, Hemodynamic Monitoring With Pulmonary Artery Catheter

43. **3** Troponin is released into the blood from cardiac muscle cells when the myocardium is damaged.

1 ALT identifies tissue destruction but it is more specific for liver injury. **2** APTT assesses blood clotting time. **4** Although potassium would be monitored, it is not diagnostic for MI.

Client Need: Reduction of Risk Potential; **Cognitive Level:** Analysis; **Nursing Process:** Assessment/Analysis; **Reference:** Ch 6, Coronary Artery Disease, Data Base

44. **3** Desired anticoagulant effect is achieved when the activated partial thromboplastin time is 1.5 to 2 times normal.

1 While anticoagulants help prevent thrombi that could block cerebral circulation, they do not increase cerebral perfusion so will not affect existing confusion. **2** Although absence of bleeding suggests that the drug has not reached toxic levels, it does not indicate its effectiveness. **4** This does not affect viscosity.

Client Need: Pharmacological and Parenteral Therapies; **Cognitive Level:** Application; **Nursing Process:** Evaluation/Outcomes; **Reference:** Ch 6, Anticoagulants

45. **2** The high vascularity of the nose, combined with its susceptibility to trauma (e.g., sneezing, nose blowing), makes it a frequent site of hemorrhage.

1, 3, 4 This adaptation usually is not associated with anticoagulant therapy.

Client Need: Pharmacological and Parenteral Therapies; **Cognitive Level:** Application; **Nursing Process:** Evaluation/Outcomes; **Reference:** Ch 6, Anticoagulants

46. **1** Coumadin is ordered day by day, based on the INR international normalized ratio of the client. This test provides a standard system to interpret prothrombin times.

2 APTT (accelerated partial thromboplastin time) is used to evaluate the effects of heparin, which acts on the intrinsic pathway. **3** Bleeding time is the time required for blood to cease flowing from a small wound; it is not used for warfarin (Coumadin)

dosage calculation. **4** Sedimentation rate is a test used to determine the presence of inflammation or infection; it does not indicate clotting ability.
Client Need: Reduction of Risk Potential; **Cognitive Level:** Analysis; **Nursing Process:** Evaluation/Outcomes;
Reference: Ch 6, Anticoagulants

47. **4** The client is up more at home, so dependent edema usually increases.
1 These should not be expected and are, in fact, signs of post-pericardotomy syndrome. **2** Serosanguineous drainage may persist after discharge. **3** These symptoms will persist longer.
Client Need: Physiological Adaptation; **Cognitive Level:** Application; **Integrated Process:** Teaching/Learning; **Nursing Process:** Planning/Implementation; **Reference:** Ch 6, Cardiac Surgery, Nursing Care

48. **1** Diuretic therapy that affects the loop of Henle generally involves the use of drugs (e.g., bumetanide [Bumex]) that directly or indirectly increase urinary sodium, chloride, and potassium excretion.
2 Sodium restriction does not necessarily accompany administration of bumetanide (Bumex). **3** Dyspnea does not directly result in a depletion of electrolytes. **4** Unless otherwise ordered, oral intake is unaffected.
Client Need: Pharmacological and Parenteral Therapies; **Cognitive Level:** Analysis; **Nursing Process:** Evaluation/Outcomes; **Reference:** Ch 6, Diuretics

49. **2** Shock may have different etiologies (e.g., hypovolemic, cardiogenic, septic, anaphylactic) but always involves a drop in BP and failure of the peripheral circulation because of sympathetic nervous system involvement. In cardiogenic shock, the failure of peripheral circulation is caused by an ineffective pump.
1 Shock can be reversed by the administration of fluids, plasma expanders, and vasoconstrictors. **3** It may be a reaction to tissue injury, but there are many different etiologies (e.g., hypovolemia, sepsis, anaphylaxis); it is not fleeting. **4** Hypovolemia is only one cause. Shock may also be septic, cardiogenic, or anaphylactic; it always involves a drop in BP.
Client Need: Physiological Adaptation; **Cognitive Level:** Comprehension; **Nursing Process:** Assessment/Analysis; **Reference:** Ch 6, Shock, Data Base

50. **4** This position is useful in treating shock because it promotes gravity-induced venous return. Warmth and fluids are also supportive to the person.
1 These are not methods used in the treatment of shock. Keeping the head of the bed elevated decreases cerebral perfusion. **2** This promotes venous pooling, which compounds shock. **3** While maintaining body temperature is important, heating pads are not indicated. They could cause burns or superficial vasodilation, which takes blood from vital organs.
Client Need: Physiological Adaptation; **Cognitive Level:** Analysis; **Nursing Process:** Planning/Implementation; **Reference:** Ch 6, Shock, Nursing Care

51. **4** In complete atrioventricular block, the ventricles take over the pacemaker function in the heart but at a much slower rate than that of the SA node. As a result there is decreased cerebral circulation, causing syncope.
1 This is not related to heart block unless decreased cerebral perfusion causes a brain attack. **2** The heart rate is usually slow because the ventricular rhythm is not initiated by the SA node. **3** This is not related to heart block.
Client Need: Physiological Adaptation; **Cognitive Level:** Application; **Nursing Process:** Assessment/Analysis; **Reference:** Ch 6, Related Procedures, Cardiac Monitoring

52. **3** Ventricular fibrillation will cause irreversible brain damage and then death within minutes because the heart is not pumping blood to the brain. Defibrillation or CPR until defibrillation is possible must be initiated immediately.
1, 2, 4 Although this condition requires prompt treatment, death is not as imminent as with ventricular fibrillation.
Client Need: Management of Care; **Cognitive Level:** Analysis; **Nursing Process:** Planning/Implementation; **Reference:** Ch 6, Related Procedures, Cardiac Monitoring

53. **1** Atropine blocks vagal stimulation of the SA node, resulting in an increased heart rate.
2 Digoxin (Lanoxin) slows the heart rate; hence it would not be indicated in this situation. **3** Lidocaine hydrochloride (Xylocaine) decreases myocardial sensitivity and would not increase heart rate. **4** Procainamide hydrochloride (Pronestyl) is an antidysrhythmic drug; it would not stimulate the heart rate.
Client Need: Pharmacological and Parenteral Therapies; **Cognitive Level:** Analysis; **Nursing Process:** Planning/Implementation; **Reference:** Ch 6, Cardiac Stimulants

54. **4** Bundle branch block interferes with the conduction of impulses from the AV node to the ventricle supplied by the affected bundle. Conduction through the ventricles is delayed, as evidenced by a widened QRS complex.
1, 3 Changes in the T waves and/or ST segments usually occur as a result of cardiac damage.
2 P waves, produced when the SA node fires to begin a cycle, are present in bundle branch block.
Client Need: Physiological Adaptation; **Cognitive Level:** Analysis; **Nursing Process:** Assessment/Analysis; **Reference:** Ch 6, Coronary Artery Disease, Data Base

55. **1** The SA node is the heart's natural pacemaker. An electronic pacemaker is used in some persons to supply an impulse that stimulates the heart to contract at a faster rate.
2 This normally receives impulses from the SA node and conducts them to the ventricular walls via the bundle of His and Purkinje's fibers. **3** This is special cardiac tissue that receives impulses from the AV node and conducts them to the ventricular walls. **4** Sympathetic fibers to the heart do not act as pacemakers to initiate and regulate the heartbeat.

Client Need: Physiological Adaptation; **Cognitive Level:** Knowledge; **Nursing Process:** Assessment/Analysis; **Reference:** Ch 6, Related Procedures, Cardiac Pacemaker Insertion

56. 3 Ventricular fibrillation reflects a rapid feeble twitching of the ventricles; it has an irregular saw-tooth configuration with unidentifiable PR intervals and QRS complexes.

1 Atrial flutter is characterized by an atrial rate of 250 to 350 beats/min and a ventricular rate of 60 to 150 beats/min; flutter to ventricular responses usually are 2:1, 3:1, or 4:1. 2 Atrial fibrillation is characterized by an atrial rate of 350 to 600 beats/min and a ventricular rate of 120 to 200 beats/min; the rhythm is grossly irregular. 4 Ventricular tachycardia has a rate of 140 to 200 beats/min; the rhythm is usually regular but may vary; P waves are unidentifiable; PR intervals are unmeasurable; QRS complexes are wide and bizarre.

Client Need: Physiological Adaptation; **Cognitive Level:** Analysis; **Nursing Process:** Assessment/Analysis; **Reference:** Ch 6, Related Procedures, Cardiac Monitoring

57. 3 Cardioversion involves administration of precordial shock, which is synchronized with the R wave to interrupt the heart rate. It is used for atrial fibrillation, paroxysmal atrial tachycardia (PAT), and ventricular tachycardia when pharmaceutical preparations fail. The heart is stopped by the electric stimulation, and it is hoped that the SA node will take over as pacemaker.

1, 2 Because there are no R waves, cardioversion would not be done. 4 Premature ventricular complexes suggest an irritable myocardium and generally respond well to antidysrhythmic agents.

Client Need: Physiological Adaptation; **Cognitive Level:** Analysis; **Integrated Process:** Teaching/Learning; **Nursing Process:** Planning/Implementation; **Reference:** Ch 6, Related Procedures, Cardioversion

58. 2 A permanent fixed (asynchronous) pacemaker is set at a predetermined rate; if a pulse rate is more or less than the preset rate, the pacemaker may be malfunctioning.

1 The client need not alter previous sleeping habits. 3 Regular activity may be resumed when healing has occurred. 4 This is the purpose of a pacemaker that provides on-demand pacing.

Client Need: Physiological Adaptation; **Cognitive Level:** Application; **Integrated Process:** Teaching/Learning; **Nursing Process:** Planning/Implementation; **Reference:** Ch 6, Related Procedures, Cardiac Pacemaker Insertion

59. 3 On-demand pacing initiates impulses when the client's pulse rate begins to fall below the preset rate. A rate below this indicates malfunction of the pacemaker.

1 The client's heart rate may still be irregular. 2 The client's heart rate may exceed the pacemaker. 4 The pacemaker affects the rate, not the volume of the pulse.

Client Need: Physiological Adaptation; **Cognitive Level:** Application; **Nursing Process:** Evaluation/Outcomes; **Reference:** Ch 6, Related Procedures, Cardiac Pacemaker Insertion

60. 2 Ventricular fibrillation is a lethal dysrhythmia and, once identified, must be terminated immediately by precordial shock (defibrillation) so the sinus node can again act as the heart's pacemaker. This is usually a standing physician's order in a coronary care unit.

1 O_2 is administered to correct hypoxia; it does not take priority over defibrillation. 3 CPR is instituted only when defibrillation fails to terminate the dysrhythmia. 4 Bicarbonate is administered to correct acidosis; it does not take priority over defibrillation.

Client Need: Physiological Adaptation; **Cognitive Level:** Application; **Nursing Process:** Planning/Implementation; **Reference:** Ch 6, Related Procedures, Cardiac Monitoring

61. 3 Amiodarone (Cardarone) decreases the irritability of the ventricles by prolonging the duration of the action potential and refractory period. It is used in the treatment of ventricular dysrhythmias.

1 Digoxin slows and strengthens ventricular contractions; it will not rapidly correct ectopic beats. 2 Furosemide (Lasix), a diuretic, does not affect ectopic foci. 4 Norepinephrine (Levophed) is a sympathomimetic and is not the drug of choice for ventricular irritability.

Client Need: Pharmacological and Parenteral Therapies; **Cognitive Level:** Analysis; **Nursing Process:** Planning/Implementation; **Reference:** Ch 6, Antidysrhythmics

62. 2 The precordial shock during cardioversion must not be delivered on the T wave or ventricular fibrillation may ensue. By placing the synchronizer in the "on" position, the machine is preset so that it will not deliver the shock on the T wave.

1 The energy level may be set from 50 to 400 W/sec. 3, 4 This will not ensure that the shock is not delivered on the T wave.

Client Need: Physiological Adaptation; **Cognitive Level:** Application; **Nursing Process:** Planning/Implementation; **Reference:** Ch 6, Related Procedures, Cardioversion

63. 1 Digoxin is used to treat atrial fibrillation, which is depicted in the strip.

2 This is a normal sinus rhythm; digoxin is not indicated. 3 This is ventricular tachycardia; digoxin is not indicated. 4 This is sinus bradycardia; digoxin is contraindicated.

Client Need: Physiological Adaptation; **Cognitive Level:** Analysis; **Nursing Process:** Assessment/Analysis; **Reference:** Ch 6, Related Procedures, Cardiac Monitoring

64. 2 Irreversible brain damage will occur if a client is anoxic for more than 4 minutes.

1 The age of the client does not affect the response by the arrest team. 3 The earlier heart rate is of minimal importance; the rhythm is more significant. 4 Although a variety of emergency medications must be available, their administration is ordered by the physician.

Client Need: Physiological Adaptation; **Cognitive Level:** Application; **Nursing Process:** Assessment/Analysis; **Reference:** Ch 6, Related Procedures, Cardiac Monitoring

65. **1** Additional help and a cardiac defibrillator must be obtained immediately.

2 The radial pulse is not used. **3** This would not be done until the airway was open, two breaths were given, and reassessment indicated that there was no carotid pulse. **4** Before cardiac compression, open the airway, pinch the nose, and give two, rather than four, full lung inflations; the client would be intubated and ventilated in the hospital setting.

Client Need: Physiological Adaptation; **Cognitive Level:** Application; **Nursing Process:** Planning/Implementation; **Reference:** Ch 6, Related Procedures, Basic Life Support (Cardiopulmonary Resuscitation [CPR]) by Health Care Providors

66. **3** The sternum must be depressed at least 3.7 to 5 cm (1½ to 2 inches) to compress the heart adequately between the sternum and vertebrae and to simulate cardiac pumping action.

1, 2, 4 This distance is ineffectual for an adult.

Client Need: Physiological Adaptation; **Cognitive Level:** Comprehension; **Nursing Process:** Planning/Implementation; **Reference:** Ch 6, Related Procedures, Basic Life Support (Cardiopulmonary Resuscitation [CPR]) by Health Care Providors

67. **4** This provides the best leverage for depressing the sternum. Thus the heart is adequately compressed, and blood is forced into the arteries. Grasping the fingers keeps them off the chest and concentrates the energy expended in the heel of the hand while minimizing the possibility of fracturing ribs.

1 Pressure spread over two hands may inadequately compress the heart and fracture the ribs. **2** Application of pressure by the fingers is less effective; this provides inadequate cardiac compression. **3** Both hands must be utilized; pressure on the lower portion of the sternum may fracture the xiphoid process, which can injure vital underlying organs.

Client Need: Physiological Adaptation; **Cognitive Level:** Application; **Nursing Process:** Planning/Implementation; **Reference:** Ch 6, Related Procedures, Basic Life Support

68. **3** Right ventricular heart failure causes increased pressure in the systemic venous system, which leads to a fluid shift into the interstitial spaces. Because of gravity, the lower extremities are first affected in an ambulatory client.

1 Pulmonary edema results in severe respiratory distress and peripheral edema. **2** Myocardial infarction itself does not cause peripheral edema. **4** Pulmonary disease would not result in varying degrees of edema.

Client Need: Physiological Adaptation; **Cognitive Level:** Analysis; **Nursing Process:** Assessment/Analysis; **Reference:** Ch 6, Heart Failure, Data Base

69. **2** Elevation of extremities promotes venous and lymphatic drainage by gravity.

1, 3 This is a dependent function of the nurse.
4 This procedure may have little effect on edema.

Client Need: Physiological Adaptation; **Cognitive Level:** Application; **Nursing Process:** Planning/Implementation; **Reference:** Ch 6, Heart Failure, Nursing Care

70. **1** Heart failure is the failure of the heart to pump adequately to meet the needs of the body, resulting in a backward buildup of pressure in the venous system. Adaptations by the body include edema, ascites, hepatomegaly, tachycardia, dyspnea, and fatigue.

2 These symptoms are generally not related to a specific disorder. **3** These symptoms might indicate coronary insufficiency or infarction. **4** These symptoms might indicate decreased fluid volume.

Client Need: Physiological Adaptation; **Cognitive Level:** Application; **Nursing Process:** Assessment/Analysis; **Reference:** Ch 6, Heart Failure, Data Base

71. **3** In right ventricular heart failure, blood backs up in the systemic capillary beds; the increase in plasma hydrostatic pressure shifts fluid from the intravascular compartment to the interstitial spaces, causing edema.

1 Increased fluid pressure in the intravascular compartment causes fluid to shift to the tissues; the tissue hydrostatic pressure does not decrease. **2** This would occur with crushing injuries or if proteins were pathologically shifting from the intravascular compartment to the interstitial spaces. **4** Although a decrease in colloid osmotic (oncotic) pressure can cause edema, it results from lack of protein intake, not increased hydrostatic pressure associated with right ventricular heart failure.

Client Need: Physiological Adaptation; **Cognitive Level:** Comprehension; **Nursing Process:** Assessment/Analysis; **Reference:** Ch 6, Heart Failure, Data Base

72. **3** Failure of the right ventricle causes an increase in pressure in the systemic circulation. To equalize this pressure, fluid moves into the tissues, causing edema, and into the abdominal cavity, causing ascites.

1 There is no loss of the cellular constituents in blood with right ventricular heart failure. **2** Ascites is the accumulation of fluid in an extracellular space, not intracellular. **4** The opposite results when there is a pressure increase in the systemic circulation.

Client Need: Physiological Adaptation; **Cognitive Level:** Comprehension; **Nursing Process:** Assessment/Analysis; **Reference:** Ch 6, Heart Failure, Data Base

73. **2** Aldactone is potassium-sparing, and therefore beverages and foods containing potassium should be limited to prevent hyperkalemia.

1 Red meat may need to be limited for other reasons not related to Aldactone. **3** Whole grains are associated with prevention of constipation and should not be avoided. **4** These foods are rich in sodium and calcium; Aldactone may cause hyponatremia.

Client Need: Pharmacological and Parenteral Therapies; **Cognitive Level:** Application; **Integrated Process:** Teaching/Learning; **Nursing Process:** Planning/Implementation; **Reference:** Ch 6, Diuretics

74. **3** Streptococcal infection can be spread through the circulation to the heart; endocarditis results and affects the valves of the heart.

1, 2, 4 This is not caused by beta-hemolytic streptococcus.

Client Need: Reduction of Risk Potential; **Cognitive Level:** Analysis; **Integrated Process:** Teaching/Learning; **Nursing Process:** Planning/Implementation; **Reference:** Ch 6, Inflammatory Diseases of the Heart, Data Base

75. 1 Irritability and restlessness associated with anxiety increase the metabolic rate, heart rate, and BP. This complicates heart failure.

2 Anxiety does not directly interfere with respirations; an increase in cardiac workload would increase respirations. 3 Anxiety can cause an increase in the amount of O_2 used and leads to an increased respiratory rate. 4 Anxiety alone usually does not elevate the body temperature.

Client Need: Physiological Adaptation; **Cognitive Level:** Comprehension; **Nursing Process:** Assessment/Analysis; **Reference:** Ch 6, Coronary Heart Disease, Nursing Care

76. 4 The orthopneic position allows maximum lung expansion because gravity reduces the pressure of the abdominal viscera on the diaphragm and lungs.

1 Elevation of the extremities should be avoided because it increases venous return, placing an increased workload on the heart. 2 Excessive coughing and mucus production is characteristic of pulmonary edema and does not need to be encouraged. 3 Positioning for postural drainage does not relieve acute dyspnea; furthermore, it increases venous return to the heart.

Client Need: Physiological Adaptation; **Cognitive Level:** Application; **Nursing Process:** Planning/Implementation; **Reference:** Ch 6, Heart Failure, Data Base

77. 2 Not adhering to the treatment regimen may interfere with effective resolution of the MI and further intervention is necessary.

1, 3, 4 This statement is an appropriate response related to teaching concerning self-care after an MI.

Client Need: Health Promotion and Maintenance; **Cognitive Level:** Analysis; **Integrated Process:** Teaching/Learning; **Nursing Process:** Evaluation/Outcomes; **Reference:** Ch 6, Coronary Artery Disease, Nursing Care

78. 2 These symptoms are associated with compromised arterial perfusion. A thrombus is a complication of a femoral arterial cardiac catheterization and must be suspected in the absence of a pedal pulse in the extremity below the entry site.

1 A circulatory assessment should be conducted first; the physician may or may not need to be notified immediately concerning the results of the assessment. 3 This is unnecessary; the symptoms indicate a local peripheral problem, not a systemic or cardiac problem. 4 These symptoms are not expected.

Client Need: Reduction of Risk Potential; **Cognitive Level:** Analysis; **Nursing Process:** Evaluation/Outcomes; **Reference:** Ch 6, Related Procedures, Cardiac Catheterization

79. 4 Because the femoral artery is large it has the potential for hematoma formation and hemorrhage after surgery.

1 The client should not be in pain after this procedure. 2 The ability to swallow is not affected

because conscious sedation, not general anesthesia, is used. 3 Although the leg used for circulatory access must be kept extended and immobile for several hours, this is not the priority.

Client Need: Reduction of Risk Potential; **Cognitive Level:** Analysis; **Nursing Process:** Evaluation/Outcomes; **Reference:** Ch 6, Related Procedures, Cardiac Catheterization

80. 4 Troponin T (cTnT) has an extraordinarily high specificity for myocardial cell injury. Cardiac troponins elevate sooner and remain elevated longer than many of the other enzymes that reflect myocardial injury.

1 ALT (alanine aminotransferase) is found predominantly in the liver; it is found in lesser quantities in the kidneys, heart, and skeletal muscles; it is used primarily to diagnose and monitor liver, not heart, disease. 2 AST (serum aspartate aminotransferase), also known as SGOT (serum glutamic-oxaloacetic transaminase), is elevated 8 hours after a myocardial infarction. 3 Total LDH (lactate dehydrogenase) levels elevate 24 to 48 hours after a myocardial infarction.

Client Need: Reduction of Risk Potential; **Cognitive Level:** Analysis; **Nursing Process:** Assessment/Analysis; **Reference:** Ch 6, Coronary Artery Disease, Data Base

81. 2 With heart failure the left ventricle is not functioning effectively, which is evidenced by an increased heart rate and crackles associated with pulmonary edema.

1 This is done after vital signs and breath sounds are obtained and the client is stabilized. 3 Although an infection would complicate heart failure, there are no signs that indicate this client has an infection. 4 This is inappropriate for immediate monitoring; it would be done after vital signs and clinical assessments have been completed.

Client Need: Reduction of Risk Potential; **Cognitive Level:** Application; **Nursing Process:** Assessment/Analysis; **Reference:** Ch 6, Heart Failure, Nursing Care

82. 4 Trauma to the artery can interfere with circulation to the accessed extremity. This is most easily assessed by checking the pulses bilaterally.

1 The client is prescribed bed rest after the procedure, so gait is not assessed. 2 The gag reflex is not affected by the test. 3 BP should not be taken in the affected arm; the increase in pressure may initiate bleeding.

Client Need: Reduction of Risk Potential; **Cognitive Level:** Application; **Nursing Process:** Evaluation/Outcomes; **Reference:** Ch 6, Related Procedures, Angiography

83. 2 Diabetes is twice as high a predictor of coronary heart disease in women than in men. Diabetes cancels the cardiac protection that estrogen provides premenopausal women.

1 This risk factor is common to both women and men. 3 An elevated C-reactive protein level, a marker of the inflammatory process, is heart-specific in predicting the likelihood of future coronary events in both women and men. 4 Low, not high, levels of

HDL-C (less than 35 mg/dL; a lipid factor) have a greater bearing on predicting CHD in women than in men.

Client Need: Health Promotion and Maintenance; **Cognitive Level:** Knowledge; **Integrated Process:** Teaching/Learning; **Nursing Process:** Planning/Implementation; **Reference:** Ch 6, Coronary Artery Disease, Data Base

84. 1 ☒ Obesity increases cardiac workload associated with vascular changes that lead to ischemia, which causes an MI.
2 ☒ Hypertension damages blood vessels and increases peripheral resistance and cardiac workload, which may lead to an MI.
3 ☐ LDL, not HDL, increases the risk for heart disease.
4 ☐ Diabetes mellitus, not insipidus, is a risk factor for an MI.
5 ☐ The risk is higher for African Americans.

Client Need: Health Promotion and Maintenance; **Cognitive Level:** Analysis; **Integrated Process:** Teaching/Learning; **Nursing Process:** Planning/Implementation; **Reference:** Ch 6, Coronary Artery Diseases, Data Base

85. 2 Although the balloon must be inflated to measure the capillary wedge pressure, leaving the balloon inflated will interfere with blood flow to the lung.
1 Bearing down will increase intrathoracic pressure and alter the reading. 3 Although a supine position is preferred, it is not essential. 4 Agency protocols relative to flushing of unused ports must be followed.

Client Need: Reduction of Risk Potential; **Cognitive Level:** Application; **Nursing Process:** Planning/Implementation; **Reference:** Ch 6, Related Procedures, Hemodynamic Monitoring With Pulmonary Artery Catheter

86. 1 ☒ The consistency of the RR interval indicates a regular rhythm.
2 ☒ A normal P wave before each complex indicates the impulse originated in the SA node.
3 ☐ Elevation of the ST segment is a sign of cardiac ischemia and is unrelated to the rhythm.
4 ☐ The number of complexes in a 6-second strip is multiplied by 10 to approximate the heart rate; normal sinus rhythm is 60 to 100 bpm.
5 ☐ The QRS duration should be less than 0.12 seconds; the PR interval should be 0.12 to 0.2 second.

Client Need: Reduction of Risk Potential; **Cognitive Level:** Analysis; **Nursing Process:** Assessment/Analysis; **Reference:** Ch 6, Related Procedures, Cardiac Monitoring

87. 4 Checking color and temperature, part of the neurovascular assessment, provides data about current perfusion of the extremity.
1 While pain assessment is essential, incisional pain does not provide data about the neurovascular status of the extremity. 2 While the presence and quality of the pedal pulse provide data about peripheral circulation, it is not necessary to count the rate. 3 Clients with peripheral arterial disease experience loss of extremity hair, which would not change suddenly because of surgery.

Client Need: Physiological Adaptation; **Cognitive Level:** Application; **Nursing Process:** Evaluation/Outcomes; **Reference:** Ch 6, Vascular Disease, Nursing Care

88. 1 ☒ Blood in the pericardial sac compresses the heart so the ventricles cannot fill; this leads to a rapid, thready pulse.
2 ☐ Tamponade causes hypotension and a narrowed pulse pressure.
3 ☒ As the tamponade increases, pressure on the heart interferes with the ejection of blood from the left ventricle, resulting in an increased pressure in the right side of the heart and the systemic circulation.
4 ☐ As the heart becomes more inefficient, there is a decrease in kidney perfusion and therefore urine output.
5 ☒ The increased venous pressure causes jugular vein distention.

Client Need: Physiological Adaptation; **Cognitive Level:** Analysis; **Nursing Process:** Evaluation/Outcomes; **Reference:** Ch 6, Cardiac Surgery, Nursing Care

89. 3 Iron is needed in the formation of hemoglobin.
1 The patient's anemia is caused by GI bleeding, not the process of RBC production. 2 Dextran is a plasma volume expander; it does not affect erythrocyte production. 4 Vitamin B_{12} is a water-soluble vitamin that must be used as a supplement when an individual has pernicious anemia.

Client Need: Pharmacological and Parenteral Therapies; **Cognitive Level:** Analysis; **Nursing Process:** Planning/Implementation; **Reference:** Ch 6, Anemias and Blood Disorders, Data Base

90. 4 In hypovolemic shock, tachycardia is a compensatory mechanism to try to increase blood flow to body organs.
1 Urine output would fall below 30 mL/hr because a decreased blood volume would cause a decreased glomerular filtration rate. 2 The BP is decreased because of the decreased blood volume. 3 This respiratory rate is within the accepted range of 12 to 20 breaths/min; the respiratory rate is rapid with hypovolemic shock.

Client Need: Physiological Adaptation; **Cognitive Level:** Application; **Nursing Process:** Assessment/Analysis; **Reference:** Ch 6, Shock, Data Base

91. 4 Baseline vital signs should be obtained immediately before administering the blood product for future comparison purposes. Two licensed nurses should confirm the verifying data between the client and the blood product. The nurse should remain with and monitor the client's vital signs during the first 15 minutes of administration of the blood product and then follow the institution's protocol to monitor for a transfusion reaction or fluid overload.
1 Vital signs must be taken immediately before the blood product infusion is begun for accurate future comparisons. 2 Blood should not be hung without following the appropriate protocol for ensuring

accuracy of the blood product for the client; the nurse should remain with and monitor the client's vital signs during the first 15 minutes of administration of the blood product to monitor for a transfusion reaction or fluid overload. **3** It is not necessary for the licensed nurse verifying the data between the client and the blood product to be a supervisor.
Client Need: Pharmacological and Parenteral Therapies; **Cognitive Level:** Analysis; **Integrated Process:** Communication/Documentation; **Nursing Process:** Planning/Implementation; **Reference:** Ch 6, Related Procedures, Blood Transfusion

92. **4** A slow rate provides time to recognize a transfusion reaction that is developing before too much blood has been administered.
1 Infusion pumps are not used routinely because the negative pressure exerted by the peristaltic or syringe-like cassette action of the device may cause RBC damage; infusion controllers that regulate flow by gravity may be used; accuracy of blood administration does not have to depend on the use of a pump. **2** Warming the blood to body temperature may cause clotting and hemolysis. **3** Blood samples may be drawn after, not before, a transfusion, but this is not routinely done.
Client Need: Pharmacological and Parenteral Therapies; **Cognitive Level:** Application; **Nursing Process:** Planning/Implementation; **Reference:** Ch 6, Related Procedures, Blood Transfusion

93. **2** Chills, headache, nausea, and vomiting are all signs of a transfusion reaction.
1 The infusion must be stopped before treatment of the symptoms begins. **3** The physician should be notified after the transfusion is stopped. **4** Slowing the infusion will continue the reaction; it may lead to kidney damage.
Client Need: Pharmacological and Parenteral Therapies; **Cognitive Level:** Application; **Nursing Process:** Planning/Implementation; **Reference:** Ch 6, Related Procedures, Blood Transfusion

94. Answer: 1000 mL.
Each bag of packed RBCs contains 250 mL for a total of 500 mL of packed RBCs. The total amount of sodium chloride received is 500 mL. 500 + 500 = 1000 mL of solution.
Client Need: Pharmacological and Parenteral Therapies; **Cognitive Level:** Application; **Integrated Process:** Communication/Documentation; **Nursing Process:** Planning/Implementation; **Reference:** Ch 6, Related Procedures, Blood Transfusion

95. **2** Massive amounts of clots formed in the microcirculation deplete platelets and clotting factors, leading to bleeding; the trauma of an injection may cause excessive bleeding.
1 This is associated with thrombophlebitis. **3** This could be traumatic and precipitate bleeding. **4** This is done to prevent thrombophlebitis.
Client Need: Reduction of Risk Potential; **Cognitive Level:** Application; **Nursing Process:** Planning/Implementation; **Reference:** Ch 6, Disseminated Intravascular Coagulation, Nursing Care

96. 1 ☒ Raisins are high in iron.
2 ☐ Although squash contains some iron, it is not the best source of iron.
3 ☐ Although carrots contain some iron, they are not the best source of iron.
4 ☒ Spinach is high in iron.
5 ☐ Although apricots contain some iron, they are not the best source of iron.
Client Need: Basic Care and Comfort; **Cognitive Level:** Analysis; **Integrated Process:** Teaching/Learning; **Nursing Process:** Planning/Implementation; **Reference:** Ch 6, Anemias and Blood Disorders, Nursing Care

97. **3** Viscosity, a measure of a fluid's internal resistance to flow, is increased as the number of red cells suspended in plasma increases.
1 The number of cells does not affect the blood pH. **2** The hematocrit would be higher. **4** RBCs do not affect immunity.
Client Need: Physiological Adaptation; **Cognitive Level:** Comprehension; **Nursing Process:** Assessment/Analysis; **Reference:** Ch 6, Review of Anatomy and Physiology, Blood

98. **2** Plasma proteins do not easily pass through the capillary endothelium. However, the leakage through the capillary endothelium is important and results in edema if not corrected (one of the lymphatic system's functions is to return "leaked" plasma proteins to the blood).
1 Blood gases (O_2 and CO_2) pass through capillary endothelium easily. **3** Glucose and ions pass through the capillary endothelium easily. **4** Amino acids and water pass through the capillary endothelium easily.
Client Need: Physiological Adaptation; **Cognitive Level:** Comprehension; **Nursing Process:** Assessment/Analysis; **Reference:** Ch 6, Review of Anatomy and Physiology, Lymphatic System

99. **2** Antibodies produced against group A beta-hemolytic streptococci sometimes interact with antigens in the heart's valves, causing damage and symptoms of rheumatic heart disease; early recognition and treatment of streptococcal infections has limited the occurrence of rheumatic heart disease.
1 Hepatitis A, an inflammation of the liver, is caused by the hepatitis A virus (HAV), not by bacteria. **3** The most common causes of meningitis, an infection of the membranes surrounding the brain and spinal cord, include *Streptococcus pneumoniae, Neisseria meningitides,* and *Haemophilus influenzae.* **4** This is thought to be an autoimmune disorder; it is not caused by microorganisms.
Client Need: Physiological Adaptation; **Cognitive Level:** Analysis; **Nursing Process:** Assessment/Analysis; **Reference:** Ch 6, Review of Microorganisms

100. **2** Although blood is screened for the antibodies, there is a period between the time a potential donor is infected and the time when antibodies are detectable; there is still a risk, but it is minimal.

1 There is no current method of destroying the virus in a blood transfusion. **3** The screening tests involve identification of the antibody, not the virus itself; the virus can be identified by the polymerase chain reaction test but is not part of routine screening. **4** Although many people consider autotransfusion for elective procedures, a trauma victim does not have this option.
Client Need: Pharmacological and Parenteral Therapies; **Cognitive Level:** Application; **Integrated Process:** Teaching/ Learning; **Nursing Process:** Planning/Implementation; **Reference:** Ch 6, Related Procedures, Blood Transfusion

101. **3** Brief pressure is generally enough to prevent bleeding.
1 No special positioning is required. **2** The site is cleansed before aspiration. **4** Frequent monitoring is unnecessary.
Client Need: Reduction of Risk Potential; **Cognitive Level:** Application; **Nursing Process:** Planning/Implementation; **Reference:** Ch 6, Related Procedures, Bone Marrow Aspiration

102. **3** Painless enlargement of the cervical lymph nodes is often the first sign of Hodgkin's disease, a malignant lymphoma of unknown etiology.
1 Axillary enlargement occurs after cervical. **2** Inguinal enlargement occurs later. **4** Mediastinal involvement follows after the disease progresses.
Client Need: Physiological Adaptation; **Cognitive Level:** Comprehension; **Nursing Process:** Assessment/Analysis; **Reference:** Ch 6, Lymphoma, Data Base

103. **3** For reasons unknown, Hodgkin's disease occurs most frequently between 15 and 30 years of age.
1 It is less common in children. **2** It is uncommon in later years. **4** It is uncommon during middle years.
Client Need: Physiological Adaptation; **Cognitive Level:** Knowledge; **Nursing Process:** Assessment/Analysis; **Reference:** Ch 6, Lymphoma, Data Base

104. **2** Radiation exposure may lead to depression of the bone marrow, with subsequent insufficient WBCs to combat infection.
1 There is no increase in the number of cells; therefore viscosity is not increased. **3** RBCs production is decreased by radiation. **4** Pathologic fractures may occur in response to disease, not treatment.
Client Need: Physiological Adaptation; **Cognitive Level:** Analysis; **Nursing Process:** Evaluation/Outcomes; **Reference:** Ch 6, Lymphoma, Data Base

105. **1** Platelets (thrombocytes) adhere to the intima of damaged vessels within seconds after injury, releasing substances that promote hemostasis.
2 Leukocytes play no role in clotting; they protect the body against microorganisms. **3** Erythrocytes are RBCs; they carry O_2 and play no role in coagulation. **4** RBCs play no role in clotting; they carry O_2 to all body cells.
Client Need: Physiological Adaptation; **Cognitive Level:** Comprehension; **Nursing Process:** Assessment/Analysis; **Reference:** Ch 6, Review of Anatomy and Physiology, Blood

106. **3** Thromboplastin is a substance released by platelets that initiates the clotting process by converting prothrombin to thrombin.
1 Bile does not contain thromboplastin. **2** Plasma does not produce thromboplastin. **4** RBCs do not produce thromboplastin.
Client Need: Physiological Adaptation; **Cognitive Level:** Comprehension; **Nursing Process:** Assessment/Analysis; **Reference:** Ch 6, Review of Anatomy and Physiology, Blood

107. **3** Fibrinogen is a soluble plasma protein that becomes the insoluble gel fibrin during the clotting process.
1 Fibrin is the insoluble gel formed from fibrinogen by the action of thrombin. **2** Thrombin is needed to convert fibrinogen to fibrin; it is also needed in platelet aggregation. **4** Prothrombin is the precursor of thrombin.
Client Need: Physiological Adaptation; **Cognitive Level:** Comprehension; **Nursing Process:** Evaluation/Outcomes; **Reference:** Ch 6, Review of Anatomy and Physiology, Blood

108. **3** Calcium acts as a catalyst to convert prothrombin to thrombin. Thrombin accelerates the formation of insoluble fibrin from the soluble fibrinogen.
1 Fluorine is a gas of the halogen group and is not involved in clotting; sodium fluoride helps harden tooth enamel. **2** Chloride is an extracellular anion that helps regulate osmotic pressure and combines with hydrogen to form hydrochloric acid; it is not involved with clotting. **4** Iron is essential for synthesis of hemoglobin; it is not involved in clotting.
Client Need: Physiological Adaptation; **Cognitive Level:** Comprehension; **Nursing Process:** Assessment/Analysis; **Reference:** Ch 6, Review of Anatomy and Physiology, Blood

109. **4** Vitamin K, synthesized by the bacterial flora of the intestine, promotes the liver's synthesis of prothrombin, an important blood clotting factor.
1, 3 This is not promoted by vitamin K. **2** Vitamin K does not affect calcium ionization.
Client Need: Physiological Adaptation; **Cognitive Level:** Comprehension; **Integrated Process:** Teaching/Learning; **Nursing Process:** Planning/Implementation; **Reference:** Ch 6, Review of Anatomy and Physiology, Blood

110. **2** Polycythemia vera results in pathologically high concentrations of erythrocytes in the blood; increased viscosity promotes thrombosis formation.
1 Hypertension is usually related to narrowing or sclerosing of arteries, not to increased number of blood cells. **3** The fragility of blood cells does not affect the viscosity of the blood. **4** Erythrocyte immaturity is not related to increased viscosity.
Client Need: Physiological Adaptation; **Cognitive Level:** Application; **Integrated Process:** Teaching/Learning; **Nursing Process:** Planning/Implementation; **Reference:** Ch 6, Anemias and Blood Disorders, Data Base

111. **1** An elevated plasma bilirubin level could indicate an increased rate of RBCs destruction (bilirubin is a product of free hemoglobin metabolism); the individual may have a hemolytic anemia (e.g., thalassemia major [Cooley's anemia], glucose-6-phosphate dehydrogenase deficiency). **2** This does not involve the destruction of red blood cells with subsequent liberation of bilirubin. **3** A decreased amount of bile pigment would be liberated. **4** O_2-carrying ability is reflected by hemoglobin level.
Client Need: Physiological Adaptation; **Cognitive Level:** Analysis; **Nursing Process:** Assessment/Analysis; **Reference:** Ch 6, Anemias and Blood Disorders, Data Base

112. **1** Because of its great blood supply and general fragility, the spleen, when ruptured, must be removed to prevent possible hemorrhage, septicemia, or peritonitis. **2** Rupturing of the spleen does not cause liver disease; it may cause hemorrhage, septicemia, or peritonitis. **3, 4** This is not the reason for performing a splenectomy.
Client Need: Physiological Adaptation; **Cognitive Level:** Application; **Nursing Process:** Assessment/Analysis; **Reference:** Ch 6, Review of Anatomy and Physiology, Lymphatic System

113. **4** Because the spleen has such vascularity, hemorrhage may occur and result in abdominal distention. **1** Although an elevated temperature is common, it is usually not the result of infection; the incidence of infection is not higher after a splenectomy, except in children, and it would not occur in the immediate postoperative period. **2, 3** The incidence of this is not higher than for other abdominal surgery.
Client Need: Physiological Adaptation; **Cognitive Level:** Application; **Nursing Process:** Evaluation/Outcomes; **Reference:** Ch 6, Anemias and Blood Disorders, Nursing Care

114. **3** Postoperative pain will cause splinting, shallow breathing, and underaeration of the lung's left lower lobe because of close proximity of the spleen to the diaphragm. **1, 2, 4** This is not specific to a splenectomy.
Client Need: Physiological Adaptation; **Cognitive Level:** Application; **Nursing Process:** Planning/Implementation; **Reference:** Ch 6, Anemias and Blood Disorders, Nursing Care

115. **2** Because of the location of the spleen, expansion of the thoracic cavity during inspiration causes pain at the operative site. **1** The presence of crackles indicates accumulation of secretions, which is not the expected outcome; the nursing care is designed to prevent this complication. **3** Because limited activity decreases oxygen consumption, shortness of breath is not a common complaint. **4** This is not to be expected; accumulation of secretions can be avoided by coughing and deep breathing.
Client Need: Physiological Adaptation; **Cognitive Level:** Application; **Nursing Process:** Evaluation/Outcomes; **Reference:** Ch 6, Anemias and Blood Disorders, Nursing Care

116. **1** ☒ Because of its great blood supply and general fragility, the spleen may hemorrhage, causing shock. **2** ☐ The immediate postoperative period is too soon for the client to exhibit signs of infection. **3** ☐ An intestinal obstruction would not occur with a splenectomy. **4** ☒ Because of its great blood supply and general fragility, the spleen may hemorrhage, causing abdominal distention. **5** ☒ Pulmonary complications may occur because the spleen is close to the diaphragm; pulmonary complications may develop because of defensive shallow breathing.
Client Need: Physiological Adaptation: **Cognitive Level:** Application; **Nursing Process:** Evaluation/Outcomes; **Reference:** Ch 6, Anemias and Blood Disorders, Nursing Care

117. **2** This is high in iron, which is necessary to produce red blood cells. **1, 3, 4** Although iron is contained in this food, it is not the best source of iron.
Client Need: Basic Care and Comfort; **Cognitive Level:** Analysis; **Integrated Process:** Teaching/Learning; **Nursing Process:** Planning/Implementation; **Reference:** Ch 6, Anemias and Blood Disorders, Nursing Care

118. **2** When the spleen ruptures, internal loss of blood may be profound, resulting in shock. **1** The nurse can assess hyperventilation if the client's breathing patterns are observed. **3** Although anxiety can cause hyperventilation, resulting in lightheadedness, the data do not indicate that the client is anxious. **4** These symptoms are not inclusive enough to indicate infection.
Client Need: Physiological Adaptation; **Cognitive Level:** Application; **Nursing Process:** Assessment/Analysis; **Reference:** Ch 6, Anemias and Blood Disorders, Nursing Care

RESPIRATORY SYSTEM

119. **4** The respiratory center in the medulla responds primarily to increased carbon dioxide concentration in the blood. **1** O_2 is normally not the primary stimulus to breathing; it functions as a primary stimulus in individuals who have chronic hypercapnia. **2** Lactic acid is not a stimulant; it is a byproduct of muscular activity. **3** Calcium ions are not stimulants for respiration; they are involved in transmission of neural impulses.
Client Need: Physiological Adaptation: **Cognitive Level:** Comprehension; **Nursing Process:** Assessment/Analysis; **Reference:** Ch 7, Review of Anatomy and Physiology, Physiology of Respiration

120. **2** The residual volume is the amount of air remaining in the lungs after maximum exhalation. **1, 3, 4** This is normally under the individual's control. The force exerted by the abdominal thrust

surpasses that which the individual is voluntarily capable of exerting.
Client Need: Physiological Adaptation; **Cognitive Level:** Comprehension; **Nursing Process:** Planning/Implementation; **Reference:** Ch 7, Related Procedures, Abdominal Thrust

121. 2 Tidal volume (TV) is defined as the amount of air exhaled after a normal inspiration.
1 This is the expiratory reserve volume (ERV).
3 The volume of air that can be forcibly inspired over and above a normal inspiration is the inspiratory reserve volume (IRV). 4 This is the residual volume (RV).
Client Need: Physiological Adaptation; **Cognitive Level:** Knowledge; **Integrated Process:** Teaching/Learning; **Nursing Process:** Assessment/Analysis; **Reference:** Ch 7, Review of Anatomy and Physiology, Physiology of Respiration

122. 4 As the diaphragm descends during inspiration, thoracic pressure is reduced because thoracic volume is increased. The pressure of the atmospheric air is higher in comparison, so air will rush into the alveoli.
1, 3 Rising pressure in the alveoli and the intrapleural space caused by relaxation of the diaphragm expels air from the alveoli. 2 Contraction of the diaphragm causes decreased pressure, leading to inspiration.
Client Need: Physiological Adaptation; **Cognitive Level:** Comprehension; **Integrated Process:** Teaching/Learning; **Nursing Process:** Assessment/Analysis; **Reference:** Ch 7, Review of Anatomy and Physiology, Physiology of Respiration

123. 1 The tidal volume is the amount of air inhaled and exhaled while breathing normally.
2 This is air that can be forcibly expired after maximum inspiration. 3 This is the maximum amount of air that can be expired after a normal expiration. 4 This is the maximum amount of air that can be inspired after a normal inspiration.
Client Need: Physiological Adaptation; **Cognitive Level:** Application; **Integrated Process:** Teaching/Learning; **Nursing Process:** Assessment/Analysis; **Reference:** Ch 7, Review of Anatomy and Physiology, Physiology of Respiration

124. 3 The lower the P_{O_2} and the higher the P_{CO_2}, the more rapidly O_2 dissociates from the oxyhemoglobin molecule.
1 The pH would be decreased with an increase in CO_2 pressure. 2 It must be associated with a decrease in O_2 pressure. 4 O_2 dissociation would be decreased in this situation.
Client Need: Reduction of Risk Potential; **Cognitive Level:** Analysis; **Nursing Process:** Assessment/Analysis; **Reference:** Ch 7, Review of Anatomy and Physiology, Physiology of Respiration

125. 3 The negative pressure from suctioning removes O_2 as well as secretions; suction should be applied only after the catheter is inserted, and it is being withdrawn.
1 Lubrication will facilitate insertion and minimize trauma; it will not prevent hypoxia. 2 The use of a sterile catheter helps prevent infection, not hypoxia. 4 This is too long; suctioning should be limited to 10 seconds.

Client Need: Physiological Adaptation; **Cognitive Level:** Application; **Nursing Process:** Planning/Implementation; **Reference:** Ch 7, Related Procedures, Suctioning of Airway

126. 2 The orthopneic position is a sitting position that permits maximum lung expansion for gaseous exchange; it also enables the client to press the lower chest or abdomen against the overbed table, which increases pressure on the diaphragm to help with exhalation, reducing residual volume.
1 This position does not permit the diaphragm to descend by gravity, and pressure of the abdominal organs against the diaphragm limits its movement.
3, 4 This position does not maximize lung expansion to the same degree as the orthopneic position.
Client Need: Physiological Adaptation; **Cognitive Level:** Application; **Nursing Process:** Planning/Implementation; **Reference:** Ch 7, Review of Anatomy and Physiology, Physiology of Respiration

127. 2 Because atelectasis involves collapsing of alveoli distal to the bronchioles, breath sounds would be diminished in the lower lobes.
1 A client would have rapid, shallow respirations to compensate for poor gas exchange. 3 Atelectasis results in a loose, productive cough. 4 Atelectasis results in an elevated temperature.
Client Need: Physiological Adaptation; **Cognitive Level:** Application; **Nursing Process:** Assessment/Analysis; **Reference:** Ch 7, Review of Anatomy and Physiology, Physiology of Respiration

128. 4 Carbon monoxide binds with hemoglobin more avidly than does oxygen. The progressive results are dyspnea, asphyxia, and death.
1 Carbon monoxide does not block CO_2 transport; it binds with hemoglobin. 2 Carbon monoxide inhibits O_2 transport, not vasodilation. 3 Carbon monoxide does not form bubbles in the blood plasma; bubbles in tissues are caused by increased nitrogen, as in decompression sickness.
Client Need: Physiological Adaptation; **Cognitive Level:** Comprehension; **Nursing Process:** Assessment/Analysis; **Reference:** Ch 7, Carbon Monoxide Poisoning, Data Base

129. 1 Air rises and is removed via a tube inserted in the upper intrapleural space.
2 This is accomplished by the tube placed at the base of the lung; fluid flows toward the base via gravity. 3 Medication will not be instilled into the intrapleural space in this situation. 4 This would cause, not prevent, a pneumothorax.
Client Need: Physiological Adaptation; **Cognitive Level:** Comprehension; **Nursing Process:** Planning/Implementation; **Reference:** Ch 7, Related Procedures, Chest Tubes

130. 3 Subcutaneous emphysema occurs when air leaks from the intrapleural space through the thoracotomy or around the chest tubes into the soft tissue; crepitus is the crackling sound heard when tissues containing gas are palpated.
1 This is related to prolonged trapping of air in the alveoli associated with emphysema, a chronic obstructive pulmonary disease. 2 Unnecessary to determine crepitus; crackles and rhonchi occur

within the lung; subcutaneous emphysema occurs in the soft tissues. **4** This is unrelated to subcutaneous emphysema, which involves gas in the soft tissues from a pleural leak.
Client Need: Physiological Adaptation; **Cognitive Level:** Application; **Nursing Process:** Planning/Implementation; **Reference:** Ch 7, Related Procedures, Chest Tubes

131. **3** Once the drainage tube is patent, the fluctuation in the water column will resume; a lack of fluctuation because of lung reexpansion is unlikely 36 hours after a traumatic open chest injury.
1 Unnecessary at this time; the chest tube is occluded and nursing intervention should be attempted first. **2** This may be done eventually, but this is not the priority at this time. **4** This would compromise aeration of the unaffected lung.
Client Need: Physiological Adaptation; **Cognitive Level:** Analysis; **Nursing Process:** Planning/Implementation; **Reference:** Ch 7, Related Procedures, Chest Tubes

132. **3** This is one method for the client to communicate after a laryngectomy; speech is produced by expelling swallowed air across constricted tissue in the pharyngoesophageal segment.
1 This is used for individuals who wish to communicate with someone who is deaf. **2** Although this may be an adjunct to verbal speech, it should not be the primary means of communication. **4** This would not allow for the spontaneous communication possible with a tracheoesophageal puncture, esophageal speech, or an electrolarynx.
Client Need: Reduction of Risk Potential; **Cognitive Level:** Application; **Integrated Process:** Teaching/Learning; **Nursing Process:** Planning/Implementation; **Reference:** Ch 7, Cancer of the Larynx, Nursing Care

133. **3** Water sports pose a severe threat; should water enter the stoma, the client will drown.
1 This is not harmful; as long as there is no obstruction, adequate O_2 will be available because the respiratory rate will increase. **2** Pillows are not contraindicated, although care should be taken not to occlude the airway by any bedding while asleep. **4** Humidity is desirable and helpful in keeping secretions liquefied.
Client Need: Reduction of Risk Potential; **Cognitive Level:** Application; **Integrated Process:** Teaching/Learning; **Nursing Process:** Evaluation/Outcomes; **Reference:** Ch 7, Cancer of the Larynx, Nursing Care

134. **2** Fluids will replace fluid loss from fever and decrease viscosity of secretions.
1 Capillary refill relates to peripheral tissue perfusion. **3** There are no data to suggest that secretions are blocking the airway; there is no support that suctioning is needed. **4** High concentrations of O_2 are generally not administered to clients with COPD; traditionally the reason given for this was clients with COPD become desensitized to CO_2 as a respiratory stimulus so that reduced O_2 levels act as the stimulus and high concentrations of O_2 would actually depress respirations. The newer

theory suggests that the hypoxic drive is valid for a small number; the majority of cases involve the Haldane effect: as hemoglobin molecules become more saturated with O_2, they are unable to transport CO_2 out of the body, leading to hypercapnia.
Client Need: Physiological Adaptation; **Cognitive Level:** Application; **Nursing Process:** Planning/Implementation; **Reference:** Ch 7, Obstructive Airway Disease, Nursing Care

135. **4** Streptococcal organisms are present on the skin, in the mucous membranes, and in the environment at all times. The most frequent portals of entry are the respiratory tract and breaks in the skin; once in the body, the organisms can be transmitted to the heart and kidneys via the circulation.
1 All are caused by streptococci. **2** Vaccinations are not available for most of these conditions; there is an antitoxin for scarlet fever, but antibiotics are now used. **3** Bacteria are not classified as parasites.
Client Need: Safety and Infection Control; **Cognitive Level:** Analysis; **Nursing Process:** Assessment/Analysis; **Reference:** Ch 7, Review of Microorganisms

136. **1** Furosemide (Lasix) acts on the loop of Henle by increasing the excretion of chloride and sodium.
2, 3 Although used in the treatment of edema and hypertension, this drug is not as potent as furosemide. **4** This is a potassium-sparing diuretic; it is less potent than thiazide diuretics.
Client Need: Pharmacological and Parenteral Therapies; **Cognitive Level:** Analysis; **Nursing Process:** Planning/Implementation; **Reference:** Ch 7, Pulmonary Edema, Data Base

137. **3** Coughing is needed to raise secretions for expectoration.
1 Oxygen will not mobilize the secretions. **2** A sitting position will allow secretions to remain in the lungs unless coughing is encouraged. **4** Rest should be encouraged only after coughing to bring up secretions mobilized by postural drainage.
Client Need: Physiological Adaptation: **Cognitive Level:** Application; **Nursing Process:** Planning/Implementation; **Reference:** Ch 7, Related Procedures, Chest Physiotherapy

138. **3** The etiology of a spontaneous pneumothorax is commonly the rupture of blebs on the lung surface. Blebs are similar to blisters, but are filled with air.
1 Pleural friction rub would result in pain on inspiration, not a pneumothorax. **2** A tracheoesophageal fistula would cause aspiration of food and saliva, resulting in respiratory distress. **4** The client had no history of trauma.
Client Need: Physiological Adaptation; **Cognitive Level:** Comprehension; **Integrated Process:** Teaching/Learning; **Nursing Process:** Assessment/Analysis; **Reference:** Ch 7, Pneumothorax, Data Base

139. **1** Retention of CO_2, after exhausting the available bicarbonate ions functioning as buffers, will cause a lower pH (respiratory acidosis).
2 Tissue necrosis results from localized tissue anoxia and will not cause the systemic response of

respiratory acidosis. **3** Increased respiratory rate may lead to respiratory alkalosis. **4** Normal O_2 saturation of hemoglobin is 95% to 100%, so this is not a sign of acidosis.
Client Need: Physiological Adaptation; **Cognitive Level:** Comprehension; **Nursing Process:** Assessment/Analysis; **Reference:** Ch 7, Obstructive Airway Disease, Data Base

140. **3** O_2 is supplied to prevent anoxia, but not in high concentrations. In an individual with emphysema a low Po_2, not high Pco_2, is often considered the respiratory stimulus. Another reason is the Haldane effect: as hemoglobin molecules become more saturated with high concentrations of O_2, they are unable to transport CO_2 out of the body, leading to hypercapnia.

1 This concentration is too high for a client with emphysema because it precipitates CO_2 narcosis. **2** This might increase the risk for mediastinal shift and interfere with expansion of the unaffected lung. **4** This dependent action would require orders as to specific electrolytes.
Client Need: Reduction of Risk Potential; **Cognitive Level:** Application; **Nursing Process:** Planning/Implementation; **Reference:** Ch 7, Obstructive Airway Disease, Data Base

141. **3** As a person with a tear in the lung inhales, air moves through that opening into the intrapleural space. This creates a positive pressure and causes partial or complete collapse of the lung.

1 Mediastinal shift occurs toward the unaffected side. **2** This is normal; with a peumothorax there is a loss of intrathoracic negative pressure. **4** This is not an impending problem.
Client Need: Physiological Adaptation; **Cognitive Level:** Analysis; **Integrated Process:** Teaching/Learning; **Nursing Process:** Assessment/Analysis; **Reference:** Ch 7, Pneumothorax, Data Base

142. **2** Sudden chest pain occurs on the affected side; it may also involve the arm and shoulder.

1 Bloody vomitus is unrelated to pneumothorax. **3** Decreased chest motion occurs because of failure to inflate the involved lung. **4** The shift toward the unaffected side results from pressure from the pneumothorax.
Client Need: Physiological Adaptation; **Cognitive Level:** Application; **Nursing Process:** Assessment/Analysis; **Reference:** Ch 7, Pneumothorax, Data Base

143. **3** The water seal chamber acts as a one-way valve to allow air from the pleural space to escape into the suction chamber but prevent a backflow of air from within the system to the client.

1 This chamber provides suction control. **2, 4** This chamber collects drainage from the client.
Client Need: Physiological Adaptation; **Cognitive Level:** Application; **Nursing Process:** Assessment/Analysis; **Reference:** Ch 7, Related Procedures, Chest Tubes

144. **3** Destruction of the alveolar walls leads to diminished surface area for gaseous exchange and an increased CO_2 level in the blood.

1 Pleural effusion occurs when there is seepage of fluid into the intrapleural space; this does not occur with emphysema. **2** Infectious obstructions occur in conditions in which microorganisms invade lung tissue; emphysema is not an infectious disease. **4** Muscle paralysis may occur in diseases affecting the neurologic system; emphysema does not affect the neurologic system; therefore it is not a neurologic disease.
Client Need: Physiological Adaptation; **Cognitive Level:** Comprehension; **Nursing Process:** Assessment/Analysis; **Reference:** Ch 7, Obstructive Airway Disease, Data Base

145. **4** Some clients with COPD (chronic obstructive pulmonary disease) respond only to the chemical stimulus of low O_2 levels. Administration of high concentrations of O_2 to these individuals will eliminate the stimulus to breathe, leading to decreased respirations and lethargy. Clients with COPD experience the Haldane effect: as hemoglobin molecules become more saturated with O_2, they are unable to transport CO_2 out of the body, leading to hypercapnia. The increased levels of CO_2 depress the CNS.

1 Cyanosis is caused by excessive amounts of reduced oxyhemoglobin; because O_2 is being administered, cyanosis may be reduced. **2** Rising CO_2 levels cause lethargy rather than anxiety. **3** High concentrations of O_2 may eliminate the stimulus to breathe, so the respiratory rate would decrease.
Client Need: Physiological Adaptation; **Cognitive Level:** Application; **Nursing Process:** Assessment/Analysis; **Reference:** Ch 7, Obstructive Airway Disease, Data Base

146. **1** Loss of elasticity causes difficult exhalation, with subsequent air trapping. Clients who have emphysema are taught to use accessory abdominal muscles and to breathe out through pursed lips to help keep the air passages open until exhalation is complete.

2 Expiration is difficult because of air trapping and poor elasticity. **3** There will be decreased vital capacity. **4** Diaphragmatic breathing is a learned mechanism that is beneficial.
Client Need: Physiological Adaptation: **Cognitive Level:** Application; **Integrated Process:** Teaching/Learning; **Nursing Process:** Planning/Implementation; **Reference:** Ch 7, Obstructive Airway Disease, Nursing Care

147. **2** These drugs cause increased heart contraction (positive inotropic effect) and increased heart rate (positive chronotropic effect). If toxic levels are reached, side effects occur and the drug should be withheld until the physician is notified.

1 This is false reassurance and a false statement. **3, 4** Controlled breathing may be helpful in allaying a client's anxiety; however, the drug may be producing side effects and should be withheld.
Client Need: Pharmacology and Parenteral Therapies; **Cognitive Level:** Analysis; **Integrated Process:** Communication/Documentation; **Nursing Process:** Planning/Implementation; **Reference:** Ch 7, Bronchodilators and Antiasthmatics

148. **2** Clients with asthma use metered-dose inhalers to administer medications prophylactically and/or during times of an asthma attack; this is an important skill to have before discharge.

1 Pulse oximetry is rarely conducted in the home; home management usually includes self-monitoring of peak expiratory flow rate. **3** Although this is important, it is not the priority; during a persistent asthma attack that does not respond to planned interventions, the client should go to the emergency department of the local hospital or call 911 for assistance. **4** Not all asthma is Associated with food allergies.

Client Need: Pharmacological and Parenteral Therapies; **Cognitive Level:** Application; **Nursing Process:** Planning/Implementation; **Reference:** Ch 7, Bronchodilators and Antiasthmatics

149. **1** Hypersecretion of the mucous glands provides an excellent warm, moist medium for microorganisms.

2 Asthma is not a disease that is voluntarily controlled. **3** Coughing must be encouraged; it prevents retention of mucus, which is an excellent medium for microorganisms. Excessive secretions also limit gaseous exchange. **4** The anesthesiologist will make recommendations about the type of anesthesia best suited for the client and the surgical procedure.

Client Need: Reduction of Risk Potential; **Cognitive Level:** Application; **Integrated Process:** Teaching/Learning; **Nursing Process:** Planning/Implementation; **Reference:** Ch 7, Obstructive Airway Disease, Nursing Care

150. **3** A peak flow meter measures the peak expiratory flow rate, the maximum flow of air that can be forcefully exhaled in 1 second; this monitors the pulmonary status of a client with asthma.

1 The peak flow measurement should be done daily in the morning before the administration of medication or when experiencing dyspnea. **2** The client should be standing or sitting straight. **4** This would interfere with an accurate test; the mouthpiece should be in the mouth between the teeth with the lips creating a seal around the mouthpiece.

Client Need: Reduction of Risk Potential; **Cognitive Level:** Application; **Integrated Process:** Teaching/Learning; **Nursing Process:** Planning/Implementation; **Reference:** Ch 7, Obstructive Airway Disease, Nursing Care

151. **3** Pressure within the pleural cavity causes a shift of the heart and great vessels to the unaffected side. This not only decreases the capacity of the unaffected lung but also impedes the filling of the right side of the heart and leads to a decreased cardiac output.

1 This complication might occur in severe chest trauma, not in mediastinal shift. **2** Infection is not caused by a mediastinal shift. **4** The volume of the unaffected lung may decrease because of pressure from the shift.

Client Need: Physiological Adaptation; **Cognitive Level:** Analysis; **Nursing Process:** Assessment/Analysis; **Reference:** Ch 7, Pneumothorax, Data Base

152. **2** Fluctuations occur with normal inspiration and expiration until the lung is fully expanded. If these fluctuations do not occur, the chest tube may be clogged or kinked; coughing should be encouraged.

1 The binder does not prevent tension on the tube; it would be contraindicated, because it limits thoracic expansion. **3** The client may not be agitated; morphine depresses respirations and is usually avoided. **4** The tube should be clamped only if ordered or if an air leak is suspected.

Client Need: Physiological Adaptation; **Cognitive Level:** Analysis; **Nursing Process:** Planning/Implementation; **Reference:** Ch 7, Related Procedures, Chest Tubes

153. **2** Leakage of air into the subcutaneous tissue is evidenced by a crackling sound when the area is gently palpated. This is referred to as crepitus.

1 Although hemostats should be readily available for any client with chest tubes in the event of a break in the drainage system, clamping the tube would not be otherwise necessary and could cause backpressure. **3** To minimize the risk for pneumothorax, the dressing is not routinely changed. **4** The system is kept closed to prevent the pressure of the atmosphere from causing a pneumothorax; drainage levels are marked on the drainage chamber to measure output. The chambers are not emptied; if they are filled, a new system will be attached.

Client Need: Physiological Adaptation; **Cognitive Level:** Analysis; **Nursing Process:** Planning/Implementation; **Reference:** Ch 7, Related Procedures, Chest Tubes

154. **1** Clients who have had joint replacement have decreased mobility; they are at risk for developing thrombophlebitis, which may lead to pulmonary embolism if the clot becomes dislodged into the circulation.

2 This leads to a decreased ability to clot so it may increase the risk of bleeding, but decrease the risk of a thrombus or embolus. **3, 4** This is not associated with an increased risk for pulmonary embolism.

Client Need: Reduction of Risk Potential; **Cognitive Level:** Analysis; **Nursing Process:** Planning/Implementation; **Reference:** Ch 7, Pulmonary Embolism and Infarction, Data Base

155. **3** Oral intake should not be attempted until return of the gag reflex because the client could aspirate.

1, 4 This is not a correct statement; there are additional factors that must be considered. **2** Although some slight irritation may occur following this test, there are usually no painful sequelae; oral intake would not be withheld because of painful swallowing, although the consistency of food may be changed.

Client Need: Reduction of Risk Potential; **Cognitive Level:** Application; **Integrated Process:** Teaching/Learning; **Nursing Process:** Evaluation/Outcomes; **Reference:** Ch 7, Related Procedures, Bronchoscopy

156. 3 With the head elevated, rather than horizontal or dependent, fluid will not collect in the interstitial spaces around the trachea.

1, 2, 4 This may cause aspiration if the gag reflex has not returned.

Client Need: Reduction of Risk Potential; **Cognitive Level:** Application; **Nursing Process:** Planning/Implementation; **Reference:** Ch 7, Related Procedures, Bronchoscopy

157. 3 Cancerous lesions in the pleural space increase the osmotic pressure, causing a shift of fluid to that space.

1 Excessive intake is usually balanced by increased urine output. **2** Inadequate chest expansion results from pleural effusion and is not the cause of it. **4** A bronchoscopy does not involve the pleural space.

Client Need: Physiological Adaptation; **Cognitive Level:** Analysis; **Nursing Process:** Assessment/Analysis; **Reference:** Ch 7, Malignant Lung Tumors, Data Base

158. 3 Cavities are evident on radiograph. Necrotic lung tissue may liquefy, leaving a cavity (cavitation), or granulose tissue can surround the lesion, become fibrous, and form a collagenous scar around the tubercle (Ghon tubercle).

1 This is determined by a positive reaction to a tuberculin skin test, not on radiograph; it only determines the presence of antibodies; it does not confirm active disease. **2** This may be determined by a sputum culture, not by radiograph. **4** Microscopic primary infection may be so small it does not appear on an radiograph.

Client Need: Physiological Adaptation; **Cognitive Level:** Comprehension; **Nursing Process:** Assessment/Analysis; **Reference:** Ch 7, Pulmonary Tuberculosis, Data Base

159. 1 ☒ The general adaptation syndrome is activated in response to *Mycobacterium tuberculosis* (a gram-positive, acid-fast bacillus) causing an infectious response, which contributes to fatigue; the altered gas exchange also contributes to fatigue because it decreases the available O_2.

2 ☐ Anorexia, not polyphagia, is a common response to most infections.

3 ☒ Hemoptysis is a response caused by damage to lung tissue; it is associated with more advanced cases.

4 ☒ Night sweats are a common symptom of infectious diseases; the infectious process influences the temperature-regulating center of the brain that promotes peripheral vasodilation and increased permeability of the peripheral blood vessels, resulting in diaphoresis.

5 ☐ A black, hairy tongue is associated with fungal infection often seen with antibiotic therapy.

Client Need: Physiological Adaptation; **Cognitive Level:** Analysis; **Nursing Process:** Assessment/Analysis; **Reference:** Ch 7, Pulmonary Tuberculosis, Nursing Care

160. 1 Rifampin (Rifadin) causes a reddish-orange discoloration of secretions such urine, sweat, and tears.

2 While liver enzymes should be monitored because of the risk of hepatitis, this action is not addressing the client's statement. **3** This is indicated for renal calculi, which is not related to rifampin (Rifadin). **4** The medication, not food, is responsible for the urine color.

Client Need: Pharmacological and Parenteral Therapies; **Cognitive Level:** Analysis; **Integrated Process:** Teaching/Learning; **Nursing Process:** Planning/Implementation; **Reference:** Ch 7, Antituberculars

161. 3 The absence of bacteria in the sputum indicates that the disease can no longer be spread by the airborne route.

1 Once an individual has been infected, the test will always be positive. **2** Treatment is over an extended period; eventually the client may not have an active disease, but still remains infected. **4** This is not evidence that the disease will not be transmitted.

Client Need: Reduction of Risk Potential; **Cognitive Level:** Analysis; **Nursing Process:** Evaluation/Outcomes; **Reference:** Ch 7, Pulmonary Tuberculosis, Nursing Care

162. 1 The phrenic nerve stimulates the diaphragm; accidental severance of one phrenic nerve would result in partial paralysis of the diaphragm.

2 Because the phrenic nerve stimulates the diaphragm, its effect on postoperative pain would be negligible. **3** The diaphragm would ascend, not descend. **4** There is less excursion because the nerve has been severed.

Client Need: Physiological Adaptation; **Cognitive Level:** Comprehension; **Nursing Process:** Evaluation/Outcomes; **Reference:** Ch 7, Review of Anatomy and Physiology, Physiology of Respiration

163. 2 A chest tube drains the leaking chyle from the thoracic area; TPN provides nutrition, boosts immune defenses, and decreases thoracic duct flow; bed rest is recommended because lymphatic flow increases with activity.

1 A gastrostomy tube will not drain fluid from the thoracic area; a high-fat diet is contraindicated but bed rest is recommended. **3** A rectal tube has no relationship to the drainage of chyle from the thoracic area; a low-fat diet and bed rest are recommended. **4** The nasogastric tube does not drain fluid from the thoracic area; a low-fat diet and bed rest are recommended; a low-fat diet of medium-chain triglycerides will reduce the production and flow of chyle.

Client Need: Physiological Adaptation; **Cognitive Level:** Analysis; **Nursing Process:** Planning/Implementation; **Reference:** Ch 7, Cancer of the Larynx, Data Base

164. 3 The client has a high risk for airway obstruction from the edema, and restlessness and dyspnea indicate hypoxia.

1 This is unimportant; the pharyngeal opening is sutured closed and a tracheal stoma is formed; the trachea is anatomically separate from the esophagus. **2** Cloudy drainage may indicate infection, which would not be an immediate postoperative

complication. **4** Crackles come from the lower airway; the surgery involves the upper airway. There is no evidence of abdominal distention.
Client Need: Physiological Adaptation; **Cognitive Level:** Application; **Nursing Process:** Evaluation/Outcomes; **Reference:** Ch 7, Cancer of the Larynx, Nursing Care

165. **4** Secretions are increased because of alterations in structure and function. A patent airway must be maintained.
1 Whispering can put tension on the suture line; initially nonverbal and written forms of communication should be encouraged. **2** The orthopneic position may cause neck flexion and block the airway. **3** The outer tube is not removed because the stoma may close.
Client Need: Physiological Adaptation; **Cognitive Level:** Application; **Nursing Process:** Planning/Implementation; **Reference:** Ch 7, Cancer of the Larynx, Nursing Care

166. **2** During suctioning of a client's secretions, negative pressure (suction) should not be applied until the catheter is ready to be drawn out because, in addition to the removal of secretions, O_2 is being depleted.
1 The sterility of the catheter can be maintained during one suctioning session; a new sterile catheter should be used for each new session of suctioning. **3** A cough reflex may be absent or diminished in some clients; the catheter should be inserted approximately 12 cm (4 to 5 inches) or just past the end of the tracheostomy tube. **4** The inner cannula is not removed during suctioning; it may be removed during tracheostomy care.
Client Need: Physiological Adaptation; **Cognitive Level:** Application; **Nursing Process:** Planning/Implementation; **Reference:** Ch 7, Related Procedures, Suctioning of Airway

167. **2** Expectoration of blood is an indication that the lung itself was damaged during the procedure; a pneumothorax or hemothorax may occur.
1 Increased lung expansion should improve cerebral oxygenation and decrease confusion if present. **3** Increased breath sounds are anticipated because the lung is closer to the chest wall after the fluid in the pleural space is removed. **4** A decreased rate may indicate improved gaseous exchange and is not evidence that the client is in danger.
Client Need: Reduction of Risk Potential; **Cognitive Level:** Application; **Nursing Process:** Evaluation/Outcomes; **Reference:** Ch 7, Related Procedures, Thoracentesis

168. **2** Suctioning also removes O_2, which can cause cardiac dysrhythmias; the nurse should try to prevent this by hyperoxygenating the client before and after suctioning.
1 To prevent trauma to the trachea, suction should only be applied while removing the catheter. **3** This kind of movement could cause tracheal damage. **4** Suction only as needed; excessive suctioning irritates the mucosa, which increases secretion production.

Client Need: Physiological Adaptation; **Cognitive Level:** Application; **Nursing Process:** Planning/Implementation; **Reference:** Ch 7, Related Procedures, Suctioning of Airway

169. **1** ☒ This is an excessive amount of drainage; 80 to 120 mL of drainage is expected in the first 24 hours postoperatively; vital signs should be taken to determine the systemic response to blood loss.
2 ☒ This is an excessive amount of drainage; the physician should be notified.
3 ☐ A fresh postoperative dressing should not be disturbed because the manipulation can cause further bleeding; it can be reinforced by the nurse if needed; the surgeon should change the first dressing.
4 ☐ It would be contraindicated to apply pressure to the neck area; it could compromise the airway or carotid circulation or cause vagal stimulation.
5 ☐ The head of the bed is kept elevated after neck surgery to decrease edema, which could compromise the airway.
Client Need: Management of Care; **Cognitive Level:** Analysis; **Nursing Process:** Evaluation/Outcomes; **Reference:** Ch 7, Cancer of the Larynx, Nursing Care

170. **1** Erosion of tissue and fever account for these classic signs of tuberculosis.
2 These are general adaptations and may be associated with a variety of respiratory conditions. **3** These are associated with excess fluid volume. **4** These are associated with a GI obstruction or cancer.
Client Need: Physiological Adaptation; **Cognitive Level:** Application; **Nursing Process:** Assessment/Analysis; **Reference:** Ch 7, Pulmonary Tuberculosis, Nursing Care

171. **2** Atelectasis with impaired gas exchange is a major complication when clients use shallow breathing to avoid pain; coughing and deep breathing help mobilize secretions.
1 This may impede deep breathing and coughing, which help prevent atelectasis. **3** Pain medication is essential in diminishing pain caused by breathing and help motivate the client to cough and deep breathe. **4** The face-down position may diminish breathing for both lungs and is contraindicated.
Client Need: Physiological Adaptation; **Cognitive Level:** Application; **Nursing Process:** Planning/Implementation; **Reference:** Ch 7, Pneumothorax/Chest Injury, Nursing Care

172. **3** Decreased O_2 to the vital centers in the brain results in restlessness and confusion.
1 This would be a late sign of respiratory failure. **2** Tachycardia, not bradycardia, would occur as a compensatory mechanism to help increase oxygen to body cells. **4** This occurs with fluid volume excess (e.g., pulmonary edema).
Client Need: Physiological Adaptation; **Cognitive Level:** Application; **Nursing Process:** Assessment/Analysis; **Reference:** Ch 7, Obstructive Airway Disease, Nursing Care

173. 1 ☐ The O₂ source does not need to be higher than the client's airway because its flow does not depend on gravity.
2 ☐ The liter flow is adjusted according to flow rate that corresponds to the percent of O₂ prescribed; this is usually identified on the base of each adaptor.
3 ☒ The adaptor's orifices allow room air to combine with the O₂ to provide a specific O₂ concentration.
4 ☐ A Venturi mask does not have a bag like a rebreather mask.
5 ☒ A Venturi mask uses one of several adaptors, which are usually color-coded, to deliver the prescribed FIO₂.
Client Need: Physiological Adaptation; **Cognitive Level:** Analysis; **Nursing Process:** Planning/Implementation; **Reference:** Ch 7, Related Procedures, Oxygen Therapy

174. 1 O₂ via nasal cannula is the most comfortable and least intrusive, because the cannula extends minimally into the nose.
2 This is intrusive and may increase anxiety.
3, 4 This method is oppressive, and clients complain of feeling "suffocated" when it is used.
Client Need: Physiological Adaptation; **Cognitive Level:** Analysis; **Nursing Process:** Evaluation/Outcomes, **Reference:** Ch 7, Related Procedures, Oxygen Therapy

175. 1 This decrease in Pao₂ indicates respiratory failure; it warrants immediate medical evaluation.
2 While this may ultimately be ordered, it is not an action the nurse would take without first notifying the physician. 3 This is inappropriate and would compound the problem; the Pao₂ is a measure of the pressure (tension) of O₂ in the plasma; this level is decreased in individuals who have perfusion difficulties, such as those with pneumonia. 4 This is negligent and dangerous; a falling Pao₂ level is a serious indication of worsening pulmonary status and must be addressed immediately; drawing another blood sample and waiting for results would take too long.
Client Need: Management of Care; **Cognitive Level:** Application; **Nursing Process:** Planning/Implementation; **Reference:** Ch 7, Acute Respiratory Distress Syndrome, Data Base

176. 4 Mechanical ventilation with PEEP will help prevent alveolar collapse and improve oxygenation.
1 Fluid is not in the pleural space so this is not indicated. 2, 3 This is contraindicated because of severe hypotension from fluid shift into the interstitial spaces in the lungs.
Client Need: Physiological Adaptation; **Cognitive Level:** Analysis; **Nursing Process:** Planning/Implementation; **Reference:** Ch 7, Related Procedures, Mechanical Ventilation

177. 3 Secretions in the airway will increase pressure by blocking air flow and must be removed.
1 ABGs are used to assess client status, but are not taken each time a pressure alarm is heard. 2 The nurse must identify/correct the problem so that the set tidal volume can be delivered. 4 Connections that are not intact would cause a low-pressure alarm.
Client Need: Physiological Adaptation; **Cognitive Level:** Application; **Nursing Process:** Planning/Implementation; **Reference:** Ch 7, Related Procedures, Mechanical Ventilation

178. 3 Like a fixed pacemaker, continuous mandatory ventilation (CMV) will trigger independently of the client's vital functions; similar to a demand pacemaker, the mandatory minute ventilation (MMV) mode will monitor the client's preset minute ventilation and will only deliver breaths as needed.
1 Both intermittent mandatory ventilation (IMV) and synchronized intermittent mandatory ventilation (SIMV) deliver mandatory breaths even though SIMV can be set to synchronize with the client's breath. 2 Expiratory positive airway pressure (EPAP) and inspiratory positive airway pressure (IPAP) refer to the expiratory and inspiratory pressures associated with bi-level positive airway pressure, and are independent of client changes. 4 Continuous positive airway pressure (CPAP) and positive end-expiratory pressure (PEEP) involve maintenance of positive pressures that are independent of client changes.
Client Need: Physiological Adaptation; **Cognitive Level:** Analysis; **Integrated Process:** Teaching/Learning; **Nursing Process:** Planning/Implementation; **Reference:** Ch 7, Related Procedures, Mechanical Ventilation

179. 1 The nurse should first assess the client's vital signs and lung sounds to determine if suctioning is needed.
2 Hyperoxygenation for 30 seconds before suctioning compensates for the removal of O₂ during the suctioning process, but it is done after auscultation of breath sounds. 3 Suctioning occurs after the lung sounds have been auscultated, the client has been preoxygenated, and the catheter is inserted into the endotracheal tube. Suctioning for less than 15 seconds is appropriate because suctioning for longer than this irritates the mucosal lining of the respiratory tract as well as induces hypoxia. 4 This is done near the end of the procedure when the catheter is rotated and removed.
Client Need: Physiological Adaptation; **Cognitive Level:** Analysis; **Nursing Process:** Planning/Implementation; **Reference:** Ch 7, Related Procedures, Suctioning

180. 2 Surveillance and containment are the first lines of defense against outbreaks of infectious disease.
1 While it is important to have adequate supplies of antibiotics to treat illness, antibiotics do not prevent illness; vaccines should be administered to protect vulnerable populations. 3 Vaccines should be used to protect all vulnerable populations such as older adults, immunocompromised individuals, those with chronic medical conditions, those caring for individuals at high risk, and health care providers, not just children; some influenza vaccines are not administered to children younger than 5 years

of age. **4** Most vaccination programs inoculate clients during the months of October and November in preparation for the influenza season, which is generally from November through March.
Client Need: Management of Care; **Cognitive Level:** Analysis; **Nursing Process:** Planning/Implementation; **Reference:** Ch 7, Pneumonia, Data Base

181. **4** Honesty and openness are essential to understand the extent of the problem so that an appropriate local and global response can be mobilized to limit emerging pandemics.
1, 2, 3 While this helps, it can only be done in response to detection and reporting of the presence of an emerging health problem. In response to the severe acute respiratory syndrome (SARS) epidemic of 2002, the International Air Transport Association began work to standardize procedures that address passenger screening and the accurate and quick tracking of passenger travel.
Client Need: Management of Care; **Cognitive Level:** Application; **Nursing Process:** Planning/Implementation; **Reference:** Ch 7, Pneumonia, Data Base

GASTROINTESTINAL SYSTEM

182. **2** In addition to this recommendation, the ACS also recommends a flexible sigmoidoscopy every 5 years or colonoscopy every 10 years or double-contrast barium enema every 5 to 10 years.
1 The ACS recommends that women have an annual mammography after age 40 years. **3** Digital rectal examinations and PSA screening should be done annually at age 50 for men. **4** The ACS recommends that breast self-examinations be performed monthly beginning at age 20 years if a person chooses to do so; it is recommended that women be instructed about the potential benefits and limitations related to breast self-examination.
Client Need: Health Promotion and Maintenance; **Cognitive Level:** Application; **Integrated Process:** Teaching/Learning; **Nursing Process:** Planning/Implementation, **Reference:** Ch 8, Cancer of the Small Intestine, Colon, or Rectum, Data Base

183. **4** Orange juice has a higher proportion of simple sugars, which are readily available for conversion to energy.
1 Milk contains fat and protein, which require a longer digesting time, and lactose, which is a disaccharide. **2** Bread contains carbohydrates, which require a longer time to digest because they must be converted to simple sugars. **3** Chocolate candy bars do not contain the high proportion of simple sugars found in orange juice; they also contain fat, which takes longer to digest.
Client Need: Basic Care and Comfort; **Cognitive Level:** Application; **Integrated Process:** Teaching/Learning;

Nursing Process: Evaluation/Outcomes; **Reference:** Ch 8, Review of Nutrients, Sources of Energy

184. **1** Glucose catabolism is the main pathway for cellular energy production.
2, 3, 4 Glucose is not used directly for this process; ATP is the energy source.
Client Need: Physiological Adaptation; **Cognitive Level:** Comprehension; **Integrated Process:** Teaching/Learning; **Nursing Process:** Planning/Implementation; **Reference:** Ch 8, Review of Anatomy and Physiology, Metabolism

185. **3** Amino acids are absorbed into the blood in the intestinal capillaries with the aid of vitamin B_6 via the energy-dependent system known as active transport.
1 Proteins are large molecules; they do not passively diffuse. **2, 4** This refers to movement across a semipermeable membrane; it does not apply to proteins.
Client Need: Basic Care and Comfort; **Cognitive Level:** Comprehension; **Integrated Process:** Teaching/Learning; **Nursing Process:** Evaluation/Outcomes; **Reference:** Ch 8, Review of Anatomy and Physiology, Absorption

186. **2** Complete proteins contain sufficient amounts of all essential amino acids and are of animal origin.
1 Not all, but rather the essential amino acids are needed. **3** Sufficient amounts of all essential amino acids must be present. **4** The body cannot make the essential amino acids; they must be present in foods ingested.
Client Need: Basic Care and Comfort; **Cognitive Level:** Comprehension; **Integrated Process:** Teaching/Learning; **Nursing Process:** Planning/Implementation; **Reference:** Ch 8, Review of Chemical Principles, Amino Acids

187. **2** Vitamin K is synthesized by intestinal bacteria but is also found in large quantities in green leafy vegetables.
1 Vitamin K is found only in specific foods, not a wide variety. **3** Vitamin K is not easily absorbed; it is fat-soluble and requires bile salts for its absorption. **4** It is synthesized by intestinal bacteria so a natural deficiency does not occur.
Client Need: Basic Care and Comfort; **Cognitive Level:** Application; **Integrated Process:** Teaching/Learning; **Nursing Process:** Evaluation/Outcomes; **Reference:** Ch 8, Review of Nutrients, Vitamins

188. **4** Vitamin C is an intercellular cement substance.
1 This is the function of vitamin K. **2** This is the function of vitamin A. **3** This is the function of vitamin D.
Client Need: Basic Care and Comfort; **Cognitive Level:** Comprehension; **Nursing Process:** Assessment/Analysis; **Reference:** Ch 8, Review of Nutrients, Vitamins

189. **1** Milk and milk products are not tolerated well because they contain lactose, a sugar that is converted to galactose by lactase.
2 This enzyme assists in the digestion of maltose, which is not a milk sugar. **3** This enzyme assists in the digestion of sucrose, which is not a milk sugar. **4** This enzyme assists in the digestion of starch, which is not a milk sugar.

Client Need: Basic Care and Comfort; **Cognitive Level:** Comprehension; **Nursing Process:** Assessment/Analysis; **Reference:** Ch 8, Review of Chemical Principles, Carbohydrates

190. 4 A triglyceride is composed of three fatty acids and a glycerol molecule. When energy is required, the fatty acids are mobilized from adipose tissue for fuel. The nurse needs to recognize that a client who is cachectic will have limited reserves to meet energy needs.

1 This is not the function of adipose tissue; its main function is storage. 2 This is not a function of adipose tissue; cholesterol is produced in the liver. 3 This is not the function of adipose tissue in fat metabolism.

Client Need: Basic Care and Comfort; **Cognitive Level:** Comprehension; **Nursing Process:** Assessment/Analysis; **Reference:** Ch 8, Functions of the Gastrointestinal System, Metabolism

191. 3 Saturated fats found in animal tissue are more dense than unsaturated fats, which are found in vegetable oils.

1, 2, 4 This characteristic of food has no bearing on fat saturation.

Client Need: Basic Care and Comfort; **Cognitive Level:** Comprehension; **Integrated Process:** Teaching/Learning; **Nursing Process:** Planning/Implementation; **Reference:** Ch 8, Review of Chemical Principles, Lipids

192. 3 Animal fats are high in dense saturated fats.

1 Fruits do not contain saturated fats. 2 Grains do not contain saturated fats. 4 Vegetable oils contain unsaturated fats.

Client Need: Basic Care and Comfort; **Cognitive Level:** Application; **Nursing Process:** Assessment/Analysis; **Reference:** Ch 8, Review of Diets

193. 1 Because triglycerides are made up of fatty acids bonded (esterified) to glycerol, their breakdown releases fatty acids as well as glycerol.

2 Triglycerides do not contain amino acids. 3 Triglycerides do not contain urea nitrogen. 4 Triglycerides do not contain simple sugars.

Client Need: Basic Care and Comfort; **Cognitive Level:** Comprehension; **Nursing Process:** Assessment/Analysis; **Reference:** Ch 8, Review of Chemical Principles, Carbohydrates

194. 4 Cholesterol is an essential structural and functional component of most cellular membranes. That it is associated with atherosclerotic plaques does not detract from its essential functions.

1 Cholesterol is not necessary for blood clotting; calcium and vitamin K are necessary. 2 Cholesterol is not essential for bone formation; calcium, phosphorus, and calciferol are necessary. 3 Cholesterol is not involved in muscle contraction; potassium, sodium, and calcium are necessary.

Client Need: Basic Care and Comfort; **Cognitive Level:** Comprehension; **Integrated Process:** Teaching/Learning; **Nursing Process:** Planning/Implementation; **Reference:** Ch 8, Review of Chemical Principles, Lipids

195. 3 A coenzyme is a nonprotein substance that, in the presence of a suitable enzyme, serves as a catalyst in chemical changes.

1 It does not form a new compound; it facilitates the process involved. 2 The vitamin or mineral is part of the process when functioning as a coenzyme. 4 The coenzyme does not neutralize the enzyme.

Client Need: Basic Care and Comfort; **Cognitive Level:** Comprehension; **Integrated Process:** Teaching/Learning; **Nursing Process:** Evaluation/Outcomes; **Reference:** Ch 8, Review of Anatomy and Physiology, Digestion

196. 1 Lipoproteins are simple proteins combined with lipids to facilitate circulation of fat in the blood.

2 Triglycerides are part of lipoproteins. 3 Phospholipids are incorporated in lipoproteins. 4 Plasma proteins do not contain fat.

Client Need: Basic Care and Comfort; **Cognitive Level:** Comprehension; **Nursing Process:** Assessment/Analysis; **Reference:** Ch 8, Review of Chemical Principles, Protein

197. 3 The body does not synthesize these amino acids; they must be ingested in the diet.

1 The essential amino acids cannot be made by the body. 2, 4 All amino acids are needed for metabolism; however, arginine and histidine are necessary for growth, but not during adulthood; amino acids cannot be synthesized by the body.

Client Need: Basic Care and Comfort; **Cognitive Level:** Application; **Integrated Process:** Teaching/Learning; **Nursing Process:** Evaluation/Outcomes; **Reference:** Ch 8, Review of Chemical Principles, Amino Acids

198. 3 Fruits contain less natural sodium than do other foods.

1 Milk is higher in natural sodium than is fruit. 2 Meat is higher in natural sodium than is fruit. 4 Vegetables are higher in natural sodium than is fruit.

Client Need: Basic Care and Comfort; **Cognitive Level:** Application; **Integrated Process:** Teaching/Learning; **Nursing Process:** Evaluation/Outcomes; **Reference:** Ch 8, Review of Diets

199. 2 Vitamin A is a fat-soluble vitamin that accumulates in the body and is not significantly excreted even if extremely large amounts are ingested. After prolonged ingestion of extremely large doses, toxic effects (irritability, increased intracranial pressure, fatigue, night sweats, severe headache) can occur.

1 Vitamin A is toxic only after prolonged large dosages. 3 Vitamin A can be stored in the liver. 4 Vitamin A cannot be synthesized by the body.

Client Need: Basic Care and Comfort; **Cognitive Level:** Application; **Nursing Process:** Assessment/Analysis; **Reference:** Ch 8, Review of Nutrients, Vitamins

200. 2 Pancreatic amylase (which enters the small intestine at the sphincter of Oddi) and sucrase, lactase, and maltase (which are released by epithelial cells covering the villi in the small intestine) are responsible for carbohydrate digestion.

1 Because ptyalin is present in saliva, some starch digestion occurs in the mouth. 3 Digestion of carbohydrates is completed before their arrival in the large intestine, which is concerned primarily with

fluid reabsorption. **4** Limited carbohydrate digestion occurs in the stomach; pepsin begins the digestion of proteins.

Client Need: Basic Care and Comfort; **Cognitive Level:** Comprehension; **Integrated Process:** Teaching/Learning; **Nursing Process:** Planning/Implementation; **Reference:** Ch 8, Review of Anatomy and Physiology, Small Intestine

201. **4** Deep green and yellow vegetables contain large quantities of the pigments alpha-, beta-, and gamma-carotene; beta-carotene is the major chemical precursor of vitamin A in human nutrition.

1 Oranges are considered a good source of both vitamin C and potassium. **2** Tomatoes are a good source of vitamin C. **3** Levels of vitamin A are higher in whole milk than in skim milk.

Client Need: Basic Care and Comfort; **Cognitive Level:** Application; **Integrated Process:** Teaching/Learning; **Nursing Process:** Planning/Implementation; **Reference:** Ch 8, Review of Nutrients, Vitamins

202. **4** Vitamin A is used in the formation of retinol, a component of the light-sensitive rhodopsin molecule.

1 Melanin is a pigment of the skin. **2** Vitamin A does not influence color vision, which is centered in the cones. **3** The cornea is a transparent part of the anterior portion of the sclera; a cataract is an opacity of the normally transparent crystalline lens. Vitamin A does not prevent cataracts.

Client Need: Physiological Adaptation; **Cognitive Level:** Application; **Nursing Process:** Assessment/Implementation; **Reference:** Ch 8, Review of Nutrients, Vitamins

203. **3** The high-Fowler's position promotes optimal entry into the esophagus aided by gravity.

1, 2 This position does not take full advantage of the effect of gravity. **4** The head of the bed should be raised, not lowered; this could contribute to aspiration.

Client Need: Basic Care and Comfort; **Cognitive Level:** Application; **Nursing Process:** Planning/Implementation; **Reference:** Ch 8, Related Procedures, Gavage (Tube Feeding)

204. **2** Small meals are not as psychologically overwhelming and do not upset the stomach easily. They are therefore better tolerated.

1 If no attempts are made to decrease portions at regular mealtimes, aversion will usually persist. **3** This does not ensure adequate nutrition; if the portion size is decreased, frequency must be increased. **4** Administration of vitamins is a dependent nursing function; vitamins do not stimulate appetite.

Client Need: Basic Care and Comfort; **Cognitive Level:** Application; **Nursing Process:** Planning/Implementation; **Reference:** Ch 8, Cancer of the Stomach, Nursing Care

205. **1** Emptying the bladder before a paracentesis prevents its accidental puncture during the procedure.

2, 4 No bowel preparation is indicated. **3** The client may eat and drink as tolerated.

Client Need: Reduction of Risk Potential; **Cognitive Level:** Application; **Integrated Process:** Teaching/Learning; **Nursing Process:** Planning/Implementation; **Reference:** Ch 8, Related Procedures, Paracentesis

206. **4** Barium salts used in a GI series and barium enemas coat the inner lining of the GI tract and then absorb x-rays passing through. They thus outline the surface features of the tract on a photographic plate.

1 Barium has no light-emitting properties. **2** Barium does not have properties of a dye. **3** Barium does not fluoresce.

Client Need: Reduction of Risk Potential: **Cognitive Level:** Comprehension; **Nursing Process:** Planning/Implementation; **Reference:** Ch 8, Related Procedures, Gastrointestinal Series

207. **1** To permit adequate visualization of the mucosa during the sigmoidoscopy, the bowel must be cleansed with a nonirritating enema before examination.

2 Because only the lower bowel is being visualized, keeping the client NPO is unnecessary; clear liquids and a laxative may be given the day before to limit fecal residue. **3** Stool should be eliminated from the colon by an enema before the examination. **4** The client does not drink such a substance in preparation for a sigmoidoscopy.

Client Need: Reduction of Risk Potential; **Cognitive Level:** Application; **Nursing Process:** Planning/Implementation; **Reference:** Ch 8, Related Procedures, Gastrointestinal Series

208. **4** To promote understanding and allay anxiety, all diagnostic tests should be explained to the client.

1, 2, 3 Preparations for tests may vary depending on the client's condition.

Client Need: Reduction of Risk Potential; **Cognitive Level:** Application; **Integrated Process:** Teaching/Learning; **Nursing Process:** Planning/Implementation; **Reference:** Ch 8, Related Procedures, Gastrointestinal Series

209. **2** For a high colonic enema, the fluid must extend higher in the colon. If the height of the enema fluid container above the anus is increased, the force and rate of flow also increase.

1 This is too low for a high cleansing enema. **3, 4** This is too high and could cause mucosal injury.

Client Need: Reduction of Risk Potential; **Cognitive Level:** Application; **Nursing Process:** Planning/Implementation; **Reference:** Ch 8, Related Procedures, Enemas

210. **3** Administration of additional fluid when a client complains of abdominal cramps adds to discomfort because of additional pressure. By clamping the tubing a few minutes, the nurse allows the cramps to subside and the enema can be continued.

1 Slowing the rate decreases pressure but does not reduce it entirely. **2** Cramps are not a reason to discontinue the enema entirely; temporary clamping of the tubing usually relieves the cramps and the procedure can be continued. **4** This will reduce the flow of the solution, which will decrease pressure but not reduce it entirely.

Client Need: Reduction of Risk Potential; **Cognitive Level:** Application; **Nursing Process:** Planning/Implementation; Reference: Ch 8, Related Procedures, Enemas

211. 1 Because the soft tissues of the GI tract lack sufficient quantities of x-ray–absorbing atoms (as are naturally present in the dense calcium salts of bone), an x-ray–absorbing coating of barium is used for radiologic studies.

2 Barium does not color the intestinal wall.

3 Barium absorbs x-rays. 4 Barium does not interact with electrolytes.

Client Need: Reduction of Risk Potential; **Cognitive Level:** Comprehension; **Integrated Process:** Teaching/Learning; **Nursing Process:** Planning/Implementation; **Reference:** Ch 8, Related Procedures, Gastrointestinal Series

212. 3 A rise in the level of formula within the tube indicates a full stomach.

1 Passage of flatus reflects intestinal motility, which does not pose a potential problem. 2 Epigastric tenderness is not necessarily caused by a full stomach. 4 A rapid inflow is the result of positioning the container too high or using a feeding tube with too large a lumen.

Client Need: Reduction of Risk Potential; **Cognitive Level:** Analysis; **Nursing Process:** Evaluation/Outcomes; **Reference:** Ch 8, Related Procedures, Gavage (Tube Feeding)

213. 1 The presence of a residual of equal to or more than the hourly rate of the feeding may indicate delayed gastric emptying or impaired absorption; if the residual is 100 mL or equal to half the ordered administration rate, the nurse should refer to the physician's order or agency policy about whether to continue with the feeding or hold the feeding for 1 hour; the American Gastrointestinal Association (1995) recommends that a tube feeding should not automatically be stopped but rather be rechecked in 1 hour; if the residual volume continues to exceed 100 mL or the hourly rate, the physician may order the rate to be reduced to decrease the risk for aspiration.

2 This evaluates fluid balance and is best performed over a 24-hour period. 3 This is a method for evaluating tube placement. 4 Although weighing the client regularly is important to evaluating overall nutritional progress, it does not provide information about absorption of a particular feeding.

Client Need: Reduction of Risk Potential; **Cognitive Level:** Application; **Nursing Process:** Evaluation/Outcomes; **Reference:** Ch 8, Related Procedures, Gavage (Tube Feeding)

214. 4 The increased osmolarity (concentration) of many formulas draws fluid into the intestinal tract, which would cause diarrhea; such feedings may need to be diluted initially until the client develops tolerance.

1 Formulas frequently have reduced fiber content. 2 Bacterial contamination is not a factor if the manufacturer's recommendations are followed. 3 Inappropriate positioning may increase the risk for aspiration, but it does not cause diarrhea.

Client Need: Reduction of Risk Potential; **Cognitive Level:** Application; **Nursing Process:** Evaluation/Outcomes; **Reference:** Ch 8, Related Procedures, Gavage (Tube Feedings)

215. 4 Because the cardiac sphincter of the stomach is slightly opened to admit the nasogastric tube, rapid feeding could result in regurgitation.

1 Distention can be diminished by avoiding the instillation of air with the feeding. 2 The speed of feeding does not cause flatulence, but the administration of air may. 3 Although indigestion may be uncomfortable, it is not hazardous to the client.

Client Need: Reduction of Risk Potential; **Cognitive Level:** Application; **Nursing Process:** Planning/Implementation; **Reference:** Ch 8, Related Procedures, Gavage (Tube Feedings)

216. 2 Vomiting may result in aspiration of vomitus, because it cannot be expelled; this could cause pneumonia or asphyxia.

1, 3, 4 This generally is not a life-threatening problem.

Client Need: Reduction of Risk Potential; **Cognitive Level:** Application; **Nursing Process:** Evaluation/Outcomes; **Reference:** Ch 8, Fracture of the Jaw, Nursing Care

217. 2 Pain and swelling should subside before 1 week postoperatively. Continued pain may indicate infection.

1 This is expected because of dried blood in the oral cavity. 3 This may occur because of generalized trauma resulting from surgery, and is expected. 4 This is expected.

Client Need: Reduction of Risk Potential; **Cognitive Level:** Application; **Integrated Process:** Teaching/Learning; **Nursing Process:** Planning/Implementation; **Reference:** Ch 8, Fracture of the Jaw, Nursing Care

218. 2 Leukoplakia are white, thickened patches that tend to fissure and become malignant; ulcerations in the mouth or on the tongue may indicate cancer.

1 Halitosis would not be an early sign of or specific to cancer of the mouth. 3 Bleeding gums occur in gingival diseases. 4 Pain associated with cancer of the tongue would not radiate to the substernal area.

Client Need: Physiological Adaptation; **Cognitive Level:** Application; **Nursing Process:** Assessment/Analysis; **Reference:** Ch 8, Cancer of the Oral Cavity, Data Base

219. 4 Heavy alcohol ingestion predisposes an individual to the development of oral cancer.

1, 2, 3 This has no effect on the development of oral cancer.

Client Need: Physiological Adaptation; **Cognitive Level:** Application; **Nursing Process:** Assessment/Analysis; **Reference:** Ch 8, Cancer of the Oral Cavity, Data Base

220. 1 Sleeping on pillows raises the upper torso and minimizes reflux of the gastric contents.

2 This would have no effect on the reflux of gastric contents. 3 Increasing the content of the stomach before lying down would aggravate the symptoms associated with gastroesophageal reflux. 4 The effect of antacids is not long-lasting enough to promote a

full night's sleep; sodium bicarbonate is not recommended as an antacid.
Client Need: Basic Care and Comfort; **Cognitive Level:** Application; **Integrated Process:** Teaching/Learning; **Nursing Process:** Planning/Implementation; **Reference:** Ch 8, Gastroesophageal Reflux Disease, Nursing Care

221. 1 Heavy lifting increases intraabdominal pressure, allowing gastric contents to move up through the lower esophageal sphincter (regurgitation), causing heartburn (pyrosis).
2 This encourages regurgitation and should be avoided. 3 Increasing fluids with meals increases gastric volume, causing distention and reflux. 4 Constrictive garments such as belts, binders, and girdles increase intraabdominal pressure and could lead to reflux.
Client Need: Basic Care and Comfort; **Cognitive Level:** Application; **Integrated Process:** Teaching/Learning; **Nursing Process:** Planning/Implementation; **Reference:** Ch 8, Gastroesophageal Reflux Disease (GERD), Nursing Care

222. 3 Approximately two thirds of clients with peptic ulcer disease have been found to have *Helicobacter pylori* infecting the mucosa and interfering with its protective function.
1, 2, 4 Antibiotics do not cause this effect.
Client Need: Physiological Adaptation; **Cognitive Level:** Application; **Integrated Process:** Teaching/Learning; **Nursing Process:** Planning/Implementation; **Reference:** Ch 8, Peptic Ulcer Disease, Data Base

223. 1 ☒ Alcohol should be avoided because it decreases esophageal sphincter pressure.
2 ☐ Coffee and tea contain caffeine, which decreases esophageal sphincter pressure, and should be avoided; milk does not have to be eliminated from the diet unless the client has lactose intolerance.
3 ☐ The head, not the foot, of the bed should be elevated to prevent nighttime reflux; at night infrequent swallowing and the recumbent position impair esophageal clearance.
4 ☐ Three large meals increase the volume pressure in the stomach, which delays gastric emptying; four to six meals are preferred.
5 ☒ These actions promote digestion and prevent eructation (belching).
6 ☒ Small, frequent meals keep the volume of food in the stomach low and facilitate gastric emptying.
Client Need: Basic Care and Comfort; **Cognitive Level:** Application; **Integrated Process:** Teaching/Learning; **Nursing Process:** Planning/Implementation; **Reference:** Ch 8, Gastroesophageal Reflux Disease, Nursing Care

224. 4 Unless diluted by the increased blood flow, the highly concentrated solution can cause injury to the veins.
1 The potential of infection is high with parenteral nutrition because of the increased glucose levels. 2, 3 This is not the primary reason, although the infusion at this site is more secure and promotes free use of the arms and hands.

Client Need: Pharmacological and Parenteral Therapies; **Cognitive Level:** Comprehension; **Nursing Process:** Planning/Implementation; **Reference:** Ch 8, Related Procedures, Parenteral Replacement Therapy

225. 2 TPN solutions are high in glucose and are administered at room temperature, factors that increase the risk of microbial growth in the solution; they should be changed daily or sooner if they appear cloudy.
1 Monitoring the blood glucose level q2h is too frequent; the client's blood glucose level should be monitored q4-6h to identify the presence of hyperglycemia, a metabolic complication of TPN. 3 The client should not breathe while the TPN catheter is changed because it could result in an air embolus; the Valsalva maneuver should be performed by the client for the few seconds it takes to switch the tubing. 4 An excess amount of glucose would be infused if the rate of the TPN were increased, and the endogenous insulin would be inadequate to meet this demand, resulting in hyperglycemia.
Client Need: Pharmacological and Parenteral Therapies; **Cognitive Level:** Application; **Integrated Process:** Teaching/Learning; **Nursing Process:** Planning/Implementation; **Reference:** Ch 8, Related Procedures, Parenteral Replacement Therapy

226. 3 The act of eating allows the hydrochloric acid in the stomach to work on and be neutralized by food rather than irritate the intestinal mucosa.
1 This symptom is not specific to duodenal ulcers. 2 This may indicate renal colic. 4 This is not specific to duodenal ulcers.
Client Need: Physiological Adaptation; **Cognitive Level:** Application; **Nursing Process:** Assessment/Analysis; **Reference:** Ch 8, Peptic Ulcer Disease, Data Base

227. 4 The vagus nerve stimulates the stomach to secrete hydrochloric acid. When it is severed, this neural pathway is interrupted and stomach secretions are decreased.
1 The portion of the vagus nerve that is severed innervates the stomach, not the heart; therefore the heart rate would not be affected. 2 The vagus nerve controls hydrochloric acid secretion, not gastric emptying; emptying is determined by the nature of foods being digested. 3 The vagus nerve is not a sensory nerve.
Client Need: Physiological Adaptation; **Cognitive Level:** Comprehension; **Integrated Process:** Teaching/Learning; **Nursing Process:** Planning/Implementation; **Reference:** Ch 8, Peptic Ulcer Disease, Data Base

228. 3 The antrum is responsible for gastrin production, which stimulates hydrochloric acid secretion; its removal reduces HCl secretion and thus reduces irritation of the gastric mucosa.
1 Removal by means of a laser beam, cryotechnique, or surgery is implemented to treat cataracts. 2 A stapedectomy, mobilization of the stapes, or a prosthetic implant is used to treat otosclerosis. 4 A resection of the fifth cranial nerve is implemented to treat trigeminal neuralgia.

Client Need: Physiological Adaptation; **Cognitive Level:** Application; **Nursing Process:** Assessment/Analysis; **Reference:** Ch 8, Peptic Ulcer Disease, Data Base

229. **3** When high-osmotic fluid passes rapidly into the small intestine, it causes hypovolemia. This results in a sympathetic response with tachycardia, diaphoresis, and dizziness. The symptoms are also attributed to a sudden rise and subsequent fall in blood glucose level.

1 The stomach is not full; its contents rapidly empty into the jejunum. **2** This could occur with intestinal obstruction; dumping syndrome is associated with increased motility originating in the jejunum. Reflux requires reverse peristalsis. **4** This is usually associated with paralytic ileus; dumping syndrome leads to increased intestinal motility.

Client Need: Reduction of Risk Potential; **Cognitive Level:** Comprehension; **Nursing Process:** Assessment/Analysis; **Reference:** Ch 8, Peptic Ulcer Disease, Nursing Care

230. **3** Nasogastric drainage is expected to be bright red during the first 12 hours after surgery and then bleeding lessens gradually within the next 12 hours after surgery in response to hemostasis in the surgical area.

1 This is unnecessary; bloody drainage is expected this soon after surgery. **2** Nasogastric suction must be working and the tube must remain patent to prevent stress on the suture line. **4** The nasogastric tube is only irrigated if the physician orders it because of the danger of injury to the suture line; generally saline at room temperature is ordered.

Client Need: Reduction of Risk Potential; **Cognitive Level:** Application; **Nursing Process:** Evaluation/Outcomes; **Reference:** Ch 8, Peptic Ulcer Disease, Nursing Care

231. **1** Patency of the tube should be maintained to ensure continued suction. Use of normal saline prevents fluid and electrolyte disturbances during irrigation.

2 The stomach is not considered a sterile body cavity, so medical asepsis is indicated. **3** Care must be taken to avoid traumatizing the mucosa. **4** Ice chips and water represent fluid intake, which must be approved by the physician; being hypotonic in nature, such intake may lower the level of serum electrolytes.

Client Need: Reduction of Risk Potential; **Cognitive Level:** Analysis; **Nursing Process:** Planning/Implementation; **Reference:** Ch 8, Peptic Ulcer Disease, Nursing Care

232. **1** Physiologic normal saline is used in gastric instillations to prevent electrolyte imbalance. Because of the fresh gastric sutures, slow and gentle instillation of saline should be performed to reestablish patency of the tube, and then the tube should be reconnected to suction to ensure stomach decompression.

2, 4 The purpose of instillation is to maintain the patency of the tube for gastric decompression; with disconnection from suction, a buildup of secretions and air can occur or the tube can become blocked

by viscous drainage. **3** Increasing the pressure may cause damage to the suture line.

Client Need: Reduction of Risk Potential; **Cognitive Level:** Analysis; **Nursing Process:** Planning/Implementation; **Reference:** Ch 8, Peptic Ulcer Disease, Nursing Care

233. **4** Fluid and electrolytes are lost through intestinal decompression; on a daily basis about 20% of the total body water is secreted into and almost completely reabsorbed by the GI tract.

1 Because the client is kept NPO, there is no stimulus to cause enzymes to be secreted into the GI tract. **2** IV dextrose supplies some carbohydrates as a source of energy; it would not be drawn from storage by intestinal decompression. **3** Because the client is being kept NPO, vitamins and minerals are not entering the GI tract and therefore are not lost.

Client Need: Reduction of Risk Potential; **Cognitive Level:** Application; **Nursing Process:** Evaluation/Outcomes; **Reference:** Ch 8, Intestinal Obstruction, Nursing Care

234. **3** Dehydration is a danger because of fluid loss with GI suction.

1, 2, 4 Based on the data provided, this symptom is not likely to occur.

Client Need: Reduction of Risk Potential; **Cognitive Level:** Application; **Nursing Process:** Evaluation/Outcomes; **Reference:** Ch 8, Intestinal Obstruction, Nursing Care

235. **4** Symptoms of dumping syndrome occur to some degree in about 50% of all individuals who have undergone a gastrectomy. They include weakness, faintness, heart palpitations, and diaphoresis. It is therefore important to explain to the client that such symptoms can be minimized by resting after meals in the semi-Fowler's position, eating small meals, and omitting concentrated and highly refined carbohydrates.

1 Gas-forming foods affect the intestines, not the stomach. **2** Modification of roughage is part of the management of intestinal rather than gastric disorders. **3** Eating habits must be modified to prevent rapid emptying of the stomach.

Client Need: Reduction of Risk Potential; **Cognitive Level:** Application; **Integrated Process:** Teaching/Learning; **Nursing Process:** Planning/Implementation; **Reference:** Ch 8, Peptic Ulcer Disease, Nursing Care

236. **3** Pernicious anemia is caused by a lack of vitamin B_{12}. Intrinsic factor, produced by the parietal cells of the gastric mucosa, is necessary for B_{12} absorption.

1 B_{12} is absorbed in the ileum. **2** The intrinsic factor is secreted by the stomach; the hemopoietic factor is the combination of B_{12} and intrinsic factor. **4** Chief cells secrete the enzymes of the gastric juice.

Client Need: Physiological Adaptation; **Cognitive Level:** Application; **Nursing Process:** Evaluation/Outcomes; **Reference:** Ch 8, Peptic Ulcer disease, Data Base

237. **2** To promote drainage of different lung regions, clients should turn every 2 hours. Deep breathing inflates the alveoli and promotes fluid drainage.

1 During physical effort, individuals with abdominal incisions often revert to shallow breathing. **2** Oxygen administration is a dependent function and is not generally required unless there is an underlying cardiac or respiratory disease. **4** The airway will be expelled once the gag reflex returns.
Client Need: Reduction of Risk Potential; **Cognitive Level:** Application; **Nursing Process:** Planning/Implementation; **Reference:** Ch 8, Peptic Ulcer Disease, Nursing Care

238. **3** Small, frequent feedings are tolerated best after a subtotal gastrectomy.
1 Roughage may be irritating to the GI tract after surgery. **2** As soon as edema subsides, the individual is generally given small amounts of fluid and then the diet is gradually progressed. **4** Recuperation from gastric surgery may take up to 3 months; allowing only food preferences does not ensure inclusion of nutrients necessary for recovery.
Client Need: Basic Care and Comfort; **Cognitive Level:** Application; **Nursing Process:** Planning/Implementation; **Reference:** Ch 8, Peptic Ulcer Disease, Nursing Care

239. **1** ☒ Calcium deficiency is a late complication of bariatric surgery because of inadequate absorption even with an intake of calcium-rich foods; calcium supplementation may be necessary.
2 ☐ This will not provide adequate calories and nutrients; six small feedings with a total of 600 to 800 calories a day is routine once the client is eating.
3 ☐ Clients need to increase, not limit, fluid intake; the dumping syndrome contributes to diarrhea, which can cause dehydration and electrolyte imbalance.
4 ☒ Foods high in protein exit the stomach more slowly than foods high in fat and carbohydrates, which minimizes the dumping syndrome.
5 ☒ Vitamin B_{12} deficiency is a late complication of bariatric surgery because of a lack of intrinsic factor, a gastric secretion necessary for the absorption of vitamin B_{12}; lifelong supplementation may be necessary.
Client Need: Reduction of Risk Potential; **Cognitive Level:** Analysis; **Integrated Process:** Teaching/Learning; **Nursing Process:** Planning/Implementation; **Reference:** Ch 8, Obesity, Nursing Care

240. **3** When ingested food rapidly enters the jejunum without having gone through the usual mixing and digestive process, the hypertonic bolus causes rapid movement of extracellular fluid into the bowel; this rapid shift decreases the circulating blood volume; also, the distended jejunum increases intestinal peristalsis and motility.
1 Backward flow of gastric contents into the esophagus causes heartburn, dysphagia, water brash, acid regurgitation, or belching (eructation). **2** This is a chronic inflammation of the lining of the stomach caused by reflux of duodenal contents; epigastric pain, nausea, vomiting, and hematemesis are

common clinical manifestations. **4** This is an inflammation of the peritoneal membrane; rigidity of abdominal muscles, abdominal pain, low-grade fever, malaise, absent bowel sounds, and shallow respirations are common clinical manifestations.
Client Need: Reduction of Risk Potential; **Cognitive Level:** Analysis; **Nursing Process:** Evaluation/Outcomes; **Reference:** Ch 8, Obesity, Nursing Care

241. **2** Clients need to be prepared emotionally for the body image changes that occur after bariatric surgery. Clients generally experience excessive abdominal skin folds after weight stabilizes, which may require a panniculectomy. Body image disturbance often occurs in response to incorrectly estimating one's size; it is not uncommon for the client to still feel fat no matter how much weight is lost.
1 The client needs to increase protein intake and avoid foods high in sugar and fat; alcohol and sweetened fluids should be avoided. **3** Barring complications, clients are ambulated and transferred to a chair within 8 hours of surgery. **4** Six small feedings for a total calorie intake of 600 to 800 calories in 24 hours plus fluids to prevent dehydration are routine once the physician orders a regular diet.
Client Need: Reduction of Risk Potential; **Cognitive Level:** Analysis; **Integrated Process:** Teaching/Learning; **Nursing Process:** Planning/Implementation; **Reference:** Ch 8, Obesity, Nursing Care

242. **1** This allows for easier digestion and absorption of medication in the stomach.
2 This client should lie on the left side for 20 to 30 minutes to delay gastric emptying. **3** This client should be ingesting a high-protein diet with limited carbohydrates and no simple sugars; this will help minimize the dumping syndrome. **4** Barring any complications, this client should be discharged in 5 days.
Client Need: Reduction of Risk Potential; **Cognitive Level:** Application; **Integrated Process:** Teaching/Learning; **Nursing Process:** Planning/Implementation; **Reference:** Ch 8, Obesity, Nursing Care

243. **2** ERCP involves the insertion of a cannula into the pancreatic and common bile ducts during an endoscopy. The test is not performed if the client's bilirubin level is greater than 3 to 5 mg/dL because cannulization may cause edema, which would increase obstruction of bile flow.
1, 3, 4 This is not directly related to this test.
Client Need: Reduction of Risk Potential; **Cognitive Level:** Analysis; **Nursing Process:** Assessment/Analysis; **Reference:** Ch 8, Cholelithiasis/Cholecystitis, Data Base

244. **4** Cholecystokinin is a widely distributed hormone whose functions include stimulation of gallbladder contraction and the release of pancreatic enzymes.
1 Gastrin stimulates the secretion of gastric juice.
2 Secretin promotes the production of bile by the liver and the secretion of pancreatic juice.

3 Enterocrinin stimulates the secretion of intestinal juice (succus entericus).
Client Need: Physiological Adaptation; **Cognitive Level:** Comprehension; **Nursing Process:** Assessment/Analysis; **Reference:** Ch 8, Review of Anatomy and Physiology, Small Intestine

245. **2** When bile does not mix with foods in the intestine, emulsification of fats cannot occur and fat digestion is retarded. Stomach motility is also reduced, because increased stomach peristalsis depends on fat digestion in the small intestine.
1 Once emulsified by bile, fatty foods are readily broken down by digestive enzymes. **3** The production of bile is unaffected. **4** Obstruction, not inadequate closure, of the ampulla of Vater causes discomfort. Bile and pancreatic secretions enter the duodenum through the ampulla of Vater. With obstruction, edema and spasm occur, blocking the flow of enzymes and causing pain.
Client Need: Physiological Adaptation; **Cognitive Level:** Analysis; **Nursing Process:** Planning/Implementation; **Reference:** Ch 8, Cholelithiasis/Cholecystitis, Data Base

246. **1** ☒ Inadequate bile flow interferes with vitamin K absorption, contributing to ecchymosis, hematuria, and other bleeding.
2 ☒ This sign results from failure of bile to enter the intestines, with subsequent backup into the biliary system and diffusion into the blood. The bilirubin is carried to all body regions including the skin and mucous membranes.
3 ☐ With obstructive jaundice the stool is clay-colored, not dark brown; the presence of bile causes stool to be brown.
4 ☐ When bile levels in the bloodstream are high, as is seen in obstructive jaundice, there is bile in the urine, causing it to have a dark color.
5 ☒ This occurs especially after eating foods high in fat and is characteristic of acute cholecystitis and biliary colic.
Client Need: Physiological Adaptation; **Cognitive Level:** Analysis; **Nursing Process:** Assessment/Analysis; **Reference:** Ch 8, Cholelithiasis/Cholecystitis, Data Base

247. **1** This sign results from failure of bile to enter the intestines, with subsequent backup into the biliary system and diffusion into the blood; the bilirubin is carried to all body regions, including the skin and mucous membranes.
2 Pain is experienced in the right upper quadrant because of spasm of the gallbladder, whether or not there is biliary obstruction. **3** The stools are not brown because the bile pigments are not present in the GI tract as a result of the obstruction of the common bile duct. **4** This indicates gastric bleeding; it is not a unique sign of cholelithiasis with obstructive jaundice; if obstruction was chronic it could interfere with vitamin K absorption and clotting.

Client Need: Physiological Adaptation; **Cognitive Level:** Analysis; **Nursing Process:** Assessment/Analysis; **Reference:** Ch 8, Cholelithiasis/Cholecystitis, Data Base

248. **2** Vitamin K is necessary in the formation of prothrombin to prevent bleeding. It is a fat-soluble vitamin and is not absorbed from the GI tract in the absence of bile.
1 Bilirubin is the bile pigment formed by the breakdown of erythrocytes. **3** Thromboplastin converts prothrombin to thrombin during the process of coagulation. **4** Cholecystokinin is the hormone that stimulates contraction of the gallbladder.
Client Need: Basic Care and Comfort; **Cognitive Level:** Comprehension; **Nursing Process:** Planning/Implementation; **Reference:** Ch 8, Review of Nutrients, Vitamins

249. **3** The location of the incision results in pain on inspiration or coughing. The subsequent reluctance to cough and deep breathe facilitates respiratory complications from retained secretions.
1 This surgery does not take a prolonged period of time. **2** Bile does not impair inflammatory or immune responses. **4** Cholelithiasis or cholecystitis is generally an inflammatory, not an infectious, process.
Client Need: Reduction of Risk Potential; **Cognitive Level:** Application; **Nursing Process:** Evaluation/Outcomes; **Reference:** Ch 8, Cholelithiasis/Cholecystitis, Nursing Care

250. **2** This is the unique function of pancreozymin, which is secreted by the duodenal mucosa. It particularly affects the production of amylase.
1 This increases intestinal juice secretion. **3** This lessens gastric secretion and motility. **4** This stimulates the flow of bile from the gallbladder.
Client Need: Physiological Adaptation; **Cognitive Level:** Knowledge; **Nursing Process:** Assessment/Analysis; **Reference:** Ch 8, Review of Anatomy and Physiology, Pancreas

251. **4** Lipase is a pancreatic enzyme that aids in the digestion of fat.
1 Lipase does not synthesize triglycerides. **2** Fat emulsification is the function of bile. **3** Lipase does not break down all dietary fat.
Client Need: Physiological Adaptation; **Cognitive Level:** Comprehension; **Nursing Process:** Assessment/Analysis; **Reference:** Ch 8, Review of Anatomy and Physiology, Pancreas

252. **4** A pseudocyst of the pancreas is an abnormally dilated space that contains blood, necrotic tissue, and enzymes and is surrounded by connective tissue.
1, 2, 3 This is an incorrect definition of a pseudocyst.
Client Need: Physiological Adaptation; **Cognitive Level:** Knowledge; **Nursing Process:** Assessment/Analysis; **Reference:** Ch 8, Pancreatitis, Data Base

253. **4** Alcohol stimulates pancreatic enzyme secretion and an increase in pressure in the pancreatic duct. The backflow of enzymes into the pancreatic interstitial spaces results in partial digestion and inflammation of the pancreatic tissue.

1 Although blockage of the bile duct with calculi may precipitate pancreatitis, this is not associated with alcohol. **2** Although the volume of secretions increases, the composition remains unchanged. **3** Alcohol does not deplete insulin stores; the demand for insulin is unrelated to pancreatitis.
Client Need: Reduction of Risk Potential; **Cognitive Level:** Comprehension; **Nursing Process:** Assessment/Analysis; **Reference:** Ch 8, Pancreatitis, Data Base

254. **3** Open communication helps to decrease anxiety.
1 Knowledge does not always reduce anxiety. **2** Antibiotics will have no direct effect on the client's anxiety. **4** This is false reassurance.
Client Need: Psychosocial Integrity; **Cognitive Level:** Application; **Integrated Process:** Caring; **Nursing Process:** Planning/Implementation; **Reference:** Ch 8, Cancer of the Pancreas, Nursing Care

255. **2** An incision close to the diaphragm (as in surgery of the pancreas) causes a great deal of pain when the client coughs and deep breathes. These clients tend to take shallow breaths, leading to inadequate expansion of the lungs, the accumulation of secretions, and infection.
1 This is unrelated to the development of respiratory tract infections. **3** The elevation of serum bilirubin level in the blood does not affect the immune mechanisms. **4** The need for pancreatic surgery generally is in response to an inflammatory, not an infectious, process.
Client Need: Reduction of Risk Potential; **Cognitive Level:** Knowledge; **Nursing Process:** Assessment/Analysis; **Reference:** Ch 8, Cancer of the Pancreas, Nursing Care

256. **4** In the liver a simple protein combines with a lipid to form a lipoprotein. Lipoproteins circulate freely in the blood and can be utilized easily and quickly in various metabolic processes.
1 Fat is stored in adipose tissue. **2** The liver does not produce phospholipids; they do not regulate metabolism. **3** The liver does not oxidize fat.
Client Need: Physiological Adaptation; **Cognitive Level:** Comprehension; **Nursing Process:** Assessment/Analysis; **Reference:** Ch 8, Review of Anatomy and Physiology, Liver

257. **1** ☒ Soft foods avoid irritation of esophageal varices if present.
2 ☐ A regular diet will not meet the dietary requirements of this client.
3 ☐ A low-protein diet would not provide enough protein to correct the severe malnutrition associated with alcoholism in the absence of an elevated serum ammonia level; in hepatic coma protein intake is reduced to 15 to 30 g.
4 ☒ A high-protein intake is necessary to correct severe malnutrition in the absence of an elevated serum ammonia level.
5 ☐ A low-carbohydrate diet will not provide for energy needs.
6 ☒ A high-carbohydrate intake provides for energy needs.

Client Need: Basic Care and Comfort; **Cognitive Level:** Analysis; **Integrated Process:** Teaching/Learning; **Nursing Process:** Planning/Implementation; **Reference:** Ch 8, Hepatic Cirrhosis, Nursing Care

258. **1** Thiamine and nicotinic acid help convert glucose for energy and therefore influence nerve activity.
2 These vitamins do not affect elimination. **3** These vitamins are not related to circulatory activity.
4 Vitamin K, not thiamine and niacin, is essential for the manufacture of prothrombin.
Client Need: Basic Care and Comfort; **Cognitive Level:** Comprehension; **Integrated Process:** Teaching/Learning; **Nursing Process:** Planning/Implementation; **Reference:** Ch 8, Review of Nutrients, Vitamins

259. **1** The liver detoxifies alcohol and is the organ most often damaged in chronic alcoholism. The high-calorie diet minimizes tissue breakdown and promotes healing.
2, 3 These organs are not involved in detoxification of alcohol. **4** This organ is not involved in detoxification of alcohol.
Client Need: Basic Care and Comfort; **Cognitive Level:** Application; **Nursing Process:** Assessment/Analysis; **Reference:** Ch 8, Hepatic Cirrhosis, Nursing Care

260. **4** The temperature during steaming is never high enough or sustained long enough to kill organisms.
1 Processing destroys the virus. **2** Because of the extremely high temperature, broiling sufficiently destroys the virus. **3** Baking would destroy the virus.
Client Need: Basic Care and Comfort; **Cognitive Level:** Application; **Integrated Process:** Teaching/Learning; **Nursing Process:** Planning/Implementation; **Reference:** Ch 8, Hepatitis, Data Base

261. **2** Contracting hepatitis B through blood transfusions can be prevented by screening donors and testing the blood.
1, 3, 4 This does not prevent transmission of hepatitis B.
Client Need: Reduction of Risk Potential; **Cognitive Level:** Application; **Nursing Process:** Assessment/Analysis; **Reference:** Ch 8, Hepatitis, Data Base

262. **3** The virus is present in the stool of clients with hepatitis A; therefore standard precautions should be followed when handling excretions. The virus may also be present in the urine and in the nasotracheal secretions.
1 Bringing food to a client requires no precautions; however, disposable utensils should be used and the utensils discarded following standard precautions because the client's nasotracheal secretions contain the virus. **2** The Centers for Disease Control and Prevention (CDC) indicate that only standard precautions are necessary when caring for a client who is positive for the presence of hepatitis A; if a client is incontinent or using an incontinence device, the CDC recommends that contact precautions be implemented. **4** Hepatitis A is not usually transmitted via the air.

Client Need: Safety and Infection Control; **Cognitive Level:** Application; **Nursing Process:** Planning/Implementation; **Reference:** Ch 8, Hepatitis, Nursing Care

263. 3 Hepatitis C (formerly called non-A, non-B hepatitis) is caused by an RNA virus that is transmitted parenterally. More effective blood screening for hepatitis C was introduced in June of 1992; this brought about a dramatic decrease in hepatitis C caused by blood transfusions; recent studies document that the risk of contracting hepatitis C from a blood transfusion is 1 in 103,000 transfusions. The incubation period is 5 to 10 weeks.

1 Hepatitis A, also known as infectious hepatitis, is caused by an RNA virus that is transmitted via the fecal-oral route. The incubation period is 2 to 6 weeks. 2 Hepatitis B is transmitted parenterally, sexually, and by direct contact with infected body secretions. The incubation period is 1 to 6 months. It is not the major cause of posttransfusion hepatitis. 4 Hepatitis D is a complication of hepatitis B.

Client Need: Safety and Infection Control; **Cognitive Level:** Comprehension; **Nursing Process:** Planning/Implementation; **Reference:** Ch 8, Hepatitis, Data Base

264. 2 Hepatitis C is a bloodborne pathogen that can be transmitted via contaminated tattoo needles.

1 Hepatitis A is not a bloodborne pathogen; it is spread through contaminated food or water. 3 Although hepatitis D is a bloodborne pathogen, it can be produced only when the hepatitis B virus is present, and hepatitis D is not the main virus associated with contaminated tattoo needles. 4 Hepatitis E is believed to be transmitted via the fecal-oral route; it is spread through contaminated food or water.

Client Need: Safety and Infection Control; **Cognitive Level:** Application; **Integrated Process:** Teaching/Learning; **Nursing Process:** Planning/Implementation; **Reference:** Ch 8, Hepatitis, Data Base

265. 3 Weight is helpful in determining the extent of ascites; 1 L of retained fluid equals approximately 2.2 lb.

1 Diet history will not help in monitoring a client's condition. 2 Bowel sounds are objective data but do not help monitor the liver. 4 Pain is subjective.

Client Need: Physiological Adaptation; **Cognitive Level:** Application; **Nursing Process:** Assessment/Analysis; **Reference:** Ch 8, Cancer of the Liver, Nursing Care

266. 1 The liver stores carbohydrates as glycogen, which is a polymer of glucose.

2 Glycerol, a byproduct of lipids, combines with three fatty acids to form a triglyceride. 3 Fat is not stored in the liver. 4 These are not a ready form of energy; combinations of amino acids form protein.

Client Need: Physiological Adaptation; **Cognitive Level:** Comprehension; **Nursing Process:** Assessment/Analysis; **Reference:** Ch 8, Review of Anatomy and Physiology, Liver

267. 3 Lipoproteins, a combination of a fat and a simple protein, have not been formed because of limited protein intake. Therefore fat accumulates in the liver.

1 Deficiency of protein results in the breakdown of tissue (catabolism) and a negative nitrogen balance. 2 Elevations of bile in the blood occur because hepatic ducts are obstructed by the enlarged liver. 4 Individuals with cirrhosis of the liver are likely to have bleeding (rather than clotting) tendencies because of the decreased synthesis of prothrombin.

Client Need: Physiological Adaptation; **Cognitive Level:** Comprehension; **Nursing Process:** Assessment/Analysis; **Reference:** Ch 8, Hepatic Cirrhosis, Data Base

268. 3 With liver failure, the protein intake is limited to 20 g daily to decrease the possibility of hepatic encephalopathy.

1 A high-fat diet is avoided because of the related cardiovascular risks and the related demand for bile. 2 Regeneration of tissue requires a high-calorie, high-carbohydrate diet. 4 Sodium usually is restricted to decrease the accumulation of fluid and help limit ascites and edema.

Client Need: Basic Care and Comfort; **Cognitive Level:** Application; **Integrated Process:** Teaching/Learning; **Nursing Process:** Planning/Implementation; **Reference:** Ch 8, Hepatic Cirrhosis, Nursing Care

269. 3 The hepatic portal vein carries blood from the capillary beds of the viscera (small and large intestinal walls, stomach, spleen, pancreas, gallbladder) to the sinusoids of the liver. The hepatic veins drain the liver sinusoids into the inferior vena cava.

1 The portal vein takes blood to the liver; the hepatic veins drain the liver sinusoids into the inferior vena cava. 2, 4 It enters the superior vena cava from the capillary beds of the viscera.

Client Need: Physiological Adaptation; **Cognitive Level:** Comprehension; **Nursing Process:** Assessment/Analysis; **Reference:** Ch 8, Hepatic Cirrhosis, Data Base

270. 4 The elevated pressure within the portal circulatory system causes elevated pressure in areas of portal systemic collateral circulation (most important, in the distal esophagus and proximal stomach). Hemorrhage is a possible complication.

1 Liver abscesses may occur as a complication of intestinal infections, not portal hypertension. 2 This may be caused by manipulation of the bowel during surgery, peritonitis, neurologic disorders, or organic obstruction, not portal hypertension. 3 Perforation of the duodenum is usually caused by peptic ulcers; it is not a direct result of portal hypertension or cirrhosis.

Client Need: Physiological Adaptation; **Cognitive Level:** Application; **Nursing Process:** Assessment/Analysis; **Reference:** Ch 8, Hepatic Cirrhosis, Data Base

271. **4** With obstruction of the portal vein there is an increase in pressure in the abdominal veins, which empty into the portal system. These veins develop collaterals to circumvent the obstruction. The collaterals are usually in the paraumbilical, hemorrhoidal, and esophageal areas.
1 Esophageal infection does not cause cirrhosis of the liver; cirrhosis of the liver can lead to portal hypertension, which can cause dilated, tortuous veins in the submucosa of the lower esophagus (esophageal varices). **2** Obstruction of this duct blocks flow of bile, causing obstructive jaundice. **3** Kupffer cells are part of the reticuloendothelial system, which helps prevent infection and does not primarily affect venous pressure.
Client Need: Physiological Adaptation; **Cognitive Level:** Application; **Nursing Process:** Assessment/Analysis; **Reference:** Ch 8, Hepatic Cirrhosis, Data Base

272. **4** In cirrhosis of the liver, fibrous scarring within the liver parenchyma compresses the portal veins and causes a backup of blood and increased pressure within the portal system. Fluid seeps into the abdominal cavity (ascites), mainly from the surface of the liver.
1 Lymph does not escape from the liver sinusoids. **2** Plasma osmotic (oncotic) pressure is decreased because of decreased albumin production. **3** Secretion of ADH and aldosterone increases as renal blood flow decreases.
Client Need: Physiological Adaptation; **Cognitive Level:** Application; **Nursing Process:** Assessment/Analysis; **Reference:** Ch 8, Hepatic Cirrhosis, Data Base

273. **3** These activities should be avoided to prevent inaccurate test results.
1 The recorder should be checked every 15 minutes. **2** This is unnecessary. **4** The capsule should be held under the tongue for 1 minute while the unit verifies that the light source is functioning.
Client Need: Reduction of Risk Potential; **Cognitive Level:** Application; **Integrated Process:** Teaching/Learning; **Nursing Process:** Planning/Implementation; **Reference:** Ch 8, Related Procedures, Gastrointestinal Series

274. **1** The increased plasma hydrostatic pressure in the extremities caused by cirrhosis and possible heart failure as a result of liver insufficiency may lead to varicose veins.
2 Toxins are not responsible for varicose veins. **3** Distention of venous walls occurs as a result of increased, rather than decreased, pressure. **4** Decreased plasma protein causes fluid to move out of the vascular compartment into the interstitial spaces.
Client Need: Physiological Adaptation; **Cognitive Level:** Application; **Nursing Process:** Assessment/Analysis; **Reference:** Ch 8, Hepatic Cirrhosis, Data Base

275. **4** This tube includes an esophageal balloon that exerts pressure on inflation, which retards hemorrhage.

1 This is used for gastric decompression, gavage, or lavage; it has one lumen. **2** This is used for gastric decompression; it has two lumens, one for decompression and one for an air vent. **3** This is used for intestinal decompression.
Client Need: Reduction of Risk Potential; **Cognitive Level:** Application; **Nursing Process:** Planning/Implementation; **Reference:** Ch 8, Hepatic Cirrhosis, Data Base

276. **1** Because the liver is unable to detoxify ammonia to urea, protein intake should be further restricted when coma is inevitable.
2, 3, 4 This relatively high intake of protein will increase blood ammonia levels.
Client Need: Basic Care and Comfort; **Cognitive Level:** Application; **Nursing Process:** Planning/Implementation; **Reference:** Ch 8, Hepatic Cirrhosis, Data Base

277. **2** Fat contains 9 kilocalories per gram; carbohydrates and proteins contain 4 kilocalories per gram; therefore 117 + 124 + 20 = 261 kilocalories.
1 This is too few calories. **3, 4** This is too many calories.
Client Need: Basic Care and Comfort; **Cognitive Level:** Application; **Nursing Process:** Evaluation/Outcomes; **Reference:** Ch 8, Review of Nutrients, Sources of Energy

278. **3** An accumulation of nitrogenous wastes in hepatic coma affects the nervous system. Flapping tremors and generalized twitching occur in the second stage of this disease.
1 Stool is often clay-colored because of lack of bile caused by biliary obstruction. **2** Elevated cholesterol levels are not necessarily present. **4** As encephalopathy progresses to coma, all reflexes are absent.
Client Need: Physiological Adaptation; **Cognitive Level:** Application; **Nursing Process:** Assessment/Analysis; **Reference:** Ch 8, Hepatic Cirrhosis, Data Base

279. **1** Bile deposits will impart a yellowish tinge (jaundice or icterus) to the skin, often first observed in the sclerae.
2 Urticaria (or hives) is generally characteristic of an allergic response. **3** Uremic frost is characteristic of kidney failure. **4** Hemangioma is a benign lesion composed of blood vessels.
Client Need: Physiologic Adaptation; **Cognitive Level:** Application; **Nursing Process:** Assessment/Analysis; **Reference:** Ch 8, Hepatic Cirrhosis, Data Base

280. **1** Increased ammonia levels indicate that the liver is unable to detoxify protein byproducts. Neomycin reduces the amount of ammonia-forming bacteria in the intestines.
2 Culture and sensitivity testing is unnecessary; cirrhosis is an inflammatory, not infectious, process. **3** White blood cells may indicate infection; however, this would have no relationship to the need for neomycin enemas. **4** Alanine aminotransferase (ALT), also called serum glutamic-pyruvic transaminase (SGPT), assesses for liver disease but has no relationship to the need for neomycin enemas.

Client Need: Reduction of Risk Potential; **Cognitive Level:** Analysis; **Nursing Process:** Assessment/Analysis; **Reference:** Ch 8, Hepatic Cirrhosis, Data Base

281. 4 One of the many functions of the liver is the manufacture of clotting factors; there is interference of this process in cirrhosis of the liver, resulting in bleeding tendencies.

1 Fat-soluble vitamins (A, D, E, and K), water-soluble vitamins (B, B$_2$, folic acid, and cobalamin), and minerals (including iron) are stored in the liver and this function is also compromised in cirrhosis; therefore these nutrients, including vitamin K, should not be limited. 2 Should the client bleed, the pulse rate may be elevated, but it is not necessary for the client to check the pulse rate several times daily. 3 A client whose prothrombin time is prolonged and platelet count is low should not be taking aspirin, even with milk.

Client Need: Reduction of Risk Potential; **Cognitive Level:** Analysis; **Integrated Process:** Teaching/Learning; **Nursing Process:** Planning/Implementation; **Reference:** Ch 8, Hepatic Cirrhosis, Data Base

282. 4 The diet should be high in protein and calories, low in fat, and gluten-free for individuals with malabsorption syndrome. Protein is needed for tissue rebuilding.

1 The client may prefer foods high in gluten, which would potentiate malabsorption. 2 IV therapy is a dependent function and does not provide all the necessary nutrients. 3 Diarrhea is caused by malabsorption, which accounts for the depressed nutritional status; once the diarrhea is corrected, it is essential to compensate by providing a nutritious diet.

Client Need: Basic Care and Comfort; **Cognitive Level:** Application; **Nursing Process:** Planning/Implementation; **Reference:** Ch 8, Malabsorption Syndrome, Data Base

283. 4 Gluten, a cereal protein, appears to be responsible for morphologic changes of the intestinal mucosa with nontropical sprue (adult celiac disease).

1 Folic acid, along with antimicrobial agents, is used to treat tropical, not celiac, sprue; it causes dramatic improvement in tropical sprue. 2 Vitamin B$_{12}$ may be administered if macrocytic anemia or achlorhydria develops; however, it does not correct the major pathology. 3 The use of corticosteroids may be advantageous with either form of sprue; however, this does not produce the dramatic effect achieved by an approach in another option.

Client Need: Basic Care and Comfort; **Cognitive Level:** Application; **Nursing Process:** Evaluation/Outcomes; **Reference:** Ch 8, Malabsorption Syndrome, Data Base

284. 3 Gluten is found in rye and should be avoided because it is irritating to the GI mucosa.

1, 2, 4 Gluten is not found in this product and does not have to be avoided.

Client Need: Basic Care and Comfort; **Cognitive Level:** Application; **Integrated Process:** Teaching/Learning; **Nursing Process:** Planning/Implementation; **Reference:** Ch 8, Malabsorption Syndrome, Data Base

285. 3 Undigested fat in the feces (steatorrhea) is associated with diseases of the intestinal mucosa (e.g., celiac sprue) or pancreatic enzyme deficiency.

1 Darkening of feces by blood pigments (melena) is related to upper GI bleeding. 2 Bright red blood in the stool is related to lower GI bleeding (e.g., hemorrhoids). 4 Stools containing blood and mucus (currant jelly stools) are associated with intussusception.

Client Need: Physiological Adaptation; **Cognitive Level:** Application; **Nursing Process:** Evaluation/Outcomes; **Reference:** Ch 8, Malabsorption Syndrome, Data Base

286. 4 Neither of these foods contains gluten, and they are permitted in a diet for a client with malabsorption syndrome.

1 The breading on the veal cutlet contains gluten and cannot be eaten by this client. 2 The bread for the sandwich contains gluten. 3 Noodles and crackers contain gluten.

Client Need: Basic Care and Comfort; **Cognitive Level:** Application; **Nursing Process:** Planning/Implementation; **Reference:** Ch 8, Malabsorption Syndrome, Data Base

287. 1 This is low in gluten and can be eaten.

2 Noodles are made of flour high in gluten and should be avoided. 3 Postum is a cereal drink high in gluten and should be avoided. 4 Bread is made with flour high in gluten and should be avoided.

Client Need: Basic Care and Comfort; **Cognitive Level:** Application; **Integrated Process:** Teaching/Learning; **Nursing Process:** Evaluation/Outcomes; **Reference:** Ch 8, Malabsorption Syndrome, Data Base

288. 3 Rebound tenderness is a classic subjective sign of appendicitis.

1 Urinary retention does not cause acute lower right quadrant pain. 2 Hyperacidity causes epigastric, not lower right quadrant, pain. 4 There is generally decreased bowel motility distal to an inflamed appendix.

Client Need: Reduction of Risk Potential; **Cognitive Level:** Application; **Nursing Process:** Assessment/Analysis; **Reference:** Ch 8, Appendicitis, Data Base

289. 4 Muscular rigidity over the affected area is a classic sign of peritonitis.

1 Malaise, rather than hyperactivity, is often associated with peritonitis. 2 Nausea, not hunger, is a common occurrence with peritonitis. 3 Urinary retention may occur following surgery as a complication of anesthesia.

Client Need: Physiological Adaptation; **Cognitive Level:** Application; **Nursing Process:** Assessment/Analysis; **Reference:** Ch 8, Peritonitis, Data Base

290. 3 The semi-Fowler's position aids in drainage and prevents spread of infection throughout the abdominal cavity.

1, 4 This position would not allow for localization of drainage. 2 The Trendelenburg position would contribute to the spread of infection throughout the abdominal cavity.

Client Need: Physiological Adaptation; **Cognitive Level:** Application; **Nursing Process:** Planning/Implementation; **Reference:** Ch 8, Peritonitis, Data Base

291. 2 A rectal catheter should be inserted approximately 4 inches to pass the rectal sphincters.

1 A catheter inserted just 2 inches will not pass beyond the rectal sphincters. 3, 4 This may damage the intestinal mucosa.

Client Need: Basic Care and Comfort; **Cognitive Level:** Comprehension; **Nursing Process:** Planning/Implementation; **Reference:** Ch 8, Related Procedures, Enemas

292. 2 The client's status requires immediate intervention; to delay treatment may prove dangerous because symptoms indicate possible perforation.

1 Diverticulitis can in most cases be treated by diet, rest, and antibiotic therapy. 3 This is not true with the diagnostic techniques presently available. 4 Age is not the factor; the symptoms indicate possible peritonitis.

Client Need: Physiological Adaptation; **Cognitive Level:** Application; **Nursing Process:** Assessment/Analysis; **Reference:** Ch 8, Diverticular Disease, Data Base

293. 4 Because the mucosa of the intestinal tract is damaged, its ability to absorb vitamins taken orally is greatly impaired.

1 Although this is true, the risks associated with IV administration will outweigh the benefits. 2 Vitamins are effective orally unless disease of the GI tract hampers absorption. 3 IV vitamins do not decrease colonic irritability.

Client Need: Pharmacological and Parenteral Therapies; **Cognitive Level:** Application; **Nursing Process:** Assessment/Analysis; **Reference:** Ch 8, Inflammatory Bowel Disease, Regional Enteritis (Crohn's Disease), Data Base

294. 2 When the diseased bowel is removed, the client's symptoms cease.

1 Surgical removal of a body part is not temporary, but permanent. 3 Ulcerative colitis does not progress to Crohn's disease; clients with ulcerative colitis have an increased risk for colorectal cancer. 4 This is not a true statement.

Client Need: Physiological Adaptation; **Cognitive Level:** Application; **Nursing Process:** Assessment/Analysis; **Reference:** Ch 8, Inflammatory Bowel Disease, Ulcerative Colitis, Data Base

295. 1 The caffeine in cola is chemically irritating to the intestinal mucosa. Caffeine also promotes secretion of gastric juice.

2 These are absorbed slowly and are not irritating. 3 These foods do not irritate the bowel and need not be restricted. 4 This is too general; except for those that contain lactose sugars, products containing sugar generally are not irritating to the mucosa.

Client Need: Basic Care and Comfort; **Cognitive Level:** Application; **Integrated Process:** Teaching/Learning; **Nursing Process:** Planning/Implementation; **Reference:** Ch 8, Irritable Bowel Syndrome, Nursing Care

296. 2 The inflammatory process tends to increase peristalsis, causing cramping and diarrhea with subsequent weight loss. As ulceration occurs, loss of blood leads to anemia.

1 Fever may or may not be a sign. 3 Hemoptysis (coughing up blood from the respiratory tract) is not a related sign. 4 Leukocytosis (increased leukocytes in the blood) is not common in this disease.

Client Need: Physiological Adaptation; **Cognitive Level:** Application; **Nursing Process:** Assessment/Analysis; **Reference:** Ch 8, Inflammatory Bowel Disease, Ulcerative Colitis, Data Base

297. 2 Occult blood in the stool could indicate active bleeding.

1 This situation does not warrant this examination. 3 There is no indication that parasites are present; the situation does not warrant this examination. 4 This situation does not warrant culturing.

Client Need: Reduction of Risk Potential; **Cognitive Level:** Application; **Nursing Process:** Assessment/Analysis; **Reference:** Ch 8, Inflammatory Bowel Disease, Ulcerative Colitis, Data Base

298. 3, 1, 4, 2

   __3__ An order of french fries has 372 calories.
   __1__ A garden salad has 95 calories.
   __4__ A Whopper with cheese has 720 calories.
   __2__ Six chicken tenders have 236 calories.

Client Need: Health Promotion and Maintenance; **Cognitive Level:** Analysis; **Integrated Process:** Teaching/Learning; **Nursing Process:** Assessment/Analysis; **Reference:** Ch 8, Review of Nutrients, Sources of Energy

299. 3 Weight loss usually is severe with Crohn's disease; therefore weight gain is a priority; this goal is specific, realistic, and measurable and has a time frame.

1, 2, 4 This is not written in terms that are measurable and it does not have a time frame; although important, it is not as high a priority as another option.

Client Need: Basic Care and Comfort; **Cognitive Level:** Application; **Nursing Process:** Evaluation/Outcomes; **Reference:** Ch 8, Inflammatory Bowel Disease, Regional Enteritis (Crohn's Disease), Nursing Care

300. 1 ☐ Table salt does not irritate the intestinal mucosa and does not need to be avoided.

   2 ☒ Cola drinks contain caffeine, which is chemically irritating to the intestinal mucosa and should be avoided.
   3 ☐ Amino acids do not irritate the intestinal mucosa.
   4 ☐ Rice products do not irritate the intestinal mucosa.
   5 ☒ Milk products are chemically irritating to the intestinal mucosa and should be avoided.

Client Need: Basic Care and Comfort; **Cognitive Level:** Analysis; **Integrated Process:** Teaching/Learning; **Nursing Process:** Planning/Implementation; **Reference:** Ch 8, Inflammatory Bowel Disease, Ulcerative Colitis, Nursing Care

301. 2 The inflammatory process associated with colitis increases peristalsis, causing abdominal cramping, diarrhea, and weight loss.

1 Coughing up blood from the respiratory tract (hemoptysis) is not associated with colitis. **3** Anemia, not polycythemia, is associated with colitis. **4** Decreased WBC count (leukopenia) is not associated with colitis.

Client Need: Physiological Adaptation; **Cognitive Level:** Application; **Nursing Process:** Assessment/Analysis; **Reference:** Ch 8, Inflammatory Bowel Disease, Ulcerative Colitis, Nursing Care

302. **2** This is low residue and is less irritating to the colon than the other choices.

1 This contains cellulose, which is not absorbed and irritates the colon. **3, 4** Milk contains lactose, which is irritating to the colon.

Client Need: Basic Care and Comfort; **Cognitive Level:** Analysis; **Integrated Process:** Teaching/Learning; **Nursing Process:** Evaluation/Outcomes; **Reference:** Ch 8, Inflammatory Bowel Disease, Ulcerative Colitis, Nursing Care

303. **3** Intussusception is the telescoping or prolapse of a segment of the bowel into the lumen of an immediately connecting part.

1 Volvulus is a twisting of the bowel onto itself. **2** Adhesions are bands of scar tissue that can compress the bowel. **4** Herniation describes protrusion of an organ through the wall that contains it.

Client Need: Physiological Adaptation; **Cognitive Level:** Comprehension; **Integrated Process:** Teaching/Learning; **Nursing Process:** Planning/Implementation; **Reference:** Ch 8, Intestinal Obstruction, Data Base

304. **4** Emotional stress of any kind can stimulate peristalsis and thereby increase the volume of drainage.

1 The client should be encouraged to eat a diet as normal as possible. **2** Ileostomy drainage is liquefied and continuous, so irrigations are not indicated. **3** The stoma will start to drain within the first 24 hours after surgery.

Client Need: Reduction of Risk Potential; **Cognitive Level:** Application; **Nursing Process:** Planning/Implementation; **Reference:** Ch 8, Inflammatory Bowel Disease, Ulcerative Colitis, Nursing Care

305. **2** Vitamin B_{12} (extrinsic factor) combines with intrinsic factor, a substance secreted by the parietal cells of the gastric mucosa, forming hemopoietic factor. Hemopoietic factor is only absorbed in the ileum, from which it travels to bone marrow and stimulates erythropoiesis.

1 This is not absorbed in the ileum. **3** Iron absorption does not occur in the ileum. **4** Trace elements of these substances are not absorbed in the ileum.

Client Need: Physiological Adaptation; **Cognitive Level:** Application; **Nursing Process:** Evaluation/Outcomes; **Reference:** Ch 8, Review of Anatomy and Physiology, Small Intestine

306. **1** Trauma to the abdominal wall and to the stoma should be avoided, so contact sports are contraindicated.

2, 3, 4 Trauma to the abdominal wall is a minimal risk in this sport.

Client Need: Reduction of Risk Potential; **Cognitive Level:** Application; **Integrated Process:** Teaching/Learning; **Nursing Process:** Planning/Implementation; **Reference:** Ch 8, Cancer of the Small Intestine, Colon, or Rectum, Nursing Care

307. **1** To take advantage of the anatomic position of the sigmoid colon and the effect of gravity, the client should be placed in a left Sims' or left side-lying position for the enema.

2, 3, 4 This position does not facilitate the flow of fluid into the sigmoid colon by gravity.

Client Need: Basic Care and Comfort; **Cognitive Level:** Application; **Nursing Process:** Planning/Implementation; **Reference:** Ch 8, Related Procedures, Enemas

308. **3** Because neomycin has limited absorption from the GI tract, it exerts its antibiotic effect on the intestinal mucosa. In preparation for GI surgery, the level of microbial organisms will be reduced.

1 Neomycin is nephrotoxic. **2** Because of limited absorption from the GI tract, the systemic effect is minimal. **4** Neomycin is mainly effective in suppression of intestinal bacteria.

Client Need: Pharmacological and Parenteral Therapies; **Cognitive Level:** Comprehension; **Nursing Process:** Assessment/Analysis; **Reference:** Ch 8, Cancer of the Small Intestine, Colon, or Rectum, Data Base

309. **2** The client must be ready to accept changes in body image and function; this acceptance will facilitate mastery of the techniques of colostomy care and optimal use of community resources.

1, 3, 4 Specific knowledge can be imparted only when an individual is ready to learn; it requires acceptance of a new body image.

Client Need: Psychosocial Integrity; **Cognitive Level:** Application; **Integrated Process:** Caring; **Nursing Process:** Assessment/Analysis; **Reference:** Ch 8, Inflammatory Bowel Disease, Ulcerative Colitis, Nursing Care

310. **2** Neomycin provides preoperative intestinal antisepsis.

1 The desired effect of this drug is unrelated to kidney function; nephrotoxicity is a side effect. **3** It will not prevent metastasis. **4** This is not the purpose of administering this medication.

Client Need: Pharmacological and Parenteral Therapies; **Cognitive Level:** Application; **Integrated Process:** Teaching/Learning; **Nursing Process:** Planning/Implementation; **Reference:** Ch 8, Cancer of the Small Intestine, Colon, or Rectum, Data Base

311. **3** This describes the stoma that has adequate vascular perfusion.

1, 2, 4 This indicates inadequate perfusion of the stoma.

Client Need: Physiological Adaptation; **Cognitive Level:** Application; **Nursing Process:** Evaluation/Outcomes; **Reference:** Ch 8, Inflammatory Bowel Disease, Ulcerative Colitis, Nursing Care

312. **3** When GI absorption is inadequate, total parenteral nutrition (TPN) is the nutritional therapy of choice because it provides needed nutrients.

1 TPN is usually used in chronic or long-term therapy, not for short-term therapy. **2** TPN is used for total, not supplemental, nutrition. **4** This is not the indication for TPN; a feeding tube would be used.
Client Need: Pharmacological and Parenteral Therapies; **Cognitive Level:** Application; **Integrated Process:** Teaching/Learning, **Nursing Process:** Evaluation/Outcomes; **Reference:** Ch 8, Related Procedures, Parenteral Replacement Therapy

313. **2** Because emotional stress can influence the progress of Crohn's disease, initially the nurse should help the client to explore self-attitudes to aid in better understanding the feelings engendered by her boyfriend dating others.
1 Initially the nurse should help the client explore the situation and the feelings it engenders rather than involve the boyfriend. **3** The client should make the decision about seeing her boyfriend. **4** This is premature; the client is not ready for a joint counseling session.
Client Need: Psychosocial Integrity; **Cognitive Level:** Application; **Integrated Process:** Caring; **Nursing Process:** Planning/Implementation; **Reference:** Ch 8, Inflammatory Bowel Disease, Regional Enteritis (Crohn's Disease), Nursing Care

314. **4** In ulcerative colitis, pathology is usually in the descending colon (left side); in Crohn's disease, it is primarily in the terminal ileum, cecum, and ascending colon on the right side.
1 Ulcerative colitis, as the name implies, affects the colon, not the small intestine. **2** There is no direct correlation of colitis with malignancy of the bowel, although psychologic, environmental, genetic, and nutritional factors, as well as preexisting disease, appear to be influential in malignancy.
3 Involvement is in the distal portion of the colon, not the proximal portion.
Client Need: Physiological Adaptation; **Cognitive Level:** Analysis; **Nursing Process:** Assessment/Analysis; **Reference:** Ch 8, Inflammatory Bowel Disease, Ulcerative Colitis, Data Base

315. **3** If medical management has failed, this is the next logical choice because it removes the affected intestine.
1 Psychotherapy might improve the client's ability to cope with the disease, but it will not solve the physical problems. **2, 4** This is a classic intervention that would have been tried during prior exacerbations and it has failed.
Client Need: Reduction of Risk Potential; **Cognitive Level:** Application; **Nursing Process:** Planning/Implementation; **Reference:** Ch 8, Inflammatory Bowel Disease, Ulcerative Colitis, Data Base

316. **1** This takes advantage of the gastrocolic reflex that occurs after eating; also, it is important to establish a time that is at the same time every day; before leaving the house for the day is the most appropriate time for a person who has a job outside the home.
2 A person working outside the house should schedule irrigations after breakfast to take advantage of the gastrocolic reflex and before

the day's activities begin. **3** This would not take advantage of the gastrocolic reflex that occurs after eating. **4** New bowel habits have to be established; irrigations take time to accomplish and need to scheduled before the day's work activities begin.
Client Need: Physiological Adaptation; **Cognitive Level:** Application; **Integrated Process:** Teaching/Learning; **Nursing Process:** Planning/Implementation; **Reference:** Ch 8, Related Procedures, Colostomy Irrigation

317. **2** The stoma of a colostomy must be dilated with a lubricated, gloved finger to prevent strictures and subsequent obstruction.
1 Clothing need not be special but should be nonconstricting. **3** Once healing has occurred, activity is not limited. **4** Diet should be as close to normal for the individual as possible; gas-forming foods should be avoided.
Client Need: Physiological Adaptation; **Cognitive Level:** Application; **Integrated Process:** Teaching/Learning; **Nursing Process:** Planning/Implementation; **Reference:** Ch 8, Cancer of the Small Intestine, Colon, or Rectum, Nursing Care

318. **3** Although foods that produce gas are generally avoided, the diet should be as close to normal as possible for optimal physiologic and psychologic adaptation.
1 A high-protein diet is important until healing occurs; but a balanced diet generally meets nutritional needs for protein. **2** There is no need to limit fiber; it provides bulk necessary for soft, formed stools. **4** Absorption of nutrients is unaffected; there is no need to increase carbohydrate intake.
Client Need: Basic Care and Comfort; **Cognitive Level:** Application; **Integrated Process:** Teaching/Learning; **Nursing Process:** Planning/Implementation; **Reference:** Ch 8, Cancer of the Small Intestine, Colon, or Rectum, Nursing Care

319. **2** Isotonic saline most closely resembles normal body fluids; it will not cause an imbalance by pulling extra fluids and electrolytes out of the circulation.
1, 3 Hypotonic solutions would allow absorption of fluid into the circulation, resulting in dilution of electrolytes and possible circulatory overload.
4 Hypertonic solutions would draw fluids out of the circulation into the GI tract; glucose provides a medium for bacterial growth.
Client Need: Reduction of Risk Potential; **Cognitive Level:** Application; **Nursing Process:** Planning/Implementation; **Reference:** Ch 8, Intestinal Obstruction, Nursing Care

320. **3** Surgery on the bowel has no direct anatomic or physiologic effect on sexual performance. However, psychologic factors could hamper this function, and the nurse should encourage verbalization.
1 There is no reason why sexual relationships must be curtailed. **2** Although it may take several months to resume satisfying sexual relationships, the surgery has no direct physiologic effect. **4** Although a

partner should understand the nature of the surgery, the focus at this time should be on the client.
Client Need: Psychosocial Integrity; **Cognitive Level:** Application; **Integrated Process:** Teaching/Learning; **Nursing Process:** Planning/Implementation; **Reference:** Ch 8, Cancer of the Small Intestine, Colon, or Rectum, Nursing Care

321. 4 A transverse colostomy is an opening created in the transverse colon. The rectal tube should be pointed to the proximal intestine, which will contain the feces.
1 A water-soluble lubricant is generally used to facilitate insertion. 2 There are no sphincters, so bearing down is unnecessary. 3 Continual force may traumatize the mucosa; lack of nerve endings diminishes sensation.
Client Need: Physiological Adaptation; **Cognitive Level:** Application; **Nursing Process:** Planning/Implementation; **Reference:** Ch 8, Related Procedures, Colostomy Irrigation

322. 3 An enema or ostomy irrigation can cause cramping. Cramping will generally subside if the tubing is clamped for a few minutes; the procedure can then be continued.
1 Discontinuing the irrigation could lead to ineffective evacuation of the colon. 2 Lowering the container will decrease the rate of flow, but fluid will continue to enter the colon if the container remains above the stoma. 4 This can injure the mucosa and does not affect cramping.
Client Need: Physiological Adaptation; **Cognitive Level:** Application; **Nursing Process:** Planning/Implementation; **Reference:** Ch 8, Related Procedures, Colostomy Irrigation

323. 2 This is far enough to direct the flow of solution into the bowel.
1 This is inadequate; fluid may leak back around the catheter. 3, 4 This may cause trauma to the mucosa.
Client Need: Physiological Adaptation; **Cognitive Level:** Comprehension; **Nursing Process:** Planning/Implementation; **Reference:** Ch 8, Related Procedures, Colostomy Irrigation

324. 3 A colostomy irrigation is much like a tap-water enema. The solution must be held high enough to allow it to flow into the bowel but not so high that it flows rapidly, or it can cause cramping or mucosal injury.
1, 2 This does not represent maximum height permitted and may not ensure flow of solution into the bowel. 4 This is too high and could cause intestinal trauma.
Client Need: Physiological Adaptation; **Cognitive Level:** Comprehension; **Integrated Process:** Teaching/Learning; **Nursing Process:** Planning/Implementation; **Reference:** Ch 8, Related Procedures, Colostomy Irrigation

325. 4 If the area is not kept both clean and dry, drainage from the colostomy can quickly cause a breakdown of the skin around the stoma. This, in combination with a warm, moist surface, also predisposes the individual to infection.
1, 2 Although oral fluids are withheld until peristalsis returns, it is essential that parenteral fluids be administered to replace the losses incurred

by surgery. 3 The client is often unable to accept the altered body image and must be given time to adjust before participating actively in self-care.
Client Need: Physiological Adaptation; **Cognitive Level:** Application; **Nursing Process:** Planning/Implementation; **Reference:** Ch 8, Cancer of the Small Intestine, Colon, and Rectum, Nursing Care

326. 3 There are few physical restraints on activity postoperatively, but the client may have emotional problems resulting from the body image changes.
1 Independence should be encouraged; however, some activities may require up to 3 months before resumption. 2 Swimming is not prohibited because water does not harm the stoma. 4 No changes in activities are necessary.
Client Need: Reduction of Risk Potential; **Cognitive Level:** Application; **Integrated Process:** Teaching/Learning; **Nursing Process:** Planning/Implementation; **Reference:** Ch 8, Cancer of the Small Intestine, Colon, or Rectum, Nursing Care

327. 3 A client with a fecal impaction has the urge to defecate but is unable to do so.
1 Flatulence may occur as a result of immobility, not just obstruction. 2 Anorexia may occur with an impaction but may also be caused by other conditions. 4 The frequency of bowel movements varies for individuals; it may be normal for this individual not to have a bowel movement for several days.
Client Need: Basic Care and Comfort; **Cognitive Level:** Analysis; **Nursing Process:** Assessment/Analysis; **Reference:** Ch 8, Intestinal Obstruction, Data Base

328. 2 When the bowel is impacted with hardened feces, there is often seepage of liquid feces around the obstruction and thus uncontrolled diarrhea.
1 The bowel may become distended if completely obstructed, but this is a late symptom if it occurs at all. 3 This is indicative of lower GI bleeding. 4 There are often frequent liquid bowel movements in the presence of an impaction.
Client Need: Basic Care and Comfort; **Cognitive Level:** Application; **Nursing Process:** Assessment/Analysis; **Reference:** Ch 8, Intestinal Obstruction, Data Base

329. 4 Prune juice and warm water can be administered prophylactically by the nurse to promote defecation. Prune juice irritates the bowel mucosa, stimulating peristalsis. Fiber in the diet increases fecal volume, which stimulates intestinal motility and the reflex for defecation.
1 This should be avoided because it can promote dependency and can result in electrolyte imbalance. 2 The routine use of laxatives promotes dependency. 3 The client is bedbound and is unable to use a commode.
Client Need: Basic Care and Comfort; **Cognitive Level:** Application; **Nursing Process:** Assessment/Analysis; **Reference:** Ch 8, Intestinal Obstruction, Nursing Care

330. 4 Fiber absorbs water, swells, and consequently stretches the bowel wall, promoting peristalsis, mass movements, and defecation. Smooth muscle tends to contract when stretched because of the reflex activity of stretch receptors.

1 Bulk caused by fiber does not irritate the bowel wall. 2 There is no chemical stimulation. 3 Bacterial action is not involved in the process by which bulk stimulates defecation.

Client Need: Basic Care and Comfort; **Cognitive Level:** Application; **Integrated Process:** Teaching/Learning; **Nursing Process:** Evaluation/Outcomes; **Reference:** Ch 8, Review of Diets

331. 3 A low-residue diet limits stool formation.

1 Bland diets are usually employed in the management of upper, not lower, GI disturbances. 2 Although a clear diet is low in residue, it does not meet normal nutritional needs. 4 A high-protein diet is indicated postoperatively to promote healing.

Client Need: Basic Care and Comfort; **Cognitive Level:** Application; **Nursing Process:** Planning/Implementation; **Reference:** Ch 8, Hemorrhoids, Data Base

332. 1 Constipation and prolonged standing may cause this problem.

2 Hypertension does not contribute to the development of hemorrhoids. 3 Spicy foods may irritate hemorrhoids but do not cause them. 4 This is unrelated to the development of hemorrhoids.

Client Need: Basic Care and Comfort; **Cognitive Level:** Application; **Integrated Process:** Teaching/Learning; **Nursing Process:** Assessment/Analysis; **Reference:** Ch 8, Hemorrhoids, Data Base

333. 4 Rectal bleeding is a common problem when hemorrhoids are present.

1 Pruritus is not a symptom that can be observed. 2 Flatulence is unrelated to hemorrhoids. 3 Anal stenosis is not a complication of hemorrhoids.

Client Need: Basic Care and Comfort; **Cognitive Level:** Application; **Nursing Process:** Assessment/Analysis; **Reference:** Ch 8, Hemorrhoids, Nursing Care

334. 2 Stool softeners are widely used to avoid straining on defecation and constipation.

1 Enemas may be ordered several days after surgery if the client has not had a bowel movement. 3 Baths are advised to promote healing and cleaning of the area. 4 Light dressings of witch hazel may be used to promote drainage and healing.

Client Need: Pharmacological and Parenteral Therapies; **Cognitive Level:** Analysis; **Nursing Process:** Planning/Implementation; **Reference:** Ch 8, Hemorrhoids, Nursing Care

335. 1 Any situation in which a needle is inserted under the skin is a potential source of hepatitis; according to the Centers for Disease Control and Prevention the range for the incubation period is 45 to 180 days; however, the average incubation period is 60 to 90 days.

2 The range for the incubation period is 45 to 180 days. 3 Hepatitis B is not transmitted by casual proximity with others. 4 Hepatitis B is not

transmitted via inadequate sanitation or a contaminated water supply.

Client Need: Physiological Adaptation; **Cognitive Level:** Analysis; **Nursing Process:** Assessment/Analysis; **Reference:** Ch 8, Hepatitis, Data Base

336. 1 The client is exhibiting classic symptoms of hyperglycemia, and simple serum glucose monitoring evaluated by a glucose monitoring machine would help guide the nurse's next action.

2 This is a useless assessment; urinary output must be evaluated in relation to intake. 3 This may be a secondary action to assess for overhydration; if headache alone were present, rather than the classic signs of hyperglycemia, taking the blood pressure might be the initial action. 4 This is unnecessary; the symptoms do not indicate infection.

Client Need: Pharmacological and Parenteral Therapies; **Cognitive Level:** Analysis; **Nursing Process:** Evaluation/Outcomes; **Reference:** Ch 8, Related Procedures, Parenteral Replacement Therapy

337. 2 This is the only vegetable listed that is included in a low-residue diet; this vegetable is low in fiber.

1, 3, 4 This vegetable contains more fiber than creamed potatoes.

Client Need: Basic Care and Comfort; **Cognitive Level:** Application; **Integrated Process:** Teaching/Learning; **Nursing Process:** Planning/Implementation; **Reference:** Ch 8, Review of Diets

338. 4 This drug is a piperidine derivative that acts directly on the intestinal muscles to decrease peristalsis.

1 This drug is a laxative, not an antidiarrheal; it increases GI motility. 2 This is not an antidiarrheal, but a bulk laxative that promotes an easier expulsion of feces. 3 This drug corrects constipation, not diarrhea; water and fat are increased in the intestine, permitting easier expulsion of feces.

Client Need: Pharmacological and Parenteral Therapies; **Cognitive Level:** Analysis; **Nursing Process:** Planning/Implementation; **Reference:** Ch 8, Antidiarrheals

339. 3 Drugs are available to help reduce viral load (antivirals), including lamivudine (Epivir HBV), interferon alfa, and adefovir dipivoxil (Hepsera).

1 Although this is a true statement, sedatives are given only PRN and do not treat the hepatitis. 2 This is used only during the incubation period. 4 Vitamins are used as adjunctive therapy and will not eliminate the hepatitis.

Client Need: Pharmacological and Parenteral Therapies; **Cognitive Level:** Analysis; **Nursing Process:** Planning/Implementation; **Reference:** Ch 8, Hepatitis, Data Base

340. 3 The diet should be high in carbohydrates with moderate to high protein and low fat content.

1, 4 This is too high in fat. 2 This is too low in carbohydrates.

Client Need: Basic Care and Comfort; **Cognitive Level:** Analysis; **Integrated Process:** Teaching/Learning; **Nursing Process:** Evaluation/Outcomes; **Reference:** Ch 8, Hepatitis, Data Base

341. 1 Hepatitis A microorganisms are transmitted via the anal-oral route; handwashing, particularly after toileting, is the most important precaution.

2 This will not deter the spread of the virus; handwashing is necessary. **3, 4** Hepatitis A microorganisms exit through the rectum, not the respiratory tract.
Client Need: Safety and Infection Control; Cognitive Level: Application; Integrated Process: Teaching/Learning; Nursing Process: Evaluation/Outcomes; Reference: Ch 8, Hepatitis, Nursing Care

342. **2** This is an expected response during the first 24 hours after a gastric resection because of oozing of blood and blood coagulation.
1 These are normal characteristics of gastric contents, which are unexpected after gastric surgery. **3** This indicates hemorrhage, which is unexpected. **4** Coffee ground material results from blood that has been digested by the gastric acid; gastric bleeding with a nasogastric tube in place will be red because gastric acids will not have time to act on the blood.
Client Need: Reduction of Risk Potential; Cognitive Level: Application; Nursing Process: Evaluation/Outcomes; Reference: Ch 8, Peptic Ulcer Disease, Nursing Care

ENDOCRINE SYSTEM

343. **4** Because water is not being reabsorbed, urine is dilute, resulting in a low specific gravity.
1 Diabetes insipidus is not a disorder of glucose metabolism; blood glucose levels are not affected. **2** As fluid is lost from the vascular compartment, serum osmolarity increases. **3** Loss of fluid may actually lower blood pressure.
Client Need: Physiological Adaptation; Cognitive Level: Application; Nursing Process: Assessment/Analysis; Reference: Ch 9, Diabetes Insipidus, Data Base

344. **3** Deficient ADH from the posterior pituitary (diabetes insipidus) can be caused by head trauma; water is not conserved by the body and excess amounts of urine are produced.
1 This would cause decreased urine production. **2** Although this could cause polyuria, it is associated with diabetes mellitus, not diabetes insipidus. **4** While this could cause dilute urine, it is unlikely that a client with head trauma would receive excess fluid because of the danger of increased intracranial pressure.
Client Need: Physiological Adaptation; Cognitive Level: Analysis; Nursing Process: Assessment/Analysis; Reference: Ch 8, Related Anatomy and Physiology, Structures of the Endocrine System

345. **1** Antidiuretic hormone aids the body in retaining fluid by causing the nephrons to reabsorb water.
2 Reabsorption of glucose is not affected, only the reabsorption of water. **3, 4** The glomeruli are not affected.
Client Need: Physiological Adaptation; Cognitive Level: Comprehension; Nursing Process: Assessment/Analysis; Reference: Ch 9, Review of Anatomy and Physiology, Pituitary Gland

346. **3** These agents are classified as antiinflammatory or immunosuppressive. Glucocorticoids interfere with the body's response to microorganisms but do not directly promote the spread of enteroviruses.
1 Immunosuppressant action causes bone marrow depression, which decreases the number of WBCs. **2** They interfere with antibody production. **4** They interfere with the release of enzymes responsible for the inflammatory response.
Client Need: Pharmacological and Parenteral Therapies; Cognitive Level: Analysis; Nursing Process: Assessment/Analysis; Reference: Ch 9, Adrenocorticoids

347. **2** Endocrine gland secretions (hormones) are inactivated by the liver and other tissues fairly rapidly; continuous hormonal secretion by the endocrine glands is regulated by immediate feedback controls, and the body's metabolism is always close to being suitable to the body's immediate needs.
1, 3, 4 This time interval does not represent secretory patterns of the endocrine glands.
Client Need: Physiological Adaptation; Cognitive Level: Knowledge; Nursing Process: Assessment/Analysis; Reference: Ch 9, Review of Anatomy and Physiology, Function of the Endocrine System

348. **4** Reabsorption of sodium and water in the kidney tubules decreases urinary output and retains body fluids.
1, 2 The opposite is true. **3** There is no effect on filtration with ADH; ADH increases reabsorption in the tubules.
Client Need: Physiological Adaptation; Cognitive Level: Comprehension; Nursing Process: Assessment/Analysis; Reference: Ch 9, Review of Anatomy and Physiology, Pituitary Gland

349. **1** ☐ Oliguria, not polyuria, occurs as ADH acts on nephrons to cause water to be reabsorbed from the glomerular filtrate.
2 ☒ Excessive levels of ADH cause inappropriate free water retention; for every liter of fluid retained, the client will gain approximately 2.2 lb.
3 ☐ Because of water reabsorption, blood volume may increase, causing hypertension, not hypotension.
4 ☒ Free water retention results in a hypoosmolar state with a dilutional hyponatremia.
5 ☐ This increases, not decreases, as a result of increased urine concentration.
Client Need: Reduction of Risk Potential; Cognitive Level: Analysis; Nursing Process: Assessment/Analysis; Reference: Ch 9, Syndrome of Inappropriate Antidiuretic Hormone Secretion, Data Base

350. **2** The hypophysis (pituitary) does not directly regulate insulin release. This is controlled by serum glucose levels. Because somatotropin release will stop after the hypophysectomy, any elevation of blood glucose level caused by somatotropin will also stop.
1 This effect may be expected after a hypophysectomy because follicle-stimulating hormone and its releasing factor will no longer be

present to stimulate spermatogenesis. **3** Thyroid-stimulating hormone will not be present; extrinsic thyroxine will have to be taken. **4** ACTH, which stimulates glucocorticoid secretion by the adrenal glands, is absent and cortisone will have to be administered.
Client Need: Physiological Adaptation; **Cognitive Level:** Analysis; **Integrated Process:** Teaching/Learning; **Nursing Process:** Evaluation/Outcomes; **Reference:** Ch 9, Hyperpituitarism, Data Base

351. 4 Because the pituitary gland is located in the brain, edema after surgery may result in increased intracranial pressure.
1 This may follow any surgery because of the effects of anesthesia and is not a specific occurrence following cranial surgery. **2** This is not an initial sign of increased intracranial pressure. This may be the result of pressure on the medulla caused by increased intracranial pressure. **3** This may occur with any surgery, not just a hypophysectomy.
Client Need: Reduction of Risk Potential; **Cognitive Level:** Application; **Nursing Process:** Evaluation/Outcomes; **Reference:** Ch 9, Hyperpituitarism, Nursing Care

352. 2 The adrenal glands, stimulated by the sympathetic nervous system, secrete epinephrine during stressful situations. The ensuing alarm reaction involves rapid adjustment of the body to meet the emergency situation.
1, 3, 4 There may be modification in secretion of hormones from this gland, but it is not directly related to meeting emergency situations.
Client Need: Physiological Adaptation; **Cognitive Level:** Comprehension; **Nursing Process:** Assessment/Analysis; **Reference:** Ch 9, Review of Anatomy and Physiology, Adrenal Gland

353. 1 Increased levels of steroids will accelerate bone demineralization.
2 Hyperparathyroidism, not hypoparathyroidism, accelerates bone demineralization. **3** Weight-bearing that occurs with strenuous activity promotes bone integrity by preventing bone demineralization. **4** Although estrogen promotes deposition of calcium into bone, high levels would not be prescribed for osteoporosis; hormone replacement therapy is associated with an increased risk for cancer of the breast.
Client Need: Pharmacological and Parenteral Therapies; **Cognitive Level:** Analysis; **Nursing Process:** Assessment/Analysis; **Reference:** Ch 9, Adrenocorticoids

354. 4 Clinical presentation of type 1 diabetes is characterized by acute onset and therefore there is no time to develop the long-term complications that are common with long-standing disease; 20% of newly diagnosed clients with type 2 diabetes demonstrate complications because the diabetes has gone undetected for an extended period of time.
1 Clinical presentation of type 1 diabetes is rapid, not slow, as pancreatic beta cells are destroyed by an autoimmune process; in type 2 diabetes, the body

is still producing some insulin, and therefore the onset of signs and symptoms is slow. **2** In type 1 diabetes, clients are generally lean or have an ideal weight; 80% to 90% of clients with type 2 diabetes are overweight. **3** Type 1 diabetes requires diet control, exercise, and subcutaneous administration of insulin, not oral agents; oral agents are used in type 2 diabetes when some insulin is still being produced.
Client Need: Physiological Adaptation; **Cognitive Level:** Analysis, **Nursing Process:** Assessment/Analysis; **Reference:** Ch 9, Diabetes Mellitus, Data Base

355. 2 Steroid therapy is usually instituted preoperatively and continued intraoperatively to prepare for the acute adrenal insufficiency that follows surgery.
1 The diet must supply ample, not high, protein and potassium; however, it must be low in calories, carbohydrates, and sodium to promote weight loss and reduce fluid retention. **3** A 24-hour urine specimen is unnecessary. **4** Glucocorticoids must be administered preoperatively to prevent adrenal insufficiency during surgery.
Client Need: Pharmacological and Parenteral Therapies; **Cognitive Level:** Analysis; **Nursing Process:** Planning/Implementation; **Reference:** Ch 9, Primary Aldosteronism, Data Base

356. 4 Excess glucocorticoids cause hyperglycemia and signs of diabetes mellitus may develop.
1 Adrenocortical hormones cause sodium retention and subsequent weight gain. **2** ACTH affects the adrenal cortex, not the pancreas. **3** Although muscle wasting is associated with excessive corticoid production, this will not cause diabetes mellitus.
Client Need: Physiological Adaptation; **Cognitive Level:** Analysis; **Nursing Process:** Assessment/Analysis; **Reference:** Ch 9, Review of Anatomy and Physiology, Pituitary Gland

357. 3 Hyperplasia of the adrenal cortex leads to increased secretion of cortical hormones, which causes signs of Cushing's syndrome.
1 This malfunction of the pituitary would result in Simmonds' disease (panhypopituitarism), which has symptoms similar to those for Addison's disease. **2** ACTH stimulates production of adrenal hormones. Inadequate ACTH would result in addisonian symptoms. **4** Cushing's syndrome results from excessive cortical hormones.
Client Need: Physiological Adaptation; **Cognitive Level:** Comprehension; **Nursing Process:** Assessment/Analysis; **Reference:** Ch 9, Cushing's Syndrome, Data Base

358. 2 Cushing's syndrome results from excess adrenocortical activity. Hypercortisolism causes fat redistribution, resulting in "buffalo hump"; it also contributes to slow wound healing, hirsutism, weight gain, hypertension, acne, moon face, thin arms and legs, and behavioral changes.
1 Menorrhagia (excessive menstrual bleeding) does not occur; menses may cease or be scanty because of virilization. **3** Edema does not occur

except when heart failure is present and severe.
4 Headaches are not caused by this syndrome.
Client Need: Physiological Adaptation; **Cognitive Level:** Application; **Nursing Process:** Assessment/Analysis; **Reference:** Ch 9, Cushing's Syndrome, Data Base

359. **1** Excess adrenocorticoids cause emotional lability, euphoria, and psychosis.

2 Increased secretion of androgens results in hirsutism. **3** Although a moon face is associated with corticosteroid therapy, ectomorphism is a term for a tall, thin, genetically determined body type and is unrelated to Cushing's syndrome. **4** Capillary fragility results in multiple ecchymotic areas.
Client Need: Physiological Adaptation; **Cognitive Level:** Application; **Nursing Process:** Assessment/Analysis; **Reference:** Ch 9, Cushing's Syndrome, Data Base

360. **2** As a result of increased cortisol levels, glucose metabolism is altered, which may contribute to an increase in blood glucose levels.

1 Increased mineralocorticoids will decrease urine output. **3** Sodium is retained by the kidneys but potassium is excreted. **4** The immune response is suppressed.
Client Need: Physiological Adaptation; **Cognitive Level:** Comprehension; **Nursing Process:** Assessment/Analysis; **Reference:** Ch 9, Review of Anatomy and Physiology, Pituitary Gland

361. **1** Depending on the purpose of the collection, a preservative to prevent breakdown of the specimen may be necessary.

2 This is not necessary. **3** The last specimen should be collected as close as possible to the end of the 24-hour period and added to the urine collected. **4** Collecting urine for the next 24 hours, not checking the I&O for the previous 24 hours, is important.
Client Need: Reduction of Risk Potential; **Cognitive Level:** Application; **Nursing Process:** Assessment/Analysis; **Reference:** Ch 9, Addison's Disease, Nursing Care

362. **4** Adrenal steroids help an individual adjust to stress. Unless received from external sources, there is no hormone available to cope with surgical stresses after an adrenalectomy.

1 Glucose stores (glycogen) will be utilized after surgery to adapt to surgery. Insulin is the hormone that facilitates conversion of glucose to glycogen. **2** Steroids do not increase inflammatory reactions. **3** Steroids would result in fluid retention, not loss.
Client Need: Pharmacological and Parenteral Therapies; **Cognitive Level:** Analysis; **Nursing Process:** Assessment/Analysis; **Reference:** Ch 9, Primary Aldosteronism, Data Base

363. **4** Hydrocortisone succinate (Solu-Cortef) is a glucocorticoid. A client undergoing bilateral adrenalectomy must be given adrenocortical hormones so that adjustment to the sudden lack of these hormones that occurs with this surgery can take place.

1 Because the adrenal glands are removed, ACTH will have no target gland on which to act. **2** Insulin

is produced by the pancreas, and its function is not altered by this surgery. **3** Because the surgery involves the adrenals, not the pituitary gland, secretion of pituitary hormones will not be affected.
Client Need: Pharmacological and Parenteral Therapies; **Cognitive Level:** Analysis; **Nursing Process:** Planning/Implementation; **Reference:** Ch 9, Adrenocorticoids

364. **1** After an adrenalectomy, adrenal insufficiency causes hypotension because of fluid and electrolyte alterations.

2 Hypoglycemia may be a problem stemming from the loss of glucocorticoids. **3** Hyponatremia may occur because of the lack of mineralocorticoid production. **4** Potassium ions may be retained because of the lack of mineralocorticoids.
Client Need: Reduction of Risk Potential; **Cognitive Level:** Application; **Nursing Process:** Evaluation/Outcomes; **Reference:** Ch 9, Primary Aldosteronism, Nursing Care

365. **3** Clients with adrenocortical insufficiency who are receiving steroid therapy usually require increased amounts of medication during periods of stress, because they are unable to produce the increased levels of glucocorticoids needed by the body at this time.

1 Although sedation may be prescribed, the major concern is the regulation of glucocorticoids in the presence of emotional or physiologic stress. **2** Increased stress requires increased glucocorticoids. **4** Although these symptoms may occur and may be minimized by an increase in glucocorticoids, the primary reason for an adjustment in dosage is to assist the body's ability to adapt to stress.
Client Need: Reduction of Risk Potential; **Cognitive Level:** Analysis; **Integrated Process:** Communication/Documentation; **Nursing Process:** Assessment/Analysis; **Reference:** Ch 9, Primary Aldosteronism, Nursing Care

366. **4** A client with Cushing's syndrome secretes excess amounts of cortisol, a corticosteroid that acts to retain sodium and water, resulting in hypernatremia and edema.

1 Hypervolemia, not hypovolemia, is caused by fluid retention. **2** Hypokalemia, not hyperkalemia, occurs because potassium is lost when there is sodium retention. **3** Hyperglycemia, not hypoglycemia, results from cortisol-induced glucose intolerance.
Client Need: Physiological Adaptation; **Cognitive Level:** Analysis; **Nursing Process:** Assessment/Analysis; **Reference:** Ch 9, Cushing's Syndrome, Data Base

367. **4** Clients with Cushing's syndrome must limit their intake of salt and increase their intake of potassium. The kidneys are retaining sodium and excreting potassium.

1 An excessive secretion of adrenocortical hormones in Cushing's syndrome, not increased or high sodium intake, is the problem. **2** Although sodium retention causes fluid retention and weight gain, the need for increased potassium must also be considered. **3** Because of steroid

therapy, excess sodium may be retained rather than excreted.
Client Need: Basic Care and Comfort; **Cognitive Level:** Comprehension; **Nursing Process:** Planning/Implementation; **Reference:** Ch 9, Cushing's Syndrome, Data Base

368. 4 Mineralocorticoids such as aldosterone cause the kidneys to retain sodium ions. With sodium, water is also retained, elevating blood pressure. Absence of this hormone thus causes hypotension.

1 Estrogen is a female sex hormone produced by the ovaries; it does not affect blood pressure. 2 Androgens are produced by the adrenal cortex; they have an effect similar to that of the male sex hormones; they do not affect blood pressure. 3 The major effect of glucocorticoids such as hydrocortisone is on glucose metabolism, not on sodium and water concentrations; absence of this hormone would not cause significant hypotension.
Client Need: Physiological Adaptation; **Cognitive Level:** Application; **Nursing Process:** Assessment/Analysis; **Reference:** Ch 9, Addison's Disease, Data Base

369. 1 Because of diminished glucocorticoid production, there is a decreased response to stress, reducing the ability to fight an infectious process.

2 Hyponatremia and hyperkalemia occur in this disorder; however, these do not alter the defense against infection. 3 Glucocorticoids are involved with metabolism; however, this does not directly affect susceptibility to infection. 4 The respiratory system is not affected.
Client Need: Physiological Adaptation; **Cognitive Level:** Application; **Nursing Process:** Assessment/Analysis; **Reference:** Ch 9, Addison's Disease, Nursing Care

370. 3 Glucocorticoids help maintain blood glucose and liver and muscle glycogen content. A deficiency of glucocorticoids causes hypoglycemia, resulting in breakdown of protein and fats as energy sources.

1 Muscular weakness and fatigue are related to fluid balance, but emaciation is not. 2 Emaciation results from diminished protein and fat stores and hypoglycemia, not from an alteration in electrolytes. 4 Masculinization does not occur in this disease.
Client Need: Physiological Adaptation; **Cognitive Level:** Analysis; **Nursing Process:** Assessment/Analysis; **Reference:** Ch 9, Addison's Disease, Data Base

371. 2 Exertion, either physical or emotional, places additional stress on the adrenal glands, which may precipitate an addisonian crisis.

1 Low levels of adrenocortical hormones will cause fatigue, and exercise may result in crisis because of increased metabolic demands. 3 This is contraindicated because of the risk for hypovolemia. 4 The nurse should assess for hyperkalemia and hyponatremia.
Client Need: Reduction of Risk Potential; **Cognitive Level:** Application; **Nursing Process:** Planning/Implementation; **Reference:** Ch 9, Addison's Disease, Nursing Care

372. 3 Lack of mineralocorticoids causes hyponatremia, hypovolemia, and hyperkalemia. Dietary modification and administration of cortical hormones are aimed at correcting these electrolyte imbalances.

1 There is no disturbance in the eosinophil count. 2 Lymphoid tissue does not change. 4 Although glucocorticoids are involved in metabolic activities, including carbohydrate metabolism, the primary aim of therapy is to restore electrolyte imbalance. Lack of electrolyte balance is life-threatening.
Client Need: Reduction of Risk Potential; **Cognitive Level:** Application; **Nursing Process:** Planning/Implementation; **Reference:** Ch 9, Addison's Disease, Data Base

373. 4 Lack of mineralocorticoids (aldosterone) leads to loss of sodium ions in the urine and subsequent hyponatremia.

1 Potassium intake is not encouraged; hyperkalemia is a problem because of insufficient mineralocorticoids. 2 This disease is caused by idiopathic atrophy of the adrenal cortex; tissue repair of the gland is not possible. 3 Vitamins are not directly energy-producing.
Client Need: Basic Care and Comfort; **Cognitive Level:** Application; **Integrated Process:** Teaching/Learning; **Nursing Process:** Planning/Implementation; **Reference:** Ch 9, Addison's Disease, Nursing Care

374. 1 Fludrocortisone acetate (Florinef) has a strong effect on sodium retention by the kidneys, which leads to fluid retention (weight gain and edema).

2 Fatigue may occur with adrenal insufficiency and is not related to cortisone therapy. 3 This commonly occurs and is not as serious a threat as the effect described in option 1. 4 Fluid retention and hence decreased urination may occur.
Client Need: Pharmacological and Parenteral Therapies; **Cognitive Level:** Application; **Integrated Process:** Teaching/Learning; **Nursing Process:** Evaluation/Outcomes; **Reference:** Ch 9, Adrenocorticoids

375. 1 Insulin functions by facilitating the transport of glucose through the cell membrane and increasing the deposits of glycogen in muscle. Both cellular glucose and muscle glycogen can be utilized for energy.

2 Thyroxine stimulates the rate of oxygen consumption and thus the rate at which carbohydrates are burned; it is not the main controlling hormone. 3 Adrenal steroids stimulate glyconeogenesis. 4 Growth hormone accelerates protein anabolism and stimulates growth.
Client Need: Physiological Adaptation; **Cognitive Level:** Comprehension; **Integrated Process:** Teaching/Learning; **Nursing Process:** Planning/Implementation; **Reference:** Ch 9, Review of Anatomy and Physiology, Pancreas

376. 1 This is excessive thirst associated with hyperglycemia; thirst is the response to osmotic diuresis and glycosuria.

2 This is excessive talking associated with mental illness, not hyperglycemia. 3 This is the excessive secretion of milk and is unrelated to hyperglycemia.

4 This is when a person has multiple developmental abnormalities and is unrelated to hyperglycemia.

Client Need: Physiological Adaptation; **Cognitive Level:** Application; **Nursing Process:** Assessment/Analysis; **Reference:** Ch 9, Diabetes Mellitus, Data Base

377. **3** Results in this range indicate prediabetes according to the American Diabetes Association.

1 Results in this range indicate hypoglycemia. **2** Results in this range are considered normal. **4** Results in this range indicate diabetes.

Client Need: Reduction of Risk Potential; **Cognitive Level:** Application; **Nursing Process:** Assessment/Analysis; **Reference:** Ch 9, Diabetes Mellitus, Data Base

378. **3** As a result of osmotic pressures created by an increased serum glucose level, the cells become dehydrated; the client must receive fluid and then insulin.

1 O₂ therapy is not necessarily indicated. **2** Carbohydrates would increase the blood glucose level, which is already high. **4** Although dietary instruction may be appropriate if the problem is related to dietary noncompliance, such instruction is inappropriate during the crisis.

Client Need: Physiological Adaptation; **Cognitive Level:** Analysis; **Nursing Process:** Planning/Implementation; **Reference:** Ch 9, Diabetes Mellitus, Data Base

379. **1** In starvation there are inadequate carbohydrates available for immediate energy and stored fats are used in excessive amounts, producing ketones.

2 There is no fat in alcohol; no fat oxidation occurs. **3** This does not require the use of great amounts of fat; calcium is deposited to form callus. **4** This does not require the use of great amounts of fat.

Client Need: Physiological Adaptation; **Cognitive Level:** Application; **Nursing Process:** Assessment/Analysis; **Reference:** Ch 9, Diabetes Mellitus, Data Base

380. **4** Oral hypoglycemics may be helpful when some functioning of the beta cells exists, as in type 2 diabetes.

1 Rapid-acting regular insulin is needed to reverse ketoacidosis. **2** Obesity does not offer enough information to determine the status of beta cell function. **3** Clients with type 1 diabetes have no functioning beta cells.

Client Need: Pharmacological and Parenteral Therapies; **Cognitive Level:** Application; **Nursing Process:** Planning/Implementation; **Reference:** Ch 9, Antidiabetic Agents

381. **1** ☐ Thirst occurs with hyperglycemia in response to dehydration associated with osmotic diuresis.

2 ☒ Palpitations, an adrenergic symptom, occur as the glucose level falls; the sympathetic nervous system is activated and epinephrine and norepinephrine are secreted, causing this response.

3 ☒ Diaphoresis is a sympathetic nervous system response that occurs as epinephrine and norepinephrine are released.

4 ☒ Slurred speech is a neuroglycopenic symptom; as the brain receives insufficient glucose, the activity of the CNS becomes depressed.

5 ☐ Hyperventilation occurs with diabetic ketoacidosis; Kussmaul respirations are an effort to counteract the effects of a buildup of ketones as the body seeks acid-base balance.

Client Need: Physiological Adaptation; **Cognitive Level:** Analysis; **Nursing Process:** Assessment/Analysis; **Reference:** Ch 9, Diabetes Mellitus, Data Base

382. **2** Ketones are produced when fat is broken down for energy.

1 Although rarely used, sodium bicarbonate may be administered to correct the acid-base imbalance resulting from ketoacidosis; acidosis is caused by excess acid, not excess base bicarbonate. **3** Diabetes does not interfere with removal of nitrogenous wastes. **4** Carbohydrate metabolism is hampered in the diabetic client.

Client Need: Physiological Adaptation; **Cognitive Level:** Comprehension; **Nursing Process:** Assessment/Analysis; **Reference:** Ch 9, Diabetes Mellitus, Data Base

383. **4** Many people are ashamed or have a distorted body image when they know they have a long-term disorder.

1 Lapses of memory are not common in diabetes unless advanced vascular changes occur in the brain. **2** Diabetes is not a valid reason for not hiring an individual. **3** This is a judgmental statement; the word "favorable" has individual interpretations.

Client Need: Psychosocial Integrity; **Cognitive Level:** Application; **Nursing Process:** Assessment/Analysis; **Reference:** Ch 9, Diabetes Mellitus, Data Base

384. **2** Infection increases the body's metabolic rate, and insulin is not available for increased demands.

1 Although emotional stress will affect glucose levels, diabetic ketoacidosis will rarely result. **3** Increased insulin dose will lead to insulin coma (hypoglycemia) if diet is not increased as well. **4** This would result in insulin coma.

Client Need: Physiological Adaptation; **Cognitive Level:** Comprehension; **Nursing Process:** Assessment/Analysis; **Reference:** Ch 9, Diabetes Mellitus, Data Base

385. **1** IV fluids are given to combat dehydration in acidosis and to keep an IV line open for administration of medications. When the electrolyte levels have been evaluated, potassium may be added if needed.

2 In acidosis potassium ions initially shift from intracellular to extracellular fluids, which results in hyperkalemia; as acidosis is corrected, hypokalemia may occur and then potassium may be administered. **3** This is an intermediate-acting insulin; rapid-acting insulin is indicated in an emergency. **4** This is not indicated; abnormally high serum potassium levels will revert once dehydration is corrected.

Client Need: Physiological Adaptations; **Cognitive Level:** Application; **Nursing Process:** Planning/Implementation; **Reference:** Ch 9, Diabetes Mellitus, Data Base

386. **2** Regular insulin is rapid-acting and should be used for diabetic coma.

1 This is intermediate-acting insulin; it is not indicated for use in an emergency. **3** This is too short-acting and must be administered concurrently with a longer-acting insulin or sulfonylurea. **4** This is a long-acting insulin, which is not indicated in an emergency.
Client Need: Pharmacology and Parenteral Therapies; **Cognitive Level:** Application; **Nursing Process:** Planning/Implementation; **Reference:** Ch 9, Diabetes Mellitus, Data Base

387. **3** Kussmaul respirations occur in diabetic coma as the body attempts to correct a low pH caused by accumulation of ketones (ketoacidosis); HHNS affects people with type 2 diabetes who still have some insulin production; the insulin prevents the breakdown of fats into ketones.
1 Fluid loss is common to both because an elevated blood glucose level ultimately leads to an polyuria. **2** Glycosuria is common to both conditions. **4** Hyperglycemia is common to both conditions.
Client Need: Physiological Adaptation; **Cognitive Level:** Analysis; **Nursing Process:** Assessment/Analysis; **Reference:** Ch 9, Diabetes Mellitus, Data Base

388. **1** The ketones produced excessively in diabetes are acetoacetic acid, beta-hydroxybutyric acid, and acetone; they are the byproducts of the breakdown of body fats and proteins for energy; this occurs when insulin is not secreted or unable to be utilized to transport glucose across the cell membrane into the cells; the major ketone, acetoacetic acid, is an alpha-ketoacid that lowers the blood pH, resulting in acidosis.
2 Glucose is not an acid; it does not change the pH. **3** Lactic acid is produced as a result of muscle contraction; it is not unique to diabetes. **4** This is a product of protein metabolism.
Client Need: Physiological Adaptation; **Cognitive Level:** Comprehension; **Nursing Process:** Assessment/Analysis; **Reference:** Ch 9, Diabetes Mellitus, Data Base

389. **2** The fingertip is preferred for glucose monitoring if hypoglycemia, not hyperglycemia, is suspected.
1 This will increase blood flow, which helps to minimize the difference between forearm and fingertip results although it does not eliminate them. **3** In a study in which rapidly fluctuating glucose levels were initiated, glucose levels at the forearm were significantly lower than samples from the fingertips; the fingertip should be used when testing before, during, and after exercising; before driving; after eating; and during illness; the fingertip most closely reflects a current glucose level. **4** Not all glucose monitors on the market can be used for AST.
Client Need: Reduction of Risk Potential; **Cognitive Level:** Application; **Integrated Process:** Teaching/Learning; **Nursing Process:** Evaluation/Outcomes; **Reference:** Ch 9, Diabetes Mellitus, Data Base

390. **3** The forearm glucose monitor is calibrated to be consistent with results obtained from a fingerstick.
1 Individuals of all ages can use these glucose monitors. **2** There is no difference in the time required to complete the test. **4** A different scale is not used for each monitor; accompanying literature will indicate if the monitor reading reflects venous blood values even though capillary blood is used.
Client Need: Reduction of Risk Potential; **Cognitive Level:** Application; **Integrated Process:** Teaching/Learning; **Nursing Process:** Planning/Implementation; **Reference:** Ch 9, Diabetes Mellitus, Data Base

391. **4** The urinary catheter and drainage bag should always remain a closed sterile system; urine should be drawn only from the catheter, not the collection bag.
1, 3 The system should remain closed so that fewer microorganisms enter the urinary system. **2** This would not yield a fresh specimen indicating present acetone levels.
Client Need: Safety and Infection Control; **Cognitive Level:** Application; **Nursing Process:** Assessment/Analysis; **Reference:** Ch 9, Diabetes Mellitus, Nursing Care

392. **2** The guidelines from the American Diabetes Association have lowered the level of an FPG that indicates whether a client has prediabetes from 110 mg/dL to 100 mg/dL; an FPG of 100 to 125 mg/dL is considered prediabetes.
1 This FPG would indicate that the client is hypoglycemic. **3, 4** An FPG of 126 mg/dL or higher indicates that the client has diabetes.
Client Need: Reduction of Risk Potential; **Cognitive Level:** Application; **Nursing Process:** Assessment/Analysis; **Reference:** Ch 9, Diabetes Mellitus, Data Base

393. **2** Because the brain requires a constant supply of glucose, hypoglycemia triggers the response of the sympathetic nervous system, which causes this sign.
1 Because blood glucose level is low, the renal threshold is not exceeded, and there is no glycosuria. **3** This is consistent with dehydration, which is often associated with hyperglycemic states. **4** This is associated with hyperglycemia; it is caused by the breakdown of fats as a result of inadequate insulin supply.
Client Need: Pharmacological and Parenteral Therapies; **Cognitive Level:** Application; **Nursing Process:** Evaluation/Outcomes; **Reference:** Ch 9, Antidiabetic Agents

394. **1** In the absence of insulin, which facilitates the transport of glucose into cells, the body breaks down proteins and fats to supply energy; ketones, a by-product of fat metabolism, accumulate, causing metabolic acidosis (pH below 7.35).
2 The opposite is true. **3** The pH of food ingested has no effect on the development of acidosis. **4** Cholesterol level has no effect on the development of acidosis.

Client Need: Physiological Adaptation; **Cognitive Level:** Comprehension; **Integrated Process:** Teaching/Learning; **Nursing Process:** Assessment/Analysis; **Reference:** Ch 9,. Diabetes Mellitus, Data Base

395. 3 The stress of an infection increases metabolism and the production of glucocorticoids, resulting in an elevated blood glucose level.

1, 2, 4 This would result in insulin coma (hypoglycemia).

Client Need: Physiological Adaptation; **Cognitive Level:** Application; **Nursing Process:** Assessment/Analysis; **Reference:** Ch 9, Diabetes Mellitus, Data Base

396. 1 ☐ As the glucose level falls, the sympathetic nervous system is activated and epinephrine and norepinephrine are secreted, causing sweating.

2 ☒ Metabolic acidosis initiates respiratory compensation in the form of Kussmaul respirations to counteract the effects of ketone buildup, resulting in a lowered P_{CO_2}.

3 ☐ Retinopathy is a long-term complication of diabetes caused by microvascular changes in the retina; it is not a sign of ketoacidosis.

4 ☒ A fruity odor to the breath (acetone breath) occurs when the ketone level is elevated in ketoacidosis.

5 ☐ With ketoacidosis plasma bicarbonate is exhausted, not elevated, in an effort to neutralize ketones when seeking acid-base balance.

Client Need: Physiological Adaptation; **Cognitive Level:** Analysis; **Integrated Process:** Communication/Documentation; **Nursing Process:** Assessment/Analysis; **Reference:** Ch 9, Diabetes Mellitus, Data Base

397. 4 In the absence of insulin, glucose cannot enter the cell or be converted to glycogen, so it remains in the blood. Breakdown of fats as an energy source causes an accumulation of ketones, which results in acidosis. The lungs, in an attempt to compensate for lowered pH, will blow off CO_2 (Kussmaul respirations).

1 This occurs in response to polyuria. **2** Hyperglycemia, not hypoglycemia, occurs. **3** High, not normal, acidity would be present.

Client Need: Reduction of Risk Potential; **Cognitive Level:** Analysis; **Nursing Process:** Assessment/Analysis; **Reference:** Ch 9, Diabetes Mellitus, Data Base

398. 1 This is an antioxidant that scavenges oxygen free radicals that are released when contrast medium causes cell death to renal tubular tissue; it also induces slight vasodilation.

2 Contrast that is renal friendly does not exist. **3** Saline alone provides better protection of the kidneys from contrast-induced nephropathy. **4** Hydration with saline, not dextrose and water, affords some protection from kidney damage caused by contrast media; dextrose would elevate the glucose level in an individual with diabetes and thus is contraindicated.

Client Need: Pharmacological and Parenteral Therapies; **Cognitive Level:** Analysis; **Nursing Process:** Planning/Implementation; **Reference:** Ch 9, Diabetes Mellitus, Data Base

399. 3 Glucagon is an insulin antagonist produced by the alpha cells in the islets of Langerhans. It causes the breakdown of glycogen and protein to glucose.

1 Acidosis occurs when there is a high serum glucose level; therefore glucagon is not indicated. **2** Diabetes mellitus involves a decreased insulin production. **4** Glucagon is not indicated in idiosyncratic reactions to insulin.

Client Need: Pharmacological and Parenteral Therapies; **Cognitive Level:** Application; **Nursing Process:** Planning/Implementation; **Reference:** Ch 9, Diabetes Mellitus, Data Base

400. 4 The bicarbonate-carbonic acid buffer system helps maintain the pH of body fluids; in metabolic acidosis there is a decrease in bicarbonate because of an increase of metabolic acids.

1 The pH is decreased. **2** The P_{O_2} is not decreased in diabetic acidosis. **3** The P_{CO_2} may be decreased by the body's attempt to eliminate CO_2 to compensate for a low pH.

Client Need: Reduction of Risk Potential; **Cognitive Level:** Analysis; **Nursing Process:** Assessment/Analysis; **Reference:** Ch 9, Diabetes Mellitus, Data Base

401. 3 Glucagon, an insulin antagonist produced by the alpha cells in the islets of Langerhans, leads to the conversion of glycogen to glucose in the liver.

1 It stimulates glycogenolysis, the conversion of glycogen to glucose. **2** It is an insulin antagonist. **4** It does not stimulate the storage of glucose but rather it stimulates the conversion of glycogen to glucose.

Client Need: Pharmacological and Parenteral Therapies; **Cognitive Level:** Comprehension; **Nursing Process:** Planning/Implementation; **Reference:** Ch 9, Diabetes Mellitus, Data Base

402. 4 Insulin stimulates cellular uptake of glucose and also stimulates the sodium/potassium pump, leading to the influx of potassium into cells. The resulting hypokalemia is offset by parenteral administration of potassium.

1 Hypokalemia may be caused by the movement of potassium back into the cells as dehydration is reversed. **2** Hypokalemia may occur because the potassium moves back into the cells as dehydration is reversed. **3** Anabolic reactions are stimulated by insulin and glucose administration; potassium is drawn into the intracellular compartment, necessitating a replenishment of extracellular potassium.

Client Need: Pharmacological and Parenteral Therapies; **Cognitive Level:** Analysis; **Nursing Process:** Planning/Implementation; **Reference:** Ch 9, Diabetes Mellitus, Data Base

403. 1 ☒ Hypoglycemia triggers the sympathetic nervous system, which releases epinephrine, in turn causing vasoconstriction and this reaction.

2 ☒ Tremors are a sympathetic nervous system response to hypoglycemia.

3 ☐ Because blood glucose concentration is low in hypoglycemia, the renal threshold is not exceeded and there is no glycosuria.
4 ☐ Acetonuria is associated with hyperglycemia; it is caused by the breakdown of fats as a result of inadequate insulin supply.
5 ☒ Diaphoresis results from the release of epinephrine by the sympathetic nervous system.
Client Need: Pharmacological and Parenteral Therapies; **Cognitive Level:** Analysis; **Nursing Process:** Evaluation/Outcomes; **Reference:** Ch 9, Diabetes Mellitus, Data Base

404. 1 Liquids containing simple carbohydrates are most readily absorbed and thus increase blood glucose level quickly.
2 Although a solution of 50% dextrose may be given if the client is comatose, 5% dextrose does not supply sufficient carbohydrates. 3 This will not alter the current situation. 4 Complex carbohydrates and protein take longer to elevate blood glucose level, so they should be administered after simple carbohydrates.
Client Need: Reduction of Risk Potential; **Cognitive Level:** Application; **Nursing Process:** Planning/Implementation; **Reference:** Ch 9, Diabetes Mellitus, Data Base

405. 2 A combination of diet, exercise, and medication is necessary to control the disease; the interaction of these therapies is reflected by the serum glucose level.
1 Weight loss may occur with inadequate insulin. 3 Acquisition of knowledge does not guarantee its application. 4 Insulin alone is not enough to control the disease.
Client Need: Physiological Adaptation; **Cognitive Level:** Analysis; **Nursing Process:** Evaluation/Outcomes; **Reference:** Ch 9, Diabetes Mellitus, Nursing Care

406. 3 A value of 258 mg/dL is above the expected range of 70 to 100 mg/dL; the nurse should administer the insulin as ordered.
1 This is unnecessary; an order for insulin exists and should be implemented. 2 This would be insufficient to lower a glucose level this high. 4 This is contraindicated because it will increase the glucose level further; orange juice, a complex carbohydrate, and a protein would be given if the glucose level were too low.
Client Need: Pharmacological and Parenteral Therapies; **Cognitive Level:** Analysis; **Nursing Process:** Planning/Implementation; **Reference:** Ch 9, Antidiabetic Agents

407. 4 A slower, longer period of time to break in new, stiff shoes will help prevent blisters and skin breakdown.
1 This will cause maceration of the skin and should be avoided. 2 The toenails should be cut by a podiatrist; they usually are cut after soaking, when the nails are softer. 3 This is too long a period of time; the client should examine the feet daily for signs of trauma.
Client Need: Reduction of Risk Potential; **Cognitive Level:** Application; **Integrated Process:** Teaching/Learning; **Nursing Process:** Evaluation/Outcomes; **Reference:** Ch 9, Diabetes Mellitus, Nursing Care

408. 2 Each client should be given an individually devised diet selecting commonly used foods from the American Diabetic Association diet; family members should be included in the diet teaching.
1 Rigid diets are difficult to obey; substitutions should be offered. 3 Nutritional requirements are different for each individual depending on many factors, such as activity level, degree of compliance, and physical status. 4 Seasonings in processed foods do not affect the management of diabetes mellitus.
Client Need: Basic Care and Comfort; **Cognitive Level:** Application; **Integrated Process:** Teaching/Learning; **Nursing Process:** Evaluation/Outcomes; **Reference:** Ch 9, Diabetes Mellitus, Data Base

409. 1, 3, 2, 4
Air should be injected into the NPH insulin vile first, which allows withdrawal of the NPH insulin at a later step in the procedure without having to instill air into the vial from a syringe that contains regular insulin. Having the syringe contain regular insulin first prevents the need to withdraw the regular insulin into a syringe that contains NPH insulin and inadvertently contaminating the regular insulin vial with the longer-acting NPH insulin; contaminating regular insulin with NPH insulin will reduce the speed at which the regular insulin functions, which in turn will delay treatment of a hyperglycemic event.
Client Need: Pharmacological and Parenteral Therapies; **Cognitive Level:** Analysis; **Nursing Process:** Planning/Implementation; **Reference:** Ch 9, Antidiabetic Agents

410. 2 Lispro has an immediate onset, a peak of 30 to 90 minutes, and a duration of 2 to 4 hours.
1 Lente is an intermediate-acting insulin with an onset of 60 to 150 minutes, a peak of 7 to 15 hours, and a duration of 24 hours. 3 Ultralente is a long-acting insulin with an onset of 4 hours and a duration of 28 hours. 4 Humulin N is an intermediate-acting insulin with an onset of 60 to 120 minutes and a duration of 18 to 24 hours.
Client Need: Pharmacological and Parenteral Therapies; **Cognitive Level:** Analysis; **Nursing Process:** Planning/Implementation; **Reference:** Ch 9, Antidiabetic Agents

411. 1 An understanding of the diet is imperative for compliance. A balance of carbohydrates, proteins, and fats usually apportioned over three main meals and two between-meal snacks needs to be tailored to the client's specific needs, with due regard for activity, diet, and therapy.
2 A total dietary regimen proportioning carbohydrates, proteins, and fats must be followed, not just sugar restriction; salt is not restricted. 3 This is true; however, indigestion is not the basis for the client's problems. 4 Total caloric intake, rather than the size of meals, is the major factor in weight gain.
Client Need: Basic Care and Comfort; **Cognitive Level:** Application; **Integrated Process:** Teaching/Learning; **Nursing Process:** Planning/Implementation; **Reference:** Ch 9, Diabetes Mellitus, Data Base

412. 3 The protein in milk and cheese may be slowly converted to glucose (gluconeogenesis), providing the body with some glucose during sleep while the Humulin N insulin is still acting.

1 The purpose of an evening snack is to cover for insulin activity during sleep. 2 The client's physical size does not indicate a need to gain weight. 4 The foods chosen are rich in protein and will be utilized slowly.

Client Need: Pharmacological and Parenteral Therapies; Cognitive Level: Application; Nursing Process: Planning/ Implementation; Reference: Ch 9, Diabetes Mellitus, Data Base

413. 3 The expected range of glycosylated hemoglobin is 4.4% to 6.4%. A value of 6% is within the normal range. Glycosylated hemoglobin measures the average blood glucose level for the 90- to 120-day period before the blood sample is collected; thus it is a reliable way to measure adherence to a therapy plan of insulin, diet, and exercise.

1 A glycosylated hemoglobin measurement does not measure rebound hyperglycemia (Somogyi effect). 2, 4 The HbA_{1c} fraction of hemoglobin is measured and its value is not affected by short-term infractions of diet or the type of insulin the client takes.

Client Need: Reduction of Risk Potential; Cognitive Level: Analysis; Nursing Process: Planning/Implementation; Reference: Ch 9, Diabetes Mellitus, Data Base

414. 1 ☒ Clients with diabetes often have peripheral neuropathies and are unaware of discomfort or pain in the feet; the feet should be examined every night for signs of trauma.

2 ☒ Well-fitting shoes prevent pressure and rubbing that can cause tissue damage and the development of ulcers.

3 ☒ Daily exercise increases the uptake of glucose by the muscles and improves insulin utilization.

4 ☐ This generally is unnecessary.

5 ☐ This may cause a pastelike residue between the toes that may macerate the skin and promote bacterial and fungal growth.

6 ☐ Clients with diabetes often have peripheral neuropathy and are unable to accurately evaluate the temperature of bath water, which can result in burns if the water is too hot.

Client Need: Reduction of Risk Potential: Cognitive Level: Analysis; Integrated Process: Teaching/Learning; Nursing Process: Planning/Implementation; Reference: Ch 9, Diabetes Mellitus, Nursing Care

415. 1 During treatment for acidosis, hypoglycemia may develop; careful observation for this complication should be made by the nurse, even without an order.

2 Withholding all glucose may cause insulin coma; monitoring for this is indicated. 3 Whole milk and fruit juices are high in carbohydrates, which are contraindicated immediately following ketoacidosis. 4 The regulation of insulin depends on the physician's orders for coverage.

Client Need: Pharmacological and Parenteral Therapies; Cognitive Level: Analysis; Nursing Process: Evaluation/ Outcomes; Reference: Ch 9, Antidiabetics, Agents

416. 1 Because the client has severe diabetes, it is essential that the blood glucose level be determined before meals to evaluate the level of control of diabetes and the possible need for insulin coverage.

2 To prevent flexion contractures of the hip, the client should not sit for a prolonged time. 3 Raising the head of the bed flexes the hips, which could result in hip flexion contractures. 4 This could result in a hip flexion contracture.

Client Need: Reduction of Risk Potential; Cognitive Level: Analysis; Nursing Process: Evaluation/Outcomes; Reference: Ch 9, Diabetes Mellitus, Nursing Care

417. 3 The abdomen is the preferred site because it is easily accessible and insulin absorption is more even and rapid than when injected in the extremities.

1, 2, 4 This is not the preferred site for the administration of insulin.

Client Need: Pharmacological and Parenteral Therapies; Cognitive Level: Application; Nursing Process: Planning/ Implementation; Reference: Ch 9, Diabetes Mellitus, Nursing Care

418. 1 The thyroid gland produces thyroxine (T_4) and triiodothyronine (T_3), which help regulate oxidation in all body cells.

2 The primary regulator is the thyroid; the adrenals influence metabolism of carbohydrates in times of stress. 3 The pituitary gland is involved in secondary regulation because it secretes TSH, which stimulates thyroid production of thyroxine and triiodothyronine. 4 The pancreas regulates glucose metabolism by secretion of insulin.

Client Need: Physiological Adaptation; Cognitive Level: Knowledge; Nursing Process: Assessment/Analysis; Reference: Ch 9, Review of Anatomy and Physiology, Thyroid Gland

419. 1 Myxedema is the severest form of hypothyroidism. Decreased thyroid gland activity means reduced production of thyroid hormones.

2 This results from excess growth hormone in adults once the epiphyses are closed. 3 This results from an excess, not a deficiency, of thyroid hormones. 4 This results from excess glucocorticoids.

Client Need: Physiological Adaptation; Cognitive Level: Analysis; Nursing Process: Assessment/Analysis; Reference: Ch 9, Hypothyroidism, Data Base

420. 3 Decreased production of thyroid hormones lowers metabolism, which leads to decreased heat production and cold intolerance.

1 Lethargy, rather than irritability, is expected. 2 Decreased metabolism requires less oxygen, so the pulse rate is generally slower. 4 The skin is dry and coarse, not moist.

Client Need: Physiological Adaptation; Cognitive Level: Application; Nursing Process: Assessment/Analysis; Reference: Ch 9, Hypothyroidism, Data Base

421. **2** Excessive thyroid hormones increase the metabolic rate, causing weight loss.

1 Listlessness occurs with hypothyroidism because of a decreased metabolic rate. **3** A slow pulse rate accompanies hypothyroidism, not hyperthyroidism, because of a decreased metabolic rate. **4** Appetite increases (polyphagia) with hyperthyroidism in an effort to meet metabolic needs.

Client Need: Physiological Adaptation; Cognitive Level: Application; Nursing Process: Assessment/Analysis; Reference: Ch 9, Hyperthyroidism, Data Base

422. **3** An individual treated for a thyroid problem by intake of radioactive iodine (^{131}I) becomes mildly radioactive, particularly in the region of the thyroid gland, which preferentially absorbs the iodine. Such clients should be treated with routine safety precautions for 48 hours (e.g., avoid prolonged contact or near-contact with others, flush toilet twice after using since radioactive iodine is excreted via the urine, and thoroughly wash hands after toileting).

1, 4 Because radioactive iodine is internalized, the client becomes the source of radioactivity. **2** The amount of radioactive iodine used is not enough to cause high radioactivity.

Client Need: Reduction of Risk Potential; Cognitive Level: Comprehension; Nursing Process: Evaluation/Outcomes; Reference: Ch 9, Hyperthyroidism, Nursing Care

423. **3** This adds iodine to the body fluids, exerting negative feedback on the thyroid tissue and decreasing its metabolism and vascularity.

1 This is an antidiuretic hormone. **2** This drug interferes with production of thyroid hormone but causes increased vascularity and size of the thyroid. **4** This is a topical antiseptic.

Client Need: Pharmacological and Parenteral Therapies; Cognitive Level: Analysis; Nursing Process: Planning/Implementation; Reference: Ch 9, Thyroid Inhibitors

424. **1** If the laryngeal nerves are injured bilaterally during surgery, the vocal cords will tighten, interfering with speech. If one cord is affected, hoarseness develops. This can be evaluated simply by having the client speak every hour.

2, 3, 4 This ability is not influenced by laryngeal nerve damage.

Client Need: Reduction of Risk Potential; Cognitive Level: Application; Nursing Process: Evaluation/Outcomes; Reference: Ch 9, Hyperthyroidism, Nursing Care

425. **2** A decreased TSH assay together with an elevated T_3 (triiodothyronine) level may indicate hyperthyroidism.

1 X-ray results would not indicate thyroid disease, and elevation of T_4 (thyroxine) level might indicate hyperthyroidism. However, this could be a false reading because of the presence of thyroid-binding globulin (TBG) and is inadequate for diagnosis when used alone. **3** Po_2 is not specific to thyroid disease, and the thyroglobulin level is most useful to monitor for recurrence of thyroid carcinoma or

response to therapy. **4** The results with the sequential multichannel autoanalyzer (SMA) are not specific to thyroid disease; the protein-bound iodine test is not definitive because it is influenced by the intake of exogenous iodine.

Client Need: Reduction of Risk Potential; Cognitive Level: Application; Integrated Process: Teaching/Learning; Nursing Process: Planning/Implementation; Reference: Ch 9, Hyperthyroidism, Data Base

426. **1** Because of the individual's increased metabolic rate, a high-calorie diet is needed to meet the energy demands of the body and prevent weight loss.

2 Sodium is not restricted because clients with hyperthyroidism perspire heavily and lose sodium. **3** GI motility is increased and does not require the additional stimulus of increased roughage. **4** Modification of consistency is unnecessary.

Client Need: Basic Care and Comfort; Cognitive Level: Application; Nursing Process: Planning/Implementation; Reference: Ch 9, Hyperthyroidism, Nursing Care

427. **4** The first and most important observation should be for respiratory obstruction. If this occurs, treatment must be instituted immediately.

1 This would be a later concern; retention would not occur in the immediate postoperative period. **2** This could result from the anesthesia; however, it is not life-threatening and usually passes. **3** The BP is not significantly affected by this type of surgery; however, surgery itself can influence BP. If the BP significantly increases, other symptoms of thyroid crisis (storm) would be present.

Client Need: Physiological Adaptation; Cognitive Level: Application; Nursing Process: Evaluation/Outcomes; Reference: Ch 9, Hyperthyroidism, Nursing Care

428. **1** Parathyroid removal eliminates the body's source of parathyroid hormone (parathormone), which increases blood calcium level. The resulting low body fluid calcium affects muscles, including the diaphragm, resulting in dyspnea, asphyxia, and death.

2 Loss of the thyroid gland would upset thyroid hormone balance and might cause myxedema. **3** The parathyroids are not involved in regulating plasma volume; the pituitary and adrenal glands are responsible. **4** The parathyroids do not regulate the adrenal glands.

Client Need: Reduction of Risk Potential; Cognitive Level: Application; Nursing Process: Evaluation/Outcomes; Reference: Ch 9, Hyperthyroidism, Nursing Care

429. **1** These signs may indicate calcium depletion as a result of accidental removal of parathyroid glands during thyroidectomy.

2 Symptoms associated with hypomagnesemia include tremor, neuromuscular irritability, and confusion. **3** Symptoms associated with metabolic acidosis include deep, rapid breathing, weakness, and disorientation. **4** Symptoms associated with hypokalemia include muscle weakness and dysrhythmias.

Client Need: Physiological Adaptation; **Cognitive Level:** Analysis; **Nursing Process:** Evaluation/Outcomes; **Reference:** Ch 9, Hyperthyroidism, Nursing Care

430. **4** Thyroid surgery sometimes results in accidental removal of the parathyroid glands. A resultant hypocalcemia may lead to contraction of the glottis, causing airway obstruction; edema also may cause obstruction.

1 A patent airway takes priority. **2** Speaking is important to determine the status of the laryngeal nerve. **3** The semi-Fowler's position is indicated to maximize respiratory excursion.

Client Need: Reduction of Risk Potential; **Cognitive Level:** Application; **Nursing Process:** Planning/Implementation; **Reference:** Ch 9, Hyperthyroidism, Nursing Care

431. **3** Soreness is to be expected. A progression to a soft diet will provide nutrients needed for healing and energy and will stimulate the return of bowel activity. Analgesics as ordered will reduce soreness during meals.

1 This is not a nursing function. **2** Soreness is to be expected; this is not an emergency necessitating medical action. **4** The soreness is not because of drying; when the client is at home, humidified air might help reduce the soreness, but it would not help the client eat the soft diet.

Client Need: Basic Care and Comfort; **Cognitive Level:** Application; **Nursing Process:** Planning/Implementation; **Reference:** Ch 9, Hyperthyroidism, Nursing Care

432. **1** This results from a decrease in the metabolic rate, which is associated with hypothyroidism.

2, 4 This is associated with hyperthyroidism because of an increase in metabolism. **3** This/is not associated with hypothyroidism; it is associated with Parkinson's disease.

Client Need: Physiological Adaptation; **Cognitive Level:** Application; **Nursing Process:** Assessment/Analysis; **Reference:** Ch 9, Hypothyroidism, Data Base

433. **4** Parathyroid hormone increases blood calcium level by accelerating calcium absorption from the intestine and kidneys and releasing calcium from bone. Vitamin D promotes calcium absorption from the intestine.

1 Phosphorus and ACTH do not interact to regulate calcium levels. Phosphorus is a component of bone; ACTH stimulates the adrenal cortex to secrete the corticosteroid hormones. **2** Vitamin A and thyroid hormone do not interact to regulate calcium levels. Vitamin A is essential for function of epithelial cells and visual purple; calcitonin (a thyroid hormone) lowers serum calcium. **3** Ascorbic acid (vitamin C) and growth hormone do not interact to regulate calcium levels. Vitamin C promotes collagen production and formation of bone matrix; growth hormone controls the rate of skeletal growth.

Client Need: Physiological Adaptation; **Cognitive Level:** Comprehension; **Nursing Process:** Assessment/Analysis; **Reference:** Ch 9, Review of Anatomy and Physiology, Parathyroid Glands

434. **1** Calcitonin, a thyroid gland hormone, prevents the reabsorption of calcium by bone. It also inhibits the release of calcium from bone. The net result is lowered serum calcium levels.

2 Aldosterone regulates fluid and electrolyte balance by promoting the retention of sodium and water and the excretion of potassium. **3** This hormone promotes the intestinal absorption of calcium and mobilizes calcium from the bones to increase blood calcium levels. **4** Calcitonin lowers serum calcium levels; the other thyroid hormones (thyroxine and triiodothyronine) control metabolic rate.

Client Need: Physiological Adaptation; **Cognitive Level:** Knowledge; **Nursing Process:** Assessment/Analysis; **Reference:** Ch 9, Review of Anatomy and Physiology, Thyroid Gland

435. **1** ☒ Tinted glasses decrease light impacting on the eyes and protect eyes that are photosensitive.

2 ☐ Cool, moist compresses are used to relieve irritation; warm compresses cause vasodilation, which could aggravate tissue congestion.

3 ☒ Elevating the head of the bed 45 degrees will promote a decrease in periorbital fluid.

4 ☒ Taping the eyelids shut at night if they do not close reduces the risk of corneal dryness, which can lead to infection or injury.

5 ☐ Artificial tears are used to moisten the eyes, not a petroleum-based jelly.

Client Need: Basic Care and Comfort; **Cognitive Level:** Analysis; **Nursing Process:** Planning/Implementation; **Reference:** Ch 9, Hyperthyroidism, Nursing Care

436. **4** Hyperparathyroidism causes calcium release from the bones, leaving them porous and weak.

1 Tetany is the result of low calcium levels; in this condition serum calcium level is high. **2** Seizures are caused by increased neural activity, a condition not related to this disease. **3** Graves' disease is the result of increased thyroid, not parathyroid, activity.

Client Need: Physiological Adaptation; **Cognitive Level:** Application; **Nursing Process:** Assessment/Analysis; **Reference:** Ch 9, Hyperparathyroidism, Data Base

437. **1** Fluids help prevent the formation of renal calculi associated with high levels of serum calcium.

2 Additional calcium intake could raise already high levels of serum calcium. **3** Seizures are associated with low, not high, levels of serum calcium. **4** Rest is contraindicated because bone destruction is accelerated.

Client Need: Physiological Adaptation; **Cognitive Level:** Application; **Nursing Process:** Planning/Implementation; **Reference:** Ch 9, Hyperparathyroidism, Nursing Care

INTEGUMENTARY SYSTEM

438. **3** The temperature range for tepid applications is approximately body temperature.

1, 2 This temperature is too cool for a tepid bath. **4** This temperature is too hot for a tepid bath.

Client Need: Safety and Infection Control; **Cognitive Level:** Knowledge; **Nursing Process:** Planning/Implementation; **Reference:** Ch 10, Burns, Data Base

439. **4** Conduction is the conveyance of energy such as heat, cold, or sound by direct contact.

1 Direct contact is not necessary to convey heat by radiation. **2** This refers to retention of heat, not its transfer. **3** This is the transfer of heat by air circulation (e.g., by fans or open windows).

Client Need: Basic Care and Comfort; **Cognitive Level:** Analysis; **Nursing Process:** Planning/Implementation; **Reference:** Ch 10, Review of Physical Principles, Heat

440. **3** O_2 perfusion is impaired during prolonged edema, leading to tissue ischemia.

1, 2, 4 This is not a complication resulting from long-term edema.

Client Need: Physiological Adaptation; **Cognitive Level:** Analysis; **Nursing Process:** Assessment/Analysis; **Reference:** Ch 10, Pressure Ulcers, Data Base

441. **1** Psoriasis is characterized by dry, scaly lesions that occur most frequently on the elbows, knees, scalp, and torso.

2 Pruritus, if present at all, is generally mild.

3 Petechiae are not characteristic. **4** Macules are erythematous flat spots on the skin as in measles; no scales are present.

Client Need: Physiological Adaptation; **Cognitive Level:** Application; **Nursing Process:** Assessment/Analysis; **Reference:** Ch 10, Skin Lesions, Secondary Skin Lesions

442. **2** Steroids are applied locally and the lesions are usually covered with plastic wrap at night to reverse the inflammatory process.

1 Solar rays may be used for treatment; other forms of ultraviolet light are preferred. **3** Potassium permanganate is an antiseptic astringent used on infected, draining, or vesicular lesions. **4** The plaques are not necrotic and therefore do not require debriding.

Client Need: Pharmacological and Parenteral Therapies; **Cognitive Level:** Analysis; **Integrated Process:** Teaching/Learning; **Nursing Process:** Planning/Implementation; **Reference:** Ch 10, Antiinflammatory Agents

443. **1** Scabies is caused by the itch mite *(Sarcoptes scabiei)*, the female of which burrows under the skin to deposit eggs. It is intensely pruritic and is transmitted by direct contact or in a limited way by soiled sheets or undergarments.

2 It is caused by the itch mite, a parasite. **3** Scabies is an acute infestation. **4** It is a disease unrelated to allergies.

Client Need: Safety and Infection Control; **Cognitive Level:** Application; **Nursing Process:** Planning/Implementation; **Reference:** Ch 10, Pediculocides/Scabicides

444. **3** Pemphigus is primarily a serious disease characterized by blisters filled with fluid. When they are less than 1 cm in diameter, they are called vesicles. When they are larger than 1 cm, they are called bullae.

1, 2, 4 Pemphigus is a disease of the skin.

Client Need: Physiological Adaptation; **Cognitive Level:** Application; **Nursing Process:** Planning/Implementation; **Reference:** Ch 10, Skin Lesions, Primary Skin Lesions

445. **1** The connective tissue degeneration of SLE leads to involvement of the basal cell layer, producing a butterfly rash over the bridge of the nose and in the malar region.

2 This occurs in scleroderma; in an advanced stage the client has the appearance of a living mummy. **3** This occurs in muscular dystrophy; it is characterized by muscle wasting and weakness. **4** This occurs in polyarteritis nodosa, a collagen disease affecting the arteries and nervous system.

Client Need: Physiological Adaptation; **Cognitive Level:** Application; **Nursing Process:** Assessment/Analysis; **Reference:** Ch 10, Systemic Lupus Erythematosus, Data Base

446. **1** Scleroderma is an immunologic disorder characterized by inflammatory, fibrotic, and degenerative changes.

2, 3, 4 This is not involved in the development of scleroderma.

Client Need: Physiological Adaptation; **Cognitive Level:** Comprehension; **Integrated Process:** Teaching/Learning; **Nursing Process:** Planning/Implementation; **Reference:** Ch 10, Scleroderma, Data Base

447. **3** The sacrum bears the most pressure because it is the focal point of the weight of the body when in the low-Fowler's position; also, shearing forces may cause local tissue trauma.

1, 2, 4 Although the other areas of the body are vulnerable, they do not bear as much body weight as the sacrum when the client is in the low-Fowler's position.

Client Need: Basic Care and Comfort; **Cognitive Level:** Application; **Nursing Process:** Assessment/Analysis; **Reference:** Ch 10, Pressure Ulcers, Data Base

448. **4** Basal cell carcinoma, the most common type of skin cancer, is most closely linked to solar ultraviolet radiation.

1 Although skin type is a genetically determined risk factor, it cannot be altered and it is influenced by solar ultraviolet radiation. **2** Diet is not a risk factor. **3** Smoking is not a risk factor.

Client Need: Physiological Adaptation; **Cognitive Level:** Application; **Nursing Process:** Assessment/Analysis; **Reference:** Ch 10, Cancer of the Skin, Data Base

449. **3** Lymphadenopathy occurs in clients with malignancies that have metastasized.

1 Skin is generally dry and itchy. **2** This occurs in clients with pemphigus. **4** This is not a symptom of melanoma.

Client Need: Physiological Adaptation; **Cognitive Level:** Application; **Nursing Process:** Assessment/Analysis; **Reference:** Ch 10, Cancer of the Skin, Data Base

450. **2** Malignant melanoma of the eye is an intraocular tumor that metastasizes rapidly; therefore enucleation (removal of the eye) is the treatment of choice.

1, 3, 4 This is only palliative at best.

Client Need: Physiological Adaptation; Cognitive Level: Application; Nursing Process: Planning/Implementation; Reference: Ch 10, Cancer of the Skin, Data Base

451. 4 Application of a solution of sodium bicarbonate (a mild alkali) after a thorough flushing with water is the best way to treat acid-splashed skin, because it will neutralize residual acid on the skin.
1 Sodium sulfate is a neutral salt, which would serve no immediate first-aid benefit. 2 Sodium chloride is a neutral salt, which would serve no immediate first-aid benefit. 3 Although this is an alkali that will neutralize an acid, it is too strong and can cause burns.
Client Need: Pharmacological and Parenteral Therapies; Cognitive Level: Analysis; Integrated Process: Teaching/Learning; Nursing Process: Planning/Implementation; Reference: Ch 10, Burns, Nursing Care

452. 1 This first-aid treatment will chemically neutralize residual alkali still on the skin. It will not reverse the chemical burns already caused by the alkali but will minimize additional chemical change.
2 A weak base will not neutralize alkaline substances. 3 This is a neutral substance; it will not neutralize a base. 4 This would not affect the pH.
Client Need: Pharmacological and Parenteral Therapies; Cognitive Level: Analysis; Integrated Process: Teaching/Learning; Nursing Process: Planning/Implementation; Reference: Ch 10, Burns, Nursing Care

453. 3 This is taken from an uninjured area of the same person's body.
1 This is skin taken from the same species. 2 A xenograft (heterograft) is skin taken from a different species. 4 This is skin taken from the same species.
Client Need: Physiological Adaptation; Cognitive Level: Knowledge; Integrated Process: Teaching/Learning; Nursing Process: Evaluation/Outcomes; Reference: Ch 10, Burns, Data Base

454. 4 A heterograft (xenograft) involves the grafting of tissues from a different species.
1 This type of graft does not exist. 2 This is skin taken from the same species. 3 This is skin taken from the same species.
Client Need: Physiological Adaptation; Cognitive Level: Knowledge; Nursing Process: Assessment/Analysis; Reference: Ch 10, Burns, Data Base

455. 3 An increased hematocrit level indicates hemoconcentration secondary to fluid loss.
1 This may be used to indicate dehydration from burns, but interpretation can be complicated by other conditions accompanying burns that also cause elevation of the BUN. 2 The pH level reflects acid-base balance. 4 This indicates the presence of an inflammatory process, not fluid loss.
Client Need: Reduction of Risk Potential; Cognitive Level: Analysis; Nursing Process: Assessment/Analysis; Reference: Ch 10, Burns, Data Base

456. 4 As the amount of tissue involved increases, there is greater extravasation of fluid into the tissues. Thus the relationship of fluid loss to body surface area is directly proportional. Several formulas (Evans, Baxter, Brooke Army Hospital) are used to estimate fluid loss based on percentage of body surface area burned.
1, 2, 3 This is incorrect; the relationship is proportional.
Client Need: Physiological Adaptation; Cognitive Level: Comprehension; Nursing Process: Assessment/Analysis; Reference: Ch 10, Burns, Data Base

457. 1 Clostridium tetani can develop in partial- and full-thickness burns that contain dead tissue.
2 Although gamma globulin provides passive immunity against certain infectious agents, it is not specifically indicated in burns. 3 Isuprel is an adrenergic drug used in the treatment of bronchospasm and heart block. 4 This drug is indicated for hypoprothrombinemia caused by the deficiency of vitamin K; it is not related to burns.
Client Need: Pharmacological and Parenteral Therapies; Cognitive Level: Analysis; Nursing Process: Planning/Implementation; Reference: Ch 10, Burns, Data Base

458. 1 The severe pain experienced by the client during debridement of burns places an emotional strain on the relationship.
2 Maintaining sterility is not a problem if the nurse understands surgical asepsis. 3 According to Maslow, basic needs of survival and safety take precedence over higher-level needs. Pain becomes all-encompassing, and the nurse must help the client cope with it. 4 This answer is not complete. The frequency with which the nurse must perform tasks is not the problem; rather, it is the pain associated with debridement and the nurse's inability to eliminate the pain.
Client Need: Physiological Adaptation; Cognitive Level: Application; Nursing Process: Planning/Implementation; Reference: Ch 10, Burns, Nursing Care

459. 1 Acceptance and a positive attitude by those in contact with the client will support the development of a positive body image by the client.
2 Eventually the client may meet with other clients with burns, but this is not the priority now. 3 Removing mirrors from the environment is unrealistic. 4 Avoidance of comments about the client's appearance is an unrealistic expectation.
Client Need: Psychosocial Integrity; Cognitive Level: Application; Integrated Process: Caring; Nursing Process: Planning/Implementation; Reference: Ch 10, Burns, Nursing Care

460. 4 A partial-thickness burn over 30% of the body is considered critical. Shock, infection, electrolyte imbalance, and respiratory distress are life-threatening complications that can occur.
1, 2, 3 Burns involving less than 30% of the body surface of older children and adults under 50 years of age are generally less severe; the condition would be rated accordingly.
Client Need: Physiological Adaptation; Cognitive Level: Comprehension; Nursing Process: Assessment/Analysis; Reference: Ch 10, Burns, Data Base

461. **4** Partial-thickness burns are very painful; this outcome is specific, realistic, and measurable.

1 This would be a priority if the burns involved the head or anterior thorax. **2** Although important, this is not the primary goal at this time. **3** Ensuring urine output is generally more of a concern with burns that involve more than 5% of the body's surface area.

Client Need: Physiological Adaptation; **Cognitive Level:** Analysis; **Nursing Process:** Planning/Implementation; **Reference:** Ch 10, Burns, Nursing Care

462. **3** In deep partial-thickness burns, destruction of the epidermis and upper layers of the dermis and injury to deeper portions of the dermis occur.

1 Eschar, a dry leathery covering of denatured protein, occurs with full-thickness burns. **2** In full-thickness burns, total destruction of the epidermis, dermis, and some underlying tissue occurs. **4** In superficial partial-thickness burns, the epidermis is destroyed or injured and a portion of the dermis may be injured.

Client Need: Physiological Adaptation; **Cognitive Level:** Analysis; **Nursing Process:** Assessment/Analysis; **Reference:** Ch 10, Burns, Data Base

463. **2** The leukocyte count would not be affected in the first few hours.

1 Pain is present in partial-thickness burns because the sensory nerves are not damaged. **3** Inhalation of hot air can cause laryngeal edema and would be a concern. **4** Replacement of fluids and electrolytes is essential in all burned clients.

Client Need: Physiological Adaptation; **Cognitive Level:** Analysis; **Nursing Process:** Assessment/Analysis; **Reference:** Ch 10, Burns, Nursing Care

464. **2** Potassium replacement is generally not indicated in the initial management of burns because hyperkalemia results from the liberation of potassium ions from the injured cells.

1, 3 This will be given to draw fluid from edematous tissue back into the bloodstream. **4** This will be given to replace fluid and electrolytes.

Client Need: Pharmacological and Parenteral Therapies; **Cognitive Level:** Analysis; **Integrated Process:** Communication/ Documentation; **Nursing Process:** Planning/Implementation; **Reference:** Ch 10, Burns, Data Base

465. **3** The pulse rate is one indicator of optimum vascular fluid volume; the pulse rate decreases as intravascular volume normalizes.

1 This would indicate hypovolemia. **2** This indicates inadequate kidney perfusion; if adequate, output should be above 30 mL/hr. **4** This would indicate hypovolemia and hemoconcentration.

Client Need: Physiological Adaptation; **Cognitive Level:** Analysis; **Nursing Process:** Evaluation/Outcomes; **Reference:** Ch 10, Burns, Nursing Care

466. **4** The circulating air bed disperses body weight over a larger surface, which reduces pressure against the capillary beds, allowing for tissue perfusion.

1 These beds are used for clients who are immobile; they do not increase mobility. **2, 3** This bed will have no effect on the development of this complication.

Client Need: Reduction of Risk Potential; **Cognitive Level:** Comprehension; **Nursing Process:** Planning/Implementation; **Reference:** Ch 10, Burns, Nursing Care

467. **2** Medical asepsis and surgical asepsis are essential for prevention of infection with the exposure method.

1 Bathing will be performed in a large tank tub. **3** Dressings are not used with the exposure method. **4** Clients are more comfortable with room temperatures of 85° F.

Client Need: Safety and Infection Control; **Cognitive Level:** Application; **Integrated Process:** Teaching/Learning; **Nursing Process:** Planning/Implementation; **Reference:** Ch 10, Burns, Data Base

468. **3** Cerebral cells require high levels of oxygen. When the partial pressure of oxygen within the circulatory system falls, the client becomes restless and cognitive functions become impaired.

1 With kidney failure the client would become progressively confused and lethargic because of the buildup of toxins in the body. **2** At this stage the client will be hypovolemic, not hypervolemic. **4** With metabolic acidosis the client would be lethargic.

Client Need: Physiological Adaptation; **Cognitive Level:** Analysis; **Nursing Process:** Assessment/Analysis; **Reference:** Ch 10, Burns, Data Base

469. **1** During the acute phase, hypokalemia results because of diuresis and the movement of potassium back into the intracellular compartment.

2 Hyperglycemia occurs during the acute phase because of lipolysis, gluconeogenesis, and glycogenolysis and a relative insulin insensitivity. **3** During the acute stage fluid shifts back into the intravascular compartment, resulting in an increased BP. **4** During the acute stage fluid shifts back into the intravascular compartment, which increases the glomerular filtration rate. When the glomerular filtration rate increases, there is an increase in the urinary output. As the urinary output increases, the urine specific gravity decreases.

Client Need: Physiological Adaptation; **Cognitive Level:** Analysis; **Nursing Process:** Assessment/Analysis; **Reference:** Ch 10, Burns, Data Base

470. **2** Necrotizing fasciitis destroys subcutaneous tissue and fascia and predisposes the client to infection and sepsis.

1, 3 Although this concern is important, it is not the primary concern at this time. **4** Necrotizing fasciitis is a problem of the integument, not the urinary system.

Client Need: Physiological Adaptation; **Cognitive Level:** Application; **Nursing Process:** Planning/Implementation; **Reference:** Ch 10, Cellulitis, Data Base

NEUROMUSCULOSKELETAL SYSTEM

471. 3 Although sympathetic impulses usually control most visceral effectors in times of stress, parasympathetic fibers likewise stimulate increased gastric contractions and increased peristalsis. Sympathetic fibers also inhibit organs such as the bladder and cause relaxation of this organ.

1, 2, 4 This statement is accurate.

Client Need: Physiological Adaptation; **Cognitive Level:** Comprehension; **Nursing Process:** Assessment/Analysis; **Reference:** Ch 11, Structures and Functions of the Nervous System, Autonomic Nervous System

472. 1 The thalamus receives sensory impulses from the spinothalamic tract and relays them to the cerebral cortex.

2 The cerebellum is involved in motor activity and coordination. **3** The hypothalamus relays messages between the cortex and autonomic centers. **4** The medulla contains the vital respiratory, cardiac, and vasomotor centers.

Client Need: Physiological Adaptation; **Cognitive Level:** Comprehension; **Nursing Process:** Assessment/Analysis; **Reference:** Ch 11, Structures and Functions of the Nervous System, Brain

473. 3 Parasympathetic nerves increase peristalsis and GI secretion.

1 The parasympathetic nervous system increases intestinal motility, which would cause diarrhea. **2** Goosebumps (piloerection), caused by contraction of the musculi arrectores pilorum, are under sympathetic control; vasoconstriction is also under sympathetic control. **4** Epinephrine is a sympathomimetic.

Client Need: Physiological Adaptation; **Cognitive Level:** Comprehension; **Nursing Process:** Assessment/Analysis; **Reference:** Ch 11, Structures and Functions of the Nervous System, Autonomic Nervous System

474. 2 Hemiplegia is paralysis of one side of the body.

1 Paresis is a weakness or partial paralysis. **3** Paraplegia is the paralysis of both lower extremities and the lower trunk. **4** This is quadriparesis.

Client Need: Physiological Adaptation; **Cognitive Level:** Application; **Nursing Process:** Assessment/Analysis; **Reference:** Ch 11, Brain Attack, Data Base

475. 1 The ache in muscles that have been vigorously worked without adequate oxygen supply is caused in part by the buildup of lactic acid. During rest, the lactic acid is oxidized completely to carbon dioxide and water, providing ATP for further muscular contraction.

2 Butyric acid is not a product of muscle contraction; it is a fatty acid occurring in feces, urine, and perspiration. **3** Acetoacetic acid is not a product of muscle contraction; it is a ketone body resulting from incomplete oxidation of fatty acids. It is also produced by the metabolism of lipids and pyruvates. **4** Hydrochloric acid is not a product of muscle contraction; it is present in the stomach to facilitate the digestive process.

Client Need: Physiological Adaptation; **Cognitive Level:** Application; **Integrated Process:** Teaching/Learning; **Nursing Process:** Assessment/Analysis; **Reference:** Ch 11, Structures and Functions of the Muscular System, Skeletal Muscles

476. 1 With an oxygen debt, a muscle would show primarily low levels of O_2 and low levels of ATP caused by the low levels of aerobic respiration, and high levels of lactic acid formation.

2 Low levels of calcium are present. **3** Low levels of glycogen are present. **4** High levels of lactic acid are present.

Client Need: Physiological Adaptation; **Cognitive Level:** Analysis; **Integrated Process:** Teaching/Learning; **Nursing Process:** Assessment/Analysis; **Reference:** Ch 11, Structures and Functions of the Muscular System, Skeletal Muscles

477. 1 The thalamus associates sensory impulses with feelings of pleasantness and unpleasantness; therefore it is partly responsible for emotions. The cortical limbic system is also involved in expression of emotions.

2 This is located in the cerebrum and controls all conscious functions. **3** This controls body temperature and serves as a neural pathway. **4** This is the outer layer of the cerebrum and controls mental functions.

Client Need: Physiological Adaptation; **Cognitive Level:** Comprehension; **Nursing Process:** Assessment/Analysis; **Reference:** Ch 11, Structures and Functions of the Nervous System, Brain

478. 2 The arteries communicating (anastomosing) at the base of the brain are referred to as the circle of Willis.

1 This is an anastomosis of blood vessels that is located in the palm of the hand. **3** This is a nerve communication network in the region of the neck and axilla. **4** This is a single large branch of the aorta.

Client Need: Physiological Adaptation; **Cognitive Level:** Knowledge; **Nursing Process:** Assessment/Analysis; **Reference:** Ch 11, Brain Attack, Data Base

479. 1 ☒ The medulla, part of the brainstem just above the foramen magnum, is concerned with vital functions such as respirations.

2 ☒ The medulla is concerned with vital functions such as the heart rate.

3 ☐ This is not controlled by the CNS.

4 ☒ The medulla is concerned with vital functions such as BP by controlling blood vessel diameter.

5 ☐ This is controlled by the hypothalamus.

Client Need: Physiological Adaptation; **Cognitive Level:** Comprehension; **Nursing Process:** Assessment/Analysis; **Reference:** Ch 11, Structures and Functions of the Nervous System, Brain

480. 1 The third cranial nerve (oculomotor) contains autonomic fibers that innervate the smooth muscle responsible for constriction of pupils.

2 The optic nerve is concerned with vision; lesions result in visual field defects and loss of visual acuity. **3** The trochlear nerve is concerned with eye movements; lesions result in diplopia, strabismus, and head tilt to the affected side. **4** The facial nerve is concerned with facial expressions; lesions result in loss of taste and paralysis of the facial muscles and the eyelids (lids remain open).
Client Need: Physiological Adaptation; **Cognitive Level:** Analysis; **Nursing Process:** Assessment/Analysis; **Reference:** Ch 11, Related Procedures, Neurologic Assessment

481. **1** The facial nerve (seventh cranial) has motor and sensory functions. The motor function is concerned with facial movement, including smiling and pursing the lips. Nonconduction of the facial nerve will cause drooping on the side of the problem.
2 Nonconduction of the facial nerve on the right side would cause that side of the face to droop. **3** Nonconduction of the left abducent nerve would prevent abduction of the left eye. **4** Nonconduction of the trigeminal nerve would cause problems in mastication.
Client Need: Physiological Adaptation; **Cognitive Level:** Analysis; **Nursing Process:** Assessment/Analysis; **Reference:** Ch 11, Related Procedures, Neurologic Assessment

482. **3** This is the space between the arachnoid and the pia mater. It is filled with cerebrospinal fluid.
1 This is the innermost of the three meninges covering the brain and spinal cord. **2** This is an opening in the atrial septum in the fetal heart. **4** This is the cerebral aqueduct, between the third and fourth ventricles, in the midbrain.
Client Need: Reduction of Risk Potential; **Cognitive Level:** Comprehension; **Integrated Process:** Teaching/Learning; **Nursing Process:** Planning/Implementation; **Reference:** Ch 11, Related Procedures, Lumbar Puncture

483. **2** Sensory impulses from temperature, touch, and pain travel via the spinothalamic pathway to the thalamus and then to the postcentral gyrus of the parietal lobe, the somatosensory area.
1 This is the area of abstract thinking and muscular movements. **3** This is the area where nerve impulses are translated into sight. **4** This is the area where nerve impulses are translated into sound.
Client Need: Physiological Adaptation; **Cognitive Level:** Comprehension; **Nursing Process:** Assessment/Analysis; **Reference:** Ch 11, Structures and Functions of the Nervous System, Brain

484. **4** A Babinski response (dorsiflexion of the first toe) is a reaction to stroking the lateral sole of the foot with a blunt object; it is indicative of damage to the corticospinal tract when seen in adults.
1 Hyperreflexia is associated with upper motor neuron damage. **2** Increased muscle tone (spasticity) is associated with upper motor neuron damage. **3** This is indicative of hypocalcemia.
Client Need: Physiological Adaptation; **Cognitive Level:** Analysis; **Nursing Process:** Assessment/Analysis; **Reference:** Ch 11, Traumatic Brain Injuries, Data Base

485. **2** The sympathetic nervous system constricts the smooth muscle of blood vessels in the skin when a person is under stress.
1 The sympathetic system stimulates, rather than inhibits, secretion by the sweat glands. **3** This is not under sympathetic control; the parasympathetic system constricts the pupils. **4** The parasympathetic system (vagus nerve) slows the pulse, and the sympathetic increases it.
Client Need: Physiological Adaptation; **Cognitive Level:** Application; **Nursing Process:** Assessment/Analysis; **Reference:** Ch 11, Structures and Functions of the Nervous System, Autonomic Nervous System

486. **4** The brachial plexus is a maze of nerves extending from the axilla to the neck in the shoulder area; trauma to the arm may injure this plexus.
1 The solar plexus, also known as the celiac plexus, is where the splanchnic nerves terminate; it is unrelated to the arms. **2** The celiac plexus (solar plexus) is where the splanchnic nerves terminate; it is unrelated to the arms. **3** The basilar plexus is a venous plexus over the basilar part of the occipital bone; it is unrelated to the arms.
Client Need: Reduction of Risk Potential; **Cognitive Level:** Analysis; **Nursing Process:** Planning/Implementation; **Reference:** Ch 11, Structures and Functions of the Nervous System, Spinal Nerves

487. **4** If there is no obstruction, pressure on the jugular vein causes increased intracranial pressure (Queckenstedt's sign). This, in turn, causes an increase in spinal fluid pressure.
1 Homans' sign is calf pain possibly elicited by dorsiflexion of the foot if thrombophlebitis is present. **2** Romberg's sign is failure to maintain balance when the eyes are closed; it indicates cerebellar pathology. **3** Chvostek's sign is twitching elicited by tapping the angle of the jaw; it occurs if hypocalcemia is present.
Client Need: Reduction of Risk Potential; **Cognitive Level:** Analysis; **Integrated Process:** Communication/Documentation; **Nursing Process:** Evaluation/Outcomes; **Reference:** Ch 11, Related Procedures, Lumbar Puncture

488. **2** This is a sign of increasing intracranial pressure, which may follow a craniotomy.
1, 3 Signs of this would take time to develop; they would not be observable immediately after surgery. **4** The pulse pressure widens with increased intracranial pressure.
Client Need: Physiological Adaptation; **Cognitive Level:** Application; **Nursing Process:** Evaluation/Outcomes; **Reference:** Ch 11, Brain Tumors, Nursing Care

489. **3** The optic chiasm is the point of crossover of some optic nerve fibers in the cranial cavity at the base of the brain. The optic tracts conduct nerve impulses through the optic chiasm to other brain regions.
1 This is the orbit. **2** Optic tracts conduct nerve impulses through the optic chiasm. **4** This is the vitreous body.
Client Need: Physiological Adaptation; **Cognitive Level:** Comprehension; **Integrated Process:** Teaching/Learning;

Nursing Process: Planning/Implementation; **Reference:** Ch 11, Structures and Functions of the Nervous System, Sense Organs

490. 3 The contraction permits the lens to return to its normal bulge, decreasing focal length and allowing focus on near objects.

1 The ciliary muscles are intrinsic (within the eyeball); the third cranial nerve (oculomotor), an extrinsic nerve, controls some movements of the eyelid. 2 In this case, the ciliary muscles would relax. 4 The rectus and oblique muscles of the eye are involved in convergence.

Client Need: Physiological Adaptation; **Cognitive Level:** Comprehension; **Nursing Process:** Assessment/Analysis; **Reference:** Ch 11, Structures and Functions of the Nervous System, Sense Organs

491. 1 Cortisone, a steroid, stabilizes lysosomal membranes, inhibiting the release of proteolytic enzymes during inflammation. This antiinflammatory drug also maximizes vasoconstrictor effects.

2, 3 An inflammatory process does not necessarily have a microbial etiology. This drug would only indirectly decrease inflammation. 4 This is not an antiinflammatory drug; it decreases secretion of aqueous humor, lowering intraocular pressure in glaucoma.

Client Need: Pharmacological and Parenteral Therapies; **Cognitive Level:** Analysis; **Nursing Process:** Planning/Implementation; **Reference:** Ch 11, Ophthalmic Agents

492. 3 Glaucoma is a disease in which there is increased intraocular pressure resulting from narrowing of the aqueous outflow channel (canal of Schlemm). This can lead to blindness, caused by compression of the nutritive blood vessels supplying the rods and cones.

1 Pupil dilation increases intraocular pressure because it narrows the canal of Schlemm. 2 Intraocular pressure is not affected by activity of the eye. 4 Although secondary infections are not desirable, the priority is to maintain vision by controlling the pressure.

Client Need: Physiological Adaptation; **Cognitive Level:** Application; **Integrated Process:** Teaching/Learning; **Nursing Process:** Planning/Implementation; **Reference:** Ch 11, Glaucoma, Data Base

493. 3 Open-angle glaucoma has an insidious onset, with increased intraocular pressure causing pressure on the retina and blood vessels in the eye. Peripheral vision is decreased as the visual field progressively diminishes.

1 This may occur with untreated acute angle-closure glaucoma. 2 Pain occurs in acute angle-closure, not open-angle, glaucoma. 4 Occlusions of the central retinal artery would cause a sudden loss of vision.

Client Need: Physiological Adaptation; **Cognitive Level:** Application; **Nursing Process:** Assessment/Analysis; **Reference:** Ch 11, Glaucoma, Data Base

494. 1 A cataract is a clouding of the crystalline lens or its capsule.

2, 3, 4 This is not included in the pathophysiology related to cataracts.

Client Need: Physiological Adaptation; **Cognitive Level:** Comprehension; **Integrated Process:** Teaching/Learning; **Nursing Process:** Planning/Implementation; **Reference:** Ch 11, Cataract, Data Base

495. 4 Activities such as rigorous brushing of hair and teeth cause increased intraocular pressure and may lead to hemorrhage in the anterior chamber.

1 This is unnecessary; clients are usually permitted to drive before this time. 2 Coughing and deep breathing can increase intraocular pressure. 3 Weakening of the eye musculature is not related to cataracts.

Client Need: Reduction of Risk Potential; **Cognitive Level:** Application; **Integrated Process:** Teaching/Learning; **Nursing Process:** Planning/Implementation; **Reference:** Ch 11, Cataract, Nursing Care

496. 4 Retinal detachment is a separation between the sensory retina and the retinal pigment epithelium. These layers are not attached by any special structures and can separate as a result of various pathologic processes.

1, 2, 3 This statement does not explain the disease process involved.

Client Need: Physiological Adaptation; **Cognitive Level:** Comprehension; **Integrated Process:** Teaching/Learning; **Nursing Process:** Planning/Implementation; **Reference:** Ch 11, Detached Retina, Data Base

497. 4 Scar formation seals the hole and promotes attachment of the two retinal surfaces.

1 The retina is part of the nervous system; it does not regenerate or grow new cells. 2 The sclera is not involved; the retina adjoins and is nourished by the choroid. 3 This is not the treatment used; treatment includes the formation of a scar by the use of lasers or surgical "buckling."

Client Need: Physiological Adaptation; **Cognitive Level:** Application; **Integrated Process:** Teaching/Learning; **Nursing Process:** Evaluation/Outcomes; **Reference:** Ch 11, Detached Retina, Data Base

498. 2 The dendrites of the cochlear nerve terminate on the hair cells of the organ of Corti in the cochlea.

1 The utricle is a membranous sac that communicates with the semicircular canals of the ear. 3 The middle ear contains bones (malleus, incus, stapes). 4 This is the part of the middle ear that contains the auditory ossicles; it is the area between the tympanic membrane and the bony labyrinth.

Client Need: Physiological Adaptation; **Cognitive Level:** Knowledge; **Integrated Process:** Teaching/Learning; **Nursing Process:** Planning/Implementation; **Reference:** Ch 11, Structures and Functions of the Nervous System, Sense Organs

499. 4 The bones in the middle ear transmit and amplify air pressure waves from the tympanic membrane to the oval window of the cochlea, which is in the inner ear. The tympanic membrane separates the outer from the middle ear.

1 The earlobe is part of the external structure of the ear. 2 The eardrum separates the outer and middle ears.

3 The organ of Corti, cochlea, and semicircular canals are in the inner ear.
Client Need: Physiological Adaptation; **Cognitive Level:** Knowledge; **Integrated Process:** Teaching/Learning; **Nursing Process:** Planning/Implementation; **Reference:** Ch 11, Structures and Functions of the Nervous System, Sense Organs

500. **2** Because the organ of hearing is the organ of Corti, located in the cochlea, nerve deafness would most likely accompany damage to the cochlear nerve.
1 The vagus nerve would affect voice production. **3** The vestibular nerve would affect balance. **4** The trigeminal nerve would affect chewing movements.
Client Need: Physiological Adaptation; **Cognitive Level:** Knowledge; **Integrated Process:** Teaching/Learning; **Nursing Process:** Planning/Implementation; **Reference:** Ch 11, Structures and Functions of the Nervous System, Sense Organs

501. **4** The labyrinth is the inner ear and consists of the vestibule, cochlea, semicircular canals, utricle, saccule, cochlear duct, and membranous semicircular canals. A labyrinthectomy is performed to alleviate the symptom of vertigo but results in deafness, because the organ of Corti and cochlear nerve are located in the inner ear.
1 Anosmia is loss of the sense of smell and would not be affected by surgery to the ear. **2** There is no pain associated with Ménière's syndrome. **3** Ménière's syndrome is not related to cerumen production.
Client Need: Reduction of Risk Potential; **Cognitive Level:** Application; **Integrated Process:** Teaching/Learning; **Nursing Process:** Evaluation/Outcomes; **Reference:** Ch 11, Ménière's Disease, Data Base

502. **2** With a partial hearing loss the auditory ossicles have not yet become fixed; as long as vibrations occur, a hearing aid may be beneficial.
1 This procedure would not be performed unless there was total hearing loss or if what was heard was useless. **3** Although the bass tones are particularly affected, all tones are affected. **4** With conduction hearing loss, bone conduction is more effective than air conduction.
Client Need: Physiological Adaptation; **Cognitive Level:** Application; **Integrated Process:** Teaching/Learning; **Nursing Process:** Planning/Implementation; **Reference:** Ch 11, Otosclerosis, Data Base

503. **2** A subjective symptom such as ringing in the ears can be felt only by the client.
1 An objective symptom refers to signs that can be assessed through direct physical examination. **3** Prodromal refers to symptoms that are early indications of a developing disease; there is insufficient information to decide this from the situation described. **4** This term generally is not used to describe a symptom; a functional disease is one in which there is an alteration in the ability to perform as intended without physiologic changes.
Client Need: Physiological Adaptation; **Cognitive Level:** Comprehension; **Nursing Process:** Assessment/Analysis; **Reference:** Ch 11, Otosclerosis, Data Base

504. **3** The middle ear contains the three ossicles—malleus, incus, and stapes—that, along with the tympanic membrane and oval window, form an amplifying system.
1 The inner ear contains both the organ of hearing (the cochlea) and the organ of balance (the vestibule). **2** The pressure of sound waves is amplified in the middle ear and transmitted to the cochlea (part of the inner ear), where it is detected by the organ of Corti and transmitted along the acoustic nerve. **4** Although the eustachian tube connects the middle ear and nasopharynx, its main purposes are to prevent organisms from entering the middle ear and to equalize pressure on both sides of the eardrum.
Client Need: Physiological Adaptation; **Cognitive Level:** Comprehension; **Nursing Process:** Assessment/Analysis; **Reference:** Ch 11, Structures and Functions of the Nervous System, Sense Organs

505. **1** Gliomas account for about 45% of all brain tumors.
2 Angiomas are tumors originating in blood vessels. **3** Meningiomas, which occur in the meninges of the brain, account for about 20% of all brain tumors. **4** Neurofibromas are tumors of nerve tissue but are more common in the peripheral nervous system.
Client Need: Physiological Adaptation; **Cognitive Level:** Knowledge; **Nursing Process:** Planning/Implementation; **Reference:** Ch 11, Brain Tumors, Data Base

506. **4** The occipital lobe is involved with visual interpretation.
1, 3 This is a function associated with the frontal lobe. **2** This is a function associated with the temporal lobe.
Client Need: Physiological Adaptation; **Cognitive Level:** Application; **Nursing Process:** Assessment/Analysis; **Reference:** Ch 11, Brain Tumors, Data Base

507. **3** The facial nerve may be damaged during surgery. Drooping of the area results from loss of muscle tone.
1 A tracheostomy is not a complication. **2** This is also called auriculotemporal syndrome; it may follow infection and suppuration of the parotid gland; it is not a surgical complication. **4** The parotid is a salivary gland; its removal would decrease salivation.
Client Need: Physiological Adaptation; **Cognitive Level:** Application; **Nursing Process:** Evaluation/Outcomes; **Reference:** Ch 11, Related Procedures, Neurologic Assessment

508. **2** Seizure disorders are usually associated with marked changes in the electrical activity of the cerebral cortex, requiring prolonged or lifelong therapy.
1 Seizures may occur despite drug therapy; the dosage may need to be adjusted. **3** A therapeutic blood level must be maintained through consistent administration of the drug irrespective of emotional stress. **4** Absence of seizures would probably result from medication effectiveness rather than from correction of the pathophysiologic condition.

Client Need: Pharmacological and Parenteral Therapies; **Cognitive Level:** Application; **Integrated Process:** Teaching/Learning; **Nursing Process:** Planning/Implementation; **Reference:** Ch 11, Anticonvulsants

509. **1** Phenytoin (Dilantin) is an anticonvulsant most effective in controlling tonic-clonic seizures. Data collection before planning nursing care for a client with a seizure disorder should always include a history of seizure incidence (type and incidence). **2** Although protection is important, the use of restraints and insertion of an object into the mouth during a seizure often cause injury as a result of tonic-clonic muscle contractions and should not be used. **3** Although these may be removed during a seizure, the client's normal routines should be respected. **4** Increased restlessness may be evidence of the prodromal phase of a seizure in some individuals, but symptoms vary so widely that the history of the client should be obtained.

Client Need: Pharmacological and Parenteral Therapies; **Cognitive Level:** Application; **Nursing Process:** Assessment/Analysis; **Reference:** Ch 11, Epilepsy, Nursing Care

510. **4** A seizure is generally self-limiting; the nurse's responsibilities include protecting the client from injury and assessing the characteristics of the seizure. **1** Nothing should be forced into the client's mouth when the teeth are clenched during a seizure; this could damage the teeth or cause an airway occlusion if improperly placed. **2** During a seizure the client loses consciousness and would be unable to discuss any aura experienced. **3** Anticonvulsants are given on a regular basis, not PRN, to achieve therapeutic levels; diazepam (Valium) may be given IV in an emergency to control status epilepticus.

Client Need: Safety and Infection Control; **Cognitive Level:** Application; **Nursing Process:** Planning/Implementation; **Reference:** Ch 11, Epilepsy, Nursing Care

511. **3** To achieve the anticonvulsant effect, therapeutic blood levels of phenytoin must be maintained. If the client is not able to take the prescribed oral preparation, the physician should be questioned about alternate routes of administration. **1** Omission would result in lowered blood levels, possibly below the necessary therapeutic level to prevent a seizure. **2** The route of administration cannot be altered without physician approval. **4** The client is being kept NPO.

Client Need: Management of Care; **Cognitive Level:** Application; **Nursing Process:** Planning/Implementation; **Reference:** Ch 11, Anticonvulsants

512. **2** The medulla contains the vital respiratory, cardiac, and vasomotor centers. **1** The pons conducts impulses; it contains reflex centers for cranial nerves V, VI, VII, and VIII (trigeminal, abducent, facial, and vestibulocochlear, respectively). **3** The midbrain deals with sensory input from the eyes and ears. **4** The thalamus relays sensory impulses to the cerebral cortex.

Client Need: Physiological Adaptation; **Cognitive Level:** Comprehension; **Nursing Process:** Assessment/Analysis; **Reference:** Ch 11, Structures and Functions of the Nervous System, Brain

513. **4** The eighth cranial nerve has two parts—the vestibular nerve and the cochlear nerve. Sensations of hearing are conducted by the cochlear nerve. **1** The frontal lobe is concerned with thinking, skeletal muscle tone, and biorhythms. **2** The occipital lobe is concerned with sight, particularly shape and color. **3** Cranial nerve VI (abducent) is concerned with abduction of the eye.

Client Need: Physiological Adaptation; **Cognitive Level:** Comprehension; **Nursing Process:** Assessment/Analysis; **Reference:** Ch 11, Related Procedures, Neurologic Assessment

514. **2** An unconscious individual loses voluntary control of the sphincters surrounding the urethra and anus. **1** This cannot be assumed; hearing is often the last sense to be lost. **3** Motion (although often purposeless) is possible in coma. **4** Unconscious clients may react to various degrees of pain.

Client Need: Physiological Adaptation; **Cognitive Level:** Application; **Nursing Process:** Assessment/Analysis; **Reference:** Ch 11, Brain Attack, Data Base

515. **1** ☐ Although this is part of a neurologic assessment, it is not part of the Glasgow Coma Scale.
   2 ☒ The scale measures best motor response.
   3 ☒ The scale measures best verbal response.
   4 ☒ The scale measures eye opening response.
   5 ☐ Although this is important to assess, it is not part of the Neurologic Assessment.

Client Need: Reduction of Risk Potential; **Cognitive Level:** Application; **Nursing Process:** Assessment/Analysis; **Reference:** Ch 11, Related Procedures, Neurologic Assessment

516. **1** This action provides reinforcement. It is important to help the client who has expressive aphasia regain maximum communicative abilities as soon as possible. **2** This approach may increase client frustration. **3** Although expectations should be realistic, improvements are possible and should be encouraged. **4** Some abilities do return, and therefore the client should be encouraged to participate.

Client Need: Psychosocial Integrity; **Cognitive Level:** Application; **Integrated Process:** Teaching/Learning; **Nursing Process:** Planning/Implementation; **Reference:** Ch 11, Brain Attack, Nursing Care

517. **2** The hypothalamus connects with the autonomic area for vasoconstriction, vasodilation, and perspiration and with the somatic centers for shivering; therefore it is an important area for regulating body temperature. **1** The thalamus receives all sensory stimuli, except taste, for transmission to the cerebral cortex; it is also involved with emotions and instinctive activities.

3 The temporal lobe is concerned with auditory stimuli; it may also be involved with the sense of smell. **4** The globus pallidus is part of the basal ganglia; it is also called the pallidum. Together with the putamen, it comprises the lenticular nucleus; it is concerned with muscle tone, which is required for specific body movements.
Client Need: Physiological Adaptation; **Cognitive Level:** Application; **Nursing Process:** Assessment/Analysis; **Reference:** Ch 11, Structures and Functions of the Nervous System, Brain

518. **1** Head injuries can cause trauma to the brain, and the client should be observed for signs of increased intracranial pressure such as headache, dizziness, and visual disturbances.

2 This is not indicated in this situation. **3** Elevating the lower extremities should be avoided because it will increase intracranial pressure. **4** The intracranial pressure may increase after trauma because of bleeding and edema. The temperature may increase because of injury to or pressure on the hypothalamus.
Client Need: Physiological Adaptation; **Cognitive Level:** Application; **Nursing Process:** Assessment/Analysis; **Reference:** Ch 11, Traumatic Brain Injuries, Nursing Care

519. **1** ☒ Increased intracranial pressure affects the hypothalamic temperature-regulating center in the brain, resulting in fever.
2 ☒ Increased intracranial pressure disrupts neurons and neurotransmitters, which results in faulty impulse transmission and an altered level of consciousness.
3 ☐ This is associated with conditions such as pulmonary edema and obstructive airway diseases.
4 ☐ Increased intracranial pressure will cause a slow, bounding pulse.
5 ☐ The BP increases with a widening pulse pressure.
Client Need: Physiological Adaptation; **Cognitive Level:** Application; **Nursing Process:** Assessment/Analysis; **Reference:** Ch 11, Brain Tumors, Nursing Care

520. **2** As an antiinflammatory agent, dexamethasone (Decadron) helps prevent cerebral edema, which generally peaks between days 3 and 5 after a brain attack; this medication may also be used following a ruptured cerebral aneurysm.

1, 4 This drug is not given for this purpose. **3** This is not the reason for giving this drug. Although blood volume may increase because dexamethasone causes sodium retention, this is not beneficial to a client after a brain attack.
Client Need: Pharmacological and Parenteral Therapies; **Cognitive Level:** Application; **Nursing Process:** Evaluation/Outcomes; **Reference:** Ch 11, Brain Attack, Data Base

521. **3** An altered level of consciousness, as determined by the Glasgow Coma Scale, precedes other changes associated with increased intracranial pressure, such as vital sign alterations.

1 Carotid circulation is not altered. **2** This would not occur in this situation. **4** Spinal reflexes generally remain intact.

Client Need: Physiological Adaptation; **Cognitive Level:** Application; **Nursing Process:** Assessment/Analysis; **Reference:** Ch 11, Brain Tumors, Nursing Care

522. **4** Residual blood from the ruptured aneurysm may have blocked the arachnoid villi, interrupting the flow of CSF, resulting in hydrocephalus.
1 Vasospasm is a protective adaptation during the active bleeding process; it does not cause hydrocephalus. **2** Broca's center is not directly affected; even if it were, there is no relationship to the development of hydrocephalus. **3** The production of CSF is not increased in this situation; increased production may result when there is a tumor of the choroid plexus.
Client Need: Physiological Adaptation; **Cognitive Level:** Comprehension; **Nursing Process:** Assessment/Analysis; **Reference:** Ch 11, Traumatic Brain Injuries, Data Base

523. **4** This is a sign of increasing intracranial pressure, which may occur after a craniotomy.
1 Bradycardia, not tachycardia, would occur. **2** The pupils will dilate, not constrict. **3** The systolic, not the diastolic, pressure would be elevated.
Client Need: Physiological Adaptation; **Cognitive Level:** Application; **Nursing Process:** Evaluation/Outcomes; **Reference:** Ch 11, Brain Tumors, Nursing Care

524. **3** Decadron is a corticosteroid that acts on the cell membrane to prevent the normal inflammatory responses; by preventing vasodilation and increased permeability, the intracranial pressure is reduced.
1, 2, 4 This is not an effect of corticosteroid therapy.
Client Need: Physiological Adaptation; **Cognitive Level:** Application; **Nursing Process:** Evaluation/Outcomes; **Reference:** Ch 11, Brain Attack, Data Base

525. **4** Transient ischemic attacks (TIAs) are temporary neurologic deficits related to cerebral hypoxia; about one third of the people who have TIAs will have a CVA within 2 to 5 years.
1, 2, 3 This is not a risk factor associated with a brain attack (CVA).
Client Need: Physiological Adaptation; **Cognitive Level:** Analysis; **Nursing Process:** Assessment/Analysis; **Reference:** Ch 11, Brain Attack, Data Base

526. **3** Bleeding into the enclosed cavity of the skull creates pressure, causing pain.
1 Seizures are not directly related to the hemorrhage; they result from abnormal electrical charges that may eventually develop as a consequence of tissue ischemia. **2** This indicates caudal deterioration with damage to the midbrain and pons. **4** As the systolic pressure increases, widening of the pulse pressure occurs because of compression of vasomotor centers.
Client Need: Physiological Adaptation; **Cognitive Level:** Application; **Nursing Process:** Assessment/Analysis; **Reference:** Ch 11, Review of Physical Principles

527. **3** A comatose client loses voluntary control of elimination.
1 Although these may occur, they are not the most common adaptations associated with brain attack and coma. **2** Because cerebral functioning is

depressed, purposeful or voluntary movement is absent. **4** Because there are different levels of coma, the individual may or may not respond to intense stimuli such as pain.
Client Need: Physiological Adaptation; **Cognitive Level:** Application; **Nursing Process:** Assessment/Analysis; **Reference:** Ch 11, Brain Attack, Data Base

528. **3** Absence of a gag reflex is common after a brain attack. To prevent aspiration, the client is positioned on the side to allow gravity to drain mucus in the nasopharyngeal area away from the trachea.
1 Chest expansion is hindered in the prone position. **2** This position allows the tongue to occlude the airway and encourages the aspiration of secretions if the gag reflex is not intact. **4** This position interferes with respiration and leads to increased intracranial pressure.
Client Need: Reduction of Risk Potential; **Cognitive Level:** Application; **Nursing Process:** Planning/Implementation; **Reference:** Ch 11, Brain Attack, Nursing Care

529. **3** Dysphagia is difficulty in swallowing.
1, 2, 4 This is unrelated to dysphagia.
Client Need: Physiological Adaptation; **Cognitive Level:** Comprehension; **Nursing Process:** Assessment/Analysis; **Reference:** Ch 11, Brain Attack, Data Base

530. **4** Clients with dysarthria have difficulty communicating verbally, and an alternate means of communication may be indicated.
1, 2, 3 This is an important aspect of care, but it is not related to dysarthria.
Client Need: Psychosocial Integrity; **Cognitive Level:** Comprehension; **Integrated Process:** Communication/ Documentation; **Nursing Process:** Assessment/Analysis; **Reference:** Ch 11, Brain Attack, Data Base

531. **1** The paralyzed side has decreased muscle tone, which may lower BP readings.
2 The return of function to the affected extremity is not influenced by taking the BP; restoration of function occurs because of resolution of inflammation or resorption of blood in the area of the infarct. **3** Taking the BP will not precipitate the formation of thrombi. **4** Although the brachial artery will be compressed when taking a BP reading, it will not cause circulatory impairment because the pressure is temporary.
Client Need: Reduction of Risk Potential; **Cognitive Level:** Application; **Nursing Process:** Planning/Implementation; **Reference:** Ch 11, Brain Attack, Nursing Care

532. **2** Passive range-of-motion exercises prevent the development of deformities and do not require any energy expenditure by the client. Instituting range-of-motion exercises is an independent nursing function.
1, 3, 4 Bed rest is prescribed to decrease oxygen demands; active exercises markedly increase oxygen consumption.
Client Need: Reduction of Risk Potential; **Cognitive Level:** Application; **Nursing Process:** Planning/Implementation; **Reference:** Ch 11, Brain Attack, Nursing Care

533. **1** Atony permits the bladder to fill without being able to empty. As pressure builds within the bladder, the urge to void occurs and just enough urine is eliminated to relieve the pressure and the urge to void. The cycle is repeated as pressure again builds. Thus small amounts are voided without emptying the bladder.
2 These might be signs of kidney failure. **3** Continual incontinence would not occur if urine were retained. **4** The total amount of urine produced would be unchanged.
Client Need: Physiological Adaptation; **Cognitive Level:** Application; **Nursing Process:** Assessment/Analysis; **Reference:** Ch 11, Brain Attack, Nursing Care

534. **3** To prevent deformity after a brain attack, the client should be positioned in functional alignment to prevent contractures.
1 Active exercises are impossible with paralyzed limbs. **2** The physician must request a consult with the physical therapist. **4** This would increase deformities and atrophy.
Client Need: Reduction of Risk Potential; **Cognitive Level:** Application; **Nursing Process:** Planning/Implementation; **Reference:** Ch 11, Brain Attack, Nursing Care

535. **2** Various types of splints or boots are available to keep the foot in a position of dorsiflexion.
1 Blocks elevate the frame of the bed and have no effect on the position of the feet. **3** Although a cradle will keep the pressure of the linen off the client's feet, which otherwise could promote footdrop, the cradle does not maintain functional alignment of the ankle. **4** Sandbags help prevent rotation of an extremity or the head.
Client Need: Basic Care and Comfort; **Cognitive Level:** Application; **Nursing Process:** Planning/Implementation; **Reference:** Ch 11, Brain Attack, Nursing Care

536. **1** Change of position at least every 1 or 2 hours helps prevent the respiratory, urinary, and cutaneous complications of immobility.
2 Too protracted a period of time in one position increases the potential for respiratory, urinary, and neuromuscular impairment; prolonged physical pressure increases the possibility of skin breakdown. **3, 4** This is an unnecessarily short time interval, resulting in inefficient use of staff time.
Client Need: Basic Care and Comfort; **Cognitive Level:** Application; **Nursing Process:** Planning/Implementation; **Reference:** Ch 11, Brain Attack, Nursing Care

537. **1** Hemiparesis creates instability. Using a cane provides a wider base of support and, therefore, greater stability.
2 Hemiparesis affects muscle strength on one side of the body; the joints are not directly affected. **3** Activity should strengthen, not injure, weakened muscles. **4** The use of a cane would not prevent involuntary movements if they were present.

Client Need: Basic Care and Comfort; **Cognitive Level:** Comprehension; **Integrated Process:** Teaching/Learning; **Nursing Process:** Planning/Implementation; **Reference:** Ch 11, Related Procedures, Mobility, Assistive Devices

538.   3 Because stomach distention after eating results in contractions of the colon (gastrocolic reflex), which promotes defecation, establishing some regularity of meals that include adequate bulk or fiber will help establish routine patterns of defecation.
   1, 2 Although increased fluid intake and activity facilitate elimination, in general they do not help establish a pattern. 4 Increased potassium is not needed for normal elimination.
Client Need: Basic Care and Comfort; **Cognitive Level:** Application; **Integrated Process:** Teaching/Learning; **Nursing Process:** Planning/Implementation; **Reference:** Ch 11, Brain Attack, Nursing Care

539.   4 As part of the rehabilitative process after a brain attack, clients must be encouraged to participate in their own care to the extent that they are able and to extend their abilities by establishing short-term goals.
   1 A client with a brain attack may or may not have dysphagia; altering the consistency of food without the need to do so may make it less palatable. 2 Making the client feel helpless discourages independence. 3 This is unrealistic; family members may not be available because of other responsibilities.
Client Need: Physiological Adaptation; **Cognitive Level:** Application; **Nursing Process:** Assessment/Analysis; **Reference:** Ch 11, Brain Attack, Nursing Care

540.   2 Bowel training is a program for the development of a conditioned reflex that controls regular emptying of the bowel. The key to success is adherence to a strict time for evacuation based on the client's individual schedule.
   1 The indiscriminate use of laxatives can result in dependency. 3 Although this should be considered, the brain attack affects the responses of the client by altering motility, peristalsis, and sphincter control despite adherence to previous habits. 4 The passage of food into the stomach does stimulate peristalsis but is only one factor that should be considered when planning a specific time for evacuation.
Client Need: Basic Care and Comfort; **Cognitive Level:** Application; **Integrated Process:** Teaching/Learning; **Nursing Process:** Planning/Implementation; **Reference:** Ch 11, Brain Attack, Nursing Care

541.   2 A full rectum may exert pressure on the urinary bladder, which may precipitate urinary incontinence.
   1 Urinary retention catheters should not be used to manage urinary incontinence initially. The use of a catheter keeps the bladder empty, which promotes atony and incontinence. 3 Caffeine acts as a diuretic and is a urinary bladder irritant; both promote urinary incontinence. 4 Carbonated beverages irritate the urinary bladder, which promotes urinary incontinence.
Client Need: Basic Care and Comfort; **Cognitive Level:** Application; **Nursing Process:** Planning/Implementation; **Reference:** Ch 11, Brain Attack, Nursing Care

542.   4 To foster communication and cooperation, family members should be involved in planning and implementing care.
   1 This intervention does not focus on the client's feelings or needs. 2 The spouse may promote dependency in the client to satisfy a need to control. 3 Although true, the family should be involved.
Client Need: Management of Care; **Cognitive Level:** Application; **Integrated Process:** Communication/Documentation; **Nursing Process:** Planning/Implementation; **Reference:** Ch 11, Brain Attack, Nursing Care

543.   2 Changes in self-image and family role can initiate a grieving process with a variety of emotional responses.
   1, 3, 4 This cannot be assumed; the client's feelings need to be elicited.
Client Need: Psychosocial Integrity; **Cognitive Level:** Application; **Integrated Process:** Caring; **Nursing Process:** Assessment/Analysis; **Reference:** Ch 11, Brain Attack, Nursing Care

544.   1 Damage to Broca's area, located in the posterior frontal region of the dominant hemisphere, causes problems in the motor aspect of speech.
   2, 3, 4 This would be associated with receptive aphasia, not expressive aphasia; receptive aphasia is associated with disease of Wernicke's area of the brain.
Client Need: Psychosocial Integrity; **Cognitive Level:** Comprehension; **Integrated Process:** Communication/Documentation; **Nursing Process:** Assessment/Analysis; **Reference:** Ch 11, Brain Attack, Data Base

545.   2 Clients with expressive aphasia must be encouraged to associate words with objects so that communication is regained.
   1 Speech can usually be improved through therapy. 3 This may cause frustration. A balance must be achieved between assisting the client to communicate and permitting time for the client to form thoughts and words independently. 4 Despite having difficulty speaking, individuals with expressive aphasia can understand what is said to them.
Client Need: Psychosocial Integrity; **Cognitive Level:** Application; **Integrated Process:** Communication/Documentation; **Nursing Process:** Planning/Implementation; **Reference:** Ch 11, Brain Attack, Nursing Care

546.   2 The pain may prevent the client from ingesting anything by mouth.
   1 Hot or cold foods or compresses should be avoided because they may trigger a painful attack. 3 Exercises may precipitate an attack. 4 This could initiate an acute attack of trigeminal neuralgia; often clients must limit oral hygiene to rinsing the mouth.
Client Need: Basic Care and Comfort; **Cognitive Level:** Application; **Nursing Process:** Planning/Implementation; **Reference:** Ch 11, Trigeminal Neuralgia, Nursing Care

547. **2** Tic douloureux, also referred to as trigeminal neuralgia, is an inflammation of the fifth cranial (trigeminal) nerve, which innervates the midline of the face and head.

1 Petechiae are minute subcutaneous hemorrhages; they are not present in this disorder. **3** Pain, not weakness, occurs in this disease. Impairment of facial muscles occurs with Bell's palsy. **4** The third (oculomotor), not fifth, cranial nerve innervates the eyelid.

Client Need: Physiological Adaptation; **Cognitive Level:** Application; **Nursing Process:** Assessment/Analysis; **Reference:** Ch 11, Trigeminal Neuralgia, Data Base

548. **1** The nurse should avoid walking swiftly past the client because drafts or even slight air currents can initiate pain.

2 The client may assume any position of comfort, but pressure on the face while in the prone position may trigger an attack. **3** Although the procedure for oral hygiene may be modified, it is not discontinued. **4** Massaging may trigger an attack and should be avoided.

Client Need: Basic Care and Comfort; **Cognitive Level:** Application; **Nursing Process:** Planning/Implementation; **Reference:** Ch 11, Trigeminal Neuralgia, Nursing Care

549. **4** Carbamazepine (Tegretol) is a nonnarcotic analgesic, anticonvulsive drug used to control pain in trigeminal neuralgia and to abort future attacks. It sometimes eliminates the need for surgery.

1 Ascorbic acid (vitamin C) may be used as an adjunct to the specific treatment for trigeminal neuralgia. Vitamin C is prescribed when the body is subject to stress, as occurs with pain. **2** Morphine is an opioid analgesic that will relieve severe pain but will not prevent its recurrence; prolonged frequent use is contraindicated because of possible addiction. **3** Allopurinol is used in the treatment of gout.

Client Need: Pharmacological and Parenteral Therapies; **Cognitive Level:** Analysis; **Nursing Process:** Planning/Implementation; **Reference:** Ch 11, Trigeminal Neuralgia, Data Base

550. **3** Severe constant pain, emotional stress, muscle tensing, and diminished nutritional intake can lead to exhaustion and fatigue.

1 Because clients are apprehensive and have pain, prolonged periods of sleep usually do not occur. **2** Pain medications do not normally cause hyperactivity. **4** The client may be very quiet for fear of precipitating an attack.

Client Need: Physiological Adaptation; **Cognitive Level:** Application; **Nursing Process:** Assessment/Analysis; **Reference:** Ch 11, Trigeminal Neuralgia, Data Base

551. **4** The client may be able to avoid stimulating the involved trigeminal nerve and thus prevent pain by chewing on the unaffected side.

1 Food that is too hot or too cold can precipitate pain. **2** Although oral hygiene may initiate pain, it cannot be avoided. It can be modified to include rinsing the mouth or using a soft swab instead of a toothbrush. **3** Warm compresses may precipitate pain.

Client Need: Basic Care and Comfort; **Cognitive Level:** Application; **Integrated Process:** Teaching/Learning; **Nursing Process:** Planning/Implementation; **Reference:** Ch 11, Trigeminal Neuralgia, Nursing Care

552. **3** Bell's palsy unilaterally affects the seventh cranial nerve, which innervates the face; the blink reflex is diminished, so corneal damage must be prevented.

1, 2, 4 This is not necessary because Bell's palsy involves the seventh cranial nerve, which innervates the facial muscles.

Client Need: Reduction of Risk Potential; **Cognitive Level:** Application; **Nursing Process:** Planning/Implementation; **Reference:** Ch 11, Bell's Palsy, Nursing Care

553. 2, 4, 3, 1

_1_ Falling should not be a problem; the client is capable of seeing clearly with the unaffected eye.

_2_ Self-esteem is a primary concern of adolescents, who are experiencing the developmental stage of identity versus role confusion.

_3_ Paralysis of one side of the face affects the ability to chew; nutrition is a basic need.

_4_ Paralysis of one side of the face affects the ability to speak clearly; communication is essential, particularly with peers.

Client Need: Physiological Adaptation; **Cognitive Level:** Analysis; **Nursing Process:** Planning/Implementation; **Reference:** Ch 11, Bell's Palsy, Nursing Care

554. **1** Diplopia and nystagmus are experienced by clients with multiple sclerosis as a result of demyelination.

2 Clients experience intention, not resting, tremors. **3** Clients experience spastic paralysis because upper motoneurons are involved. **4** Although emotional affect and speech are affected, intelligence remains intact.

Client Need: Physiological Adaptation; **Cognitive Level:** Application; **Nursing Process:** Assessment/Analysis; **Reference:** Ch 11, Multiple Sclerosis, Data Base

555. **2** This tends to increase symptoms and may result in burns because of decreased sensation.

1 Using a straw gives the client more control of liquid intake, preventing aspiration. **3** Although a bladder regimen to maintain control is preferable, the use of pads can avoid embarrassment. **4** The disease does have periods of remission and exacerbation.

Client Need: Reduction of Risk Potential; **Cognitive Level:** Analysis; **Integrated Process:** Teaching/Learning; **Nursing Process:** Evaluation/Outcomes; **Reference:** Ch 11, Multiple Sclerosis, Nursing Care

556. **2** Spacing activities will encourage maximum functioning within the limits of strength and fatigue.

1 Bed rest and limited activity may lead to muscle atrophy and calcium depletion. **3** Strengths, rather than limitations, should be stressed. **4** This is

unnecessary. It is nursing's responsibility to maintain client safety and meet client needs.
Client Need: Basic Care and Comfort; **Cognitive Level:** Application; **Nursing Process:** Planning/Implementation; **Reference:** Ch 11, Multiple Sclerosis, Nursing Care

557. 3 As a result of muscle weakness, the vital capacity is reduced, leading to increased risks of respiratory complications; impaired swallowing can also lead to aspiration.
1 Although ALS is progressive, clients with myasthenia gravis may be stable with treatment and clients with Guillain-Barré syndrome may experience a complete recovery. 2 None of these diseases are caused by a lack of neurotransmitters; only myasthenia gravis is associated with a decreased number of receptor sites. 4 Twitching is not expected with myasthenia gravis or Guillain-Barré syndrome.
Client Need: Physiological Adaptation; **Cognitive Level:** Analysis; **Nursing Process:** Assessment/Analysis; **Reference:** Ch 11, Myasthenia Gravis, Data Base

558. 2 Guillain-Barré syndrome is a progressive paralysis beginning with the lower extremities and moving upward; therefore the client probably will not sense the need to void and would require an indwelling catheter to monitor urinary output.
1 The use of a straw would not be an effective stimulant for the facial muscles; oral intake may be contraindicated depending on the extent of the paralysis because of the risk for aspiration. 3 With progressive paralysis, the client will not be able to perform aerobic exercises. 4 Antibiotics are not given prophylactically; antibiotics will not help if pneumonia is caused by etiologies that are not bacterial.
Client Need: Basic Care and Comfort; **Cognitive Level:** Analysis; **Nursing Process:** Assessment/Analysis; **Reference:** Ch 11, Guillain-Barré, Nursing Care

559. 3 Myasthenia gravis is a degenerative disease that occurs slightly more often in females during young adulthood.
1, 2, 4 This does not represent the incidence of myasthenia gravis.
Client Need: Physiological Adaptation; **Cognitive Level:** Knowledge; **Integrated Process:** Teaching/Learning; **Nursing Process:** Planning/Implementation; **Reference:** Ch 11, Myasthenia Gravis, Data Base

560. 3 One of the pathologic changes is electron microscopic evidence of fewer AChR sites; also, antibodies cause destruction and blockade at the AChR sites.
1 There is no genetic defect in the production of ACh; rather than a genetic cause, it is thought that myasthenia gravis has an autoimmune etiology. 2 Although the defect is at the neuromuscular junction, it is not an inefficiency in the use of ACh, but a decrease in the number of receptor sites for ACh. 4 This enzyme is inhibited by anticholinesterase drugs used to treat myasthenia

gravis, leaving more ACh available to the damaged or decreased ACh receptors.
Client Need: Physiological Adaptation; **Cognitive Level:** Comprehension; **Integrated Process:** Teaching/Learning; **Nursing Process:** Planning/Implementation; **Reference:** Ch 11; Myasthenia Gravis, Data Base

561. 3 Myasthenia gravis is a chronic disorder with exacerbations that are precipitated by emotional stress, ingestion of alcohol, and physiologic stress such as infection.
1 The prognosis is not excellent; there is no cure. 2 The disease is characterized by exacerbations and remissions. 4 The disease is chronic. Death does not occur within a short period, but usually after the muscles of respiration are affected.
Client Need: Physiological Adaptation; **Cognitive Level:** Comprehension; **Integrated Process:** Teaching/Learning; **Nursing Process:** Planning/Implementation; **Reference:** Ch 11, Myasthenia Gravis, Data Base

562. 4 Raising the head of the bed allows gravity to assist in the swallowing of saliva, fluid, and food, thus decreasing the chance for aspiration. This should be done before the meal.
1 Alerting the physician to the problem is necessary, but only after client safety is ensured. 2 O_2 will not assist in the management of dysphagia or the prevention of aspiration. 3 This is unnecessary, unless the client has aspirated.
Client Need: Basic Care and Comfort; **Cognitive Level:** Application; **Nursing Process:** Planning/Implementation; **Reference:** Ch 11, Myasthenia Gravis, Nursing Care

563. 3 Weakened muscles result in ineffective coughing; secretions are retained and provide a medium for bacterial growth.
1 The airways are not narrowed. 2 Immune mechanisms are not impaired directly. 4 Viscosity of secretions depends on fluid intake and humidity.
Client Need: Physiological Adaptation; **Cognitive Level:** Comprehension; **Nursing Process:** Assessment/Analysis; **Reference:** Ch 11, Myasthenia Gravis, Data Base

564. 2 Neostigmine, an anticholinesterase, inhibits the breakdown of ACh, thus prolonging neurotransmission.
1 Neostigmine's action is at the myoneural junction, not the cerebral cortex. 3 Neostigmine prevents neurotransmitter breakdown but is not a neurotransmitter. 4 Neostigmine's action is at the myoneural junction, not the sheath.
Client Need: Pharmacological and Parenteral Therapies; **Cognitive Level:** Application; **Nursing Process:** Planning/Implementation; **Reference:** Ch 11, Cholinesterase Inhibitors

565. 1 Tensilon improves muscle strength in myasthenic crisis; weakness persists if symptoms are caused by cholinergic crisis, which can result from toxic levels of neostigmine.
2 Tensilon is not used for synergistic effects; the duration of effect is brief. 3 This is the same type of drug as neostigmine; no resistance

is indicated. **4** The diagnosis has already been established and treatment initiated.

Client Need: Pharmacological and Parenteral Therapies; **Cognitive Level:** Analysis; **Nursing Process:** Planning/Implementation; **Reference:** Ch 11, Cholinesterase Inhibitors

566. **4** Parkinson's disease involves destruction of the neurons of the substantia nigra, caudate nucleus, and globus pallidus of the basal ganglia. The cause of this destruction is unknown.

1 This pathologic condition is associated with multiple sclerosis. **2** This condition would result in auditory and visual problems; it is not associated with Parkinson's disease. **3** This condition is associated with myasthenia gravis.

Client Need: Physiological Adaptation; **Cognitive Level:** Comprehension; **Integrated Process:** Teaching/Learning; **Nursing Process:** Assessment/Analysis; **Reference:** Ch 11, Parkinson's Disease, Data Base

567. **3** The onset of this disease is not sudden, but insidious, with a prolonged course and gradual progression.

1, 2 The onset is slow and gradual. **4** The onset is not irregular; there is a gradual, regular progression of symptoms.

Client Need: Physiological Adaptation; **Cognitive Level:** Comprehension; **Nursing Process:** Assessment/Analysis; **Reference:** Ch 11, Parkinson's Disease, Data Base

568. **3** This is the best response to the client's question. The client with this disease cannot execute automatic involuntary movements and has difficulty swallowing saliva.

1 It is known that bradykinesia and muscular weakness cause difficulty in swallowing saliva. **2** There is no true paralysis or loss of sensation with this disease. **4** Muscular rigidity occurs with this disease but is not the cause of drooling.

Client Need: Physiological Adaptation; **Cognitive Level:** Application; **Integrated Process:** Teaching/Learning; **Nursing Process:** Planning/Implementation; **Reference:** Ch 11, Parkinson's Disease, Data Base

569. **1** Destruction of the neurons of the basal ganglia results in decreased muscle tone. The masklike appearance and monotonous speech patterns can be interpreted as a flat affect.

2 Rigidity is caused by sustained muscle contractions. Movement is jerky in quality (cogwheel rigidity). **3, 4** This is not associated with Parkinson's disease.

Client Need: Physiological Adaptation; **Cognitive Level:** Application; **Nursing Process:** Assessment/Analysis; **Reference:** Ch 11, Parkinson's Disease, Data Base

570. **1** The client with Parkinson's disease (PD) often has a stooped posture because of the tendency of the head and neck to be drawn down; this shift away from the center of support causes instability.

2 Hesitation is part of the disease; clients may use a marching rhythm to help maintain a more fluid gait. **3** The tremors of PD occur at rest (resting tremors).

4 The client must consciously attempt to maintain a natural arm swing for balance.

Client Need: Basic Care and Comfort; **Cognitive Level:** Application; **Integrated Process:** Teaching/Learning; **Nursing Process:** Planning/Implementation; **Reference:** Ch 11, Parkinson's Disease, Nursing Care

571. **4** Levodopa (L-dopa) is the precursor of dopamine. It is converted to dopamine in the brain cells, where it is stored until needed by axon terminals; it functions as a neurotransmitter.

1, 3 This is not an action of L-dopa. **2** This is not an action of L-dopa; neurons do not regenerate.

Client Need: Pharmacological and Parenteral Therapies; **Cognitive Level:** Comprehension; **Nursing Process:** Evaluation/Outcomes; **Reference:** Ch 11, Antiparkinson Agents

572. **1** Because of pressure on the sciatic nerve, pain radiating to the hip and leg is common.

2, 4 This is not associated with this disorder. **3** Although weakness (paresis) may occur, paralysis is not common.

Client Need: Physiological Adaptation; **Cognitive Level:** Application; **Nursing Process:** Assessment/Analysis; **Reference:** Ch 11, Degenerative Disk Disease, Data Base

573. **1** These actions, as well as lifting and straining, cause an increase in the intraspinal pressure, resulting in pain.

2 This does not affect the intraspinal pressure and should not cause pain. **3** Although pain may increase as a result of compression of the vertebrae, the increase is gradual, not sudden. **4** Flexing the knees and hips relieves pressure and pain.

Client Need: Physiological Adaptation; **Cognitive Level:** Application; **Nursing Process:** Assessment/Analysis; **Reference:** Ch 11, Degenerative Disk Disease, Nursing Care

574. **3** Inflammation from the trauma of intravertebral disk surgery could lead to injury of the nerve root, with consequent motor or sensory dysfunction.

1 Cerebral edema does not occur. **2** Rather than spasticity, urinary retention may develop if pressure on the nerve root occurs as a result of edema or bleeding. **4** Pain is usually experienced at the operative site and in the legs as a result of edema around the cord.

Client Need: Reduction of Risk Potential; **Cognitive Level:** Application; **Nursing Process:** Evaluation/Outcomes; **Reference:** Ch 11, Degenerative Disk Disease, Nursing Care

575. **2** Log-rolling maintains the alignment of the vertebral column.

1 Coughing will increase the pressure of the CSF surrounding the spinal cord and intensify the pain; incentive spirometry and turning should be used to prevent respiratory complications. **3** Peritonitis is not a danger because the abdominal cavity is not opened. **4** Flexion of the knees is avoided postoperatively because it alters intervertebral pressure.

Client Need: Reduction of Risk Potential; **Cognitive Level:** Application; **Nursing Process:** Planning/Implementation; **Reference:** Ch 11, Degenerative Disk Disease, Nursing Care

576. 2 Increased oral secretions and a sore throat that limits the ability to cough are expected responses after a cervical laminectomy.
1 To prevent strain on the operative site, flexion of the head is avoided. 3 The head of the bed may be only slightly elevated after a cervical laminectomy. 4 Limited range of motion occurs after both operations.
Client Need: Reduction of Risk Potential; Cognitive Level: Analysis; Nursing Process: Planning/Implementation; Reference: Ch 11, Degenerative Disk Disease, Nursing Care

577. 1 To avoid additional spinal cord damage, the individual should be moved only with a backboard. Moving a person whose spinal cord has been injured could cause irreversible paralysis.
2 A back injury precludes changing the person's position. 3 A back injury is suspected; therefore the person should not be moved. 4 A flat board would be indicated; however, one rescuer should not move the person without help.
Client Need: Physiological Adaptation; Cognitive Level: Application; Integrated Process: Communication/ Documentation; Nursing Process: Planning/Implementation; Reference: Ch 11, Spinal Cord Injury, Nursing Care

578. 2 Both legs and generally the lower part of the body are paralyzed in paraplegia.
1 There is no term to describe this condition; all parts below an injury are affected. 3 This is hemiplegia. 4 This is quadriplegia.
Client Need: Physiological Adaptation; Cognitive Level: Comprehension; Integrated Process: Teaching/Learning; Nursing Process: Planning/Implementation; Reference: Ch 11, Spinal Cord Injury, Data Base

579. 1 Because of the location of the micturition reflex center (in the sacral region of the spinal cord), bladder function may be impaired with lower spinal cord injuries.
2 This client's ability to ingest, digest, or metabolize is not affected; therefore nutrition is less of a problem than bladder control. 3 These exercises require motor control, which the client does not have. 4 Because there is no voluntary control over the lower extremities, mobility is usually accomplished through the use of a wheelchair rather than ambulation.
Client Need: Basic Care and Comfort; Cognitive Level: Application; Nursing Process: Assessment/Analysis; Reference: Ch 11, Spinal Cord Injury, Data Base

580. 4 Correct positioning maintains functional alignment, which helps prevent contracture formation.
1 Deep massage may dislodge thrombi that have formed as a result of venous stasis. 2 Because the client is paralyzed, active exercises are not possible. 3 The tilt board is used primarily to prevent orthostatic hypotension or bone demineralization.
Client Need: Basic Care and Comfort; Cognitive Level: Application; Nursing Process: Planning/Implementation; Reference: Ch 11, Spinal Cord Injury, Nursing Care

581. 1 Pressure ulcers easily develop when a particular position is maintained; the body weight, directed continuously in one region, restricts circulation and results in tissue necrosis.
2 Clients often state that they are comfortable and wish to remain in one position. 3 Proper positioning with supportive devices and range of motion are more effective measures to prevent contractures. 4 Because turning is usually done laterally, the circulation to the lower extremities is not dramatically affected.
Client Need: Basic Care and Comfort; Cognitive Level: Application; Nursing Process: Planning/Implementation; Reference: Ch 11, Spinal Cord Injury, Nursing Care

582. 4 Clients in the early stages of spinal cord damage experience an atonic bladder, which is characterized by the absence of muscle tone, an enlarged capacity, no feeling of discomfort with distention, and overflow with a large residual. This leads to urinary stasis and infection. High fluid intake limits urinary stasis and infection by diluting the urine and increasing urinary output.
1 Dehydration is not a major problem after spinal cord injury. 2 Pressure-relieving devices and interventions are most essential in preventing skin breakdown. 3 An electrolyte imbalance is not a major problem after spinal cord injury.
Client Need: Basic Care and Comfort; Cognitive Level: Application; Nursing Process: Planning/Implementation; Reference: Ch 11, Spinal Cord Injury, Nursing Care

583. 3 Spinal shock is immediate after a transection of the spinal cord; it usually lasts from 1 to 6 weeks and results in flaccid paralysis of all skeletal muscles.
1 This occurs after spinal shock has subsided. 2 During the acute phase, retention of urine and feces occurs as a result of decreased tone of the bladder and bowel; thus incontinence is unusual. 4 Respirations are labored, but spontaneous breathing continues, indicating that the level of injury is below C4 and respirations are not affected.
Client Need: Physiological Adaptation; Cognitive Level: Application; Nursing Process: Assessment/Analysis; Reference: Ch 11, Spinal Cord Injury, Data Base

584. 2 Muscles are flaccid during spinal shock but develop spasticity with recovery; these movements are entirely involuntary.
1 Once nervous tissue is transected, it does not regenerate and paralysis therefore remains. 3 Although thrombophlebitis could occur, the client would not have any sensation of pain. 4 Although edema may be subsiding, motor function will not return if the cord is transected; paralysis remains below the level of the injury.
Client Need: Physiological Adaptation; Cognitive Level: Analysis; Integrated Process: Teaching/Learning; Nursing Process: Planning/Implementation; Reference: Ch 11, Spinal Cord Injury, Data Base

585. 1 These are symptoms of autonomic dysreflexia, which are commonly precipitated by a distended bladder.

2, 3 These are not associated with the symptoms of autonomic dysreflexia. 4 BP rises suddenly with autonomic dysreflexia.

Client Need: Basic Care and Comfort; **Cognitive Level:** Analysis; **Nursing Process:** Assessment/Analysis; **Reference:** Ch 11, Spinal Cord Injury, Data Base

586. 4 During prolonged inactivity, bone resorption proceeds faster than bone formation, and lack of therapeutic weight-bearing on bone results in demineralization. A tilt table provides gradual progressive weight-bearing, which counters these effects.

1 Lateral turning is possible and necessary if a client is immobile, but a tilt table does not make this possible. 2 The tilt table is used for scheduled periods in physical therapy. The nursing care required to prevent pressure ulcers must be consistently performed frequently throughout the day and night. 3 The tilt table does not cause hyperextension of the spine; the spine remains in functional body alignment.

Client Need: Basic Care and Comfort; **Cognitive Level:** Comprehension; **Integrated Process:** Teaching/Learning; **Nursing Process:** Planning/Implementation; **Reference:** Ch 11, Spinal Cord Injury, Nursing Care

587. 2 Clients with quadriplegia do not have and never will have the muscle innervation, strength, or balance needed for ambulation.

1 Bracing and crutch-walking require muscle strength and coordination that an individual with quadriplegia does not have. 3 Quadriplegia refers to paralysis of all four extremities. 4 Orthostatic hypotension can be prevented by any upright positioning and does not necessarily require a wheelchair.

Client Need: Basic Care and Comfort; **Cognitive Level:** Application; **Integrated Process:** Teaching/Learning; **Nursing Process:** Planning/Implementation; **Reference:** Ch 11, Spinal Cord Injury, Data Base

588. 3 Synovial fluid minimizes friction at joints by providing lubrication for the moving parts.

1 Synovial fluid increases the efficiency of joint movements. 2 Synovial fluid increases work output. 4 Synovial fluid increases the speed of movements.

Client Need: Physiological Adaptation; **Cognitive Level:** Comprehension; **Integrated Process:** Teaching/Learning; **Nursing Process:** Planning/Implementation; **Reference:** Ch 11, Structures and Functions of the Muscular System

589. 4 The greater density of compact bone makes it stronger than cancellous bone. Compact bone forms from cancellous bone by the addition of concentric rings of bone substance to the marrow spaces of cancellous bone. The large marrow spaces are reduced to haversian canals.

1 Overall size does not determine strength. 2 Weight alone is not a factor. 3 Volume is not related to strength.

Client Need: Physiological Adaptation; **Cognitive Level:** Comprehension; **Integrated Process:** Teaching/Learning; **Nursing Process:** Planning/Implementation; **Reference:** Ch 11, Structures and Functions of the Skeletal System, Bone Formation

590. 3 Allopurinol interferes with the final steps in uric acid formation by inhibiting the production of xanthine oxidase.

1 This drug prevents the formation of uric acid; it does not affect bone density. 2 Allopurinol has no effect on swelling of the synovial membranes. 4 This medication prevents the synthesis of uric acid, not its crystallization.

Client Need: Pharmacological and Parenteral Therapies; **Cognitive Level:** Application; **Integrated Process:** Teaching/Learning; **Nursing Process:** Planning/Implementation; **Reference:** Ch 11, Antigout Agents

591. 1 Colchicine decreases the formation of lactic acid, which may promote the deposition of uric acid in the joints. It also decreases the inflammatory response.

2 Hydrocortisone is an antiinflammatory agent; it is not used to treat gout. 3 Ibuprofen is a nonsteroidal antiinflammatory agent; it does not prevent the formation of uric acid. 4 Benemid acts to inhibit the resorption of urate in the kidneys and therefore decreases uric acid in the blood; it is not useful in the treatment of acute gout but rather of chronic gout.

Client Need: Pharmacological and Parenteral Therapies; **Cognitive Level:** Analysis; **Nursing Process:** Planning/Implementation; **Reference:** Ch 11, Antigout Agents

592. 2 Like other organ meats, liver is a high-purine food (range of 150 to 1000 mg/100 g) and should be avoided.

1 Eggs have insignificant amounts of purine and are unrestricted. 3 Cheese has insignificant amounts of purine and is unrestricted. 4 Foods that contain a moderate amount of purine (50 to 150 mg/dL), such as salmon, may be eaten 4 times a week.

Client Need: Reduction of Risk Potential; **Cognitive Level:** Comprehension; **Integrated Process:** Teaching/Learning; **Nursing Process:** Planning/Implementation; **Reference:** Ch 11, Arthritis, Nursing Care

593. 4 Warm compresses (at or slightly above body temperature) dilate blood vessels, increasing blood flow to the area and decreasing edema.

1, 2, 3 This temperature is too cool to increase blood flow to the area.

Client Need: Basic Care and Comfort; **Cognitive Level:** Application; **Nursing Process:** Planning/Implementation; **Reference:** Ch 11, Arthritis, Nursing Care

594. 2 Elevated tissue pressure restricts blood flow, causing increasing ischemia and increasing pain; it is the cardinal early symptom of compartment syndrome.

1 The arm would feel cool, not warm, because of a decrease in circulation. 3 Sluggish capillary refill, not rapid, is a sign of compartment syndrome. 4 The pulse would be diminished, not bounding; increasing edema impairs circulation.

Client Need: Physiological Adaptation; **Cognitive Level:** Application; **Nursing Process:** Assessment/Analysis; **Reference:** Ch 11, Fractures of the Extremities, Nursing Care

595. 1 This is not a priority at this point. The client is too traumatized to learn. It will assume priority as the client's recovery progresses.

2 The nurse must closely monitor hemoglobin level because blood loss is a major problem 3 Maintaining a pressure dressing helps to prevent edema and bleeding, and to shape the residual limb for a prosthesis 4 The client has experienced a major life event; the nurse will need to be empathetic and use interviewing skills to encourage expression of feelings.

Client Need: Physiological Adaptation; **Cognitive Level:** Analysis; **Nursing Process:** Planning/Implementation; **Reference:** Ch 11, Amputation, Nursing Care

596. 3 The hips are in extension when the client is prone; this keeps the hips from flexing.

1 In the left side-lying position the right hip will be flexed, promoting contracture formation. 2 This promotes flexion contracture formation. 4 This is not related to the prevention of hip-flexion contractures.

Client Need: Reduction of Risk Potential; **Cognitive Level:** Application; **Integrated Process:** Teaching/Learning; **Nursing Process:** Planning/Implementation; **Reference:** Ch 11, Amputation, Nursing Care

597. 3 Elastic bandages compress the residual limb, preventing edema and promoting residual limb shrinkage and molding; the bandage must be rewrapped when it loosens.

1, 2 This would have a systemic effect on fluid balance; edema of the residual limb is a localized response to inflammation. 4 Prolonged immobilization of the residual extremity in one position can lead to a flexion contracture of the hip.

Client Need: Reduction of Risk Potential; **Cognitive Level:** Application; **Nursing Process:** Planning/Implementation; **Reference:** Ch 11, Amputation, Nursing Care

598. 4 Preparing muscles that will do the work in crutch-walking is imperative.

1 The biceps are not the major muscles required for crutch-walking. 2 Contractures of the limb will not have a great influence on the ability to use crutches. 3 Strengthening the hamstring muscles will not assist in the use of crutches.

Client Need: Basic Care and Comfort; **Cognitive Level:** Application; **Integrated Process:** Teaching/Learning; **Nursing Process:** Planning/Implementation; **Reference:** Ch 11, Related Procedures, Mobility: Assistive Devices

599. 4 Flexion contracture of the hip can be prevented by routinely placing the client in a prone position to extend the hip.

1, 2 This can cause flexion of the hip, which will result in a hip contracture and affect balance. 3 Lying in this position does not allow for full extension of the hip.

Client Need: Basic Care and Comfort; **Cognitive Level:** Application; **Nursing Process:** Planning/Implementation; **Reference:** Ch 11, Amputation, Nursing Care

600. 3 Because capillary perfusion is blocked by the pulmonary embolus, O_2 saturation drops and the client experiences shortness of breath, dyspnea, and tachypnea.

1, 2 This is not a classic sign of pulmonary embolus. 4 The pain associated with pulmonary embolus is generally sudden in onset, severe, and located in the chest, not the hip.

Client Need: Reduction of Risk Potential; **Cognitive Level:** Application; **Nursing Process:** Evaluation/Outcomes; **Reference:** Ch 11, Fracture of the Hip, Nursing Care

601. 1 This position offsets the development of hip deformities resulting from contractures. It also maintains the correct center of gravity when the client is upright.

2 This promotes flexion contracture of the hip. 3 A prosthesis may be applied early in the postoperative period, but requires a rigid dressing (cast) to prevent edema; ambulation can be facilitated by the use of a walker, crutches, parallel bars, or cane. 4 This may alter the center of gravity and cause a loss of balance.

Client Need: Basic Care and Comfort; **Cognitive Level:** Application; **Integrated Process:** Teaching/Learning; **Nursing Process:** Planning/Implementation; **Reference:** Ch 11, Amputation, Nursing Care

602. 2 A continuous passive motion device is most commonly used after knee replacement to gradually increase knee flexion without weight-bearing or strain.

1 Because it provides passive range of motion, muscle tone is not affected. 3 A continuous passive motion device is not used to prevent tissue breakdown. 4 Since muscles are not contracting, venous stasis is not prevented.

Client Need: Basic Care and Comfort; **Cognitive Level:** Application; **Integrated Process:** Teaching/Learning; **Nursing Process:** Evaluation/Outcomes; **Reference:** Ch 11, Related Procedures, Continuous Passive Motion Device

603. 1 Rehabilitation should begin immediately. This includes preoperative discussion of the nature of the operation and rehabilitation techniques.

2, 3, 4 This is too late; valuable rehabilitation time has been wasted.

Client Need: Reduction of Risk Potential; **Cognitive Level:** Application; **Integrated Process:** Teaching/Learning; **Nursing Process:** Planning/Implementation; **Reference:** Ch 11, Amputation, Nursing Care

604. 4 The neural endings that innervated the limb are still intact and may be stimulated within the residual limb.

1 Severed blood vessels are not involved in phantom limb sensation. 2 Although an individual must grieve over a lost body part, the grieving is unrelated to phantom limb sensation. 3 Although

phantom limb sensation is a hallucinatory-type experience, it is not part of a psychotic process.
Client Need: Basic Care and Comfort; **Cognitive Level:** Comprehension; **Nursing Process:** Evaluation/Outcomes; **Reference:** Ch 11, Amputation, Nursing Care

605. **1** A four-point gait provides for weight-bearing on all points that touch the floor and maximum support during ambulation.
2, 3 A three-point gait is used when one extremity cannot bear weight. **4** A swing-through gait does not simulate ambulation; it is used when the individual can bear weight but lacks the muscular control needed for ambulation without an assistive device.
Client Need: Basic Care and Comfort; **Cognitive Level:** Application; **Integrated Process:** Teaching/Learning; **Nursing Process:** Planning/Implementation; **Reference:** Ch 11, Related Procedures, Mobility: Assistive Devices

606. **3** In the four-point gait the client brings the left crutch forward first, followed by the right foot; then the right crutch is brought forward, followed by the left foot. Thus both legs must be able to bear some weight.
1 Although the arms are extended to allow the hands to bear weight, the elbows are not maintained in this position. **2** Pressure on the axillae may damage nerves in the area. **4** Both extremities must be able to bear weight.
Client Need: Basic Care and Comfort; **Cognitive Level:** Application; **Integrated Process:** Teaching/Learning; **Nursing Process:** Planning/Implementation; **Reference:** Ch 11, Related Procedures, Mobility: Assistive Devices

607. **3** This response explains why the traction may not be released; a continuous pull must be maintained.
1 Reducing the weight requires a physician's order; removing half the weights will not maintain the bone in alignment. **2** This ignores the client's request to release the traction; further assessment is needed. **4** Although this is a true statement, it does not provide the rationale as to why the weights cannot and should not be released.
Client Need: Basic Care and Comfort; **Cognitive Level:** Application; **Integrated Process:** Teaching/Learning; **Nursing Process:** Planning/Implementation; **Reference:** Ch 11, Fractures of the Extremities, Nursing Care

608. **2** Constriction of circulation decreases venous return and increases pressure within the vessels. Fluid then moves into the interstitial spaces, causing edema.
1, 3, 4 This would indicate infection.
Client Need: Reduction of Risk Potential; **Cognitive Level:** Application; **Nursing Process:** Evaluation/Outcomes; **Reference:** Ch 11, Fractures of the Extremities, Nursing Care

609. **4** In crutch-walking the client uses the triceps, trapezius, and latissimus muscles. A client who has been in bed may need to implement an exercise program to strengthen these shoulder and upper arm muscles before initiating crutch-walking.
1 This activity does not strengthen muscles used in crutch-walking. **2** Keeping the leg in abduction alters

the center of gravity, which impedes ambulation.
3 Back muscles are not used in crutch-walking.
Client Need: Basic Care and Comfort; **Cognitive Level:** Application; **Integrated Process:** Teaching/Learning; **Nursing Process:** Planning/Implementation; **Reference:** Ch 11, Related Procedures, Mobility: Assistive Devices

610. **3** The paraplegic client is unable to exercise the lower extremities actively.
1 Changing a position involves moving the extremities; contractures develop as a result of prolonged immobility. **2** The use of pillows, splints, and other supportive devices helps maintain alignment and prevent the shortening of muscle fibers associated with contractures. **4** Passive range-of-motion exercises help maintain joint mobility and prevent contractures.
Client Need: Basic Care and Comfort; **Cognitive Level:** Application; **Integrated Process:** Teaching/Learning; **Nursing Process:** Planning/Implementation; **Reference:** Ch 11, Spinal Cord Injury, Nursing Care

611. **4** Calcium that has left the bones as a response to prolonged inactivity enters the blood and may precipitate in the kidneys, forming calculi.
1 Increased fluid intake is helpful in avoiding this condition by preventing urinary stasis. **2** Calculi may develop despite adequate kidney function; kidney function may be impaired by the presence of calculi and urinary tract infections associated with urinary stasis or repeated catheterizations. **3** Calcium intake is usually limited to prevent the increased risk for calculi.
Client Need: Basic Care and Comfort; **Cognitive Level:** Application; **Integrated Process:** Teaching/Learning; **Nursing Process:** Planning/Implementation; **Reference:** Ch 11, Spinal Cord Injury, Nursing Care

612. **4** Calcium leaves the long bones during periods of prolonged bed rest. The tilt table places the client in an upright position, which provides for weight-bearing.
1 The tilt table is used to prevent orthostatic hypotension by gradually allowing an individual who has been immobilized to adjust to an upright position. **2** The client is carefully strapped to the table so that mobility is actually impaired to ensure safety. **3** Although the pressure on bony prominences is altered, the use of the tilt table is not frequent enough to prevent the development of pressure ulcers.
Client Need: Basic Care and Comfort; **Cognitive Level:** Comprehension; **Integrated Process:** Teaching/Learning; **Nursing Process:** Planning/Implementation; **Reference:** Ch 11, Spinal Cord Injury, Nursing Care

613. **3** Rehabilitating exercises carried out under water minimize strain on the body. The buoyant force of the water enables the limbs to move more easily.
1 Vapors are produced above water as a result of evaporation; they do not facilitate exercise.
2 Exercises are carried out near the surface of the water

where the water pressure would have little effect. **4** Water temperature would not assist movement.
Client Need: Basic Care and Comfort; **Cognitive Level:** Application; **Integrated Process:** Teaching/Learning; **Nursing Process:** Planning/Implementation; **Reference:** Ch 11, Review of Physical Principles

614. **3** As a result of contraction and pulling of the muscles on the two bone fragments, there is a characteristic shortening of the femur with external rotation of the extremity.
1 Lateral motion of the leg does not occur; the leg externally rotates. **2** Lateral motion of the leg does not occur. **4** The extremity externally rotates as the muscles contract; shortening, not lengthening, occurs.
Client Need: Physiological Adaptation; **Cognitive Level:** Application; **Nursing Process:** Assessment/Analysis; **Reference:** Ch 11, Fracture of the Hip, Data Base

615. **1** Traction is frequently used in the treatment of a fractured hip to align the bones (reduction of fracture). If such traction were not employed, the muscles would go into spasm, shifting the bone fragments and causing pain.
2 Traction is usually a temporary measure before surgery; contractures result from a shortening of the muscles by prolonged immobility. **3** Although the affected extremity must be properly aligned, turning and moving the client is still necessary. **4** External rotation is contraindicated and prevented by the use of sandbags or trochanter rolls.
Client Need: Basic Care and Comfort; **Cognitive Level:** Application; **Integrated Process:** Teaching/Learning; **Nursing Process:** Planning/Implementation; **Reference:** Ch 11, Fracture of the Hip, Data Base

616. **1** A fracture in the neck of the femur will cause shortening of the femur and external rotation. To correct this misalignment, the client's leg should be extended and maintained in slight internal rotation.
2 To reduce the fracture, it is necessary to maintain the leg in extension, counteracting the contraction of the quadriceps that may cause overriding of bone fragments. **3** To reduce the fracture, it is necessary to maintain the leg in extension, counteracting the contraction of the quadriceps that may cause overriding of bone fragments. **4** External rotation of the thigh as a result of muscle contraction tends to misalign the bone fragments; therefore slight internal rotation or functional alignment is preferred.
Client Need: Basic Care and Comfort; **Cognitive Level:** Application; **Nursing Process:** Planning/Implementation; **Reference:** Ch 11, Fracture of the Hip, Data Base

617. **1** After a fractured hip, the muscle spasms and the client's tendency to flex the hips can lead to flexion contractures of the hip.
2 The hip will tend to adduct. **3** Contractures most often involve flexor, not extensor, muscles. **4** The hip will tend to be externally rotated.
Client Need: Basic Care and Comfort; **Cognitive Level:** Application; **Nursing Process:** Planning/Implementation; **Reference:** Ch 11, Fracture of the Hip, Data Base

618. **4** After a fracture, if blood supply is cut off or impaired, necrosis of the bone may occur from lack of oxygen and nutrient perfusion.
1 The word aseptic indicates that infection is not present. **2** Early weight-bearing at the fracture site might result in trauma to bone; circulation would not be impaired. **3** Immobilization does not cut off circulation to the bone; it may cause contractures.
Client Need: Physiological Adaptation; **Cognitive Level:** Analysis; **Nursing Process:** Assessment/Analysis; **Reference:** Ch 11, Fracture of the Hip, Data Base

619. **3** Elevating the foot of the bed uses gravity and the client's weight for countertraction.
1 This would not increase countertraction. **2** This would increase traction rather than countertraction. **4** This would have no effect on countertraction.
Client Need: Basic Care and Comfort; **Cognitive Level:** Application; **Nursing Process:** Planning/Implementation; **Reference:** Ch 11, Fracture of the Hip, Data Base

620. **2** Intramedullary nails are used to maintain bone alignment and provide support along the femur's length.
1, 3, 4 Because this orthopedic problem does not affect the shaft of a long bone, an intramedullary nailing device is not appropriate.
Client Need: Basic Care and Comfort; **Cognitive Level:** Application; **Nursing Process:** Planning/Implementation; **Reference:** Ch 11, Fractures of the Extremities, Data Base

621. **3** This position involves hip flexion greater than 90 degrees. This puts stress on the operative site and could dislodge the prosthesis.
1, 2, 4 This is acceptable because little stress is placed on the operative site.
Client Need: Reduction of Risk Potential; **Cognitive Level:** Application; **Nursing Process:** Planning/Implementation; **Reference:** Ch 11, Fracture of the Hip, Data Base

622. **2** Ankle movement, particularly dorsiflexion of the foot, allows muscle contraction, which compresses veins, reducing venous stasis and risk for thrombus formation.
1 Because the client is being turned, the client's muscles are not contracting to compress the veins and prevent venous stasis. The client must be turned at least every 2 hours to help prevent skin breakdown and pneumonia. **3** The client is generally not allowed out of bed until at least 1 day postoperatively. **4** Sitting for long periods is contraindicated because pressure on the popliteal space and the dependent position of the lower extremities increase venous stasis.
Client Need: Reduction of Risk Potential; **Cognitive Level:** Application; **Nursing Process:** Planning/Implementation; **Reference:** Ch 11, Fracture of the Hip, Nursing Care

623. **3** Assessment of the pedal pulse should include the strength of the pulse. Symmetry, the correspondence of homologous parts on opposite sides of the body, indicates whether the pulses are equal.
1 Contractility is not a characteristic of a pulse but of the heart; rate is not measured with pedal pulses.

2 Color of skin is not a pulse characteristic; rhythm relates to the heart; it does not reflect a peripheral problem. **4** Local temperature is not a characteristic of the pedal pulse; pulsations are not visible in pedal pulses.
Client Need: Reduction of Risk Potential; **Cognitive Level:** Application; **Nursing Process:** Planning/Implementation; **Reference:** Ch 11, Fracture of the Hip, Nursing Care

624. **3** Because of the recumbent position, drainage may flow under the client and not be noticed.
1 This should be done more frequently; however, the site is a more reliable indicator of hemorrhage. **2** The girth of the thigh is not an indicator of hemorrhage. **4** Dressings impede accurate assessment.
Client Need: Reduction of Risk Potential; **Cognitive Level:** Application; **Nursing Process:** Planning/Implementation; **Reference:** Ch 11, Fracture of the Hip, Nursing Care

625. **1** This supports the site; the involved leg must be maintained in alignment, avoiding adduction to prevent dislocation of the prosthesis.
2 The pillow will not affect venous return, which relates to thrombus formation. **3** Adduction, not flexion contractures, is of most concern after surgery. **4** Although friction is decreased when skin does not interface with skin, this is not the reason for separating the thighs and lower limbs.
Client Need: Basic Care and Comfort; **Cognitive Level:** Application; **Nursing Process:** Planning/Implementation; **Reference:** Ch 11, Fracture of the Hip, Nursing Care

626. **1** Placing the feet apart creates a wider base of support and brings the center of gravity closer to the ground. This improves stability.
2 Bending at the waist should be avoided because it strains the lower back muscles; the power for lifting should be supplied by the muscles of the thighs and buttocks. **3** Pressure on the abdomen is prevented by tightening the abdominal and gluteal muscles to form an internal girdle; keeping the body straight does not reduce strain on the abdominal musculature. **4** Relaxing the abdominal muscles with physical activity increases back strain.
Client Need: Basic Care and Comfort; **Cognitive Level:** Application; **Nursing Process:** Planning/Implementation; **Reference:** Ch 11, Review of Physical Principles

627. **1** ☒ An increase in body temperature may indicate the presence of an infection.
2 ☐ Flexion of the hip is contraindicated until permitted because it could dislodge the head of the femur from the acetabulum.
3 ☒ This assesses the neural integrity distal to the surgical site.
4 ☐ No external pins are present with an internal fixation.
5 ☒ This assesses the circulatory integrity distal to the surgical site.
Client Need: Physiological Adaptation; **Cognitive Level:** Analysis; **Nursing Process:** Evaluation/Outcomes; **Reference:** Ch 11, Fracture of the Hip, Nursing Care

628. **2** Weight-bearing on the uninvolved leg helps maintain its muscle tone while limiting the stress on the involved extremity.
1 When the legs are in a dependent position, venous return is reduced. **3** Speed is not important when moving a client from the bed to a chair. **4** This is an unacceptable rationale for care.
Client Need: Basic Care and Comfort; **Cognitive Level:** Application; **Integrated Process:** Teaching/Learning; **Nursing Process:** Planning/Implementation; **Reference:** Ch 11, Fracture of the Hip, Nursing Care

629. **4** The pelvis is elevated by actions involving the unaffected upper extremities and unoperated leg.
1 It is impossible to lift the pelvis with this movement. **2** The involved leg should not be used because it could dislodge the prosthesis. **3** The client should not turn on the operative side immediately after surgery.
Client Need: Reduction of Risk Potential; **Cognitive Level:** Application; **Integrated Process:** Teaching/Learning; **Nursing Process:** Planning/Implementation; **Reference:** Ch 11, Fracture of the Hip, Nursing Care

630. **3** The three-point gait, which requires considerable arm strength, is used when a limb cannot bear weight. The affected leg and crutches are advanced together, and the strong leg swings through.
1, 2 This requires weight-bearing on both feet.
4 This is used for individuals who cannot move their lower extremities; it does not simulate ambulation.
Client Need: Basic Care and Comfort; **Cognitive Level:** Application; **Integrated Process:** Teaching/Learning; **Nursing Process:** Planning/Implementation; **Reference:** Ch 11, Related Procedures, Mobility: Assistive Devices

631. **3** To prevent nerve damage in the axillary area, the palms should bear all the weight.
1 This is unsafe and next to impossible to perform. **2** Pressure in the axillary area causes nerve damage to the brachial plexus. **4** Weight-bearing on the affected lower extremity is initially contraindicated.
Client Need: Basic Care and Comfort; **Cognitive Level:** Application; **Integrated Process:** Teaching/Learning; **Nursing Process:** Planning/Implementation; **Reference:** Ch 11, Related Procedures, Mobility: Assistive Devices

632. **3** Excessive flexion of the hip can cause dislocation.
1 Climbing stairs does not cause undue stress on the operative site. **2** This would be encouraged as long as no extremes of position are used. **4** This would be encouraged because it prevents hip flexion contractures.
Client Need: Reduction of Risk Potential; **Cognitive Level:** Application; **Integrated Process:** Teaching/Learning; **Nursing Process:** Evaluation/Outcomes; **Reference:** Ch 11, Fracture of the Hip, Nursing Care

633. **2** Because pain is an all-encompassing and often demoralizing experience, the client should be kept as pain-free as possible.
1 Surgery is used to correct deformities and facilitate movement; relief of pain is the priority.
3 Concentration is difficult when a client is in

severe pain; relief of pain is the priority. **4** Motivation is difficult when a client is in severe pain; relief of pain is the priority.
Client Need: Basic Care and Comfort; **Cognitive Level:** Analysis; **Nursing Process:** Planning/Implementation; **Reference:** Ch 11, Arthritis, Nursing Care

634. **3** An antinuclear antibody test (ANA) may be positive in clients with autoimmune disorders such as rheumatoid arthritis and systemic lupus erythematosus.

1 Pancreatic lipase is an enzyme that catalyzes the breakdown of lipids; this is a test used to diagnose pancreatic problems. **2** Bence Jones protein is a urine test helpful in diagnosing multiple myeloma. **4** Alkaline phosphatase is a blood test to determine phosphorus activity; it is used in diagnosing liver and biliary tract disorders and identifying periods of active bone growth or metastasis of cancer to bone.
Client Need: Reduction of Risk Potential; **Cognitive Level:** Analysis; **Nursing Process:** Assessment/Analysis; **Reference:** Ch 11, Arthritis, Data Base

635. **1** Active exercises, alternated with periods of rest, offer the best chance at avoiding the joint deformities associated with rheumatoid arthritis because they move each involved joint through its full range of motion.

2 Massage affects the muscles, not the joints, and would do little to prevent deformities. **3** Immobilization of joints by bracing would promote the formation of contractures and deformities. **4** Isometric exercise will promote muscle, not joint, function.
Client Need: Basic Care and Comfort; **Cognitive Level:** Application; **Nursing Process:** Planning/Implementation; **Reference:** Ch 11, Arthritis, Nursing Care

636. **3** ROM exercises must be instituted to maintain mobility of joints. Balanced activity and rest will promote resolution of the inflammation.

1 Pain may persist but cannot be allowed to legitimize inactivity. **2** Activity will not prevent the inflammatory process; it may aggravate it. **4** Severely damaged joints may require prosthetic replacement.
Client Need: Basic Care and Comfort; **Cognitive Level:** Application; **Integrated Process:** Teaching/Learning; **Nursing Process:** Planning/Implementation; **Reference:** Ch 11, Arthritis, Nursing Care

637. **1** Osteoarthritis affects the hips and knees first because they are the weight-bearing joints and undergo the most stress. The resulting joint damage causes a series of physiologic responses (e.g., release of cytokines and proteolytic enzymes) that lead to more damage.

2 Although these are weight-bearing joints and eventually are affected, normal motion is not as great as in the hips and knees; thus there is less degeneration. **3** Although the distal interphalangeal joints are frequently affected, the remaining

interphalangeal joints and metacarpals are not. **4** Although the spine may be affected, shoulder joints are not the most likely to be involved first unless there was an injury or a history of repetitive motions; these are not weight-bearing joints.
Client Need: Physiological Adaptation; **Cognitive Level:** Application; **Nursing Process:** Assessment/Analysis; **Reference:** Ch 11, Arthritis, Data Base

638. **2** Steroids have an antiinflammatory effect that can reduce arthritic pannus formation.

1 This will not provide lubrication. **3** Ankylosis refers to fusion of joints. It is only indirectly influenced by steroids, which exert their major effect on the inflammatory process. **4** Injection of a drug is not physiotherapy.
Client Need: Pharmacological and Parenteral Therapies; **Cognitive Level:** Comprehension; **Integrated Process:** Teaching/Learning; **Nursing Process:** Planning/Implementation; **Reference:** Ch 11, Arthritis, Data Base

639. **2** Ossification of cartilage, particularly of the spine, causes fixation of the involved joints.

1 Inflammation and thickening of the synovial membrane are characteristics of arthritis. **3** Although rest is essential, complete immobility would result in a loss of joint motion. **4** Redness and swelling are symptoms of local inflammation; they do not indicate irreversible damage.
Client Need: Physiological Adaptation; **Cognitive Level:** Application; **Nursing Process:** Assessment/Analysis; **Reference:** Ch 11, Arthritis, Data Base

640. **2** Heberden nodules are the bony or cartilaginous enlargements of the distal interphalangeal joints that are associated with osteoarthritis.

1, 3, 4 These deformities occur with rhematoid arthritis.
Client Need: Physiological Adaptation; **Cognitive Level:** Analysis; **Integrated Process:** Teaching/Learning; **Nursing Process:** Planning/Implementation; **Reference:** Ch 11, Arthritis, Data Base

641. **3** Inactivity over an extended time increases stiffness and pain in joints.

1 Assistive exercises help maintain joint mobility. **2** This is not a factor; cold packs may decrease joint discomfort. **4** The latex fixation test is positive when the rheumatoid factor is found in blood serum; this factor is present in many conditions, including rheumatoid arthritis, aging, narcotic addiction, and SLE.
Client Need: Physiological Adaptation; **Cognitive Level:** Application; **Nursing Process:** Assessment/Analysis; **Reference:** Ch 11, Arthritis, Data Base

642. **4** There are no dietary restrictions, but iron and vitamins should be encouraged to treat any underlying nutritional deficiencies.

1 These nutritional restrictions are not indicated. **2** A high-calorie diet would increase the client's weight; this is contraindicated because it would increase the strain on weight-bearing joints.

3 A balanced diet protein intake should fulfill nutritional needs; there is no need to increase protein or restrict calcium.
Client Need: Basic Care and Comfort; **Cognitive Level:** Analysis; **Nursing Process:** Planning/Implementation; **Reference:** Ch 11, Arthritis, Nursing Care

643. **2** Because of its antiinflammatory effect, aspirin is useful in treating arthritis symptoms.
1 Xanax is an antianxiety, not an antiinflammatory, agent. **3, 4** Opioids should be avoided because they promote drug dependency and do not affect the inflammatory process.
Client Need: Pharmacological and Parenteral Therapies; **Cognitive Level:** Analysis; **Nursing Process:** Planning/Implementation; **Reference:** Ch 11, Nonsteroidal Antiinflammatory Drugs

644. **1** Exercise of involved joints is important to maintain optimal mobility and prevent buildup of calcium deposits.
2, 3, 4 Immobilization causes loss of joint mobility and contractures.
Client Need: Basic Care and Comfort; **Cognitive Level:** Application; **Nursing Process:** Planning/Implementation; **Reference:** Ch 11, Arthritis, Nursing Care

645. **3** Heat and cold applications reduce inflammation and discomfort.
1 This will depend on the client's tolerance. **2** Avoiding exercise will increase the destructive effects of immobility. **4** Exercises are necessary to prevent contractures and permanent joint damage, but cannot be gradually increased unless the client is able to tolerate them.
Client Need: Basic Care and Comfort; **Cognitive Level:** Analysis; **Nursing Process:** Planning/Implementation; **Reference:** Ch 11, Arthritis, Nursing Care

646. **4** There is no special diet for arthritis. A balanced diet, consisting of foods from all levels of the MyPyramid diet, is essential in maintaining nutrition.
1, 2 Limiting the diet to particular foods does not provide all essential nutrients. **3** If nutritional intake is adequate, large doses of multivitamins are unnecessary and dangerous.
Client Need: Basic Care and Comfort; **Cognitive Level:** Application; **Nursing Process:** Planning/Implementation; **Reference:** Ch 11, Arthritis, Nursing Care

647. **1** Laminar air flow decreases the risk for bone infection, because potentially contaminated air continuously flows away from the sterile field, decreasing the concentration of airborne pathogens.
2 The procedure is performed at one time. **3** Surgery is generally considered when destruction of the femoral head and acetabulum is extensive. **4** The lithotomy position is used for gynecologic procedures; the side-lying position is generally used for hip surgery.
Client Need: Reduction of Risk Potential; **Cognitive Level:** Application; **Nursing Process:** Planning/Implementation; **Reference:** Ch 11, Arthritis, Data Base

URINARY/REPRODUCTIVE SYSTEMS

648. **1** Primitive sex cells, called spermatogonia, are present in newborn males. At puberty these cells mature and form spermatozoa (spermatogenesis).
2 Spermatogenesis does not occur until puberty. **3** Spermatogonia are found at this time. **4** Only immature cells are found during this period.
Client Need: Physiological Adaptation; **Cognitive Level:** Knowledge; **Nursing Process:** Assessment/Analysis; **Reference:** Ch 12, Review of Anatomy and Physiology of the Reproductive System

649. **3** Sperm cells are fragile and can be destroyed by heat, causing sterility.
1 Sperm do not move through the urine; they are found in semen. **2** Sperm achieve motion from their flagella; they move from the epididymis to the vas deferens to the ejaculatory ducts to the urethra. **4** During embryonic development the testes are not suspended.
Client Need: Physiological Adaptation; **Cognitive Level:** Comprehension; **Nursing Process:** Assessment/Analysis; **Reference:** Ch 12, Review of Anatomy and Physiology of the Reproductive System

650. **3** Condylomata acuminata are variably sized cauliflower-like warts occurring principally on the genitals or the anogenital skin or mucosa of both females and males; they are transmitted by sexual activity.
1 Scabies is an infestation of the skin by *Sarcoptes scabiei* (itch mite). **2** Herpes zoster is an acute vesicular skin infection caused by the varicella-zoster virus. **4** The epididymis is part of the male reproductive system and cancer in this area is not called condylomata acuminata.
Client Need: Physiological Adaptation; **Cognitive Level:** Knowledge; **Nursing Process:** Assessment/Analysis; **Reference:** Ch 12, Review of Microorganisms

651. **3** *Trichomonas vaginalis* is a protozoan that favors an alkaline environment.
1 This does not cause trichomonal infections. A yeast is a unicellular, usually oval, nucleated fungus. **2** This does not cause trichomonal infections. A fungus is a simple parasitic plant. **4** This does not cause trichomonal infections. A spirochete is a motile spiral-shaped bacterium.
Client Need: Physiological Adaptation; **Cognitive Level:** Comprehension; **Nursing Process:** Assessment/Analysis; **Reference:** Ch 12, Review of Microorganisms

652. **4** The PSA is an indication of cancer of the prostate; the higher the level, the greater the tumor burden.
1 Elevated creatinine levels may be caused by impaired renal function as a result of blockage by an enlarged prostate but do not indicate that metastasis has occurred. **2** Elevated BUN levels may be caused by impaired renal function as a result of blockage by an enlarged prostate but do not indicate that metastasis has occurred. **3** Nonprotein nitrogen refers to waste

products from metabolism of protein and includes urea, creatinine, uric acid, and ammonia.
Client Need: Reduction of Risk Potential; **Cognitive Level:** Analysis; **Nursing Process:** Planning/Implementation; **Reference:** Ch 12, Cancer of the Prostate, Data Base

653. **3** Inability to empty the bladder, as a result of pressure exerted by the enlarging prostate on the urethra, causes a backup of urine into the ureters and finally the kidneys (hydronephrosis).
1 BPH develops over the client's life span; it is not congenital. **2** It is uncommon for BPH to become malignant. **4** This level is elevated in prostatic carcinoma.
Client Need: Physiological Adaptation; **Cognitive Level:** Comprehension; **Nursing Process:** Assessment/Analysis; **Reference:** Ch 12, Benign Prostatic Hyperplasia, Data Base

654. **2** The kidneys are ultimately responsible for maintaining fluid and electrolyte balance by excretion or retention based on the body's needs.
1 Aldosterone will cause retention of sodium ions by the nephrons and subsequent fluid retention. **3** The lungs eliminate water and CO_2 only if excess carbonic acid is present; their role in fluid and electrolyte balance is less extensive than that of the kidneys. **4** Antidiuretic hormone has a direct effect on the nephrons, resulting in water retention.
Client Need: Physiological Adaptation; **Cognitive Level:** Analysis; **Nursing Process:** Assessment/Analysis; **Reference:** Ch 12, Review of Anatomy and Physiology of the Urinary System

655. **1** Osmosis is the diffusion of water through a selectively permeable membrane. Such membranes include cellular membranes and capillary walls. Osmosis occurs in the kidney tubules and in all capillary beds.
2 Diffusion is the process by which particulate matter in a fluid moves from an area of greater concentration to an area of lesser concentration. **3** Dialysis is the diffusion of small molecules, other than water, down their concentration gradients through a selectively permeable membrane. **4** Active transport is the movement of molecules against a concentration gradient and requires energy input; osmosis and diffusion are passive processes.
Client Need: Physiological Adaptation; **Cognitive Level:** Analysis; **Nursing Process:** Assessment/Analysis; **Reference:** Ch 12, Review of Anatomy and Physiology of the Urinary System

656. **2** The prostate gland is a tubuloalveolar gland shaped like a ring, with the urethra passing through its center.
1 The epididymis lies along the top and sides of the testes. **3** The seminal vesicles are on the posterior surface of the bladder. **4** This gland lies below the prostate.
Client Need: Physiological Adaptation; **Cognitive Level:** Comprehension; **Integrated Process:** Teaching/Learning; **Nursing Process:** Assessment/Analysis; **Reference:** Ch 12, Review of Anatomy and Physiology of the Reproductive System

657. **4** Because the female's urethra is closer to the anus than the male's, it is at greater risk for becoming contaminated.

1 Urinary pH is within the same range in both males and females. **2** Hormonal secretions have no effect on the development of bladder infections. **3** The position of the bladder is the same in males and females.
Client Need: Physiological Adaptation; **Cognitive Level:** Comprehension; **Nursing Process:** Assessment/Analysis; **Reference:** Ch 12, Urinary Tract Infections, Data Base

658. **2** Refrigeration retards the growth of bacteria and may preserve the specimen for several hours.
1, 3 Growth of bacteria will alter the pH and the glucose and protein levels in the urine; it must be refrigerated to retard growth. **4** This represents an unnecessary waste of time, effort, and money.
Client Need: Reduction of Risk Potential; **Cognitive Level:** Application; **Nursing Process:** Planning/Implementation; **Reference:** Ch 12, Urinary Tract Infections, Nursing Care

659. **3** This ensures drainage and prevents bladder distention and other complications. Patency of the catheter should be established before notifying the physician.
1 Assessment is necessary before consultation with the physician. **2** Patency of the catheter should be assessed first. This may be necessary if the catheter is clogged. This usually is required when the drainage is viscous rather than liquid. **4** Irrigation is avoided if possible because of the associated risk for infection.
Client Need: Reduction of Risk Potential; **Cognitive Level:** Application; **Nursing Process:** Assessment/Analysis; **Reference:** Ch 12, Related Procedures, Urinary Catheterization

660. **4** An indwelling catheter dilates the urinary sphincters, keeps the bladder empty, and short-circuits the reflex mechanism based on bladder distention. When the catheter is removed, the body must adapt to functioning once again.
1, 3 Although this could cause difficulty in voiding, there are no data presented to draw this conclusion. **2** This would not cause this problem.
Client Need: Basic Care and Comfort; **Cognitive Level:** Comprehension; **Nursing Process:** Assessment/Analysis; **Reference:** Ch 12, Related Procedures, Urinary Catheterization

661. **3** An enlarged prostate constricts the urethra, interfering with urine flow and causing retention. When the bladder fills and approaches capacity, small amounts can be voided but the bladder never empties completely.
1 Edema does not cause the client to void frequently in small amounts because there is a decreased production of urine. **2** Dysuria is painful or difficult urination, which is not part of the client's symptoms. **4** The urge to void is caused by stimulation of the stretch receptors as the bladder fills with urine; in suppression, little or no urine is produced.
Client Need: Physiological Adaptation; **Cognitive Level:** Analysis; **Nursing Process:** Assessment/Analysis; **Reference:** Ch 12, Cancer of the Prostate, Data Base

662. 4 Cleansing the urinary meatus and adjacent skin removes accumulated bacteria, limiting the possible introduction of microbes into the urinary tract.
1 Although cleansing the perineal area is helpful, it is actually the organisms closest to the meatus that gain entry to the urinary tract first. 2 Although encouraging fluids helps prevent urinary stasis and subsequent infection, the most common source of infection is microorganisms from around the meatus. 3 Irrigations require opening the closed drainage system and allowing the entry of microorganisms; this increases the risk for infection.
Client Need: Safety and Infection Control; **Cognitive Level:** Application; **Nursing Process:** Planning/Implementation; **Reference:** Ch 12, Related Procedures, Urinary Catheterization

663. 2 The total amount of irrigation solution instilled into the bladder is eliminated with urine and therefore must be subtracted from the total output to determine the volume of urine excreted.
1 An accurate specific gravity cannot be obtained when irrigating solutions are being instilled into the bladder. 3 Hourly outputs are indicated only if there is concern about renal failure or oliguria. 4 A 24-hour urine test is not accurate if the client is receiving continuous irrigations.
Client Need: Basic Care and Comfort; **Cognitive Level:** Application; **Nursing Process:** Planning/Implementation; **Reference:** Ch 12, Related Procedures, Continuous Bladder Irrigation

664. 3 The length of the urethra is shorter in females than in males; therefore microorganisms have a shorter distance to travel to reach the bladder. The proximity of the meatus to the anus in females also increases the incidence of urinary tract infections.
1 Fluid intake may or may not be adequate in both males and females and would not account for the difference. 2 The anatomic length of the urethra in females predisposes them to infection. Hygienic practices can be inadequate in males or females. 4 Mucous membranes are continuous in both males and females.
Client Need: Physiological Adaptation; **Cognitive Level:** Comprehension; **Integrated Process:** Teaching/Learning; **Nursing Process:** Planning/Implementation; **Reference:** Ch 12, Urinary Tract Infections, Data Base

665. 4 The causative organism should be isolated before starting antibiotic therapy.
1 This test will not determine the infective organisms causing the problem. 2 Catheterization is not routine for urethritis. 3 Although client teaching is important, at this time it is not the priority.
Client Need: Reduction of Risk Potential; **Cognitive Level:** Application; **Nursing Process:** Assessment/Analysis; **Reference:** Ch 12, Urinary Tract Infections, Nursing Care

666. 1 Cloudy urine usually indicates purulent drainage (pyuria) associated with infection.
2 Viscosity is a subjective characteristic that is not measurable. 3 Specific gravity yields information

related to fluid balance. 4 Urinary glucose and acetone levels are not affected by urinary tract infections.
Client Need: Physiological Adaptation; **Cognitive Level:** Application; **Nursing Process:** Assessment/Analysis; **Reference:** Ch 12, Urinary Tract Infections, Nursing Care

667. 4 Changes in the amount of blood in the urine may indicate progressive increases in kidney damage.
1, 3 This is unrelated to hematuria. 2 This is unrelated to hematuria; it is associated with breakdown of adipose tissue.
Client Need: Physiological Adaptation; **Cognitive Level:** Comprehension; **Nursing Process:** Assessment/Analysis; **Reference:** Ch 12, Urinary Tract Infections, Data Base

668. 4 Hemolytic streptococci, common in throat infections, can initiate an immune reaction that damages the glomeruli.
1 Baths may be linked to urethritis, not glomerulonephritis. 2 Fluid restriction is moderated as the client improves; fluid helps prevent urinary stasis. 3 Activity helps prevent urinary stasis.
Client Need: Health Promotion and Maintenance; **Cognitive Level:** Application; **Integrated Process:** Teaching/Learning; **Nursing Process:** Planning/Implementation; **Reference:** Ch 12, Glomerulonephritis, Data Base

669. 1 Sharp, severe pain (renal colic) radiating toward the genitalia and thigh is caused by ureteral distention. The priority is to relieve the pain.
2 Although the client is overweight and weight loss would be desirable, it is a long-term goal. 3 Although this may occur, blood loss is usually not massive. 4 Hypertension is not specific to urinary calculi.
Client Need: Physiological Adaptation; **Cognitive Level:** Application; **Nursing Process:** Planning/Implementation; **Reference:** Ch 12, Urolithiasis, Nursing Care

670. 2 Urine is strained to determine whether any calculi or calcium gravel has been passed.
1 Fluids should be encouraged to promote dilute urine and facilitate passage of the calculi. 3 Blood pressure assessment is of no particular importance to the patient with kidney stones. 4 Administration of analgesics is based on the physician's order.
Client Need: Reduction of Risk Potential; **Cognitive Level:** Application; **Nursing Process:** Assessment/Analysis; **Reference:** Ch 12, Urolithiasis, Nursing Care

671. 3 Uric acid stones are controlled by a low-purine diet; foods high in purine, such as organ meats and meat extracts, should be avoided.
1, 2, 4 This is not high in purine and need not be avoided.
Client Need: Basic Care and Comfort; **Cognitive Level:** Application; **Integrated Process:** Teaching/Learning; **Nursing Process:** Planning/Implementation; **Reference:** Ch 12, Urolithiasis, Data Base

672. 4 Output should be at least more than 30 mL/hr; these clients usually receive an intake of 2000 to 3000 mL/24 hr.
1 Blood, tinting the urine pink, is expected.
2 Drainage may be pink; bright red drainage should

be reported. **3** This intake is adequate; however, a higher intake is usually preferred.
Client Need: Management of Care; **Cognitive Level:** Analysis; **Integrated Process:** Communication/Documentation; **Nursing Process:** Planning/Implementation; **Reference:** Ch 12, Urolithiasis, Nursing Care

673. **4** Cystolithectomy refers to the removal of calculi in the bladder.
1 Cystometry is the process of measuring the bladder's pressure and capacity. **2** Cystolithiasis denotes the presence of calculi in the bladder. **3** Cryoextraction refers to the use of subfreezing temperatures for the removal of tissue.
Client Need: Physiological Adaptation; **Cognitive Level:** Comprehension; **Integrated Process:** Teaching/Learning; **Nursing Process:** Planning/Implementation; **Reference:** Ch 12, Urolithiasis, Data Base

674. **2** Calcium and phosphorus are components of these stones; foods high in calcium and phosphorus should be avoided.
1, 4 This diet is indicated for clients with gout. **3** Diets high in this element must be avoided.
Client Need: Basic Care and Comfort; **Cognitive Level:** Application; **Integrated Process:** Teaching/Learning; **Nursing Process:** Planning/Implementation; **Reference:** Ch 12, Urolithiasis, Data Base

675. **4** Uric acid stones are controlled by a low-purine diet. Foods high in purine, such as organ meats and extracts, should be avoided.
1 Milk should be avoided with calcium, not uric acid, stones. **2** Cheese should be avoided with cystine, not uric acid, stones. **3** Only organ meats must be avoided.
Client Need: Basic Care and Comfort; **Cognitive Level:** Application; **Integrated Process:** Teaching Learning; **Nursing Process:** Planning/Implementation; **Reference:** Ch 12, Urolithiasis, Data Base

676. **3** This is an increase in nitrogenous waste, particularly urea, in the blood, common to end-stage renal disease.
1 Excessive nephron damage in end-stage renal disease causes oliguria, not polyuria; excessive urination is common in early kidney insufficiency from an inability to concentrate urine. **2** This is common with biliary obstruction, not end-stage renal disease. **4** Hypotension does not occur in end-stage renal disease; BP may be elevated as a result of increased total body water.
Client Need: Physiological Adaptation; **Cognitive Level:** Application; **Nursing Process:** Assessment/Analysis; **Reference:** Ch 12, Chronic Kidney Failure, Data Base

677. **1** An output of 50 mL/hr is adequate. When output drops below 30 mL/hr, it may indicate renal failure and the physician should be notified.
2 This is contraindicated. The client would probably still be under the influence of anesthesia and have no gag reflex. **3** This is unnecessary and would require a physician's order. **4** The physician should be notified if hourly output drops below 30 mL/hr.

Client Need: Reduction of Risk Potential; **Cognitive Level:** Application; **Integrated Process:** Communication/Documentation; **Nursing Process:** Planning/Implementation; **Reference:** Ch 12, Adenocarcinoma of the Kidney, Nursing Care

678. **4** Preoperative cleansing of the bowel is mandated before surgical resection and formation of a urinary conduit.
1 Fluids should not be restricted until after midnight of the operative day. **2** These exercises have no direct effect on this procedure. **3** An ileal conduit is not irrigated.
Client Need: Reduction of Risk Potential; **Cognitive Level:** Application; **Nursing Process:** Planning/Implementation; **Reference:** Ch 12, Bladder Tumors, Nursing Care

679. **3** The ureters are implanted in a segment of the ileum, and urine drains continually because there is no sphincter; continent catheterizable stomal reservoirs do not continually drain but are accessed with a catheter approximately every 4 hours.
1 Ileal conduits are not neurologically innervated; therefore no peristalsis exists. **2** No feces are present in an ileal conduit. **4** Absorption of nutrients is not affected by an ileal conduit.
Client Need: Physiological Adaptation; **Cognitive Level:** Comprehension; **Nursing Process:** Evaluation/Outcomes; **Reference:** Ch 12, Bladder Tumors, Data Base

680. **1** Because of the anatomic position of the incision, drainage would flow by gravity and accumulate under the client lying in the supine position.
2 Nail beds would indicate peripheral perfusion, not early hemorrhage. **3** Respiratory hemorrhage is not common after kidney surgery. **4** BP decreases in hemorrhage, and pulse rate increases.
Client Need: Physiological Adaptation; **Cognitive Level:** Application; **Nursing Process:** Evaluation/Outcomes; **Reference:** Ch 12, Adenocarcinoma of the Kidney, Nursing Care

681. **1** Postoperatively the client has a suprapubic cystostomy tube to instill a GU irrigant to dilute the urine and limit clot formation, as well as an indwelling catheter under tension to limit bleeding and drain urine.
2 This would not be expected. **3** The kidneys are not involved in this surgery. **4** The ureters are not involved in this surgery.
Client Need: Physiological Adaptation; **Cognitive Level:** Application; **Nursing Process:** Planning/Implementation; **Reference:** Ch 12, Benign Prostatic Hypertrophy, Nursing Care

682. **2** The catheter must be reinserted by the physician to ensure bladder emptying, maintain pressure at the operative site, and prevent hemorrhage.
1 Because of the danger of further trauma to the urethra and surgical site, the surgeon should insert the catheter. **3** Irrigations require a physician's order. **4** In addition to urinary drainage, the balloon of the urethral catheter exerts pressure against the prostate to help control bleeding and should be reinserted.

Client Need: Management of Care; **Cognitive Level:** Application; **Integrated Process:** Communication/Documentation; **Nursing Process:** Planning/Implementation; **Reference:** Ch 12, Benign Prostatic Hypertrophy, Nursing Care

683. **1** The bladder is a sterile body cavity; when introducing a solution/catheter, surgical asepsis is required.

2 Excessive pressure can traumatize the lining of the urinary tract. **3** The solution is generally administered at room temperature. **4** This is done if the fluid does not return by gravity; the negative pressure exerted during aspiration may cause trauma.

Client Need: Safety and Infection Control; **Cognitive Level:** Comprehension; **Nursing Process:** Planning/Implementation; **Reference:** Ch 12, Related Procedures, Urinary Catheterization

684. **3** Because the urine and irrigant are mixed, the amount of infused irrigant must be measured accurately and subtracted from the total output to determine the urinary output.

1 The bedside drainage bag contains both irrigant and urine. **2** The purpose of continuous bladder irrigation is to prevent obstruction of the catheter; stopping the irrigation would increase the risk for obstruction. **4** Both urine and irrigant mix in the bladder and drain from the same port.

Client Need: Basic Care and Comfort; **Cognitive Level:** Application; **Nursing Process:** Planning/Implementation; **Reference:** Ch 12, Related Procedures, Continuous Bladder Irrigation

685. **1** Bicarbonate buffering is limited, hydrogen ions accumulate, and acidosis results.

2 The rate of respirations increases in metabolic acidosis to compensate for a low pH. **3** The fluid balance does not significantly alter the pH. **4** The retention of sodium ions is related to fluid retention and edema rather than to acidosis.

Client Need: Physiological Adaptation; **Cognitive Level:** Analysis; **Nursing Process:** Assessment/Analysis; **Reference:** Ch 12, Acute Kidney Failure, Data Base

686. **3** The amount of protein permitted in the diet (usually below 50 g) depends on the extent of kidney function; excess protein causes an increase in urea concentration, which should be avoided; adequate calories are provided to prevent tissue catabolism that also results in an increase in metabolic waste products.

1 In kidney failure the kidneys are unable to eliminate the waste products of a high-protein diet. **2** The body is able to synthesize the nonessential amino acids. **4** Urea is a waste product of protein metabolism; the body is able to synthesize the nonessential amino acids.

Client Need: Basic Care and Comfort; **Cognitive Level:** Comprehension; **Nursing Process:** Planning/Implementation; **Reference:** Ch 12, Acute Kidney Failure, Data Base

687. **2** In kidney failure, as the glomerular filtration rate decreases, phosphorus is retained. As hyperphosphatemia occurs, calcium is excreted. Calcium depletion (hypocalcemia) causes tetany.

1, 3, 4 The symptoms described are not characteristic of this condition.

Client Need: Physiological Adaptation; **Cognitive Level:** Analysis; **Integrated Process:** Teaching/Learning; **Nursing Process:** Assessment/Analysis; **Reference:** Ch 12, Acute Kidney Failure, Data Base

688. **3** An elevated blood urea nitrogen level, indicating uremia, is toxic to the CNS and causes mental cloudiness and confusion and can result in a loss of consciousness.

1 Hyperkalemia is associated with muscle weakness, irritability, nausea, and diarrhea. **2** Hypernatremia is associated with firm tissue turgor, oliguria, and agitation. **4** Dehydration can cause fatigue, dry skin and mucous membranes, along with rapid pulse and respiratory rates.

Client Need: Physiological Adaptation; **Cognitive Level:** Analysis; **Nursing Process:** Assessment/Analysis; **Reference:** Ch 12, Acute Kidney Failure, Data Base

689. **3** This adaptation results from excess nitrogenous wastes.

1 Extensive nephron damage causes oliguria, not polyuria. **2** Hypotension does not occur; the BP is within the expected range or elevated as a result of increased total body fluid. **4** Metabolic, not respiratory, acidosis occurs because of the kidneys' inability to excrete hydrogen and regulate sodium and bicarbonate levels.

Client Need: Physiological Adaptation; **Cognitive Level:** Application; **Nursing Process:** Assessment/Analysis; **Reference:** Ch 12, Chronic Kidney Failure, Data Base

690. **4** Diffusion moves particles from an area of greater concentration to an area of lesser concentration; osmosis moves fluid from an area of lesser to an area of greater concentration of particles, thereby removing waste products into the dialysate, which is then drained from the abdomen.

1 The principle of ultrafiltration involves a pressure gradient, which is associated with hemodialysis, not peritoneal dialysis. **2** Peritoneal dialysis cleanses the peritoneal cavity directly and the blood indirectly.

3 Dialysate does not clear toxins in a short time; exchanges may occur four or five times a day.

Client Need: Physiological Adaptation; **Cognitive Level:** Comprehension; **Integrated Process:** Teaching/Learning; **Nursing Process:** Evaluation/Outcomes; **Reference:** Ch 12, Chronic Kidney Failure, Data Base

691. **4** Peritoneal dialysis uses the peritoneum as a selectively permeable membrane for diffusion of toxins and wastes from the blood into the dialyzing solution.

1 Peritoneal dialysis acts as a substitute for kidney function; it does not reestablish kidney function. **2** The dialysate does not clean the peritoneal membrane; the semipermeable membrane allows toxins and wastes to pass into the dialysate within the abdominal cavity. **3** Fluid in the abdominal cavity does not enter the intracellular compartment.

Client Need: Physiological Adaptation; **Cognitive Level:** Comprehension; **Integrated Process:** Teaching/Learning; **Nursing Process:** Evaluation/Outcomes; **Reference:** Ch 12, Chronic Kidney Failure, Data Base

692. 4 Protein breakdown liberates cellular potassium ions, leading to hyperkalemia, which can cause cardiac dysrhythmia and standstill. The failure of the kidneys to maintain a balance of potassium is one of the main indications for dialysis.

1 Ascites occurs in liver disease and is not an indication for dialysis. 2 Dialysis is not the usual treatment for acidosis; usually this responds to administration of alkaline drugs. 3 Dialysis is not a treatment for hypertension; this is usually controlled by antihypertensive medication and diet.

Client Need: Physiological Adaptation; **Cognitive Level:** Application; **Nursing Process:** Assessment/Analysis; **Reference:** Ch 12, Chronic Kidney Failure, Data Base

693. 1 Sodium is the most abundant cation in the extracellular fluid and functions as part of the sodium/potassium pump. In the presence of a deficit, the client will exhibit confusion, lethargy, headache, and muscle cramps.

2 Spasm of the facial muscles following a tap over the facial nerve (Chvostek's sign) indicates hypocalcemia. 3 Cardiac dysrhythmias are associated with increases or decreases in potassium and calcium. 4 An increase in body temperature reflects a possible infection, not an electrolyte imbalance.

Client Need: Physiological Adaptation; **Cognitive Level:** Analysis; **Nursing Process:** Evaluation/Outcomes; **Reference:** Ch 12, Chronic Kidney Failure, Nursing Care

694. 3 Because an external shunt provides circulatory access to a major artery and vein, special safety precautions must be taken to prevent disconnection of the cannula. Disconnection can cause unimpeded excessive blood loss and death. Clamps should be carried at all times by the client and the client should know how to use them in preparation for this emergency.

1, 2, 4 Although a potential complication, this does not pose the same immediate threat to life as does exsanguination.

Client Need: Physiological Adaptation; **Cognitive Level:** Application; **Nursing Process:** Evaluation/Outcomes; **Reference:** Ch 12, Chronic Kidney Failure, Nursing Care

695. 3 Insertion of an arteriovenous shunt represents a break in the first line of defense against infection, the skin. An infection of an arteriovenous shunt can be avoided by strict aseptic (sterile) technique.

1 An elastic bandage would interfere with examination of the site. 2 This is expected; a bruit can be auscultated because of the increased arterial pressure in the area. 4 Taking a BP measurement in the affected arm could damage the shunt.

Client Need: Physiological Adaptation; **Cognitive Level:** Application; **Nursing Process:** Planning/Implementation; **Reference:** Ch 12, Chronic Kidney Failure, Nursing Care

696. 2 Turning from side to side will change the position of the catheter, thereby freeing the drainage holes of the tubing, which may be obstructed.

1, 3 This does not influence drainage of dialysate from the peritoneal cavity. 4 The position of the catheter should be changed only by the physician.

Client Need: Physiological Adaptation; **Cognitive Level:** Application; **Nursing Process:** Planning/Implementation; **Reference:** Ch 12, Chronic Kidney Failure, Nursing Care

697. 1 Radiation may damage the bowel mucosa, causing bleeding.

2 BP changes are not expected during radiation therapy. 3 Enemas are contraindicated with lower abdominal radiation because of the damaged intestinal mucosa. 4 Diarrhea, not constipation, occurs with radiation that influences the intestine.

Client Need: Physiological Adaptation; **Cognitive Level:** Application; **Nursing Process:** Evaluation/Outcomes; **Reference:** Ch 12, Bladder Tumors, Nursing Care

698. 3 The expected serum creatinine range is 0.5 to 1.2 mg/dL. The nurse should obtain additional information that may indicate acute rejection; therefore the nurse must first assess for decreased urine output and changes in vital signs.

1 Once additional data are collected (such as urine output, current blood work reports) and the IV infusions are checked, the nurse should contact the physician, explain the situation, and implement further orders. 2 Eventually the nurse should ensure that proper infusion rates, along with IV medications, are being maintained after the client is first assessed for decreased urine output and for changes in vital signs. 4 Current blood work reports should be obtained after the client is assessed for decreased urine output and changes in vital signs.

Client Need: Reduction of Risk Potential; **Cognitive Level:** Analysis; **Nursing Process:** Evaluation/Outcomes; **Reference:** Ch 12, Chronic Kidney Failure, Nursing Care

INFECTIOUS DISEASES

699. 1 Malaria is caused by the protozoan *Plasmodium falciparum*, which is carried by mosquitoes.

2, 3, 4 This will not prevent protozoa from entering the bloodstream.

Client Need: Health Promotion and Maintenance; **Cognitive Level:** Application; **Integrated Process:** Teaching/Learning; **Nursing Process:** Planning/Implementation; **Reference:** Ch 13, Malaria, Data Base

700. 3 Parasites invade the erythrocytes, subsequently dividing and causing the cell to burst. The spleen enlarges from the sloughing of RBCs.

1 Oliguria, not polyuria, occurs in malaria-induced kidney failure. 2, 4 This does not occur.

Client Need: Physiological Adaptation; **Cognitive Level:** Analysis; **Nursing Process:** Assessment/Analysis; **Reference:** Ch 13, Malaria, Data Base

701. **4** Maintaining adequate nutritional and fluid balance is essential to life and must be accomplished during periods when intestinal motility is not excessive so that absorption can occur.

1 Although shaking chills may occur, seizures do not generally occur. **2** This is not used in the treatment of malaria. **3** Infection may occur only through direct serum contact or a bite from an infected *Anopheles* mosquito.

Client Need: Basic Care and Comfort; **Cognitive Level:** Analysis; **Nursing Process:** Planning/Implementation; **Reference:** Ch 13, Malaria, Nursing Care

702. **3** Quinine sulfate is used for malaria when the plasmodia are resistant to the less toxic chloroquine. However, a new strain of *Plasmodium*, resistant to quinine, must be treated with a combination of quinine (quick acting), pyrimethamine, and sulfonamide (slow acting).

1 The aim of therapy is to eliminate, not control, the parasite. **2** Reinfestation can occur with a different species or strain of *Plasmodium*. **4** The immunity is permanent if drug therapy is successful.

Client Need: Pharmacological and Parenteral Therapies; **Cognitive Level:** Application; **Integrated Process:** Teaching/Learning; **Nursing Process:** Planning/Implementation; **Reference:** Ch 13, Malaria, Data Base

703. **1** *Plasmodium falciparum* in persons who have chronic malaria can cause hemoglobinuria, intravascular hemolysis, and renal failure as a result of destruction of RBCs.

2, 3, 4 This is unrelated to the development of blackwater fever.

Client Need: Physiological Adaptation; **Cognitive Level:** Application; **Nursing Process:** Assessment/Analysis; **Reference:** Ch 13, Malaria, Data Base

704. **1** The client has a weakened immune response. Instructions regarding rest, nutrition, and avoidance of unnecessary exposure to people with infections help reduce the risk for infection.

2 Clients can be taught cognitive strategies to cope with, but not prevent. **3** The client may experience social isolation as a result of society's fears and misconceptions; these are beyond the client's control. **4** Although Kaposi's sarcoma is related to HIV infection, there are no specific measures to prevent its occurrence.

Client Need: Health Promotion and Maintenance; **Cognitive Level:** Application; **Integrated Process:** Teaching/Learning; **Nursing Process:** Planning/Implementation; **Reference:** Ch 13, Acquired Immunodeficiency Syndrome, Nursing Care

705. **2** Epidemiologic evidence has identified breast milk as a source of HIV transmission.

1 This behavior is not believed to transmit HIV. **3** This is unrelated to transmission of HIV. **4** HIV transmission does not occur from this type of contact.

Client Need: Safety and Infection Control; **Cognitive Level:** Application; **Nursing Process:** Assessment/Analysis; **Reference:** Ch 13, Acquired Immunodeficiency Syndrome, Nursing Care

706. **1** A person cannot contract HIV by eating from dishes previously used by an individual with AIDS; routine care is adequate.

2, 3, 4 This is unnecessary.

Client Need: Safety and Infection Control; **Cognitive Level:** Application; **Integrated Process:** Teaching/Learning; **Nursing Process:** Planning/Implementation; **Reference:** Ch 13, Acquired Immunodeficiency Syndrome, Data Base

707. **3** Vaseline (petroleum jelly) breaks down condom integrity and would increase the risk for condom failure.

1 Using Vaseline instead of a water-soluble lubricant shows a lack of knowledge about condom use, a form of safer sex. **2** Although the person is attempting to be responsible, there is a lack of knowledge and the behavior is unsafe. **4** Condom use shows the client has some understanding about the transmission of HIV.

Client Need: Safety and Infection Control; **Cognitive Level:** Analysis; **Integrated Process:** Teaching/Learning; **Nursing Process:** Evaluation/Outcomes; **Reference:** Ch 13, Acquired Immunodeficiency Syndrome, Nursing Care

708. **3** Irritation of the mucosa may cause increased bleeding or perforation and therefore should be avoided.

1 All clients' diets should be nutritionally balanced; this is not specific to this client's problem. **2** Bulk and roughage may irritate the mucosa and should be decreased. **4** Psychologic support is not the primary goal; efforts should be made to include foods that are psychologically beneficial, but do not include foods that are irritating to the mucosa.

Client Need: Basic Care and Comfort; **Cognitive Level:** Analysis; **Nursing Process:** Planning/Implementation; **Reference:** Ch 13, Viral and Bacterial Infectious Gastroenteritis, Data Base

709. **4** *Clostridium welchii* (*C. perfringens*) is a spore-forming bacterium that produces a toxin that decays muscle, releasing a gas; it is one of the major causative agents for gas gangrene.

1 *Clostridium tetani* enters the body via puncture of the skin and affects the nervous system; gas gangrene does not occur with this organism. **2** This disease is caused by *Bacillus anthracis*, not *Clostridium*. **3** *Clostridium botulinum* contaminates food that is then ingested, causing botulism.

Client Need: Physiological Adaptation; **Cognitive Level:** Knowledge; **Nursing Process:** Assessment/Analysis; **Reference:** Ch 13, Tetanus, Data Base

710. **3** Infection is caused by viral contact with the dermal layer of skin; cleansing the wound with soap and water helps remove superficial contaminants.

1 Antivenins are not effective against microbiologic stresses. **2** A pressure dressing will not prevent

infection. **4** Application of a tourniquet may impair circulation and will not prevent infection.
Client Need: Physiological Adaptation; **Cognitive Level:** Application; **Nursing Process:** Planning/Implementation; **Reference:** Ch 13, Rabies, Data Base

711. **1** *Toxoplasma gondii*, a protozoan, can be transmitted by exposure to infected cat feces or by ingestion of undercooked contaminated meat.
2 Toxoplasmosis is not related to heavy metals. **3** *Toxoplasma gondii* is a parasite of warm-blooded animals; fish are not considered the source of contamination. **4** Toxoplasmosis is not related to radiation.
Client Need: Health Promotion and Maintenance; **Cognitive Level:** Application; **Integrated Process:** Teaching/Learning; **Nursing Process:** Planning/Implementation; **Reference:** Ch 13, Toxoplasmosis, Data Base

712. **2** Toxins from the bacillus invade nervous tissue; respiratory spasms may result in respiratory failure.
1, 3, 4 This generalized condition is not life-threatening.
Client Need: Physiological Adaptation; **Cognitive Level:** Application; **Nursing Process:** Assessment/Analysis; **Reference:** Ch 13, Tetanus, Nursing Care

713. **4** Painful pharyngeal spasms when swallowing or even looking at water are responsible for the use of the term hydrophobia to refer to rabies.
1 The CNS is affected; diarrhea is not a concern. **2** Memory is not affected by this disease. **3** Urinary stasis is not the expected problem; catheterization can be employed.
Client Need: Physiological Adaptation; **Cognitive Level:** Application; **Nursing Process:** Assessment/Analysis; **Reference:** Ch 13, Rabies, Nursing Care

714. **1** Massive doses of penicillin may limit CNS damage if treatment is started before neural deterioration from syphilis occurs.
2 Tranquilizers are used to modify behavior, not to treat general paresis. **3** Behavior, not paresis, is treated with behavior modification. **4** Electroconvulsive therapy is used to treat certain psychiatric disorders.
Client Need: Pharmacological and Parenteral Therapies; **Cognitive Level:** Application; **Nursing Process:** Planning/Implementation; **Reference:** Ch 13, Syphilis, Data Base

715. **3** Inflammation associated with gonorrhea may lead to destruction of the epididymis in males and tubal mucosal destruction in females, causing sterility.
1 Many gonococci have become penicillin resistant and difficult to treat. **2** Gonorrhea is a common sexually transmitted disease. **4** *Neisseria gonorrhoeae* will invade internal structures, particularly the epididymis in males and the fallopian tubes in females.
Client Need: Physiological Adaptation; **Cognitive Level:** Application; **Nursing Process:** Assessment/Analysis; **Reference:** Ch 13, Gonorrhea, Data Base

716. **3** Ceftriaxone (Rocephin) inhibits the synthesis of bacterial cell walls. It is effective against *Neisseria gonorrhoeae*, a gram-negative diplococcus.
1 Acyclovir interferes with DNA synthesis, causing decreased viral replication, and is used to treat herpes. **2** Colistin sulfate is effective against most gram-negative enteric pathogens such as *Escherichia coli*. **4** Dactinomycin is an antineoplastic agent.
Client Need: Pharmacological and Parenteral Therapies; **Cognitive Level:** Analysis; **Nursing Process:** Planning/Implementation; **Reference:** Ch 13, Gonorrhea, Data Base

717. **3** Once people become sexually active, they usually remain sexually active; a condom, although not 100% effective, is the best protection against gonorrhea in a sexually active person.
1 This has no proven protective effect against sexually transmitted infections; excessive douching can alter the vaginal environment and may promote an ascending infection. **2** This is not the most realistic response to a sexually active person. **4** Spermicidal cream has no protective effect against sexually transmitted infections.
Client Need: Safety and Infection Control; **Cognitive Level:** Application; **Integrated Process:** Teaching/Learning; **Nursing Process:** Evaluation/Outcomes; **Reference:** Ch 13, Gonorrhea, Nursing Care

718. **3** Gonorrhea frequently is an ascending infection and affects the fallopian tubes.
1 Syphilis, if untreated, may spread to the nervous system via the blood; it does not usually cause ascending infection of the fallopian tubes. **2** Abortion should not cause inflammation of the fallopian tubes. **4** This is an aberrant growth; it would not cause inflammation of the fallopian tubes.
Client Need: Physiological Adaptation; **Cognitive Level:** Knowledge; **Nursing Process:** Assessment/Analysis; **Reference:** Ch 13, Gonorrhea, Data Base

719. **3** The exudate from herpes virus type 2 is highly contagious; gown, gloves, and a facial shield provide a barrier.
1 The organism is not in respiratory tract secretions; the organism is present in the exudate from active lesions. **2** This is unnecessary. **4** This is not an airborne infectious disease.
Client Need: Safety and Infection Control; **Cognitive Level:** Application; **Nursing Process:** Planning/Implementation; **Reference:** Ch 13, Herpes Genitalis, Nursing Care

720. **3** Although the usual incubation period of syphilis is about 3 weeks, clinical symptoms may appear as early as 9 days or as long as 3 months after exposure.
1, 2, 4 The usual incubation period is 21 days.
Client Need: Safety and Infection Control; **Cognitive Level:** Knowledge; **Integrated Process:** Teaching/Learning; **Nursing Process:** Planning/Implementation; **Reference:** Ch 13, Syphilis, Data Base

721. **2** The tertiary stage is noncontagious; tertiary lesions contain only small numbers of treponemes.

1 The primary stage lasts 8 to 12 weeks; the chancre is teeming with spirochetes, and the individual is contagious. **3** The incubation stage lasts 2 to 6 weeks; spirochetes proliferate at the entry site, and the individual is contagious. **4** The duration of the secondary stage is variable (about 5 years); skin and mucosal lesions contain spirochetes, and the individual is highly contagious.

Client Need: Safety and Infection Control; **Cognitive Level:** Comprehension; **Integrated Process:** Teaching/Learning; **Nursing Process:** Planning/Implementation; **Reference:** Ch 13, Syphilis, Data Base

722. **1** Gonorrhea is a highly contagious disease transmitted through sexual intercourse. The incubation period varies, but symptoms usually occur 2 to 10 days after contact. Early effective treatment prevents complications.

2 The parents may be unaware that their child has gonorrhea. **3** Contracting venereal infection is not necessarily indicative of promiscuity. **4** Most birth control measures do not protect against the transmission of sexually transmitted infections.

Client Need: Health Promotion and Maintenance; **Cognitive Level:** Application; **Nursing Process:** Planning/Implementation; **Reference:** Ch 13, Gonorrhea, Nursing Care

723. **1** Ceftriaxone (Rocephin) followed by doxycycline (Vibramycin) is specific for *Neisseria gonorrhoeae* and eradicates the microorganism; other treatment regimens are available for resistant strains.

2 If the disease progresses before the diagnosis is made, complications such as sterility, valve damage, or joint degeneration may occur. **3** Transmission is not controlled; the organism is eliminated. **4** If tubal structures, valves, or joints degenerate, the pathologic changes will not be reversed by antibiotic therapy.

Client Need: Pharmacology and Parenteral Therapies; **Cognitive Level:** Knowledge; **Integrated Process:** Teaching/Learning; **Nursing Process:** Planning/Implementation; **Reference:** Ch 13, Gonorrhea, Data Base

DRUG-RELATED RESPONSES

724. **4** Tumor necrosis factor (TNF) is produced mainly by macrophages in the synovium; over time, through various mechanisms, the presence of TNF causes inflammation of the synovium, destruction of bone and cartilage, joint stiffness, and pain; TNF inhibitors or blockers neutralize TNF, thereby interrupting the inflammatory cascade; this inhibits the inflammatory response and other mechanisms, thereby slowing tissue damage.

1, 2, 3 TNF inhibitors are not ordered for a client with this disease.

Client Need: Pharmacological and Parenteral Therapies; **Cognitive Level:** Application; **Nursing Process:** Evaluation/Outcomes; **Reference:** Ch 11, Arthritis, Data Base

725. **3** Povidone-iodine (Betadine) is an effective bactericidal compound that helps eliminate surface bacteria that would contaminate culture results.

1 Betadine does not have this property. **2** Alcohol is not used because it is bacteriostatic; it inhibits, not eliminates, microorganisms. **4** Although Betadine may provide a cool feeling, this not the reason for its use.

Client Need: Pharmacological and Parenteral Therapies; **Cognitive Level:** Application; **Nursing Process:** Planning/Implementation; **Reference:** Ch 3, General Nursing Care of Clients at Risk for Infection

726. **2** Acetazolamide (Diamox) is a carbonic anhydrase inhibitor that decreases inflow of aqueous humor and controls intraocular pressure in an attack of acute angle-closure glaucoma.

1, 3 This diuretic has no effect on the eye. **4** This strong miotic does not affect the production of aqueous humor.

Client Need: Pharmacological and Parenteral Therapies; **Cognitive Level:** Analysis; **Nursing Process:** Planning/Implementation; **Reference:** Ch 11, Ophthalmic Agents

727. **4** Methyldopa is associated with acquired hemolytic anemia and should be discontinued to prevent progression and complications.

1 Ferrous sulfate is an iron supplement to correct, not cause, the symptoms of anemia. **2** This is not associated with RBC destruction. **3** Famotidine (Pepcid) would not cause these symptoms; it decreases gastric acid secretion, which would decrease the risk of gastrointestinal bleeding.

Client Need: Pharmacological and Parenteral Therapies; **Cognitive Level:** Application; **Nursing Process:** Evaluation/Outcomes; **Reference:** Ch 6, Antihypertensives

728. **3** Aldactone is a potassium-sparing diuretic; hyperkalemia is an adverse effect.

1, 2, 4 This diuretic generally causes hypokalemia.

Client Need: Pharmacological and Parenteral Therapies; **Cognitive Level:** Application; **Nursing Process:** Evaluation/Outcomes; **Reference:** Ch 6, Diuretics

729. **2** Albuterol's sympathomimetic effect causes cardiac stimulation that may result in tachycardia and palpitations.

1 Albuterol may cause restlessness, irritability, and tremors, not lethargy. **3** Albuterol may cause dizziness, not visual disturbances. **4** Albuterol will cause tachycardia, not bradycardia.

Client Need: Pharmacological and Parenteral Therapies; **Cognitive Level:** Application; **Nursing Process:** Evaluation/Outcomes; **Reference:** Ch 7, Bronchodilators and Antiasmatics

730. **2** Intrathecal morphine can depress respiratory function depending on the level it reaches within the spinal column; hourly assessments during the first 12 to 24 hours will allow for early intervention with naloxone (Narcan) if respiratory depression needs to be corrected.

1 Bradycardia and hypotension occur. **3** Central nervous system depression occurs secondary to hypoxia. **4** This is too long a time between doses if the client's respirations are depressed. The recommended adult dosage usually is 0.4 to 2 mg every 2 to 3 minutes if indicated.
Client Need: Pharmacological and Parenteral Therapies; **Cognitive Level:** Application; **Nursing Process:** Evaluation/Outcomes; **Reference:** Ch 3, Pain, Opioid Analgesics

731. **2** Changing positions slowly will help prevent the side effect of orthostatic hypotension.
1 This drug can relax the esophagus and lead to acid reflux; lying down after meals could intensify this effect. **3, 4** This is not necessary.
Client Need: Pharmacological and Parenteral Therapies; **Cognitive Level:** Application; **Integrated Process:** Teaching/Learning; **Nursing Process:** Planning/Implementation; **Reference:** Ch 6, Antidysrhythmics

732. **2** Nitroglycerin tablets are affected by light, heat, and moisture. A loss of potency can occur after 3 months, reducing the drug's effectiveness in relieving pain. A new supply should be obtained routinely.
1 This indicates the tablets have retained their potency. **3, 4** This does not necessarily indicate a loss of potency.
Client Need: Pharmacological and Parenteral Therapies; **Cognitive Level:** Application; **Integrated Process:** Teaching/Learning; **Nursing Process:** Planning/Implementation; **Reference:** Ch 6, Coronary Vasodilators

733. **2** Warfarin depresses prothrombin activity and inhibits the formation of several of the clotting factors by the liver. Its antagonist is vitamin K, which is involved in prothrombin formation.
1 Heparin is an anticoagulant. **3** Protamine sulfate is the antidote for heparin overdose. **4** Imferon is an iron supplement, not an antidote for warfarin.
Client Need: Pharmacological and Parenteral Therapies; **Cognitive Level:** Analysis; **Nursing Process:** Planning/Implementation; **Reference:** Ch 6, Anticoagulants

734. **3** Metoprolol is a beta blocker; it will decrease the heart rate and thus is contraindicated with bradycardia.
1 Metoprolol is an antihypertensive agent. **2, 4** By reducing cardiac output, metoprolol reduces myocardial O_2 consumption, which helps prevent ischemia and anginal pain.
Client Need: Pharmacological and Parenteral Therapies; **Cognitive Level:** Analysis; **Integrated Process:** Communication/Documentation; **Nursing Process:** Planning/Implementation; **Reference:** Ch 6, Antidysrhythmics

735. **1** Beta blockers reduce cardiac output, so they are contraindicated for clients with uncontrolled heart failure.
2 Beta blockers are used to treat hypertension because they cause vasodilation and decrease cardiac contractility. **3** Beta blockers lower heart rate. **4** Beta blockers are used to treat coronary artery disease because they decrease myocardial O_2 demand

by reducing peripheral resistance and cardiac contractility.
Client Need: Pharmacological and Parenteral Therapies; **Cognitive Level:** Analysis; **Integrated Process:** Communication/Documentation; **Nursing Process:** Planning/Implementation; **Reference:** Ch 6, Antidysrhythmics

736. **3** Therapeutic effects of simvastatin include decreased levels of serum triglycerides, LDL, and cholesterol.
1 This is not related to simvastatin; it is a measure used to evaluate blood coagulation. **2, 4** This is not related to simvastatin.
Client Need: Pharmacological and Parenteral Therapies; **Cognitive Level:** Application; **Nursing Process:** Evaluation/Outcomes; **Reference:** Ch 6, Antilipidemics

737. **3** Because furosemide (Lasix) and aspirin compete for the same renal excretory sites, salicylate toxicity may occur even with lower dosages.
1 Aspirin does not affect furosemide metabolism. **2** This response does not take into account the other drug that the client is receiving. **4** Although furosemide has a hyperuricemic effect similar to that of the thiazide diuretics, it is not potentiated by aspirin.
Client Need: Pharmacological and Parenteral Therapies; **Cognitive Level:** Application; **Nursing Process:** Evaluation/Outcomes; **Reference:** Ch 6, Diuretics

738. **3** Nitroglycerin is sensitive to light and moisture and must be stored in a dark, airtight container.
1 This medication usually is taken PRN. The daily number may be as high as 12 to 15 tablets; if more than 3 tablets are necessary in a 15-minute period, the person should be taken to the hospital emergency department. **2** This may be an expected side effect and the medication should not be discontinued. **4** Dizziness indicates the physician may need to decrease the dosage.
Client Need: Pharmacological and Parenteral Therapies; **Cognitive Level:** Application; **Integrated Process:** Teaching/Learning; **Nursing Process:** Planning/Implementation; **Reference:** Ch 6, Coronary Vasodilators

739. **4** This is a nonopioid analgesic that inhibits prostaglandins, which serve as mediators for pain; it does not impact platelet function.
1, 2, 3 This is a nonselective nonsteroidal antiinflammatory drug (NSAID) that is contraindicated for a client undergoing surgery; nonselective NSAIDs have an inhibitory effect on thromboxane, which is a strong aggregating agent, and can result in bleeding.
Client Need: Pharmacological and Parenteral Therapies; **Cognitive Level:** Analysis; **Integrated Process:** Communication/Documentation; **Nursing Process:** Planning/Implementation; **Reference:** Ch 6, Other Nonopioid Analgesics

740. **2** As renal perfusion increases, urinary output also should increase; doses greater than 10 mcg/kg/min can cause renal vasoconstriction and decreased urinary output.
1 A change in BP is not a direct predictor of the effectiveness of dopamine given at a level of

2 mcg/kg/min; at 10 mcg/kg/min a client will experience an increased cardiac output and increased BP. **3** Body temperature does not indicate improved renal perfusion. **4** In this situation an improvement of renal perfusion is not directly related to the client's level of consciousness.

Client Need: Pharmacological and Parenteral Therapies; **Cognitive Level:** Analysis; **Nursing Process:** Evaluation/Outcomes; **Reference:** Ch 6, Medications to Manage Hypotension in Shock

741. **4** Antiemetics should be administered prophylactically to decrease nausea and enhance appetite.

1 The diet should provide maximum protein and carbohydrates to meet demands related to restoration of body cells and energy. **2** This would not alter the client's nutrition. **3** Small, frequent feedings are more appropriate because they are best tolerated.

Client Need: Pharmacological and Parenteral Therapies; **Cognitive Level:** Application; **Nursing Process:** Planning/Implementation; **Reference:** Ch 6, General Nursing Care of Clients With Neoplastic Disorders

742. **1** Visual disturbances are a sign of toxicity because retinopathy can occur with this drug.

2, 3, 4 This is not a sign of toxicity.

Client Need: Pharmacological and Parenteral Therapies; **Cognitive Level:** Application; **Integrated Process:** Teaching/Learning; **Nursing Process:** Evaluation/Outcomes; **Reference:** Ch 11, Arthritis, Nursing Care

743. **1** Toxic levels of digoxin stimulate the medullary chemoreceptor trigger zone, resulting in nausea and subsequent anorexia.

2, 3, 4 Although anorexia, nausea, and vomiting may be side effects of this drug, they do not indicate toxicity.

Client Need: Pharmacological and Parenteral Therapies; **Cognitive Level:** Analysis; **Nursing Process:** Evaluation/Outcomes; **Reference:** Ch 6, Cardiac Glycosides

744. **2** Most chemotherapeutic agents interfere with mitosis. The bone marrow consists of rapidly dividing cells, and therefore its activity is depressed.

1 Because of bone marrow depression, leukopenia—not leukocytosis—can occur. **3** The ESR generally increases in the presence of tissue inflammation or necrosis. **4** The hemoglobin and hematocrit levels may be decreased.

Client Need: Pharmacological and Parenteral Therapies; **Cognitive Level:** Application; **Nursing Process:** Evaluation/Outcomes; **Reference:** Ch 3, Neoplastic Disorders, Related Pharmacology, Major Side Effects

745. **3** Visual disturbances such as blurred and/or yellow vision may be evidence of digitalis toxicity.

1, 2, 4 This is not a symptom of digitalis toxicity.

Client Need: Pharmacological and Parenteral Therapies; **Cognitive Level:** Application; **Integrated Process:** Teaching/Learning; **Nursing Process:** Evaluation/Outcomes; **Reference:** Ch 6, Cardiac Glycosides

746. **2** A low serum potassium level when digoxin (Lanoxin) is administered can contribute to toxicity. Digoxin inhibits sodium-potassium ATPase.

1 Digoxin should be given over a 5-minute, not 1-minute, period through a Y-tube or 3-way stopcock. **3** There are many syringe, Y-site, and additive incompatibilities; manufacturers of digoxin recommend that the medication should not be administered with other drugs. **4** The apical and radial pulses, not the BP, should be assessed before administering digoxin.

Client Need: Pharmacological and Parenteral Therapies; **Cognitive Level:** Application; **Nursing Process:** Evaluation/Outcomes; **Reference:** Ch 6, Cardiac Glycosides

747. **4** The dosage of Coumadin is adjusted according to INR results; if the client fails to take the drug as prescribed, the tests are not reliable in monitoring the response to therapy.

1 Although some medications can affect the absorption or metabolism of Coumadin and also should be investigated, this is less likely to be a cause of fluctuations in laboratory values. **2, 3** This does not affect the absorption of Coumadin.

Client Need: Pharmacological and Parenteral Therapies; **Cognitive Level:** Application; **Nursing Process:** Assessment/Analysis; **Reference:** Ch 6, Anticoagulants

748. **4** Warfarin anticoagulants are administered orally and take 2 or 3 days to achieve the desired effect on the INR. Heparin, which must be administered parenterally, has immediate effects.

1 These drugs do not dissolve clots already present. **2** Because each drug affects a different part of the coagulation mechanism, dosages must be adjusted separately. **3** This does not account for the reason for the administration of both drugs; warfarin will not exert an immediate therapeutic effect.

Client Need: Pharmacological and Parenteral Therapies; **Cognitive Level:** Application; **Integrated Process:** Teaching/Learning; **Nursing Process:** Planning/Implementation; **Reference:** Ch 6, Anticoagulants

749. **1** Warfarin derivatives cause an increase in the prothrombin time and INR, leading to an increased risk for bleeding. Any abnormal or excessive bleeding must be reported, because it may indicate toxic levels of the drug.

2, 3, 4 This is not a sign of bleeding, the primary concern with Coumadin.

Client Need: Pharmacological and Parenteral Therapies; **Cognitive Level:** Application; **Integrated Process:** Teaching/Learning; **Nursing Process:** Planning/Implementation; **Reference:** Ch 6, Anticoagulants

750. **2** Aspirin can cause decreased platelet aggregation, increasing the risk for undesired bleeding that may occur with administration of anticoagulants.

1 Ferrous sulfate does not affect Coumadin; it is used for RBC synthesis. **3** Isoxsuprine hydrochloride is a vasodilator; it does not affect bleeding. **4** Chlorpromazine is a neuroleptic; it does not affect bleeding.

Client Need: Pharmacological and Parenteral Therapies; **Cognitive Level:** Analysis; **Integrated Process:** Teaching/Learning; **Nursing Process:** Planning/Implementation; **Reference:** Ch 6, Anticoagulants

751. **3** Assessment for bleeding is a priority when administering a thrombolytic agent because it may lead to hemorrhage.

1 The heart rate is not affected. **2** Electrolyte levels are not affected. **4** This is not necessary.

Client Need: Pharmacological and Parenteral Therapies; **Cognitive Level:** Application; **Nursing Process:** Evaluation/Outcomes; **Reference:** Ch 6, Thrombolytics (Fibrinolytics)

752. **3** INH (isoniazid) often leads to pyridoxine (vitamin B_6) deficiency because it competes with the vitamin for the same enzyme. This is most often manifested by peripheral neuritis, which can be controlled by regular administration of vitamin B_6.

1 Pyridoxine does not enhance INH effects.

2 Vitamin B_6 does not improve immune status.

4 Pyridoxine does not destroy organisms.

Client Need: Pharmacological and Parenteral Therapies; **Cognitive Level:** Comprehension; **Integrated Process:** Teaching/Learning; **Nursing Process:** Planning/Implementation; **Reference:** Ch 6, Antituberculars

753. **1** ☐ Morphine does not increase urine output.

2 ☒ The CNS depressant effect of morphine causes lethargy.

3 ☒ The CNS depressant effect of morphine causes bradycardia.

4 ☐ Morphine causes constriction of the pupils.

5 ☒ The CNS depressant effect of morphine causes bradypnea.

Client Need: Pharmacological and Parenteral Therapies; **Cognitive Level:** Application; **Nursing Process:** Evaluation/Outcomes; **Reference:** Ch 3, Opioid Analgesics

754. **2** Morphine sulfate binds with the same receptors as natural opioids. However, it has a rapid onset, lowers BP, decreases pulmonary reflexes, and produces sedation.

1 Chloral hydrate is a hypnotic that is not appropriate for the acute situation described.

3 Phenobarbital has a slower onset than morphine and does not affect respirations and BP to the same extent as morphine. **4** Hydroxyzine hydrochloride (Atarax) is generally used to control anxiety associated with less acute situations.

Client Need: Pharmacological and Parenteral Therapies; **Cognitive Level:** Analysis; **Nursing Process:** Planning/Implementation; **Reference:** Ch 7, Pulmonary Edema, Data Base

755. **4** The glucosamine molecule is glucose-based and may be unsafe for a client who has an impaired glucose tolerance; also, it may increase resistance to insulin and interfere with antidiabetic medication.

1 Studies suggest that glucosamine helps to slow the progression of osteoarthritis and even regenerate damaged cartilage; this results in improved joint function and reduction of joint pain and stiffness.

2, 3 Glucosamine does not appear to be harmful to clients with this health problem.

Client Need: Pharmacological and Parenteral Therapies; **Cognitive Level:** Analysis; **Integrated Process:** Teaching/Learning; **Nursing Process:** Planning/Implementation; **Reference:** Ch 11, Arthritis, Data Base

756. **4** Levodopa is the metabolic precursor of dopamine. It reduces sympathetic outflow by limiting vasoconstriction, which may result in orthostatic hypotension.

1 Levodopa should be administered with food to minimize gastric irritation. **2** Although periodic tests to evaluate hepatic, renal, and cardiovascular status are required for prolonged therapy, whether these tests should be done on a weekly basis has not been established. **3** Levodopa may produce either symptom, but no established pattern of such responses exists.

Client Need: Pharmacological and Parenteral Therapies; **Cognitive Level:** Application; **Nursing Process:** Evaluation/Outcomes; **Reference:** Ch 11, Antiparkinson Agents

757. **1** Gingival hyperplasia is an adverse effect of long-term phenytoin (Dilantin) therapy. The incidence can be decreased by maintaining therapeutic blood levels and meticulous oral hygiene.

2 Alkalinity is not related to Dilantin or to the gingival hyperplasia caused by Dilantin. **3** These are not direct effects of Dilantin. **4** Plaque and bacterial growth at the gum line are unrelated to Dilantin or to the hyperplasia caused by it.

Client Need: Pharmacological and Parenteral Therapies; **Cognitive Level:** Application; **Integrated Process:** Teaching/Learning; **Nursing Process:** Planning/Implementation; **Reference:** Ch 11, Anticonvulsants (Antiseizure)

758. **4** Tensilon, an anticholinesterase drug, causes temporary relief of symptoms of myasthenia gravis in clients who have the disease and is therefore an effective diagnostic aid.

1 There is a decrease in symptoms. **2** Consciousness is not affected. **3** Hypotension may occur.

Client Need: Reduction of Risk Potential; **Cognitive Level:** Application; **Nursing Process:** Evaluation/Outcomes; **Reference:** Ch 11, Cholinesterase Inhibitors

759. **2** Warfarin sodium (Coumadin) has been shown to inhibit the metabolism of phenytoin (Dilantin), which results in an accumulation of this drug in the body.

1 By potentiating the anticoagulant, phenytoin decreases clotting potential. **3** This is true only if the client is receiving phenytoin to control the seizure disorder. **4** Seizures do not have a significant effect on the metabolism of Coumadin.

Client Need: Pharmacological and Parenteral Therapies; **Cognitive Level:** Analysis; **Nursing Process:** Assessment/Analysis; **Reference:** Ch 11, Anticonvulsants (Antiseizure)

760. **1** Phenytoin inhibits folic acid absorption and potentiates effects of folic acid antagonists. Folic acid is helpful in correcting certain anemias that can result from administration of phenytoin. The dosage must be carefully adjusted because folic acid diminishes the effects of phenytoin.

2, 3, 4 This is not an effect of folic acid.
Client Need: Pharmacological and Parenteral Therapies; **Cognitive Level:** Analysis; **Nursing Process:** Assessment/Analysis; **Reference:** Ch 11, Anticonvulsants (Antiseizure)

761. **1** Carbamazepine (Tegretol) is administered to control pain by reducing the transmission of nerve impulses in clients with trigeminal neuralgia.

2 Liver function is monitored to detect an adverse reaction to carbamazepine, not to determine therapeutic effectiveness. **3** This medication is not given to influence cardiac output. **4** Tegretol is not administered to clients with trigeminal neuralgia (tic douloureux) for its anticonvulsant properties because seizures are not present with this disorder.
Client Need: Pharmacological and Parenteral Therapies; **Cognitive Level:** Analysis; **Nursing Process:** Evaluation/Outcomes; **Reference:** Ch 11, Anticonvulsants (Antiseizure)

762. Answer: 5 mL
Calculate the dosage by using ratio and proportion.

$5\,g : 10\,mL = 2.5\,g : x\,mL$
$5x = 25$
$x = 5\,mL$

Client Need: Pharmacological and Parenteral Therapies; **Cognitive Level:** Application; **Nursing Process:** Planning/Implementation; **Reference:** Ch 2, Nursing Responsibilities Related to Medication Administration

763. **2** Two tablets every 3 hours over 24 hours equals a total of 16 tablets daily. Since each tablet has 650 mg, then $650 \times 16 = 10,400$ mg. This is more than twice the recommended maximum dose of 4000 mg/24 hr for short-term use.

1 5200 mg is less than the amount of Darvocet the client is taking. **3** 15,500 mg is more than the amount of Darvocet the client is taking. **4** 18,800 mg is more than the amount of Darvocet the client is taking.
Client Need: Pharmacological and Parenteral Therapies; **Cognitive Level:** Application; **Nursing Process:** Planning/Implementation; **Reference:** Ch 2, Nursing Responsibilities Related to Medication Administration

764. Answer: 1.5 mL
First convert the 500 mg to its equivalent in grams. Use the "desired over have" formula of ratio and proportion:

$$\frac{Desired}{Have}\frac{500\,mg}{1000\,mg} \times \frac{x\,gram}{1\,gram}$$

$1000x = 500$
$x = \dfrac{500}{1000}$
$x = 0.5,$

therefore 500 mg is equivalent to 0.5 grams

Now use the "desired over have" formula of ratio and proportion to solve the problem:

$$\frac{Desired}{Have}\frac{0.5\,gram}{1\,gram} \times \frac{x\,mL}{3\,mL}$$

$x = 0.5 \times 3$
$x = 1.5\,mL,$

therefore 1.5 mL of the antibiotic should be added to the 50-mL IVPB bag
Client Need: Pharmacological and Parenteral Therapies; **Cognitive Level:** Application; **Nursing Process:** Planning/Implementation; **Reference:** Ch 2, Nursing Responsibilities Related to Medication Administration

765. **3** Mafenide (Sulfamylon) interferes with the kidneys' role in hydrogen ion excretion, resulting in metabolic acidosis.

1, 2, 4 This is not an adverse effect of this drug.
Client Need: Pharmacological and Parenteral Therapies; **Cognitive Level:** Application; **Nursing Process:** Evaluation/Outcomes; **Reference:** Ch 10, Antiinfectives

766. **2** Quinine administered orally can cause gastric irritation, resulting in nausea and vomiting. By administering such a medication immediately after meals, the nurse minimizes its irritating effect.

1 Absorption of the drug is not significantly affected by administration after meals. **3** The appetite is not affected by this drug as long as gastric irritation is avoided. **4** Quinidine sulfate or gluconate, not quinine, is given for its antidysrhythmic effect.
Client Need: Pharmacological and Parenteral Therapies; **Cognitive Level:** Application; **Nursing Process:** Evaluation/Outcomes, **Reference:** Ch 13, Malaria, Nursing Care

767. **2** Potassium iodide, which aids in decreasing the vascularity of the thyroid gland, decreases the risk for hemorrhage.

1 Thyroid hormone substitutes will regulate the body's metabolism. **3** Calcium is needed to maintain parathyroid function. **4** Radioactive iodine, not potassium iodide, ablates thyroid tissues.
Client Need: Pharmacological and Parenteral Therapies; **Cognitive Level:** Comprehension; **Integrated Process:** Teaching/Learning; **Nursing Process:** Assessment/Analysis; **Reference:** Ch 9, Hyperthyroidism, Data Base

768. **4** Antacids interfere with absorption of drugs such as anticholinergics, barbiturates, tetracycline, and digoxin.

1 Antacids should be given 1 or 2 hours after meals and at bedtime. **2** Liquid antacids are faster in onset of action. **3** They may be taken as frequently as every 1 to 2 hours without adverse effects.
Client Need: Pharmacological and Parenteral Therapies; **Cognitive Level:** Application; **Integrated Process:** Teaching/Learning; **Nursing Process:** Planning/Implementation; **Reference:** Ch 8, Antacids

769. **3** Any product containing aluminum, magnesium, or calcium ions should not be taken in the hour before or after an oral dose, because it decreases absorption by as much as 25% to 50%.

1 Food interferes with absorption; it should be given 1 hour before or 2 hours after meals. **2** Citrus juice has no influence on this drug. **4** Antacids will interfere with absorption.

Client Need: Pharmacological and Parenteral Therapies; **Cognitive Level:** Application; **Nursing Process:** Planning/Implementation; **Reference:** Ch 3, Infection, Antibiotics

770. **3** This interferon immune modifier causes flulike symptoms such as fever, muscle aches, and lethargy.

1 An integumentary response to this drug is sweating, not lack of perspiration (anhidrosis). **2** This drug may cause hypocalcemia, not hypercalcemia. **4** This drug may cause tachycardia, not bradycardia.

Client Need: Pharmacological and Parenteral Therapies; **Cognitive Level:** Application; **Integrated Process:** Teaching/Learning; **Nursing Process:** Planning/Implementation; **Reference:** Ch 11, Multiple Sclerosis, Nursing Care

771. **3** Hydrocortisone is a glucocorticoid that has antiinflammatory action and aids in metabolism of carbohydrate, fat, and protein, causing elevation of blood glucose level. Thus it enables the body to adapt to stress.

1 Potassium salts are retained in Addison's disease. **2** Cardiac dysrhythmias are caused by electrolyte imbalances, and dyspnea is caused by hypovolemia and decreased O_2 supply; neither is affected by hydrocortisone. **4** Lack of angiotensin II is not the cause of hypotension in this disorder.

Client Need: Pharmacological and Parenteral Therapies; **Cognitive Level:** Analysis; **Integrated Process:** Teaching/Learning; **Nursing Process:** Planning/Implementation; **Reference:** Ch 9, Addison's Disease, Data Base

772. **2** DDAVP replaces the ADH, facilitating reabsorption of water and consequent return of normal urine output and thirst.

1 The mechanisms that regulate pH are not affected. **3** DDAVP does not alter serum glucose level; diabetes mellitus, not diabetes insipidus, results in hyperglycemia. **4** Although a correction of tachycardia is consistent with correction of dehydration, the client is not dehydrated if the fluid intake is adequate; respirations are unaffected.

Client Need: Pharmacological and Parenteral Therapies; **Cognitive Level:** Application; **Nursing Process:** Evaluation/Outcomes; **Reference:** Ch 9, Diabetes Insipidus, Nursing Care

773. **3** Naloxone (Narcan) is an opioid (narcotic) antagonist and will reverse respiratory depression caused by opiates.

1, 2, 4 This is not needed; naloxone will correct the respiratory depression.

Client Need: Pharmacological and Parenteral Therapies; **Cognitive Level:** Analysis; **Nursing Process:** Planning/Implementation; **Reference:** Ch 7, Opioid Antagonist

774. **1** To prevent crystal formation, the client should have sufficient intake to produce 1000 to 1500 mL of urine daily while taking this drug.

2 Straining urine is not indicated when a client is taking a urinary antiinfective. **3** Urinary decrease is of concern, because it may indicate renal failure. If fluids are encouraged, the client's output should increase. **4** The drug need not be taken at a strict time daily.

Client Need: Pharmacological and Parenteral Therapies; **Cognitive Level:** Application; **Integrated Process:** Teaching/Learning; **Nursing Process:** Planning/Implementation; **Reference:** Ch 12, Kidney-Specific Antiinfectives

775. **2** Salicylates can cause ototoxicity, which can manifest as tinnitus or muffled hearing.

1, 3, 4 This is not an effect of salicylate intoxication.

Client Need: Pharmacological and Parenteral Therapies; **Cognitive Level:** Application; **Integrated Process:** Teaching/Learning; **Nursing Process:** Planning/Implementation; **Reference:** Ch 3, Pain, Nonsteroidal Antiinflammatory Drugs

776. **1** ☐ Calcium levels are not affected.

2 ☒ Changing positions slowly helps reduce orthostatic hypotension.

3 ☒ Peripheral edema may occur as a result of heart failure and must be reported.

4 ☐ Hair loss does not occur.

5 ☒ Grapefruit juice affects the metabolism of calcium channel blockers.

Client Need: Pharmacological and Parenteral Therapies; **Cognitive Level:** Analysis; **Integrated Process:** Teaching/Learning; **Nursing Process:** Planning/Implementation; **Reference:** Ch 6, Antidysrhythmics

777. **3** Adverse reactions include blood dyscrasias, such as eosinophilia, thrombocytopenia, aplastic anemia, and leukopenia, which can be life-threatening.

1, 4 This is not an adverse reaction to a gold compound. **2** Although cutaneous lesions can occur, they (unlike thrombocytopenia) are not life-threatening.

Client Need: Pharmacological and Parenteral Therapies; **Cognitive Level:** Analysis; **Nursing Process:** Evaluation/Outcomes; **Reference:** Ch 11, Arthritis, Nursing Care

778. **3** Although most chemotherapy causes diarrhea, vincristine can cause severe constipation, impaction, or paralytic ileus.

1, 2, 4 This side effect is shared with most other chemotherapeutic agents.

Client Need: Pharmacological and Parenteral Therapies; **Cognitive Level:** Application; **Nursing Process:** Planning/Implementation; **Reference:** Ch 3, General Nursing Care of Clients With Neoplastic Disorders

779. **4** Prolonged chemotherapy may slow the production of leukocytes in bone marrow, thus suppressing the activity of the immune system. Antibiotics may be required to help counter infections that the body can no longer handle easily.

1 The liver does not produce leukocytes. **2, 3** Although leukocytes are in both blood and lymph nodes, these cells are more mature than those found in the bone marrow and thus more resistant to the effects of chemotherapy.

Client Need: Pharmacological and Parenteral Therapies; **Cognitive Level:** Analysis; **Nursing Process:** Assessment/Analysis; **Reference:** Ch 3, Neoplastic Disorders, Related Pharmacology, Major Side Effects

780. 3 Many chemotherapeutic agents function by interfering with DNA replication associated with cellular reproduction (mitosis). The rapid mitosis of the stratified squamous epithelium of the mouth and anus results in these areas being powerfully affected by the drugs.

1 Anorexia is not the cause of stomatitis. 2 This effect is not caused by direct irritation; most agents are administered parenterally. 4 Chemotherapeutic agents affect the cells that are most rapidly proliferating, which include not only the cells of the GI epithelium but also those of the bone marrow and hair follicles.

Client Need: Pharmacological and Parenteral Therapies; **Cognitive Level:** Comprehension; **Nursing Process:** Evaluation/ Outcomes; **Reference:** Ch 3, Neoplastic Disorders, Related Pharmacology, Basic Concepts

781. 2 Methotrexate is a folic acid antagonist that can cause depression of bone marrow. This serious toxic effect is sometimes prevented by administration of folic acid. Some physicians advocate its administration after a course of methotrexate therapy so as not to interfere with methotrexate activity.

1, 3 Folic acid is a metabolite and does not destroy cancer cells. 4 Leucovorin calcium does not increase the production of phagocytes.

Client Need: Pharmacological and Parenteral Therapies; **Cognitive Level:** Comprehension; **Integrated Process:** Teaching/ Learning; **Nursing Process:** Evaluation/Outcomes; **Reference:** Ch 3, Neoplastic Disorders, Related Pharmacology, Miscellaneous Agents

782. 2 Hormone therapy must be withdrawn slowly to allow the appropriate organ to adjust and resume production of the hormone.

1, 3, 4 This is not the reason for gradual withdrawal of the drug.

Client Need: Pharmacological and Parenteral Therapies; **Cognitive Level:** Comprehension; **Nursing Process:** Evaluation/ Outcomes; **Reference:** Ch 9, Adrenocorticoids

783. 3 Prolonged use of steroids may cause leukopenia as a result of bone marrow depression.

1, 2 This elevates in acute inflammatory diseases; steroids help decrease it. 4 Serum glucose levels increase with steroid use.

Client Need: Pharmacological and Parenteral Therapies; **Cognitive Level:** Application; **Nursing Process:** Evaluation/ Outcomes; **Reference:** Ch 9, Adrenocorticoids

784. 2 Secretions and drainage are tested to determine the antibiotics to which the organism is particularly sensitive or resistant (sensitivity).

1 This is a test for antibody content. 3 This test provides data about fluid and electrolyte balance. 4 The erythrocyte sedimentation rate (ESR) is a nonspecific test for the presence of inflammation.

Client Need: Pharmacological and Parenteral Therapies; **Cognitive Level:** Analysis; **Nursing Process:** Assessment/Analysis; **Reference:** Ch 3, Infection General Nursing Care of Clients at Risk for Infection

785. 4 Streptomycin is ototoxic and may cause damage to the auditory and vestibular portions of the eighth cranial nerve.

1, 2, 3 This is not affected by streptomycin.

Client Need: Pharmacological and Parenteral Therapies; **Cognitive Level:** Analysis; **Nursing Process:** Evaluation/ Outcomes; **Reference:** Ch 7, Antituberculars

786. 3 Nonsystemic antacids are not readily absorbed, so they do not alter acid-base balance. Sodium bicarbonate is absorbed and can alter the acid-base balance.

1 These preparations do contain sodium. 2 Nonsystemic antacids are insoluble and not readily absorbed. 4 These are side effects of nonsystemic antacids.

Client Need: Pharmacological and Parenteral Therapies; **Cognitive Level:** Analysis; **Integrated Process:** Teaching/Learning; **Nursing Process:** Assessment/Analysis; **Reference:** Ch 8, Antacids

787. 4 It decreases gastric secretion by inhibiting histamine at H_2 receptors.

1, 2, 3 This is not the action of ranitidine.

Client Need: Pharmacological and Parenteral Therapies; **Cognitive Level:** Comprehension; **Nursing Process:** Planning/ Implementation; **Reference:** Ch 8, Antisecretory Agents

788. 3 Over time clients receiving morphine develop tolerance and require increasing doses to relieve pain, thus requiring continuing reassessments.

1 This would not meet the client's need for relief from pain. 2 The client is terminal and the risk for addiction is of no concern. 4 The respiratory, not the heart, rate is the significant vital sign to be monitored; morphine depresses the CNS, specifically the respiratory center in the brain.

Client Need: Pharmacological and Parenteral Therapies; **Cognitive Level:** Application; **Nursing Process:** Assessment/ Analysis; **Reference:** Ch 3, Pain, General Nursing Care of Clients in Pain

789. 1 ☐ The prophylactic drug therapy will be continued for 6 to 12 months.

2 ☒ The children are at an increased risk because the client's spouse has tuberculosis; the children should be screened as members of the household.

3 ☐ Pyridoxine should be taken to prevent neuritis, which is associated with INH.

4 ☒ The positive skin test indicates that the client has been exposed to the bacilli and developed antibodies, not necessarily the disease itself; further diagnostic studies are indicated.

5 ☒ Both wine and aged cheese contain tyramine and histamine, which can cause headache, flushing, and a drop in BP and should be avoided when taking INH.

Client Need: Pharmacological and Parenteral Therapies; **Cognitive Level:** Analysis; **Integrated Process:** Teaching/Learning;

Nursing Process: Evaluation/Outcomes; **Reference:** Ch 7, Antituberculars

790. **2** Rifamin (Rifadin) increases the metabolism of oral contraceptives, which may result in an unplanned pregnancy.

1, 3, 4 Rifampin (Rifadin) does not interact with this medication.

Client Need: Pharmacological and Parenteral Therapies; **Cognitive Level:** Analysis; **Nursing Process:** Assessment/Analysis; **Reference:** Ch 7, Antituberculars

791. **3** These drugs are incompatible in the same IV and therefore they must be administered separately. By instituting a second line for the antibiotic, the heparin can continue to infuse.

1 Twice a day both drugs must run concurrently. Also, flushing the line may not eliminate remnants of the heparin, which is incompatible with vancomycin. **2** This is unsafe because heparin and vancomycin are incompatible and should not be administered via the same intravenous line. **4** The client has two medications ordered and it is the nurse's responsibility, not the practitioner's, to administer them safely.

Client Need: Pharmacological and Parenteral Therapies; **Cognitive Level:** Analysis; **Nursing Process:** Planning/Implementation; **Reference:** Ch 3, Infection Antibiotics

792. **4** Angiotensin II receptor antagonists, such as valsartan (Diovan), block vasoconstrictor and aldosterone-producing effects of angiotensin II at receptor sites, including vascular smooth muscle, thus reducing the BP; dizziness, orthostatic hypotension, and excessive hypotension may occur.

1 Diarrhea, not constipation, may occur with Diovan. **2** Hyperkalemia, not hypokalemia, may occur with Diovan. **3** Diovan does not cause an alteration in visual acuity.

Client Need: Pharmacological and Parenteral Therapies; **Cognitive Level:** Application; **Nursing Process:** Evaluation/Outcomes; **Reference:** Ch 6, Antihypertensives

793. **2** Constipation is a side effect of this non-nitrate antidysrhythmic because of its anticholinergic properties.

1 A thin, watery discharge from the nose (rhinorrhea) does not occur with this medication because of its anticholinergic properties. **3** Hypoglycemia, not hyperglycemia, may occur. **4** Urinary hesitancy and retention, rather than stress incontinence, occur.

Client Need: Pharmacological and Parenteral Therapies; **Cognitive Level:** Application; **Integrated Process:** Teaching/Learning; **Nursing Process:** Planning/Implementation; **Reference:** Ch 6, Antidysrhythmics

794. **2** Timolol (Blocadren) should not be taken at night because the BP usually drops when sleeping. This medication blocks beta-adrenergic receptors in the heart, which ultimately lowers the BP. Therefore the drug should be taken early in the morning to maximize its therapeutic effect.

1 Orthostatic hypotension is a side effect of Blocadren and the client should change positions slowly to prevent dizziness and falls. **3** Drowsiness is a side effect of Blocadren and the client should be taught precautions to prevent injury. **4** The pulse rate should be taken before administration because ventricular dysrhythmias and heart block may occur with Blocadren.

Client Need: Pharmacological and Parenteral Therapies; **Cognitive Level:** Analysis; **Integrated Process:** Teaching/Learning; **Nursing Process:** Evaluation/Outcomes; **Reference:** Ch 6, Antidysrhythmics

795. **4** Zyloprim can potentiate the effect of oral hypoglycemics, causing hypoglycemia; the blood glucose level should be monitored more frequently.

1 NSAIDs can be taken concurrently with Zyloprim. **2** A daily fluid intake of 2500 to 3000 mL will limit the risk of developing renal calculi. **3** Zyloprim should be taken with milk or food to decrease GI irritation.

Client Need: Pharmacological and Parenteral Therapies; **Cognitive Level:** Analysis; **Integrated Process:** Teaching/Learning; **Nursing Process:** Planning/Implementation; **Reference:** Ch 9, Antidiabetics

796. **1** Bright yellow urine is an expected, insignificant side effect of vitamin B complex.

2 There is no need to increase oral fluids. The client may consume the usual daily intake of fluid. **3** The vitamin may precipitate nausea when taken on an empty stomach; therefore the vitamin should be taken with food. **4** Vitamin B complex is a water-soluble vitamin and excess amounts are excreted in the urine.

Client Need: Pharmacological and Parenteral Therapies; **Cognitive Level:** Application; **Integrated Process:** Teaching/Learning; **Nursing Process:** Planning/Implementation; **Reference:** Ch 8, Review of Nutrients, Vitamins

797. **2** Rapid administration of Lasix can cause tinnitus, loss of hearing, and ear pain.

1 Lasix has a diuretic effect; urinary retention does not occur. **3** Lasix does not affect the heart. **4** Lasix does not cause peripheral neuropathy.

Client Need: Pharmacological and Parenteral Therapies; **Cognitive Level:** Analysis; **Nursing Process:** Evaluation/Outcomes; **Reference:** Ch 6, Diuretics

798. **1** Human B-type natriuretic peptide binds to the receptor in vascular smooth muscle and endothelial cells, leading to smooth muscle relaxation. Dyspnea will decrease as a result of the action of this drug.

2 Hypotension will not decrease. Hypotension is a side effect of Natrecor. **3** Natrecor is not used for unstable angina. **4** Natrecor is not an antidysrhythmic.

Client Need: Pharmacological and Parenteral Therapies; **Cognitive Level:** Analysis; **Nursing Process:** Evaluation/Outcomes; **Reference:** Ch 6, Heart Failure, Data Base

799. **3** The home environment is safer than the hospital environment because the client has previously

been exposed to the microorganisms in the home and the hospital environment contains more resistant, virulent pathogens.

1, 2, 4 This is a correct statement that indicates that the teaching was successful.

Client Need: Pharmacological and Parenteral Therapies; **Cognitive Level:** Application; **Integrated Process:** Teaching/Learning; **Nursing Process:** Evaluation/Outcomes; **Reference:** Ch 3, General Nursing Care of Clients With Neoplastic Disorders

800. 1 The client is most likely experiencing fat embolism syndrome (FES). The average time of onset of FES is 18 to 24 hours after injury to long bones or crushing injury. Fat globules and tissue thromboplastin exit from the bone marrow and local tissue as a result of the injury. Fat molecules enter the venous circulation, move to the lungs, and embolize small capillaries. Petechial rash on the neck, chest, conjunctivae, or axillae is a classic sign of FES (occurs in 50% to 60% of clients with FES). The elevated temperature, pulse rate, and respirations are associated with FES; 75% of clients with FES exhibit neurologic signs such as altered mental state, restlessness, agitation, lethargy, confusion, or coma.

2 The client is not experiencing urinary retention because the output indicates adequate hourly output of at least 50 mL/hr. **3** The client is not experiencing hypovolemic shock. Although the client may experience tachypnea, tachycardia, and an elevated temperature with hypovolemic shock, the blood pressure will decrease and urine output will decrease below 30 mL/hr. **4** The client is not experiencing a pulmonary embolism. This is more likely to occur 4 to 10 days after trauma. Although tachypnea, tachycardia, an elevated temperature, restlessness, and agitation are common with pulmonary embolism, the client is not exhibiting sudden chest pain, dyspnea, cough or hemoptysis, or areas of dullness or crackles when auscultating breath sounds.

Client Need: Physiological Adaptation; **Cognitive Level:** Analysis; **Nursing Process:** Evaluation/Outcomes; **Reference:** Ch 11, Fracture of the Extremities, Nursing Care

Foundations of Mental Health/Psychiatric Nursing

DEVELOPMENT OF THE PERSONALITY

OVERVIEW

A. Sum of all traits that differentiate one individual from another
B. Total behavior pattern of an individual through which the inner interests are expressed
C. The individual's unique and distinctive way of perceiving, behaving, and interacting with the environment and other people
D. Constellation of defense mechanisms for dealing with inner and outer pressures
E. A functional role within a family system
F. Emergence of personality occurs around 2 years of age

FACTORS INVOLVED IN PERSONALITY DEVELOPMENT

A. Behavior is a learned response that develops as a result of past experiences and genetic and psychologic factors
B. To protect the individual's emotional well-being, these experiences are organized in the psyche on three different levels
  1. Conscious: composed of past experiences, easily recalled
  2. Subconscious: composed of material that has been deliberately pushed out of the conscious but can be recalled with some effort
  3. Unconscious: contains the largest body of material; greatly influences behavior
    a. This material cannot be deliberately brought back into awareness because usually it is unacceptable and painful to the individual
    b. If recalled, usually it is disguised or distorted, as in dreams or slips of the tongue; however, it is still capable of producing high levels of anxiety
    c. According to Freud, the personality consists of three parts: the id, ego, and superego
      (1) Id is the inborn unconscious instincts, impulses, and urges; it is totally self-centered
      (2) Ego is the conscious self, the "I" that deals with reality; the part of the personality that is shown to the environment; ego strengths enable an individual to cope with frustration

and delay gratification; ego begins to develop during infancy
      (3) Superego is the part of the personality that, mainly on an unconscious level, controls, inhibits, and regulates impulses and instincts whose uncontrolled expression would endanger the emotional well-being of the individual and the stability of the society; incorporates parental, religious, and societal values; it develops between the ages of 3 to 6 years

FORMATION OF THE PERSONALITY

A. Personality of an individual develops in overlapping stages that shade and merge together
  1. Particular conflicts and tasks must be mastered during each stage of development from infancy to maturity if needs are to be met and mental health maintained/enhanced
  2. Successful resolution of the conflicts and acquisition of the tasks associated with each stage is essential to development
  3. If these tasks are not acquired at specific periods, the basic structure of the personality will be weakened
  4. Factors in each stage persist as a permanent part of the personality
  5. Childhood identifications are integrated with basic drives, native endowments, and opportunities offered in social roles
  6. Unresolved conflicts remain in the unconscious and may, at times, result in maladaptive behavior
  7. Personality is capable of change throughout life; as one ages there may be a decreased ability to cope
B. Psychodynamic theory (Freud)
  1. Psychodynamic theories propose that human behavior is largely governed by motives and drives that are internal and often unconscious
  2. Freud believed that development proceeds best when children's psychosexual needs at each stage are met, but not exceeded; the stages are
    a. Oral (birth to 1 year)—psychosexual needs gratified orally; unable to delay gratification; begins to develop self-concept from the responses of others

b. Anal (1 to 3 years)—bladder and bowel training occurs; this interferes with instinctual impulses; struggle of giving of self and breaking the symbiotic ties to mother; as the ties are broken, the child learns independence; struggle with toilet training creates conflict between child's needs and parents' desires

c. Phallic (3 to 5 years)—psychosexual energy directed to genitals (oedipal); values and rules learned from parents; guilt and self-esteem develop; incestuous desire for opposite sex parent develops and creates fear and guilt feelings; desires are repressed, and introjection and role identification with parent of the same sex occurs

d. Latency (6 to 12 years)—mastery of learning; relationships with same-sex peers develop; sexual instincts are relatively quiet

e. Genital (12 years and beyond)—period of sexual maturity in which psychosexual needs are directed toward heterosexual relationships; sexual activity increases; sexual identity is strengthened or attacked

C. Psychosocial theory (Erikson)

1. Psychosocial theory attributes development to social interactions and relationships that occur throughout the life span

2. Erikson believed that development results from social aims or conflicts arising from feelings, parent-child interactions, and social relationships

3. Eight major crises or conflicts need to be faced during a lifetime; each stage is marked by a struggle between two opposing tendencies, both of which are experienced by the individual. Stages are

a. Trust versus mistrust (birth to 1 year)—infant develops a sense of whether the world can be trusted; child learns to depend on satisfaction that is derived from attention to needs; and when needs are met, trust develops; psychosocial strength—hope

b. Autonomy versus shame and doubt (1 to 3 years)—child develops first sense of self as independent or as shameful and doubtful; the struggle of holding on to or letting go; an internal struggle for self-identity; love versus hate; psychosocial strength—will

c. Initiative versus guilt (3 to 6 years)—child learns ability to try new things and learns how to handle failure; period of intensive activity, play, and consuming fantasies where child interjects parents' social consciousness; psychosocial strength—purpose

d. Industry versus inferiority (6 to 12 years)—child learns how to make things with others and strives to achieve success; psychosocial strength—self-worth

e. Identity versus confusion (puberty to young adulthood)—adolescent determines own sense of self; psychosocial strength—fidelity

f. Intimacy versus isolation (young adulthood)—person makes commitment to another; moves from the relative security of self-identity to the relative insecurity involved in establishing intimacy with another; isolation and self-absorption occur if unsuccessful; psychosocial strength—love

g. Generativity versus stagnation (middle adulthood)—person seeks to guide the next generation or risks feelings of personal incompleteness; psychosocial strength—care

h. Integrity versus despair (late life)—older adult seeks a sense of personal accomplishment, adapts to triumphs and disappointments with a certain ego integrity and accepts death, or falls into despair; psychosocial strength—wisdom

D. Interpersonal theory (Sullivan)

1. Development results from interpersonal relationships with others in maximizing satisfaction of needs while minimizing insecurity

2. Believed that development results from interpersonal relationships in the infancy, childhood, juvenile, preadolescent, adolescent, and late adolescent stages

a. Infancy (0 to 2 years): learns to differentiate self from others; through trial and error, learns from parental interactions to rely on others to gratify needs and satisfy wishes; develops a sense of basic trust, security, and self-worth when this occurs; ends with language development

b. Childhood (2 to 6 years): language development allows for education; development of body image and self-perception; self-esteem develops with sublimation; child learns to communicate needs through the use of words and to accept delayed gratification and interference with wish fulfillment; expresses impulses in socially acceptable ways or develops a feeling of living among enemies

c. Juvenile (6 to 10 years): relations with peers allow child to see self objectively; develops conscience; behavior is connected to others' opinions; organizes and uses experiences in terms of approval and disapproval received; begins using selective inattention and disassociates those experiences that cause physical or emotional discomfort and pain

d. Preadolescent (10 to 13 years): develops same-sex friends; moves from egocentrism to love; able to form satisfying relationships and work with peers; uses competition, compromise, and cooperation

e. Adolescent (13 to 17 years): interest in sexual activity; learns how to establish satisfactory relationships with members of the opposite sex; if attractions are severely discouraged or thwarted by adults, the adolescent will feel insecure and lonely

    f. Late adolescent (17 to 19 years): personality integration; able to integrate the needs of society without becoming overwhelmed with anxiety; inability to achieve personality integration results in regression and egocentrism for life

    g. Young adult: becomes economically, intellectually, and emotionally self-sufficient

    h. Older adult: learns to be interdependent and assumes responsibility for others

    i. Senescence: develops an acceptance of responsibility for what life is and was and of its place in the flow of history

E. Cognitive development theory (Piaget)
1. Sensorimotor stage (infancy-toddler): infant develops physically with a gradual increase in the ability to think and use language; progresses from simple reflex responses through repetitive behaviors to deliberate and imaginative activity
2. Preoperational thought stage (preschool): child learns to imitate and play; begins to use symbols and language although interpretation is literal
3. Preoperational thought stage continues (school age): child begins to understand relationships and develops basic conceptual thought and intuitive reasoning
4. Concrete operational thought stage (preadolescent): thinking is more socialized and logical with increased intellectual and conceptual development; begins problem solving by use of inductive reasoning and logical thought
5. Formal operational stage (adolescent): develops true abstract thought by application of logical tests; achieves conceptual independence and problem-solving ability

PHYSIOLOGY, COGNITION, EMOTIONS, AND BEHAVIOR

OVERVIEW

A. Feelings, thoughts, physiology, and behaviors are all interactive and each influences the others
B. Life is a continually changing process, and when these changes occur in areas of significance, they often produce distinct emotional responses including
1. Resistance to change: the individual hesitates to accept or adapt to the change and may attempt to deny its occurrence or reject its outcome
2. Regression: the individual returns to an earlier type of behavior that, at the time, provided some satisfaction and gratification and now provides an escape from the unacceptable or anxiety-producing situation
3. Acceptance and progression: the individual adapts to the change and expends energy on outside objects rather than self-centered aims
C. Many therapists use a variety of therapeutics approaches based on client need

NEUROPHYSIOLOGIC THEORETICAL BASIS OF BEHAVIOR

A. There is general acceptance that there is no real division between mind and body, mental and physical, brain and thought
B. Research into the neurophysiologic basis for behavior focuses on the anatomy and physiology of the brain and nervous system and their relationship to health and illness
1. Structural differences such as changes in ventricle size or cerebral atrophy are identified by neuroimaging methods such as MRI and CT scans
2. Physiologic differences, such as hyperactivity in certain areas of the brain, are identified by electroencephalogram (EEG) studies and positron emission tomography (PET) scans
C. An understanding of the anatomy and physiology of the central nervous system is essential
1. The brain weighs about 3 lb and is composed of trillions of cells, 100 billion neurons, and the cells that support their function
2. Neurons do not touch each other but communicate across the synapse that separates them via chemical messengers called neurotransmitters
3. Neurons will be receptive to some neurotransmitters and not to others
4. Major excitatory and inhibitory neurotransmitters include dopamine, norepinephrine, serotonin, acetylcholine, and gamma-aminobutyric acid (GABA)
5. The level of neurotransmitters that will excite or inhibit neural activity is influenced by their production, metabolism/inactivation, and reuptake/storage
6. Abnormalities in the level of various neurotransmitters have been linked to many psychiatric illnesses (e.g., excess of dopamine to schizophrenia; decreased serotonin levels to depression), and most psychotropic medications work by altering levels of neurotransmitters
D. Considerable knowledge gaps still exist as to the specific pathophysiology of psychiatric disorders, but research continues, especially in the area of neurotransmitters
E. Research is examining the importance of other factors such as genetics, infections, sleep deprivation, toxins, nutrition, hormonal shifts, and stress as influences on neurobiology and behavior
F. Only a few diseases have identified genetic markers, including Huntington's disease and a rare form of Alzheimer's disease

PSYCHOBIOLOGIC HEALTH

A. Category of psychophysiologic disruptions in which organic impairment is evident
B. Anxiety stimulates the autonomic nervous system, and the nervous and endocrine impulses appear to center

on one particular organ, creating actual physical illness and changes in tissue structure

C. Selye's stress theory has helped to identify mental-physical interactions

D. Predisposing factors are described from biologic, psychologic, and sociocultural perspectives; precipitating stressors include any experience the individual interprets as stressful

E. The stress is often unrecognized consciously; if recognized, individuals are unable to relate this to the physical symptoms of the psychophysiologic disorder

F. Efforts to match specific stressors to specific diseases have not been successful

G. Psychologic diseases have both physical stressors (e.g., dietary changes, physical exertion, allergic immune responses, infectious agents) and psychologic (e.g., anxiety, fear, tension) stressors, which combine to produce pathophysiology and signs and symptoms

H. Common psychobiologic diseases/disorders include migraine headaches, primary hypertension, angina, neck and back pain, asthma, irritable bowel, neurodermatitis, impotence, and frigidity

I. In many autoimmune disorders (e.g., systemic lupus erythematosus, ulcerative colitis, myasthenia gravis, multiple sclerosis) there is also an exacerbation of symptoms or relapse during periods of psychologic stress; stress also may diminish the immune response

J. Therapy: must be directed toward both the physical and emotional problems

COGNITIVE THEORY

A. Cognitive theorists believe that
1. Patterns of thinking, mindsets, and belief systems will greatly influence feelings and behavior
2. Dysfunctional cognitive patterns and cognitive distortions (e.g., pessimism, overgeneralizing, unrealistic expectations) lead to alterations in mood and behavior

B. Cognitive therapy is most effective in treating clients with anxiety and mood disorders

C. Interventions are focused on the identification of dysfunctional thought patterns and replacement with healthier, more reality-based thinking

D. Examples of cognitive therapy include
1. Thought journals: client records situations in which cognitive distortions occurred, and the thoughts and feelings that followed
2. Cognitive restructuring through the development of positive self-talk and rational mindset: when a cognitive distortion/negative thought occurs the client replaces it with more positive rational thoughts
3. Cognitive rehearsal: client prepares mental script to deal with situations that usually trigger cognitive distortions

BEHAVIORAL THEORY

A. Behavioral theorists believe that
1. All behavior is motivated and learned
2. Automatic or habitual behavior patterns develop over time through reinforcement, but can be unlearned

B. Behavioral therapy is effective in working with client populations with limited cognitive skills (children, mentally retarded) and for disorders with significant behavioral components (phobias, compulsions)

C. Consistency in nursing response is essential for behavioral interventions

D. Examples of behavioral therapy include
1. Contracting: client agrees, orally or in writing, to change dysfunctional behavior; contracts include specific behavior to be modified, the positive reinforcers, and the consequences if contract is broken
2. Token/reward system: desired behavior receives concrete positive reinforcement (e.g., colorful stickers during toilet training for child)
3. Desensitization: client is exposed to slowly increasing experiences with anxiety-producing stimulus while practicing behavioral techniques such as relaxation or deep breathing
4. Flooding: client is exposed to anxiety-producing stimulus continuously in a supportive environment until intensity of response diminishes

MASLOW'S HUMANISTIC THEORY

A. Maslow's humanistic theory, a nondevelopmental theory, postulates that people are guided by a variety of needs, from basic physiologic ones to self-actualization, the need to achieve one's full potential

B. The existence of unmet needs and the desire to achieve optimum self-potential are fundamental sources of human motivation. Needs are
1. Physiologic—satisfying needs for oxygen, water, food, shelter, sleep, and relief of sexual tension
2. Safety—avoiding harm and achieving security and safety
3. Love and belonging—giving and receiving affection, developing companionship, group acceptance
4. Esteem and recognition—achieving recognition from others leads to self-esteem, prestige, and work success
5. Self-actualization—achieving one's own unique potential

C. With the gratification of basic needs, other higher needs emerge, driving one toward self-potential

D. People may simultaneously be working to achieve needs on more than one level

ANXIETY AND COPING BEHAVIORS

OVERVIEW

A. Anxiety (see Chapter 19, Nursing Care of Clients With Disorders Related to Anxiety and Alterations in Mood)
  1. Diffuse feeling of uneasiness, uncertainty, and helplessness that occurs as a result of a threat to an individual's self-concept, esteem, identity, or safety
  2. Usual response to a threat or stressors
  3. Different from fear, which has a specific source or object that can be identified and described
  4. An emotion that is subjective in nature and without a specific object
  5. Related to one's culture, because culture influences one's values
  6. Causes are uncertain, but research indicates a combination of physical, psychosocial, and environmental factors
B. Levels of anxiety
  1. Mild—alertness level: automatic response of the CNS that prepares the body for danger by regulating internal processes and concentrating all energies for internal activity; perceptual field is increased
  2. Moderate—apprehension level: response to anticipation of short-term threat that prepares the individual for efficient performance; perceptual field is narrowed since focus is on the immediate concern
  3. Severe—high anxiety level: focus is on a specific detail, and behavior is aimed at relieving anxiety; needs much direction by others to focus on another detail or area; marked reduction in the perceptual field limits cognitive abilities
  4. Panic—extreme level: involves the disorganization of the personality and is associated with dread and terror; communication abilities and problem solving are nonexistent; even with direction, the person has great difficulty following commands; perceptual field is distorted; prolonged period of panic results in exhaustion and death; intervention is essential
C. Behavioral defenses against anxiety (Table 15-1: Coping Skills: Affective and Problem Solving)
  1. Consciously directed, task-oriented behaviors that are deliberate attempts to problem solve, resolve conflicts, and gratify; they tend to involve the individual's deliberate effort to maintain control, reduce tension, and limit anxiety; they include attack, withdrawal, and compromise behaviors
    a. Attack behavior: an attempt to overcome obstacles to satisfy a need
      (1) Constructive behaviors reflect use of problem solving
      (2) Destructive behaviors usually are accompanied by feelings of anger and hostility and may violate rights, property, and well-being of others

Table 15-1 Coping Skills: Affective and Problem Solving

Affective	Problem Solving
Pray	Seek advice
Daydream	Obtain another's perspective
Eat, drink, and smoke	Learn new information/skill
Exercise	Set goals
Seek comfort from others	Ask for help
Meditate and do yoga	Do research
Withdraw	Delegate responsibilities
Bathe	Seek alternatives
Sleep	Brainstorm ideas
Make a joke	Draw on past experiences
Cry	Develop new resources
Watch TV or go to a movie	
Take a drive	

    b. Withdrawal behavior: can be expressed physically or psychologically
      (1) Physical withdrawal involves removing oneself from the source of threat
      (2) Psychologic withdrawal occurs when one admits defeat, becomes apathetic, or lowers aspirations; when this behavior isolates the person or interferes with work production, it causes additional problems
    c. Compromise is essential in situations that cannot be resolved through attack or withdrawal; it occurs by changing usual methods of operating, altering goals, or adjusting personal needs
      (1) Compromise behaviors usually are constructive and are noted in approach-approach and avoidance-avoidance situations
      (2) Compromise solutions can later offer opportunities for renegotiation or adapting different coping mechanisms
  2. Task-oriented reactions and effective problem solving are influenced by the expectation of some degree of success and drawing on one's past successes to deal with current stressful situations
  3. Problem-solving perseverance and the belief that one can endure the discomfort help one find the courage to cope with anxiety
  4. Task-oriented reactions are not always successful in coping with stressful situations; therefore ego-oriented reactions (defense mechanisms) are often used to protect the self

DEFENSE MECHANISMS

A. Defense mechanisms are unconscious cognitive responses that provide protection for the personality from overwhelming anxiety
B. Defense mechanisms are most helpful in coping with mild and moderate levels of anxiety because they offer protection from feelings of inadequacy and worthlessness; when used, the individual may have a clear, slightly distorted, or more distorted perception

Table 15-2 The Use of Defense Mechanisms in Relation to the Perception of Reality

Clear Perception of Reality	Slightly Distorted Perception of Reality	More Distorted Perception of Reality
Fantasy	Compensation	Denial
Identification	Conversion	Dissociation
Introjection	Displacement	Regression
Rationalization	Intellectualization	Repression
Sublimation	Projection	
Substitution	Reaction formation	
Suppression	Splitting	
	Undoing	

of reality; defense mechanism if used to extreme may impede interpersonal relationships and limit productivity (Table 15-2: The Use of Defense Mechanisms in Relation to the Perception of Reality)
C. Identifiable patterns of response begin to form when individuals respond to most situations they encounter with the same type of behavior
D. Commonly used defense mechanisms that help an individual to cope with reality include
 1. Compensation: the individual makes up for a perceived lack in one area by emphasizing capabilities in another
 2. Identification: the individual internalizes characteristics of an idealized person
 3. Rationalization: the individual makes acceptable excuses for behavior, feelings, outcomes; attempts to explain behavior by logical reasoning but does not address underlying feelings
 4. Sublimation: a socially acceptable behavior is substituted for an unacceptable instinct; this mechanism is used when the expression of these instincts would prove a threat to the self
 5. Substitution: the individual replaces an unacceptable emotion or goal by another that is more acceptable
E. In addition to the commonly used defenses, all individuals may use compensatory-type defenses in times of stress; these, when used in moderation, are adaptive; if used to excess, frequently they create greater emotional problems
 1. As the use of these compensatory defenses increases and encompasses more of the individual's life, contact with reality is interrupted and distortions begin
 2. These patterns of behavior are considered deviations and usually are viewed as signs of emotional stress and problems
  a. Conversion: emotional conflict is unconsciously changed into a physical symptom that can be expressed openly and without anxiety
  b. Denial: emotional conflict is blocked from the conscious mind, and the individual cannot recognize its existence
  c. Displacement: emotions related to an emotionally charged situation or object are shifted to a relatively safe substitute situation or object

  d. Dissociation: separation of any group of mental or behavioral processes from the rest of the individual's consciousness or identity
  e. Fantasy: conscious distortion of unconscious wishes and needs to obtain gratification and satisfaction
  f. Intellectualization: use of thinking, ideas, or intellect to avoid emotions
  g. Introjection: complete acceptance of another's opinions and values as one's own
  h. Projection: unconscious denial of unacceptable feelings and emotions in oneself while attributing them to others
  i. Reaction formation: the individual unconsciously reverses unacceptable feelings and behaves in the exact opposite manner
  j. Regression: return to an earlier stage of behavior when stress creates problems at the present stage of development
  k. Repression: involuntary exclusion from consciousness of those ideas, feelings, and situations that are creating conflict and causing discomfort
  l. Splitting: viewing others or situations as either all good or all bad; failure to integrate the positive and negative qualities in oneself
  m. Suppression: voluntary exclusion from consciousness of those ideas, feelings, and situations that are creating conflict and causing discomfort
  n. Undoing: act or communication that attempts to compensate for or negate a previous one

DYSFUNCTIONAL PATTERNS OF BEHAVIOR

A. Various theories (psychoanalytic, developmental, neurobiologic, sociocultural, behavioral, cognitive) identify factors that lead to patterns of behavior that are dysfunctional
 1. Psychoanalytic theories focus on interpersonal relationships and communication patterns that are especially influenced by childhood experiences
 2. Developmental theories focus on the ability to accomplish age-related tasks
 3. Neurobiologic theories focus on brain structure and/or neurochemistry
 4. Sociocultural theories focus on learned values, beliefs, norms, and rituals that reinforce behavior
 5. Behavioral theories focus on behaviors as learned patterns that have been positively reinforced
 6. Cognitive theories focus on the relationship among beliefs, mindsets, and behavior
B. Most dysfunctional behavior is the result of multiple stressors
C. Dysfunctional behavior increases with increased severity of stressors as the ability of an individual to cope is overwhelmed

D. Dysfunctional patterns of behavior usually reflect long-term problems in ability to cope with reality; continued use of these patterns impairs the individual's ability to grow and change and therefore creates further stress

E. Dysfunctional patterns of behavior and specific psychiatric diagnoses that can be correlated to certain patterns of dysfunctional behavior include
  1. Withdrawn behavior
     a. Pathologic retreat from, or an avoidance of, people and reality; withdrawn behavior can range from poor socialization to retreat into a private world of delusion, hallucination, and fantasy
     b. Associated with autism, schizophrenia, and other psychotic disorders, depression, anxiety, dementia
  2. Projective behavior
     a. Denial of one's own feelings, faults, and failures while attributing them to other people or objects; projective behavior can range from displacing anger onto a less threatening person to blaming others for one's own addiction or aggressive behavior
     b. Associated with substance abuse, antisocial personality, paranoid personality, phobias
  3. Aggressive behavior
     a. Physical, symbolic, or verbal behavior that is forceful or hostile and enacted to intimidate others; aggression occurs on a continuum ranging from angry body language to physical violence
     b. Associated with substance abuse, conduct disorders, mania, delirium, dementia
  4. Self-destructive behavior
     a. Indulging in actions that could lead to self-harm (e.g., noncompliance with medical regimens, substance abuse, engaging in high-risk activities) or violence against self (e.g., cutting, overdose); self-destructive behaviors can range from a client with a cardiac problem who fails to follow dietary restrictions to a client who attempts or commits suicide
     b. Associated with depression, mania, borderline personality
  5. Addictive behavior
     a. Repeated or chronic use of a substance (e.g., alcohol, drugs, cigarettes) with a resulting dependency on the substance; continued use of the substance despite the occurrence of related problems; behaviors such as gambling addiction and compulsive overeating that continue despite occurrence of related problems have not been classified in the *DSM-IV-TR* but usually are viewed as addictive disorders
     b. Associated with substance abuse, antisocial personality

CHAPTER

16 The Practice of Mental Health/Psychiatric Nursing

LEGAL CONCEPTS RELATED TO MENTAL HEALTH/PSYCHIATRIC NURSING

OVERVIEW

A. A fundamental component of psychiatric nursing is to understand the legal framework used to regulate the care and treatment of clients with mental illness; each state has its own mental health code that delineates the law in this area; case law may also set precedents that guide care

B. Adherence to the Patient Care Partnership (formerly The Patient's Bill of Rights) is essential

C. All civil rights are maintained

D. Clients have the right to be treated in the least restrictive environment; any curtailment of autonomy must be substantiated by documentation supporting the need to limit the client's freedom; clients retain the right to a lawyer and the right to request a court hearing; clients may execute a psychiatric advance directive stating treatment preferences

E. Types of hospital admissions
   1. Voluntary admission: client of lawful age may apply in writing to be admitted for treatment to a mental health facility; written notice of intent to leave may be required with a waiting period during which the psychiatrist may choose to change admission status to involuntary
   2. Involuntary admission (commitment): client who has not agreed to treatment is placed in a mental health facility; criteria for involuntary admission in some states are very circumscribed—danger to self or others; in other states requirements are more liberal—mentally ill and in need of treatment and/or unable to provide for own basic needs; most states have various routes for involuntary admission that may include
      a. Emergency hospitalization: used to intervene when there is an immediate threat by a client to self or others; this short-term (48 to 72 hours) commitment is allowed for the assessment of the client and to determine if more long-term commitment is needed or the client can be discharged to outpatient treatment
      b. Court ordered observational admission: used to assess the mental status of a person in relation to legal activities (e.g., competency to stand trial)

   c. Formal commitment: used to treat clients with chronic mental illnesses over a prolonged period; periodic reviews may be made at 3, 6, or 12 months
   d. Two-psychiatrist commitment: two psychiatrists document that the client has met the state's criteria for involuntary care; most states provide for an intermediate length of time (1 to 6 weeks) admission
   e. Physician's Emergency Certificate: allows the facility to keep the person against their will

F. Seclusion and restraint: a client who is a threat to self or others may be placed in a seclusion room or in four-point restraints to prevent injury or harm
   1. A physician must give an order for seclusion or restraint for each incidence and renew it every few hours as determined by state mental health law; PRN seclusion and restraint orders are not acceptable
   2. The nurse must document the initial and continued need for seclusion or restraint; client must be observed constantly if in restraints and checked every 15 minutes if in seclusion; hourly physical assessment must be performed if client's condition permits
   3. Hydration, nutrition, and elimination needs must be met while the client is in seclusion or restraint
   4. When it is determined that the client is no longer a threat to self or others, the client must be released from seclusion or restraint
   5. Chemical restraint: the nurse may administer a PRN medication without the client's consent if the client is dangerous to self or others

G. Court-ordered medication: a client's right to refuse treatment may be overruled, and the client may be court mandated to take medication to decrease the threat of injury to self or others

H. Psychiatric advance directive: a client with a recurrent/chronic psychiatric disease may establish an advance directive to guide treatment during a future episode of mental illness when judgment is impaired

THE NURSE'S RESPONSIBILITIES IN RELATION TO THE LAW

A. Implement care that meets the Scope and Standard of Psychiatric-Mental Health Clinical Nursing Practice as described by the ANA and nursing practice laws of the state where practicing (e.g., health promotion, case management, treatment of human responses)

B. Remain current with skills and knowledge base

C. Keep accurate and concise client records

D. Maintain client/family confidentiality; an exception must be made to notify others (e.g., police, intended victim) if a credible threat against another person is made by the client

E. Know the laws governing practice within the state, the rights and duties of the nurse, and the rights of the client

F. Maintain current malpractice liability insurance coverage

COMMUNITY HEALTH SERVICES

OVERVIEW

A. Purposes
   1. Provide prevention, treatment, and rehabilitation services for individuals with emotional problems; also support for families
   2. Maintain individuals and families in the community
   3. Provide hospital care within the community in those instances when the individual cannot be maintained on an outpatient basis
   4. Emphasize managed care mandates that shift care from costly inpatient treatment to community and home health visits

B. Types of settings in which services are provided
   1. Outpatient services
      a. Storefront clinics, daycare centers, mobile units, intensive outpatient programs, partial hospitalization programs, or day treatment centers
      b. Walk-in clinics in hospitals and psychiatric emergency departments
      c. Emergency services
      d. Crisis intervention centers, including hot-line phone centers and the Internet
      e. Private community practice, schools, and shelters
      f. Dual-diagnoses programs (mental health and chemical dependency)
      g. Mental health home nursing
      h. Forensic settings
   2. Inpatient services
      a. Specialized psychiatric hospitals, both long-term and short-term care
      b. General hospital psychiatric units
      c. Short-term placement (provide respite for caregivers, provide safe environment during episodes of aggressive acting-out)
   3. Aftercare services
      a. Foster homes
      b. Halfway houses
      c. Sheltered workshops
      d. Daycare centers

C. Types of services
   1. Observation, diagnosis, and determination of client needs
   2. Crisis intervention
   3. Direct care services to clients, including
      a. Individual, family, and group therapy
      b. Pharmacologic therapy
      c. Electroconvulsive therapy
      d. Occupational therapy
      e. Recreational therapy
   4. Therapeutic milieu
      a. Supports the individual during the period of crisis
      b. Helps the individual learn new ways of coping with problems
   5. Referral to other community agencies for necessary services
   6. Vocational counseling
   7. Health screening
   8. Education for professionals and consumers of mental health care

THE NURSE'S ROLE IN COMMUNITY NURSING

A. Case finding

B. Assessment of the individual's needs

C. Establishment of the therapeutic milieu

D. Consultation and collaboration with other professionals including the interdisciplinary team (e.g., physicians, psychologists, social workers, school teachers, clergy, nursing home and managed adult residential facility staff)

E. Active participation with the health team, including the individual and family

F. Involvement in individual, family, and group therapy

G. Supervision of unlicensed staff

H. Coordination of health services for the individual and family; referral and preparation of client for scheduled appointments

I. Education of groups within the community

J. Function as client advocate including seeking health insurance parity for reimbursement of costs for psychiatric treatment

THERAPEUTIC NURSE-CLIENT RELATIONSHIP

OVERVIEW

A. Phases of a therapeutic nurse-client relationship (see The Nurse-Client Relationship under Communication in Chapter 2)

B. Themes of communication (see The Communication Process under Communication in Chapter 2)

C. Therapeutic communication requires a basic understanding and use of interviewing techniques (see The Nurse-Client Relationship under Communication in Chapter 2)

Table 16-1 Differences Between a Social and a Professional Relationship	
Social	Professional
Unstructured time frame	Structured time
Not goal directed	Goal directed
Focus on mutual needs	Focus on client's needs
Nontheoretical	Theory-based interaction
Independent relationships	Part of a treatment team
Informal duties	Legal and ethical duties
No financial concerns	Financial issues
	Confidentiality
	Documentation

Table 16-2 Types of Crises	
Type of Crisis	Description
Maturational	Transitions in development require new behaviors and skills (basis of Erikson's theory); considered normal and often are predictable so that preventive strategies can be implemented (e.g., retirement planning)
Situational	Specific common external events that are not anticipated and create stress (e.g., job loss, amputation of a limb)
Adventitious	Disaster type events that affect groups (e.g., tornado) or unpredictable unusual individual event (e.g., rape) Some theorists believe that crisis intervention immediately after an adventitious crisis can reduce the incidence of posttraumatic stress disorder

D. Issues that interfere with a therapeutic relationship during the working phase of a therapeutic relationship
   1. Transference: the client superimposes feelings from other relationships onto the nurse-client relationship (e.g., client gets angry easily at nurse who resembles a former significant other with whom the client had a contentious relationship)
   2. Countertransference: the nurse superimposes feelings from other relationships onto the nurse-client relationship (e.g., older nurse treats a younger client like a son or daughter)
   3. Resistance: client fails to engage in or sabotages treatment (e.g., forgets appointments, keeps changing subject)
   4. Blurring of a professional versus a social relationship (see Table 16-1: Differences Between a Social and Professional Relationship)

GENERAL NURSING CARE OF CLIENTS WITH MENTAL HEALTH/PSYCHIATRIC PROBLEMS

A. Help people to prevent mental health problems and assist clients to cope with mental health problems
B. Accept and respect people as individuals and strive to separate the person from behavior that may be dysfunctional
C. Reorient client to person, place, time, and situation
D. Limit or reject inappropriate behavior without rejecting the individual
E. Help individuals set appropriate limits for themselves or set limits for them when they are unable to do so
F. Recognize that all behavior has meaning and is meeting the needs of the person performing it, regardless of how distorted or meaningless it appears to others
G. Accept the dependency needs of individuals while supporting and encouraging moves toward independence; build on ego strengths
H. Create a nonjudgmental environment that encourages individuals to express their feelings
I. Recognize that individuals need to use their dysfunctional defenses until other healthier defenses can be substituted

Table 16-3 Caplan's Phases of Crisis Development	
Phase	Description
Phase 1	Exposure to stressor (can be real or imagined) causes increasing anxiety as usual coping skills do not bring resolution to the problem.
Phase 2	Utilization of more dysfunctional coping behaviors occurs as high level of anxiety impedes problem solving.
Phase 3	Anxiety reaches panic level when effective coping is lost.
Phase 4	Anxiety overwhelms the individual, who feels immobilized or acts out with violence and self-destructive behaviors; personality disorganization occurs.

J. Recognize how feelings, behavior, and thoughts are interactive and influence relationships
K. Recognize that individuals frequently respond to the behavioral expectations of others: family, peers, and authority figures (e.g., health team members)
L. Recognize that all individuals have a potential for movement toward higher levels of emotional health
M. Include family members in the health care team when they can be supportive; recognize that in the Latino-American culture family bonds and support are important

CRISIS INTERVENTION

OVERVIEW

A. A crisis is an acute, time-limited emotional response to a stressful event or series of stressful events that can be real, potential, or imagined; a crisis can overwhelm a person's coping abilities (Table 16-2: Types of Crises)
B. Crises progress through four distinct phases (Table 16-3: Caplan's Phases of Crisis Development)
C. Continuing stress increases vulnerability and causes anxiety and physical discomfort (review anxiety content) and threatens the person's self-esteem, integrity, and safety
D. The response to a stressor varies from person to person and will be determined by perception of the situation, prior coping skills, and psychologic and physical health (e.g., some may experience a mid-life crisis or empty-nest syndrome and others may not)

E. As the individual tries to regain psychologic equilibrium, there is the opportunity for personal growth by learning new coping skills and developing additional resources

F. Ineffective coping during a crisis can lead to personality disorganization and long-term maladaptive behaviors

G. Crises are usually self-limiting and last between 4 and 6 weeks

H. Crisis intervention is a focused short-term therapy for clients in situations in which their usual coping has been overwhelmed

Nursing Care of Clients in Crisis

A. Interventions are directive and goal oriented because of the short time frame. They focus on present problem and immediate crisis issues only

B. Interventions progress through stages: intervening immediately, stabilizing the client, facilitating a realistic understanding of the event, facilitating use of resources, encouraging self-reliance

C. Assessment includes client's developmental level, perception of the event, past and current coping skills, resources and support systems, and potential for violence/suicide

D. The client is encouraged to express feelings and develop healthier coping skills

E. Referrals for more long-term care treatment, support groups, and social services may be needed

NURSING CARE IN RELATION TO VIOLENCE

DOMESTIC VIOLENCE

Overview

A. Includes child abuse, partner abuse, and elder abuse

B. Abuse can be physical, emotional, sexual, and financial; with children and dependent adults, neglect (failure to provide reasonable care and supervision) is far more common than abuse

C. The incidence of psychiatric illness and addiction disorders is higher in families where there is domestic violence

D. Families where abuse occurs are often isolated, with few support systems, have a history of abusive behaviors, and experience stressors such as unemployment or illness (see content of Crisis Intervention)

E. The child who is most likely to be abused has a physical or mental handicap, was born prematurely or at a difficult time in the family's history; such children become scapegoats and are blamed for the family's problems

F. Societal influences of violence, sexual imagery, cultural norms about family roles and the use of physical punishment to discipline may increase the tendency toward domestic violence

Nursing Care of Situations of Domestic Violence/Neglect

A. Identify signs of violence/neglect
   1. Unexplained or frequent injuries, accidents; conflicting stories about injuries, delayed treatment for injuries
   2. Failure to thrive; delayed growth and development
   3. Inadequate hygiene and inappropriate dress, eating and sleeping disorders
   4. Depression
   5. Sexually transmitted infections; inappropriate (premature) sexual knowledge

B. Report suspicions of child and elder abuse to the appropriate governmental agency, which is a requirement for nursing licensure in most states; the nurse does not need to be absolutely certain and provide proof; there only needs to be a reasonable suspicion

C. Nursing interventions
   1. Interventions for elder and child abuse include education about usual growth and development, methods of discipline of children, referral to support groups and social services, anger management, assertiveness training, and relaxation therapy
   2. Removal of at-risk children; dependent adults may be removed from the home for their safety
   3. Victims of partner abuse usually require several attempts before successfully leaving an abusive situation; victims should be helped to develop strategies for exiting an abusive situation, which include identifying financial resources, safe houses, and support groups; nurses should guard against expressing frustration to victims who choose to remain in their current situations

ANGER MANAGEMENT

Overview

A. A form of therapy that focuses on clients with a history of hostile/aggressive behavior

B. Teaches clients to assume responsibility for hostile actions, identify anger triggers, and learn new methods of responding

The Nurse's Role in Anger Management Therapy

A. Teach clients enhanced communication skills

B. Teach clients relaxation techniques

C. Encourage cognitive therapy strategies to redefine anger triggers and responses

ASSERTIVENESS TRAINING

Overview

A. Clients learn the difference between aggressive, nonassertive, passive-aggressive, and assertive communication and behavior

B. Role playing and cognitive restructuring are used

C. A form of therapy often recommended for clients with depression and dependent personality disorder

The Nurse's Role in Assertiveness Training

A. Teach differences between aggressive, nonassertive, passive-aggressive, and assertive communication and behavior
B. Role model assertive communication and behavior
C. Provide positive reinforcement for assertive behavior

RAPE COUSELING

Overview

A. Rape counseling is a form of therapy directed to victims of sexual assault; sexual assault occurs when there is lack of consent regarding the event; minors and people with cognitive impairments are regarded as being unable to give consent; sexual activity between a minor or a cognitively impaired adult and a competent adult is a form of sexual assault
B. Sexual assaults may include actions such as fondling or indecent exposure
C. Although most victims of rape are women, men also can be victims of rape
D. Myths such as the woman must have done something to provoke the rape often keep women from reporting rapes
E. The acute reaction to rape is often shock, disbelief, and dissociation from the event
F. Somatic problems, sleep disorders, phobias, social withdrawal, and depression may occur as later responses, especially if therapy is not sought and given

Nursing Care of Clients Who Have Experienced Sexual Assault

A. Acute interventions include treatment of physical injuries, protection against sexually transmitted infections, offering of pregnancy prevention and emotional support
B. Creating a safe environment in which victim may express feelings and regain some sense of choice and control is important
C. Family and friends of the victim may also need to be given support and directed in how to appropriately support the victim
D. Assistance from rape counselors and referrals to rape counseling centers should be made
E. Assistance with gathering evidence for criminal prosecution may be needed, but nursing focus should remain on the provision of physical care and emotional support
F. There should be long-term follow-up with a rape counseling center

NURSING CARE IN RELATION TO THERAPEUTIC MODALITIES

GROUP THERAPY

Overview

A. Group therapy uses the dynamics of the group to achieve results less likely to occur in a one-to-one

Table 16-4 Comparison of Group Effectiveness

Factor	Effective Group	Ineffective Group
Atmosphere	Relaxed and interested	Tense and bored
Goal setting	Clearly defined and accepted Modified as needed	Vague and not supported
Goal emphasis	Process and task functions balanced	Tasks and process needs are not balanced
Cohesiveness	Built through trust and mutual support	Too close and overcontrolling or limited connection among members
Conflict	Accept differences Work to resolve conflicts	Avoid facing conflicts or unresolved ongoing conflicts
Power	Shared Determined by ability	Based on position only
Leadership	Based on needs and ability Delegates appropriately	Overcontrolling or weak
Communication	Open and two-way	Closed and one-way Dominated by a few members
Decision making	Consensus when appropriate	From leader down with little input from members
Problem solving	Encourage constructive criticism	Limited by inflexibility
Creativity	Open to new ideas	New ideas discouraged
Self-evaluation	Open to all members Frequently performed	Performed by only a few members infrequently

nurse-client relationship (e.g., decreasing sense of isolation, instilling hope through example of others, providing opportunities to help others)
B. Group process describes how the group is functioning; group content describes what topics or tasks are addressed
C. Groups can be effective or ineffective (see Table 16-4: Comparison of Group Effectiveness)

The Nurse's Role in Group Therapy

A. Selecting clients suitable for the group (level of attention and communication skills)
B. Orienting group members to the group process
C. Maintaining individual member's psychologic and physical safety
D. Facilitating group process when necessary
E. Assisting the group to achieve therapeutic goals by encouraging member participation; all communication has value

THERAPEUTIC MILIEU

Overview

A. Therapeutic milieu is the provision of an environment that consistently encourages the highest level of functioning of clients
B. The environment supports client independence and responsibility, as well as improves social interactions (e.g., daily schedule of activities, communal dining, wearing street clothes) while maintaining safety

C. Clients and health team members interact and work together to improve clients' functions

The Nurse's Role in Maintaining a Therapeutic Milieu

A. Develop and maintain schedule of unit activities
B. Encourage client independence in daily activities as appropriate
C. Provide opportunities for healthy socialization
D. Maintain client safety

RELAXATION THERAPY

Overview

A. Promotes relaxation through meditation, progressive relaxation, deep breathing, guided imagery, and biofeedback
B. Integrated into many types of treatment for clients who need to develop healthier methods for coping with stress

The Nurse's Role in Relaxation Therapy

A. Teach and reinforce relaxation techniques
B. Lead relaxation groups

FAMILY THERAPY

Overview

A. Family therapy is derived from systems theory and group therapy
B. The guiding principle is that treating the individual in isolation from the family allows dysfunctional interpersonal patterns to continue once the client returns to the family environment, which often undermines progress made in individual therapy
C. Many of the problems identified in an individual may in actuality be responses to dysfunctional family interactions
D. Family therapy may be used for a variety of clients and may be the best type of intervention for domestic violence

RELATED PHARMACOLOGY: PSYCHOTROPIC MEDICATIONS

OVERVIEW

A. Chemicals that produce profound effects on the mind, emotions, and body
B. Within one decade (the 1950s) three major classes of psychotropic drugs—antimanic, antipsychotic, and antidepressant—were developed
C. These compounds significantly advanced the treatment of bipolar illness, psychosis, and depression
D. The decrease in state hospital census has been attributed to the introduction of psychotropic drugs
E. Psychotropic drugs include antianxiety or anxiolytic agents; antipsychotic or neuroleptic agents; antidepressants, antimanic, and mood-stabilizing agents; and sedative and hypnotic agents

F. The safety of psychotropic drugs during pregnancy is of concern; consult with psychiatrist and pharmacist before administration
G. Response to psychotropic medications, both therapeutic and side effects, varies greatly from person to person
H. The goal of psychopharmacology is to administer the medication and dosage that will maximize therapeutic effects and minimize side effects
I. Medication is only one component of treatment; used to increase client's ability to engage in other forms of therapy
J. Relapse in the client with a psychiatric problem most often is related to failure to adhere to medication regimen

Antianxiety/Anxiolytic Medications
Description

A. Used in the treatment of anxiety, for alcohol withdrawal, and in the induction of sleep
B. Exert a general depressing effect on the CNS; many also exert skeletal muscle-relaxant and antiseizure effects
C. Anxiolytics are available in oral and parenteral (IM, IV) preparations
D. Intended for short-term use when the individual has difficulty in coping with environmental stresses and accomplishing daily activities
E. Benzodiazepines enhance the gamma-aminobutyric acid (GABA) activity (the primary inhibitory neurotransmitter in the brain), resulting in further opening of the chloride ion channel and a further inhibition of neuronal activity; a decrease in the firing rate of neurons results in lowering of anxiety

Types

A. Benzodiazepines
  1. Short-acting
     a. Alprazolam (Xanax)
     b. Midazolam (Versed)
     c. Oxazepam (Serax)
     d. Triazolam (Halcion)
  2. Medium-acting
     a. Estazolam (ProSom)
     b. Lorazepam (Ativan)
     c. Temazepam (Restoril)
  3. Long-acting
     a. Chlordiazepoxide (Librium)
     b. Clonazepam (Klonopin)
     c. Clorazepate (Tranxene)
     d. Diazepam (Valium)
     e. Flurazepam (Dalmane)
B. Nonbarbiturates
  1. Buspirone (BuSpar)
  2. Chloral hydrate (Noctec)
  3. Diphenhydramine (Benadryl)
  4. Eszopiclone (Lunesta)
  5. Hydroxyzine (Atarax, Vistaril)
  6. Ramelteon (Rozerem)

7. Zaleplon (Sonata)
8. Zolpidem (Ambien)

C. Antidepressants indicated for anxiety
   1. Clomipramine (Anafranil)
   2. Fluoxetine (Prozac)
   3. Fluvoxamine (Luvox)
   4. Paroxetine (Paxil)
   5. Sertraline (Zoloft)
   6. Venlafaxine (Effexor XR)

Precautions

A. Drug interactions: these drugs potentiate depressant effects of alcohol or sedatives
B. Adverse effects: related to diminished mental alertness; caution about driving or operating hazardous machinery until tolerance develops
C. Tolerance to the sedative and hypnotic effects develops eventually with all these drugs, although it develops more slowly with the benzodiazepines than other drugs; tolerance can contribute to self-medication and dosage escalation
D. Overdose of benzodiazepines: flumazenil (Romazicon) is the drug of choice to counter effects
E. All of these drugs, if taken in large enough doses or for extended time periods, can lead to physical and emotional dependence
F. A drop in BP of 20 mm Hg (systolic) on standing warrants withholding the drug and notifying the physician
G. Benzodiazepine use should not be abruptly discontinued to avoid a withdrawal syndrome; discontinue drug if receiving electroconvulsive therapy (ECT)
H. Physical withdrawal symptoms can occur any time these drugs are taken continuously for more than 2 weeks; signs and symptoms closely resemble the original sleep or anxiety complaints
I. Clients treated with BuSpar need education regarding the fact that antianxiety effects are not apparent for 3 to 6 weeks; this is a longer lag time than other drugs in this category
J. Caffeine can worsen symptoms of anxiety; it is thought to interfere with medications used to treat these disorders

Nursing Care of Clients Receiving Antianxiety/Anxiolytic Medications

A. Assess the client's medication history, knowledge level, and use of current medications (prescribed, OTC, and illicit drugs), medication allergies, and pattern of alcohol, tobacco, and herbal use because all may interfere with anxiolytics
B. Explore the client's perceptions and feelings about medications; clarify misinformation and concerns
C. Review psychotropic drug references for current information
D. Plan for client education regarding benzodiazepines should include

1. OTC drugs may increase potency
2. Driving or working with machinery should be avoided while sedative side effects are present
3. CNS depressants and alcohol potentiate effects
4. Drug should not be discontinued abruptly
5. If prior assessment reveals use of herbal or related products (St. John's wort, kava, ginseng, etc.), consult with psychiatrist and pharmacist

E. Monitor the effects of medication (effects on target symptoms, side effects, and adverse reactions)
F. Administer medications exactly as prescribed
G. Teach the client about the medication; desired effect; side effects; food, herbal, and activity restrictions; and lag period between onset of treatment and symptom remission
H. Supplement verbal teaching with appropriate written or audiovisual materials
I. Administer controlled substances according to schedule restrictions
J. Evaluate client's response to medications and understanding of teaching
K. Encourage client involvement in therapy to decrease stressors and improve coping to limit long-term need for antianxiety medication

Neuroleptics (Antipsychotic Agents)
Description

A. Used to treat agitated behavior and psychotic symptoms, that is, symptoms of being out of touch with reality; makes client better able to participate in therapy
B. Act by blocking dopamine receptors in the CNS; they also block the muscarinic receptors for acetylcholine and the alpha receptors for norepinephrine
   1. Positive (type I) symptoms of schizophrenia (e.g., hallucinations, delusions) respond to traditional and newer antipsychotic drugs
   2. Negative (type II) symptoms (e.g., apathy, flat affect) are more responsive to the newer atypical antipsychotic drugs
C. Available in oral and parenteral (IM, IV) preparations
D. Effective in treating symptoms of psychosis noted in schizophrenia, schizophreniform disorder, schizoaffective disorder, and delusional disorder
E. May be prescribed in conjunction with benzodiazepines, which is thought to minimize the dose of neuroleptics and diminish the potential for tardive dyskinesia
F. Antipsychotic effects usually occur within 1 to 2 weeks after initiating treatment, but sedative effect can be immediate

Types

A. Traditional drugs (first-generation drugs)—phenothiazines
   1. Chlorpromazine (Thorazine)
   2. Thioridazine (Mellaril)
   3. Fluphenazine (Prolixin, Permitil)
   4. Perphenazine (Trilafon)
   5. Prochlorperazine (Compazine)
   6. Trifluoperazine (Stelazine)

B. Traditional drugs (first-generation drugs)—
nonphenothiazines
1. Haloperidol (Haldol)
2. Thiothixene (Navane)
3. Loxapine (Loxitane)
4. Molindone (Moban)
5. Pimozide (Orap)
C. Atypical drugs (second-generation drugs)
1. Aripiprazole (Abilify)
2. Clozapine (Clozaril)
3. Olanzapine (Zyprexa, Zydis)
4. Quetiapine (Seroquel)
5. Risperidone (Risperdal)
6. Ziprasidone (Zeldox, Geodon)

Precautions

A. Drug interactions
1. Potentiate the action of alcohol, barbiturates, antihypertensives, and anticholinergics
2. Concomitant use should be avoided if possible
3. Antipsychotic medications should be temporarily discontinued when spinal or epidural anesthesia is necessary
B. Adverse effects
1. Agranulocytosis (manifested by cold or sore throat)
2. Jaundice (hepatotoxicity)
3. Drowsiness (highest incidence in initial days of therapy because of CNS depression)
4. Orthostatic hypotension (CNS depression)
5. Constipation and urinary retention (anticholinergic effects)
6. Anorexia (depressed appetite center)
7. Hypersensitivity reactions (tissue fluid accumulation, visual changes, impotence, cessation of menses or ovulation)
8. Cardiac toxicity (direct toxic effect)
9. Extrapyramidal side effects (EPS)
   a. Dystonia: occurs early in treatment, possibly after initial dosage; involves grimacing, torticollis, intermittent muscle spasms
   b. Pseudoparkinsonism: resembles true parkinsonism (tremor, masklike facies, drooling, restlessness, festinating gait, rigidity)
   c. Akathisia: motor agitation (restless legs, "jitters," nervous energy); most common of all EPS
   d. Akinesia: fatigue, weakness (hypotonia), painful muscles, lack of energy (anergia)
   e. Tardive dyskinesia: late-appearing after prolonged use of antipsychotic drugs; not related to dopamine-acetylcholine imbalance; most severe effect characterized by involuntary movements of face, jaw, and tongue; lip smacking, grinding of teeth, rolling or protrusion of tongue, tics, diaphragmatic movements that may impair breathing; condition disappears during sleep; antiparkinsonian drugs ineffective and condition is usually irreversible; all antipsychotics should be discontinued to see if symptoms subside

f. Neuroleptic malignant syndrome: infrequent yet extreme life-threatening condition occurring in severely ill clients and is thought to be the result of dopamine blockage in the hypothalamus; associated with high-potency antipsychotic drugs, especially when given in a large loading dose; symptoms are hyperthermia (cardinal symptom), muscular rigidity, tremors, impaired ventilation, muteness, altered consciousness, unstable blood pressure, and autonomic hyperactivity
g. Weight gain and metabolic syndrome (abdominal obesity, dyslipidemia, hypertension, and insulin resistance)
C. Antiparkinsonian drugs are given to block the EPS that are related to dopamine and acetylcholine imbalance
1. Anticholinergics: benztropine (Cogentin); biperiden (Akineton); procyclidine (Kemadrin); trihexyphenidyl (Artane); a missed dose should be taken up to 2 hours before next dose
2. Antihistamine: diphenhydramine (Benadryl)
3. Others
   a. Treat neuroleptic malignant syndrome: amantadine (Symmetrel) and bromocriptine (Parlodel)
   b. Treat akinesia and akathisia: benzodiazepines (lorazepam [Ativan], diazepam [Valium], clonazepam [Klonopin])
   c. Treat EPS: clonidine (Catapres) and propranolol (Inderal)
   d. Treat acute dystonic reactions: ethopropazine (Parsidol)
   e. Treat tardive dyskinesia: nifedipine (Procardia) and verapamil (Calan)

Nursing Care of Clients Receiving Neuroleptics (Antipsychotic Agents)

A. Monitor for signs of hepatic toxicity (e.g., jaundice)
B. Monitor for signs of infection (e.g., sore throat)
C. Monitor BP in supine and standing positions
1. Assist client to rise from bed slowly and sit on bed before ambulating
2. Assess for hypotension and tachycardia, which usually are a response to hypotension
3. If hypotension occurs, monitor by measuring BP before each dose is given
4. Consult physician as to safe BP systolic/diastolic parameters for each client
D. Offer sugar-free chewing gum or hard candy to increase salivation and relieve dry mouth
E. Assist with ambulation as necessary; keep side rails up when nonambulatory
F. Assess for EPS (antiparkinsonism agent may be prescribed to decrease symptoms)
G. Monitor blood work during long-term therapy (periodic CBCs, liver function tests, lipid profiles, glucose tolerance, blood glucose levels, and chemistry

analysis; weekly WBC count if administering clozapine)

H. Monitor dietary intake to avoid weight loss resulting from caloric expenditure caused by EPS or weight gain associated with metabolic syndrome

I. Instruct client to
   1. Avoid administration with other CNS depressants, including concurrent use of alcohol
   2. Avoid engaging in potentially hazardous activities
   3. Avoid exposure to direct sunlight; wear protective clothing and sunglasses outdoors
   4. Recognize EPS and report their occurrence to the physician immediately
   5. Avoid changing positions rapidly
   6. Notify physician if sore throat, fever, or weakness occurs; avoid crowded, potentially infectious places
   7. Increase water intake and eat high-fiber diet to avoid constipation
   8. Expect weight gain; control weight with appropriate diet
   9. Avoid mixing neuroleptics with certain juices or liquids (e.g., coffee, tea, or cola beverages), which may decrease effectiveness of drug
   10. Avoid antacids or take them 1 to 2 hours after antipsychotic drug is taken because antacids decrease absorption of antipsychotics
   11. Avoid smoking because it decreases serum levels of antipsychotics

J. Use precautions to avoid drug contact with skin; can cause contact dermatitis

K. Recognize that drug noncompliance is common; monitor clients during administration to ensure medication is taken to prevent "cheeking" (client may discard tablet or save tablets to attempt overdose); consult physician about use of longer-acting drugs (such as fluphenazine decanoate [Prolixin], haloperidol decanoate [Haldol], or risperidone [Risperdal]); liquid forms of medications; or rapidly dissolving tablets (such as olanzapine [Zyprexa, Zydis])

L. Evaluate client's response to medication and understanding of teaching

Antidepressants
Description

A. The primary clinical indication for use of antidepressant drugs is major depressive illness; also used in the treatment of panic disorder, other anxiety disorders, posttraumatic stress disorder, narcolepsy, attention deficit disorders, and enuresis in children; atypical antidepressant bupropion (Wellbutrin) also is used as an adjunctive treatment for smoking cessation

B. Selective serotonin reuptake inhibitors, with their low side effect profile, are being used to treat eating disorders and obsessive-compulsive disorder

C. Antidepressant drugs affect the neurotransmitters norepinephrine and/or serotonin by partially blocking their reuptake; roles for other neurotransmitters are unclear and under study

D. Available in oral and parenteral (IM) preparations

E. Psychopharmacologic treatment is based on the restoration of acceptable levels of neurotransmitter systems by blocking the uptake in the presynaptic nerve ending, inhibiting breakdown, stimulating the release, and reducing stimulation at the site of the postsynaptic beta receptors (i.e., down-regulation)

F. All antidepressant drugs may need to be taken for 2 to 4 weeks before therapeutic response occurs; side effects may occur with initial doses

G. Monoamine oxidase inhibitors (MAOIs) elevate norepinephrine levels in brain tissues by interfering with the enzyme MAO; act as psychic energizers; rarely used because of serious drug and food interactions that cause hypertensive crisis

Types

A. Tricyclic drugs (TCAs) or nonselective cyclic drugs
   1. Amitriptyline (Elavil, Endep)
   2. Clomipramine (Anafranil)
   3. Desipramine (Norpramin)
   4. Doxepin (Sinequan, Triadapin)
   5. Imipramine (Tofranil)
   6. Nortriptyline (Aventyl, Pamelor)
   7. Protriptyline (Vivactil, Triptil)
   8. Trimipramine (Surmontil)

B. Monoamine oxidase inhibitors (MAOIs)
   1. Isocarboxazid (Marplan)
   2. Phenelzine sulfate (Nardil)
   3. Selegiline (Eldepryl, Emsam)
   4. Tranylcypromine sulfate (Parnate)

C. Selective serotonin reuptake inhibitors (SSRIs)
   1. Citalopram (Celexa)
   2. Fluoxetine (Prozac, Prozac Weekly, Sarafem)
   3. Fluvoxamine (Luvox)
   4. Escitalopram (Lexapro)
   5. Paroxetine (Paxil)
   6. Sertraline (Zoloft)

D. Atypical new generation drugs
   1. Amoxapine (Ascendin)
   2. Bupropion (Wellbutrin)
   3. Bupropion SR (Wellbutrin SR, Zyban)
   4. Duloxetine (Cymbalta)
   5. Maprotiline (Ludiomil)
   6. Mirtazapine (Remeron)
   7. Trazodone (Desyrel)
   8. Venlafaxine (Effexor)
   9. Venlafaxine XR (Effexor XR)

Precautions

A. Tricyclic antidepressants (TCAs)
   1. Drug interactions: potentiate effects of anticholinergic drugs and CNS depressants (e.g., alcohol and sedatives)
   2. Adverse effects
      a. Orthostatic hypotension, skin rash, drowsiness, dry mouth, blurred vision, constipation, urine retention, and tachycardia

b. CNS stimulation in older adults (excitement, restlessness, incoordination, fine tremor, nightmares, delusions, disorientation, insomnia)
3. TCAs should not be given to clients with narrow-angle glaucoma
4. TCAs are contraindicated during recovery phase of myocardial infarction or when client's history indicates cardiac dysrhythmias and cardiac conduction defects
5. There should be a minimum of 14 days between switching the TCA-resistant client to MAOIs to avoid hypertensive crisis
6. Abrupt discontinuation of TCAs can cause nausea, headache, and malaise
B. Monoamine oxidase inhibitors (MAOIs)
1. Drug interactions: MAOIs potentiate the effects of alcohol, barbiturates, anesthetic agents, cocaine, antihistamines, narcotics, corticoids, anticholinergics, and sympathomimetic drugs
2. Drug-food interactions: hypertensive crisis with vascular rupture, occipital headache, palpitations, stiffness of neck muscles, emesis, sweating, photophobia, and cardiac dysrhythmias may occur when neurohormonal levels are elevated by ingestion of foods with high tyramine content (e.g., pickled herring, beer, wine, chicken livers, aged or natural cheese, chocolate, caffeine, cola, licorice, avocados, bananas, and bologna); processed cheeses and fresh cheese (e.g., cottage cheese) are low in tyramine
3. Adverse effects
a. Orthostatic hypotension (CNS effect)
b. Skin rash (hypersensitivity)
c. Drowsiness (CNS depression)
d. Dry mouth, blurred vision, urinary retention, tachycardia (anticholinergic effect)
e. Sexual dysfunction (autonomic effect)
f. Nightmares, delusions, disorientation, insomnia (CNS stimulation)
C. Selective serotonin reuptake inhibitors (SSRIs)
1. Drug interactions: may interact with tryptophan; question concomitant use of diazepam, warfarin, and digoxin; should be discontinued 4 to 6 weeks before switching to MAOIs
2. Adverse effects: insomnia, headache, dry mouth, sexual dysfunction, anxiety, diarrhea and other GI complaints
3. Usually these drugs are administered before noon to avoid insomnia or sleep disturbances
4. Serotonin syndrome: confusion, coma, agitation, tachycardia, BP changes, nausea, myoclonus, hyperreflexia, tremors, ataxia, hyperpyrexia; usually resolves with elimination of SSRIs and supportive care
D. Atypical new-generation drugs
1. Adverse effects: increased appetite, weight gain, and sleep disturbances; mild anticholinergic side effects noted

2. Bupropion (Wellbutrin) is thought to affect dopamine reuptake and agitation is sometimes produced

Nursing Care of Clients Receiving Antidepressants
A. Monitor for self-destructive behavior, particularly during the second week of drug therapy when suicidal ideation remains and energy increases; maintain suicide precautions
B. Monitor serum glucose levels in clients with diabetes mellitus
C. Instruct client to
1. Change positions slowly
2. Avoid engaging in hazardous activities
3. Use sugar-free chewing gum or hard candy to stimulate salivation
4. Check with physician before taking all OTC preparations, alcohol, and cough or herbal medicines (e.g., St. John's wort)
5. Expect therapeutic effect to be delayed; may take up to 3 weeks with MAOIs and 2 to 4 weeks with other antidepressants
D. Avoid concurrent administration of adrenergic drugs; limit or eliminate caffeine use to prevent exacerbation of depression
E. MAOIs
1. Maintain dietary restrictions; avoid foods containing tyramine; provide for nutritional education
2. Monitor client for occurrence of hypertensive crisis (occipital headache, palpitations, and stiff neck)
F. Recommend Prozac, weekly capsule (90 mg), to treat noncompliant clients
G. Evaluate client's response to medication and understanding of teaching

Antimanic and Mood-Stabilizing Agents
Description
A. Used to control the manic episode of mood disorders and for maintenance in clients with a history of mania
B. Lithium affects the neurotransmitters of multiple systems including dopamine, norepinephrine, serotonin, acetylcholine, and GABA
C. Improves productivity by decreasing psychomotor activity or response to environmental stimuli
D. Antimanic agents are available in oral capsules and tablets, both regular and sustained-release forms, and in concentrates
Types
A. Antimanic agents and mood stabilizers
1. Lithium carbonate (Eskalith, Lithotabs, Lithane, Lithonate)
2. Lithium carbonate sustained release (Eskalith C-R, Lithobid)
3. Lithium citrate concentrate (Cibalith-S)
B. Alternative antimanic agents and mood stabilizers
1. Carbamazepine (Tegretol)
2. Gabapentin (Neurontin)

3. Lamotrigine (Lamictal, Lamictal CD)
4. Topiramate (Topamax)
5. Valproates (Depakene, Depakote, Depakote ER, Depacon, Deproic, Epival)

C. Some antipsychotic agents (e.g., aripiprazole and ziprasidone) may be used during the acute manic phase of bipolar illness to assist with symptom control until therapeutic levels of other antimanic medications are achieved

Precautions

A. Drug interactions: diuretics increase the reabsorption of lithium, resulting in possible toxic effects; haloperidol and thioridazine, when given with these drugs, can result in encephalopathic syndrome; sodium bicarbonate or sodium chloride increases the excretion of lithium

B. Drug-food interaction: restriction of sodium intake increases drug substitution for sodium ions, which causes signs of hyponatremia (nausea, vomiting, diarrhea, muscle fasciculations, stupor, seizures); therefore salt intake must be maintained; daily intake of over 250 mg of caffeine with lithium decreases effect of antianxiety drugs

C. Adverse effects: excess voiding and extreme thirst caused by drug suppression of respiratory depression and coma are toxic side effects; toxic effects can easily occur because the difference between the therapeutic level and toxic level is slight

D. To achieve a clinical response, 1 to 2 weeks of treatment will be necessary; antipsychotic agents or benzodiazepines may be used in combination with lithium to control manic symptoms initially until antimanic clinical response occurs

Nursing Care of Clients Receiving Antimanic and Mood-Stabilizing Agents

A. Recognize that therapeutic effects will be delayed for several weeks

B. Check concurrent medications for potential interactions

C. Administer with meals to reduce GI irritation; ensure that drug is not crushed or chewed; liquid forms are available

D. Encourage avoidance of hazardous activities

E. Teach that medication should not be discontinued abruptly and that if it is discontinued, it should be done with medical supervision

F. Provide nursing care specific to lithium
1. Maintain sodium and fluid intake because dehydration and hyponatremia predispose to lithium toxicity
2. Monitor weight and for signs of dependent edema
3. Assess therapeutic blood levels (0.5 to 1.5 mEq/L) weekly for 1 month and then at 2- to 3-month intervals
4. Teach about side effects: headache, drowsiness, dizziness, dry mouth, anorexia, nausea, hypotension, edema

5. Teach about signs of toxicity: vomiting, diarrhea, tremors, weakness, lassitude, severe thirst, tinnitus, dilute urine
6. Refer pregnant woman to health care provider; cessation of lithium during pregnancy is recommended to avoid teratogenic effects during first trimester

G. Provide nursing care specific to valproate
1. Administer elixir alone; do not dilute with carbonated beverages
2. Teach about side effects: sedation, drowsiness, nausea, vomiting, diarrhea, constipation, heartburn
3. Teach about signs of toxicity: visual disturbances, rash, diarrhea, light-colored stools, jaundice, protracted vomiting

H. Evaluate client's response to medication and understanding of teaching

Sedative and Hypnotic Agents
Description

A. Benzodiazepines have almost entirely replaced the barbiturates in the treatment of anxiety and sleep disorders; sedative and hypnotic agents are primarily used in general medicine rather than psychiatry

B. Insomnia, hypersomnia, narcolepsy, parasomnias, periodic leg movements (nocturnal myoclonus), and sleep apnea are among the disorders that are responsive to these agents

C. Specific psychiatric conditions do predispose clients to insomnia (mood disorders, anxiety, and dementias)

D. CNS depressants have antianxiety effects in low dosages, produce sleep in high dosages, and have general anesthetic-like states in very high dosages

E. All hypnotic drugs probably alter either the character or the duration of REM sleep

F. Sedatives reduce nervousness, excitability, and irritability without causing sleep, but a sedative can become a hypnotic in large doses

G. Hypnotics cause sleep and have a more potent effect on the CNS than sedatives

H. Sedative-hypnotics are classified chemically into three groups: barbiturates, benzodiazepines, and nonbenzodiazepines

Types

A. Benzodiazepines (see Antianxiety/Anxiolytic Medications)

B. Barbiturates: amobarbital (Amytal); butabarbital (Butisol); pentobarbital (Nembutal); phenobarbital (Luminal); secobarbital (Seconal)

C. Antidepressant: trazodone (Desyrel)

D. Chloral derivative: chloral hydrate (Noctec)

E. Antihistamines: diphenhydramine (Benadryl); hydroxyzine (Atarax)

F. Beta-adrenergic blocker: propranolol (Inderal)

G. Anxiolytic: buspirone (BuSpar)

H. Nonbenzodiazepine hypnotics: see Antianxiety/Anxiolytic Medications

Precautions

A. Sedative-hypnotic preparations are generally intended for either occasional or short-term use

B. Hypnotic drugs have undesirable effects (physiologic addiction, fatal overdose potential, and dangerous interactions with other drugs and alcohol)

C. Barbiturate sedatives increase the metabolism of anticoagulants because they induce liver enzyme synthesis

D. Buspirone appears to be a potent antianxiety agent with no identified addictive potential; it is not effective in the management of drug or alcohol abuse

E. Chloral hydrate and paraldehyde are not used for treatment of alcohol withdrawal because of toxic effects; paraldehyde is sometimes used for treating status epilepticus when other drugs have failed

F. The sedative-hypnotics are CNS depressants

G. Tolerance develops to sedative and hypnotic agents; therefore the client in the outpatient setting may resort to increasing doses to produce the desired effect

H. If taken in large dosages or for a long time period, physical and emotional dependence occurs

I. Once physical dependence has developed, abrupt discontinuation of sedative-hypnotics leads to withdrawal
1. Withdrawal characteristics: insomnia, weakness, muscle tremors, anxiety, irritability, sweating, anorexia, fever, nausea and vomiting, headache, incoordination, and restlessness
2. After several days, severe symptoms of withdrawal may develop: postural hypotension, tinnitus, incoherence, delirium, psychosis, seizures, status epilepticus, cardiovascular collapse, loss of temperature regulation, and/or death

J. To avoid withdrawal, it is important to slowly and gradually taper the dose with the same drug or one that is cross-tolerant

K. Excess ingestion
1. Any of the sedative-hypnotics may cause unconsciousness, coma, cardiorespiratory depression, and death
2. Treatment/removal of the drug from the stomach by aspiration, resuscitative measures (assisted ventilation, cardiac massage), hemodialysis of diffusible drug, vasopressor administration to counteract vascular collapse, and correction of acidosis
3. Follow-up drug supervision to avoid repetition of the problem
4. Initiation of psychotherapy for depressed clients

L. Refer to Precautions under Antianxiety/Anxiolytic Medications for additional information

Nursing Care of Clients Receiving Sedative and Hypnotic Agents

A. Assess for history of drug or alcohol abuse or suicide attempts by overdose because of the increased risk for abuse

B. Assess for pregnancy and breastfeeding, as safe use has not been established

C. Explore the client's perceptions and feelings about medications; clarify any misinformation and concerns

D. Plan for client teaching about specific sedative-hypnotic agents; institute safety precautions

E. Supplement verbal teaching with appropriate written or audiovisual materials

F. Administer controlled substances according to schedule restrictions

G. Assess for undesired effects (e.g., respiratory depression, increased sedation, and hypotension)

H. Review methods to improve sleep hygiene: minimize daytime napping, increase physical activity except just before bedtime, eliminate caffeine intake after dinner, establish bedtime routines, maintain regular sleep schedule

I. Evaluate client's response to medication and understanding of teaching

J. Refer to Nursing Care of Clients Receiving Antianxiety/Anxiolytic Medications

17 Nursing Care of Clients With Disorders Usually First Evident in Infancy, Childhood, or Adolescence

OVERVIEW

A. These disorders may be characterized by physical as well as psychologic symptoms and must be distinguished from expected variances in growth and development

B. The *DSM-IV-TR* criteria for diagnosis are behavioral manifestations that are not age appropriate, deviate from cultural norms, and create deficits or impairments in adaptive functioning

C. Psychiatric care of the child or adolescent is a subspecialty within psychiatric nursing. Although there is a wide range of deficits with these disorders, there are fundamental principles that apply

D. All care should be based on the child's developmental level and directed toward helping the child grow emotionally. Recognize that all children, especially these children, require the following
   1. Protection from danger, including impulsive acts and self-destructive behavior
   2. Love and acceptance
   3. Basic physiologic needs to be met
   4. Meaningful trusting relationships
   5. Opportunities to explore the environment

GENERAL NURSING CARE RELATED TO DISORDERS FIRST EVIDENT IN INFANCY, CHILDHOOD, OR ADOLESCENCE

Assessment/Analysis
A. Attainment or delay of developmental milestones (e.g., motor, language, social, etc.)
B. Parental behavior and attitude (e.g., expectations, acceptance/rejection, encouragement/pressure)
C. Personal and family medical history (e.g., vision, hearing, general health, perinatal history, familial disorders)
D. Onset, characteristics, and pattern of speech; ability to communicate with others
E. Level of anxiety, frustration, self-esteem
F. Behavioral manifestations (e.g., ability to perform ADLs, hyperactivity, distractibility, attention span, impulsiveness, repetitive behaviors, tics)

G. Social abilities (e.g., ability to connect with others/environment, aggressiveness, ability to follow directions/rules, respect for others and their belongings)

Planning/Implementation
A. Develop a trusting relationship with the child and family
   1. Be as truthful as possible when caring for the child
   2. Provide consistent caregivers
   3. Make all explanations as clear as possible and at the appropriate cognitive level
B. Help the child to see self as worthwhile
   1. Encourage verbalization of feelings
   2. Accept child and focus on strengths to raise self-esteem
   3. Foster independence by emphasizing abilities and achievements rather than limitations
   4. Provide opportunities so the child can experience success and satisfaction
   5. Use positive reinforcement for child's strengths and abilities
   6. Teach and model more adaptive coping behaviors
   7. Increase sense of empathy through role modeling, role playing, group therapy
   8. Support and encourage the child's movement toward independence but allow dependency when necessary
C. Establish a favorable environment in which the child can gain or regain a favorable equilibrium
   1. Set realistic, attainable goals
   2. Maintain routines based on the child's usual schedule; maintain safety
   3. Manage hyperactivity and aggressive behaviors: progress from avoiding situations that precipitate unacceptable behavior to monitoring behavior for rising anxiety, signaling child to use self-control, and finally to placing child in time out when appropriate
   4. Set limits that are as realistic as possible but as firm as necessary, avoiding manipulation
   5. Provide for consistency both in approach and in rules and regulations
   6. Use a firm system of rewards and punishments within set limits
   7. Point out reality, but accept the child's views of it
   8. Recognize that the maladaptive behavior has meaning for the child or may be beyond the child's control (e.g., tic disorder)

9. Plan activities to provide a balance between energy expenditure and quiet time
10. Introduce the child to new situations gradually; permit the child to bring a familiar, comforting object
11. Engage in parallel play to connect with withdrawn child in a nonthreatening manner

D. Involve family in parenting education and management training
1. Assist the parents to gain an accurate understanding of their child's strengths and weaknesses
2. Help parents cope with feelings such as guilt, failure, or anger
3. Help parents and child to identify triggers to maladaptive behaviors
4. Involve family in multifamily therapy to work through problems of daily life and to gain new information and more adaptive coping skills
5. Teach parents to provide firm and consistent discipline and ignore temper tantrums
6. Provide parents with a list of available community resources
7. Assist family with placement of child when home care can no longer be provided because of changes in child or ability of caregivers

E. Minimize long-term consequences
1. Identify and treat deficits early, including sensorimotor deficits
2. Provide psychotherapy: play, group, or individual therapy
3. Support, depending on age and degree of disability, attendance at a school, therapeutic nursery program, a day treatment program, or special education
4. Treat associated problems (e.g., sensory losses)
   a. Provide activities consistent with disorder
   b. Refer for physical therapy
   c. Refer infant for child stimulation therapy and early intervention program to help prepare child physically and socially for school
   d. Refer for occupational therapy
   e. Refer for speech therapy, allow time to verbalize, not completing words or sentences, avoid nonverbal behavior that implies impatience and use picture boards
   f. Provide ongoing assistance to promote social and academic success

F. Administer prescribed medication
1. Pervasive developmental disorders: neuroleptics, stimulants
2. Attention deficit hyperactivity disorder: methylphenidate (Ritalin, Concerta); give after breakfast to ensure dietary intake and, if given a second dose before 6 PM to limit insomnia
3. Tic disorders: sedatives, anticonvulsives (antiseizure); prescribed but usually have minimal effect

4. Enuresis: desmopressin (DDAVP, Stimulate); tricyclic antidepressants for children more than 5 years old
5. Anxiety disorders: stimulants, antianxiety agents

MAJOR DISORDERS FIRST EVIDENT IN INFANCY, CHILDHOOD, OR ADOLESCENCE

❋ MENTAL RETARDATION

See Cognitive Impairment (Mental Retardation) in Chapter 31, Nursing Care of Toddlers

❋ LEARNING DISORDERS

Data Base
A. Learning disorders (LDs) are frequently found in association with a variety of medical conditions (lead poisoning, fetal alcohol syndrome); genetic predisposition, perinatal injury, neurologic, and general medical conditions may also be associated
B. Behavioral/clinical findings
1. Achievement on individually administered, standardized tests in reading, mathematics, or written expression is substantially below (defined as 2 or more standard deviations between achievement and IQ) that expected for age, schooling, and level of intelligence; LDs must be differentiated from normal variations in academic attainment and from scholastic difficulties resulting from lack of opportunity, inadequate teaching, cultural factors, or impaired vision or hearing
2. Demoralization, lower self-esteem, and deficits in social skills may be associated
3. Employment difficulties and social adjustment are noted in adolescence and adulthood

Nursing Care of Children With Learning Disorders
(See General Nursing Care Related to Disorders First Evident in Infancy, Childhood, or Adolescence for Assessment/Analysis and Planning/Implementation)
A. Evaluation/Outcomes
1. Participates in school and home activities
2. Follows directions
3. Carries tasks to completion
4. Benefits from remediation

❋ MOTOR SKILLS DISORDERS

Data Base
A. No definitive cause has been identified for developmental motor and coordination disorders that interfere with academic achievement or activities of daily living; no specific neurologic disorders are present
B. Behavioral/clinical findings: lack of coordination that may continue through adolescence and adulthood

Nursing Care of Children With Motor Skills Disorders

(See General Nursing Care Related to Disorders First Evident in Infancy, Childhood, or Adolescence for Assessment/Analysis and Planning/Implementation)

A. Evaluation/Outcomes
  1. Maintains or increases mobility/agility
  2. Engages in activities suitable to interests, capabilities, and developmental level

COMMUNICATION DISORDERS

Data Base

A. Developmental type: inability to begin or interruption in normal patterns of speech in the absence of physiologic causes

B. Acquired type: impairment in expressive language from a physiologic cause (e.g., brain tumor, brain attack, head trauma); may occur at any age, with sudden onset or presence of faulty speech patterns that are persistent and increased by stress

C. Behavioral/clinical findings
  1. Two common types
     a. Cluttering: abnormally rapid, erratic, dysrhythmic speech patterns that make communication very difficult to follow
     b. Stuttering: frequent repetition of sounds or syllables that impairs speech fluency although child has normal laryngeal skills; usually occurring at the beginning of a word or phrase
  2. Communication disorders are associated with anxiety, avoidance of social situations, and loss of self-esteem

Nursing Care of Children With Communication Disorders

(See General Nursing Care Related to Disorders First Evident in Infancy, Childhood, or Adolescence for Assessment/Analysis and Planning/Implementation)

A. Evaluation/Outcomes
  1. Demonstrates a decrease in speech pattern disturbances
  2. Demonstrates increased participation in social and public situations

PERVASIVE DEVELOPMENTAL DISORDERS (INCLUDING AUTISTIC DISORDER AND ASPERGER'S DISORDER)

Data Base

A. Autism is viewed as a behavioral disorder caused by abnormal brain function, resulting in an alienation or withdrawal from reality; signs may be evident before 2 years of age but it usually is diagnosed by 3 years of age

B. Asperger's disorder is similar to but differs from autism in that it has a later onset and has no delay in cognitive and language development; problems with social relationships become evident when child enters school

C. Interference with intellect may be so profound that child appears mentally retarded; turns to inanimate objects and self-centered activity for security

D. Puberty can be a crucial stage for showing improvement or further deterioration

E. Behavioral/clinical findings
  1. Severe and pervasive impairment in reciprocal social interaction (e.g., indifferent or aversion to affection and physical contact)
  2. Severe and pervasive impairment of communication skills (verbal: e.g., misuse of pronouns; nonverbal: e.g., lack of eye contact)
  3. Above behaviors usually accompanied by stereotypical behavior, interests, and activities (e.g., adheres to routines and rituals with aversion to minor changes; repetitive motor mannerisms)
  4. Disinterest in eating; bizarre, unpredictable, uncontrolled behavior

Nursing Care of Children With Pervasive Developmental Disorders

(See General Nursing Care Related to Disorders First Evident in Infancy, Childhood, or Adolescence for Assessment/Analysis and Planning/Implementation)

A. Evaluation/Outcomes
  1. Remains safe from injury
  2. Decreases inappropriate behavior (e.g., self-destructive behavior)
  3. Uses fewer stereotypical/repetitive motor behaviors
  4. Increases use of first-person speech

ATTENTION DEFICIT HYPERACTIVITY DISORDER (ADHD)

Data Base

A. Thought to have a neurobiologic basis (e.g., genetic, perinatal stress); sometimes complicated by family dynamics and progressive consequences of related learning problems

B. Symptoms persist in less severe form into adulthood

C. Behavioral/clinical findings
  1. Inappropriately inattentive; short attention span; easily distracted; learning disabilities
  2. Excessive talking and impulsiveness (e.g., cannot take turns, interrupts)
  3. Difficulty organizing tasks and activities; does not complete tasks
  4. Squirming and fidgeting; hyperactivity may or may not be present

Nursing Care of Children With Attention Deficit Hyperactivity Disorder

(See General Nursing Care Related to Disorders First Evident in Infancy, Childhood, or Adolescence for Assessment/Analysis and Planning/Implementation)

A. Evaluation/Outcomes
  1. Participates in home and school activities
  2. Carries tasks to completion
  3. Follows directions

UNSPECIFIED CONDUCT DISORDER/ OPPOSITIONAL DEFIANT DISORDER

Data Base

A. Disregard for society's rules/norms and rights of others

B. Disregard and lack of empathy for the feelings of others

C. Onset may occur as early as age 5 or 6, but usually is in late childhood or early adolescence; often diagnosed as having an antisocial personality as an adult

D. Behavior is repeated despite rational arguments and punishment and causes significant impairment in social, academic, or work performance

E. Behavioral/clinical findings
   1. Aggression toward people and animals
   2. Unfeeling toward others
   3. Destruction of property
   4. Deceitfulness or theft
   5. Serious violations of rules

Nursing Care of Children With Unspecified Conduct Disorder/Oppositional Defiant Disorder

(See General Nursing Care Related to Disorders First Evident in Infancy, Childhood, or Adolescence for Assessment/Analysis and Planning/Implementation)

A. Evaluation/Outcomes
   1. Decreases destructive acts at self or others
   2. Demonstrates an increased ability to delay gratification

TIC DISORDERS

Data Base

A. Imbalance in neurotransmitters is thought to be the underlying cause; familial or autosomal-dominant patterns exist in high percentage of tic disorders; more common in males

B. Diagnosis based on the duration, variety of tics, and age of onset

C. Behavioral/clinical findings
   1. Tourette's disorder: evidence of multiple motor tics (e.g., involuntary, uncontrolled, multiple, rapid movements of muscles such as eye blinking, twitching, and head shaking that occur in episodes throughout the day) and at least one vocal tic (e.g., involuntary production of sounds such as throat clearing, grunting, barking, or the utterance of socially unacceptable words [coprolalia])
   2. Chronic motor or vocal disorder: evidence of single or multiple motor or vocal tics, but not both
   3. Transient disorder: evidence of motor and/or vocal tics lasting for at least 1 month, but no more than 12 consecutive months
   4. Can be controlled for short duration; not usually present during sleep; increased during times of stress
   5. Serious violations of rules

Nursing Care of Children With Tic Disorders

(See General Nursing Care Related to Disorders First Evident in Infancy, Childhood, or Adolescence for Assessment/Analysis and Planning/Implementation)

A. Evaluation/Outcomes
   1. Demonstrates a decrease in tic behavior
   2. Functions socially despite presence of tic

ELIMINATION DISORDERS

Data Base

A. Incontinence of feces or urine in inappropriate places

B. No identifiable physical problems are present

C. Chronologic age is at least 4 years or equivalent developmental level

D. Behavioral/clinical findings
   1. Functional encopresis: involuntary or intentional defecation in inappropriate places, including clothing
   2. Functional enuresis: involuntary or intentional micturition in inappropriate places, including clothing (nocturnal bedwetting is most frequent; child may or may not be aware of voiding or recall a dream about the act of urinating)
   3. Avoidance of social situations (e.g., school, play groups) because of loss of self-esteem, anxiety, and/ or rejection by peers

Nursing Care of Children With Elimination Disorders

(See General Nursing Care Related to Disorders First Evident in Infancy, Childhood, or Adolescence for Assessment/Analysis and Planning/Implementation)

A. Evaluation/Outcomes
   1. Demonstrates a decrease in encopresis or enuresis
   2. Exhibits an increase in self-esteem

ANXIETY DISORDERS OF INFANCY, CHILDHOOD, OR ADOLESCENCE

Data Base

A. Some anxiety is expected in childhood and adolescence because fears and worries are part of development

B. Anxiety becomes a problem when the individual fails to move beyond the fears of a particular developmental stage

C. Behavior interferes with daily functioning and educational, social, and occupational achievement

D. Behavioral/clinical findings
   1. Separation anxiety: excessive anxiety centered on harm befalling self, family, or those to whom child has attachment
      a. Occurs most often between 6 and 30 months of age
      b. Refusal to attend school or activities that lead to temporary parental separation
      c. Physical complaints when separation is anticipated
      d. Problems with sleeping

2. School phobia: Severe anxiety about attending school
   a. Overwhelming shyness and insecurity
   b. Psychophysiologic symptoms used to justify nonattendance
   c. Anxiety increases in response to attempts to force attendance
   d. Nonattendance at school has emotional and legal implications
3. Selective mutism: persistent failure to speak in specific social situations
   a. Social involvement limited to family members or people who are familiar to the child
   b. Excessive shyness or timidity with strangers
4. Reactive attachment disorder: disturbed or developmentally inappropriate behavior that leads to psychosocial deprivation; begins before age 5

a. Failure to initiate or respond to most social interactions
b. Difficulty in choice of attachment figures

Nursing Care of Children With Anxiety Disorders of Infancy, Childhood or Adolescence
(See General Nursing Care Related to Disorders First Evident in Infancy, Childhood, or Adolescence for Assessment/Analysis and Planning/Implementation)
A. Evaluation/Outcomes
   1. States a decrease in anxiety and worry
   2. Demonstrates a decrease in physiologic symptoms
   3. Develops relationships outside of family members
   4. Attends school on a consistent basis

Nursing Care of Clients With Disorders Related to Alterations in Cognition and Perception

OVERVIEW

A. The primary initial deficit occurs in cognition, although there may be changes in the client's mood and behavior

B. Includes disorders associated with
1. Temporary or permanent changes in brain tissue that were historically labeled organic brain syndrome or organic mental disorders
2. Persistent disturbances in memory resulting from a medical condition or substance use
3. Psychosis that may be acute and short-term or chronic and debilitating; includes schizophrenia, delusional paranoid, and schizoaffective disorders; brief psychotic and shared psychotic disorders; and psychotic disorders caused by medical conditions or substance use

GENERAL NURSING CARE OF CLIENTS WITH DISORDERS RELATED TO ALTERATIONS IN COGNITION AND PERCEPTION

A. Provide a safe, familiar environment; provide direct supervision as necessary; provide a consistent caregiver to foster trust

B. Reorient the client to time, place, person, and situation (e.g., clocks, calendar, incorporation of statements into ordinary conversation that reorient the client); excessive use of reorientation may cause anxiety; keep statements short, simple, and concrete and use nonverbal cues

C. Keep client involved in reality-based activities and in the home situation as long as possible

D. Allow client to assume as much responsibility for self-care as possible

E. Provide a quiet environment but do not understimulate; reduce unfamiliar stimuli; help client maintain relationships

F. Plan care so that the staff approaches these clients when they appear receptive

G. Attempt to follow familiar routines; keep the schedule of activities flexible to make use of the client's lability of mood and easy distractibility

H. Encourage adequate nutritional intake; set limits on hyperorality; monitor I&O

I. Provide diversional activities including exercises that the client enjoys and can handle

J. Observe for changing physiologic and neurologic symptoms

K. Prevent physical harm related to confusion, aggression, or fluid and electrolyte imbalance

L. Support and educate family caregivers; maintain nonjudgmental attitude

M. Encourage periodic relief from responsibility of total care; refer to community agencies that provide homecare helpers or respite care if appropriate

N. Support the family's decision to place client in a nursing home

MAJOR DISORDERS RELATED TO ALTERATIONS IN COGNITION AND PERCEPTION

✿ DELIRIUM

Data Base

A. Etiologic factors
1. Syndromes from which the client usually recovers, because the changes may be reversible and temporary if identified and treated promptly
2. Delirium is always secondary to some physical disorder or drug response
3. Clinical manifestations develop over a short period (hours or days), and cognitive impairment fluctuates during a 24-hour period
4. Stressors
   a. Infection
      (1) Intracranial or nervous system (e.g., meningitis or encephalitis)
      (2) Systemic (e.g., AIDS, acute or chronic respiratory disorders)
   b. Trauma to the head
   c. Circulatory disturbances resulting in impairment of blood flow to the brain
   d. Metabolic disorders: electrolyte imbalance resulting from dehydration, diarrhea, and vomiting; fever; endocrine imbalances
   e. Ingestion of psychoactive substances, accumulative CNS effect of prescribed medications or street drugs, or withdrawal syndromes (e.g., delirium tremens from alcohol withdrawal)

Table 18-1 Comparison of Clinical Findings of Delirium and Dementia

Delirium	Dementia
Acute onset (hours/days)	Chronic
Rapidly progressive	Insidious
Intense anxiety and irritability	Short attention span
Tremors/hyperreflexia	Memory loss
Insomnia	Impaired new learning
Hyperactivity	Lack of initiative/apathy
Fever and tachycardia	Blunted or labile affect
Hypertension	Loss of judgment
Hallucinations and delusions	Motor disturbances
Convulsions	Exaggeration of traits
Death	Lower personal standards

    f. Multiple etiologies (e.g., combination of medical condition and substance interaction)

B. Behavioral/clinical findings (Table 18-1: Comparison of Clinical Findings of Delirium and Dementia)
  1. Delirium accompanied by confusion, hallucinations (a perception in absence of an external stimulus), illusions (misinterpretations of an actual stimulus), and delusions (fixed false beliefs)
  2. Disorientation and confusion as to time, place, person, and situation
  3. Memory defects for both recent and remote events and facts
  4. Slurring or rapid speech that may occur concurrently with an indistinct pronunciation or use of words
  5. Tremors, incoordination, imbalance, and incontinence may develop
  6. Physical symptoms such as hyperthermia, tachycardia, and GI changes (e.g., anorexia, nausea, vomiting, diarrhea)
  7. Agitation and irritability
  8. Insomnia

C. Therapeutic interventions
  1. Reduction of causative agent such as fever or toxins
  2. Prevention of further damage
  3. Provision of diet high in calories, protein, and vitamins; increase in fluid intake; elimination of caffeine
  4. Prescription of mild sedatives if necessary
  5. Provision of a safe, quiet environment with increased supervision
  6. Reorientation to time, place, person, and situation
  7. Communication with simple direct statements in calm voice; use nonverbal cues
  8. Channel agitation into safe activities

Nursing Care of Clients With Delirium

A. Assessment/Analysis
  1. History of onset and progression of symptoms from family members
  2. Orientation to time, place, person, and situation
  3. Occurrence of memory defects
  4. Mood swings or behavior associated with delirium
  5. State of consciousness
  6. Vital signs and physical symptoms

B. Planning/Implementation
  1. Refer to Nursing Care of Clients With Delirium, Nursing Care of Clients With Dementia, Nursing Care of Clients With Amnestic Disorders, and other sections in this chapter referring to nursing care of clients with cognitive disorders
  2. Implement measures as ordered to reduce causative factors
  3. If appropriate, reassure family members that symptoms associated with delirium may subside with treatment
  4. Provide one-to-one caregiver assignment during restless or agitated periods

C. Evaluation/Outcomes
  1. Remains free from injury
  2. Remains oriented ×4 to time, place, person, and situation
  3. Assumes increased responsibility for self-care
  4. Maintains a diet high in calories, protein, and vitamins
  5. Avoids intake of pharmacologic substance associated with delirium
  6. Continues to visit health care provider for treatment and amelioration of underlying cause

DEMENTIA

Data Base

A. Etiologic factors
  1. Differs from expected aging process
  2. Alzheimer's disease and vascular disease are the two most common causes; death occurs after years of decline mentally and physically; Alzheimer's disease is the fourth leading cause of death in the United States
  3. Stressors
    a. Anatomic changes in the brain from trauma, tumors, and degenerations of tissue (e.g., atrophy, widening ventricles, senile plaques caused by deposits of amyloid protein, neurofibrillary tangles)
    b. Infections such as tertiary syphilis and AIDS
    c. Circulatory disturbances causing anoxia and permanent brain damage (e.g., cerebral arteriosclerosis, brain attack)
    d. Nutritional deprivation of brain cells (e.g., pellagra)
    e. Toxins including chronic alcohol abuse
    f. Decreased level of neurotransmitters, especially acetylcholine
    g. Chromosomal defects (e.g., Huntington's disease)
    h. Immunologic defects creating prolonged inflammatory response in brain tissue

B. Behavioral/clinical findings (Table 18-1: Comparison of Clinical Findings of Delirium and Dementia)
  1. Dementia has an insidious onset with symptoms following a progressively downhill course

2. Early recognition of cognitive deficits may lead to anger, anxiety, and depression. As cognitive deficits progress and self-awareness declines, these symptoms may be replaced by apathy and social withdrawal; anxiety may still occur when cognitive abilities are overwhelmed and confusion increases

3. Progression moves from mild forgetfulness for recent events and mild expressive aphasia to inability to perform ADLs and mutism
   a. Aphasia (language disturbance)
   b. Apraxia (impaired motor activities)
   c. Agnosia (inability to recognize familiar objects)
   d. Amnesia
   e. Ataxia (impaired coordination)
   f. Disturbance in planning, organizing, sequencing, and abstracting (executive function)
   g. Emotional lability or flatness
   h. Hallucinations, illusions, and delusions
   i. Sundowning phenomenon: agitated behaviors of physical aggression peak between 2 and 9 PM; disquieted behaviors of nighttime sleeplessness and wandering peak between midnight and 6 AM

C. Therapeutic interventions
   1. The same as those for delirium with greater emphasis on preventing further damage (see Therapeutic interventions under Delirium)
   2. Anti-Alzheimer's agents: donepezil (Aricept), rivastigmine (Exelon), memantine (Namenda)

Nursing Care of Clients With Dementia

A. Assessment/Analysis
   1. History of onset and progression of symptoms from family
   2. Physical and emotional status in relation to needs associated with nutrition, fluid and electrolyte status, hygiene and toileting capabilities, and safety
   3. History of premorbid personality, abilities, and level of functioning from family
   4. History of impaired memory
   5. History of hallucinations (visual) and delusions (persecution)
   6. Identification of caregivers and their ability to provide adequate care
   7. Existence of advance directives
   8. Results of the Mini-Mental State Exam (MMSE) that are less than 23, which is indicative of cognitive impairment; maximum score on MMSE is 30; MMSE assesses orientation (e.g., identifying year, date, location), registration (e.g., repeating names of objects), attention and calculation (e.g., identifying serial numbers, spelling a word backward), recall (e.g., restating words previously said by examiner), language (e.g., naming objects, following a three-stage command, reading and obeying a command)

B. Planning/Implementation
   1. Refer to Nursing Care of Clients With Delirium, Nursing Care of Clients With Dementia, Nursing

Care of Clients With Amnestic Disorders, and other sections in this chapter referring to nursing care of clients with cognitive disorders
   2. Toilet client frequently
   3. Feed the client who is not able to feed self
   4. Protect client from self and environment; modify residence to prevent injury and wandering; increase supervision
   5. Support client's attempts at independence when appropriate
   6. Support family's decisions regarding present and future care of client; encourage completion of advance directives while client has capacity
   7. Assess effectiveness of medication to delay progression of cognitive symptoms
   8. Support caregivers as necessary (e.g., respite care, home health aides, long-term residence for clients with dementia, support groups)

C. Evaluation/Outcomes
   1. Remains free from injury
   2. Maintains maximal potential for as long as possible
   3. Family utilizes community resources as necessary

AMNESTIC DISORDERS

Data Base
A. Etiologic factors
   1. Disturbance in memory related to medical condition (e.g., head trauma, brain attack)
   2. Disturbance in memory related to persistent effects of substance (e.g., drug abuse, medication, or toxin exposure)

B. Behavioral/clinical findings
   1. Impaired ability to learn new information
   2. Difficulty recalling previously learned information or past events
   3. No evidence of anxiety related to a traumatic event
   4. Impaired social and occupational functions

C. Therapeutic interventions: see Dementia

Nursing Care of Clients With Amnestic Disorders

A. Assessment/Analysis
   1. History of onset and progression of symptoms from family
   2. Physical and emotional status
   3. History of previous functioning level

B. Planning/Implementation
   1. Refer to Nursing Care of Clients With Delirium, Nursing Care of Clients With Dementia, Nursing Care of Clients With Amnestic Disorders, and other sections in this chapter referring to nursing care of clients with cognitive disorders
   2. Maintain the client in a safe environment
   3. Support the client's attempts at independence when appropriate
   4. Assist with health care team's efforts to identify causative agent

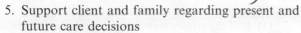

5. Support client and family regarding present and future care decisions

C. Evaluation/Outcomes
1. Demonstrates remission of amnesia
2. Returns to previous level of functioning
3. Family utilizes community resources

❀ SUBSTANCE-INDUCED AMNESTIC DISORDERS

Data Base

A. Etiologic factors
1. Nervous system, particularly the CNS, directly affected by medications, drugs, and toxins
2. Occurs in individuals with substance-abuse disorders
3. Behavioral changes may be related to a vitamin deficiency such as thiamine, especially in long-term alcohol abuse such as Korsakoff's syndrome
4. Memory disturbance persists long after drug or toxin exposure has ended

B. Behavioral/clinical findings
1. Specific neurologic and psychologic signs and maladaptive behavior such as euphoria; dysphoria; apathy; confabulation; psychomotor agitation, excitement, or depression; hypervigilance; and violent behavior
2. Symptoms of dementia or delirium may be present depending on the substance used
3. Physical symptoms such as depressed respirations, cardiac irregularities, and GI changes may occur
4. Memory disturbance causes significant impairment in social and work activities and represents a decline in previous level of function
5. Impairment in ability to learn new information or to recall previously learned information

C. Therapeutic interventions: see Delirium

Nursing Care of Clients With Substance-Induced Amnestic Disorders

A. Assessment/Analysis
1. History, physical examination, or laboratory findings related to drug abuse or toxin exposure
2. History of symptom onset (rapid/slow)
3. Orientation to time, place, person, and situation
4. Ability to have short-term and long-term recall
5. Level of consciousness and stimulation necessary to evoke a response
6. Physiologic status

B. Planning/Implementation
1. Refer to Nursing Care of Clients With Delirium, Nursing Care of Clients With Dementia, Nursing Care of Clients With Amnestic Disorders, and other sections in this chapter referring to nursing care of clients with cognitive disorders
2. Refer to Planning/Implementation under Nursing Care of Clients With Dementia and Nursing Care of Clients With Delirium

C. Evaluation/Outcomes
1. Abstains from injurious substances
2. Reduces maladaptive behavior
3. Remains free from injury
4. Remains cognitively stable or slightly improves

❀ SCHIZOPHRENIC DISORDERS

Data Base

A. Etiologic factors
1. Foremost etiology today is the biologic perspective (e.g., neuroanatomy, genetics, endocrinology, and immunology all produce symptoms; trauma and disease as causation continue to be researched)
2. Biologic components
   a. Heredity and genetics
   b. Neuroanatomic differences and neurochemicals (e.g., dopamine hyperactivity)
      (1) Structure and function of nervous system
      (2) Teratogenic drug exposure
      (3) Neuroanatomic differences in brain (e.g., enlarged ventricles)
   c. Neurotransmitter function: abnormal neurotransmitter-endocrine interactions
   d. Immunologic factors: viral exposure during pregnancy
   e. High arousal levels from stress, disease, drugs, and trauma
      (1) Stress such as bombardment of stimuli from life events may contribute to relapse and return of symptoms
      (2) Diseases such as prenatal virus exposure; encephalitis
      (3) Trauma from birth complications, head trauma, childhood accidents
      (4) Drugs such as cannabis and cocaine
3. Psychosocial considerations are significant; causative models postulate that biologic vulnerability interacts with stressful environmental influences to produce the symptoms of schizophrenia
4. Onset in men usually is between ages 18 and 25 years; onset for women is later, between 25 and 35 years; incidence of schizophrenia slightly higher in men
5. Chronic insecurity and failure in interpersonal relationships impair functioning
6. Regardless of the ultimate etiology, a disturbed relationship with the environment and the family is an almost universal characteristic
7. Course of the disease: either acute or chronic; some will demonstrate almost normal functioning with intermittent psychotic episodes; others have diminished functioning with intermittent psychotic episodes; about 10% to 25% demonstrate severely diminished functioning with ongoing psychotic symptoms

B. Types
1. Although historically much time and effort were directed toward identifying types of schizophrenia,

it should be recognized that the classification is not static; there is overlapping symptomatology; individuals diagnosed as being in one classification frequently are diagnosed at a later time in another classification

2. Paranoid type: exhibits delusions of persecution or grandiosity, or both; less often noted are delusional themes of jealousy, religiosity, or somatization

3. Disorganized type: exhibits disorganized speech and behavior; exhibits childlike affect and uninhibited sexual behaviors; socially inept

4. Catatonic type: features marked psychomotor disturbance that may involve motor immobility (waxy flexibility), excessive motor activity, extreme negativism, mutism, posturing, echolalia, or echopraxia

5. Undifferentiated type: demonstrates delusions, hallucinations, disorganized speech, disorganized behavior; does not demonstrate behaviors usually observed in paranoid, disorganized, or catatonic types

6. Residual type: criteria for schizophrenia and subtypes listed above are not met; there is continuing evidence of negative symptoms and two or more of these characteristic symptoms (e.g., delusions, hallucinations, disorganized speech, and gross disorganization); develops later in the course of the disease

C. Behavioral/clinical findings
1. Primary symptoms are often referred to as "the 4 As"
   a. Disturbances in association, affect (flattened affect), ambivalence, and autistic thinking
   b. Additional "As" include attention deficits and activity disturbances
2. Characteristic symptoms generally fall into two broad categories (Table 18-2: Schizophrenia: Symptom Categorization)
   a. Positive symptoms (additional behaviors)
      (1) Include disorganized or bizarre alterations in thinking, speech, perception (altered reality testing), behavior, and mood
      (2) More apparent during acute relapses
      (3) More responsive to medication and interactive therapies

Table 18-2 Schizophrenia: Symptom Categorization

Type I Symptoms	Type II Symptoms
Hallucinations	Apathy
Delusions	Social withdrawal
Loose association	Flat affect
Concrete thinking	Poor ADLs
Neologisms	Anhedonia
Catatonia	Paucity of ideas
Agitation/violence	Paucity of speech

b. Negative symptoms (deficits of behaviors)
   (1) Include affect flattening, apathy/avolition, anhedonia, and attention deficit
   (2) More apparent during nonacute periods
   (3) Less responsive to therapy; more complex and difficult to treat
3. Problems in cognitive functioning involve attention deficits, abstract concept formation, decision making, and problem solving
4. Alterations in mood: symptoms are dysphoria, suicidiality, and hopelessness; approximately 15% commit suicide
5. Social and occupational role dysfunction
6. Duration of at least 6 months

D. Therapeutic interventions
1. Psychotherapy (individual, family, and group counseling)
2. Motivational therapy
3. Occupational and vocational therapy
4. Daycare treatment programs in community settings that foster interpersonal relationships
5. Pharmacologic therapy: positive symptoms respond to traditional antipsychotic drugs; negative symptoms respond more effectively to atypical drugs (see Related Pharmacology, Psychotropic Medications in Chapter 16)
6. Paranoid schizophrenia appears to be the most responsive to treatment when compared to responses typical of other subtypes; clients appear to be at a higher functioning level

Nursing Care of Clients With Schizophrenic Disorders

A. Assessment/Analysis
1. History of start of disorder from client and family if available
2. Presence of delusional ideation (fixed false belief) and/or hallucinations (perceived stimuli without external stimuli); specific assessment for command hallucinations (voices telling client to do something)
3. Presence of suspiciousness and/or feelings of paranoia; presence and extent of fear of other clients and staff
4. History of work and social functioning
5. Presence of precipitating or current stress factors
6. Unclear or incomplete client and family communication patterns; double-bind communication (contradictory invalidating messages)
7. Physiologic status

B. Planning/Implementation
1. Respect the client as a human being with both dignity and worth; establish a therapeutic relationship
2. Accept clients at their present level of functioning; meet basic physiologic needs; first focus on nonthreatening topics when communicating
3. Avoid trying to argue the client out of delusions or hallucinations

4. Accept that the hallucinations and delusions are real to the client and possibly frightening; stay with and support the client; focus on feelings, not the misperceptions of reality
5. Encourage the development of interpersonal relationships between the client and others; help client learn to trust through consistency in interactions
6. Point out reality to the client but do not impose staff's concept of reality; involve client in reality-based activities such as ADLs
7. Monitor nutritional status and hygiene
8. Set limits on inappropriate or unsafe behavior or use distraction
9. Clarify unclear communication such as neologisms (words invented by the client that have meaning only to the client)
10. Encourage the client to follow a plan of organized activity and the prescribed drug regimen
11. Observe for adverse drug reactions whenever large doses of antipsychotic medications are being administered
12. Teach client to recognize and report extrapyramidal side effects (EPS) to avoid physical discomfort
13. Administer antiparkinsonian agents to minimize EPS
14. Encourage the client to continue medications even after symptoms abate
15. Recognize that the client's ability to test reality is distorted by psychopathology
16. Maintain safety of the client, especially during acute phase; safety remains the highest priority because of impaired judgment and/or command hallucinations

C. Evaluation/Outcomes
1. Remains free from adverse side effects of psychotropic drug regimen
2. Continues taking prescribed medications
3. Exhibits a decrease in hallucinations
4. Differentiates between hallucinations and reality
5. Remains free from injury to self and others
6. Demonstrates a reduction in anxiety through verbalization or body language
7. Demonstrates improved functioning with activities of daily living and socialization
8. Continues therapy after discharge

✾ DELUSIONAL (PARANOID) DISORDERS

Data Base

A. Etiologic factors
1. Individuals who demonstrate the suspiciousness and fixed false beliefs (delusions) common to paranoid conditions but do not exhibit the thinking and behavioral disorganization or the personality disintegration found in the other psychoses
2. Premorbid personality: uses the compensatory mechanisms of the projective pattern of behavior

3. Paranoid defenses considered by some to be a protective mechanism against unconscious homosexuality or overt hostility
4. Neurobiologic perspective
   a. The exact nature of the physiologic disruption is not well-defined; it is thought that psychotic disorders involve an abnormality in the transmission of neural impulses, and that the difficulty occurs at the synaptic level and involves neurochemicals such as dopamine, serotonin, and norepinephrine
   b. Neurologic and cognitive impairments are less and prognosis seems better
   c. See Biologic components under Schizophrenic Disorders
5. Cultural and religious background must be taken into account because variations exist in cultures and subcultures

B. Behavioral/clinical findings
1. Exhibits a rather elaborate, highly organized paranoid delusional system while preserving other functions of the personality
2. Apart from the impact of the delusions, there is no interference with thinking and functioning; nor are the delusions bizarre
3. Delusions are drawn from real-life situations and have a coherent theme
4. Hallucinations are not prominent; if present they usually are auditory and are related to the delusional theme
5. Predominant theme of delusions determines type of paranoia (e.g., grandiose, jealous, persecutory)
6. Intellectual and occupational functioning less impaired than social or marital relationships

C. Types
1. Erotomanic: delusion that another person is in love with the client; idealized, romantic love or spiritual union, rather than sexual attraction, is basic to this type
2. Grandiose: delusion that the client has some great (but unrecognized) talent or insight or has made an important discovery; less commonly, the individual claims a special relationship with a prominent person or claims to be a prominent person
3. Jealous: delusion of unfaithfulness by one's spouse or lover based on incorrect inferences is the central theme of this type
4. Persecutory: delusion that one is being conspired against, spied upon, cheated, followed, poisoned or drugged, maligned, harassed, or obstructed in the pursuit of long-term goals
5. Somatic: delusion involving bodily functions or sensations

D. Therapeutic interventions
1. Pharmacotherapy with neuroleptics considered most helpful; see Neuroleptics (Antipsychotic Medications) under Related Pharmacology in Chapter 16

2. Individual psychotherapy may provide some relief of symptoms
3. The course of paranoid disorders varies but is more hopeful than other psychotic disorders, because they are most responsive to treatment

Nursing Care of Clients With Delusional (Paranoid) Disorders

A. Assessment/Analysis
   1. History of start of disorder from client and family if available
   2. Presence of hallucinations and delusional ideation; may constitute a danger to self or others
   3. Presence of suspiciousness; paranoid feelings usually are limited to specific areas in the client's life
   4. Absence of odd or bizarre behavior and other criteria related to schizophrenia
   5. Social and marital functioning
B. Planning/Implementation
   1. Provide an environment with some intellectual challenges that do not threaten security
   2. Avoid counteraggression and retaliation against the client
   3. Accept and recognize the client's need for a superior attitude
   4. Meet sarcasm and ridicule in a matter-of-fact manner
   5. Set limits on inappropriate behaviors that are derived from delusions
   6. Accept the client's misinterpretations of events as the client's perception of the events
   7. Point out reality but do not challenge the client's delusions directly
   8. Foster the development of social interaction with consistency in staff and gradual integration into unit activities

C. Evaluation/Outcomes
   1. Continues to function in society
   2. Avoids factors that stimulate delusional thinking

SCHIZOAFFECTIVE DISORDER

Data Base

A. Etiologic factors
   1. This disturbance is unrelated to the direct physiologic effects of a substance or medication or a general medical condition
   2. An uninterrupted period of illness including a major depressive episode or manic episode concurrent with symptoms of schizophrenia (delusions or hallucinations, disorganized speech or behavior, and negative symptoms)
   3. Occurs in early adulthood
B. Behavioral/clinical findings
   1. Demonstrates a mixture of symptoms from both schizophrenia and mood disorders
   2. The thought processes and bizarre behavior appear schizophrenic, but there is usually marked elation or depression
C. Therapeutic interventions
   1. Antipsychotic and/or antidepressant agents may be used to treat symptoms
   2. Therapy depends on the type and severity of the symptoms exhibited

Nursing Care of Clients With a Schizoaffective Disorder

See Nursing Care of Clients With Schizophrenic Disorders in this chapter and Bipolar Disorders in Chapter 19

19 Nursing Care of Clients With Disorders Related to Anxiety and Alterations in Mood

OVERVIEW

A. The primary initial deficit occurs in mood or ability to handle anxiety, although there may be changes in the client's cognition and behavior
B. Anxiety disorders are the most common of all psychiatric disorders, resulting in considerable distress and functional impairment; rarely treated in inpatient psychiatric settings unless the anxiety is extreme with greatly impaired functioning or if treated concurrently with another psychiatric disorder
C. Anxiety and depressed mood may find expression in the physical complaints and symptoms associated with somatoform and dissociative disorders

MAJOR DISORDERS ASSOCIATED WITH ANXIETY

GENERAL NURSING CARE OF CLIENTS WITH ANXIETY DISORDERS

A. Provide an environment that limits demands on the client and permits attention to resolution of conflicts; establish a trusting relationship
B. Accept symptoms as real to the client
C. Attempt to limit the use of defenses, but do not try to stop them until the client is ready to give them up
D. Encourage the client to develop a balance between work and relaxation
E. Help the client develop better ways of handling anxiety-producing situations through problem solving and cognitive/behavioral therapies; assist client to expand supportive network; assist significant others to understand what is happening to the client
F. Accept physical symptoms but do not emphasize or call attention to them
G. Reduce demands on the individual as much as possible; help client to identify ways to reduce stresses in life; plan a routine schedule of activities
H. Recognize when anxiety interrupts ability to think clearly
 I. Intervene to protect client from acting out on impulses that may be harmful to self or others; recognize that the client is acting out because of fear, not to be antisocial

J. Determine comorbidity (cooccurrence) of anxiety disorders and depression because they frequently occur simultaneously
K. Be aware that anxiety is contagious to other clients and staff

GENERALIZED ANXIETY DISORDER (GAS)

Data Base
A. Etiologic factors
1. Psychologic, behavioral, and psychobiologic theories are all offered; the latter theory is most promising
2. Development of the anxiety usually permits some measure of social adjustment
3. Commonly begins in early adulthood as a result of environmental factors in childhood
4. Early life rigid and orderly
5. Pressures of decision making regarding lifestyle that occur in the early adult years seem to act as precipitating factors
6. Excessive anxiety and worry about at least two life situations
B. Behavioral/clinical findings
1. Excessive anxiety and worry about a number of events or activities for a 6-month duration
2. Inability to control the worry
3. Anxiety and worry associated with three or more of the following symptoms: restlessness (akathisia) or feeling on-edge, easily fatigued, difficulty concentrating, irritability, muscle tension, and sleep disturbance
4. Impairment in social or occupational relationships caused by anxiety, worry, and physical symptoms
5. Anxiety is not due to direct physiologic effects of substances or a medical condition
6. Symptoms of autonomic hyperarousal (tachycardia, tachypnea, dizziness, and dilated pupils) are less prominent than in other anxiety disorders
C. Therapeutic interventions: same as those for Panic Disorders

Nursing Care of Clients With Generalized Anxiety Disorder
A. See General Nursing Care of Clients With Anxiety Disorders
B. See Nursing Care of Clients With Panic Disorder

✤ PANIC DISORDER

Data Base

A. Etiologic factors
   1. Biochemical and genetic theories are most often cited as the underlying cause of anxiety disorders; no one gene or biochemical dysfunction has been singled out
   2. Recurrent attacks of severe anxiety may not be associated with a stimulus but can occur spontaneously
   3. Development of symptoms usually permits some measure of social adjustment
   4. Onset varies, most often noted between late adolescence and mid-30s; a small number of cases begin in childhood, or after age 45
   5. Early life rigid and orderly
   6. Pressures of decision making regarding lifestyle that occur in the early adult years seem to act as precipitating factors
   7. Discrete periods of intense discomfort or fear for more than 1 month in duration

B. Behavioral/clinical findings
   1. Acute, brief attacks of intense fear or discomfort that can be overwhelming
   2. Four or more of the following symptoms: palpitations or accelerated heart rate, sweating, trembling or shaking, shortness of breath, feelings of choking, chest pain or discomfort, nausea or abdominal distress, depersonalization, fear of losing control, fear of dying, paresthesias, and chills or hot flashes

C. Therapeutic interventions
   1. Complete medical workup to reassure the individual and rule out physical illness
   2. Psychotherapy, family therapy, group therapy; cognitive/behavioral therapies
   3. Sedatives, antidepressants, and antianxiety agents useful short term when client is unable to cope or accomplish daily activities and until healthier coping emerges

Nursing Care of Clients With Panic Disorder

A. Assessment/Analysis
   1. Progression of somatic symptoms and complaints
   2. Interference in ADLs and social and occupational functioning
   3. Situational triggers that may or may not precipitate the onset of an attack
   4. Determination whether panic symptoms relate to an agoraphobic situation

B. Planning/Implementation
   1. See General Nursing Care of Clients With Anxiety Disorders
   2. Remain with client during an attack
   3. Do not get caught up in client's panic; remain calm and in control of the situation
   4. Recognize that clients usually have less anxiety in private rooms with decreased environmental stimulation

C. Evaluation/Outcomes
   1. Identifies situations that increase anxiety
   2. Demonstrates increased use of anxiety-reducing behaviors
   3. Follows prescribed treatment regimen
   4. Reports a decreased number of panic attacks

✤ PHOBIC DISORDERS

Data Base

A. Etiologic factors
   1. Multiple theories as to the cause (genetic, psychologic, developmental, and environmental) are being studied; etiology remains unverified
   2. Onset begins in childhood; traumatic phobias can occur throughout the life span
   3. Pressures of decision making regarding lifestyle that occur in the early adult years seem to act as precipitating factors
   4. Anxiety unconsciously transferred to an inanimate object or situation, which then symbolically represents the conflict and can be avoided
   5. Anxiety is severe if the object, situation, or activity cannot be avoided

B. Behavioral/clinical findings
   1. Anxiety appears when clients find themselves in places that threaten their sense of security
   2. Attempts are made to avoid these distressing situations
   3. Depending on the phobic object, the individual's lifestyle is often greatly limited
   4. Fear of being trapped, embarrassed, or humiliated in social situations
   5. Adults recognize that the fear is excessive or unreasonable but cannot control it

C. Types
   1. Agoraphobia: fear of being alone or in public places where help would not be immediately available if necessary; includes tunnels, bridges, crowds, buses, and trains
   2. Social phobia: fear of doing something in public that could be embarrassing or cause negative evaluations (e.g., speaking, dancing, eating in front of others)
   3. Specific phobia: fear of a specific object, animal, or situation

D. Therapeutic interventions
   1. Same as those for Panic Disorders
   2. Behavior modification: a counter-conditioning technique to overcome fears by gradually increasing exposure to the feared object, situation, or animal (desensitization) or by continuous exposure to the point of exhaustion of anxiety (flooding)
   3. Pharmacologic and cognitive therapies

Nursing Care of Clients With Phobic Disorders

A. Assessment/Analysis
   1. Behaviors associated with anxiety disorders
   2. Presence, type, and duration of phobia (at least 6 months)

3. Interference in activities of daily living and social and occupational functioning
4. Behaviors used to avoid phobic object or stress-producing situations
5. Pervasive anxiety and fear

B. Planning/Implementation
1. See General Nursing Care of Clients With Anxiety Disorders
2. Recognize client's feelings about phobic object or situation
3. Provide constant support if exposure to phobic object or situation cannot be avoided
4. Assist with relaxation and cognitive/behavioral techniques to control or diminish anxiety levels

C. Evaluation/Outcomes
1. Tolerates desensitization process
2. Copes with anxiety-producing object or situation effectively
3. Follows prescribed treatment regimen
4. Utilizes relaxation techniques to diminish anxiety
5. Decreases anxiety's impacts on ability to function

❀ OBSESSIVE-COMPULSIVE DISORDER (OCD)

Data Base

A. Etiologic factors
1. Decreased levels of serotonin
2. OCD is a chronic anxiety disorder that responds to different treatment strategies
3. Symptoms worsen with stress
4. Pressures of decision making regarding lifestyle that occur in the early adult years seem to act as precipitating factors
5. Unconscious control of anxiety by the use of rituals and thoughts
6. Obsessions or compulsions are recognized as excessive and interfere with daily activities but cannot be controlled
7. Some evidence that early life patterns were rigid and orderly

B. Behavioral/clinical findings
1. Major defensive mechanisms utilized are isolation, undoing, and reaction formation
2. Thoughts persist and become repetitive and obsessive
3. Some research notes that compulsive behavior precedes obsessive thinking
4. Client is indecisive and demonstrates a striving for perfection and superiority
5. Intellectual and verbal defenses are used
6. Anxiety and depression may be present in various degrees, particularly if rituals are prevented
7. Adults experiencing this disorder usually recognize that obsessions or compulsions are excessive or unreasonable; children do not have this insight
8. Obsessions or compulsions may consume most of client's waking hours (at minimum more than 1 hour per day) and therefore interfere with ADLs, occupation, social activities, or relationships
9. OCD symptoms are similar in adults and children

C. Therapeutic interventions
1. Similar to those for Panic Disorders
2. Behavior modification to attempt to limit the length and/or frequency of ritual
3. Cognitive therapy
4. Pharmacologic treatment: clomipramine (Anafranil) and fluvoxamine (Luvox) to control symptoms

Nursing Care of Clients With Obsessive-Compulsive Disorders

A. Assessment/Analysis
1. Behavior associated with anxiety disorders
2. Type and use of ritual or obsession
3. Level of interference in lifestyle
4. Degree of anxiety experienced by the client
5. Extent of danger inherent in the ritual or obsession

B. Planning/Implementation
1. See General Nursing Care of Clients With Anxiety Disorders
2. Recognize that the client understands that the ritual has no rational basis but cannot control it
3. Allow the client to continue the ritual but attempt to limit the length and frequency of the ritual unless ritual causes harm and must be stopped (e.g., excessive handwashing causing skin damage); interrupting the ritual increases anxiety
4. Support clients in their attempt to reduce dependency on the ritual
5. Role model appropriate behavior and discuss adaptive responses with client

C. Evaluation/Outcomes
1. Demonstrates decrease in need to perform ritual or continue obsession
2. Controls anxiety without ritual or obsession
3. Follows prescribed treatment regimen
4. Learns new adaptive coping responses
5. Decreases use of anxiety-binding activities and increases time in completing tasks of daily living and social/recreational activities

❀ POSTTRAUMATIC STRESS DISORDER (PTSD)

Data Base

A. Etiologic factors
1. Follows a devastating event that is outside the range of usual human experience (e.g., rape, assault, military combat, hostage situations, natural or precipitated disasters)
2. Neurobiology of PTSD does not follow the usual fight-or-flight stress response; studies indicate a complex interaction of neuroendocrinology, neuroanatomy, genetics, and traumatic stress

3. Individual's response must involve intense fear, helplessness, or horror; in children the response must involve disorganized or agitated behaviors
4. The traumatic event is persistently reexperienced as flashbacks, distressing dreams, sense of reliving the experience, or exposure to situations that foster recall of the event (including anniversaries)

B. Behavioral/clinical findings
  1. Exposure to a traumatic event resulting in actual death, threatened death, or serious injury to others or self and/or responding to the event with intense fear, confusion, helplessness, horror, or denial; onset at any age
  2. Feelings of isolation and detachment
  3. Difficulty sleeping
  4. Violent outbursts of anger
  5. Depression
  6. Interrupted concentration
  7. Hypervigilance
  8. Avoidance of associated stimuli
  9. Substance abuse in attempt to control symptoms
  10. Duration of disturbance more than 1 month

C. Therapeutic interventions
  1. Same as those for panic disorders
  2. Behavior modification to provide controlled exposure to recall of the event
  3. Supportive therapy
  4. Use of eye movement, desensitization, reprocessing techniques (EMDR)
  5. Imagery, relaxation, and meditation may also be useful

Nursing Care of Clients With Posttraumatic Stress Disorder

A. Assessment/Analysis
  1. Behavior associated with anxiety disorders
  2. History of traumatic experience
  3. Sleep-pattern disturbances
  4. Screening for symptoms of major depression, phobias, and substance abuse
  5. Presence of depression, outbursts of anger, and/or decreased concentration

B. Planning/Implementation
  1. See General Nursing Care of Clients With Anxiety Disorders
  2. Stay with client when memory of the event returns to the conscious level
  3. Protect client from acting out violently with disregard for safety of self or others

C. Evaluation/Outcomes
  1. Uses coping mechanisms to more realistically deal with the traumatic event and flashbacks
  2. Verbalizes decrease in dreams or flashbacks regarding the traumatic event
  3. Follows prescribed treatment regimen
  4. Demonstrates new adaptive ways of coping with anxiety

MAJOR SOMATOFORM DISORDERS

GENERAL NURSING CARE OF CLIENTS WITH SOMATOFORM DISORDERS

A. Establish a trusting relationship
B. Provide an environment that limits demands on the client and permits attention to resolution of conflicts
C. Recognize a pattern of multiple recurring clinically significant somatic complaints; symptoms are real to client
D. Attempt to limit the use of defenses, but do not try to stop them until the individual is ready to give them up
E. Encourage the individual to develop a balance between work and relaxation
F. Help the individual develop better ways of handling anxiety-producing situations through problem solving and cognitive therapies
G. Accept physical symptoms but do not talk about, emphasize, or call attention to them
H. Minimize sick-role behavior
I. Help client identify and label needs met by symptoms

CONVERSION DISORDERS

Data Base

A. Etiologic factors
  1. Anxiety unconsciously converted to physical symptoms that are not under voluntary control; usually localized to one area of the body; these symptoms permit the individual to avoid some unacceptable activity
  2. Development of symptoms usually permits some measure of social adjustment
  3. Generally begins before 30 years of age; may recur
  4. Early life often rigid and orderly; physical illness frequently used by the family as an excuse for problems
  5. Pressures of decision making regarding lifestyle in the early adult years seem to be precipitating factors

B. Behavioral/clinical findings
  1. Presence of symptoms or deficits affecting voluntary motor or sensory function
  2. Conflicts or stressors, usually dependence versus independence, precede the initiation or exacerbation of symptoms or deficits (paralysis, blindness, deafness)
  3. Noticeable lack of concern about the problem; this lack of concern has been labeled "la belle indifference"
  4. Impairment may vary over different episodes and does not follow anatomic structure; paralysis or numbness may circle the foot or arm instead of beginning at the joint and is known as stocking-and-glove anesthesia
  5. The individual appears relieved by symptoms and demonstrates little anxiety when observed

6. The symptom or deficit is not related to an underlying medical condition, to substances, or to a cultural norm; this distinguishes conversion from psychophysiologic disorders that are associated with tissue changes

C. Therapeutic interventions
1. Complete medical workup to rule out medical problems
2. Psychotherapy, family therapy, group therapy as necessary to resolve severe emotional problems
3. Pharmacologic approach: antianxiety agents rarely helpful; antidepressants (SSRIs) appear to be more effective

Nursing Care of Clients With Conversion Disorders

A. Assessment/Analysis
1. Presence of physical symptoms with no physiologic basis
2. Level of concern regarding physical symptoms
3. Degree of impairment
4. Level of anxiety

B. Planning/Implementation
See General Nursing Care of Clients With Somatoform Disorders

C. Evaluation/Outcomes
1. Reduces need to develop physical symptoms to decrease anxiety
2. Uses problem solving rather than physical symptoms to handle anxiety-producing situations

✿ BODY DYSMORPHIC DISORDERS

Data Base

A. Etiologic factors
1. Preoccupied with a defect in appearance, either imagined or exaggerated if a slight defect is present (not of delusional intensity)
2. Onset usually during adolescence, but can begin in childhood; lasts for several years
3. No predisposing factor in early life or family patterns has been identified

B. Behavioral/clinical findings
1. History of multiple visits to plastic surgeons to correct imagined defects
2. Preoccupation with imagined deficit causes avoidance or impairment in social and occupational relationships
3. Often exhibits symptoms of depression or obsessive-compulsive personality traits

C. Therapeutic interventions
1. Same as those for conversion disorder

Nursing Care of Clients With Body Dysmorphic Disorders

A. Assessment/Analysis
1. Preoccupation with imagined physical defects
2. History of medical and surgical therapies to correct imagined defects

3. Ability to handle stressful situations
4. Level of anxiety

B. Planning/Implementation
See General Nursing Care of Clients With Somatoform Disorders

C. Evaluation/Outcomes
1. Recognizes that emphasis on physical defect is exaggerated
2. Uses problem solving rather than physical defect to handle anxiety-producing situations
3. Accepts and is comfortable with self

✿ HYPOCHONDRIASIS

Data Base

A. Etiologic factors
1. Preoccupation with the belief that one has a serious illness because of how physical symptoms are interpreted
2. A positive medical evaluation does not allay fears
3. Knowledge of symptoms associated with a given disease aids in the client's developing a similar set of symptoms, leading the client to conclude that the disease is present
4. Psychosocial stresses are believed to lead to development of this disorder
5. Usually begins between 20 and 30 years of age; can occur across the life span

B. Behavioral/clinical findings
1. Misinterpretation and exaggeration of physical symptoms
2. Inability to accept reassurance even after exhaustive testing and therapy; leads to "doctor shopping"
3. History of repeated absences from work
4. Duration of disturbance is at least 6 months
5. Adoption of sick role and invalid lifestyle

C. Therapeutic interventions
1. Same as those for conversion disorder

Nursing Care of Clients With Hypochondriasis

A. Assessment/Analysis
1. Level of preoccupation with symptoms
2. Past and present degree of interference with functioning related to symptoms
3. Duration and degree of disability associated with symptoms
4. History of psychosocial precipitant stressors

B. Planning/Implementation
See General Nursing Care of Clients With Somatoform Disorders

C. Evaluation/Outcomes
1. Accepts that there is no physical basis for the symptoms
2. Uses more effective coping mechanisms to deal with anxiety
3. Accepts need to continue therapy even after condition has improved

❋ DISSOCIATIVE DISORDERS

Data Base

A. These disorders are characterized by either a sudden or a gradual disruption in the usual integrated functions of consciousness, memory, identity, or perception of the environment
B. The disruption may be transient or may become a well-established pattern
C. Etiologic factors: related to increased stress or traumatic event(s) such as sexual abuse during childhood
D. Types
   1. Dissociative amnesia: characterized by an inability to recall important personal information, usually of a traumatic or stressful nature as distinguished from ordinary forgetfulness
   2. Dissociative fugue: characterized by sudden, unexpected travel accompanied by an inability to recall one's past, identity confusion, or the assumption of a new identity
   3. Dissociative identity disorder (also know as multiple personality disorder): characterized by coexistence of two or more distinct personalities within an individual
   4. Depersonalization disorder: characterized by persistent or recurrent feeling of being detached from one's mental processes or body that is accompanied by intact reality testing
E. Behavioral/clinical findings
   1. Inability to recall important personal information usually of a traumatic or stressful nature
   2. Gaps in recalling aspects of an individual's life history; usually related to traumatic episodes
F. Therapeutic interventions
   1. Complete medical workup to rule out possibility of organic causes (e.g., brain tumor)
   2. Psychotherapy, individual and family
   3. Development of more effective and satisfying ways to handle anxiety

Nursing Care of Clients With Dissociative Disorders

A. Assessment/Analysis
   1. Identity
   2. Memory
   3. Consciousness
   4. Physical condition
   5. Psychosocial component to discover fundamental anxiety source
   6. History of emotional trauma in childhood from client (if possible) and family
   7. Suicidal risk
   8. Recent use of alcohol or drugs
B. Planning/Implementation
   1. See General Nursing Care of Clients With Anxiety Disorders
   2. Assist with treatment plan to alleviate the troublesome symptoms

   3. Reinforce effective coping skills
   4. Provide for family therapy
   5. Assist with problem solving
   6. Encourage involvement in long-term therapy
C. Evaluation/Outcomes
   1. Recalls and identifies past experiences correctly
   2. Verbalizes increased satisfaction with family and work relationships
   3. Ceases incidents of being absent without explanation
   4. Develops more effective coping mechanisms to deal with anxiety

MAJOR DISORDERS RELATED TO ALTERATIONS IN MOOD

GENERAL NURSING CARE OF CLIENTS WITH MOOD DISORDERS

A. Monitor nutritional intake and elimination
B. Keep the environment nonchallenging and with decreased stimuli; avoid boredom; focus on feelings
C. Observe children and adolescents for irritable mood; observe adults for depressive episodes
D. Protect the client from suicide or violent acting out during the entire episode; keep under constant observation if necessary; keep communication open and direct; ask if client has a specific plan to commit suicide
E. Keep activities simple, uncomplicated, and repetitive in nature; they should be of short duration and require little concentration; activities should be based on client's status: psychomotor retardation in depression and hyperactivity in mania; initial interaction should be with the nurse and then expanded to one or two other people
F. Observe for adverse effects of drugs; monitor therapeutic blood levels if appropriate
G. Encourage the client to continue medications even after symptoms abate
H. Caution and teach the client regarding special dietary precautions when taking certain medications (e.g., monoamine oxidase inhibitors [MAOIs])
I. Assist with developing coping strategies; plan for follow-up support and supervision

❋ BIPOLAR DISORDER

Data Base

A. Characterized by a cyclical disturbance of mood, encompassing emotional extremes: episodes of the vehement energy of mania, the despair and lethargy of depression, or a mixture of both
B. Presence of one or more manic or hypomanic episodes in a client with a history of depressive episodes; the predominant mood is elevated or irritable, accompanied by one or more of these symptoms: hyperactivity, lack of judgment with no regard for consequences, pressured speech, flight of ideas,

distractibility, inflated self-esteem, risky behavior, and hypersexuality
  1. Hypomanic: mood elation with higher than usual activity and social interaction, but not as expansive as full mania; a distinct period of elevated or irritable mood that is clearly different from mania; duration at least 4 days
  2. Mania: an elevated, expansive, or irritable mood accompanied by hyperactivity, grandiosity, and loss of reality
C. Neurobiologic perspective
  1. Neurotransmitters, or certain chemicals in the brain that regulate mood, have been identified (serotonin, dopamine, norepinephrine, and gamma-aminobutyric acid [GABA])
  2. Research suggests this disorder results from complex interactions among chemicals, including neurotransmitters and hormones
  3. Family and twin studies suggest a genetic component, but no gene has at this time been identified except in rare, familial forms of the disorder
  4. Biologic rhythms and physiology related to depression show abnormal sleep EEGs, sensitivity to absence of sunlight, and circadian rhythm disturbance
  5. Physiologic theory postulates that mood also may respond to drugs or a variety of physical illnesses
    a. Drugs associated with depressive status: alcohol, sedative-hypnotics, amphetamine withdrawal, glucocorticoids, propranolol, resperidone, and steroid contraceptives
    b. Drugs associated with manic status: cocaine, MAOIs, tricyclic antidepressants, steroids, and levodopa
    c. Physical illness, such as brain attack (cerebrovascular accident, and some endocrine disorders (e.g., Cushing's disease and hypothyroidism) can lead to depressive episodes
D. Generally occurs between 20 and 40 years of age, although it has been reported in clients older than 50 years, and is increasingly diagnosed in children and adolescents
E. May be a response to loss (dysfunctional grieving), increased stress, or change in life events, role, and sleeping and/or eating patterns; contemplation of suicide may be a severe overreaction to the stress
F. Increased levels of norepinephrine, dopamine, and serotonin in acute mania
G. Decreased levels of norepinephrine, dopamine, and serotonin in depression
H. Resumption of customary activities between episodes
I. Obesity is a related factor; depressed mood may be altered by dietary modifications (e.g., increase intake of tryptophan, omega-3 fatty acids, and B complex vitamins, especially folic acid)

✣ DEPRESSIVE EPISODE OF A BIPOLAR DISORDER

Data Base
A. Etiologic factors: see Data Base under Bipolar Disorder
B. Behavioral/clinical findings
  1. Prime symptoms are either a depressed mood or loss of interest or pleasure, occurring during a 2-week period, with a change in level of functioning, plus five or more of the following:
    a. Change in weight
    b. Insomnia (especially early morning awakening)
    c. Psychomotor agitation or retardation
    d. Fatigue
    e. Worthless feelings or inappropriate guilt
    f. Somatic complaints
    g. Diminished hygiene
    h. Concentration difficulties
    i. Inability to make decisions
    j. Social withdrawal
    k. Suicidal behavior progresses from suicidal ideation, suicide threats, suicide gestures, suicide attempts, to successful suicides; presuicidal behaviors include no interest in the future, giving away personal possessions
  2. Orientation and logic unaffected
  3. Sex drive (libido) decreased
  4. Constipation and urinary retention may occur
  5. Depression and suicidal gestures may increase as anniversary of loss of loved object nears
C. Therapeutic interventions
  1. Electroconvulsive therapy (ECT)
    a. A brief electrical stimulus is applied to the brain, resulting in a seizure that alters brain chemistry and eventually alters mood
    b. Used most often for clients with recurrent depressions, delusions, suicidal ideation, and those who are resistant to drug therapy
    c. Drugs such as succinylcholine chloride (Anectine), a depolarizing muscle relaxant causing paralysis, are used to reduce the intensity of muscle contractions during the tonic/clonic stage and are given after a short-acting barbiturate or other sedative/anesthetic
    d. Side effects include fatigue, muscle soreness, mild temporary confusion and temporary short-term memory loss; side effects should resolve in a few weeks after treatment ends
  2. High-protein, high-carbohydrate diet to provide for energy; dietary supplements may be necessary
  3. Psychotherapy, cognitive and behavioral therapies
  4. Pharmacologic approach in depressive phase: antidepressant drugs that increase the level of norepinephrine at subcortical neuroeffector sites

Nursing Care of Clients During a Depressive Episode of a Bipolar Disorder

A. Assessment/Analysis
   (Table 19-1: Bipolar Disorder: Symptoms of Depression)
   1. Presence of feelings of worthlessness, guilt, and suicidal ideation or acting out; presence of a plan increases the danger of suicide
   2. Presence of depressed mood, loss of interest or pleasure, and slowing of psychomotor activity
   3. Weight for recent changes and to establish a baseline
   4. Changes in sleep patterns
   5. Changes in the ability to concentrate

B. Planning/Implementation
   1. See General Nursing Care of Clients With Mood Disorders
   2. Accept client's inability to carry out daily routines; assist with ADLs
   3. Set expectations that can be achieved by the client
   4. Provide realistic praise whenever possible
   5. Involve client in simple repetitious tasks and activities
   6. Accept client's feelings of worthlessness as real; client's feelings should not be denied, condoned, or approved
   7. Protect client from suicidal acting out, especially when the depression begins to lift; suicide is a real and ever-present danger throughout the entire illness
   8. Spend time with client to demonstrate staff's recognition of client's worth
   9. Recognize that client has ambivalence about suicide and is fearful of feelings
   10. Teach client about ECT treatments; stay with client after treatment; orient as necessary
   11. Refer for grief counseling, assertiveness training, and anger management

C. Evaluation/Outcomes
   1. Avoids acting out suicidal ideation
   2. Verbalizes feelings
   3. Verbalizes increased feelings of self-worth

4. Continues prescribed treatment regimen
5. Returns to preillness level of function

MANIC EPISODE OF A BIPOLAR DISORDER

Data Base

A. Etiologic factors: see Data Base under Bipolar Disorder
B. Behavioral/clinical findings
   1. Abnormally and persistently elevated, expansive, or irritable mood for a duration of 1 week, plus three or more of the following symptoms:
      a. Grandiosity
      b. Insomnia
      c. Verbosity (pressured speech)
      d. Flight of ideas
      e. Hypersexuality
      f. Distractibility
      g. Social intrusiveness
      h. Psychomotor agitation
      i. Excessive involvement in pleasurable activities without regard for consequences
   2. Marked impairment in functioning, occupational and social activities and relationships
   3. Extreme overactivity requires hospitalization to prevent harm to self or others
   4. Symptoms are unrelated to a general medical condition or physiologic effects of a substance
C. Therapeutic interventions
   1. High-protein, high-carbohydrate diet is provided for energy; hand-held foods should be available; adequate fluids
   2. Psychotherapy once medication has decreased mania
   3. Pharmacologic approach: improves productivity by decreasing psychomotor activity or response to environmental stimuli

Nursing Care of Clients During a Manic Episode of a Bipolar Disorder

A. Assessment/Analysis
   (Table 19-2: Bipolar Disorder: Symptoms of Mania)

Table 19-1 Bipolar Disorder: Symptoms of Depression			
Affect	**Cognition**	**Physiology**	**Behavior**
Apathy	Pessimism	Anorexia	Decreased ADLs
Anhedonia	Worry	Insomnia	Irritability
Anxiety	Poor concentration	Early morning awakening	Agitation
Anger	Slowed thinking	Fatigue	Psychomotor retardation
Guilt	Indecisiveness	Constipation	Social withdrawal
Helplessness	Hypochondriasis	Impotence	Crying
Loneliness	Suicidal ideation	Decreased libido	Self-abusive acts
Low self-esteem	Negative self-appraisal	Initially some clients experience hypersomnia	Substance abuse
Sadness	Psychosis	and compulsive eating; this changes as	
Emptiness		depression worsens to anorexia and	
Flat expression		insomnia	

1. Progression of manic behavior
2. Extent of elevated mood
3. Extent of psychomotor agitation
4. Impairment in functioning, including activities of daily living
5. Feelings of grandiosity and euphoria
6. Nutrition, hygiene, and rest patterns
7. Danger to self or others
8. Physiologic status

B. Planning/Implementation
   1. See General Nursing Care of Clients With Mood Disorders
   2. Accept client while rejecting objectionable behavior
   3. Permit expression of hostility and ambivalence without reinforcement of guilt feelings; usually precipitated by anxiety
   4. Approach in a calm, collected manner and maintain self-control
   5. Set limits for behavior; channel excess energy into safe, nonstrenuous, noncompetitive activities
   6. Communicate in a nonargumentative manner
   7. Use client's easy distractibility to interrupt hyperactive behavior, which may avoid injury and exhaustion
   8. Advise all caregivers to approach client in a consistent manner
   9. Prevent physical exhaustion and maintain physical health; provide foods that can be eaten on the run
   10. Maintain environmental safety for client, other clients, and staff
   11. Direct and channel client's energy into safe, controlled activities
   12. Maintain client's contact with reality by helping with grooming and dressing
   13. Monitor medications and side effects
   14. Educate family as to early symptoms of hypomanic episode

C. Evaluation/Outcomes
   1. Exhibits a decrease in manic behavior
   2. Verbalizes feelings of increased self-worth
   3. Displays improvement in judgment
   4. Relaxes more readily
   5. Maintains adequate nutrition

6. Adheres to medication regimen
7. Demonstrates an absence of destructive behaviors

MAJOR DEPRESSION

Data Base
A. Etiologic factors
   1. See Data Bases under Bipolar Disorder and Depressive Episode of a Bipolar Disorder
   2. Neurotransmitter dysregulation includes serotonin, norepinephrine, dopamine, acetylcholine, and GABA systems; neuropeptides are also altered, including corticotropin-releasing hormones
   3. Individuals with chronic or severe medical conditions are at increased risk
   4. Psychosocial stressors associated with a major loss play a significant role in first or second depressive onset
   5. Familial history among close biologic relatives increases risk for this disorder
   6. Onset usually occurs in late 20s, but may occur across the life span
B. Behavioral/clinical findings
   1. Diminished interest or pleasure in all activities; apathy and anhedonia
   2. Decreased appetite with weight loss or overeating with weight gain
   3. Psychomotor retardation; anergia; constipation
   4. Anxiety, somatic complaints, tearfulness, fearfulness, and hopelessness
   5. Insomnia or hypersomnia
   6. Feelings of worthlessness
   7. Inappropriate guilt
   8. Interruption in thinking and concentration that may interfere with occupational and social functioning; difficulty in making decisions
   9. Recurrent pessimistic thoughts; suicidal ideation with or without a plan (Table 19-3: Suicide: Stressors and Risk Factors and Lethality of Means Chosen)
C. Therapeutic interventions
   1. See Depressive Episode of a Bipolar Disorder, Data Base, Therapeutic interventions)

Nursing Care of Clients With Major Depression
A. See General Nursing Care of Clients With Mood Disorders
B. See Nursing Care of Clients During a Depressive Episode of a Bipolar Disorder

CYCLOTHYMIC DISORDER

Data Base
A. Etiologic factors
   1. There are numerous hypomanic episodes dispersed with periods of depressed mood and lack of interest in pleasurable activities
   2. No evidence of true manic or major depressive episodes

Table 19-2 Bipolar Disorder: Symptoms of Mania			
Affect	Cognition	Physiology	Behavior
Extroverted	Poor insight	Weight loss	Pressured speech
Irritable/brittle	Impulsive	Dehydration	Increased libido
Overly optimistic	Poor judgment	Poor nutrition	Spending sprees
Euphoric/high	No introspection	Lack of sleep	Restlessness
Labile	Poor concentration	Does not feel tired	Wastes energy
Lack of shame or guilt	Flight of ideas		Legal troubles
Overly humorous	Loose association		Aggressive
Low intimacy	Poor reality testing		Irresponsible
	Very distractible		Inappropriate attire
	Grandiose and persecutory delusions		Socially intrusive
	Weak ego boundaries		

Table 19-3 Suicide: Stressors and Risk Factors and Lethality of Means Chosen

Stressors and Risk Factors

Older adults
Male gender
Single status
Social isolation
Chronic and painful illnesses
Substance abuse (including overdose, intoxication, withdrawal)
History of attempts
Specific plan
Availability of means to commit suicide
Recent stressors
Psychiatric illness (especially depression and schizophrenia)
Inadequate coping skills
Religious/cultural attitudes
Lethality of intended means of suicide

LETHALITY OF MEANS CHOSEN

Higher	Lower
Hanging	Overdose
Guns	Wrist cutting
Jumping	

People die from "lower lethality" methods. All suicidal threats, gestures, and attempts must be taken seriously.

3. Symptom-free intervals are generally shorter than 2 months duration
4. The mood disturbance is not due to physiologic effects of substances or to a medical condition
5. Duration: at least 2 years in adults; in children/adolescents, mood can be irritable for at least 1 year
B. Behavioral/clinical findings
 1. Alternating mood swings between elation and sadness; apparently unrelated to external environment
 2. Individual is regarded as temperamental, moody, unpredictable, inconsistent, or unreliable
 3. Mood swings do not demonstrate great emotional intensity
 4. Refer to Data Base under Bipolar Disorder for hypomanic symptoms
C. Therapeutic interventions
 1. Often unnecessary; if required, same as those for Depressive or Manic Episode of a Bipolar Disorder
 2. Medication often unnecessary; if required, same as those for Depressive or Manic Episode of a Bipolar Disorder

Nursing Care of Clients With a Cyclothymic Disorder

A. See General Nursing Care of Clients with Mood Disorders
B. See Nursing Care of Clients During a Depressive Episode of a Bipolar Disorder
C. See Nursing Care of Clients During a Manic Episode of a Bipolar Disorder

DYSTHYMIC DISORDER

Data Base

A. Etiologic factors
 1. Biochemical theories continue to be researched
 2. Genetic transmission theories of mood disorders are derived from family studies
 3. Depression is real and suicide can occur
 4. Feelings of guilt or brooding about the past
B. Behavioral/clinical findings
 1. Depressed mood for most of day
 2. Duration: at least 2 years in adults; in children and adolescents, mood can be irritable for at least 1 year
 3. Two or more of the following: depressed appetite or overeating, insomnia, low energy or fatigue, low self-esteem, concentration/problem-solving difficulties, feelings of hopelessness; anergia
 4. Impairment in social, occupational, and other roles
 5. No evidence of manic or hypomanic episodes in present or past history
 6. In children/adolescents the symptoms noted are irritability and depression; low self-esteem, poor social skills, and pessimism; school performance and social interactions are impaired
C. Therapeutic interventions
 1. Often unnecessary; if required, same as those for Depressive Episode of a Bipolar Disorder
 2. Medications often unnecessary; if required, same as those for Depressive Episode of a Bipolar Disorder

Nursing Care of Clients With a Dysthymic Disorder

A. See General Nursing Care of Clients With Mood Disorders
B. See Nursing Care of Clients During a Depressive Episode of a Bipolar Disorder

20

OVERVIEW

A. The primary/initial deficit occurs in behavior, although there will be changes in the client's mood and cognition
B. Includes disorders with dysfunctional behaviors
1. Sleep disorders
2. Eating disorders
3. Personality disorders
4. Adjustment disorders
5. Substance abuse
6. Factitious disorders (although not classified as psychiatric illnesses in the *DSM-IV-TR*, they are also maladaptive behaviors and will be presented here)

MAJOR DISORDERS RELATED TO ALTERATIONS IN BEHAVIOR

✿ SLEEP DISORDERS

Data Base
A. Basic information
1. A common problem in adults, rarely treated in an inpatient psychiatric setting, can present as a symptom of depressive, manic, or anxiety disorders
2. Sleep consists of two distinct states: REM (rapid eye movement), also called dream sleep, and NREM (non-REM) sleep, which is divided into four stages
3. Sleep is a cyclic phenomenon with restorative qualities
4. The dreaming that occurs during sleep is also helpful to gain insights, solve problems, work through emotional reactions, and prepare for the future
5. Sleep disorders are conditions that repeatedly disrupt the pattern of sleep, leading to diminished performance
B. Etiologic factors
1. The sleep cycle evolves throughout the life cycle and becomes decreased with age
2. It is a disorder from which the client usually recovers, because the changes may be reversible and temporary if treated
3. Neuroendocrine arousal system thought to release corticosteroids by the hypothalamic-pituitary-adrenal axis, as well as stimulate the neurotransmitter system, producing norepinephrine and serotonin
4. Genetic factors show a biologic tendency may be inherited (e.g., light sleepers in a family); no single gene has been identified
5. Environmental factors thought to contribute to sleep disturbances, such as jet lag, shift work, fast pace of life, stress, and noise
6. Biologic factors such as cardiovascular, endocrine, psychiatric, infections, cough related to pulmonary disease, pain, use of stimulants including caffeine, and side effects or drug interactions of many medications all contribute to sleep-related problems
7. Impaired function results from sleep deprivation
C. Types
1. Primary
   a. Insomnia—disorder of initiating or maintaining sleep; anxiety and depression are major causes
   b. Parasomnias—disorders associated with sleep stages (sleepwalking, night terrors, nightmares, restless leg syndrome, and enuresis); most common in children
   c. Narcolepsy—disorder of repeated irresistible attacks of refreshing sleep
2. Secondary
   a. Sleep disorders related to mental disorders—noted in this category are anxiety-related disorders, depressive disorders, and manic episodes
   b. Substance-induced sleep disorders—included in this subclass are conditions related to intoxication, periods of withdrawal, use of stimulants, and side effects of many medications
   c. Sleep disorders related to general medical conditions—etiology must be established through history, physical examination, or laboratory findings in this subclass
D. Behavioral/clinical findings
1. Onset usually begins in young adulthood; more prevalent with increasing age
2. Difficulty initiating or maintaining sleep, or nonrestorative sleep, for at least 1 month
3. Depression is usually associated with fragmented sleep patterns
4. Sleeplessness is a cardinal feature noted in manic disorders; it is an early sign of impending mania in bipolar disorders

5. Abuse of alcohol or stimulants, heavy smoking, and use of OTC cold remedies cause decreased total sleep time
6. Insomnia precipitated by anxiety
E. Therapeutic interventions
1. Relaxation techniques
2. Sleep hygiene practices (e.g., use bed just for sleep, interrupt racing thoughts)
3. Sedative/hypnotic agents (see Sedative and Hypnotic Agents under Related Pharmacology in Chapter 16); used judiciously, particularly in older adults; used short-term, not long-term

Nursing Care of Clients With Sleep Disorders
A. Assessment/Analysis
1. History of onset, duration, and sleep patterns
2. Daily routines, night rituals
3. Diet and physical activity
4. Stressors
5. Level of daytime alertness, nap patterns
6. Restless leg movement, snoring
7. Drug, alcohol, caffeine, nicotine use
8. Pharmacologic or herbal remedies
B. Planning/Implementation
1. Provide a quiet, restful environment; demonstrate relaxation techniques
2. Plan care when client is receptive
3. Obtain a diet recall (diary) to assess food/liquid intake and caffeine consumption; instruct client to avoid stimulants (coffee, tea, chocolate, nicotine, and OTC cold remedies) at bedtime
4. Establish a daily exercise regimen during the day hours to reduce stress
5. Provide diversional activities during the day to avoid napping
6. Instruct client to eat a larger meal at noon rather than at dinner
7. Establish set sleep patterns and promote effective sleep hygiene practices
8. Promote comfort and control physical disturbances at night; provide a private room if necessary
9. Instruct to limit bedroom activities to sleep and sex; leave the bedroom if unable to sleep
10. Assist with ruling out medical conditions that contribute to sleep-related problems
C. Evaluation/Outcomes
1. Copes with anxiety-producing situations effectively
2. Uses relaxation techniques
3. Limits use of stimulants
4. Reports restorative sleep
5. Reports improved sense of well-being

EATING DISORDERS
Overview
A. Eating behaviors and perceptions of body shape and weight are severely disturbed
B. Anorexia and bulimia nervosa may be present in the same client or exist separately

C. Compulsive overeating, although not currently classified as an eating disorder, is another maladaptive behavior involving eating

General Nursing Care of Clients With Eating Disorders
A. Recognize that the adolescent or adult requires
1. Basic physiologic and safety needs to be met
2. Acceptance
3. Meaningful relationships
4. Limit setting of manipulative behavior
5. Monitoring during and after mealtime
6. An awareness of type, amount, and patterns of food eaten (food diary)
7. Consultation with nutritionist to determine adequate dietary regimen
B. Direct care toward helping the individual to mature
1. Establishing a relationship based on trust
2. Promoting self-worth
3. Setting limits that are realistic
4. Being consistent in approach and in rules and regulations
5. Supporting and encouraging independence
6. Teaching more effective ways of coping
7. Encouraging participation in individual and family therapy

ANOREXIA NERVOSA
Data Base
A. Etiologic factors
1. Decreased levels of norepinephrine, serotonin, and dopamine
2. Combination of genetic, neurochemical, developmental, psychologic, social, cultural, and familial factors cited
3. More common in females
4. Avoidance of food may result from excessive concern with obesity
5. Apparent failure to separate from mother and become autonomous; unconscious fear of growing up
6. Onset usually during adolescence through young adulthood; less common in older adults but is increasing in perimenopausal women
B. Behavioral/clinical findings
1. Subtypes
   a. Restricting type: weight loss is accomplished through dieting, fasting, or excessive exercise
   b. Binge eating/purging type: weight loss is accomplished through binge eating or purging (or both); use of self-induced vomiting and misuse of laxatives, diuretics, or enemas on weekly basis
2. Weight less than 85% of expected weight
3. Distorted self-image; appear fat to themselves even when emaciated
4. Intense fear of becoming fat, even though underweight

5. May have history of compulsive traits such as rigidity, ritualistic behavior, and meticulousness; need to control or prove control
6. Usually very manipulative
7. Usually high achievers academically
8. Frequent discord in family relationships, especially with mother
9. Often interested in food and cooking in general; serves as a control strategy
10. Cessation of menses in females
11. Inability to sustain self-starvation may result in bulimic episodes (bingeing of food followed by self-induced vomiting)
12. Fatigue or hyperactivity
13. Feeling of fullness after small intake
14. Nausea
15. Constipation
16. Emaciation
17. Hypotension; fluid and electrolyte disturbances; dependent edema
18. Low blood glucose level
19. Anemia
20. Erosion of tooth enamel (if vomiting)
21. Lanugo (fine, brittle body hair)
C. Therapeutic interventions
1. Unified team approach
2. Behavior modification techniques that focus on client's responsibility for weight gain
3. Time limit on meals
4. Use of nasogastric tube if weight loss is so great or fluid and electrolyte imbalance is so severe that it causes a threat to life
5. Psychotherapy focusing on self-image
6. Group and cognitive therapy
7. Family therapy with all members of family involved
8. Gradual increase in calories and protein under guidance of nutritionist
9. Antidepressants have been helpful especially with comorbid depression

Nursing Care of Clients With Anorexia Nervosa

A. Assessment/Analysis
1. Complete physical and dental examination to rule out associated medical complications of eating disorder
   a. Involved systems are CNS, renal, hematologic, gastrointestinal, endocrine, and cardiovascular
   b. Skin, hair (lanugo—fine, brittle body hair), and nutritional status
2. Weight and height
3. Signs of fluid and electrolyte imbalance
4. History of amenorrhea
5. Indulgence in excessive exercise
6. Behavior reflecting obsessiveness with food
7. History of stringent control of intake of food
8. Depressive mood
9. Motivation to change maladaptive eating patterns

B. Planning/Implementation
1. Refer to General Nursing Care of Clients With Eating Disorders
2. Develop a therapeutic environment
3. Establish a behavior modification program
4. Help client identify feelings
5. Briefly discuss dietary modification with the client in a nonthreatening manner
6. Provide diet high in nutrient-dense foods
7. Do not focus on eating or weight loss
C. Evaluation/Outcomes
1. Maintains dietary intake adequate to meet daily caloric requirements
2. Reaches and maintains appropriate body weight
3. Develops realistic body image
4. Identifies and verbalizes feelings
5. Accepts age-appropriate role
6. Resolves separation and individuation issues

✿ BULIMIA NERVOSA

Data Base

A. Etiologic factors
1. Most common in adolescent through 30-year-old population
2. More common in females but seen in males who need to maintain low weights, such as jockeys
3. Obesity is frequently found in parents or siblings
4. Predisposition to depression
5. Discord in family relationships
6. Obsession with food results from a morbid fear of obesity and the pathologic need to binge
B. Behavioral/clinical findings
1. Subtypes
   a. Purging type: engages in purging behaviors
   b. Nonpurging type: uses fasting or excessive exercise, not purging
2. Compulsive eating binges characterized by rapid consumption of excessive amounts of high-caloric foods in brief periods followed by induced purging (vomiting, enemas, laxatives, or diuretics)
3. Periods of severe dieting or fasting between binges
4. Sporadic vigorous exercising between binges
5. Weight may be within expected range with frequent fluctuations above or below expected range because of alternating binges and fasts
6. Lack of control over eating during episode
7. Depression and self-deprecating thoughts follow binges
8. Bingeing and purging patterns occurring at least biweekly, for past 3 months
9. Extroverted
10. Possible intermittent substance abuse
11. Very concerned with body image and appearance
12. Repeated attempts to control or lose weight
C. Therapeutic interventions
1. See Therapeutic Interventions under Anorexia Nervosa, except for the use of a nasogastric tube

2. Treatment of depression, which is the most frequently observed psychologic concomitant condition associated with bulimia

Nursing Care of Clients With Bulimia Nervosa

A. Assessment/Analysis
   1. Behavior indicative of purging such as self-induced vomiting and use of enemas, laxatives, and/or diuretics
   2. Obsession with excessive exercise
   3. Pattern and duration of bingeing
   4. Undue concern with body weight and shape
   5. Physiologic changes such as dental caries, chipped teeth, enlarged parotid glands, calluses, or scars on knuckles from induced vomiting
   6. Signs of fluid and electrolyte imbalances
   7. Weight and height
   8. History of consuming tremendous amounts of calories in a short period of time
   9. Symptoms of depression or obsessive-compulsive behaviors
   10. Substance abuse (drug[s], pattern, duration)
B. Planning/Implementation
   1. See General Nursing Care of Clients With Eating Disorders
   2. Provide a nonjudgmental, accepting environment
   3. Set realistic limits; keep client under close observation to prevent purging
   4. Encourage verbalization of feelings
   5. Help client to identify feelings associated with bingeing and purging
   6. Shift focus from food, eating, and exercise to emotional issues
C. Evaluation/Outcomes
   1. Limits dietary intake to caloric requirements
   2. Reduces episodes of bingeing
   3. Reduces episodes of purging
   4. Identifies feelings
   5. Verbalizes emotions and needs
   6. Reports no depressive symptoms

PERSONALITY DISORDERS

Data Base

A. Basic information
   1. These disorders are extreme exaggerations of personality traits or styles that often define the uniqueness of the individual
   2. Under stress, individuals manifest patterns of inflexibility, maladaptive emotional responses, and functioning impairments
   3. A personality disorder, according to the *DSM-IV-TR*, is an "enduring pattern of inner experiences and behavior that deviates markedly from the expectations of the individual's culture, is pervasive and inflexible, has an onset in adolescence or early adulthood, is stable over time, and leads to distress or impairment."

B. Etiologic factors
   1. Psychodynamic theory postulates that individuals with personality disorders have deficits in psychosexual development or failure to achieve object constancy
   2. Neurobiologic perspective
      a. Research evidence suggests that the development of major personality disorders is determined by environmental factors that interact with biologic factors such as inability to tolerate anxiety, aggressiveness, and genetic vulnerability to certain affects
      b. Family and twin studies are demonstrating a strong genetic influence; this suggests some connection between biologic factors and personality organization
      c. Study findings suggest a structural brain deficit in antisocial personality disorder that may cause low arousal, low fear, lack of conscience, and deficits in decision making
      d. Further research is needed to clarify the role of inheritance in relation to brain structure and function in the development of personality disorders
   3. Sociocultural factors (isolation and family instability) can influence the ability to establish and maintain relationships
   4. Relationship problems develop early in life, and often move through predictable stages ranging from idealization and overevaluation and ending with rationalization, devaluation, and rejection of others person
   5. Premorbid personality of individuals demonstrating any of these disorders resembles the compensatory mechanisms associated with the pathologic counterpart
C. Types and behavioral/clinical findings
   1. Antisocial personality disorder
      a. Chronic lifelong disturbance that conflicts with society's laws and customs
      b. Inability to postpone gratification; lives only for the moment
      c. Randomly acts out aggressive egocentric impulses on society
      d. Does not profit from past experiences or punishment; does not take responsibility for actions and blames others for problems
      e. Has the ability to ingratiate self but wears down others
      f. Is in contact with reality but does not seem to care about it or people
      g. More common in men
   2. Avoidant personality disorder
      a. Social discomfort and timidity
      b. Loner; unwilling to get involved with others
      c. Fear of negative evaluation from others
   3. Borderline personality disorder
      a. Unstable and intense interpersonal relationships
      b. Impulsive, unpredictable behavior that is potentially self-destructive

c. Marked mood shifts

d. Identity disturbance

e. Chronic feeling of emptiness

f. History of parental abuse or neglect in early childhood; sexual abuse by nonparents

g. More common in women

4. Dependent personality disorder

a. Unable to make decisions

b. Lack of self-confidence

c. Dependent and submissive

d. Induces others to assume responsibility

5. Histrionic personality disorder

a. Emotional instability and hyperexcitability

b. Extroverted and directed toward gaining attention

c. Vain and deliberately manipulative

6. Narcissistic personality disorder

a. Overblown sense of importance

b. Strong need for attention and admiration

c. Relationships marked by ambivalence

d. Preoccupation with appearance

7. Obsessive-compulsive personality disorder

a. Rigidity, overconscientiousness, inordinate capacity for work

b. Driven by obsessive concerns

c. Behavior contains many rituals that the client cannot control

8. Paranoid personality disorder

a. Frequent use of projective mechanisms

b. Suspiciousness, fear, irritability, and stubbornness

c. Reality testing not greatly impaired

9. Schizoid personality disorder

a. Avoidance of meaningful interpersonal relationships; prefers solitary activities

b. Use of autistic thinking, emotional detachment, and daydreaming

c. Introverted since childhood but maintaining fair contact with reality

d. Asexual

10. Schizotypal personality disorder

a. Unattached, withdrawn

b. Affectively and intellectually diminished

c. Frequently part of the vagabond or transient groups of society

d. Behavior or appearance that is eccentric or peculiar

11. Personality disorder not otherwise specified (components of mixed disorders, passive-aggressive, or depressive personality disorder)

a. Does not meet criteria for a specific personality disorder

b. Generally has features of more than one specific type (mixed disorders)

c. Causes clinically significant distress of functional impairment beginning in early adulthood

d. Also included are depressive and passive-aggressive personality disorders

(1) Depressive personality disorder characteristics include several of the following

(a) Usual mood dominated by dejection, gloom, unhappiness

(b) Low self-esteem

(c) Critical and negativistic toward others

(d) Pessimistic

(e) Prone to feelings of guilt and remorse

(2) Passive-aggressive personality disorder characteristics include several of the following

(a) Passively resists fulfilling social and occupational tasks

(b) Complains of not being understood or appreciated

(c) Is sullen and argumentative

(d) Envious and resentful of others more fortunate

(e) Exaggerates and complains of personal misfortune

(f) Alternates between hostile defiance and contrition

(3) Both of these disorders deleted from *DSM-IV-TR* for further study; included here as a reminder of negativistic traits

D. Therapeutic interventions

1. Individual, group, and family psychotherapy

2. Crisis intervention when necessary

3. Vocational and occupational therapy

4. Psychotropic drugs have a limited role

5. Dialectical behavioral therapy

Nursing Care of Clients With Personality Disorders

A. Assessment/Analysis

1. Level of social and occupational functioning

2. Individual's perception of problem

3. Why client is seeking treatment at this time

4. Level of anxiety

5. Pending criminal charges

6. Drug and alcohol abuse

7. History of suicidal gestures and present risk

B. Planning/Implementation

1. Maintain consistency, concern, and a professional relationship

2. Accept the individual as is; do not retaliate if provoked

3. Protect the individual from others while protecting others from the individual

4. Place realistic limits on behavior; make known what those limits are

5. Strive for consistency among health team members; avoid splitting of staff

6. Initiate cognitive and behavioral strategies

C. Evaluation/Outcomes

1. Demonstrates decreased episodes of acting out

2. Verbalizes decrease in anxiety

3. Accepts and continues long-term therapy

4. Recognizes and functions within limits of personality

✳ ADJUSTMENT DISORDERS

Data Base

A. Etiologic factors
1. These disorders are characterized by a short-term disturbance in mood or behavior with nonpsychotic manifestations resulting from identifiable stressors
2. The severity of the reaction is not predictable by the severity of the stressors
3. Problematic response to life events, either developmental or situational
4. Interaction of personality, crisis, developmental factors, and cultural influences should be considered
5. No apparent underlying mental disorder, but client may have low self-esteem and present behavior may be extremely disturbed
6. Exhibits capacity to adapt to the overwhelming stress when given the time to do so
7. Problems with distortions or interruptions in thinking processes and decision making tend to resolve themselves

B. Behavioral/clinical findings
1. Infancy: extremely upset; demonstrating grief when separated from mother
2. Childhood: regression to an earlier level of development when a new sibling arrives; intense anxiety on entering school
3. Adolescence: struggle for independence; leads to hypersensitivity and frequent episodes of heightened anxiety
4. Adult life: heightened anxiety in response to the stressors associated with events such as marriage, pregnancy, divorce, change of employment, purchase of a house
5. Later life: menopause and climacteric, "loss" of children to marriage, retirement, and death of a mate produce extreme stress
6. Onset begins within 3 months of stressors
7. Significant impairment in social and occupational functioning
8. Duration of disorder lasts no longer than 6 months after stress has ceased
9. Onset may occur at any age; commonly noted in children and adolescents

C. Therapeutic interventions
1. See Therapeutic interventions under Panic Disorders in Chapter 19

Nursing Care of Clients With Adjustment Disorders

A. Assessment/Analysis
1. Individual's perception of problem
2. Factors impinging on current situation
3. Individual's personal strengths and support systems
4. Level of anxiety
5. Identification of type(s) of stressors and onset

B. Planning/Implementation
1. Help the client and/or parents recognize and accept that a problem exists

2. Maintain client safety
3. Encourage the identification and use of support systems
4. Attempt to minimize environmental pressures
5. Allow the client time to recover personal resources

C. Evaluation/Outcomes
1. Reorganizes defenses
2. Utilizes support systems
3. Verbalizes a decrease in anxiety
4. Develops more effective coping

✳ SUBSTANCE ABUSE

Overview

A. Substance refers to a drug of abuse, a medication, or a toxin
B. Substance abuse: maladaptive pattern of drug use leading to impairment or distress, as manifested by one or more of the following occurring within a 12-month period
1. Failure to fulfill major roles
2. Use in hazardous situations
3. Recurring related legal problems
4. Continued use despite social or interpersonal problems
C. Although not currently classified as addiction diagnoses in the *DSM-IV-TR*, behaviors such as compulsive gambling, compulsive sexual activity, and compulsive overeating are now being treated as addictive disorders similar to substance-related disorders
D. Substance intoxication: a reversible substance-specific syndrome caused by recent ingestion of, or exposure to, a substance resulting in maladaptive behavior or psychologic changes from effect on the CNS
E. Substance withdrawal: development of a substance-specific syndrome resulting from cessation or reduction in substance use that has been heavy or prolonged
1. Impairment in role functioning (social, school, or occupational)
2. Symptoms are not from another mental disorder
F. Substance tolerance: the need for greatly increased amounts of the substance to achieve the desired effects or a markedly diminished effect with the continued use of the same amount of substance
G. Polysubstance abuse: abuse of two or more drugs or of alcohol and drugs
H. Potentiation: two or more substances interact in the body to produce an effect greater than the sum of the effects of each substance taken alone
I. Substance dependence: the continued use of a substance despite significant related problems in cognitive, physiologic, and behavioral components; spending more time in getting, taking, and recovering from the substance; continuous abuse despite knowledge of physical or psychologic problems or awareness of complications resulting from continued use of the substance

✤ ALCOHOL ABUSE

Data Base

A. Etiologic factors
   1. Depression of major brain functions (mood, cognition, attention, concentration, insight, judgment, memory, affect) resulting in diminished emotional rapport with others
   2. Alcohol is a CNS depressant that is dose-dependent and ranges from lethargy, unconsciousness, coma, respiratory distress, to death
   3. Causation theories range from genetic, stress, or environmental factors to interpersonal factors; none fully explains causation
   4. Neurobiologic perspective
      a. The biologic or genetic theory continues to be researched
      b. Some research has identified subtypes of alcoholism; one type is associated with early onset, inability to abstain, and an antisocial personality; another type is associated with later onset (after age 25), inability to stop drinking once started, and a passive-dependent personality; this latter type seems more to be influenced by the environment
      c. Some researchers subscribe to the single genetic transmission; others think that complex genetic factors are involved in alcoholism
      d. Biologic differences in the response to alcohol may influence susceptibility
B. Behavioral/clinical findings
   1. Intoxication: state in which coordination or speech is impaired and behavior is altered
   2. Episodic excessive drinking: becoming intoxicated as infrequently as four times a year; episodes may vary in length from hours to days or weeks; may be called binge drinking
   3. Habitual excessive drinking: becoming intoxicated more than 12 times a year or being recognizably under the influence of alcohol more than once a week even though not considered intoxicated
   4. Alcohol addiction: direct or strong presumptive evidence of dependence on alcohol; demonstrated by withdrawal symptoms (e.g., nausea, hypertension, anorexia) or by the inability to go for a day without drinking; when there is a history of heavy drinking for 3 or more months, the individual is considered addicted to alcohol
   5. Rationalization and denial are often used defense mechanisms; may fill in gaps in memory with fabricated information (confabulation)
   6. Early symptoms of alcoholism: frequent drinking sprees, increased intake, drinking alone or in the early morning
   7. Chronic excessive alcohol consumption leads to multisystem physiologic impairments including cardiomyopathy, peripheral neuropathy, blackouts, Wernicke's encephalopathy, and Korsakoff's syndrome

C. Therapeutic interventions
   1. Should be multifaceted (social and medical); involves psychotherapy (group, family, and individual counseling); clients can be assisted only when they admit they need help
   2. Self-help groups such as Alcoholics Anonymous provide support; most effective intervention to change destructive behaviors
   3. Pharmacologic therapies
      a. Negative conditioning with disulfiram (Antabuse) appears to help but never given without the client's full knowledge, understanding, and consent
      b. Naltrexone hydrochloride (Trexan, ReVia) to help overcome the craving for alcohol
      c. Thiamine given to support neurologic functioning and limit peripheral neuropathies
   4. Relaxation therapy
   5. Physical needs must be met because dietary needs have often been ignored for long periods
   6. Assist family with effects of alcoholism and issues of codependency and enabling; self-help groups such as Al-Anon and Adult Children of Alcoholics

Nursing Care of Clients Who Abuse Alcohol

A. Assessment/Analysis
   1. History of alcohol use/abuse from client and family if available
   2. Use of the CAGE questionnaire
      a. Have you ever felt that you ought to Cut down on your drinking?
      b. Have people Annoyed you by criticizing your drinking?
      c. Have you ever felt Guilty about your drinking?
      d. Have you ever had a drink first thing in the morning (Eye opener) to steady your nerves or get rid of a hangover?
   3. Blood alcohol level (BAL); people with high tolerance to alcohol will appear less intoxicated despite having elevated blood alcohol levels (Table 20-1: Effects of Blood Alcohol Levels)
   4. Data collection pertaining to substance dependence and psychiatric impairment
   5. Client's perception of the problem
   6. Sleep patterns
   7. Use of the Clinical Institute Withdrawal Assessment for Alcohol (CIWA-Ar) Scale to assess withdrawal and evaluate medication used to limit withdrawal symptoms (Table 20-2: Clinical Institute Withdrawal Assessment for Alcohol [CIWA-Ar] Scale)
   8. Physical and emotional status in relation to needs associated with nutrition, fluid and electrolyte status, and safety
   9. Factors influencing the client's decision to seek treatment at this time
B. Planning/Implementation
   1. Supervise and prevent injury if client is intoxicated
   2. Monitor for CNS and respiratory depression

Table 20-1 Effects of Blood Alcohol Levels

Blood Alcohol Level	Effect on Body
0.02	Slight mood changes
0.06	Lowered inhibition, impaired judgment, decreased rational decision-making abilities
0.08	Legally drunk, deterioration of reaction time and control
0.15	Impaired balance, movement, and coordination Difficulty standing, walking, talking
0.20	Decreased pain and sensation Erratic emotions
0.30	Diminished reflexes Semiconsciousness
0.40	Loss of consciousness Very limited reflexes Anesthetic effects
0.50	Death

Table 20-2 Clinical Institute Withdrawal Assessment for Alcohol [CIWA-Ar] Scale

Nausea and vomiting	None to constant nausea Frequent dry heaves Vomiting
Tremors	None to severe
Paroxysmal sweats	None to drenching sweats
Anxiety	None to equivalent to acute panic states
Agitation	None to pacing back and forth constantly Thrashing about
Tactile disturbances	None to continuous tactile hallucinations (itching, burning, numbness)
Auditory disturbances	None to continuous auditory hallucinations
Visual disturbances	None to continuous visual hallucinations
Headache	None to extremely severe
Orientation	Oriented to disoriented to place and/or person

Modified form Sullivan JT, Sykora K, Schneiderman J, et al: Assessment of alcohol withdrawal: the revised Clinical Institute Withdrawal Assessment for Alcohol Scale (CIWA-Ar). *Br J Addict* 84:1353-1357, 1989.

3. Provide a well-controlled, alcohol-free environment; explain unit routines
4. Plan a full program of activities but provide for adequate rest; environment should be well lit and quiet
5. Support the client without criticism or judgment
6. Expect and accept lapses as client is changing a long-term habit; accept failures without judgment or punishment; teach how to handle relapses
7. Avoid attempting to talk client out of the problem or making client feel guilty
8. Accept the smooth facade that the client may present while approaching the lonely and fearful individual behind it
9. Monitor visitors because they may supply the client with alcohol
10. Prevent the development of delirium tremens (DTs), hallucinations, and illusions; stay with and support client if DTs occur; point out reality if illusions or hallucinations occur
11. Accept hostility and acting-out behaviors without criticism or retaliation; set appropriate limits if hostility is physical or escalates
12. Recognize ambivalence and limit the need for decision making
13. Maintain the client's interest in a therapy program
14. Provide education on alcohol and negative physical and mental health
15. Refer to an appropriate 12-step group such as Alcoholics Anonymous
16. Provide family counseling to address effects of drinking and sobriety on the family

C. Evaluation/Outcomes
1. Recognizes, accepts, and seeks treatment for problem
2. Accepts responsibility for problem without blaming others
3. Achieves optimal physiologic and nutritional status
4. Learns new, more self-preserving coping mechanisms
5. Verbalizes feelings and situations that pose increased risk for alcohol use
6. Enters into and continues with community-based self-help program
7. Maintains abstinence from alcohol and chemical substances
8. Demonstrates responsibility in meeting own health care needs

✦ DRUG ABUSE

Data Base
A. Etiologic factors
1. Misuse of drugs, usually by self-administration, in such a way as to bring about physical, emotional, or behavioral changes and a blurring of reality
2. Stressors: premorbid personality, utilizing compensatory mechanisms of the addictive pattern of behavior
B. Addictive capacity depends on the drug, from lowest potential to highest potential (e.g., progressing from codeine, alcohol, and barbiturates to heroin); concurrent use of multiple drugs is called polysubstance use and usually includes alcohol
C. Behavioral/clinical findings
1. Physical examination may reveal an underweight, malnourished individual with multiple dental caries and depressed CNS functioning
2. Job or academic failure; marital conflicts; poor reality testing; personality change
3. History of violent acting out with total disregard for human life or suffering
4. History of stealing to support habit
5. Inability to maintain activities of daily living or fulfill role obligations
6. Marked tolerance with a progressive need for higher doses to achieve desired effects
7. Opiates (opioids)
   a. Needle marks (track marks), particularly on limbs or between toes, can lead to infections

(e.g., endocarditis, hepatitis, or HIV); wearing long-sleeved shirts, even in warm weather

b. Constricted pupils, drowsiness, slurred speech, psychomotor retardation

c. Yawning, lacrimation, rhinorrhea, and perspiration appear 10 to 15 hours after the last opiate injection; unrealistic high; pronounced depression

d. Severe abdominal cramps if too much time has elapsed between use

8. Cocaine

a. Hypervigilance, increased sexual activity, paranoid ideation, and cocaine-induced psychosis with hallucinations

b. Snorting leads to nasal septum destruction, hoarseness, and throat infections

c. Marked letdown with progression to severe depression after use

9. Techno drugs: ecstasy (MDMA, methylenedioxymethamphetamine) and ketamine resemble amphetamine effects; they are also known as recreational drugs

a. Adverse effects of psychostimulants can cause hyperthermia, acute renal failure, depression, panic, psychosis, and cardiovascular collapse

b. Sleep disorders, depression, high anxiety levels, hostility, and impulsiveness are all associated with recreational drug use

c. Sexual assault/rape drug flunitrazepam (Rohypnol) produces disinhibition and voluntary muscle relaxation along with anterograde amnesia; alcohol potentiates the effects

D. Therapeutic interventions

1. Treatment for drug overdose

a. Opioid (narcotic) antagonists

(1) Nalorphine (Nalline), a partial antagonist, and naloxone (Narcan), a pure antagonist, will improve respiratory rate, although they may not affect level of consciousness; respiratory depression can recur when these drugs are metabolized before the narcotic has been metabolized to a safe level

(2) Nalline will increase respiratory depression if barbiturates have also been used, so Narcan is the drug of choice when in doubt about the substance used

(3) These antagonists completely or partially reverse opioid (narcotic) depression and may produce an acute abstinence (withdrawal) syndrome by blocking the euphoric and physiologic effects of the opioid

b. Gastric lavage may be done if substance had been taken orally within the past several hours

2. Treatment for withdrawal symptoms

a. Antidepressants seem to block the "high" from stimulant abuse and diminish the craving for the substance

b. Clonidine (Catapres) suppresses opiate (narcotic) withdrawal symptoms and decreases adrenergic excess while opiate receptors return to normal levels

(1) Heroin addicts who are first stabilized on methadone before detoxification do better than those who go directly from heroin to Catapres

(2) Catapres should not be used in those individuals who also abuse alcohol or those who have unstable psychiatric or cardiovascular conditions

3. Methadone maintenance for opiate addiction: programs do not treat addiction, but change the addiction from an illegal drug to a legal drug, which is administered under supervision; has proven successful only in individuals with long-standing addictions

a. Reduction in dosage can cause withdrawal symptoms

b. Withdrawal symptoms begin to develop in 8 hours and may last as long as 2 weeks

c. Methadone is approved for treatment of pregnant opioid addicts

d. Lα-Acetylmethadol (LAAM) is an alternative to methadone; its 3-day effectiveness increases independence; it is an addictive opioid (narcotic) with effects similar to morphine

4. High-calorie, high-protein diet with vitamin supplements because of inadequate eating habits

5. Treatment in groups run by former addicts

6. Therapeutic community setting

7. Psychotherapy and family therapy on an outpatient basis

8. Vocational counseling

Nursing Care of Clients Who Abuse Drugs

A. Assessment/Analysis

1. History of drugs being used

2. Urine toxicology screen and HIV test

3. Drug abuse screening test

4. History of length and pattern of drug dependence

5. Time since last dose was taken

6. Physical status of the client for signs and symptoms of drug dependence; nutritional status

7. Signs of drug overdose or withdrawal; use of established scales (e.g., Clinical Institute Narcotic Assessment [CINA] Scale or Clinical Opiate Withdrawal Scale [COWS]) to help with completeness and consistency of assessment

8. Degree of difficulty sustaining role in relation to family members, job, school, etc.

9. Why client is seeking treatment at this time

10. Pending criminal charges

11. Presence of hallucinations, paranoid ideation, and depression (often associated with cocaine use)

12. Potential for violence toward others or self

13. Relationship between substance use and psychiatric disorders (known as dual diagnosis)
14. Potential for recurrence of drug abuse after period of withdrawal

B. Planning/Implementation
1. Set firm controls and keep area drug-free when the client is hospitalized
2. Keep atmosphere pleasant and cheerful but not overly stimulating
3. Contribute to the client's self-confidence, self-respect, and security in a realistic manner; focus on feelings
4. Walk the fine line between a relatively permissive and a firm attitude
5. Expect and accept evasion, manipulative behavior, and negativism, but require the client to shoulder certain standards of responsibility
6. Accept the client without approving the behavior
7. Do not permit the client to become isolated
8. Introduce the client to group activities as soon as possible; evaluate client's response to group interaction
9. Protect clients from themselves and others
10. Refer to appropriate 12-step group such as Alcoholics Anonymous and Narcotics Anonymous
11. Treat physical effects of substance abuse
12. Provide education related to the disease process and health effects

C. Evaluation/Outcomes
1. Recognizes, accepts, and seeks treatment for problem
2. Accepts responsibility for problem without blaming others
3. Achieves optimal physiologic and nutritional status
4. Learns new, more self-preserving coping mechanisms
5. Verbalizes feelings and emotions
6. Enters into and continues with community-based self-help program
7. Abstains from all mood-altering chemicals

❋ FACTITIOUS DISORDERS

Data Base
A. The *DSM-IV-TR* does not classify specific factitious disorders, but falling within this category are
1. Malingering: making a conscious attempt to deceive others by pretending to be sick
2. Munchausen syndrome: intentionally causing own illness; this may involve self-mutilation, fever, hemorrhage, hypoglycemia, seizures, nonhealing wounds, and abdominal or back pain
3. Munchausen syndrome by proxy: parent creates an illness in the child through simulation or production of illness; frequent symptoms include bleeding, seizures, apnea, diarrhea, vomiting, fever, and rash

B. Etiologic factors
1. Manipulation of the health care system for personal gain
2. No predisposing factor has been identified
3. People with health care knowledge may use it to aid in deception

C. Behavioral/clinical findings
1. Physical or psychologic symptoms that are intentionally produced or feigned to enable one to assume the sick role and for other secondary gains; back pain and recurrent headaches are two chief complaints
2. "Doctor shopping," seeking treatment in multiple emergency departments; commonly, little or no improvement is made in comfort or symptom management
3. Must be distinguished from a true medical condition through a medical workup
4. When under supervision of other caretakers, the child who is abused by Munchausen syndrome by proxy exhibits no symptoms
5. The somatoform disorders may be useful to help distinguish physiologic from intentional conditions

D. Therapeutic interventions
1. Psychiatric treatment
2. Supervision of child who is victim of Munchausen syndrome by proxy
3. Munchausen syndrome by proxy reported to child protective services

Nursing Care of Clients With Factitious Illness
A. Assessment/Analysis
1. Level of preoccupation with symptoms that keep recurring despite treatment
2. Absence of symptoms when client is closely observed
3. Past and present degree of interference with functioning related to symptoms
4. Duration and degree of disability associated with symptoms
5. History of psychosocial precipitant stressors

B. Planning/Implementation
1. Report suspected situations of Munchausen syndrome by proxy to child protective services
2. Recognize negative feelings toward the client for deception and remain nonjudgmental while establishing nurse-client relationship
3. Keep lines of communication open and direct
4. See General Nursing Care for Clients With Somatoform Disorders, Chapter 19

C. Evaluation/Outcomes
1. Uses more effective coping mechanisms to deal with anxiety than feigning illness
2. Accepts need for psychotherapy
3. Avoids causing harm to self or others

21 Nursing Care of Clients With Sexual and Gender Identity Disorders

OVERVIEW

A. Changing social and cultural mores have caused many of the sexual behaviors that were once considered deviations to be removed from the list of "abnormal practices"
B. Today sexual activities are considered abnormal only if they are directed toward anyone or anything other than consenting adults or are performed under unusual circumstances

GENERAL NURSING CARE OF CLIENTS WITH SEXUAL AND GENDER IDENTITY DISORDERS

A. Reflect on own sexual values and mores
B. Accept the individual as a person in emotional pain
C. Create a safe, nonjudgmental environment that permits open communication
D. Begin with less sensitive topics and move gradually to more personal issues
E. Avoid punitive or judgmental remarks or responses; speak in matter-of-fact manner
F. Provide for privacy and protect the individual from others
G. Set limits on the individual's sexual acting out
H. Report suspected child or elder abuse to appropriate protective service agencies

MAJOR DISORDERS ASSOCIATED WITH SEXUAL AND GENDER IDENTITY DISORDERS

❁ PARAPHILIAS

Data Base
A. Etiologic factors
   1. Paraphilias: sexual urges or fantasies that are directed toward nonhuman objects or infliction of pain to self, partner, children, or other nonconsenting individuals
   2. Behavior continues for at least 6 months; concurrent overt or covert emotional problems
B. Behavioral/clinical findings are based on type of paraphilia and include
   1. Exhibitionism: sexual pleasure by exposing the genitals

   2. Pedophilia: attraction to children as sex objects; acting on impulses results in child abuse
   3. Voyeurism: sexual gratification by watching the sexual play of others
   4. Sadism: sexual gratification by cruelty to others; acting on impulses may result in abuse of vulnerable person (child, older adult, significant other)
   5. Masochism: sexual gratification obtained from self-suffering
C. Therapeutic interventions
   1. Usually unsuccessful unless individual really wants to change
   2. Psychotherapy, cognitive and behavioral therapy may be effective if change is desired

Nursing Care of Clients With Paraphilias

A. Assessment/Analysis
   1. History of sexual behavior
   2. Presence of other psychosocial difficulties
   3. Level of anxiety regarding sexual behavior
   4. Pending criminal charges
   5. Why client is seeking treatment at this time
   6. Potential for violence toward others or self
B. Planning/Implementation
   See General Nursing Care for Clients With Sexual and Gender Identity Disorders
C. Evaluation/Outcomes
   1. Ceases socially unacceptable behavior
   2. Seeks and continues long-term therapy
   3. Limits paraphiliac behavior to consenting adults
   4. Utilizes safer sex practices

❁ SEXUAL DYSFUNCTION

Data Base
A. Etiologic factors
   1. Inhibition or interference with the desire, excitement, orgasm, or resolution phases of the sexual response cycle
   2. Dysfunction is often a combination of psychogenic and physiologic factors
   3. Dysfunction can be lifelong or acquired
   4. Dysfunction can be generalized or situational
B. Types and behavioral/clinical findings
   1. Sexual desire disorders: deficient, absent, or extreme aversion to and avoidance of sexual activity

2. Sexual arousal disorders: partial or complete failure to achieve a physiologic or psychologic (subjective) response to sexual activity
3. Orgasm disorders: delay in or absence of orgasm or premature ejaculation
4. Sexual pain disorders: recurrent or persistent genital pain before, during, or after sexual activity

C. Therapeutic interventions
1. Treatment of underlying physiologic cause if present
2. Sexual counseling for client and partner
3. Vacuum constriction device for males
4. Pharmacologic therapy: sildenafil (Viagra), tadalafil (Cialis), alprostadil (Muse, Caverject)
5. Surgical intervention: semi-rigid or inflatable penile prosthesis

Nursing Care of Clients With Sexual Dysfunction

A. Assessment/Analysis
1. Feelings about difficulties in functioning sexually
2. Expectations regarding sexual ability
3. Effect of sexual dysfunction on relationship with significant other

B. Planning/Implementation
1. See General Nursing Care for Clients With Sexual and Gender Identity Disorders
2. Recognize that the problem is real to the client regardless of age
3. Recognize that the desire to function sexually does not diminish with age
4. Teach about techniques and treatments (e.g., avoid alcohol, recreational drug use, and sedatives/hypnotics; use penile vacuum constrictive device)
5. Teach side effects of erectile agents such as sildenafil (Viagra): headache, flushing, dizziness, hypotension, diarrhea, dyspepsia; avoid concurrent use with nitroglycerin because it can cause cardiovascular collapse

C. Evaluation/Outcomes
1. Reports an increased satisfaction in sexual functioning
2. Reports sexual ability approaches sexual expectations

✳ GENDER IDENTITY DISORDERS

Data Base

A. Etiologic factors
1. Origins are unknown

2. Most children are firmly committed to gender role expectations as early as 18 months

B. Behavioral/clinical findings
1. Persistent discomfort with one's assigned gender and a feeling that it is inappropriate or inaccurate
2. Persistent preference for cross-sex roles
3. Cross-dressing

C. Therapeutic interventions
1. Individual or group psychotherapy
2. Antianxiety or antidepressant medication if necessary
3. Monitoring of children/adolescents over an extended period of time to aid in diagnosing
4. Surgical sex reassignment and hormone therapy

Nursing Care of Clients With Gender Identity Disorders

A. Assessment/Analysis
1. Distress about assigned sex role
2. Behaviors, social habits, and cross-dressing inappropriate for sexual gender
3. Preoccupation with becoming, being, or behaving as the opposite sex
4. History of sexual orientation (asexual, homosexual, bisexual, heterosexual)
5. Presence of depressive behaviors and suicidal ideation

B. Planning/Implementation
1. See General Nursing Care for Clients With Sexual and Gender Identity Disorders
2. Accept own feelings about client's cross-dressing
3. Accept and understand client's discomfort with gender
4. Encourage client to become involved with support groups
5. Be aware that if discomfort or depression is severe, self-mutilation and suicide are possibilities
6. Assist client to sort out solution (acceptance, suppression, information regarding surgical sex reassignment)

C. Evaluation/Outcomes
1. Verbalizes increased comfort with self
2. Ultimately accepts gender or explores surgical options
3. Participates in support groups

22 Mental Health/Psychiatric Nursing Review Questions With Answers and Rationales

QUESTIONS

FOUNDATIONS OF MENTAL HEALTH/ PSYCHIATRIC NURSING

1. The nurse understands that Freud's phallic stage of psychosexual development, which compares with Erikson's psychosocial phase of initiative versus guilt, is seen best at:
   1. Adolescence
   2. 6 to 12 years
   3. 3 to 5½ years
   4. Birth to 1 year

2. Which relationship is of most concern to the nurse because of its importance in the formation of the personality?
   1. Peer
   2. Sibling
   3. Parent-child
   4. Heterosexual

3. The nurse identifies that a client is using displacement. Which client behavior has the nurse identified?
   1. Ignoring unpleasant aspects of reality
   2. Resisting any demands made by others
   3. Using imaginative activity to escape reality
   4. Directing pent-up emotions to other than the primary source

4. In the process of development, the individual strives to maintain, protect, and enhance the integrity of the self. The nurse understands that this usually is accomplished through the use of:
   1. Affective reactions
   2. Withdrawal patterns
   3. Ritualistic behaviors
   4. Defense mechanisms

5. A client diagnosed with major depression tells the nurse, "No matter what I do, everything turns out bad." The nurse understands that this is an example of the client:
   1. Utilizing a cognitive distortion
   2. Seeking sympathy from the nurse
   3. Looking to avoid responsibility for actions
   4. Regressing to an earlier developmental level

6. A male college student, who is smaller than average and unable to participate in sports, becomes the life of the party and a stylish dresser. The nurse identifies this as an example of the defense mechanism of:
   1. Introjection
   2. Sublimation
   3. Compensation
   4. Reaction formation

7. A nursing assistant complains to the nurse that an older female client with dementia will complete tasks, but only when she feels like it, and wonders how one can deal with this. The nurse's response to the staff member should be based on the understanding that in addition to the dementia in this client, older adults:
   1. Lose their ability to cooperate
   2. Cannot perform step procedures
   3. Are ambivalent toward authority
   4. Have a decreased ability to cope

8. About a month after their toddler is diagnosed as moderately retarded, the parents discuss the toddler's future, reflecting specifically on plans for their child's independent functioning. The nurse recognizes that the parents:
   1. Are using denial
   2. Accept the child's diagnosis
   3. Are using intellectualization
   4. Accept their child's limitations

9. The nurse bases care on the generally accepted concept of personality development that states:
   1. By 2 years of age the personality is firmly set
   2. The personality is capable of change and modification throughout life
   3. The capacity for personality change decreases rapidly after adolescence
   4. By the end of the first 6 years, the personality has reached its adult parameters

10. One day a male client with the diagnosis of borderline personality disorder describes a situation that happened at work when his immediate supervisor reprimanded him for not completing an assignment. He explains that it was not his fault and states, "people get angry and take it out on me." Which defense mechanism identified by the nurse was the client using in this situation?
    1. Denial
    2. Projection

3. Displacement

4. Intellectualization

11. The nurse understands that problems with dependence versus independence develop during the stage of growth and development known as:

1. Infancy

2. School age

3. Toddlerhood

4. Preschool age

12. When planning to teach about the stages of growth and development, what stage does the nurse indicate as basically concerned with role identification?

1. Oral stage

2. Genital stage

3. Oedipal stage

4. Latency stage

13. The nurse utilizes play when interacting with children based on the understanding that play for the preschool-age child is necessary for the emotional development of:

1. Projection

2. Introjection

3. Competition

4. Independence

14. The nurse knows that the resolution of the Oedipus complex takes place when the child:

1. Rejects the parent of the same sex

2. Introjects behaviors of both parents

3. Identifies with the parent of the same sex

4. Identifies with the parent of the opposite sex

15. Surgery can be a very traumatic event for a child. The nurse, when performing preoperative preparation, knows that according to Piaget's stages of cognitive development, children will experience the greatest fear during the:

1. Sensorimotor stage

2. Preoperational stage

3. Formal operational stage

4. Concrete operational stage

16. A client is habitually expressing anxiety through physical symptoms. Which defense mechanism identified by the nurse is being used by this client?

1. Projection

2. Regression

3. Conversion

4. Hypochondriasis

17. The nurse understands that evidence of the existence of the unconscious is best demonstrated by:

1. Ease of recall

2. Slips of the tongue

3. Déjà vu experiences

4. Free-floating anxiety

18. The nurse on the psychiatric unit identifies that a client has an increased ability to tolerate frustration. The nurse knows that, according to psychoanalytic theory, the ability to tolerate frustration is an example of one of the functions of the:

1. Id

2. Ego

3. Superego

4. Unconscious

19. A male client experiencing delusions of persecution and auditory hallucinations is admitted for psychiatric evaluation. Later, the nurse on the unit greets the client by saying, "Good evening. How are you?" The client, who has been referring to himself as "man," answers, "The man is bad." This is an example of:

1. Dissociation

2. Transference

3. Displacement

4. Reaction formation

20. The nurse understands that the superego is that part of the psyche that:

1. Contains the instinctual drives

2. Is the source of creative energy

3. Develops from internalizing the concepts of parents and significant others

4. Operates on the pleasure principle and demands immediate gratification

21. A client with a diagnosis of borderline personality disorder has negative feelings toward the other clients on the unit and considers them all to be "bad." Which defense was being used by the client when the client made this statement?

1. Splitting

2. Ambivalence

3. Passive aggression

4. Reaction formation

22. In response to a question posed during a group meeting, the nurse explains that the superego is that part of the self that says:

1. "I like what I want."

2. "I want what I want."

3. "I should not want that."

4. "I can wait for what I want."

23. The nurse identifies that a person has a mature personality when the:

1. Ego conforms to the demands of the superego

2. Society sets demands to which the ego responds

3. Superego has replaced and increased all the controls of the parents

4. Ego acts as a balance between the pressures of the id and the superego

24. Incidents of child molestation often are revealed years later when the victim is an adult. The nurse teaches that this can best be explained by the ego defense mechanism of:

1. Repression

2. Regression

3. Rationalization

4. Reaction formation

25. A client with diabetes is able to discuss in great detail the metabolic process in diabetes while eating a piece of chocolate cake topped with butter frosting. What defense mechanism does the nurse identify when evaluating this behavior?

1. Projection

2. Dissociation

3. Displacement

4. Intellectualization

26. An older adult tells the nurse, "I regret many of the choices I have made during my life." Which of Erikson's developmental tasks does the nurse recognize that the client has probably failed to accomplish?
   1. Ego integrity versus despair
   2. Identity versus role diffusion
   3. Generativity versus stagnation
   4. Autonomy versus shame and doubt

27. A client states, "I get down on myself when I make a mistake." Using a cognitive therapy approach, what intervention is most appropriate by the nurse?
   1. Teach the client relaxation exercises to diminish stress
   2. Provide the client with mastery experiences to boost self-esteem
   3. Explore with the client past experiences that caused the client's distress
   4. Help the client modify the belief that anything less than perfection is horrible

28. Which of these techniques should the nurse teach a client to eliminate intrusive, unwanted thoughts?
   1. Reflecting
   2. Clouding/fogging
   3. Thought stopping
   4. Verbalizing the implied

29. A psychiatric unit uses a behavioral approach to determine clients' level of privileges. Which factor should the nurse use to determine an increase in privileges?
   1. A lifting of depression
   2. An improved short-term memory
   3. Performing hygiene activities independently
   4. Verbalizing a desire to change the response to stress

30. When teaching about child abuse, the nurse includes the fact that the defense mechanism most often used by the physically abusive individual is:
   1. Transference
   2. Manipulation
   3. Displacement
   4. Reaction formation

31. The nurse teaches a client that the level of anxiety that best enhances an individual's power of perception is:
   1. Mild
   2. Panic
   3. Severe
   4. Moderate

32. A client attending a mental health daycare unit is scheduled for several diagnostic studies. Which client behavior best indicates to the nurse that the client has received adequate preparation for these studies?
   1. The client requests that the tests be reexplained
   2. The client checks the appointment card repeatedly
   3. The client paces the hallway the morning before the tests
   4. The client arrives early, waiting quietly to be called for the tests

33. Before discharge, the nurse should teach the family of an anxious client that anxiety can be recognized as:
   1. A totally unique feeling
   2. Consciously motivated thoughts and wishes
   3. Fears that are related to the total environment
   4. A behavior pattern observed in ourselves and others

34. The nurse knows that sublimation is a defense mechanism that helps the individual:
   1. Act-out in reverse something already done or thought
   2. Return to an earlier, less mature, stage of development
   3. Channel unacceptable impulses into socially approved behavior
   4. Exclude from consciousness things that are psychologically disturbing

35. Strict toilet training before a child is ready will cause problems in personality development because at this age a child is learning to:
   1. Satisfy own needs
   2. Identify own needs
   3. Satisfy parents' needs
   4. Live up to society's expectations

THE PRACTICE OF MENTAL HEALTH/ PSYCHIATRIC NURSING

36. A nurse working on a unit in a psychiatric hospital is responsible for performing a variety of functions. Which are the ones that a registered nurse is legally permitted to perform? Identify all that apply.
   1. ☐ Psychotherapy
   2. ☐ Health promotion
   3. ☐ Case management
   4. ☐ Prescribing medication
   5. ☐ Treating human responses

37. The psychiatrist orders "Restraints PRN" for a client who has a history of violent behavior. The nurse should:
   1. Utilize the restraint order if the client begins to act-out
   2. Ask the psychiatrist to clarify the type of restraint order
   3. Ensure that the entire staff is aware of the restraint order
   4. Recognize that PRN orders for restraints are unacceptable

38. A client on the psychiatric unit asks the nurse about psychiatric advance directives (PAD). The nurse explains that these advance directives:
   1. Make the appointment of a surrogate decision maker unnecessary
   2. Permit the client to dictate what treatments will be given during future hospitalizations
   3. Eliminate the need for involuntary admissions when the client is a threat to self or others

4. Allow the client, while having the capacity, to consent or refuse potential psychiatric treatments in the event of a future incapacitating mental health crisis

39. The statement that best describes the practice of psychiatric nursing is:
   1. Helps people with present or potential mental health problems
   2. Ensures clients' legal and ethical rights by acting as a client advocate
   3. Focuses interpersonal skills on people with physical or emotional problems
   4. Acts in a therapeutic way with people who are diagnosed as having a mental disorder

40. A 45-year-old physician is admitted to the psychiatric unit of a community hospital. The client is restless, loud, aggressive, and resistive during the admission procedure and states, "I will take my own blood pressure." What is the most therapeutic response by the nurse?
   1. "Right now, doctor, you are just another client."
   2. "If you would rather, doctor, I'm sure you will do it OK."
   3. "If you do not cooperate, I will get the attendants to hold you down."
   4. "I am sorry, but I cannot allow that. I must take your blood pressure."

41. For most nurses the most difficult part of the nurse-client relationship is:
   1. Remaining therapeutic and professional
   2. Being able to understand and accept the client's behavior
   3. Developing an awareness of self and the professional role in the relationship
   4. Accepting responsibility in identifying and evaluating the real needs of the client

42. The father of a 16-year-old boy who has just been diagnosed with Hodgkin's disease tells the nurse he does not want his son to know the diagnosis. What response by the nurse is best in this situation?
   1. "It is best if he knows the diagnosis."
   2. "The cure rate for Hodgkin's disease is high."
   3. "Would you like someone with Hodgkin's to talk to you?"
   4. "Let's talk about why you don't want him to know."

43. A male nurse is caring for a client. The client states, "You know, I've never had a male nurse before." The nurse's best reply should be:
   1. "Does it bother you to have a male nurse?"
   2. "There aren't many of us; we're a minority."
   3. "How do you feel about having a male nurse?"
   4. "You sound upset. I will get a female nurse to care for you."

44. A male nurse reminds a client that it is time for group therapy. The client responds by yelling at the nurse, "You are always telling me what to do, just like my father." This client's response is an example of:
   1. Regression
   2. Transference

3. Reaction formation
4. Countertransference

45. In psychiatric nursing, the most important tool the nurse brings to a helping relationship is:
   1. Oneself and a desire to help
   2. Knowledge of psychopathology
   3. Advanced communication skills
   4. Years of experience in psychiatric nursing and milieu management

46. A Latino American client with schizophrenia is admitted to an emergency department crisis unit in an aggravated and disheveled state after failing to take prescribed medications for the last 5 days. When developing a plan of care that incorporates the client's cultural background, the nurse gives priority to:
   1. Inclusion of the family in the client's plan of care
   2. The client's need to control personal and social space
   3. The meaning and attention the client places on the future
   4. Socioeconomic considerations regarding hospitalization

47. A 30-year-old woman is brought to the local community hospital by a family member because the woman "has been acting strange." When the nurse assesses this client, which statements meet involuntary hospitalization criteria? Select all that apply.
   1. ☐ "I cry all the time I am so depressed."
   2. ☐ "I would like to end it all with sleeping pills."
   3. ☐ "The voices say it is okay for me to kill all prostitutes."
   4. ☐ "My boss is always picking on me and it makes me angry."

48. The nurse encourages a client to join a self-help group after being discharged from a mental health facility. The purpose of having people work in a group is to provide:
   1. Support
   2. Confrontation
   3. Psychotherapy
   4. Self-awareness

49. As depression begins to lift, a client is asked to join a small discussion group that meets every evening on the unit. The client is reluctant to join because, "I have nothing to talk about." What is the best response by the nurse?
   1. "Maybe tomorrow you will feel more like talking."
   2. "Could you start off by talking about your family?"
   3. "A person like you has a great deal to offer the group."
   4. "You feel you will not be accepted unless you have something to say?"

50. During a group meeting a male client tells everyone of his fear of his impending discharge from the hospital. It is most appropriate for the nurse leading the group to respond:
   1. "You ought to be happy that you're leaving."
   2. "Maybe you're not ready to be discharged yet."

3. "Maybe others in the group have similar feelings that they would share."
4. "How many in the group feel that this member is ready to be discharged?"

51. When a psychiatric nurse uses the family systems theory in practice, which statement by the nurse is most typical of this theory?
1. "Describe for me in your own words what caused this situation."
2. "You need to abide by the unit rules and attend the community meetings."
3. "Whenever someone permanently leaves the home, the boundaries are upset."
4. "You're doing better; let's talk to the doctor about lowering your medication dosage."

52. A week after the admission of a client with the diagnosis of paranoid schizophrenia, the client stands up in the lounge and throws a chair across the room and starts yelling at the other clients. Several of the other clients have frightened expressions, one starts to cry, and another begins to pace. After removing the agitated client from the room, what should the nurse do next?
1. Refocus clients' negative comments to more positive topics
2. Arrange a unit meeting to discuss what just happened
3. Continue the unit's activities as if nothing has happened
4. Have a private talk with the clients who cried and started to pace

53. A female client, whose long-term live-in lover has just terminated their relationship, comes to the emergency service in severe crisis. After being seen by the nurse, the client agrees to call the local mental health clinic for short-term counseling. Which client behavior helps the nurse evaluate whether the nursing intervention was effective? The client:
1. Is seeking out assistance for help with coping
2. Has returned to her precrisis level of functioning
3. Has learned new methods of coping with her loss
4. Is demonstrating diminished symptoms of anxiety

54. The nurse is aware that a co-worker's mother died 16 months ago. The co-worker cries every time someone mentions the word "mother" or if the mother's name is mentioned. Which should the nurse understand in this situation?
1. Everyone cries when their mother dies
2. This behavior is an expected response
3. This person should seek help with grieving
4. The co-worker was extremely attached to the mother

55. During a staff development program, the nurse educator emphasizes that nurses caring for middle-aged adults who are experiencing midlife crisis should understand that this crisis is most often a result of the:
1. Many role changes adults experience at this time
2. Individual's perception of his or her life situation

3. Anticipation of negative changes associated with old age
4. Lack of support from family members who are busy with their own lives

56. A 35 year old is admitted for an amputation of the left leg. Before surgery the nurse observes that the client is diaphoretic, voiding frequently, having difficulty understanding what is being said, and complaining of palpitations. What should the nurse do first after making these assessments?
1. Have a stat ECG done on the client
2. Ask the client to talk about feelings
3. Obtain a urine specimen for culture and sensitivity
4. Ask the physician for a stat order for an IM tranquilizer

57. During a staff development program, when discussing the reaction of middle-aged women to their children leaving home, the nurse educator reminds the group that recent studies have demonstrated that today's women most commonly experience a feeling of:
1. Anxiety
2. Depression
3. Satisfaction
4. Hopelessness

58. The nurse identifies that the main goal in planning care for a client in crisis is to:
1. Schedule follow-up counseling for the client
2. Restore the client's psychologic equilibrium
3. Have the client gain insight into the problems
4. Refer the client for occupational and physiotherapy

59. A 30 year old who has been in a gay relationship for the past 3 years comes to the emergency department in a near panic state. He tells the nurse that his lover of many years has just terminated their relationship. What should the nurse do to help the client cope with this loss?
1. Identify his support system
2. Explore his psychotic thoughts
3. Reinforce his current self-image
4. Suggest he explore his sexual orientation

60. Which approach should the nurse use during crisis intervention?
1. Passive and reflective
2. Active and goal-directed
3. Future-oriented and passive
4. Interpretative and analytical

61. The nurse understands that the outcome that is unrelated to a client in a crisis state is:
1. Decompensating to a lower level of functioning
2. Learning and using more constructive coping skills
3. Adapting and returning to a prior level of functioning
4. Continuing a high level of anxiety for more than 3 months

62. Which is the most important assessment data for the nurse to gather from the client in crisis?
1. The client's work habits
2. Any significant physical health data

3. A history of any emotional problems in the family
4. The specific circumstances surrounding the client's perceived crisis situation

63. An extremely anxious client enters a crisis center and asks for help. Which response by the nurse best reflects the nurse's role in crisis intervention?
1. "Tell me what you have done to help yourself."
2. "Can you tell me about what is bothering you?"
3. "I understand in the past you have had problems."
4. "I will be here for you to help you figure things out."

64. When assisting clients to cope with a crisis, the professional care provider should follow the principles of intervention. Place the following interventions in order of priority when caring for a person experiencing a crisis.
1. _____ Stabilize the victim
2. _____ Intervene immediately
3. _____ Encourage self-reliance
4. _____ Utilize available resources
5. _____ Facilitate understanding of the event.

65. A child in the first grade is murdered, and counseling is planned for the other children in the child's school. Which should the nurse identify first to understand a child's response to a crisis?
1. Developmental level of the child
2. Quality of the child's peer relationships
3. Child's perception of the crisis situation
4. Child's communication patterns with family members

66. One of the initial goals of anger management is to have clients:
1. Express remorse over aggressive actions
2. Take responsibility for their hostile behavior
3. Develop alternative methods to release feelings
4. Teach others how to avoid triggering their anger

67. A nurse leads an assertiveness training program for a group of clients. Which statement demonstrates that the treatment has been effective?
1. "I know I should put the needs of others before mine."
2. "I don't like to be called 'Dearie,' so I told him not to do it anymore."
3. "I won't stand for it. I told my boss he's a jerk and to get off my back."
4. "I find it easier to agree up front and then just do enough so that no one notices."

68. A newly licensed primary nurse is working with a married woman who has come to the emergency department several times with injuries that appear to be related to domestic violence. When talking with the nurse manager, the primary nurse expresses disgust that the woman returns to the same situation. The best response by the nurse manager is:
1. "She must not have the financial resources to leave her husband."
2. "The woman is free to choose her own life and there is nothing the staff can do."
3. "Most woman attempt to leave about six times before they are able to do so."
4. "The woman should be told how foolish she is to remain in her current situation."

69. What is the most important information the nurse should teach to prevent relapse in a client with a psychiatric illness?
1. Develop a close support system
2. Create a stress-free environment
3. Refrain from activities that cause anxiety
4. Follow the prescribed medication regimen

70. A depressed client has been prescribed a tricyclic antidepressant. The nurse teaches the client to expect to notice a significant change in the depression within:
1. 4 to 6 days
2. 2 to 4 weeks
3. 5 to 6 weeks
4. 12 to 16 hours

71. The nurse teaches clients that they should follow their diet restrictions while taking a monoamine oxidase inhibitor. What will develop if they do not follow these restrictions?
1. Occipital headaches
2. Generalized urticaria
3. Severe muscle spasms
4. Sudden drop in blood pressure

72. A client is receiving lithium carbonate. While this medication is being administered, it is important that the nurse:
1. Restrict the client's daily sodium intake
2. Test the client's urine specific gravity weekly
3. Monitor the client's drug blood level regularly
4. Withhold the client's other medications for 1 week

73. A client in the hyperactive phase of a mood disorder, bipolar type, is receiving lithium carbonate. The nurse identifies that the client's lithium blood level is 1.8 mEq/L. It is most appropriate for the nurse to:
1. Continue the usual dose of lithium and note any adverse reactions
2. Discontinue the drug until the lithium serum level drops to 0.5 mEq/L
3. Ask the physician to increase the dose of lithium because the blood lithium level is too low
4. Hold the drug and notify the physician immediately because the blood lithium level may be toxic

74. The nurse understands that neuroleptics are the drugs of choice to relieve symptoms of:
1. Psychosis
2. Depression
3. Excessive activity
4. Narcotic withdrawal

75. The nurse understands that a common manageable side effect of neuroleptics is:
1. Jaundice
2. Melanocytosis
3. Drooping eyelids
4. Unintentional tremors

76. What medication should the nurse expect to administer to actively reverse the overdose sedative effects of benzodiazepines?
1. Lithium
2. Methadone

3. Romazicon
4. Chlorpromazine

77. The nurse is caring for a client who abruptly withdrew from barbiturate use. The nurse should expect the client to experience:
   1. Ataxia
   2. Seizures
   3. Diarrhea
   4. Urticaria

78. The nurse understands that the theory that anxiety has a biologic basis, and therefore antianxiety agents are effective, is contingent on the concept that:
   1. Degeneration of myelin will increase anxiety
   2. An excess of dopamine is found in anxious clients
   3. Decreased amounts of norepinephrine and serotonin cause anxiety
   4. Drugs with an inhibitory effect that activate GABA receptors can calm anxiety

79. A client with schizophrenia, who has type II (negative) symptoms, is prescribed risperidone (Risperdal). The nurse should evaluate that the medication has minimized the type II symptoms when the client:
   1. Is less agitated
   2. Has fewer delusions
   3. Shows interest in unit activities
   4. Reports that the hallucinations have stopped

80. A 52-year-old male client with a diagnosis of schizophrenia is about to be discharged to a halfway house. This is his fifth admission in less than 1 year. He improves while in the hospital, but after discharge he forgets to take his medication, is unable to function, and must be rehospitalized. A medication that can be administered IM by the nurse to this client on an outpatient basis every 2 to 3 weeks is:
   1. Haldol
   2. Valium
   3. Lithium carbonate
   4. Prolixin decanoate

81. A client is scheduled for a 6-week electroconvulsive therapy treatment program. What intervention by the nurse is important to maintain safety of the client during the 6-week treatment program?
   1. Tyramine-free meals
   2. Avoidance of exposure to the sun
   3. Maintenance of a steady sodium intake
   4. Elimination of benzodiazepines for nighttime sedation

82. The physician orders imipramine (Tofranil), 75 mg three times per day, for a client. What nursing action is appropriate when administering this drug to a client?
   1. Avoid administration of barbiturates or steroids with this drug
   2. Warn the client not to eat cheese, fermenting products, and chicken liver
   3. Observe the client for increased tolerance so that the therapeutic dosage is maintained
   4. Have the client checked for intraocular pressure and provide instructions to be alert for symptoms of glaucoma

83. A client is to be discharged from a psychiatric unit with orders for haloperidol (Haldol) therapy. As part of the teaching plan concerning this medication, the nurse should teach the client to avoid:
   1. Driving at night
   2. Staying in the sun
   3. Ingesting aged cheeses
   4. Taking medications containing aspirin

84. A nurse is evaluating the medication regimens of a group of clients to determine whether the therapeutic level has been achieved. For which medication should the nurse review the client's serum blood level?
   1. Sertraline (Zoloft)
   2. Lorazepam (Ativan)
   3. Olanzapine (Zyprexa)
   4. Valproic acid (Depakene)

85. A client with depression is to receive fluoxetine (Prozac). A precaution that the nurse must remember when initiating treatment with this drug is that:
   1. It must be given with milk and crackers to avoid hyperacidity and discomfort
   2. Eating cheese or pickled herring or drinking wine may cause a hypertensive crisis
   3. The blood level may not be sufficient to cause noticeable improvement for 2 to 4 weeks
   4. Blood levels will need to be obtained weekly for 3 months to check for appropriate levels

86. A client with diabetes, who has been taking insulin, is psychotic and now is to receive haloperidol (Haldol). The nurse should be concerned with this drug combination because it may:
   1. Depress respirations
   2. Decrease control of the diabetes
   3. Intensify the action of both drugs
   4. Increase the danger of extrapyramidal side effects

87. Drugs such as trihexyphenidyl (Artane), biperiden (Akineton), or benztropine (Cogentin) are often prescribed in conjunction with:
   1. Barbiturates
   2. Antidepressants
   3. Antianxiety agents/anxiolytics
   4. Antipsychotic agents/neuroleptics

88. After examining a client who continues to exhibit negative symptoms (flat affect, isolation, poverty of speech, and lack of motivation) of schizophrenia, the physician writes an order to change the client's drug therapy from haloperidol (Haldol) to risperidone (Risperdal). The dosage ordered is 1 mg twice per day for 3 days. What is the most important safety measure for the nurse to take?
   1. Monitor the client for mood changes and suicidal tendencies, especially during early therapy
   2. Determine if the morning dosage of Haldol had been given and then start the initial dose of Risperdal at bedtime
   3. Assess for the side effects of sedation, restlessness, and muscle spasm after the drug has been administered

4. Review the medication sheet to determine the time of the last dose of Haldol before administering the correct dosage of Risperdal at 2 PM

89. The psychiatric nurse teaches clients in a medication education group that photosensitization is a side effect associated with the use of:
   1. Sertraline (Zoloft)
   2. Lithium carbonate (Lithane)
   3. Methylphenidate hydrochloride (Ritalin)
   4. Chlorpromazine hydrochloride (Thorazine)

90. After 2 weeks of neuroleptic drug therapy, the nurse notices that the client has become jaundiced. The nurse continues to give the neuroleptic until the psychiatrist can be consulted. In situations such as this:
   1. Jaundice is a benign side effect and has little significance
   2. Jaundice is sufficient reason to discontinue the neuroleptic
   3. The blood level of neuroleptics must be maintained once established
   4. The psychiatrist's order for the neuroleptic should be reduced by the nurse

91. An acting-out, older client has been receiving fluphenazine (Prolixin) for several months. After identifying that the client sits rigidly in a chair, the nurse assesses the client closely for other evidence of adverse effects of the drug, including:
   1. Inability to concentrate, excess salivation
   2. Uncoordinated movement of extremities, tremors
   3. Reluctance to converse, nonverbal clues indicating fear
   4. Minimal use of nonverbal expression, rambling speech

92. The nurse monitors a client with chronic undifferentiated schizophrenia for the side effects of an antipsychotic drug. For which potentially irreversible extrapyramidal side effect should the nurse monitor the client?
   1. Torticollis
   2. Oculogyric crisis
   3. Tardive dyskinesia
   4. Pseudoparkinsonism

93. A monoamine oxidase inhibitor (MAOI) is prescribed. What should the nurse teach the client to avoid?
   1. Prolonged exposure to the sun
   2. Ingesting wines and aged cheeses
   3. Engaging in active physical exercise
   4. Over-the-counter NSAID medications

94. For the past 5 days, a client has been receiving tranylcypromine (Parnate) 10 mg po twice a day for treatment of a major depressive episode. This morning, the client refuses the medication, stating, "It doesn't help, so what's the use of taking it?" What response by the nurse best demonstrates an understanding of the action of this monoamine oxidase inhibitor (MAOI)?
   1. "It takes 6 to 8 weeks for this medication to have an effect."
   2. "Sometimes it takes 2 to 4 weeks to see an improvement."

   3. "You should have felt a response by now. I'll notify your physician."
   4. "I'll talk to the physician about increasing the dosage, and that will help."

95. The nurse understands that the most potentially dangerous side effect of tricyclic antidepressants is:
   1. Mydriasis
   2. Dry mouth
   3. Constipation
   4. Urinary retention

96. A client with schizophrenia is actively psychotic, and a new medication regimen is prescribed. The client's spouse wants to know which of the prescribed medications will be most helpful to treat the psychosis. The nurse should tell the client that the drug most helpful to reduce psychotic symptoms is:
   1. Citalopram (Celexa)
   2. Benztropine mesylate (Cogentin)
   3. Ziprasidone hydrochloride (Geodon)
   4. Acetaminophen with hydrocodone (Lortab)

97. A psychotic client is receiving olanzapine (Zyprexa). When administering this drug, it is important that the nurse understand that this medication:
   1. Can be given only intramuscularly
   2. Requires a special tyramine-free diet
   3. Should be taken on an empty stomach
   4. Will dissolve instantly after placement in the client's mouth

98. Antipsychotic drugs can cause extrapyramidal side effects. Which responses should the nurse document as indicating pseudoparkinsonism? Select all that apply.
   1. ☐ Rigidity
   2. ☐ Tremors
   3. ☐ Mydriasis
   4. ☐ Photophobia
   5. ☐ Bradykinesia

99. A male client with schizophrenia is receiving benztropine mesylate (Cogentin) in conjunction with an antipsychotic. When at the clinic, the client tells the nurse that occasionally he forgets to take the Cogentin. The nurse should teach him that if this should happen again, he should:
   1. Notify the physician immediately
   2. Use 2 pills at the next regularly scheduled dose
   3. Skip the dose, but take the next regularly scheduled dose 2 hours early
   4. Take the pill as soon as possible, up to 2 hours before the next dose

100. The physician prescribes olanzapine (Zyprexa) for a client with bipolar disorder, manic episode. What cautionary advice should the nurse give the client?
   1. Sit up slowly
   2. Report double vision
   3. Expect increased salivation
   4. Take the medication on an empty stomach

101. Neuroleptic malignant syndrome is a potentially fatal reaction to antipsychotic therapy. The nurse must

identify the signs and symptoms of this syndrome. Select all that apply.
1. ☐ Jaundice
2. ☐ Diaphoresis
3. ☐ Hyperrigidity
4. ☐ Hyperthermia
5. ☐ Photosensitivity

NURSING CARE OF CLIENTS WITH DISORDERS USUALLY FIRST EVIDENT IN INFANCY, CHILDHOOD, OR ADOLESCENCE

102. The nurse is caring for a preschool-age child with a history of physical and sexual abuse. What is the most advantageous therapy for this child?
1. Play
2. Group
3. Family
4. Psychodrama

103. A 3-year-old child is diagnosed with autism. Which should the nurse expect when assessing this child? Check all that apply.
1. ☐ Imitates others
2. ☐ Seeks physical contact
3. ☐ Avoids eye-to-eye contact
4. ☐ Engages in cooperative play
5. ☐ Performs repetitive activities
6. ☐ Displays interest in children rather than adults.

104. The nurse uses behavior modification to foster toilet training efforts in a cognitively impaired child. What reward should the nurse provide to reinforce appropriate use of the toilet by the child?
1. Candy bar
2. Piece of fruit
3. Hug with praise
4. Choice of rewards

105. When planning care for a group of children, the nurse understands that the problem of separation anxiety becomes most problematic for children hospitalized during the age of:
1. 5 to 11½ years
2. 12 to 18 years
3. 6 to 30 months
4. 36 to 59 months

106. The nurse teaches that autism is a form of a pervasive developmental disorder (PDD) that can be differentiated from other forms of PDD in that autism:
1. Has less severe linguistic handicaps
2. Has an early onset before 36 months of age
3. Is the only form that does not include seizures
4. Is the only form that does not include mental retardation

107. What is the prognosis for a normal productive life for a child diagnosed with autism?
1. Dependent on an early diagnosis
2. Often related to the child's overall temperament

3. Emphasized with the parents regardless of child's level of functioning
4. Unlikely because of interference with so many parameters of functioning

108. The nurse knows that most common characteristic of autistic children is that they:
1. Respond to any stimulus
2. Respond to physical contact
3. Seem unresponsive to the environment
4. Are totally involved with the environment

109. The nurse teaches that the signs of autism initially may be evident when the child is about:
1. 2 years of age
2. 6 years of age
3. 6 months of age
4. 1 to 3 months of age

110. For which clinical indication should the nurse observe the child suspected of being autistic?
1. Not wanting to eat
2. Crying for attention
3. Catatonic-like rigidity
4. Enjoying being with people

111. A 6-year-old girl with autism is nonverbal and has limited eye contact. What should the nurse do initially to promote social interaction?
1. Engage in parallel play while sitting next to the child
2. Encourage the child to vocalize through sound games and songs
3. Provide play opportunities for the child to play with other children
4. Use therapeutic holding when the child does not respond to verbal interactions

112. A 10-year-old boy, who was diagnosed with autism at the age of 3, attends a school for developmentally disabled children and lives with his parents. He has frequent episodes of biting his arms and banging his head and needs help with feeding and toileting. The priority nursing goal for this child is, "The child will:
1. Be able to feed himself."
2. Control repetitive behaviors."
3. Remain safe from self-inflicted injury."
4. Develop control of urinary elimination."

113. When planning activities for a child with autism, the nurse must remember that autistic children respond best to:
1. Large-group activity
2. Loud, cheerful music
3. Individuals in small groups
4. Their own self-stimulating acts

114. The nurse understands that one of the major behavioral characteristics of children with attention deficit disorder is their:
1. Overreaction to stimuli
2. Continued use of rituals
3. Delayed speech development
4. Inability to use abstract thought

115. The nurse teaches parents of a child with attention deficit hyperactivity disorder (ADHD) that ADHD usually is treated with:
    1. Lorazepam (Ativan)
    2. Haloperidol (Haldol)
    3. Methylphenidate (Ritalin)
    4. Methocarbamol (Robaxin)

116. A hyperactive 9-year-old child, with a history of attention deficit hyperactivity disorder, is admitted for observation after a motor vehicle accident. What should be the focus of nursing actions to meet the goal of personal safety?
    1. Requesting the child write at least three safety rules
    2. Asking the child to verbalize as many safety rules as possible
    3. Talking with the child about the importance of using a seat belt
    4. Encouraging the child to talk with other children about their opinions of safety rules

117. A 4-year-old boy is diagnosed with attention deficit hyperactivity disorder. When obtaining a history from the parents, what information about the child should the nurse expect? Select all that apply.
    1. ❑ Is impulsive
    2. ❑ Talks excessively
    3. ❑ Is spiteful and vindictive
    4. ❑ Annoys others deliberately
    5. ❑ Plays video games for hours
    6. ❑ Does not follow through or finish tasks

118. The nurse is caring for a child with school phobia. The nurse teaches the parents that the best treatment is to:
    1. Accompany the child to the classroom
    2. Return the child to school immediately
    3. Explain why attendance at school is necessary
    4. Allow the child to enter the classroom before other children

119. The nurse understands that the childhood problem that has legal as well as emotional aspects and cannot be ignored is:
    1. School phobias
    2. Fear of animals
    3. Fear of monsters
    4. Sleep disturbances

120. The mother of a boy with a tentative diagnosis of attention deficit hyperactivity disorder (ADHD) arrives at the pediatric clinic insisting that the doctor give her a prescription for medication that will control his behavior. The nurse's best response is:
    1. "It must be so frustrating to deal with your son's behavior."
    2. "Have you considered any alternatives to using medication?"
    3. "Perhaps you are looking for an easy solution to the problem."
    4. "Are you aware of the side effects of medications used for ADHD?"

121. The nurse understands that children with attention deficit hyperactivity disorder may be learning-disabled. This means that these children:
    1. Will probably not be self-sufficient as adults
    2. Have intellectual deficits that interfere with learning
    3. Experience perceptual difficulties that interfere with learning
    4. Are performing usually two grade levels below their age norm

122. The physician orders methylphenidate (Ritalin) once a day for a child with an attention deficit hyperactivity disorder. The nurse should teach the parents to administer the daily dose:
    1. Before breakfast
    2. Just after breakfast
    3. Immediately before lunch
    4. As soon as the child awakens

123. A child is diagnosed with attention deficit hyperactivity disorder (ADHD). The nurse teaches the parents strategies to assist their child to cope with this disorder. These strategies should include:
    1. Orienting the child to reality
    2. Rewarding appropriate conduct
    3. Suppressing feelings of frustration
    4. Using restraints when behavior is out of control

124. An 8-year-old boy is diagnosed with oppositional defiant disorder. When the nurse assesses the child, the behavior that supports this diagnosis is the fact that the boy:
    1. Is easily distracted
    2. Argues with adults
    3. Lies to obtain favors
    4. Initiates physical fights

125. A 16-year-old male adolescent, with the diagnosis of conduct disorder since the age of 10, is placed in a residential facility because the parents can no longer manage his behavior. He has a history of fighting, stealing, vandalizing property, and running away from home. He is aggressive, has no friends, and has been suspended from school repeatedly. When developing a plan of care for this client, what should be the nurse's priority?
    1. Preventing violence
    2. Supporting self-esteem
    3. Limiting defensive coping
    4. Promoting social interaction

126. The nurse is working with school-age children who have the diagnosis of conduct disorder, childhood-onset type. The nurse understands that these children are at risk for having their conduct disorder progress to an additional disorder during adolescence; therefore in the future the nurse should assess these clients for signs of:
    1. Oppositional defiant disorder
    2. Antisocial personality disorder
    3. Pervasive developmental disorder
    4. Attention deficit hyperactivity disorder

127. A child with the diagnosis of attention deficit hyper-activity disorder often becomes frustrated and loses control. The nurse should use a variety of graduated techniques to manage disruptive behaviors. List the numbers of the following interventions in order from the least invasive technique to the most invasive technique.
    1. _____ Place the child in time-out
    2. _____ Monitor behavior for cues of rising anxiety
    3. _____ Use a signal to remind the child to use self-control
    4. _____ Avoid situations that usually precipitate frustration

128. The nurse is caring for an adolescent with the diagnosis of conduct disorder who is receiving behavioral therapy to attempt to limit activities that violate societal norms. A specific outcome criterion unique for adolescents with this problem is, "The client will:
    1. Exhibit increased impulse control."
    2. Identify two positive personal attributes."
    3. Demonstrate respect for the rights of others."
    4. Use age-appropriate play activities with at least one peer."

129. A client with the diagnosis of Tourette's syndrome has demonstrated a combination of motor tics and involuntary vocal utterances. When the client engages in verbal utterances that are often obscene, the nurse understands that this behavior is known as:
    1. Palilalia
    2. Coprolalia
    3. Echokinesis
    4. Agoraphobia

NURSING CARE OF CLIENTS WITH DISORDERS RELATED TO ALTERATIONS IN COGNITION AND PERCEPTION

130. When conducting a mini-mental status exam on an older client, the nurse should test specifically for short-term memory by asking the client to:
    1. Subtract serial 7s from 100
    2. Copy a simple geometric figure
    3. State three random words mentioned earlier in the exam
    4. Name two common objects when the nurse points to them

131. The nurse recognizes that dementia of the Alzheimer's type is characterized by:
    1. Aggressive acting-out behavior
    2. Periodic remissions and exacerbations
    3. Hypoxia of selected areas of brain tissue
    4. Areas of brain destruction called senile plaques

132. A 75-year-old man with the diagnosis of dementia has been cared for by his wife for 5 years. For the past 2 years he has not spoken and is incontinent of urine and feces. During the last month he has changed from being placid and easygoing to agitated and aggressive. He is admitted to a psychiatric hospital for treatment with psychopharmacology. Which is the priority nursing care while this client is in the psychiatric facility?
    1. Managing his behavior
    2. Preventing further deterioration
    3. Focusing on the needs of the wife
    4. Establishing an elimination retraining program

133. Which nursing intervention is most helpful in meeting the needs of an older adult hospitalized with the diagnosis of dementia of the Alzheimer's type?
    1. Providing a nutritious diet high in carbohydrates and proteins
    2. Simplifying the environment as much as possible while eliminating the need for choices
    3. Developing a consistent nursing plan with fixed time schedules to provide for emotional needs
    4. Providing an opportunity for many alternative choices in the daily schedule to stimulate interest

134. When attempting to understand the behavior of an older adult diagnosed with vascular dementia, the nurse recognizes that the client is probably:
    1. Not capable of using any defense mechanisms
    2. Using one method of defense for every situation
    3. Making exaggerated use of old, familiar mechanisms
    4. Attempting to develop new defense mechanisms to meet the current situation

135. Which should the nurse include in the plan of care for the client with vascular dementia?
    1. A reeducation program
    2. Details for supportive care
    3. An introduction of new leisure-time activities
    4. Plans to involve the client in group therapy sessions

136. The nurse is assessing a client and attempting to distinguish between dementia and delirium. Which factors are unique to delirium? Check all that apply.
    1. ☐ Slurred speech
    2. ☐ Lability of mood
    3. ☐ Long-term memory loss
    4. ☐ Visual or tactile hallucinations
    5. ☐ Insidious deterioration in cognition
    6. ☐ Fluctuating levels of consciousness

137. A delirious client sees a design on the wallpaper and perceives it as an animal. The nurse should report this as an example of:
    1. A delusion
    2. An illusion
    3. A hallucination
    4. An idea of reference

138. The nurse's best approach when caring for a confused, older client is to provide an environment with:
    1. Space for privacy
    2. Group involvement
    3. Trusting relationships
    4. Activities that are varied

139. An older male client on the psychiatric unit becomes upset while in the day room. When attempting to help the client, what should be the nurse's initial intervention?
    1. Instruct the client to be quiet
    2. Allow the client to act-out until he tires
    3. Give directions in a firm, low-pitched voice
    4. Lead the client from the room by taking him by his arm

140. An older adult is admitted to a psychiatric hospital with the diagnosis of dementia. The nurse recognizes that it would be most unusual for this client to demonstrate:
    1. Resistance to change
    2. Preoccupation with personal appearance
    3. A tendency to dwell on the past and ignore the present
    4. The inability to concentrate on new activities or interests

141. When answering questions from the family of a client with Alzheimer's disease, the nurse explains, "This disease is:
    1. A slow and relentless deterioration of the mind."
    2. A functional disorder that occurs in the later years."
    3. A disease that first emerges in the fourth decade of life."
    4. Easily diagnosed through laboratory and psychologic tests."

142. It is important for nurses working with clients who have a diagnosis of dementia to adopt a common approach of care because these clients need to:
    1. Relate in a consistent manner to staff
    2. Learn that the staff cannot be manipulated
    3. Accept controls that are concrete and fairly applied
    4. Have sameness and consistency in their environment

143. A nurse is assessing a client with dementia. Which client assessment is unexpected?
    1. Acts pessimistic
    2. Appears agitated
    3. Has a short attention span
    4. Exhibits disordered reasoning

144. The nursing goal of the therapeutic psychiatric environment for the confused client is to:
    1. Assist the client to relate to others
    2. Make the hospital atmosphere more homelike
    3. Help the client become popular in a controlled setting
    4. Maintain the highest level of safe, independent functioning

145. What is the most appropriate nursing intervention when working with clients who exhibit mild cognitive impairment?
    1. Reality orientation
    2. Behavioral confrontation
    3. Reflective communication
    4. Reminiscence group therapy

146. Geriatric clients with behavioral changes are often admitted to the psychiatric unit for screening and evaluation. As part of the nursing assessment, it is important to observe for signs of dementia. The four "As" of Alzheimer's disease are:
    1. Amnesia, apraxia, agnosia, aphasia
    2. Avoidance, aloofness, asocial, asexual
    3. Autism, loose association, apathy, affect
    4. Aggressive, amoral, ambivalent, attractive

147. A 78-year-old male has been brought to the clinic by his family because they believe he has become increasingly confused over the past week. What can the nurse ask the client to assess his orientation?
    1. Explain a proverb
    2. State where he was born
    3. Identify the name of the hospital
    4. Recall what he had eaten for breakfast

148. A nurse is assigned to care for a regressed 19-year-old college student recently admitted to the psychiatric unit with a 1-month history of talking to unseen people and refusing to get out of bed, go to class, or get involved in daily grooming activities. The nurse's initial efforts should be directed toward helping the client by:
    1. Providing frequent rest periods and avoiding exhaustion
    2. Facilitating the client's social relationships with a peer group
    3. Reducing environmental stimuli and maintaining dietary intake
    4. Attempting to establish a meaningful relationship with the client

149. A client diagnosed with schizophrenia is experiencing auditory hallucinations. The nurse makes the following statements when interacting with this client. Place these statements in the order in which they should occur.
    1. _____ "I do not hear any voices."
    2. _____ "Come with me for a walk."
    3. _____ "Hearing voices must be frightening."
    4. _____ "The voices you hear are part of your illness."

150. The nurse understands that projection, rationalization, denial, and distortion by hallucinations and delusions are examples of a disturbance in:
    1. Logic
    2. Association
    3. Reality testing
    4. Thought processes

151. A male client with schizophrenia has a history of hearing voices that tell him he is a bad person. While having a conversation with a nurse with whom he has been working, the client states that he is starting to hear the voices again. What is the best response by the nurse?
    1. "Try to ignore the voices."
    2. "What are the voices saying to you?"
    3. "Don't believe what the voices are saying."
    4. "Try not to be afraid because they are only voices."

152. When caring for a client whose behavior is characterized by pathologic suspicion, the nurse should:
1. Remove the client from environmental stress
2. Help the client realize the suspicions are unrealistic
3. Ask the client to explain the reasons for the feelings
4. Help the client to feel accepted by the staff on the unit

153. One evening the nurse finds a client, who has been experiencing persecutory delusions, trying to get out the door. The client states, "Please let me go. I trust you. The Mafia is going to kill me tonight." Which response is most therapeutic?
1. "You are frightened. Come with me to your room and we can talk about it."
2. "Nobody here wants to harm you, you know that. I'll come with you to your room."
3. "Come with me to your room. I'll lock the door and no one will get in to harm you."
4. "Thank you for trusting me. Maybe you can trust me when I tell you no one can kill you while you're here."

154. A delusional client refuses to eat because of a belief that the food is poisoned. One of the most appropriate ways for the nurse to initially intervene is to:
1. Taste the food in the client's presence
2. Simply state that the food is not poisoned
3. Show the client that other people are eating without being harmed
4. Tell the client that tube feedings will be started if eating does not begin

155. A client with schizophrenia is admitted to an acute care psychiatric unit. Which positive signs and symptoms exhibited by this client should the nurse document?
1. Withdrawal, poverty of speech, inattentiveness
2. Flat affect, decreased spontaneity, asocial behavior
3. Hypomania, labile mood swings, episodes of euphoria
4. Hyperactivity, auditory hallucinations, loose associations

156. An acutely ill client with the diagnosis of schizophrenia has just been admitted to the mental health unit. When working with this client initially, the nurse's most therapeutic action should be to:
1. Spend time with the client to build trust and demonstrate acceptance
2. Involve the client in occupational therapy and use diversional activity
3. Delay one-to-one interactions until medications reduce the psychotic symptoms
4. Involve the client in multiple small-group discussions to distract attention from the fantasy world

157. A client with the diagnosis of schizophrenia plans an activity schedule with the help of the treatment team. After agreement by all, a written copy is posted in the client's room. When it is time for the client to go for a walk, what should the nurse say when approaching the client?
1. "It's time for you to go for a walk now."
2. "Do you want to take your scheduled walk now?"
3. "When would you like to go for your walk today?"
4. "You are supposed to be going for your walk now."

158. During the admission procedure, a client appears to be responding to voices. The client cries out at intervals, "No, no, I didn't kill him. You know the truth; tell that policeman. Please help me!" The nurse should:
1. Listen attentively and assume a facial expression of disbelief
2. Sit there quietly and not respond to the client's statements
3. Respond by saying, "I want to help you. I realize you must be very frightened."
4. Say, "Do not become so upset. No one is talking to you; the accusing voices are part of your illness."

159. The nurse has been observing a client for some time. The client is delusional, talking about people who are plotting to do harm. The staff notices that the client is pacing more than usual. The nurse decides that the client is beginning to lose control. What is the best nursing intervention?
1. Encourage the client to use a punching bag
2. Move the client to a quiet place on the unit
3. Suggest that the client sit down for a while
4. Allow the client to continue pacing with supervision

160. A male client with a history of schizophrenia comes to the mental health clinic for a regularly scheduled group therapy session. When the client enters the office, he is agitated and exhibits behaviors that indicate he is hearing voices. When the nurse begins to walk toward the client from across the room, the client pulls out a large knife. Which is the best approach to use with this client?
1. Firm
2. Passive
3. Empathetic
4. Confrontational

161. The nurse knows that prominent symptoms lasting for at least 1 month that are diagnostic for paranoid schizophrenia are:
1. Delusions and hallucinations
2. Poverty of speech with apathy
3. Bizarre behaviors associated with drug use
4. Disturbed relationships and poor grooming

162. While the nurse is talking with a client, a female client comes up and yells, "I hate you. You're talking about me again," and throws a glass of juice at the nurse. What is the best nursing approach to respond to this situation?
1. Repeat the client's words and ask for clarification
2. Remove the client to her room because she needs to have limits placed on her behavior.
3. Ignore both the behavior and the client, clean up the juice, and talk to her when she is better.
4. Verbalize feelings of annoyance as an example to the client that it is more acceptable to verbalize feelings than to act-out.

163. As the nurse enters a room and approaches a male client who has been diagnosed with schizophrenia, the client states, "Get out of here before I hit you! Go away!" The nurse recognizes that this client's aggressive behavior was probably related to the fact that he:

1. Felt hallucinating and the voices were directing his response
2. Was afraid that he might harm the nurse if the nurse came nearer
3. Was reminded of someone who was frightening and threatening to him
4. Felt hemmed in and trapped when the nurse came around the bed toward him

164. A client who experiences auditory hallucinations agrees to discuss with the nurse alternative coping strategies. For the next 3 days when the nurse attempts to focus on alternative strategies, the client gets up and leaves the interaction. It is most therapeutic for the nurse to state:

1. "Come back; you agreed that you would discuss other ways to cope."
2. "You seem very uncomfortable every time I bring up a new way to cope."
3. "Did you agree to talk about other ways to cope because you thought that was what I wanted?"
4. "You walk out each time I start to discuss the hallucinations; does that mean you've changed your mind?"

165. What is the nurse's most appropriate action when a client is seen openly masturbating in the recreation room?

1. Restraining the client's hands
2. Putting the client in seclusion
3. Stating that such behavior is unacceptable
4. Demonstrating no reaction to the behavior

166. To achieve one of the primary objectives of providing a therapeutic daycare environment for a client who is withdrawn and seclusive, the nurse should:

1. Foster a trusting relationship
2. Administer medications on time
3. Involve the client in a group with peers
4. Remove the client from the family home

167. A client experiencing hallucinations tells the nurse, "The voices are telling me I'm no good." The client asks whether the nurse hears the voices. Which is the most appropriate response by the nurse?

1. "It is the voice of your conscience, which only you can control."
2. "No, I do not hear your voices, but I believe you can hear them."
3. "The voices are coming from within you; only you can hear them."
4. Hearing "the voices are a symptom of your illness; don't pay any attention to them."

168. The nurse enters a client's room and notes that the client appears preoccupied. Then, turning to the nurse, the client states, "They are saying terrible things about me. Can't you hear them?" The most therapeutic response by the nurse is:

1. "It seems you heard them before?"
2. "Try to get control of your feelings."
3. "There is no one here but me, and I don't hear anything."
4. "I don't hear what you say you hear, but I can see you are upset."

169. The nurse observes a regressed, emotionally disturbed client using the hands to eat soft foods. The nurse can best intervene by:

1. Placing a spoon in the client's hand and suggesting it be used
2. Saying in a joking way, "Well, I guess fingers were made before forks."
3. Ignoring the behavior and observing several additional meals before intervening
4. Removing the food while saying, "You can't have any more until you use your spoon."

170. The most serious indication of impending assaultive behavior is when the client:

1. Uses profane language
2. Touches people excessively
3. Exhibits a sudden withdrawal
4. Experiences command hallucinations

171. While watching TV in the day room, a female client who has demonstrated withdrawn, regressed behavior suddenly screams, bursts into tears, and runs out of the room to the far end of the hallway. What is the most therapeutic action for the nurse to take?

1. Walk to the end of the hallway where the client is standing
2. Accept the action as just being impulsive behavior of a sick person
3. Document the incident in the client's record while the memory is fresh
4. Ask another client who was in the day room what made the client act as she did

172. When a regressed, emotionally disturbed client voids on the floor in the sitting room of the psychiatric unit, the nurse should intervene by:

1. Making the client mop the floor
2. Restricting the client's fluids throughout the day
3. Toileting the client more frequently with supervision
4. Withholding privileges each time the client voids on the floor

173. A regressed, emotionally disturbed client who has been watching the nurse for a few days suddenly walks up and shouts, "You think you're so damned perfect and good. I think you stink!" Which is the most appropriate response by the nurse?

1. "Do you mean I smell?"
2. "You seem angry with me."
3. "Boy, you're in a bad mood."
4. "I can't be all that bad, can I?"

174. A client is experiencing auditory hallucinations. The client tells the nurse, "I am a terrible, evil person; the

voices are telling me that God needs to punish me." The most therapeutic initial response by the nurse is:
1. "God is loving and will not punish you."
2. "The voices you are hearing are just a fantasy."
3. "Tell me what you are thinking about yourself."
4. "You aren't a wicked person; God and I both love you."

175. The most appropriate way for the nurse to help a withdrawn, emotionally disturbed adolescent client to accept the realities of daily living is to:
1. Assist the client to care for personal hygiene needs
2. Encourage the client to keep up with school studies
3. Encourage the client to join the other clients in group singing
4. Leave the client alone when there appears to be a disinterest in the activities at hand

176. Which is the best nursing intervention to encourage a withdrawn, noncommunicative client to talk?
1. Focus on nonthreatening subjects
2. Try to get the client to discuss feelings
3. Sit and look through magazines with the client
4. Ask questions that require "yes" or "no" answers

177. When caring for clients exhibiting psychotic patterns of thinking and behavior, an important aspect of nursing care is to:
1. Help keep the client oriented to reality
2. Involve the client in activities throughout the day
3. Help the client understand that it is harmful to withdraw from situations
4. Encourage the client to discuss why mixing with other people is being avoided

178. Observation is an important aspect of nursing care. It is especially important in the care of the withdrawn client because it:
1. Is useful in making a diagnosis
2. Tells the staff how ill the client is
3. Indicates the degree of depression
4. Helps in understanding the client's behaviors

NURSING CARE OF CLIENTS WITH DISORDERS RELATED TO ANXIETY AND ALTERATIONS IN MOOD

179. When the nurse is reviewing the record of a client who was recently admitted to a residential psychiatric facility, it indicates that the client was exhibiting akathisia. To determine whether this adaptation is still present, the nurse should assess whether the client:
1. Exhibits facial tics
2. Displays motor restlessness
3. Maintains a body position for hours
4. Repeats the movements of another person

180. The nurse recognizes that an excellent indicator of improvement in a client with the diagnosis of generalized anxiety disorder is when the client:
1. Learns to avoid anxiety
2. Participates in activities

3. Takes medication as prescribed
4. Identifies when anxiety is developing

181. The nurse is caring for a client with a generalized anxiety disorder. When the nurse assesses the client, which is one of the best indicators of the client's present condition?
1. Memory
2. Behavior
3. Judgment
4. Responsiveness

182. An obviously distraught client arrives at the mental health clinic. The client is disheveled, is agitated, and demands that someone "do something to end this feeling." The nurse identifies that the client has:
1. A feeling of panic
2. Suicidal tendencies
3. Narcissistic ideation
4. A demanding personality

183. A client's severe anxiety and panic is often considered to be "contagious." When the nurse identifies that personal feelings of anxiety are increasing, the nurse should:
1. Refocus the conversation on some pleasant topics
2. Say to the client, "Calm down, you are making me anxious, too."
3. Say, "I have to leave for awhile. I'll send someone in and I'll be back later."
4. Remain quiet so that personal feelings of anxiety do not become apparent to the client

184. The nurse understands that a phobic reaction rarely will occur unless the person:
1. Thinks about the feared object
2. Is in an unfamiliar environment
3. Is seeking attention from others
4. Comes into contact with the feared object

185. The nurse has explored the modalities available for the treatment of phobias. Which treatment should the nurse tell the client has the highest success rate for people with phobias?
1. Systematic desensitization using relaxation techniques
2. Insight therapy to determine the origin of the anxiety and fear
3. Psychotherapy aimed at rearranging psychotic thought processes
4. Psychoanalytic exploration of repressed conflicts of an earlier developmental phase

186. When speaking with the client who has just experienced a panic attack, the nurse can best address the client's concerns most therapeutically by stating:
1. "I would have been upset too."
2. "Episodes like this can be upsetting, but they do end."
3. "You are concerned that this might happen again."
4. "Your family was concerned that you were having a heart attack."

187. People who are involved in a bioterrorism attack exhibit immediate responses to the traumatic event. Which adaptations can the nurse expect in survivors during the immediate period after a traumatic event? Select all that apply.
1. ☐ Guilt
2. ☐ Denial
3. ☐ Altruism
4. ☐ Confusion
5. ☐ Helplessness

188. The parents of a man who is experiencing posttraumatic stress disorder has decided to care for their son at home. The priority intervention that the psychiatric home care nurse must include in the plan of care for the parents is to:
1. Help the parents keep the client within the home environment
2. Work to resolve the problems that cause the parents to be fearful
3. Discuss the parents' feelings of ambivalence about what the client is enduring
4. Assist the parents to understand that the client may avoid emotional attachments

189. A client with a general anxiety disorder says to the nurse, "What can I do to prevent over-responding to stress in the future?" What is the nurse's best response?
1. "Hone your problem-solving skills."
2. "Improve your time management skills."
3. "Ignore situations that you cannot change."
4. "Develop a wide variety of coping strategies."

190. The nurse understands that it is unusual for an individual with an anxiety disorder to handle the anxiety by:
1. Acting-out with antisocial behavior
2. Converting it into a physical symptom
3. Regressing to earlier levels of adjustment
4. Displacing it onto less-threatening objects

191. How should the nurse expect a client's anxiety to be manifested physiologically?
1. Dilated pupils, dilated bronchioles, increased pulse rate, hyperglycemia, and peripheral vasoconstriction
2. Constricted pupils, dilated bronchioles, increased pulse rate, hypoglycemia, and peripheral vasodilation
3. Constricted pupils, constricted bronchioles, increased pulse rate, hypoglycemia, and peripheral vasodilation
4. Dilated pupils, constricted bronchioles, decreased pulse rate, hypoglycemia, and peripheral vasoconstriction

192. The most appropriate way the nurse can decrease a client's anxiety is by helping the client:
1. Avoid unpleasant objects and events
2. Prolong exposure to fearful situations
3. Acquire skills with which to face stressful events
4. Introduce an element of pleasure into fearful situations

193. A young client is admitted with a severe anxiety disorder. The client is crying, wringing the hands, and pacing. What should be the first nursing intervention?
1. Stay physically close to the client
2. Gently ask what is bothering the client
3. Tell the client to try to relax by sitting quietly
4. Get the client involved in a nonthreatening activity

194. The nurse understands that in a conversion disorder pseudoneurologic symptoms such as paralysis or blindness:
1. Are unconscious methods for getting attention
2. Will subside if the client is helped to focus on getting healthy
3. Are generally necessary for the client to cope with a stressful situation
4. Will usually resolve when the client learns to deal with ongoing family conflicts

195. A client newly diagnosed with a conversion disorder is manifesting paralysis of the leg. The nurse can expect this client to:
1. Demonstrate a spread of paralysis to other body parts
2. Require continuous psychiatric treatment to maintain individual functioning
3. Recover the use of the affected leg but, under stress, again develop similar symptoms
4. Follow a rather unpredictable emotional course in the future, depending on exposure to stress

196. The nurse is caring for a client who has a diagnosis of conversion disorder with paralysis of the lower extremities. Which is the most therapeutic intervention for the nurse to implement?
1. Encouraging the client to try to walk
2. Telling the client that there is nothing wrong
3. Avoiding focusing on the client's physical symptoms
4. Helping the client follow through with the physical therapy plan

197. The nurse understands that for a client with a diagnosis of conversion disorder, anxiety is:
1. Diffuse and free floating
2. Consciously felt by the client
3. Projected onto the environment
4. Localized and relieved by the symptom

198. The nurse understands that the basic difference between psychophysiologic disorders and somatoform disorders is that in psychophysiologic disorders there is:
1. A feeling of illness
2. An emotional cause
3. An initial tissue change
4. A restriction of activities

199. A 20-year-old female client believes that doorknobs are contaminated and refuses to touch them, except with a paper tissue. What nursing intervention is most therapeutic for this client?
1. Supply the client with paper tissues to help her function until her anxiety is reduced

2. Encourage the client to scrub the doorknobs with a strong antiseptic so that she does not need to use tissues

3. Explain to the client that her idea about doorknobs being contaminated is part of her illness and her precaution is not necessary

4. Encourage the client to touch doorknobs by removing all available paper tissue until she learns to deal with the situation

200. The nurse understands that compulsive symptoms, such as using paper towels to open doors, develop because the clients are:
1. Unconsciously controlling unacceptable impulses or feelings
2. Consciously using this method to punish themselves
3. Listening to voices that tell them the doorknobs are unclean
4. Fulfilling a need to punish others by carrying out an annoying procedure

201. The nurse is developing a care plan for a client with an obsessive-compulsive behavior disorder. Which nursing intervention will most likely increase the client's anxiety?
1. Permitting the client's ritualistic acts three times a day
2. Involving the client in establishing the therapeutic plan
3. Helping the client understand the nature of the anxiety
4. Providing the client with a nonjudgmental environment

202. Why is the hospital or day-treatment center often indicated for the treatment of the client with an obsessive-compulsive disorder? This setting:
1. Prevents the client from completing symptomatic rituals
2. Allows the staff to exert control over the client's activities
3. Resolves the client's anxiety because decision making is minimal
4. Provides the neutral environment the client needs to work through conflicts

203. What should the nurse include in the initial nursing plan of care for a 40-year-old client with the long-standing, obsessive-compulsive behavior of hand and body washing?
1. Denying the client time for ritualistic behavior
2. Determining the purpose of the ritualistic behavior
3. Providing the client with a routine schedule of activities
4. Suggesting a symptom substitution technique to refocus the behavior

204. A client with a history of obsessive-compulsive behaviors has been attending a psychiatric day-treatment center. There has been a marked decrease in symptoms, and the client expresses a wish to obtain a part-time job. On the day of a job interview the client comes to the center fretful and displaying symptoms. Which is the nurse's best response in this situation?
1. "I know you're anxious, but make yourself go to the interview and conquer your fear."
2. "If going to an interview makes you this anxious, it seems like you're not ready to work."
3. "It must be that you really don't want that job after all. I think you should think more about it."
4. "Going for your interview triggered some feelings in you. Perhaps you could call a friend to drive you to your appointment."

205. To give effective nursing care to a client who is using ritualistic behavior, the nurse must first understand that the client:
1. Should be prevented from performing the rituals
2. Needs to realize that the ritual serves no purpose
3. Must immediately be diverted when performing the ritual
4. Does not want to repeat the ritual, but feels compelled to do so

206. What is the priority discharge criterion for a female client who is using ritualistic behaviors? The client is able to:
1. Verbalize positive aspects about herself
2. Follow the rules of the therapeutic milieu
3. Recognize that her hallucinations occur at times of extreme anxiety and can be controlled
4. Verbalize signs and symptoms of increasing anxiety and intervene to maintain it at a manageable level

207. A psychiatrist prescribes an antiobsessional agent for a client who is using ritualistic behavior. A common antiobsessional medication that the nurse can expect the practitioner to order for this client is:
1. Fluvoxamine (Luvox)
2. Benztropine (Cogentin)
3. Amantadine (Symmetrel)
4. Diphenhydramine (Benadryl)

208. A client is using ritualistic behaviors. Why does the nurse allow the client ample time for the performance of the ritual?
1. Denial of this activity may precipitate panic levels of anxiety
2. Anger turned inward on the self should be allowed to be expressed
3. Successful performance of independent activities enhances self-esteem
4. Provides an opportunity to point out that the behavior is inappropriate

209. Although the nurse becomes tense as the client with an obsessive-compulsive personality disorder carries out a ritual, the nurse understands that a compulsive act is one that:
1. Has a purpose but is useless
2. Is performed after long urging
3. Appears to be performed willingly
4. Seems absurd but is necessary to the person

210. The nurse understands that a therapeutic treatment of a female client with ritualistic behavior should be directed toward helping her to:
    1. Redirect her energy into activities to help others
    2. Learn that her behavior is not serving a realistic purpose
    3. Forget her fears by administering antianxiety medications
    4. Understand her behavior is caused by maladaptive coping to increased anxiety

211. Which is the best nursing intervention to meet the needs of individuals who demonstrate obsessive-compulsive behavior?
    1. Restricting their movements
    2. Calling attention to their behavior
    3. Keeping them busy to distract them
    4. Supporting but limiting their behavior

212. A client with a somatoform disorder is well-known to the nurse from prior hospitalizations. When planning care for the client the nurse must be aware that this client is prone to:
    1. Ask the nurse to make a recommendation for palliative care
    2. Write down conversations in order to remember information
    3. Monopolize conversations about the anxiety being experienced
    4. Redirect the conversation with the nurse to physical symptoms

213. A client is admitted to the mental health unit with the diagnosis of bipolar disorder, depressed. During the assessment interview when the client avoids eye contact, responds in a very low voice, and is tearful, it is most therapeutic for the nurse to state:
    1. "You'll find that you'll get better faster if you try to help us to help you."
    2. "Hold my hand; I know you are frightened. I will not allow anyone to harm you."
    3. "I'm your nurse. I'll take you to the day room as soon as I get some information."
    4. "I know this is difficult, but as soon as we are finished, I'll take you to your room."

214. An older adult has not been eating well since admission. The client repeatedly states, "No one cares." What is the most appropriate response by the nurse?
    1. "We all care about you; now please eat."
    2. "You know you have to eat; it will keep you alive."
    3. "I care about you. What foods do you especially like?"
    4. "I care about you. Will you please eat some of this food for me?"

215. A client is admitted to the mental health unit because of a progressively increasing depression over the past month. During the initial assessment, the nurse should expect the client to display:
    1. Elated affect related to reaction formation
    2. Loose associations related to thought disorder

3. Physical exhaustion resulting from decreased physical activity
    4. Paucity of verbal expression caused by slowed thought processes

216. When the nurse is developing a plan of care for a depressed client, which approach by the nurse is most therapeutic?
    1. Allowing time for the client's slowness when planning activities
    2. Helping the client focus on family strengths and support systems
    3. Encouraging the client to perform menial tasks to meet the need for punishment
    4. Telling the client repeatedly that the staff views the client as worthwhile and important

217. Which statement is most appropriate for the nurse to use when interviewing a newly admitted 35-year-old depressed client whose thoughts focus on feelings of unworthiness and failure?
    1. "Tell me how you feel about yourself."
    2. "Tell me what has been bothering you."
    3. "Why do you feel so bad about yourself?"
    4. "What can we do to help you during your stay with us?"

218. A female client whose depression is beginning to lift remains aloof from the other clients on the psychiatric unit. The nurse with whom the client has developed a relationship may help her participate in some activity by:
    1. Finding solitary pursuits that the client can enjoy
    2. Speaking to the client about the importance of entering into activities
    3. Asking the physician to speak to the client about participating in activities
    4. Inviting another client to take part in a joint activity with the nurse and the client

219. Which activity is most appropriate for the nurse to introduce to a depressed client during the early part of hospitalization?
    1. Game of Trivial Pursuit
    2. Project involving drawing
    3. Small aerobic exercise group
    4. Card game with three other clients

220. A withdrawn client refuses to get out of bed and becomes upset. What action is most therapeutic for the nurse to take?
    1. Require the client to get out of bed at once
    2. Stay with the client until the client calms down
    3. Give the client the PRN neuroleptic that is ordered
    4. Allow the client to stay in bed for now without company

221. A female client with the diagnosis of bipolar disorder, depressive episode, has been hospitalized on a psychiatric unit for 1 week. When scheduling activities for this client, it is most appropriate to plan for the client to:
    1. Complete a jigsaw puzzle by herself
    2. Play a game of cards with several other clients

3. Talk with the nurse several times during the day
4. Engage in a game of Ping-Pong with another client

222. During a special meeting to discuss the unexpected suicide of one of the female clients while on a weekend pass, the nurse overhears another client moan softly, "I'm next. Oh, my God, I'm next. They couldn't prevent hers and they can't protect me." What is the most therapeutic response by the nurse?
1. "You seem to be afraid you will hurt yourself"
2. "The other client was a lot sicker than you are."
3. "It's different. The other client was home; you are here."
4. "There is no need to worry. Passes will be canceled for a while."

223. An older depressed client is concerned about many fears that are upsetting and frightening and expresses a feeling of having committed the "unpardonable sin." The nurse can best reassure the client by stating:
1. "Your family loves you very much."
2. "You know that you are not a bad person."
3. "You know, those ideas of yours are in your imagination."
4. "Your ideas, which are part of your illness, will change as you improve."

224. A client who attempted suicide by slashing her wrists is transferred from the emergency department to the psychiatric unit of a community hospital. When the client arrives on the unit, the priority nursing intervention should be to:
1. Obtain the client's vital signs
2. Initiate a therapeutic relationship
3. Inspect the bandages for signs of bleeding
4. Institute continuous observation of the client

225. After admission, the nurse needs to evaluate a depressed client's potential for suicide. The approach that best gains this information is for the nurse to ask:
1. The client about plans for the future
2. The client whether suicide is now being considered
3. Other clients about suicide while the client is in the group
4. Family members whether the client has ever attempted suicide

226. A middle-aged female client with major depression feels all her family members have been killed because she has been sinful and needs to be punished. The prime responsibility of the nurse caring for this client should be to:
1. Protect the client against any suicidal impulses
2. Keep up the client's interest in the outside world
3. Help the client handle her concern for family members
4. Reassure the client that past behaviors are not being punished

227. A client is admitted to the mental health unit after attempting suicide. When the nurse approaches, the client is tearful and silent. Which is the nurse's best initial response?
1. Note the behavior, record it, and notify the attending physician
2. Sit quietly next to the client and wait until the client begins to speak
3. Say, "You are crying; that means you feel badly about attempting suicide and really want to live."
4. Say, "I notice you are tearful and seem sad. Tell me what it's like for you and perhaps we can begin to work it out together."

228. A nurse has been assigned to work with a depressed client on a one-to-one basis. The next morning the client refuses to get out of bed, stating, "I'm too sick to be helped and I don't want to be bothered." What is the best response the nurse can make?
1. "You will not feel better unless you make the effort to get up and get dressed."
2. "I know you will feel better again if you only make the attempt to help yourself."
3. "Everyone feels this way in the beginning as they confront repressed feelings. I'll sit down with you."
4. "I know you don't feel like getting up, but you probably will feel better if you do. Let me help you get started."

229. An older, depressed client frequently paces the halls, becoming physically tired from the activity. To help the client reduce this activity, the nurse should:
1. Supply the client with simple, monotonous tasks
2. Request a sedative order from the client's physician
3. Restrain the client in a chair, reducing the opportunity to pace
4. Place the client in a single room, thus limiting pacing to a smaller area

230. The nurse sits with an older depressed client twice a day, although there is little verbal communication. One afternoon, the client asks, "Do you think they'll ever let me out of here?" The nurse's best reply should be:
1. "Maybe you should ask your doctor."
2. "Everyone says you're doing just fine."
3. "Why, do you think you are ready to leave?"
4. "You have the feeling that you might not leave?"

231. The nurse develops a long-term therapy goal for a female client hospitalized for a major depressive episode. The goal states the client will:
1. Talk openly about her depressed feelings
2. Identify and use new defense mechanisms
3. Discuss the unconscious source of her anger
4. Verbalize realistic perceptions of herself and others

232. A depressed client states, "I am no good. I'm better off dead." Which intervention by the nurse is a priority?
1. Stating, "I think you're good; you should think of living."
2. Alerting the staff to provide 24-hour observation of the client

3. Responding, "I will stay with you until you are less depressed."
4. Unobtrusively removing those articles that may be used in a suicide attempt

233. What is a positive nursing action when caring for a middle-aged, depressed client?
   1. Play a game of chess with the client
   2. Allow the client to make personal decisions
   3. Sit down next to the client at frequent intervals
   4. Provide the client with frequent periods of time for reflection

234. A teenager recently committed suicide. The school community was saddened by the event and grief counselors have been working with students. The school nurse understands that other students may attempt to copy the behavior. When observing the student body, the nurse should monitor for presuicide behavior, which includes:
   1. Giving away prized possessions
   2. Memorializing the dead teenager
   3. Talking excessively about the event
   4. Becoming involved in student activities

235. A client with a diagnosis of major depression refuses to participate in unit activities because of being "just too tired." What nursing approach best expresses an understanding of this client's needs?
   1. Planning a rest period for the client during activity time
   2. Explaining why the staff believes the activities are therapeutic
   3. Helping the client express negative feelings about the activities
   4. Accepting the client's behavior calmly while setting firm limits

236. The nurse stops by the room of a tearfully depressed newly admitted client and offers to walk the client to the evening meal. The client looks intently at the nurse, saying nothing. Which is the best response by the nurse?
   1. "I'll be at the desk if you need me."
   2. "You must tell me what you are feeling now."
   3. "It must be very difficult for you to be on a psychiatric unit."
   4. "We will walk together to dinner when you pull yourself together."

237. A client is admitted to the psychiatric hospital after many self-inflicted nonlethal injuries over the last month. The nurse identifies that these injuries are documented on the admission history as suicidal:
   1. Threats
   2. Gestures
   3. Attempts
   4. Ideations

238. During individual sessions designed to help the depressed client with a history of suicide attempts explore alternative coping strategies, it is most appropriate for the nurse to ask:
   1. "How have you managed your problems in the past?"

2. "What do you feel you have learned from this suicide attempt?"
3. "How will you manage the next time your problems start piling up?"
4. "Were there other things going on in your life that made you want to die?"

239. The nurse is assigned to care for a middle-aged, depressed female client on a day when the client seems more withdrawn and depressed than usual. Which intervention by the nurse is most appropriate?
   1. Remain visible to the client
   2. Get the client involved in group activities
   3. Ask the client if it would help to sit with her a while
   4. Spend a few extra minutes with the client throughout the day

240. The nurse is to discharge a client from the psychiatric unit who has been treated for major depression. Which statement by the nurse demonstrates the most understanding at this time?
   1. "Call the unit night or day if you have problems."
   2. "I am going to miss you; we have become good friends."
   3. "I know you are really going to be all right when you go home."
   4. "This is my phone number; call me to let me know how you are doing."

241. On the second day after admission, a suicidal client asks the nurse, "Why am I being observed around the clock, and why is my freedom to move around the unit restricted?" Which reply by the nurse is most appropriate?
   1. "Why do you think we are observing you?"
   2. "What makes you think that we are observing you?"
   3. "We are concerned that you might try to harm yourself."
   4. "Your doctor has ordered it so the doctor is the one you should ask about it."

242. After 4 days on the inpatient psychiatric unit, a client on suicidal precautions tells the nurse, "Hey, look! I was feeling pretty depressed for a while, but I'm certainly not going to kill myself." The nurse's best response to this statement is:
   1. "Kill yourself? I don't understand."
   2. "You do seem to be feeling better."
   3. "Suppose we talk some more about this."
   4. "We have to observe you until your psychiatrist tells us to stop."

243. During a group discussion, it is learned that a female group member masked her depression and suicidal urges and indeed committed suicide several days ago. The nurse leading the group should be prepared primarily to deal with the:
   1. Guilt that group members feel because they could not prevent another's suicide
   2. Lack of concern over the member's act of suicide expressed by some of the group

3. Guilt, and anger of the co-leaders that they failed to anticipate and prevent the suicide

4. Anxiety and fear by some members of the group that their own suicidal urges may go unnoticed and unprotected

244. The nurse should anticipate that the treatment plan for a client admitted with a severe, persistent, intractable depression and suicidal ideation will probably include:
1. Electroconvulsive therapy
2. Short-term psychoanalysis
3. Nondirective psychotherapy
4. High doses of anxiolytic drugs

245. A severely depressed client is to have electroconvulsive therapy. When discussing this therapy, what should the nurse tell the client?
1. Sleep will be induced and treatment will not cause pain
2. With new methods of administration, treatment is totally safe
3. It is better not to talk about it, but you can ask any question you like
4. There may be some permanent memory loss as a result of the treatment

246. An extremely depressed client is to begin electroconvulsive therapy and expresses anxiety about the procedure. When explaining this procedure, the nurse should emphasize that:
1. Answers to any questions will be provided
2. Periods of amnesia will follow the treatment
3. The treatments will make the client feel better
4. The client will not be alone during the treatment

247. The nurse understands that a side effect of electroconvulsive therapy that a client may experience is:
1. Loss of appetite
2. Postural hypotension
3. Complete loss of memory for a time
4. Confusion immediately after the treatment

248. When the nurse sits next to a depressed client and begins to talk, the client says to the nurse, "I'm stupid and useless. Talk with the other people who are more important." Which response by the nurse is most therapeutic?
1. "Everyone is important."
2. "Do you feel that you are not important?"
3. "Why do you feel you are not important?"
4. "I want to talk with you because you are important to me."

249. A client is admitted to a mental health facility for depression. In an effort to promote a positive self-regard, the nurse should:
1. Set limits on the client's negative behaviors
2. Praise the client's efforts at every opportunity
3. Involve the client in activities that promote success
4. Encourage the client to participate in activities with other clients

250. During an interaction, a depressed client says, "I want to die." Which is the most therapeutic response by the nurse?
1. "You would rather not live."
2. "You are not alone in feeling this way."

3. "When was the last time you felt this way?"
4. "Do you believe that there is life after death?"

251. A hyperactive client exhibiting manic behavior is admitted to the hospital. In view of the client's elated state, the nurse should arrange for the client to be in a room:
1. That has basic simple furnishings
2. With another client who is very quiet
3. That will provide a great deal of stimuli
4. With another client exhibiting similar behavior

252. During the orientation tour for three new staff members, a young, hyperactive manic client greets them by saying, "Welcome to the funny farm. I'm Jo-Jo, the head yo-yo." Which meaning can the nurse assign to the client's statement? The client is:
1. Trying to fill the "life-of-the-party" role
2. Looking for attention from the new staff
3. Unable to distinguish fantasy from reality
4. Anxious over the arrival of the new staff members

253. When the language of a client in the manic phase of a bipolar disorder becomes vulgar and profane, what is the best intervention by the nurse?
1. State, "We do not like that kind of talk around here."
2. Ignore it, since the client is using it only to get attention
3. Recognize the language as part of the illness, but set limits on it
4. State, "When you can talk in an acceptable way, we will talk to you."

254. A client with the diagnosis of bipolar I disorder, manic episode, has a superior, authoritative manner and is constantly instructing the other clients on the unit about how to dress, what to eat, and where to sit. The nurse intervenes in these behaviors because they will eventually make the other clients feel:
1. Angry
2. Dependent
3. Inadequate
4. Ambivalent

255. A client with the diagnosis of bipolar disorder, manic episode, is extremely active, talks constantly, and tends to badger the other clients, some of whom are now becoming agitated. What is the best strategy for the nurse to use with this client?
1. Humor
2. Sympathy
3. Distraction
4. Confrontation

256. What nursing intervention may redirect a hyperactive, manic client therapeutically?
1. Asking the client to guide other clients as they clean their rooms
2. Suggesting the client initiate social activities on the unit for the client group
3. Encouraging the client to tear pictures out of magazines for a scrap book
4. Providing a pencil and paper to encourage the client to write a short story

257. The nurse is assigned to care for a 39-year-old, hyperactive, manic client who exhibits flight of ideas. The client is not eating. The nurse recognizes this may be because the client:
    1. Feels undeserving of the food
    2. Is too busy to take the time to eat
    3. Wishes to avoid the clients in the dining room
    4. Believes that at this time there is no need for food

258. A physician has been a client of the psychiatric service for the past 3 days. The client has questioned the authority of the treatment team, has advised other clients that their treatment plans are wrong, and has been generally disruptive in group therapy. The nurse's most appropriate response should be to:
    1. Ignore the client and hope the disruptive behavior will stop
    2. Restrict the client's contact with other clients until the disruptive behavior ceases
    3. Tell the other clients that they should not pay attention to what the client says
    4. Understand that the client is unable to control this behavior and that limits must be set

259. During a client's periods of extreme mania and hyperactivity, how should the nursing staff provide for the client's nutritional needs?
    1. Accept the fact that the client will eat if hungry.
    2. Follow the client around the dining room with a tray.
    3. Allow the client to prepare own meals to eat when desired.
    4. Provide the client with frequent, high-calorie feedings that can be hand-held.

260. A 23-year-old client has been admitted to a psychiatric hospital after a month of unusual behavior that included eating and sleeping very little, talking and singing constantly, and going on frequent shopping sprees. In the hospital, the client is demanding, bossy, and sarcastic. The nurse understands that the adaptations the client is exhibiting usually are found in clients with the diagnosis of:
    1. Major depression
    2. Bipolar disorder, manic phase
    3. Antisocial personality disorder
    4. Chronic undifferentiated schizophrenia

261. When approaching a client during a period of great overactivity, it is essential for the nurse to:
    1. Use a firm and warm, consistent approach
    2. Allow the client to choose the activities in which to participate
    3. Anticipate and physically control the client's hyperactivity
    4. Let the client know the staff will not tolerate destructive behavior

262. When developing the plan of care for a client in the manic phase of bipolar disorder, the nurse should plan to:
    1. Focus the client's interest in reality
    2. Encourage the client to talk as much as needed

    3. Persuade the client to complete any task that has been started
    4. Provide constructive channels for redirecting the client's excess energy

263. Clients with the diagnosis of bipolar disorder, manic episode, most likely will exhibit signs of:
    1. Passivity
    2. Dysphoria
    3. Anhedonia
    4. Grandiosity

264. Depressed clients often have the primary characteristic of early morning awakening. Which nursing intervention in the day time is best for the staff to implement for this client?
    1. Restrict the client's access to the bedroom
    2. Offer the client a series of relaxation tapes
    3. Reschedule the client's bedtime to an earlier hour
    4. Suggest that the client exercise before going to bed

NURSING CARE OF CLIENTS WITH DISORDERS RELATED TO ALTERATIONS IN BEHAVIOR

265. The nurse on a psychiatric unit can begin to help an extremely anxious client with a sleep problem who has been assigned to a four-bed room since admission by saying:
    1. "You seem unable to sleep at night"
    2. "I'm going to move you to a private room"
    3. "Don't worry; you'll sleep when you're tired"
    4. "I'll get you the sedative your doctor ordered"

266. During an intake interview, the client relates experiencing overwhelming irresistible attacks of sleep. Which sleep disorder does the nurse identify after this interview?
    1. Insomnia
    2. Narcolepsy
    3. Sleep apnea
    4. Sleep terror

267. A female client verbalizes that she has been having trouble sleeping and feels wide awake as soon as she gets into bed. The nurse teaches the client about interventions that promote sleep. Check all that apply.
    1. ☐ Eat a heavy snack near bedtime
    2. ☐ Read in bed before shutting out the light
    3. ☐ Leave the bedroom if you are unable to sleep
    4. ☐ Drink a cup of warm tea with milk at bedtime
    5. ☐ Exercise in the afternoon rather than in the evening
    6. ☐ Count backward from 100 to 0 when your mind is racing

268. A client has a diagnosis of primary insomnia. Before assessing this client, the nurse recalls the numerous causes of this disorder. Select all that apply.
    1. ☐ Chronic stress
    2. ☐ Severe anxiety
    3. ☐ Generalized pain
    4. ☐ Excessive caffeine

5. ❒ Chronic depression

6. ❒ Environmental noise

269. A female client, age 16, is admitted to the psychiatric service with the diagnosis of anorexia nervosa. She has lost 20 pounds in 6 weeks. She is very thin but excessively concerned about being overweight. Her daily intake is 10 cups of coffee. What is the most important initial nursing intervention for this client?

1. Compliment her on her lovely figure

2. Explain the value of adequate nutrition

3. Explore the reasons why she does not eat

4. Attempt to establish a relationship of trust

270. The nurse determines that an appropriate behavior modification goal for a client with anorexia nervosa is that the client will:

1. Eat every meal for a week

2. Gain a pound of weight a week

3. Attend group therapy every day

4. Talk about food for 1 hour a day

271. Evaluation of clients with anorexia nervosa requires reassessment of behaviors after admission. The nursing assessment that indicates that the therapy is beginning to become effective is when the client:

1. Is hiding food in pockets of clothing

2. States that the admission has been helpful

3. Has gained 6 pounds since admission 3 weeks ago

4. Is the last to leave the dining room table after meals

272. A 16-year-old cachectic adolescent, with the diagnoses of anorexia nervosa, dehydration, and electrolyte imbalances, is admitted to a mental health facility. The adolescent is obsessed with her weight, exercises for hours every day, takes enemas and laxatives several times a week, and engages in self-induced vomiting. Which is a priority when the nurse plans care for this client?

1. Identifying personal strengths

2. Controlling impulsive behavior

3. Correcting electrolyte imbalances

4. Establishing a contract for treatment goals

273. The nurse understands that the major difference between anorexia nervosa and bulimia nervosa is that the individual with bulimia nervosa:

1. Is obese and is attempting to lose weight

2. Has a distorted body image and sees the body as fat

3. Has behaviors and an appearance that appear more normal

4. Is struggling with a conflict of dependence versus independence

274. When creating a therapeutic environment for clients with bulimia nervosa, the nurse should strive for one that is:

1. Controlling

2. Empathetic

3. Focused on food

4. Based on realistic limits

275. A 20-year-old college student is brought to the psychiatric hospital by her parents. Her admitting diagnosis is borderline personality disorder. When talking with the parents, which information can the nurse expect to be included in the client's history? Select all that apply.

1. ❒ Impulsiveness

2. ❒ Lability of mood

3. ❒ Ritualistic behavior

4. ❒ Self-destructive behavior

5. ❒ Psychomotor retardation

276. A hospitalized client, diagnosed with a borderline personality disorder, consistently breaks the unit's rules. This behavior should be confronted because it will help the client:

1. Control anger

2. Reduce anxiety

3. Set realistic goals

4. Become more self-aware

277. A client with a personality disorder tells the nurse, "I want to tell you something, but you must promise to keep it a secret." Which response may impair the therapeutic relationship? "I would like to hear what you have to say:

1. And as a client advocate, I will respect your right to confidentiality."

2. But I am part of a team that shares important information about clients."

3. But I cannot promise to keep what you say confidential from the rest of the staff."

4. And I hope that you will trust me to do what is in your best interests with the information."

278. An adult client with a borderline personality disorder becomes nauseated and vomits immediately after drinking 2 ounces of shampoo as a suicide gesture. Which is the most appropriate initial response by the nurse?

1. Promptly notify the attending physician

2. Immediately institute suicide precautions

3. Assess the client's vital signs and administer syrup of ipecac

4. Sit quietly with the client until nausea and vomiting subside

279. When working with the nurse during the orientation phase of the relationship, a client with a borderline personality disorder will probably have the most difficulty in:

1. Controlling anxiety

2. Terminating the session on time

3. Accepting the psychiatric diagnosis

4. Setting mutual goals for the relationship

280. A young adult is diagnosed with a schizotypal personality disorder. How might the nurse describe the client's behavior?

1. Rigid and controlling

2. Submissive and immature

3. Arrogant and attention seeking

4. Introverted and emotionally withdrawn

281. Which action should the nurse take when caring for a client with the diagnosis of schizotypal personality disorder?
    1. Set limits on manipulative behavior
    2. Encourage participation in group therapy
    3. Respect the client's need for social isolation
    4. Understand that seductive behavior is expected

282. A client has the diagnosis of histrionic personality disorder. Which behavior can the nurse expect when assessing this client?
    1. Dramatic and theatrical
    2. Boastful and egotistical
    3. Rigid and perfectionistic
    4. Aggressive and manipulative

283. Which are most important for the nurse to implement when working with a client with the diagnosis of antisocial personality disorder?
    1. Teach and role-model assertiveness
    2. Use a gentle and reassuring approach
    3. Provide clear boundaries and consequences
    4. Present an empathetic and democratic approach

284. When formulating a nursing plan of care for a client with an antisocial personality disorder, the nurse should take into consideration that this client:
    1. Suffers from a great deal of anxiety
    2. Rapidly learns by experience if punished
    3. Is generally unable to postpone gratification
    4. Has a great sense of responsibility toward others

285. The nursing staff is discussing the best way to develop a relationship with a new client who has an antisocial personality disorder. People with this disorder have difficulty relating to others because they:
    1. Will not count on others
    2. Cannot empathize with others
    3. Never learned to be dependent on others
    4. Have difficulty communicating socially with others

286. A young, handsome man with a diagnosis of antisocial personality disorder is being discharged from the hospital next week. He asks the nurse for her phone number so that he can call her for a date. Which is the nurse's best response?
    1. "We are not permitted to date clients."
    2. "No, you are a client and I am a nurse."
    3. "I like you, but our relationship is professional."
    4. "It is against my professional ethics to date clients."

287. The nurse identifies that a client is pretending to be ill. The nurse understands that this behavior is usually thought to be:
    1. Psychotic
    2. Malingering
    3. Out of contact with reality
    4. Using conversion defenses

288. A nurse is orienting a new client to the unit when another client rushes down the hallway and asks the nurse to sit down to talk. The client requesting the nurse's attention is extremely manipulative and uses socially acting-out behaviors when demands are unmet. How should the nurse intervene?
    1. Suggest that the client requesting attention speak with another staff member
    2. Leave the new client and talk with the other client to avoid precipitating acting-out behavior
    3. Introduce the two clients and suggest that the client join the new client and the nurse on the tour
    4. Tell the interrupting client to sit down and be patient, stating, "I'll be back as soon as possible."

289. A client with a diagnosis of narcissistic personality disorder has been given a day pass from the psychiatric hospital. The client is due to return at 6 PM. At 5 PM the client telephones the nurse in charge of the unit and says, "Six o'clock is too early. I feel like coming back at 7:30." To be most therapeutic, the nurse should tell the client to:
    1. Return immediately, to demonstrate control
    2. Return on time or restrictions will be imposed
    3. Come back by 6:45, as a compromise to set limits
    4. Come back as soon as possible or the police will be sent

290. A client has been diagnosed with an adjustment disorder with mixed anxiety and depression. What is the primary problem for a client with an adjustment disorder?
    1. Deficient memory
    2. Impaired self-esteem
    3. Intolerance to activity
    4. Disturbed personal identity

291. The nurse understands that the most important factor in rehabilitation of a client addicted to alcohol is the:
    1. Availability of community resources
    2. Accepting attitude of the client's family
    3. Client's emotional or motivational readiness
    4. Qualitative level of the client's physical state

292. The nurse expects that clients with a history of alcoholism with Wernicke's encephalopathy associated with Korsakoff's syndrome will be treated initially by:
    1. Providing a low-fat diet
    2. Judicious use of neuroleptics
    3. Oral administration of Thorazine
    4. Intramuscular injections of thiamine

293. A client with an alcohol abuse problem asks whether the nurse can see the bugs that are crawling on the bed. Which should be the nurse's initial reply?
    1. "No, I don't see any bugs."
    2. "I will get rid of them for you."
    3. "I will stay here until you are calmer."
    4. "Those bugs are a part of your sickness."

294. A recovering alcoholic joins Alcoholics Anonymous to help maintain sobriety. The nurse knows that AA is classified as a:
    1. Social group
    2. Self-help group
    3. Resocialization group
    4. Psychotherapeutic group

295. Clients addicted to alcohol use denial as one of their prime defense mechanisms. The nurse further understands that these clients use denial to:
    1. Reduce their feelings of guilt
    2. Live up to others' expectations
    3. Make them seem more independent
    4. Have them look better in the eyes of others

296. When a client makes up stories to fill in blank spaces of memory, the nurse should document this as:
    1. Lying
    2. Denying
    3. Rationalizing
    4. Confabulating

297. When discussing plans with a client seeking help, the nurse knows that the most effective treatment of alcoholism is accomplished by:
    1. Individual or group psychotherapy
    2. Admission to an alcoholic unit in a hospital
    3. Active membership in Alcoholics Anonymous
    4. The daily administration of disulfiram (Antabuse)

298. To determine the potential an individual has for a drinking problem, the nurse uses the CAGE Screening Test for Alcoholism. Which is one of the four questions included in this test?
    1. "Do you feel you are a normal drinker?"
    2. "Have you ever felt bad or guilty about your drinking?"
    3. "Are you always able to stop drinking when you want to?"
    4. "How often did you have a drink containing alcohol in the past year?"

299. A client undergoing alcohol detoxification asks whether attendance at Alcoholics Anonymous (AA) is required. Which is the nurse's best reply?
    1. "You'll find you'll need their support."
    2. "No, it is best to wait until you feel you really need them."
    3. "What feelings do you have about going to those meetings?"
    4. "Yes, because you will learn how to cope with your problem."

300. A client is attending AA after withdrawing from alcohol. The nurse understands that the ultimate purpose of self-help groups such as AA is to help members:
    1. Change destructive behavior
    2. Develop functional relationships
    3. Identify how they present themselves to others
    4. Understand their patterns of interacting within the group

301. A client who has just begun attending Alcoholics Anonymous asks the nurse whether it is really necessary to go to meetings. Which is the nurse's best response?
    1. "Yes, if you really want to get well."
    2. "It's your decision about whether or not you want to attend."
    3. "You think that attending these meetings may not be helpful?"

    4. "It sounds like you think attending meetings is too much effort."

302. A client with a long history of alcohol abuse spends 28 days in the detoxification unit. When planning for the client's discharge, the nurse understands that an essential component of the discharge plan is a referral to a:
    1. Halfway house
    2. Family therapist
    3. Psychoanalytic therapy group
    4. Community-based self-help group

303. The nurse understands that a key indicator that a client with a long history of alcohol abuse is ready for treatment is evidenced by the client's:
    1. Drinking only socially
    2. Not drinking for 2 weeks
    3. Self-admission for detoxification
    4. Verbalizing an honest desire for help

304. The nurse evaluates that a male client has accepted his drinking as a problem when he:
    1. Attends scheduled inpatient group meetings
    2. Takes his Antabuse each morning as ordered
    3. Attends Alcoholics Anonymous meetings daily
    4. Volunteers to be a sponsor for another alcoholic

305. A client who is a polysubstance abuser is mandated to seek drug and alcohol counseling. When working with the client, the nurse identifies that the priority outcome criterion for this client is, "The client will:
    1. Verbalize that a substance abuse problem exists."
    2. Discuss the effect of drug use on self and others."
    3. Express negative feelings about the present life situation."
    4. Explore the use of substances and problematic behaviors."

306. In considering how addictive certain drugs are, the nurse understands that some have a higher potential for causing addiction than others. List the addiction potential of the following drugs in order, from the drug with the lowest potential to cause addiction to the drug with the highest potential for addiction.
    1. _____ Heroin
    2. _____ Alcohol
    3. _____ Codeine
    4. _____ Barbiturates

307. The nurse is caring for a young client who is a narcotic addict and has had surgery to repair a laceration of the heart caused by a bullet. The client is receiving methadone hydrochloride. The nurse understands that this medication is given because it:
    1. Allows symptom-free termination of narcotic addiction
    2. Converts narcotic use from an illicit to a legally controlled drug
    3. Provides postoperative pain control without causing narcotic dependence
    4. Counteracts the depressive effects of long-term opiate use on cardiac and thoracic muscles

308. When methadone hydrochloride dosage is lowered, the nurse must observe the surgical client who is addicted to narcotics for evidence of:
   1. Piloerection, lack of interest in surroundings
   2. Agitation, attempts to escape from the hospital
   3. Skin dryness, scratching under incisional dressing
   4. Lethargy, refusal to participate in therapeutic exercise

309. A female client has been receiving oxycodone (OxyContin) for moderate pain associated with multiple injuries sustained in a motor vehicle accident. The client has returned three times for refills of the prescription. What assessment by the nurse, in addition to the client's slurred speech, leads the nurse to suspect opioid intoxication?
   1. Hypervigilance
   2. Lability of mood
   3. Constricted pupils
   4. Increased respirations

310. The nurse identifies the presence of drug abuse when the client exhibits:
   1. A physiologic need for a drug
   2. A psychologic dependence on a drug
   3. Compulsive drug use on either a continuous or periodic basis
   4. Excessive drug use inconsistent with acceptable medical practice

311. Within an hour of receiving naloxone hydrochloride (Narcan) to combat an overdose of heroin, a client is responding. The nurse should continue close observation of the client's status because:
   1. The drug may cause peripheral neuropathy
   2. When combined, Narcan and heroin cause cardiac depression
   3. The narcotic effect may cause a return of symptoms after the drug is metabolized
   4. Hyperexcitability and amnesia may cause the client to thrash about and become abusive

312. When thinking about alcohol and drug abuse, the nurse understands that:
   1. Most polydrug abusers also abuse alcohol
   2. Most alcoholics become polydrug abusers
   3. Addictive individuals tend to use hostile, abusive behavior
   4. An unhappy childhood is a causative factor in many addictions

313. A client is brought to the emergency department by friends because of increasingly bizarre behavior. When assessing the client, which adaptations indicate that the client probably was using cocaine? Check all that apply.
   1. ☐ Euphoria
   2. ☐ Agitation
   3. ☐ Panic attacks
   4. ☐ Slurred speech
   5. ☐ Hypervigilance
   6. ☐ Impaired judgment

314. Shortly after admission, an adolescent male client falls to the floor and has tonic-clonic movements. He does not respond verbally, but the nurse notes that he is still chewing gum. The nurse should:
   1. Remove the chewing gum
   2. Document the observations
   3. Send another client for help
   4. Insert a tongue blade between the teeth

315. A client who has been an inpatient on a medical unit for more than 6 days continues to complain of severe abdominal symptoms. Nursing staff members are deeply concerned because there has been no response to treatment. All tests are negative. The client finally is diagnosed with Munchausen syndrome. Which feeling will the nurses probably experience?
   1. Pity
   2. Anger
   3. Annoyance
   4. Indifference

316. A child has been hospitalized repeatedly for illnesses with unknown etiologies. Finally, the practitioner makes the diagnosis of Munchausen's syndrome by proxy. The nurse's most therapeutic approach with the involved parent is:
   1. Confrontation
   2. Open communication
   3. Health teaching about child rearing
   4. Validation of the child's physical status

NURSING CARE OF CLIENTS WITH SEXUAL AND GENDER IDENTITY DISORDERS

317. Which is a frequent finding in clients with paraphiliac sexual disorders?
   1. Other covert or overt emotional problems are present
   2. Gonadal and pituitary hormone deficiencies are involved
   3. Overassociation with society's fringe groups has thwarted judgment
   4. An inadequate physical development of the sexual organs has occurred

318. A 43-year-old, well-dressed man charged with molesting a 7-year-old child is admitted for psychiatric evaluation. When the nurse asks him to come to dinner, he refuses and states, "I don't want anyone to see me. Leave me alone." What is the nurse's best response?
   1. "Certainly, I respect your wishes."
   2. "You sound upset; let's talk about it."
   3. "It will be easier to face other people right away."
   4. "Only the staff members know why you are here."

319. A 4-year-old girl tells the school nurse that her father has been getting into bed with her at night and touching her. The nurse should:
   1. Ask the child to describe the touching
   2. Tell the teacher to report any inappropriate behavior

3. Report the child's conversation to child protective services
4. Contact the father to come to the school immediately

320. A male client with the diagnosis of gender identity disorder has been dressing and functioning in society as a woman for 2 years and has decided to have sex reassignment surgery. He tells the nurse that all his life he has considered himself to be female. Place the following nursing interventions in order of priority when caring for this client.
1. _____ Treat the client with respect
2. _____ Investigate own feelings about sexuality
3. _____ Encourage the client to explore his feelings
4. _____ Accept the decision to have sex reassignment surgery
5. _____ Explore ways that the decision can be shared with significant others

321. The physician orders sildenafil (Viagra) for a male client with erectile dysfunction. The nurse should teach the client about the common side effects of this drug. Indicate all that apply.
1. ☐ Flushing
2. ☐ Headache
3. ☐ Dyspepsia
4. ☐ Constipation
5. ☐ Hypertension

322. A male client with the diagnosis of pedophilia is admitted to the psychiatric hospital because of repeated episodes of exhibitionism. In the recreation room the client exposes himself to the nurse and begins to masturbate. The nurse should:
1. Turn away from the client and ignore the behavior
2. Tell the client that the behavior is unacceptable and to stop
3. Remove the client from the recreation room and escort him to his own room
4. Recognize that the behavior is part of his illness and obtain an order for a libido-lowering medication

323. During a routine yearly physical an older adult says to the nurse, "I have not had sex lately because I can no longer get it up!" The nurse's initial response should be:
1. "Let's discuss this concern a little more."
2. "Be sure to tell the physician about this problem."
3. "This is an expected physiological response to getting older."
4. "There is medication available for erectile dysfunction."

324. The nurse identifies that a male client may have a sexual arousal disorder when during a yearly physical the client states:
1. "I have no interest in sex."
2. "I don't get very hard anymore."
3. "I climax almost before we even get started."
4. "I take forever before I finally have an orgasm."

325. A 25-year-old woman with the diagnosis of bipolar disorder, manic episode, is admitted to the psychiatric unit. The nurse on the psychiatric unit reviews the admission information provided by the client's husband and assesses the client. Based on the information in the chart below, what is an appropriate nursing intervention?
1. Assigning the client to a private room
2. Suggesting the client play cards with several other clients
3. Encouraging the development of insight through introspection
4. Having the client sit at the communal dining table during meals

CLIENT CHART

Admission Information
Interview with client's husband
"My wife is 25 years old and we have been married for 3 years. She always had a lot of energy, but lately she is constantly on the go and is acting crazy. She hardly ever sleeps, has been giving away her clothes and buying all new sexy clothes, and rarely eats. She became furious when I took the credit card away from her. She demands sex constantly, and I found out she has been having multiple affairs. Finally I couldn't take it any more, and I brought her to the hospital."

Client Assessment
Client is talking loudly and jumps from one topic to another; exhibiting constant motor activity. Client is wearing skimpy clothing without undergarments. Client states, "I like wearing my new clothes because I get turned on when people look at me." At times uses profanity, particularly when talking about how her husband took away her credit card. Client not exhibiting combative or physically assaultive behavior.

ANSWERS AND RATIONALES

FOUNDATIONS OF MENTAL HEALTH/ PSYCHIATRIC NURSING

1. **3** This is the age of Freud's phallic stage and Erikson's stage of initiative versus guilt.

   1 This age is Freud's genital stage and Erikson's stage of identity versus role confusion. **2** This age is Freud's latency stage and Erikson's stage of industry versus inferiority. **4** This age is Freud's oral stage and Erikson's stage of trust versus mistrust.
   Client Need: Health Promotion and Maintenance; **Cognitive Level:** Comprehension; **Nursing Process:** Assessment/Analysis; **Reference:** Ch 15, Formation of the Personality

2. **3** Children view their own worth by the response received from their parents. This sense of worth sets the basic ego strengths and is vital to the formation of the personality.

   1 Peer groups come later in a child's development, but the parent-child relationship is still the most important. **2** Although important, it is not as important as the parent-child relationship. **4** This comes later in life, after the basic personality has been formed.
   Client Need: Health Promotion and Maintenance; **Cognitive Level:** Comprehension; **Nursing Process:** Assessment/Analysis; **Reference:** Ch 15, Formation of the Personality

3. **4** When acting-out against the primary source of anxiety creates even further anxiety or danger, the individual may use displacement to express feelings on a safer person or object.

   1 This is an example of denial. **2** This reflects an inability to mature and accept responsibility. **3** This is fantasy.
   Client Need: Psychosocial Integrity; **Cognitive Level:** Application; **Nursing Process:** Assessment/Analysis; **Reference:** Ch 15, Defense Mechanisms

4. **4** When the individual experiences a threat to self-esteem, anxiety increases and defense mechanisms are used to protect the self.

   1 Affective reactions are mood disorders. **2** Withdrawal patterns are an abnormal way of coping with stress; if carried to an extreme, behavior can become pathologic. **3** Ritualistic behaviors are not an aspect of the developmental process.
   Client Need: Psychosocial Integrity; **Cognitive Level:** Analysis; **Nursing Process:** Assessment/Analysis; **Reference:** Ch 15, Defense Mechanisms

5. **1** This client is using the cognitive distortions of overgeneralization and pessimism. Negative events are magnified and become the focus while contrary positive experiences are minimized and ignored. By focusing on the negative, the depressive mood is reinforced.

   2, 3, 4 There are no data to support this conclusion.
   Client Need: Psychosocial Integrity; **Cognitive Level:** Analysis; **Nursing Process:** Assessment/Analysis; **Reference:** Ch 15, Cognitive Theory

6. **3** By developing skills in one area, the individual compensates or makes up for a real or imagined deficiency, thereby maintaining a positive self-image.

   1 If the student incorporated the qualities of the college athlete, that would be introjection. **2** This deals more with unacceptable impulses that may pose a threat. **4** This person is not trying to make amends for unacceptable feelings (reaction formation) but rather for a believed deficiency and an inadequate self-image.
   Client Need: Psychosocial Integrity; **Cognitive Level:** Analysis; **Nursing Process:** Assessment/Analysis; **Reference:** Ch 15, Defense Mechanisms

7. **4** Fears and anxieties about themselves and their possessions are common in older adults because of a decreased self-concept and an altered body image; these changes result in a decreased ability to cope.

   1 Aging need not necessarily bring about losing one's ability to cooperate. **2** This behavior is noted in the middle stage of Alzheimer's disease; usually it is not observed in older adults. **3** The attitude of older adults about authority or others in their environment is set; indecision about life situations may be due to insecurity.
   Client Need: Health Promotion and Maintenance; **Cognitive Level:** Analysis; **Integrated Process:** Teaching/Learning; **Nursing Process:** Planning/Implementation; **Reference:** Ch 15, Formation of the Personality

8. **1** Use of denial involves failure to acknowledge the reality of a situation.

   2, 4 This is not demonstrated in this situation.
   3 Intellectualization involves discussing the child's problem in a technical manner; this is not demonstrated in this situation.
   Client Need: Psychosocial Integrity; **Cognitive Level:** Analysis; **Nursing Process:** Assessment/Analysis; **Reference:** Ch 15, Defense Mechanisms

9. **2** Any behavioral therapy or learning of new methods of coping with situations requires modifications of approach and attitudes; hence personality is always capable of change.

   1 Certain personality traits are established by age 2, but not the total personality. **3** The capacity for change exists throughout the life cycle. **4** Accepting this theory closes the door on all future growth and development.
   Client Need: Health Promotion and Maintenance; **Cognitive Level:** Comprehension; **Nursing Process:** Assessment/Analysis; **Reference:** Ch 15, Formation of the Personality

10. **2** Attributing unacceptable feelings or attributes to others is the mechanism known as projection; the data demonstrate use of this defense mechanism.

    1 Denial is the unconscious refusal to recognize the reality of an anxiety-producing situation; the data do not demonstrate use of this defense mechanism.
    3 Displacement is the shifting of feelings from an emotionally charged situation to a substitute person

or object; the data do not demonstrate use of this defense mechanism. **4** Intellectualization is the use of reasoning to avoid confronting an objectionable impulse; the data do not demonstrate use of this defense mechanism.

Client Need: Psychosocial Integrity; **Cognitive Level:** Analysis; **Nursing Process:** Assessment/Analysis; **Reference:** Ch 15, Defense Mechanisms

11. **3** The toddler is learning autonomy, but because of the nature of development, there is still physical and emotional dependence on the parents.

1 The major task during infancy is the development of trust. **2** This stage deals with the task of industry and developing skills for working in and relating to the world. **4** This stage deals with developing a sense of initiative.

Client Need: Health Promotion and Maintenance; **Cognitive Level:** Comprehension; **Nursing Process:** Assessment/Analysis; **Reference:** Ch 15, Formation of the Personality

12. **3** The child resolves oedipal conflicts by learning to identify with the parent of the same sex and accomplishes this by mimicking the role of this parent.

1 This is the earliest stage of development and operates solely on the pleasure principle, largely id oriented; this stage is concerned with development of trust. **2** Interest shifts from the anal region to the genital region, and questions about sexuality arise during this stage. **4** There is increasing sex-role development; this stage is concerned with peer-group identification.

Client Need: Health Promotion and Maintenance; **Cognitive Level:** Comprehension; **Nursing Process:** Assessment/Analysis; **Reference:** Ch 15, Formation of the Personality

13. **2** Values and beliefs from parents and society are expressed through the child's play world. These values become part of the child's system through the process of internalization (introjection).

1 If this happens, children will learn to blame others for their own faults. **3** This occurs at a later age. **4** The environment and others in it, rather than play, influence independence.

Client Need: Health Promotion and Maintenance; **Cognitive Level:** Analysis; **Nursing Process:** Assessment/Analysis; **Reference:** Ch 15, Formation of the Personality

14. **3** The child realizes that the parent of the same sex cannot be bested in a struggle for the affection of the parent of the opposite sex. The role and behavior of the same-sex parent are therefore assumed by the child to attract the parent of the opposite sex.

1 This is a conflict, not a resolution. **2** Doing this gives rise to greater conflict and leaves a fragmented self. **4** This is in conflict with heterosexual drives.

Client Need: Health Promotion and Maintenance; **Cognitive Level:** Application; **Nursing Process:** Assessment/Analysis; **Reference:** Ch 15, Formation of the Personality

15. **2** Children 2 to 7 years old have difficulty distinguishing reality from fantasy; this presents the greatest challenge to the nurse.

1 Children from birth to 1 year of age focus on "in the moment" thinking; preoperative preparation most likely will not be recalled. **3** Children 12 to 16 years of age can think in the abstract and have the ability to solve complex problems; children in this stage usually do not pose difficulties in preoperative teaching. **4** Children 7 to 11 years of age have the ability to comprehend and visualize a series of events and can think about the past and present; this stage provides less of a challenge to absorb preoperative teachings.

Client Need: Health Promotion and Maintenance; **Cognitive Level:** Application; **Integrated Process:** Teaching/Learning; **Nursing Process:** Planning/Implementation; **Reference:** Ch 15, Formation of the Personality

16. **3** The development of physical symptoms without a physical cause is an anxiety-reducing mechanism known as conversion.

1 Blaming others in the environment for failure and mistakes is not converting anxiety into physical symptoms. **2** Going back to an earlier state when one felt safer and more secure is not converting anxiety into physical symptoms. **4** This is a continued concern about health characterized by anxiety and an unrealistic interpretation of real or imaginary symptoms as an indication of serious illness.

Client Need: Psychosocial Integrity; **Cognitive Level:** Analysis; **Nursing Process:** Assessment/Analysis; **Reference:** Ch 15, Defense Mechanisms

17. **2** Slips of the tongue, also called "Freudian slips," are material from the unconscious that slips out in unguarded moments.

1 Material in the unconscious cannot deliberately be brought back to awareness. **3** There is no evidence linking déjà vu experiences (paramnesia) to the unconscious. Déjà vu is the feeling of having witnessed or experienced a new situation previously. **4** Although free-floating anxiety is linked to the unconscious, the best evidence of the unconscious is slips of the tongue.

Client Need: Psychosocial Integrity; **Cognitive Level:** Application; **Nursing Process:** Assessment/Analysis; **Reference:** Ch 15, Factors Involved in Personality Development

18. **2** Mediating frustration within the real world is an ego function and requires ego strengths.

1 The id is unable to tolerate frustration because it is totally involved with gratification. **3** The superego is involved with putting pressure on the ego because the id does not tolerate frustration. **4** The unconscious does not deal with frustration.

Client Need: Health Promotion and Maintenance; **Cognitive Level:** Application; **Nursing Process:** Assessment/Analysis; **Reference:** Ch 15, Factors Involved in Personality Development

19. **1** Talking in the third person reflects poor ego boundaries and a dissociation from the real self.

2 Transference is the movement of emotional energy and feelings that one has for one person to another person. **3** Displacement is the attempt to reduce anxiety by transferring the emotions

associated with one object or person to another. **4** Reaction formation is the expression of an emotion opposite the one felt.
Client Need: Psychosocial Integrity; **Cognitive Level:** Analysis; **Integrated Process:** Communication/Documentation; **Nursing Process:** Assessment/Analysis; **Reference:** Ch 15, Defense Mechanisms

20. **3** The superego incorporates all experiences and learning from external environments (society, family, etc.) into the internal environment.
1, 4 This is the function of the id. **2** With its drives the id is a source of creative energy.
Client Need: Health Promotion and Maintenance; **Cognitive Level:** Application; **Nursing Process:** Assessment/Analysis; **Reference:** Ch 15, Factors Involved in Personality Development

21. **1** Splitting is the compartmentalization of opposite-affect states and failure to integrate the positive and negative aspects of self or others.
2 Ambivalence is the experience of feeling opposite emotions at the same time. **3** Passive aggression is the expression of hostility toward another in an indirect, nonassertive way. **4** Reaction formation is the expression of unacceptable desires by the adoption of opposite behaviors in an exaggerated way.
Client Need: Psychosocial Integrity; **Cognitive Level:** Analysis; **Nursing Process:** Assessment/Analysis; **Reference:** Ch 15, Defense Mechanisms

22. **3** Conscience and a sense of right and wrong are expressed in the superego, which acts to counterbalance the id's desire for immediate gratification.
1 This does not reflect any part of the self. **2** This is the id seeking satisfaction. **4** A healthy ego can delay gratification and is in balance with reality.
Client Need: Health Promotion and Maintenance; **Cognitive Level:** Analysis; **Integrated Process:** Teaching/Learning; **Nursing Process:** Planning/Implementation; **Reference:** Ch 15, Factors Involved in Personality Development

23. **4** The mature personality does not respond to the immediate gratification demands of the id or the oppressive control of the superego because the ego is strong enough to maintain a balance between them.
1 There would be no healthy resolution of conflicts if the superego were always in control. **2** With society in control there would be chaos, rather than maturity. **3** This creates a rigid personality that makes impossible demands on the self.
Client Need: Health Promotion and Maintenance; **Cognitive Level:** Analysis; **Nursing Process:** Assessment/Analysis; **Reference:** Ch 15, Factors Involved in Personality Development

24. **1** Repression is a coping mechanism in which unacceptable feelings are kept out of conscious awareness; later, under stress or anxiety, thoughts or feelings surface and come into one's conscious awareness.
2 Regression is the use of an unconscious coping mechanism through which a person avoids anxiety by

returning to an earlier, more satisfying, or comfortable time in life. **3** Rationalization does not address the delay factor; it is an attempt to falsify an experience by constructing logical or socially approved explanations. **4** Reaction formation is defined as disguising unacceptable feelings and exhibiting the opposite feelings.
Client Need: Psychosocial Integrity; **Cognitive Level:** Analysis; **Nursing Process:** Assessment/Analysis; **Reference:** Ch 15, Defense Mechanisms

25. **4** Intellectualization occurs when a painful emotion is avoided by means of a rational explanation that removes the event from any personal significance.
1 Projection is the blaming of others as a means of dealing with one's own shortcomings. **2** Dissociation is a means of handling conflict by a temporary alteration of consciousness or identity; amnesia is an example. **3** Displacement is the discharging of a pent-up feeling, generally hostility, on an object or person perceived to be weaker than the person who aroused the feelings.
Client Need: Psychosocial Integrity; **Cognitive Level:** Analysis; **Nursing Process:** Assessment/Analysis; **Reference:** Ch 15, Defense Mechanisms

26. **1** The sense of ego integrity comes from satisfaction with life and acceptance of what has been and what is. Despair is due to guilt or remorse over what might have been.
2 During puberty adolescents attempt to find themselves and integrate values with those of society; an inability to solve conflict results in confusion and hinders mastery of future roles. **3** During early and middle adulthood the individual is concerned with the ability to produce and to care for that which is produced or created; failure during this stage leads to self-absorption or stagnation. **4** Autonomy is developed during the toddler period and corresponds to the child's ability to control the body and environment; doubt can result when made to feel ashamed or embarrassed.
Client Need: Health Promotion and Maintenance; **Cognitive Level:** Application; **Nursing Process:** Assessment/Analysis; **Reference:** Ch 15, Formation of the Personality

27. **4** Cognitive therapy seeks to find underlying self-defeating beliefs and replace them with more reality-based positive beliefs.
1, 2 This reflects a behavioral approach. **3** This reflects a more psychoanalytic approach.
Client Need: Psychosocial Integrity; **Cognitive Level:** Analysis; **Integrated Process:** Caring; **Nursing Process:** Planning/Implementation; **Reference:** Ch 15, Cognitive Theory

28. **3** Thought-stopping was developed by Joseph Wolpe for this purpose.
1 Reflecting is referring feelings back to the client so that they can be recognized and dealt with effectively. **2** Clouding/fogging is an assertiveness technique that concurs with another's statement without being defensive or agreeing to change. **4** Verbalizing the implied is putting into words what the client has inferred.

Client Need: Psychosocial Integrity; **Cognitive Level:** Analysis; **Integrated Process:** Teaching/Learning; **Nursing Process:** Planning/Implementation; **Reference:** Ch 15, Cognitive Theory

29. 3 These behaviors are evidence of the client's ability to act responsibly.

1, 2 Although this shows an improvement, it is not related to the critical element of behavioral therapy. 4 Verbalizations without actions do not show the improvement in behavior sought in behavioral therapy.
Client Need: Psychosocial Integrity; **Cognitive Level:** Application; **Nursing Process:** Evaluation/Outcomes; **Reference:** Ch 15, Behavioral Theory

30. 3 Displacement is a defense mechanism in which one's pent-up feelings toward a threatening person are discharged on less-threatening others.

1 Transference is a mechanism by which affects or emotional tones are shifted from one individual to another; it is unrelated to child abuse. 2 Manipulation is a mechanism by which individuals attempt to manage, control, or use others to suit their own purpose or to gain an advantage; it is unrelated to child abuse. 4 Reaction formation is a mechanism by which unacceptable feelings are repressed while the exact opposite feelings are expressed; it is unrelated to child abuse.
Client Need: Psychosocial Integrity; **Cognitive Level:** Analysis; **Nursing Process:** Assessment/Analysis; **Reference:** Ch 15, Defense Mechanisms

31. 1 Mild anxiety motivates one to action, such as learning or making changes. Higher levels of anxiety tend to blur the individual's perceptions and interfere with functioning.

2 Attention is severely reduced by panic. 3 The perceptual field is greatly reduced with severe anxiety. 4 The perceptual field is narrowed with moderate anxiety.
Client Need: Psychosocial Integrity; **Cognitive Level:** Application; **Integrated Process:** Teaching/Learning; **Nursing Process:** Assessment/Analysis; **Reference:** Ch 15, Anxiety and Coping Behaviors, Overview

32. 4 The client's early arrival indicates an expected degree of anxiety; the quiet waiting indicates that the client has been told what to expect.

1 This indicates an inadequate explanation or the inability of the client to remember the explanation that had been given. 2, 3 This indicates a high degree of anxiety that may denote a fear of the tests because they were not adequately explained.
Client Need: Psychosocial Integrity; **Cognitive Level:** Analysis; **Integrated Process:** Teaching/Learning; **Nursing Process:** Evaluation/Outcomes; **Reference:** Ch 15, Anxiety and Coping Behaviors, Overview

33. 4 Anxiety is a human response, causing both physical and emotional changes that everyone experiences when faced with stressful situations.

1 Anxiety is experienced to a greater or lesser degree by every person. 2 Anxiety does not operate from the conscious level. 3 The fear may be related to a specific aspect of, rather than the total, environment.

Client Need: Psychosocial Integrity; **Cognitive Level:** Comprehension; **Integrated Process:** Teaching/Learning; **Nursing Process:** Planning/Implementation; **Reference:** Ch 15, Anxiety and Coping Behaviors, Overview

34. 3 The individual using sublimation attempts to fulfill desires by selecting a socially acceptable activity rather than one that is socially unacceptable.

1 This is reaction formation. 2 This is regression. 4 This is repression.
Client Need: Psychosocial Integrity; **Cognitive Level:** Analysis; **Nursing Process:** Assessment/Analysis; **Reference:** Ch 15, Defense Mechanisms

35. 2 Toddlers struggle to identify their own needs. Too early and too strict toilet training results in ambivalence because toddlers' needs and physical abilities are in conflict with parental demands. Toddlers are faced with giving up these needs or risking parental disapproval.

1 Children are involved from birth in satisfying their own needs. 3 Children are involved from birth in satisfying their parents' needs, but toilet training is really the first time a conflict develops. 4 A child has no interest in society's expectations.
Client Need: Health Promotion and Maintenance; **Cognitive Level:** Application; **Nursing Process:** Assessment/Analysis; **Reference:** Ch 15, Formation of the Personality

THE PRACTICE OF MENTAL HEALTH/ PSYCHIATRIC NURSING

36. 1. ☐ Registered nurses may use counseling interventions but may not perform psychotherapy; psychotherapy may be performed by psychiatric/mental health clinical nurse specialists or psychiatric/mental health nurse practitioners.

2 ☒ Health promotion is within the legal scope of nursing practice.

3 ☒ Case management is within the legal scope of nursing practice.

4 ☐ Only those who are legally licensed to prescribe medications, such as psychiatric nurse practitioners, may do so.

5 ☒ Treating human responses is within the legal scope of nursing practice.
Client Need: Management of Care; **Cognitive Level:** Analysis; **Nursing Process:** Planning/Implementation; **Reference:** Ch 16, The Nurse's Responsibilities in Relation to the Law

37. 4 New orders must be written each time a client requires restraints. When a client is acting-out, the nurse may use restraints or a seclusion room and then obtain the necessary order.

1, 2, 3 PRN restraint orders are not permitted.
Client Need: Management of Care; **Cognitive Level:** Application; **Nursing Process:** Planning/Implementation; **Reference:** Ch 16, Legal Concepts Related to Mental Health/Psychiatric Nursing, Overview

38. 4 The purpose of a PAD is to allow psychiatric clients the opportunity to provide input into future treatment decisions.
1 Having a surrogate decision maker can assist in ensuring the client's wishes are followed. A client can have both a PAD and a health care proxy. 2 The client cannot dictate what treatments will be offered or given. The physician and treatment team will decide on a plan of care, which the client may accept or reject. 3 If the client is a threat to self or others, involuntary admission may be required whether a PAD exists or not.
Client Need: Management of Care; **Cognitive Level:** Comprehension; **Integrated Process:** Teaching/Learning; **Nursing Process:** Planning/Implementation; **Reference:** Ch 16, Legal Concepts Related to Mental Health/Psychiatric Nursing, Overview

39. 1 An important aspect of the role of the psychiatric nurse is primary, secondary, and tertiary interventions to promote emotional equilibrium.
2, 3 This is only a small part of the role of the psychiatric nurse, a role usually shared with others on the health team. 4 This is only a part of the role of the psychiatric nurse, since psychiatry is concerned with people with varying degrees of mental and emotional disorders.
Client Need: Psychosocial Integrity; **Cognitive Level:** Analysis; **Integrated Process:** Caring; **Nursing Process:** Assessment/Analysis; **Reference:** Ch 16, General Nursing Care of Clients with Mental Health/Psychiatric Problems

40. 4 This simply states facts without getting involved in role conflict.
1 Being a doctor is a big part of this client's self-esteem, and by this remark the nurse is threatening that self-esteem. 2 This will confuse the client's role on the unit. A client who is a physician cannot be responsible for checking vital signs. 3 Threats will only make the situation worse and set the tone for future negative nurse-client interactions.
Client Need: Psychosocial Integrity; **Cognitive Level:** Analysis; **Integrated Process:** Communication/Documentation; **Nursing Process:** Planning/Implementation; **Reference:** Ch 16, Therapeutic Nurse-Client Relationship, Overview

41. 3 The nurse's major tool in psychiatric nursing is the therapeutic use of self. Psychiatric nurses must learn to identify their own feelings and understand how they affect the situation.
1, 2 Although this may be difficult, an awareness of self is still the most difficult. 4 This implies that the nurse is working alone in caring for the client.
Client Need: Management of Care; **Cognitive Level:** Analysis; **Nursing Process:** Assessment/Analysis; **Reference:** Ch 16, Therapeutic Nurse-Client Relationship, Overview

42. 4 This statement does not prejudge the father; it encourages communication.
1 This response disregards the father's feelings and cuts off further communication. 2 This statement may stop communication and does not recognize the father's concerns. 3 This statement is premature and does not recognize the father's concerns.
Client Need: Psychosocial Integrity; **Cognitive Level:** Analysis; **Integrated Process:** Caring, Communication/Documentation; **Nursing Process:** Planning/Implementation; **Reference:** Ch 16, Therapeutic Nurse-Client Relationship, Overview

43. 3 This statement encourages the client to express and explore feelings; also, it is open and nonjudgmental.
1, 4 This puts the client on the defensive rather than encouraging verbalization of feelings. 2 This does not encourage further conversation and the client will not have the opportunity to express feelings; this response focuses on the nurse rather than on the client.
Client Need: Psychosocial Integrity; **Cognitive Level:** Application; **Integrated Process:** Caring, Communication/Documentation; **Nursing Process:** Planning/Implementation; **Reference:** Ch 16, Therapeutic Nurse-Client Relationship, Overview

44. 2 With transference a client assigns to someone the feelings and attitudes originally associated with an important significant other.
1 With regression a client reverts to past levels of coping to reduce anxiety. 3 With reaction formation a client displays the exact opposite behavior, attitude, or feeling to that which is demonstrated in a given situation. 4 With countertransference the professional provider of care exhibits an emotional reaction to a client based on a previous relationship or on unconscious needs or conflicts.
Client Need: Psychosocial Integrity; **Cognitive Level:** Analysis; **Nursing Process:** Assessment/Analysis; **Reference:** Ch 16, Therapeutic Nurse-Client Relationship, Overview

45. 1 The nurse brings to a therapeutic relationship the understanding of self and basic principles of therapeutic communication; this is the unique aspect of the helping relationship.
2, 3, 4 This supports the psychotherapeutic management model, but it is not the most important tool used by the nurse in a therapeutic relationship.
Client Need: Psychosocial Integrity; **Cognitive Level:** Application; **Integrated Process:** Caring; **Nursing Process:** Planning/Implementation; **Reference:** Ch 16, Therapeutic Nurse-Client Relationship, Overview

46. 1 In the Latino American culture, usually there is a strong family bond, and the support of the family is essential during problematic times.
2 Latino American clients do not have a need for personal and social space that is different from the predominant American culture. 3 Latino American clients tend to be present, not future, time oriented. 4 Socioeconomic status does not play more than the usual role in deciding on appropriate health care options.
Client Need: Psychosocial Integrity; **Cognitive Level:** Application; **Integrated Process:** Caring, Communication/Documentation; **Nursing Process:** Planning/Implementation; **Reference:** Ch 16, General Nursing Care of Clients With Mental Health/Psychiatric Problems

47. 1 ☐ This statement does not indicate that the client plans to harm herself or another.
2 ☒ This statement indicates a suicide threat; it is a direct expression of intent but without action.

3 ☒ The threat to harm others must be heeded; the client must be protected from harming herself as well as harming others.

4 ☐ This statement reflects the client's feelings of anger and the cause, but does not indicate a threat to self or others.

Client Need: Psychosocial Integrity; **Cognitive Level:** Analysis; **Nursing Process:** Assessment/Analysis; **Reference:** Ch 16, Legal Concepts Related to Mental Health/Psychiatric Nursing, Overview

48. 1 Self-help group members share similar experiences and can provide valuable understanding and support to each other.

2, 4 Although this may occur, it is not the primary purpose of self-help groups. **3** Self-help groups provide an opportunity for people to interact, not engage in professional psychotherapy.

Client Need: Psychosocial Integrity; **Cognitive Level:** Analysis; **Integrated Process:** Caring; **Nursing Process:** Assessment/Analysis; **Reference:** Ch 16, Group Therapy

49. 4 This reflective statement allows the client to either validate or correct the nurse.

1 This delays confronting the problem and avoids exploring feelings. **2** This is a response that gives advice and does not allow the client to explore feelings. **3** This denies the client's statement and does not allow the exploration of feelings.

Client Need: Psychosocial Integrity; **Cognitive Level:** Analysis; **Integrated Process:** Communication/Documentation; **Nursing Process:** Planning/Implementation; **Reference:** Ch 16, Group Therapy

50. 3 This permits the client to see that personal feelings are not unique but are shared by others.

1 This statement makes the client worry about not feeling happy. **2** This is a nonsupportive response to a realistic fear of leaving the safe hospital and going back to where problems must be confronted. **4** How the others feel about whether the client is ready to be discharged is totally irrelevant

Client Need: Psychosocial Integrity; **Cognitive Level:** Application; **Integrated Process:** Caring, Communication/Documentation; **Nursing Process:** Planning/Implementation; **Reference:** Ch 16, Group Therapy

51. 3 Boundaries relate to family systems theory.

1 This statement is reflective of crisis theory, because it addresses the client's perspective of the precipitating event. **2** This statement is reflective of milieu theory. **4** This statement is reflective of biologic theory.

Client Need: Psychosocial Integrity; **Cognitive Level:** Analysis; **Integrated Process:** Communication/Documentation; **Nursing Process:** Planning/Implementation; **Reference:** Ch 16, Family Therapy

52. 2 This provides an opportunity for the other clients to voice and share feelings and to identify and separate real from imaginary fears; an open expression of feelings allows the nurse to deal with clients' fears and provide reassurance.

1 This denies clients' concerns, which may increase their anxiety and fear. **3** Ignoring the situation denies

reality and may precipitate or reinforce feelings of vulnerability and fear in the other clients. **4** This may meet the needs of these two clients but ignores the needs of the other clients.

Client Need: Psychosocial Integrity; **Cognitive Level:** Application; **Integrated Process:** Communication/Documentation; **Nursing Process:** Planning/Implementation; **Reference:** Ch 16, Therapeutic Milieu, Overview

53. 1 Going for counseling demonstrates the client's recognition that assistance is needed.

2, 3, 4 There are no data to support this conclusion.

Client Need: Psychosocial Integrity; **Cognitive Level:** Application; **Nursing Process:** Evaluation/Outcomes; **Reference:** Ch 16, Crisis Intervention, Overview

54. 3 Crying is a release, but the individual should have developed effective coping mechanisms by this time.

1 Not necessarily; people express grief in a variety of ways. **2** Excessive crying 16 months after the death of a loved one is not considered an expected response. **4** This is an assumption and is not a valid assessment.

Client Need: Psychosocial Integrity; **Cognitive Level:** Application; **Integrated Process:** Caring; **Nursing Process:** Planning/Implementation; **Reference:** Ch 16, Crisis Intervention, Nursing Care

55. 2 The most significant factor in either precipitating or avoiding crisis is not the events but how the individual perceives them.

1 Changes in role may occur, but again, the individual's perception of these changes is most influential. **3** This may be a factor, but perception is most important. **4** This is not a significant factor; the family may provide support and a crisis can still occur.

Client Need: Psychosocial Integrity; **Cognitive Level:** Application; **Nursing Process:** Assessment/Analysis; **Reference:** Ch 16, Crisis Intervention, Overview

56. 2 The symptoms presented are indicative of a severe anxiety reaction related to a crisis; the client has a need to vent feelings.

1 This is a premature action that requires a physician's order. **3** The symptoms presented are not indicative of a urinary tract infection. **4** An order for a mild tranquilizer may be necessary later; this will be too soon.

Client Need: Psychosocial Integrity; **Cognitive Level:** Application; **Integrated Process:** Caring; **Nursing Process:** Planning/Implementation; **Reference:** Ch 16, Crisis Intervention, Nursing Care

57. 3 Studies demonstrate that as more women enter the work force, they experience fewer negative responses to the "empty nest" created by children leaving home.

1, 2, 4 This may occur for some women but not many.

Client Need: Health Promotion and Maintenance; **Cognitive Level:** Application; **Nursing Process:** Assessment/Analysis; **Reference:** Ch 16, Crisis Intervention, Overview

58. 2 Crisis intervention is short-term therapy with the major goal of restoring clients to their precrisis state.

1 This is not the goal of crisis intervention, although it may be necessary if psychologic equilibrium cannot be restored. **3** This is not always necessary for clients to be able to function effectively. **4** This is not a goal but an action to help achieve a goal; it is not part of crisis intervention.
Client Need: Psychosocial Integrity; **Cognitive Level:** Comprehension; **Nursing Process:** Planning/Implementation; **Reference:** Ch 16, Crisis Intervention, Overview

59. **1** A client in crisis needs to rely on available support systems for assistance; therefore it is vital for the nurse to identify the client's support system.
2 Nothing in the history demonstrates psychotic thoughts are present. **3** The client's self-image is fairly negative at this time and should not be reinforced. **4** This will add to the client's anxiety and not help the client cope with the loss.
Client Need: Psychosocial Integrity; **Cognitive Level:** Application; **Integrated Process:** Caring; **Nursing Process:** Planning/Implementation; **Reference:** Ch 16, Crisis Intervention, Nursing Care

60. **2** During crisis intervention the nurse should be goal-directed and active in assessing the current situation and handling the interview with authority.
1 These are not appropriate; the client cannot move without direction. **3** These are not appropriate to crisis intervention. **4** This approach might be more appropriate for long-term therapy.
Client Need: Psychosocial Integrity; **Cognitive Level:** Analysis; **Integrated Process:** Caring; **Nursing Process:** Planning/Implementation; **Reference:** Ch 16, Crisis Intervention, Nursing Care

61. **4** This is not an expected outcome of a crisis because by definition a crisis is resolved in 6 weeks.
1 Although this is not the most ideal outcome for a crisis situation, it is a possible outcome. **2, 3** This is a desirable outcome of a crisis situation.
Client Need: Psychosocial Integrity; **Cognitive Level:** Application; **Nursing Process:** Assessment/Analysis; **Reference:** Ch 16, Crisis Intervention, Overview

62. **4** This assessment assists the nurse to determine what the situation means to the client.
1, 2, 3 This is not as important but should be included in a later assessment.
Client Need: Psychosocial Integrity; **Cognitive Level:** Application; **Nursing Process:** Assessment/Analysis; **Reference:** Ch 16, Crisis Intervention, Nursing Care

63. **4** Clients in crisis need assistance with coping; the nurse must be involved with problem solving.
1, 2, 3 Although a positive interview statement, this does not focus on the nurse's involvement with problem solving.
Client Need: Psychosocial Integrity; **Cognitive Level:** Application; **Integrated Process:** Caring, Communication/Documentation; **Nursing Process:** Planning/Implementation; **Reference:** Ch 16, Crisis Intervention, Nursing Care

64. 2, 1, 5, 4, 3

___2___ The sooner a client who has experienced a crisis receives professional intervention, the sooner the individual can be helped to cope effectively.
___1___ Clients must then be stabilized to ensure that order has been reestablished to their physical and emotional status.
___5___ Understanding the event helps the individual to move from shock and disbelief to the next stage of coping.
___4___ Utilizing resources helps the individual to move from shock and disbelief to the next stage of coping.
___3___ Eventually the client can move toward self-reliance.
Client Need: Psychosocial Integrity; **Cognitive Level:** Analysis; **Nursing Process:** Planning/Implementation; **Reference:** Ch 16, Crisis Intervention, Nursing Care

65. **1** Developmental level is essential to understanding a child's response to a crisis situation; the variety of coping abilities usually increases as the child progresses through the stages of growth and development.
2, 4 Although this is important and eventually should be done, it is not an initial assessment. **3** This should be assessed after the child's developmental level is identified.
Client Need: Psychosocial Integrity; **Cognitive Level:** Application; **Nursing Process:** Assessment/Analysis; **Reference:** Ch 16, Crisis Intervention, Nursing Care

66. **2** Before progress can be made in treating anger, clients need to take responsibility for their behavior. As long as they blame others, they will not be motivated to change.
1 Clients may express remorse but continue to blame others and not feel the need for change. **3** This is a worthwhile goal but it is more appropriate later in therapy. It is not an initial goal. **4** These clients need to change themselves, not teach others to change.
Client Need: Psychosocial Integrity; **Cognitive Level:** Application; **Nursing Process:** Planning/Implementation; **Reference:** Ch 16, Anger Management, Overview

67. **2** This is an assertive statement; it clearly states what the problem is and sets limits on undesired behavior without being demeaning.
1 This is a nonassertive or passive statement that denies the individual's own needs and desires. **3** This is an aggressive statement that is demeaning and intimidating. **4** This is a passive aggressive response that avoids direct, honest confrontation for devious manipulation.
Client Need: Psychosocial Integrity; **Cognitive Level:** Analysis; **Integrated Process:** Teaching/Learning; **Nursing Process:** Evaluation/Outcomes; **Reference:** Ch 16, Assertiveness Training

68. **3** Nurses who work with clients who are victims of partner abuse need to be supportive and patient. It takes time and several attempts for most victims to be able to leave abusive relationships.
1 This may or may not be true. There is not enough information to support this conclusion. **2** The staff

can encourage the woman to make plans for addressing various potential events. Information about social services and help lines can be beneficial. **4** Shaming the woman will only make her less likely to seek help.
Client Need: Psychosocial Integrity; **Cognitive Level:** Analysis; **Integrated Process:** Teaching/Learning; **Nursing Process:** Planning/Implementation; **Reference:** Ch 16, Domestic Violence, Nursing Care

69. **4** This is important because side effects and denial of illness may cause clients to stop taking their medications; this is a common cause of relapse.
1 Although this is beneficial, this may not always be possible to achieve. **2** It is impossible to create a stress-free environment; clients need to learn better ways to cope with stress. **3** Refraining from any activity that may cause anxiety is too restrictive.
Client Need: Pharmacological and Parenteral Therapies; **Cognitive Level:** Analysis; **Integrated Process:** Teaching/Learning; **Nursing Process:** Planning/Implementation; **Reference:** Ch 16, Related Pharmacology: Psychotropic Medications, Overview

70. **2** It takes this long for the drug to reach therapeutic blood levels.
1, 4 This is much too short a time for therapeutic levels to be achieved. **3** Improvement in depression should be demonstrated earlier than this.
Client Need: Pharmacological and Parenteral Therapies; **Cognitive Level:** Comprehension; **Integrated Process:** Teaching/Learning; **Nursing Process:** Planning/Implementation; **Reference:** Ch 16, Antidepressants

71. **1** Occipital headaches are the beginning of a hypertensive crisis that results from excessive tyramine.
2 This is unrelated to the ingestion of tyramine. **3** These are unrelated to the ingestion of tyramine. **4** Excessive tyramine causes an increase, not a decrease, in blood pressure.
Client Need: Pharmacological and Parenteral Therapies; **Cognitive Level:** Application; **Integrated Process:** Teaching/Learning; **Nursing Process:** Planning/Implementation; **Reference:** Ch 16, Antidepressants

72. **3** Lithium carbonate alters sodium transport in nerve and muscle cells and causes a shift toward intraneuronal metabolism of catecholamines. Since the range between therapeutic and toxic levels is very small, the client's serum lithium level should be monitored closely.
1 Sodium restriction may cause electrolyte imbalance and lithium toxicity. **2** This is not necessary or useful. **4** This may or may not be necessary; it depends on what the client is receiving.
Client Need: Pharmacological and Parenteral Therapies; **Cognitive Level:** Application; **Nursing Process:** Planning/Implementation; **Reference:** Ch 16, Antimanic and Mood-Stabilizing Agents

73. **4** The lithium level should be maintained between 0.5 and 1.5 mEq/L.

1, 3 This is unsafe. **2** The lithium level is currently unsafe but it does not need to drop to 0.5 mEq/L before being resumed.
Client Need: Pharmacological and Parenteral Therapies; **Cognitive Level:** Analysis; **Nursing Process:** Planning/Implementation; **Reference:** Ch 16, Antimanic and Mood-Stabilizing Agents

74. **1** The neuroleptics modify the behavior of psychotic clients so they can cope more effectively with the environment and benefit from therapy.
2 Antidepressants, not antipsychotics, are used for depression. **3** Ritalin is used to treat children with attention-deficit hyperactivity disorders; neuroleptics decrease the severity of psychotic symptoms. **4** Neuroleptics are contraindicated during narcotic withdrawal.
Client Need: Pharmacological and Parenteral Therapies; **Cognitive Level:** Comprehension; **Nursing Process:** Evaluation/Outcomes; **Reference:** Ch 16, Neuroleptics (Antipsychotic Agents)

75. **4** Unintentional tremors are one of the extrapyramidal side effects of the neuroleptics and are considered common and manageable.
1 This is a severe but not a common occurrence; periodic liver function tests should be done. **2** An excessive number of melanocytes is not a side effect of neuroleptics. **3** This is not a common side effect.
Client Need: Pharmacological and Parenteral Therapies; **Cognitive Level:** Application; **Nursing Process:** Planning/Implementation; **Reference:** Ch 16, Neuroleptics (Antipsychotic Agents)

76. **3** Flumazenil (Romazicon) is the drug of choice in the management of overdose when a benzodiazepine is the only agent ingested by a client not at risk for seizure activity. This medication competitively inhibits activity at benzodiazepine recognition sites on GABA/benzodiazepine receptor complexes.
1 This drug is used in the treatment of mood disorders. **2** This drug is used for narcotic addiction withdrawal. **4** This drug is contraindicated in the presence of central nervous system depressants.
Client Need: Pharmacological and Parenteral Therapies; **Cognitive Level:** Analysis; **Nursing Process:** Planning/Implementation; **Reference:** Ch 16, Antianxiety/Anxiolytic Medications

77. **2** This is a serious side effect that may happen with abrupt withdrawal from barbiturates.
1, 3, 4 This is not associated with barbiturate withdrawal.
Client Need: Pharmacological and Parenteral Therapies; **Cognitive Level:** Application; **Nursing Process:** Evaluation/Outcomes; **Reference:** Ch 16, Sedative and Hypnotic Agents

78. **4** GABA, a neurotransmitter, promotes a balance between dopamine and glutamate; it is effective in reducing anxiety.
1 This is unrelated to anxiety; a degeneration of myelin is associated with multiple sclerosis. **2** An

excess of dopamine is found in clients with schizophrenia. **3** Decreased amounts of norepinephrine and serotonin are related to depression.
Client Need: Pharmacological and Parenteral Therapies; **Cognitive Level:** Analysis; **Nursing Process:** Assessment/Analysis; **Reference:** Ch 16, Antianxiety/Anxiolytic Medications

79. **3** Apathy is a common type II (negative) symptom; flat affect and lack of socialization also are common.
1, 2, 4 This is a type I (positive) symptom.
Client Need: Pharmacological and Parenteral Therapies; **Cognitive Level:** Analysis; **Nursing Process:** Evaluation/Outcomes; **Reference:** Ch 16, Neuroleptics (Antipsychotic Agents)

80. **4** This medication can be given IM every 2 to 3 weeks for clients who are unreliable in taking oral medications; it allows them to live in the community while keeping the symptoms under control.
1 Haloperidol (Haldol) IM has a duration of 4 to 8 hours. **2, 3** This drug is not given for schizophrenia.
Client Need: Pharmacological and Parenteral Therapies; **Cognitive Level:** Analysis; **Nursing Process:** Planning/ Implementation; **Reference:** Ch 16, Neuroleptics (Antipsychotic Agents)

81. **4** The use of these drugs can raise the seizure threshold, which is counterproductive.
1 A tyramine-free diet is required with MAOI therapy, not after electroconvulsive therapy. **2** Photosensitivity is not a side effect of electroconvulsive therapy. **3** A stable sodium level is necessary with lithium, not electroconvulsive, therapy.
Client Need: Pharmacological and Parenteral Therapies; **Cognitive Level:** Analysis; **Nursing Process:** Planning/ Implementation; **Reference:** Ch 16, Antianxiety/Anxiolytic Medications

82. **4** The development of glaucoma is one of the side effects of imipramine (Tofranil), and the client should be taught the symptoms.
1 This is true of monoamine oxidase inhibitors (MAOIs). **2** Tofranil is not an MAOI. **3** This is essential for a person being treated with lithium.
Client Need: Pharmacological and Parenteral Therapies; **Cognitive Level:** Analysis; **Nursing Process:** Planning/ Implementation; **Reference:** Ch 16, Antidepressants

83. **2** Haldol causes photosensitivity. Severe sunburn can occur on exposure to the sun.
1 There is no known side effect that affects night driving. **3** This is true if the client were taking an MAO inhibitor. However, people taking psychotropic medications should avoid alcohol. **4** Aspirin is not contraindicated.
Client Need: Pharmacological and Parenteral Therapies; **Cognitive Level:** Application; **Integrated Process:** Teaching/ Learning; **Nursing Process:** Planning/Implementation; **Reference:** Ch 16, Neuroleptics (Antipsychotic Agents)

84. **4** Valproic acid (Depakene) must reach a therapeutic level to be effective, and the serum level must be

monitored for therapeutic and toxic levels of the drug.
1, 2, 3 The serum drug levels are not monitored with this medication.
Client Need: Pharmacological and Parenteral Therapies; **Cognitive Level:** Analysis; **Nursing Process:** Planning/ Implementation; **Reference:** Ch 16, Antimanic and Mood-Stabilizing Agents

85. **3** This drug does not produce an immediate effect; nursing measures must be continued to decrease the risk for suicide.
1 This precaution is not necessary. **2** These food precautions are taken with the MAO inhibitors. **4** This is not necessary with Prozac.
Client Need: Pharmacological and Parenteral Therapies; **Cognitive Level:** Application; **Nursing Process:** Planning/ Implementation; **Reference:** Ch 16, Antianxiety/Anxiolytic Medications

86. **2** Haldol alters the effectiveness of exogenous insulin, and the combination of Haldol and insulin must be used with caution.
1 The occurrence of respiratory depression is more likely with a combination of antipsychotics and barbiturates. **3** This is more likely to occur if the antipsychotic were fluoxetine (Prozac). **4** There are no data to support this statement.
Client Need: Pharmacological and Parenteral Therapies; **Cognitive Level:** Analysis; **Nursing Process:** Evaluation/ Outcomes; **Reference:** Ch 16, Neuroleptics (Antipsychotic Agents)

87. **4** These drugs are used to control the extrapyramidal (parkinsonism-like) symptoms that often develop as a side effect of neuroleptic therapy.
1 Barbiturates do not have extrapyramidal side effects that respond to these drugs.
2 Antiparkinsonian drugs usually are not prescribed in conjunction with antidepressants because antidepressants do not cause parkinsonism-like symptoms. **3** There is no documented use of these drugs with antianxiety agents because they do not have extrapyramidal side effects.
Client Need: Pharmacological and Parenteral Therapies; **Cognitive Level:** Analysis; **Nursing Process:** Planning/ Implementation; **Reference:** Ch 16, Neuroleptics (Antipsychotic Agents)

88. **2** It is important that the nurse discontinue previous antipsychotic medications before starting risperidone to minimize the period of overlap and therefore avoid a drug interaction.
1 Although safety is of concern, it is more important to monitor for mood change and suicidal tendencies after the drug's therapeutic level has been reached, when the client will have clearer thought processes and more energy. **3** The symptoms of extrapyramidal reactions are not likely to occur with this low dosage of Risperdal. **4** This will not allow enough of a lag period between the two drugs and may precipitate a drug reaction.

Client Need: Pharmacological and Parenteral Therapies; **Cognitive Level:** Analysis; **Nursing Process:** Planning/Implementation; **Reference:** Ch 16, Neuroleptics (Antipsychotic Agents)

89. 4 Clients taking chlorpromazine should be told to stay out of the sun. Photosensitivity makes the skin more susceptible to burning.

1, 2, 3 Photosensitivity is not a side effect of this drug.

Client Need: Pharmacological and Parenteral Therapies; **Cognitive Level:** Analysis; **Integrated Process:** Teaching/Learning; **Nursing Process:** Planning/Implementation; **Reference:** Ch 16, Neuroleptics (Antipsychotic Agents)

90. 2 Liver damage is a well-documented toxic side effect of neuroleptics. By continuing to administer the drug, the nurse failed to use professional knowledge in the performance of responsibilities as outlined in the Nurse Practice Act.

1 Liver damage, indicated by jaundice, is a well-documented side effect. **3** Blood levels must be reduced when signs of liver damage are present.

4 The neuroleptic should be stopped, not reduced; liver damage is a well-documented toxic side effect.

Client Need: Pharmacological and Parenteral Therapies; **Cognitive Level:** Analysis; **Nursing Process:** Planning/Implementation; **Reference:** Ch 16, Neuroleptics (Antipsychotic Agents)

91. 2 Acute dystonic reactions, parkinsonian syndrome, dyskinesia, and akathisia are observable side effects of fluphenazine (Prolixin) therapy.

1 After the first few days of treatment, Prolixin has no effect on concentration or other mental abilities; there is a decrease, not an increase, in salivation. **3, 4** These are not side effects of the drug Prolixin.

Client Need: Pharmacological and Parenteral Therapies; **Cognitive Level:** Application; **Nursing Process:** Planning/Implementation; **Reference:** Ch 16, Neuroleptics (Antipsychotic Agents)

92. 3 This occurs as a late and persistent extrapyramidal complication of long-term antipsychotic therapy. It can take many forms (e.g., torsion spasm, opisthotonos, oculogyric crisis, drooping of the head, protrusion of the tongue).

1, 2, 4 This is reversible with administration of drugs such as Cogentin and Benadryl.

Client Need: Pharmacological and Parenteral Therapies; **Cognitive Level:** Analysis; **Nursing Process:** Evaluation/Outcomes; **Reference:** Ch 16, Neuroleptics (Antipsychotic Agents)

93. 2 The monoamine oxidase inhibitors can cause a hypertensive crisis if food or beverages that are high in tyramine are ingested.

1 This is important for clients taking one of the phenothiazines. **3** This is not contraindicated.

4 NSAIDs are not prohibited with MAOI medications.

Client Need: Pharmacological and Parenteral Therapies; **Cognitive Level:** Application; **Integrated Process:** Teaching/

Learning; **Nursing Process:** Planning/Implementation; **Reference:** Ch 16, Antidepressants

94. 2 It usually takes 2 to 4 weeks to attain a therapeutic blood level of this monoamine oxidase inhibitor (MAOI).

1, 4 This medication works within 2 to 4 weeks. **3** The client may need a longer time to see an effect from this medication.

Client Need: Pharmacological and Parenteral Therapies; **Cognitive Level:** Analysis; **Integrated Process:** Teaching/Learning; **Nursing Process:** Planning/Implementation; **Reference:** Ch 16, Antidepressants

95. 1 Mydriatic action can precipitate an acute attack of glaucoma, which may result in blindness.

2, 3, 4 Although this is a side effect, it is not serious and can be resolved.

Client Need: Pharmacological and Parenteral Therapies; **Cognitive Level:** Application; **Nursing Process:** Evaluation/Outcomes; **Reference:** Ch 16, Antidepressants

96. 3 Ziprasidone hydrochloride (Geodon) is a neuroleptic, which will reduce psychosis by affecting the action of both dopamine and serotonin.

1 Citalopram (Celexa) is a selective serotonin reuptake inhibitor (SSRI) antidepressant.

2 Benztropine mesylate (Cogentin) is an anticholinergic. **4** Acetaminophen with hydrocodone (Lortab) is an analgesic/opioid.

Client Need: Pharmacological and Parenteral Therapies; **Cognitive Level:** Analysis; **Nursing Process:** Planning/Implementation; **Reference:** Ch 16, Neuroleptics (Antipsychotic Agents)

97. 4 Olanzapine (Zyprexa, Zydis) is an oral disintegrating tablet, which will instantly dissolve on contact with moisture.

1 This medication can be given only orally.

2 Tyramine-free diets are necessary with MAOIs, not antipsychotics. **3** This is not necessary with this medication.

Client Need: Pharmacological and Parenteral Therapies; **Cognitive Level:** Comprehension; **Nursing Process:** Planning/Implementation; **Reference:** Ch 16, Neuroleptics (Antipsychotic Agents)

98. 1 ☒ Because of the effect of antipsychotics on the postsynaptic dopamine receptors in the brain, antipsychotic medications may cause this response.

2 ☒ Same as answer 1.

3 ☐ This is a side effect of anticholinergic, not antipsychotic, drugs.

4 ☐ Same as answer 3.

5 ☒ Same as answer 1.

Client Need: Pharmacological and Parenteral Therapies; **Cognitive Level:** Analysis; **Integrated Process:** Communication/Documentation; **Nursing Process:** Evaluation/Outcomes; **Reference:** Ch 16, Neuroleptics (Antipsychotic Agents)

99. 4 This is the advised intervention when a dose is missed; interruption of the medication may precipitate signs of withdrawal such as anxiety and tachycardia.

1 This is unnecessary. **2** This provides an excessive amount of the medication at one time. **3** Skipping a dose is not advised unless taking it is too close to the next regularly scheduled dose.

Client Need: Pharmacological and Parenteral Therapies; **Cognitive Level:** Analysis; **Integrated Process:** Teaching/Learning; **Nursing Process:** Planning/Implementation; **Reference:** Ch 16, Neuroleptics (Antipsychotic Agents)

100. **1** Zyprexa, a thienobenzodiazapine, can cause orthostatic hypotension.

2 Blurred, not double, vision may occur. **3** An anticholinergic effect of Zyprexa is decreased salivation. **4** Zyprexa may cause nausea and other GI upsets; it should be taken with fluid or food.

Client Need: Pharmacological and Parenteral Therapies; **Cognitive Level:** Application; **Integrated Process:** Teaching/Learning; **Nursing Process:** Planning/Implementation; **Reference:** Ch 16, Neuroleptics (Antipsychotic Agents)

101. **1** ☐ This is not associated with neuroleptic malignant syndrome.

2 ☒ This occurs with neuroleptic malignant syndrome as a result of dopamine blockade in the hypothalamus.

3 ☒ Same as answer 2.

4 ☒ Same as answer 2.

5 ☐ Same as answer 1.

Client Need: Pharmacological and Parenteral Therapies; **Cognitive Level:** Analysis; **Nursing Process:** Evaluation/Outcomes; **Reference:** Ch 16, Neuroleptics (Antipsychotic Agents)

NURSING CARE OF CLIENTS WITH DISORDERS USUALLY FIRST EVIDENT IN INFANCY, CHILDHOOD, OR ADOLESCENCE

102. **1** It is the most effective method for the child to play out feelings; when feelings are allowed to surface, the child can then learn to face them by controlling, accepting, or abandoning them.

2, 3, 4 This is not child-specific and generally is more suited for adolescents, young adults, and adults.

Client Need: Health Promotion and Maintenance; **Cognitive Level:** Analysis; **Integrated Process:** Caring; **Nursing Process:** Planning/Implementation; **Reference:** Ch 17, General Nursing Care Related to Disorders First Evident in Infancy, Childhood, or Adolescence

103. **1** ☐ Impairments in communication and imaginative activity result in a failure to imitate others.

2 ☐ Children with autism are indifferent to or have an aversion to affection and physical contact.

3 ☒ Impairments in social interaction are manifested by a lack of eye contact, a lack of facial responses, and a lack of responsiveness to and interest in others.

4 ☐ Impairments in social interaction and imaginative activity are manifested by failure to engage in cooperative or imaginative play with others.

5 ☒ Children with autism display obsessive ritualistic behaviors, such as rocking, spinning, dipping, swaying, walking on toes, head banging, or hand biting, because of their self-absorption and need to stimulate themselves.

6 ☐ Children with autism are unable to establish meaningful relationships with adults or children because of their lack of responsiveness to others.

Client Need: Psychosocial Integrity; **Cognitive Level:** Analysis; **Nursing Process:** Assessment/Analysis; **Reference:** Ch 17, Pervasive Developmental Disorders, Data Base

104. **3** Secondary reinforcers involve the use of social approval; behaviors such as a hug meet this requirement.

1, 2 Food is a primary reinforcer and should not be associated with behavior modification. **4** The child may not select an appropriate secondary reinforcer.

Client Need: Health Promotion and Maintenance; **Cognitive Level:** Application; **Integrated Process:** Caring; **Nursing Process:** Planning/Implementation; **Reference:** Ch 17, General Nursing Care Related to Disorders First Evident in Infancy, Childhood, or Adolescence

105. **3** Infants and toddlers 6 to 30 months of age experience separation anxiety; it is this age-group's major stressor and is most traumatic to the child and parent.

1 The school-age child is more accustomed to periods of separation from parents. **2** Adolescents are often ambivalent about whether they want their parents with them when hospitalized. Peer group separation may pose more anxiety for the adolescent. **4** Separation anxiety occurs in this age group, but it is less obvious and less serious than in the toddler.

Client Need: Health Promotion and Maintenance; **Cognitive Level:** Comprehension; **Nursing Process:** Assessment/Analysis; **Reference:** Ch 17, Anxiety Disorders of Infancy, Childhood, and Adolescence, Data Base

106. **2** Autism impairs bonding and communication and therefore becomes apparent early in life.

1 Autism has both delayed and deviant linguistic problems. **3** About 25% of children with autism have a seizure disorder. **4** Autism may, and often does, include mental retardation.

Client Need: Psychosocial Integrity; **Cognitive Level:** Comprehension; **Nursing Process:** Assessment/Analysis; **Reference:** Ch 17, Pervasive Developmental Disorders, Data Base

107. **4** Research studies have shown that the prognosis for normal productive functioning in autistic people is guarded, particularly if there are delays in language development.

1 Early accurate diagnosis has not been shown to affect prognosis to any extent. **2** While temperament may affect the child's response to treatment, it does not affect prognosis to any extent. **3** This is false reassurance and is not helpful.

Client Need: Psychosocial Integrity; **Cognitive Level:** Application; **Nursing Process:** Assessment/Analysis; **Reference:** Ch 17, Pervasive Developmental Disorders, Data Base

108. **3** Poor interpersonal relationships, inappropriate behavior, and learning disabilities prevent these children from emotionally adapting or responding to the environment despite a possible high level of intelligence.

1 It is the lack of response to stimuli that is the clue to a child's being emotionally disturbed. **2** They have an aversion to physical contact. **4** The exact opposite is true.

Client Need: Psychosocial Integrity; **Cognitive Level:** Application; **Nursing Process:** Assessment/Analysis; **Reference:** Ch 17, Pervasive Developmental Disorders, Data Base

109. **1** By 2 years of age the child should demonstrate an interest in others, communicate verbally, and possess the ability to learn from the environment. Before these skills develop, autism is difficult to diagnose. Usually by 3 years the signs of autism become more profound.

2 Autism can be diagnosed long before this age. **3, 4** Infantile autism can occur at this age but is difficult to diagnose.

Client Need: Psychosocial Integrity; **Cognitive Level:** Comprehension; **Nursing Process:** Assessment/Analysis; **Reference:** Ch 17, Pervasive Developmental Disorders, Data Base

110. **1** From infancy the child is nonresponsive. Not wanting to eat demonstrates a further withdrawal.

2, 3, 4 This is not indicative of an autistic child.

Client Need: Psychosocial Integrity; **Cognitive Level:** Application; **Nursing Process:** Assessment/Analysis; **Reference:** Ch 17, Pervasive Developmental Disorders, Data Base

111. **1** Entering the child's world in a nonthreatening way helps to promote trust and eventual interaction with the nurse.

2, 3 This is unrealistic at this time; this is a long-term goal. **4** This may be necessary when the child initiates self-mutilating behaviors.

Client Need: Psychosocial Integrity; **Cognitive Level:** Application; **Nursing Process:** Planning/Implementation; **Reference:** Ch 17, Pervasive Developmental Disorders, Data Base

112. **3** The priority is safety; the child must be protected from self-harm.

1 Although this is a basic need that may be attained, it is not the priority. **2** Repetitive behaviors are comforting and unless they are harmful their limitation is not a priority. **4** Clients who need help with toileting are not necessarily incontinent; in addition, this is not the priority.

Client Need: Safety and Infection Control; **Cognitive Level:** Application; **Nursing Process:** Planning/Implementation; **Reference:** Ch 17, Pervasive Developmental Disorders, Nursing Care

113. **4** Autistic behavior turns inward. These children do not respond to the environment but attempt to maintain emotional equilibrium by rubbing and manipulating themselves and displaying a compulsive need for behavioral repetition.

1 Large-group (or small-group) activity has little effect on the autistic child's response. **2** These children do seem to respond to music, but not necessarily loud, cheerful music. **3** Part of the autistic pattern is the inability to interact with others in the environment.

Client Need: Psychosocial Integrity; **Cognitive Level:** Application; **Nursing Process:** Assessment/Analysis; **Reference:** Ch 17, Pervasive Developmental Disorders, Data Base

114. **1** A practically universal characteristic of these children is distractibility. They are highly reactive to any extraneous stimuli, such as noise and movement, and are unable to inhibit their responses to such stimuli.

2 Rituals are uncommon, but the use of repetition in language or movement may be seen. **3** Delayed development of language skills is not the major problem but children with attention deficit disorder may exhibit dyslexia (reading difficulty), dysgrammatism (speaking difficulty), dysgraphia (writing difficulty), or delayed talking. **4** Loss of abstract thought is not a universal characteristic associated with children with attention deficit disorder.

Client Need: Psychosocial Integrity; **Cognitive Level:** Application; **Nursing Process:** Assessment/Analysis; **Reference:** Ch 17, Attention Deficit Hyperactivity Disorder, Data Base

115. **3** Ritalin appears to act by stimulating release of norepinephrine from nerve endings in the brainstem.

1 Ativan is a benzodiazepine used to treat anxiety and insomnia. **2** Haldol is an antipsychotic medication. **4** Robaxin is a muscle relaxant.

Client Need: Pharmacological and Parenteral Therapies; **Cognitive Level:** Analysis; **Integrated Process:** Teaching/Learning; **Nursing Process:** Planning/Implementation; **Reference:** Ch 17, General Nursing Care of Children With Disorders First Evident in Infancy, Childhood, or Adolescence

116. **3** Focusing on specifics is important for children who are easily distracted.

1 Focusing on more than one item at a time might be difficult for an easily distracted child. **2** Hyperactive children respond best to concrete tasks; this is not a concrete task. **4** A child who is easily distracted has difficulty talking to a group of children regarding a particular topic.

Client Need: Health Promotion and Maintenance; **Cognitive Level:** Application; **Integrated Process:** Teaching/Learning; **Nursing Process:** Planning/Implementation; **Reference:** Ch 17, General Nursing Care Related to Disorders First Evident in Infancy, Childhood, or Adolescence

117. **1** ☒ Impulsivity, the inability to limit or control words or actions, results in spontaneous, irresponsible verbalizations or behaviors.

2 ☒ Hyperactivity occurs with both words and actions.

3 ☐ This is associated with oppositional defiant disorder and is reflective of negativistic, hostile, defiant behavior toward others.

4 ☐ This is associated with oppositional defiant disorder and is reflective of insubordinate, hostile behavior toward authority; children with attention deficit hyperactivity can be annoying but the behavior is not deliberate.

5 ☒ Games that are fun, engaging, and interactive often maintain the focus of the child with attention deficit hyperactivity disorder.

6 ☒ Inattention and distractibility result in an inability to focus long enough to complete tasks.

Client Need: Psychosocial Integrity; **Cognitive Level:** Analysis; **Nursing Process:** Assessment/Analysis; **Reference:** Ch 17, Attention Deficit Hyperactivity Disorder, Data Base

118. 2 The longer these children stay out, the more difficult it is to get them to return to school because more fantasies and fears develop.

1 This will feed into the child's fear that the phobia is realistic. 3 The use of this approach rarely accomplishes anything. 4 This will increase, not decrease, the child's fear.

Client Need: Psychosocial Integrity; **Cognitive Level:** Application; **Integrated Process:** Teaching/Learning; **Nursing Process:** Planning/Implementation; **Reference:** Ch 17, General Nursing Care Related to Disorders First Evident in Infancy, Childhood, or Adolescence

119. 1 School phobia is a symptom that cannot legally be ignored for long because children must attend school. It requires intervention to alleviate the separation anxiety and/or to promote the child's increasing independence.

2, 3, 4 This symptom requires the parents to comfort, to reorient to reality, and to help the child regain self-control. Legally there are no requirements mandating treatment for this common childhood problem.

Client Need: Management of Care; **Cognitive Level:** Application; **Nursing Process:** Assessment/Analysis; **Reference:** Ch 17, Anxiety Disorders of Infancy, Childhood, and Adolescence, Data Base

120. 1 This response acknowledges the mother's distress and encourages her to verbalize her feelings.

2 This response is insensitive to the mother's feelings; it may be more appropriate later when the mother's stress has diminished. 3 Although this may be true, this response is confrontational and may close off communication. 4 This response is insensitive to the mother's feelings; it may be more appropriate later if medication is prescribed and health teaching is started.

Client Need: Psychosocial Integrity; **Cognitive Level:** Analysis; **Integrated Process:** Caring, Communication/Documentation; **Nursing Process:** Planning/Implementation; **Reference:** Ch 17, General Nursing Care Related to Disorders First Evident in Infancy, Childhood, or Adolescence

121. 3 This disorder interferes with the ability to perceive and respond to sensory stimuli, which causes a

deficit in interpreting new sensory data, makes learning difficult, and results in learning disabilities.

1, 4 This is not necessarily true. 2 This is not true; there is no mental retardation present.

Client Need: Psychosocial Integrity; **Cognitive Level:** Application; **Nursing Process:** Assessment/Analysis; **Reference:** Ch 17, Attention Deficit Hyperactivity Disorder, Data Base

122. 2 Ritalin is an appetite suppressant; it should be given after meals.

1, 3, 4 Ritalin at this time may suppress the child's appetite.

Client Need: Pharmacological and Parenteral Therapies; **Cognitive Level:** Application; **Integrated Process:** Teaching/Learning; **Nursing Process:** Planning/Implementation; **Reference:** Ch 17, General Nursing Care Related to Disorders First Evident in Infancy, Childhood, and Adolescence

123. 2 External rewards can motivate as well as increase self-esteem.

1 This is unnecessary because children with attention deficit hyperactivity disorder are alert and oriented. 3 Feelings of frustration should not be suppressed but rather the child should learn how to cope with these feelings in an acceptable manner. 4 The use of restraints is contraindicated because they are restrictive and punitive.

Client Need: Psychosocial Integrity; **Cognitive Level:** Application; **Integrated Process:** Teaching/Learning; **Nursing Process:** Planning/Implementation; **Reference:** Ch 17, General Nursing Care of Clients With Disorders First Evident in Infancy, Childhood, or Adolescence

124. 2 Oppositional defiant disorder is a repeated pattern of negativistic, disobedient, hostile, defiant behavior toward authority figures usually exhibited before 8 years of age.

1 This is associated with attention deficit hyperactivity disorder and reflects an inability to sustain focus on a task. 3 This is associated with conduct disorder and reflects a violation of a societal norm. 4 This is associated with conduct disorder and reflects a violation of the rights of another.

Client Need: Psychosocial Integrity; **Cognitive Level:** Application; **Nursing Process:** Assessment/Analysis; **Reference:** Ch 17, Unspecified Conduct Disorder/Oppositional Defiant Disorder, Data Base

125. 1 Clients with conduct disorder are at risk for physically, emotionally, or sexually harming themselves or others; safety of the client and others is the priority.

2, 3, 4 Although this is important, it is not the priority.

Client Need: Safety and Infection Control; **Cognitive Level:** Application; **Nursing Process:** Planning/Implementation; **Reference:** Ch 17, Unspecified Conduct Disorder/Oppositional Defiant Disorder, Nursing Care

126. 2 Children who exhibit behaviors associated with conduct disorder before the age of 10, rather than during adolescence, have a higher incidence of

developing antisocial personality disorder during adolescence.

1 If an oppositional defiant disorder persists for at least 6 months, it may be a precursor of a conduct disorder. **3** Pervasive developmental disorders are characterized by impairments in reciprocal social interaction and communication skills; types include autistic, Asperger's, Rett, and childhood disintegrative disorders; they are not preceded by a conduct disorder. **4** Attention deficit hyperactivity disorder is often dually diagnosed with oppositional defiant disorder or conduct disorder and may precede the development of Tourette's syndrome.

Client Need: Health Promotion and Maintenance; **Cognitive Level:** Comprehension; **Nursing Process:** Assessment/Analysis; **Reference:** Ch 17, Unspecified Conduct Disorder/Oppositional Defiant Disorder, Data Base

127. 4, 2, 3, 1

___4___ Situations that promote inattention, hyperactivity, and impulsivity should be avoided

___2___ Monitor behavior for cues of rising anxiety.

___3___ When cues of increasing frustration are noted, the child should be sent a word, gesture, or eye contact as a reminder to maintain control.

___1___ Strategic removal, such as a time-out, should be used as a last resort because it may afford status or make the child a scapegoat.

Client Need: Psychosocial Integrity; **Cognitive Level:** Analysis; **Nursing Process:** Planning/Implementation; **Reference:** Ch 17, General Nursing Care Related to Disorders First Evident in Infancy, Childhood, or Adolescence

128. **3** This outcome is specific for children with a risk for violence directed at others; children with the diagnosis of conduct disorder typically present with a repetitive and persistent pattern of behavior that violates the basic rights of others or major age-appropriate societal norms or rules.

1 This is a short-term goal for children with a variety of mental disorders of childhood such as attention deficit hyperactivity disorder and oppositional defiant disorder. **2** This is a short-term goal for children who have disturbed self-esteem. **4** This is a short-term goal for children who have impaired social interaction.

Client Need: Psychosocial Integrity; **Cognitive Level:** Analysis; **Nursing Process:** Evaluation/Outcomes; **Reference:** Ch 17, Unspecified Conduct Disorder/Oppositional Defiant Disorder, Data Base

129. **2** Coprolalia is the use of involuntary vocalizations that are often obscene, socially unacceptable, or profane.

1 Palilalia is repeating one's own sounds or words. **3** Echokinesis is imitating someone else's movements. **4** Agoraphobia is the fear of being alone in a public place.

Client Need: Psychosocial Integrity; **Cognitive Level:** Analysis; **Nursing Process:** Assessment/Analysis; **Reference:** Ch 17, Tic Disorders, Data Base

NURSING CARE OF CLIENTS WITH DISORDERS RELATED TO ALTERATIONS IN COGNITION AND PERCEPTION

130. **3** This technique tests the client's ability to recall from short-term memory.

1 This part of the exam tests the ability to calculate and pay attention. **2** This part of the exam tests visual comprehension. **4** This part of the exam tests verbal skills for aphasia.

Client Need: Psychosocial Integrity; **Cognitive Level:** Application; **Nursing Process:** Planning/Implementation; **Reference:** Ch 18, Dementia, Nursing Care

131. **4** When an older person's brain atrophies, some unusual deposits of iron are scattered on nerve cells. Throughout the brain, areas of deeply staining amyloid, called senile plaques, can be found; these plaques are end stages in the destruction of brain tissue.

1 This may or may not be part of the disorder. **2** It is a chronic deterioration, not one with remissions and exacerbations. **3** This is typical of vascular dementia, not dementia of the Alzheimer's type.

Client Need: Psychosocial Integrity; **Cognitive Level:** Comprehension; **Nursing Process:** Assessment/Analysis; **Reference:** Ch 18, Dementia, Data Base

132. **1** The client must be kept from harming himself or others; he needs a calm, supportive environment that meets his needs and maintains his dignity.

2 Dementia usually is characterized by progressive deterioration that is not preventable; however, some drugs such as tacrine (Cognex) and donepezil (Aricept) may slow mild to moderate dementia. **3** Although addressing the needs of family members is important, the focus of care primarily is on the client. **4** This may be unrealistic and is not the priority.

Client Need: Psychosocial Integrity; **Cognitive Level:** Application; **Nursing Process:** Planning/Implementation; **Reference:** Ch 18, Dementia, Nursing Care

133. **2** Clients with this disorder need a simple environment. Because of brain cell destruction, they are unable to make choices.

1 A well-balanced diet is important throughout life, not just during senescence; a diet high in carbohydrates and protein may be lacking other nutrients such as fats. **3** Emotional needs must be met on a continuous basis, not just at a fixed time. **4** The client may be incapable of making choices; providing many alternative choices will only increase anxiety.

Client Need: Psychosocial Integrity; **Cognitive Level:** Application; **Nursing Process:** Planning/Implementation; **Reference:** Ch 18, Dementia, Nursing Care

134. **3** These clients attempt to utilize defense mechanisms that have worked in the past but use them in an exaggerated manner. Because of brain cell destruction, these clients are unable to develop new defense mechanisms.

1 Clients with dementia will depend on old, familiar defense mechanisms. **2** The client is not capable of focusing on one defense mechanism. **4** The client is incapable of developing new defense mechanisms at this time.

Client Need: Psychosocial Integrity; **Cognitive Level:** Application; **Nursing Process:** Assessment/Analysis; **Reference:** Ch 18, Dementia, Nursing Care

135. **2** Damaged brain cells do not regenerate. Care is therefore directed toward preventing further damage and providing protection and support.

1 The deterioration of the brain cells makes an extensive reeducation program unrealistic. **3** A client with this disorder may not be able to grasp, understand, or enjoy new leisure activities. **4** It is beyond the scope of the client's ability to function in a group therapy session.

Client Need: Psychosocial Integrity; **Cognitive Level:** Application; **Integrated Process:** Caring; **Nursing Process:** Planning/Implementation; **Reference:** Ch 18, Dementia, Nursing Care

136. **1** ☒ Delirium, a transient cognitive disorder caused by global dysfunction in cerebral metabolism, causes sparse or rapid speech that may be slurred and incoherent.

2 ☐ Clients with delirium consistently are irritable, anxious, and fearful; lability of mood is associated with dementia.

3 ☐ Short-term memory loss is associated with both delirium and dementia; eventually long-term memory loss is associated with dementia.

4 ☒ Visual or tactile hallucinations and illusions may occur with delirium because of altered cerebral functioning; hallucinations are not prominent with dementia.

5 ☐ The onset of delirium is abrupt (hours to days) and has an organic basis; it is often precipitated by drugs such as anesthesia, analgesics, and antibiotics or by conditions such as infections, end-stage renal disease, and substance abuse or withdrawal; the onset of dementia is slow and insidious (years).

6 ☒ Clients with delirium fluctuate from hyperalert to difficult to arouse; they may lose orientation to time and place; clients with dementia do not have fluctuating levels of consciousness, but they may be confused and disoriented.

Client Need: Psychosocial Integrity; **Cognitive Level:** Analysis; **Nursing Process:** Assessment/Analysis; **Reference:** Ch 18, Delirium, Data Base

137. **2** An illusion is a misperception or misinterpretation of an actual external stimulus.

1 This is a false belief that cannot be changed even by evidence; it is associated with psychoses. **3** This results from an imaginary, not real, stimulus. **4** A belief that others are talking about the person

is not a visual distortion, but rather an idea of reference.

Client Need: Psychosocial Integrity; **Cognitive Level:** Application; **Integrated Process:** Communication/Documentation; **Nursing Process:** Assessment/Analysis; **Reference:** Ch 18, Delirium, Data Base

138. **3** A one-to-one trusting relationship is essential to help the client become more involved and interested in interpersonal relationships.

1 Privacy usually is not an issue for a confused client who requires increased supervision. **2** A very confused individual needs to start with a one-to-one relationship before progressing to group involvement. **4** Selected activities, rather than a large variety of activities, are best.

Client Need: Psychosocial Integrity; **Cognitive Level:** Application; **Integrated Process:** Caring; **Nursing Process:** Planning/Implementation; **Reference:** Ch 18, Dementia, Nursing Care

139. **3** Clients who are out of control are seeking control and frequently respond to simple directions stated in a firm voice.

1 "Be quiet" is an order that is nontherapeutic; furthermore, this is demeaning behavior on the part of the nurse. **2** This will not help the client gain control of actions and might be frightening to other clients in the day room. **4** This is done only after an attempt at calming the client has failed.

Client Need: Psychosocial Integrity; **Cognitive Level:** Application; **Integrated Process:** Communication/Documentation; **Nursing Process:** Planning/Implementation; **Reference:** Ch 18, Dementia, Nursing Care

140. **2** The client with delirium, dementia, or another cognitive disorder rarely expresses any concern about personal appearance. The staff must meet most of the client's needs in this area.

1 Resistance to change is a symptom of this disorder. **3** The past is where these clients feel more comfortable rather than the threatening present. **4** A short attention span and little or no interest in new activities are typical of dementia.

Client Need: Psychosocial Integrity; **Cognitive Level:** Application; **Nursing Process:** Assessment/Analysis; **Reference:** Ch 18, Dementia, Data Base

141. **1** This is a true statement; clients become progressively worse over time.

2 Alzheimer's disease is an organic, not a functional, disorder. **3** Alzheimer's disease usually appears in people 60 years and older. **4** At this time there are no diagnostic tools other than autopsy that can provide a definite confirmation of Alzheimer's disease.

Client Need: Psychosocial Integrity; **Cognitive Level:** Comprehension; **Integrated Process:** Communication/Documentation; **Nursing Process:** Planning/Implementation; **Reference:** Ch 18, Dementia, Data Base

142. **4** A consistent approach and consistent communication from all members of the health team help the client who has dementia remain a bit more reality-oriented.

1 It is the staff members who need to be consistent. **2** Clients who have this disorder do not attempt to manipulate the staff. **3** This is not needed when working with clients who have this disorder; consistency is most important.
Client Need: Psychosocial Integrity; **Cognitive Level:** Application; **Nursing Process:** Planning/Implementation; **Reference:** Ch 18, Dementia, Nursing Care

143. **1** A client who acts apathetic and pessimistic is demonstrating characteristics of depression, not dementia.
2 The behavior of clients with dementia tends to be inappropriate, restless, and agitated. **3** Cognitive abilities are impaired, evidenced by a short attention span, limited ability to focus, and limited judgment and insight. **4** Cognitive abilities are impaired, evidenced by disordered reasoning; speech may be incoherent; memory, particularly short-term memory, is impaired.
Client Need: Psychosocial Integrity; **Cognitive Level:** Application; **Nursing Process:** Assessment/Analysis; **Reference:** Ch 18, Dementia, Data Base

144. **4** The therapeutic milieu is directed toward helping the client develop effective ways of functioning safely independently.
1 This is only one small part of the overall goal. **2** The therapeutic milieu allows some items from home to make the client less anxious; however, the goal is not to duplicate a home situation. **3** This accomplishes nothing in regard to a long-term goal of functioning in society.
Client Need: Psychosocial Integrity; **Cognitive Level:** Analysis; **Nursing Process:** Planning/Implementation; **Reference:** Ch 18, Dementia, Nursing Care

145. **1** Reality orientation is generally helpful to clients exhibiting mild cognitive impairment; these clients are aware of their impairment, and orientation then reduces anxiety.
2 Behavioral confrontation is not therapeutic, because it may cause frustration and increase psychomotor agitation in a client with cognitive impairment. **3** Reflective communication is a technique in which the nurse restates or repeats the client's statements; it can be used to clarify thoughts but can also lead to frustration when the approach is overdone. **4** Reminiscence group therapy is helpful with severely confused, disorganized clients because it reinforces identity, acknowledges what was significant, and often compensates for the dullness of the present.
Client Need: Psychosocial Integrity; **Cognitive Level:** Application; **Nursing Process:** Planning/Implementation; **Reference:** Ch 18, Dementia, Nursing Care

146. **1** Neurofibrillary tangles in the hippocampus cause recent memory loss (amnesia); temporoparietal deterioration causes cognitive deficiencies in speech (aphasia), purposeful movements (apraxia), and comprehension of visual, auditory, and other sensations (agnosia).

2 These characteristics are related to schizoid personality. **3** These characteristics are related to schizophrenia. **4** These characteristics are related to antisocial personality.
Client Need: Psychosocial Integrity; **Cognitive Level:** Analysis; **Nursing Process:** Assessment/Analysis; **Reference:** Ch 18, Dementia, Data Base

147. **3** Orientation to place refers to an individual's awareness of the objective world in its relation to the self; orientation to time, place, and person is part of the assessment of cerebral functioning.
1 This requires abstract thinking, which involves a higher integrative function than orientation to place. **2** This assesses remote memory, not orientation. **4** This assesses recent memory, not orientation.
Client Need: Psychosocial Integrity; **Cognitive Level:** Analysis; **Nursing Process:** Assessment/Analysis; **Reference:** Ch 18, Dementia, Nursing Care

148. **4** The first step in a plan of care should be the establishment of a meaningful relationship because it is through this relationship that the client can be helped.
1 Encouraging frequent rest periods isolates the client, and this is not therapeutic. **2** This is a long-term goal. **3** Reduction of stimuli may limit the hallucinations, but there is no evidence that the client is not eating meals.
Client Need: Psychosocial Integrity; **Cognitive Level:** Application; **Integrated Process:** Caring; **Nursing Process:** Planning/Implementation; **Reference:** Ch 18, Schizophrenic Disorders, Nursing Care

149. 3, 4, 1, 2
   3   The nurse should then point out reality.
   4   Finally, the nurse should attempt to distract the client from the hallucination.
   1   The nurse should first identify the client's feelings.
   2   After identifying the client's feelings, the nurse should then simply explain why the voices occur.
Client Need: Psychosocial Integrity; **Cognitive Level:** Analysis; **Integrated Process:** Communication/Documentation; **Nursing Process:** Planning/Implementation; **Reference:** Ch 18, Schizophrenic Disorders, Nursing Care

150. **3** When individuals use these defense mechanisms, they are unable to test out their feelings or differentiate the real world from their personal intrapsychic perceptions.
1, 2, 4 This is only one part of reality testing.
Client Need: Psychosocial Integrity; **Cognitive Level:** Analysis; **Nursing Process:** Assessment/Analysis; **Reference:** Ch 18, Schizophrenic Disorders, Data Base

151. **1** Clients can sometimes learn to push voices aside, particularly within the framework of a trusting relationship; it may provide the client with a sense of power to manage the hallucinatory voices.
2 Once it has been established that the voices are not issuing commands to harm self or others, focusing on the content of the hallucinations is not

therapeutic. **3, 4** This is a useless statement; clients believe and are frightened by hallucinations.
Client Need: Psychosocial Integrity; **Cognitive Level:** Analysis; **Integrated Process:** Communication/Documentation; **Nursing Process:** Planning/Implementation; **Reference:** Ch 18, Schizophrenic Disorders, Nursing Care

152. **4** Delusions are protective and can be abandoned only when the individual feels secure and adequate. This response is the only one directed at building the client's security and reducing anxiety.
1 This is helpful but almost impossible. **2** Clients cannot be argued out of a delusion. **3** The client is unable to explain the reason for the feelings.
Client Need: Psychosocial Integrity; **Cognitive Level:** Application; **Integrated Process:** Caring; **Nursing Process:** Planning/ Implementation; **Reference:** Ch 18, Delusional (Paranoid) Disorders, Nursing Care

153. **1** This response recognizes the client's feelings and provides assurance that the staff member will be present.
2 The client does not know this; if the client did, delusions would not be present. **3** Locking the client in a room will only increase the fear and delusion. **4** The client is not ready to accept this and really believes danger is imminent.
Client Need: Psychosocial Integrity; **Cognitive Level:** Analysis; **Integrated Process:** Caring; Communication/Documentation; **Nursing Process:** Planning/Implementation; **Reference:** Ch 18, Delusional (Paranoid) Disorders, Nursing Care

154. **2** Clients cannot be argued out of delusions, so the best approach is a simple statement of reality.
1 This is a form of entering into the client's delusions; the client may only feel that a particular part was free of poison. **3** This is trying to argue the client out of the delusion. It will not work. The client can make up a reason ("They have the antidote") to continue in the false belief. **4** Threats are always inappropriate nursing interventions.
Client Need: Psychosocial Integrity; **Cognitive Level:** Analysis; **Integrated Process:** Communication/Documentation; **Nursing Process:** Planning/Implementation; **Reference:** Ch 18, Delusional (Paranoid) Disorders, Nursing Care

155. **4** These are positive symptoms associated with schizophrenia; positive symptoms reflect a distortion or excess of normal functions.
1, 2 These are negative symptoms associated with schizophrenia; negative symptoms reflect a lessening or absence of normal functions. **3** These symptoms are associated with bipolar disorder, manic episode.
Client Need: Psychosocial Integrity; **Cognitive Level:** Analysis; **Integrated Process:** Communication/Documentation; **Nursing Process:** Assessment/Analysis; **Reference:** Ch 18, Schizophrenic Disorders, Data Base

156. **1** The initial goal should be to demonstrate acceptance and work toward developing trust; spending time with the client best meets this initial goal.
2 This will increase the anxiety of a psychotic client; it is a correct action in the working phase of the

nurse-client relationship. **3** This delays the initial stage of the nurse-client relationship. **4** This will increase anxiety; it is an acceptable action in the ongoing working, not initial, phase of a therapeutic relationship.
Client Need: Psychosocial Integrity; **Cognitive Level:** Analysis; **Integrated Process:** Caring; **Nursing Process:** Assessment/ Analysis; **Reference:** Ch 18, Schizophrenic Disorders, Nursing Care

157. **1** This message is concise and does not require decision making; it is less likely to increase anxiety.
2 This asks the client to make a decision when a "no" answer is unacceptable. **3** Forcing the client to make a decision when acutely ill may increase anxiety; also, this permits the unacceptable answer of "never." **4** This is somewhat accusatory; it may increase anxiety by placing responsibility on the client.
Client Need: Psychosocial Integrity; **Cognitive Level:** Analysis; **Integrated Process:** Communication/Documentation; **Nursing Process:** Planning/Implementation; **Reference:** Ch 18, Schizophrenic Disorders, Nursing Care

158. **3** This response demonstrates an understanding of the client's feelings and encourages the client to share feelings, which is an immediate need.
1 This is judgmental and demeaning to the client. **2** This probably will increase the client's fears. **4** Although this statement points out reality, it gives a command that is unrealistic and closes the communication process.
Client Need: Psychosocial Integrity; **Cognitive Level:** Analysis; **Integrated Process:** Caring, Communication/Documentation; **Nursing Process:** Planning/Implementation; **Reference:** Ch 18, Schizophrenic Disorders, Nursing Care

159. **2** Clients losing control feel frightened and threatened. They need external controls and a reduction in external stimuli.
1 This is helpful for pent-up aggressive behavior but not for agitation associated with delusions. **3** The client is unable, at this time, to sit in one place; the client's agitation is building. **4** The client may get completely out of control if allowed to continue pacing.
Client Need: Psychosocial Integrity; **Cognitive Level:** Application; **Integrated Process:** Caring; **Nursing Process:** Planning/ Implementation; **Reference:** Ch 18, Schizophrenic Disorders, Nursing Care

160. **1** A firm approach prevents anxiety transference and provides structure and control for a client who is out of control.
2 A passive approach for a client who may be out of control does not provide structure, which may increase the client's anxiety. **3** Although the nurse should always base a therapeutic response on empathy, an obviously empathetic response may indicate to the client that his behavior is acceptable. **4** A confrontational approach in this situation may escalate the client's agitation and precipitate further acting-out.

Client Need: Psychosocial Integrity; **Cognitive Level:** Application; **Nursing Process:** Planning/Implementation; **Reference:** Ch 18, Schizophrenic Disorders, Nursing Care

161. 1 Diagnostic criteria for paranoid schizophrenia include two or more symptoms such as delusions and hallucinations; other less prominent criteria are disorganized behavior and negative symptoms.
    2, 4 These behaviors are not prominent for paranoid schizophrenia but fit other subtypes of schizophrenia. **3** Bizarre behavior related to drug use does not fit these diagnostic criteria.

Client Need: Psychosocial Integrity; **Cognitive Level:** Application; **Nursing Process:** Assessment/Analysis; **Reference:** Ch 18, Schizophrenic Disorders, Data Base

162. 2 The client's behavior is escalating and unsafe. She needs to be brought to her room, where there is decreased environmental stimulation and less chance for her to act-out against others.
    1 The nurse will be accepting physical abuse, which should never be done. **3** The behavior and the client should never be ignored; the client needs limits set on behavior now. **4** When a client is already acting-out, the nurse must intervene to stop the behavior. Discussing the client's feelings can come later when the client is exhibiting more control.

Client Need: Psychosocial Integrity; **Cognitive Level:** Application; **Integrated Process:** Caring; **Nursing Process:** Planning/Implementation; **Reference:** Ch 18, Schizophrenic Disorders, Nursing Care

163. 4 Clients acutely ill with schizophrenia frequently do not trust others; feeling hemmed in may be frightening, causing them to lash out.
    1 There is no indication that voices are speaking to the client in this instance. **2** Clients acutely ill with schizophrenia usually are more concerned with what is happening to them and are not able to be concerned with others. **3** Although this may be true, it is not the primary motivation for this behavior.

Client Need: Psychosocial Integrity; **Cognitive Level:** Analysis; **Nursing Process:** Assessment/Analysis; **Reference:** Ch 18, Schizophrenic Disorders, Data Base

164. 2 This response focuses on a feeling that the client may be experiencing and provides an opportunity to validate the nurse's statement.
    1 This response demands that the client stay in an uncomfortable situation without offering any support. **3** This response fails to recognize the part anxiety plays in changing behavior. **4** This response seems like an attack on the client; also, although it offers an explanation for the behavior, it fails to convey an understanding that changing behavior is anxiety-producing.

Client Need: Psychosocial Integrity; **Cognitive Level:** Analysis; **Integrated Process:** Caring; Communication/Documentation; **Nursing Process:** Planning/Implementation; **Reference:** Ch 18, Schizophrenic Disorders, Nursing Care

165. 3 The nurse should set limits on this behavior when it is not performed in a private area; this accepts the client but rejects the behavior. Also, limits

may need to be set on this behavior when it is excessive.
    1 This is unrealistic and violates the client's rights. **2** This is a punishment rather than a setting of limits. **4** The nurse has a responsibility to the other clients to limit the behavior.

Client Need: Psychosocial Integrity; **Cognitive Level:** Application; **Nursing Process:** Planning/Implementation; **Reference:** Ch 18, Schizophrenic Disorders, Nursing Care

166. 1 An interpersonal relationship based on trust must be established before clients can be helped back to reality.
    2 This is an important part of the treatment and care, but it is of lesser importance than a trusting relationship. **3** Socialization comes at a later time in therapy. **4** There is nothing to indicate an urgency to remove the client from the home.

Client Need: Psychosocial Integrity; **Cognitive Level:** Application; **Integrated Process:** Caring; **Nursing Process:** Planning/Implementation; **Reference:** Ch 18, Schizophrenic Disorders, Nursing Care

167. 2 The nurse, demonstrating knowledge and understanding, accepts the client's perceptions even though they are hallucinatory.
    1 This may increase the client's guilt and fear. **3** This may increase the client's fear. **4** This presents reality but negates the client's feelings and asks for unrealistic responses.

Client Need: Psychosocial Integrity; **Cognitive Level:** Analysis; **Integrated Process:** Caring; **Nursing Process:** Planning/Implementation; **Reference:** Ch 18, Schizophrenic Disorders, Nursing Care

168. 4 This is the most therapeutic option; it interjects reality and focuses on the client's behavior.
    1 This response elicits a yes or no answer. **2** This is a directive response by the nurse and it will be perceived as threatening by a disturbed client experiencing hallucinations. **3** Although this interjects reality, it is not the most therapeutic response.

Client Need: Psychosocial Integrity; **Cognitive Level:** Analysis; **Integrated Process:** Caring, Communication/Documentation; **Nursing Process:** Planning/Implementation; **Reference:** Ch 18, Schizophrenic Disorders, Nursing Care

169. 1 The client needs limits to be set. This response sets limits and rejects the behavior but accepts the client.
    2 This does not help raise the client to a functioning level. **3** This serves no useful purpose; inappropriate behavior should be dealt with when first noted. **4** This is a punishing action; it shows no support or acceptance of the client.

Client Need: Psychosocial Integrity; **Cognitive Level:** Application; **Integrated Process:** Caring, **Nursing Process:** Planning/Implementation; **Reference:** Ch 18, Schizophrenic Disorders, Nursing Care

170. 4 Command hallucinations are dangerous because they may influence the client to engage in behavior dangerous to self or others.

1 Although profane language may be a cause for concern, it is not as dangerous as command hallucinations. **2** Although excessive touching of others may be a cause for concern, it is not as dangerous as command hallucinations. **3** Although withdrawn behavior may be a cause for concern, it is not as dangerous as command hallucinations.

Client Need: Safety and Infection Control; **Cognitive Level:** Analysis; **Nursing Process:** Assessment/Analysis; **Reference:** Ch 18, Schizophrenic Disorders, Nursing Care

171. **1** This lets the client know the nurse is available. It also demonstrates an acceptance of the client.

2 This is an avoidance technique; it shows a lack of acceptance of the client as a person. **3** Although it is important to document the incident on the client's record, it does not take precedence over letting the client know the nurse is there if needed. **4** Another client's perception of the incident may or may not be valid.

Client Need: Psychosocial Integrity; **Cognitive Level:** Application; **Integrated Process:** Caring; **Nursing Process:** Planning/Implementation; **Reference:** Ch 18, Schizophrenic Disorders, Nursing Care

172. **3** The client is voiding on the floor not to express hostility, but because of confusion. Taking the client to the toilet frequently limits voiding in inappropriate places.

1 This is a form of punishment for something the client cannot control. **2** This is not realistic; it will have no effect on the problem and may lead to physiologic problems. **4** If the client were doing this to express hostility, such action is useful, but not when the client is unable to control the behavior.

Client Need: Basic Care and Comfort; **Cognitive Level:** Application; **Nursing Process:** Planning/Implementation; **Reference:** Ch 18, Schizophrenic Disorders, Nursing Care

173. **2** This response reflects on the client's feelings rather than focusing on the verbalization.

1 This response focuses on the statement rather than on the feeling behind it. **3** This response dismisses the client and the client's feelings. **4** This response puts the client on the defensive and asks for verification that the nurse is indeed a good person; it fails to focus on the feeling behind the statement.

Client Need: Psychosocial Integrity; **Cognitive Level:** Analysis; **Integrated Process:** Communication/Documentation; **Nursing Process:** Planning/Implementation; **Reference:** Ch 18, Schizophrenic Disorders, Nursing Care

174. **3** Encouraging the client to focus on the self will facilitate communication and foster self-perception.

1 This denies the client's feelings and provides false reassurance. **2** This is inaccurate information and does not focus on the client's feelings. **4** This denies the client's feelings and provides false reassurance.

Client Need: Psychosocial Integrity; **Cognitive Level:** Analysis; **Integrated Process:** Caring, Communication/Documentation;

Nursing Process: Planning/Implementation; **Reference:** Ch 18, Schizophrenic Disorders, Nursing Care

175. **1** Assisting clients with grooming keeps them in contact with reality and allows them to see that staff members care enough to help. It also places value on appearance.

2 This is not as important as grooming at this time. **3** A one-to-one relationship is best initially. **4** The client may withdraw even more.

Client Need: Psychosocial Integrity; **Cognitive Level:** Application; **Integrated Process:** Caring; **Nursing Process:** Planning/ Implementation; **Reference:** Ch 18, Schizophrenic Disorders, Nursing Care

176. **1** Nursing care involves a steady attempt to draw the client into some response. This can best be accomplished by focusing on nonthreatening subjects that do not demand a specific response.

2 The client is not ready yet to discuss feelings, so the first step is to focus on nonthreatening subjects. **3** By doing this, the nurse is showing acceptance of the client but is doing nothing to encourage communication. **4** Questions like these do not encourage a person to speak.

Client Need: Psychosocial Integrity; **Cognitive Level:** Application; **Integrated Process:** Communication/Documentation; **Nursing Process:** Planning/Implementation; **Reference:** Ch 18, Schizophrenic Disorders, Nursing Care

177. **1** Keeping the withdrawn client oriented to reality prevents the client from withdrawing even further into a private world.

2 A gradual involvement in selected activities is best. **3** This is futile at this time. **4** The client is unable to tell anyone why this is so.

Client Need: Psychosocial Integrity; **Cognitive Level:** Application; **Nursing Process:** Planning/Implementation; **Reference:** Ch 18, Schizophrenic Disorders, Nursing Care

178. **4** By observing the client, the nurse is better able to understand the client's behavior, which can be an indication of feelings.

1 It is only one of the many aspects that are part of making a diagnosis; this is true in the care of all clients, not just the withdrawn individual. **2** Observation alone is insufficient to make this judgment; however, it allows the staff to individualize the plan of care to suit the client's needs. **3** It is more important to have insight into what the person may be feeling rather than the degree of depression.

Client Need: Psychosocial Integrity; **Cognitive Level:** Application; **Nursing Process:** Assessment/Analysis; **Reference:** Ch 18, Schizophrenic Disorders, Nursing Care

NURSING CARE OF CLIENTS WITH DISORDERS RELATED TO ANXIETY AND ALTERATIONS IN MOOD

179. **2** With akathisia the client exhibits a constant state of movement; this is characterized by restlessness and difficulty sitting still, including constant jiggling of the arms and/or legs.

1 The distortion of voluntary movements, such as tics, spasms, or myoclonus, is known as dyskinesia. **3** This is a form of catatonia known as waxy flexibility. **4** This is known as echopraxia.

Client Need: Psychosocial Integrity; **Cognitive Level:** Comprehension; **Nursing Process:** Assessment/Analysis; **Reference:** Ch 19, Generalized Anxiety Disorder, Data Base

180. **4** Recognition of anxiety or symptoms of increasing anxiety is an indication that the client is improving.

1 Avoidance of anxiety is not a good indication of improvement; there is no guarantee that anxiety can always be avoided. **2, 3** This does not indicate improvement or recognition of feelings; the client may just be doing what others expect.

Client Need: Psychosocial Integrity; **Cognitive Level:** Analysis; **Nursing Process:** Evaluation/Outcomes; **Reference:** Ch 19, Generalized Anxiety Disorder, Nursing Care

181. **2** The client's current behavior is the best indicator of the client's current level of functioning; all behavior has meaning.

1, 3, 4 This is important and should be assessed, but it is not the best indicator of current level of functioning.

Client Need: Psychosocial Integrity; **Cognitive Level:** Application; **Nursing Process:** Assessment/Analysis; **Reference:** Ch 19, Generalized Anxiety Disorder, Nursing Care

182. **1** The client can no longer control or tolerate feelings and attempts to disregard reality as a means of avoiding it.

2 The client has not indicated plans for self-harm; the client is asking others to do something to help relieve the feeling. **3** The client is experiencing panic and is crying for help; this behavior is not typical of a narcissistic personality. **4** The client is in a state of panic and is crying for help; this behavior does not indicate a demanding personality.

Client Need: Psychosocial Integrity; **Cognitive Level:** Application; **Nursing Process:** Assessment/Analysis; **Reference:** Ch 19, Panic Disorders, Data Base

183. **3** The nurse who is anxious should leave the situation after providing for continuity of care; the client will be aware of the nurse's anxiety, and the nurse's presence will be nonproductive and nontherapeutic.

1, 2 This meets the nurse's need; this response may make the client feel guilty that something was said that upset the nurse; the client will be aware of the nurse's anxiety, which will increase the client's own anxiety. **4** The client will probably sense the nurse's anxiety through nonverbal channels, if not through verbal responses.

Client Need: Psychosocial Integrity; **Cognitive Level:** Analysis; **Integrated Process:** Communication/Documentation; **Nursing Process:** Assessment/Analysis; **Reference:** Ch 19, General Nursing Care of Clients With Anxiety Disorders

184. **4** With phobias the individual transfers anxiety to a safer inanimate object or situation. Therefore the anxiety and resulting feelings will be precipitated only when in direct contact with the object or situation.

1 It is not thinking about the feared object that causes anxiety; it is the possibility of having to come into contact with it. **2** It is the presence of the phobic object or situation that triggers the anxiety, not the unfamiliarity of the environment. **3** Phobias are severe anxiety reactions and are not attention-seeking actions.

Client Need: Psychosocial Integrity; **Cognitive Level:** Comprehension; **Nursing Process:** Assessment/Analysis; **Reference:** Ch 19, Phobic Disorders, Data Base

185. **1** The most successful therapy for clients with phobias involves behavior modification techniques using desensitization.

2 Insight into the origin of the phobia will not necessarily help the client overcome the problem. **3** This may increase understanding of the phobia but may not help the client to deal with the fear; there is no psychotic thought process associated with phobias. **4** Psychoanalysis may increase understanding of the phobia, but may not help the client deal successfully with the unreasonable fear.

Client Need: Psychosocial Integrity; **Cognitive Level:** Analysis; **Nursing Process:** Planning/Implementation; **Reference:** Ch 19, Phobic Disorders, Data Base

186. **3** Recurrence of attacks is a common concern.

1 This is not therapeutic. **2** Although this response initially focuses on feelings, it then cuts off communication. **4** The client will be focused on own needs, not what the family says.

Client Need: Psychosocial Integrity; **Cognitive Level:** Analysis; **Integrated Process:** Communication/Documentation; **Nursing Process:** Planning/Implementation; **Reference:** Ch 19, Panic Disorders, Data Base

187. **1** ☐ Feelings of guilt may emerge later when the individual moves from focusing on the self to an increased interaction with others.

2 ☒ Shock and disbelief are the initial responses to a traumatic experience; a situational crisis usually is unexpected and its impact causes disequilibrium.

3 ☐ Concern for others emerges later after the individual is able to set aside or resolve own needs.

4 ☒ A crisis causes disequilibrium and the individual experiences confusion, disorganization, and difficulty making decisions.

5 ☒ When a person is unable to cope, helplessness and regression often emerge; a crisis occurs when a painful, frightening event occurs that is so overwhelming an individual's usual coping mechanisms are inadequate.

Client Need: Psychosocial Integrity; **Cognitive Level:** Analysis; **Nursing Process:** Assessment/Analysis; **Reference:** Ch 19, Posttraumatic Stress Disorder, Data Base

188. 4 The client will tend to avoid emotional attachment to significant others because this is a common way to protect the self from the experience of potential future losses. The priority at this time is to have family members develop an understanding of what is happening to the client.

1 Although it is important to keep the client safe and secure when in the home, the family should not restrict the client to the home environment. 2 Although issues need to be resolved, this is not the priority. 3 Although this discussion may be necessary, it is not the priority.

Client Need: Psychosocial Integrity; **Cognitive Level:** Application; **Integrated Process:** Caring; **Nursing Process:** Planning/Implementation; **Reference:** Ch 19, General Nursing Care of Clients With Anxiety Disorders

189. 4 This increases the individual's ability to cope with stress; different defenses can be used in various situations.

1 The client already has identified the problem. 2 This may or may not be helpful. 3 People should not ignore situations that impact them.

Client Need: Psychosocial Integrity; **Cognitive Level:** Application; **Integrated Process:** Communication/Documentation; **Nursing Process:** Planning/Implementation; **Reference:** Ch 19, General Nursing Care of Clients With Anxiety Disorders

190. 1 Acting-out anxiety with antisocial behavior is most commonly found in individuals with personality rather than anxiety disorders.

2 This is an example of a conversion disorder, which decreases anxiety. 3 Regression is an attempt during periods of stress to return to behavior that has been satisfying and is appropriate at an earlier stage of development. 4 This is typical of a phobic disorder, which decreases anxiety.

Client Need: Psychosocial Integrity; **Cognitive Level:** Analysis; **Nursing Process:** Assessment/Analysis; **Reference:** Ch 19, General Anxiety Disorders, Data Base

191. 3 The "fight or flight" responses of the autonomic nervous system are stimulated and result in these findings.

1 The pupils dilate, not constrict, and the blood glucose level increases, not decreases. 2 The "fight or flight" response is not characterized by constricted pupils, constricted bronchioles, and hypoglycemia. 4 The pulse rate increases, and the blood glucose level increases, not decreases.

Client Need: Psychosocial Integrity; **Cognitive Level:** Analysis; **Nursing Process:** Assessment/Analysis; **Reference:** Ch 19, General Anxiety Disorder, Data Base

192. 3 Learning a variety of coping mechanisms helps reduce anxiety in stressful situations.

1 A person must learn to cope with unpleasant objects and events and cannot avoid all unpleasant objects and events. 2 Prolonged exposure may increase anxiety to possibly uncontrollable levels. 4 Fearful situations can never be viewed as pleasurable.

Client Need: Psychosocial Integrity; **Cognitive Level:** Application; **Nursing Process:** Planning/Implementation; **Reference:** Ch 19, General Nursing Care of Clients With Anxiety Disorders

193. 1 By staying physically close, the nurse conveys to the client the message that someone cares enough to be there and that the client is a person worthy of care.

2 The client is incapable of telling anyone what the problem is. 3 Sitting still will increase the tension the client is experiencing. 4 This is not an initial nursing intervention.

Client Need: Psychosocial Integrity; **Cognitive Level:** Application; **Integrated Process:** Caring; **Nursing Process:** Planning/Implementation; **Reference:** Ch 19, Panic Disorders, Nursing Care

194. 3 The client is caught between two equally compelling needs, and movement or sight is impossible. Paralysis or blindness justifies to the client the inability to move in any direction.

1 It is an unconscious method of solving a conflict. 2 It is necessary for the client to focus on the problem causing the disorder, not on other things. 4 It is more important that the client learn how to deal with personal feelings before dealing with family conflicts that may or may not exist.

Client Need: Psychosocial Integrity; **Cognitive Level:** Comprehension; **Nursing Process:** Assessment/Analysis; **Reference:** Ch 19, Conversion Disorders, Data Base

195. 3 The conversion type of defense tends to be a learned behavioral response that the individual will use when put under stress.

1 This is not a likely occurrence. 2 Psychiatric treatment may be needed at different times throughout life but usually not on a continuous basis. 4 Based on studies of this disorder, it usually returns when the client is under severe stress.

Client Need: Psychosocial Integrity; **Cognitive Level:** Analysis; **Nursing Process:** Assessment/Analysis; **Reference:** Ch 19, Conversion Disorders, Data Base

196. 3 The physical symptoms are not the client's major problem and therefore should not be the focus for care. This is a psychologic problem, and the focus should be on this level.

1 This is focusing on the physical symptoms of the conflict; the client is not ready to give up the symptom. 2 The disorder operates on an unconscious level but is very real to the client; this response denies feelings. 4 Psychotherapy has to come before physical therapy.

Client Need: Psychosocial Integrity; **Cognitive Level:** Application; **Nursing Process:** Planning/Implementation; **Reference:** Ch 19, Conversion Disorders, Nursing Care

197. 4 The client's anxiety results from being unable to choose psychologically between two conflicting actions. The conversion to a physical disability removes the choice and therefore reduces the anxiety.

1 The anxiety is not diffuse and free-floating but rather localized and converted to a physical

disability. **2** The conversion of the anxiety to a physical disability occurs on an unconscious level; the original anxiety no longer exists and the client generally is not anxious about the physical disability. **3** The anxiety is internalized into a physical symptom, not projected onto the environment.
Client Need: Psychosocial Integrity; **Cognitive Level:** Comprehension; **Nursing Process:** Assessment/Analysis; **Reference:** Ch 19, Conversion Disorder, Data Base

198. **3** The psychophysiologic response (hyperfunction or hypofunction) creates actual tissue change. Somatoform disorders are unrelated to organic changes.
1 There is a feeling of illness in both instances. **2** There is an emotional component in both instances. **4** There may be a restriction of activities in both instances.
Client Need: Psychosocial Integrity; **Cognitive Level:** Analysis; **Nursing Process:** Assessment/Analysis; **Reference:** Ch 19, Conversion Disorders, Data Base

199. **1** The client is using this compulsive behavior to control anxiety and needs to continue with it until the anxiety is reduced and more acceptable methods are developed to handle it.
2, 3 This will not change the client's behavior; she cannot stop the compulsive act because it reduces anxiety. **4** This will greatly increase anxiety; compulsive behavior is a defense that cannot be interrupted until new defenses are learned.
Client Need: Psychosocial Integrity; **Cognitive Level:** Application; **Integrated Process:** Caring; **Nursing Process:** Planning/Implementation; **Reference:** Ch 19, Obsessive-Compulsive Disorders, Nursing Care

200. **1** By carrying out the compulsive ritual, the client unconsciously tries to control the situation so that she will not act on unacceptable impulses and feelings.
2 This mechanism does not operate on a conscious level. **3** Hallucinations are not part of a phobic disorder. **4** They feel no need to punish others.
Client Need: Psychosocial Integrity; **Cognitive Level:** Analysis; **Nursing Process:** Assessment/Analysis; **Reference:** Ch 19, Obsessive-Compulsive Disorders, Data Base

201. **1** This sets an unrealistic limit that will increase anxiety by removing a defense the client needs.
2 This will increase self-esteem and self-control, not increase anxiety. **3** This is done in therapy as the client's condition improves. Insight is slowly developed to minimize anxiety. **4** This will reduce, not increase, anxiety, because the client will feel free to express feelings.
Client Need: Psychosocial Integrity; **Cognitive Level:** Analysis; **Nursing Process:** Evaluation/Outcomes; **Reference:** Ch 19, Obsessive-Compulsive Disorders, Nursing Care

202. **4** These clients can work through their underlying conflicts more easily or productively when demands are reduced and the routine is simple.

1 Preventing these clients from carrying out rituals can precipitate panic reactions. **2** The intent of therapy should be to help the client gain control, not to enable others to do the controlling. **3** Since anxiety stems from unconscious conflicts, a controlled environment alone is not enough to effect resolution.
Client Need: Psychosocial Integrity; **Cognitive Level:** Comprehension; **Nursing Process:** Planning/Implementation; **Reference:** Ch 19, Obsessive-Compulsive Disorders, Nursing Care

203. **3** The initial action is to avoid hurrying the client because this increases anxiety and the performance of the ritual. Routines will also decrease anxiety and the need for the ritual.
1 Taking away all of the client's ritualistic behaviors will be ineffective and serve to increase anxiety. **2** This is one of the goals to be accomplished late during the client's hospitalization, not in the initial phase. Some clients will never be able to identify the purpose of their ritual beyond the fact that it helps decrease their anxiety. **4** This action is an appropriate intervention during the working phase of the nurse-client intervention, not the initial phase.
Client Need: Psychosocial Integrity; **Cognitive Level:** Application; **Nursing Process:** Planning/Implementation; **Reference:** Ch 19, Obsessive-Compulsive Disorders, Nursing Care

204. **4** The symptoms are a defense against anxiety resulting from decision making, which triggers old fears; the client needs support.
1 This denies the client's overwhelming anxiety and lacks realistic support. **2** This is judgmental; the client should be encouraged to work through symptoms, not avoid risk. **3** This is judgmental; an increase in anxiety does not necessarily mean the client does not want to attain the goal.
Client Need: Psychosocial Integrity; **Cognitive Level:** Analysis; **Integrated Process:** Communication/Documentation; **Nursing Process:** Planning/Implementation; **Reference:** Ch 19, Obsessive-Compulsive Disorders, Nursing Care

205. **4** The repeated thought or act defends the client against even higher, more severe levels of anxiety.
1, 3 To deny the client the ritual may precipitate panic levels of anxiety. **2** The client already recognizes that the ritual serves little purpose.
Client Need: Psychosocial Integrity; **Cognitive Level:** Application; **Nursing Process:** Assessment/Analysis; **Reference:** Ch 19, Obsessive-Compulsive Disorders, Data Base

206. **4** This outcome will result from teaching the client to recognize situations that provoke ritualistic behavior and from the client learning how to interrupt the pattern.
1, 2 This is not a priority; the client probably had little difficulty in this area. **3** No evidence was presented to indicate the client was hallucinating.
Client Need: Psychosocial Integrity; **Cognitive Level:** Analysis; **Nursing Process:** Evaluation/Outcomes; **Reference:** Ch 19, Obsessive-Compulsive Disorders, Nursing Care

207. 1 This drug blocks the uptake of serotonin, which leads to a decrease in obsessive-compulsive behaviors.

2, 3 This is an antiparkinsonian agent, not an antidepressant. 4 This is an antihistamine, not an antianxiety agent.

Client Need: Pharmacological and Parenteral Therapies; **Cognitive Level:** Analysis; **Nursing Process:** Planning/Implementation; **Reference:** Ch 19, Obsessive-Compulsive Disorders, Data Base

208. 1 The repeated act defends the client against severe anxiety; interruption of the ritual will result in increased anxiety.

2 The performance of a ritual is not anger turned inward on the self; the ritual reduces anxiety. 3 Rituals are not activities that enhance self-esteem; they control anxiety. 4 Pointing out that the behavior is inappropriate will further increase anxiety. The client does not want to perform the ritual, but feels compelled to do so to keep anxiety at a controllable level.

Client Need: Psychosocial Integrity; **Cognitive Level:** Application; **Nursing Process:** Planning/Implementation; **Reference:** Ch 19, Obsessive-Compulsive Disorders, Nursing Care

209. 4 The client's exact compliance in carrying out the compulsive ritual relieves anxiety, at least temporarily. Furthermore, it meets a need and is necessary to the client.

1 The compulsive act is purposeless repetition and useful only in that it temporarily decreases anxiety for the client. 2 Urging has no effect on trying to have the client start or stop the ritualistic behavior. 3 The person cannot stop the activity; it is not under voluntary control.

Client Need: Psychosocial Integrity; **Cognitive Level:** Application; **Nursing Process:** Assessment/Analysis; **Reference:** Ch 19, Obsessive-Compulsive Disorders, Nursing Care

210. 4 Helping clients understand that a behavior is being used to control anxiety usually makes them more amenable to psychotherapy.

1 Treatment includes activities to help the client, not others. 2 The client usually understands this already. 3 This will only mask symptoms and will not get at the root of what is bothering the client.

Client Need: Psychosocial Integrity; **Cognitive Level:** Application; **Nursing Process:** Planning/Implementation; **Reference:** Ch 19, Obsessive-Compulsive Disorders, Nursing Care

211. 4 Accepting these clients and their symptomatic behavior sets the foundation for the nurse-client relationship. Setting limits provides external controls and helps lower anxiety.

1 Restricting movements will have no effect other than to increase anxiety. 2 This will only increase their anxiety and increase their use of the behavior. 3 This is unrealistic.

Client Need: Psychosocial Integrity; **Cognitive Level:** Application; **Integrated Process:** Caring; **Nursing Process:** Planning/Implementation; **Reference:** Ch 19, Obsessive-Compulsive Disorders, Nursing Care

212. 4 Clients with a somatoform disorder are preoccupied with the symptoms that are being experienced and usually do not want to talk about their emotions or relate them to their present situation.

1 These clients want and seek treatment, not palliative care. 2 A problem with memory is not associated with somatoform disorders. 3 Clients with a somatoform disorder do not seek opportunities to discuss their feelings.

Client Need: Psychosocial Integrity; **Cognitive Level:** Application; **Nursing Process:** Planning/Implementation; **Reference:** Ch 19, General Nursing Care of Clients With Somatoform Disorders

213. 4 This recognizes feelings and tells what is expected.

1 This is threatening and gives false reassurance; it puts the responsibility on the client and does not allow for expression of feelings. 2 This may lead the client to think that the environment is unsafe, which may increase insecurity and anxiety. 3 Being with other people in a strange situation will add more stress to the new and already frightening experience of hospitalization.

Client Need: Psychosocial Integrity; **Cognitive Level:** Analysis; **Integrated Process:** Caring, Communication/Documentation; **Nursing Process:** Planning/Implementation; **Reference:** Ch 19, Depressive Episode of a Bipolar Disorder, Nursing Care

214. 3 This provides a direct response to the client's concern and allows some exploration of food choices.

1 Focusing on several caretakers does little to meet the client's basic security needs. 2 This does not address the client's comment that "No one cares." 4 This encourages dependency on the nurse; the message is clearly, "Do it for me, not because it is important for you."

Client Need: Psychosocial Integrity; **Cognitive Level:** Application; **Integrated Process:** Caring, Communication/Documentation; **Nursing Process:** Planning/Implementation; **Reference:** Ch 19, Depressive Episode of a Bipolar Disorder, Nursing Care

215. 4 As depression increases, thought processes become more slowed and verbal expression decreases.

1 The affect of the depressed person usually is one of sadness, or it may be blank. 2 Loose associations are seen most often in clients with schizophrenia, not depressed clients. 3 Decreased physical activity will not produce physical exhaustion.

Client Need: Psychosocial Integrity; **Cognitive Level:** Application; **Nursing Process:** Assessment/Analysis; **Reference:** Ch 19, Major Depression, Data Base

216. 1 Routines should be kept simple and no demands should be made that the client cannot meet. The client is depressed, and all reactions will be slow. Putting pressure on the client will only increase anxiety and feelings of worthlessness.

2 The client will have to focus on personal strengths, not on family strengths. 3 This feeds into the client's feelings of unworthiness and frustration. 4 Feelings of worth must come from within the individual; the

nurse must reassure the client through actions, not words.
Client Need: Psychosocial Integrity; **Cognitive Level:** Application; **Nursing Process:** Planning/Implementation; **Reference:** Ch 19, Depressive Episode of a Bipolar Disorder, Nursing Care

217. 1 Because major depression is due to the client's feelings of self-rejection, it is important for the nurse to have the client initially identify these feelings before a plan of action can be taken. Later discussion should be on other topics so as not to reinforce negative thoughts and feelings.
2 This is asking the client to draw a conclusion; the client may be unable to do so at this time. Also, many depressions are not related to external events but may be related to the client's psychobiology. 3 Asking "why" does not let a client explore feelings; it usually elicits an "I don't know" response. 4 This is beyond the scope of the client's abilities now; clients will rather have the nurse tell them how staff can help them than help themselves.
Client Need: Psychosocial Integrity; **Cognitive Level:** Analysis; **Integrated Process:** Communication/Documentation; **Nursing Process:** Planning/Implementation; **Reference:** Ch 19, Depressive Episode of a Bipolar Disorder, Nursing Care

218. 4 Bringing another client into a set situation is the most therapeutic, least-threatening approach.
1 At this point in time, it will not be therapeutic to allow the client to remain with solitary pursuits.
2 Explanations will not necessarily change behavior.
3 This transfers nursing responsibility to the physician.
Client Need: Psychosocial Integrity; **Cognitive Level:** Analysis; **Nursing Process:** Planning/Implementation; **Reference:** Ch 19, General Nursing Care of Clients With Mood Disorders

219. 2 An art-type project that may be worked on successfully at one's own pace is appropriate for a depressed client.
1, 4 This requires too much concentration and may increase the client's feelings of despair. 3 This client is probably experiencing psychomotor retardation and at this point this activity may not be appropriate for this client.
Client Need: Psychosocial Integrity; **Cognitive Level:** Analysis; **Nursing Process:** Planning/Implementation; **Reference:** Ch 19, General Nursing Care of Clients With Mood Disorders

220. 2 This provides support and security without rejecting the client or placing value judgments on behavior.
1 Limits will have to be set in giving care, but staying with the client and showing acceptance are immediate nursing actions. 3 This only calms the client down; it does not try to deal with the problem. 4 This ignores the problem; isolation implies punishment.
Client Need: Psychosocial Integrity; **Cognitive Level:** Application; **Integrated Process:** Caring; **Nursing Process:** Planning/Implementation; **Reference:** Ch 19, General Nursing Care of Clients With Mood Disorders

221. 3 Involving the client in a one-on-one conversation provides individualized, low-anxiety-producing

attention and gives the message that the client is important, which supports self-esteem.
1 This may require too much concentration for a depressed client. 2 This may require too much concentration for a depressed client; also, it involves competition, which is not therapeutic at this time.
4 A depressed client does not have the energy to engage in a game of Ping-Pong; also, this is a competitive game, which is not therapeutic at this time.
Client Need: Psychosocial Integrity; **Cognitive Level:** Application; **Nursing Process:** Planning/Implementation; **Reference:** Ch 19, Depressive Episode of a Bipolar Disorder, Nursing Care

222. 1 This statement identifies the importance of feelings and provides an opening so that the client may talk about them.
2 The client is not going to believe this, and it is not helping the client express feelings. 3 The nursing goal is to help people function outside the hospital environment and not be afraid to leave the hospital.
4 A statement like this avoids the real issue and solves nothing.
Client Need: Psychosocial Integrity; **Cognitive Level:** Analysis; **Integrated Process:** Caring, Communication/Documentation; **Nursing Process:** Planning/Implementation; **Reference:** Ch 19, Depressive Episode of a Bipolar Disorder, Nursing Care

223. 4 This statement points out reality while accepting the fact that the client believes the feelings and thoughts are real.
1 This is false reassurance that the nurse does not know as fact. 2 The client does not know this and believes the opposite to be true. 3 This is reality but it is not a supportive response.
Client Need: Psychosocial Integrity; **Cognitive Level:** Analysis; **Integrated Process:** Caring, Communication/Documentation; **Nursing Process:** Planning/Implementation; **Reference:** Ch 19, Depressive Episode of a Bipolar Disorder, Nursing Care

224. 4 This action protects the client from acting on suicidal thoughts and provides a sense of security.
1 Although this may be done eventually, it is not the priority. 2, 3 Although this is important, it is not the priority.
Client Need: Psychosocial Integrity; **Cognitive Level:** Application; **Nursing Process:** Planning/Implementation; **Reference:** Ch 19, General Nursing Care of Clients With Mood Disorders

225. 2 Directness is the best approach at the first interview, because this sets the focus and concern and lets the nurse know what the client is feeling now.
1 At this point the client is most likely unable to think past the present, much less deal with future plans. 3 This is an indirect approach, but initially the direct approach with the client is best. 4 This is one resource for input; but regarding suicide, it is best to approach the client directly.
Client Need: Psychosocial Integrity; **Cognitive Level:** Analysis; **Integrated Process:** Communication/Documentation; **Nursing Process:** Planning/Implementation; **Reference:** Ch 19, General Nursing Care of Clients With Mood Disorders

226. 1 Suicidal impulses take priority, and the client must be stopped from acting on them while treatment is in progress.

2 This has a very low order of priority. 3 This is a secondary concern. 4 Reassurance will not necessarily decrease the client's feeling; safety is the priority.

Client Need: Psychosocial Integrity; Cognitive Level: Application; Nursing Process: Planning/Implementation; Reference: Ch 19, General Nursing Care of Clients With Mood Disorders

227. 4 This response recognizes feelings and behavior and encourages the client to share feelings; it also promotes trust, which is essential to a therapeutic relationship.

1 While it is important to record behavior and notify the physician, it is not enough and does not meet the client's needs. 2 This will not meet the depressed client's needs. 3 This assumes too much and may be inaccurate.

Client Need: Psychosocial Integrity; Cognitive Level: Analysis; Integrated Process: Caring, Communication/Documentation; Nursing Process: Planning/Implementation; Reference: Ch 19, General Nursing Care of Clients With Mood Disorders

228. 4 This acknowledges the client's feelings, offers hope, and assists the client to a higher level of functioning.

1, 2, 3 This is not necessarily true; it ignores the client's feelings and closes off the opportunity for further discussion of feelings.

Client Need: Psychosocial Integrity; Cognitive Level: Application; Integrated Process: Caring, Communication/Documentation; Nursing Process: Planning/Implementation; Reference: Ch 19, Depressive Episode of a Bipolar Disorder, Nursing Care

229. 1 These clients can usually be fairly easily distracted by planned involvement in repetitious, simple tasks.

2 This should be employed only if the client's restlessness cannot be controlled with other measures and the physical exhaustion creates a danger for the client. 3 This is abusive treatment for a client with a need to pace and reinforces the client's belief that punishment is required for redemption. 4 The client may perceive this isolation as a punishment, and it will not allow for observation by the staff.

Client Need: Psychosocial Integrity; Cognitive Level: Application; Nursing Process: Planning/Implementation; Reference: Ch 19, General Nursing Care of Clients With Mood Disorders

230. 4 The nurse's response urges the client to reflect on feelings and encourages communication.

1 This is shifting responsibility from the nurse to the doctor; it is an evasion technique. 2 This is not what the client is asking the nurse; it closes the door to further communication. 3 "Why" asks the client to draw a conclusion, which this client may not be able to do.

Client Need: Psychosocial Integrity; Cognitive Level: Analysis; Integrated Process: Communication/Documentation; Nursing Process: Planning/Implementation; Reference: Ch 19, General Nursing Care of Clients With Mood Disorders

231. 4 A major part of depression involves an inability to accept the self as it is, which leads to making demands on others to meet unrealistic needs.

1 A short-term goal is to talk about the client's depressed feelings; a long-term goal is to look at what is causing those feelings. 2 Developing new defense mechanisms is not the priority because they tend to help the client avoid reality. 3 This is not important or crucial to the client's recovery.

Client Need: Psychosocial Integrity; Cognitive Level: Analysis; Nursing Process: Planning/Implementation; Reference: Ch 19, Depressive Episode of a Bipolar Disorder, Nursing Care

232. 2 This is the most therapeutic approach to prevent suicide. The staff member also provides special attention to help the client meet dependency needs and reduce a self-defeating attitude.

1 This response negates client's feelings and cuts off further communication. 3 This is unrealistic because the nurse cannot be with the client constantly until the depression lifts. 4 The priority is 24-hour observation of the client; removing articles that may provide a means for suicide should also be done.

Client Need: Psychosocial Integrity; Cognitive Level: Analysis; Integrated Process: Caring, Communication/Documentation; Nursing Process: Planning/Implementation; Reference: Ch 19, Depressive Episode of a Bipolar Disorder, Nursing Care

233. 3 This gives the client the nonverbal message that someone cares and views the client as being worthy of attention and concern.

1 The concentration required for chess is too much for the client at this time. 2 The client is incapable of making decisions at this time. 4 Depressed clients often have too much thinking time.

Client Need: Psychosocial Integrity; Cognitive Level: Analysis; Integrated Process: Caring; Nursing Process: Planning/Implementation; Reference: Ch 19, Depressive Episode of a Bipolar Disorder, Nursing Care

234. 1 This behavior indicates that the student expects no future.

2 It is typical to pay tribute to dead friends. 3 Talking about the event helps to resolve the conflict involved. 4 Becoming involved in school activities demonstrates a return to usual life patterns.

Client Need: Psychosocial Integrity; Cognitive Level: Application; Nursing Process: Assessment/Analysis; Reference: Ch 19, Depressive Episode of a Bipolar Disorder, Data Base

235. 4 Fatigue and apathy are symptoms of depression. If members of the staff criticize, it will only increase the client's negative feelings.

1 This allows the client to manipulate the environment. 2 This will not change the client's mind about the activities. This response does not show an understanding of the client's needs. 3 This will only reinforce negative feelings about the activities.

Client Need: Psychosocial Integrity; Cognitive Level: Application; Integrated Process: Caring; Nursing Process: Planning/Implementation; Reference: Ch 19, Depressive Episode of a Bipolar Disorder, Nursing Care

236. 3 This statement lets the client know the nurse realizes the client is having difficulty without asking direct questions or focusing on specific behavior.

1 This is an avoidance technique. 2 This response is stated more like an order than an offering of an opportunity to express feelings. 4 This is negating the client's feelings.

Client Need: Psychosocial Integrity; **Cognitive Level:** Application; **Integrated Process:** Caring, Communication/Documentation; **Nursing Process:** Planning/Implementation; **Reference:** Ch 19, Major Depression, Nursing Care

237. 2 Suicidal gestures involve superficial nonlethal injuries; the client has no intent to die as a result of the injuries.

1 Suicidal threats are a person's verbal statement of intent to commit suicide; there are threats but no action. 3 Suicidal attempts are actual implementations of severe self-injurious acts; there is an attempt to cause serious self-harm or death. 4 Suicidal ideations are a person's thoughts regarding suicide; there is no definitive intent or action expressed.

Client Need: Psychosocial Integrity; **Cognitive Level:** Analysis; **Integrated Process:** Communication/Documentation; **Nursing Process:** Assessment/Analysis; **Reference:** Ch 19, Depressive Episode of a Bipolar Disorder, Data Base

238. 3 This question focuses the interaction toward the future and invites the client to explore alternative coping strategies.

1 This question explores past coping strategies and should have been asked as a part of the initial assessment of the client. 2 This question attempts to explore the client's insight into present coping strategies, which should have been done before discussing the alternatives with the client. 4 This question asks the client once more to ensure that all the precipitating stressors have been identified; this should have been done in the initial assessment.

Client Need: Psychosocial Integrity; **Cognitive Level:** Analysis; **Integrated Process:** Communication/Documentation; **Nursing Process:** Planning/Implementation; **Reference:** Ch 19, General Nursing Care of Clients With Mood Disorders

239. 4 Spending extra time with the client demonstrates that the client is worthy of the nurse's time and that the nurse cares.

1 This does not show the acceptance and care that sitting with the client would. 2 The client may be unable, at this point, to expend energy on anything outside the self. 3 It is unlikely that the client will respond to the nurse because the client feels unworthy and depressed.

Client Need: Psychosocial Integrity; **Cognitive Level:** Analysis; **Integrated Process:** Caring; **Nursing Process:** Planning/Implementation; **Reference:** Ch 19, Depressive Episode of a Bipolar Disorder, Nursing Care

240. 1 This statement demonstrates an understanding that the newly discharged client needs to have the support of the therapeutic unit when discharged. The client needs to feel that in a crisis the staff will be there for support.

2 The role of the nurse was not to become a good friend but to aid the client in becoming a functioning being again. 3 This response provides false reassurance; the nurse may not know this. 4 This is unprofessional and blurs the roles of nurse and client.

Client Need: Psychosocial Integrity; **Cognitive Level:** Analysis; **Integrated Process:** Caring, Communication/Documentation; **Nursing Process:** Planning/Implementation; **Reference:** Ch 19, General Nursing Care of Clients With Mood Disorders

241. 3 This statement is honest and helps establish trust. Also, the client may realize that staff members care and feel that the client is worthy of care.

1 This is a response that places the client on the defensive. 2 This is an inappropriate response to a rather obvious situation. 4 This is an evasive tactic by the nurse.

Client Need: Psychosocial Integrity; **Cognitive Level:** Analysis; **Integrated Process:** Communication/Documentation; **Nursing Process:** Planning/Implementation; **Reference:** Ch 19, General Nursing Care of Clients With Mood Disorders

242. 3 This encourages the client to talk about feelings without the nurse setting the focus for the discussion.

1 This will make the client wonder where the nurse had been for 4 days. 2 This cuts further communication of feelings; the client's statement may indicate a desire to act on suicidal ideation. 4 This shifts the responsibility of care to the psychiatrist rather than dealing with it directly.

Client Need: Psychosocial Integrity; **Cognitive Level:** Analysis; **Integrated Process:** Communication/Documentation; **Nursing Process:** Planning/Implementation; **Reference:** Ch 19, General Nursing Care of Clients With Mood Disorders

243. 4 Ambivalence about life and death plus the introspection commonly found in clients with emotional problems can lead to increased anxiety and fear in the group members.

1 This probably will be a secondary concern of the group leader. 2 It is not a primary concern; but this indifference also should be explored later to see what is behind such apparent indifference, which may be a mask to cover feelings. 3 These feelings must be handled within the support and supervisory systems for the staff; the other group members are the primary concern.

Client Need: Psychosocial Integrity; **Cognitive Level:** Analysis; **Nursing Process:** Planning/Implementation; **Reference:** Ch 19, General Nursing Care of Clients With Mood Disorders

244. 1 Electroconvulsive therapy, which interrupts established patterns of behavior, helps relieve symptoms and limits possible suicide attempts in clients with severe, intractable

depressions that do not respond to antidepressant medication.
2 The client's depressed mood greatly limits participation in psychotherapy; feelings precipitated by therapy may lead to suicidal acting-out. **3** Psychotherapy is directed toward helping the person learn new coping mechanisms and better ways of dealing with problems; the depressed client needs direction to accomplish this. **4** These are antianxiety medications that are not ordinarily used for clients with depression.
Client Need: Psychosocial Integrity; **Cognitive Level:** Analysis; **Nursing Process:** Planning/Implementation; **Reference:** Ch 19, Depressive Episode of a Bipolar Disorder, Data Base

245. **1** Clients fear this therapy because of the expected pain. If they are reassured that they will be asleep and have no pain, there will be less anxiety and more cooperation.
2 No treatment requiring anesthesia is totally safe. **3** Clients may not realize their own fears and not know what questions to ask; this statement cuts off further communication. **4** Temporary, not permanent, loss occurs.
Client Need: Psychosocial Integrity; **Cognitive Level:** Application; **Integrated Process:** Communication/Documentation; **Nursing Process:** Planning/Implementation; **Reference:** Ch 19, Depressive Episode of a Bipolar Disorder, Data Base

246. **4** The staff's presence provides continued emotional support and helps relieve anxiety.
1 This will be part of explaining the treatments; the focus should be on having someone present, not on fear. **2** Not all clients experience amnesia, and the amnesia passes; placing emphasis on amnesia will increase fear. **3** The treatments may not make the client feel better; this is false reassurance.
Client Need: Psychosocial Integrity; **Cognitive Level:** Application; **Integrated Process:** Teaching/Learning; **Nursing Process:** Planning/Implementation; **Reference:** Ch 19, Depressive Episode of a Bipolar Disorder, Nursing Care

247. **4** The electrical energy passing through the cerebral cortex during ECT results in a temporary state of confusion after treatment.
1, 2, 3 This is not a usual or expected side effect.
Client Need: Psychosocial Integrity; **Cognitive Level:** Application; **Nursing Process:** Evaluation/Outcomes; **Reference:** Ch 19, Depressive Episode of a Bipolar Disorder, Data Base

248. **4** This statement expresses the nurse's positive thoughts about the client while letting the client know that the nurse is concerned.
1 This demonstrates the nurse's positive thoughts about all people and does not focus on the client specifically. **2** Although this statement may promote verbalization of feelings, it does not communicate the nurse's positive regard for the client, which might support a more positive self-esteem. **3** The client may not be aware of what caused feelings of insignificance and may not be able to answer this question.

Client Need: Psychosocial Integrity; **Cognitive Level:** Analysis; **Integrated Process:** Caring; **Nursing Process:** Planning/Implementation; **Reference:** Ch 19, Depressive Episode of a Bipolar Disorder, Nursing Care

249. **3** Self-esteem and feelings of competence are increased when a person experiences success.
1 Although this is a necessary intervention when a depressed client attempts to commit self-harm, it will not promote feelings of self-esteem. **2** Clients recognize unwarranted praise and often interpret these responses as a form of belittlement or pity. **4** This may or may not increase self-esteem; also, the client may not have the physical or emotional energy to interact with other clients.
Client Need: Psychosocial Integrity; **Cognitive Level:** Application; **Nursing Process:** Planning/Implementation; **Reference:** Ch 19, Depressive Episode of a Bipolar Disorder, Nursing Care

250. **1** This response uses paraphrasing to demonstrate to the client that it is all right to talk about these feelings; it recognizes the client's sense of hopelessness without intensifying the feeling while providing an opportunity to verbalize further.
2 Although this may be a true statement, it takes the focus away from the client. **3** This information is insignificant at this time; this question might be appropriate after the client's feelings have been validated and discussed at the feeling level. **4** This takes the focus off the client's feelings and places it on a philosophical level.
Client Need: Psychosocial Integrity; **Cognitive Level:** Analysis; **Integrated Process:** Caring; **Nursing Process:** Planning/Implementation; **Reference:** Ch 19, General Nursing Care of Clients With Mood Disorders

251. **1** Overactive individuals are stimulated by environmental factors. A responsibility of the nurse is to simplify their surroundings as much as possible.
2 The quiet client may become the target of this client's overactivity. **3** During this phase the client needs a decrease in stimuli. **4** During this phase the client needs a decrease in stimuli; two overactive clients together may produce excessive stimuli.
Client Need: Psychosocial Integrity; **Cognitive Level:** Application; **Nursing Process:** Planning/Implementation; **Reference:** Ch 19, Manic Episode of a Bipolar Disorder, Nursing Care

252. **4** The client's behavior demonstrates increased anxiety. Since it was directed toward the new staff, it was probably precipitated by their arrival.
1 The client is not filling the "life-of-the-party" role; the client is resorting to previous coping behavior in the face of extreme stress. **2** This is possible, but the remark is more indicative of increased anxiety. **3** The client is aware of what is going on and who everyone is at this time.
Client Need: Psychosocial Integrity; **Cognitive Level:** Analysis; **Nursing Process:** Assessment/Analysis; **Reference:** Ch 19, Manic Episode of a Bipolar Disorder, Data Base

253. **3** Recognizing the language as part of the illness makes it easier to tolerate, but limits must be set for the benefit of the staff and other clients. Setting limits also shows the client that the nurse cares enough to stop the behavior. **1** This statement shows little understanding or tolerance of the illness. **2** Ignoring the behavior is a form of rejection; the client is not using the behavior for attention. **4** This statement demonstrates a rejection of the client and little understanding of the illness.

Client Need: Psychosocial Integrity; **Cognitive Level:** Application; **Integrated Process:** Caring; **Nursing Process:** Planning/ Implementation; **Reference:** Ch 19, Manic Episode of a Bipolar Disorder, Nursing Care

254. **1** A person with a condescending, bossy attitude frequently evokes feelings of anger in others as a means to decrease their anxiety.

2 It is unlikely that a condescending, bossy attitude will produce feelings of dependency in others.

3 It is unlikely that a condescending, bossy attitude will produce feelings of inadequacy in others.

4 It is unlikely that a condescending, bossy attitude will produce feelings of ambivalence in others.

Client Need: Psychosocial Integrity; **Cognitive Level:** Analysis; **Nursing Process:** Assessment/Analysis; **Reference:** Ch 19, Manic Episode of a Bipolar Disorder, Nursing Care

255. **3** During periods of hyperactivity, the client has a short attention span and can be distracted easily; this is a therapeutic intervention for all the clients. **1, 4** This approach may increase anxiety, activity, and aggressive behavior. **2** The nurse should be empathetic, not sympathetic.

Client Need: Psychosocial Integrity; **Cognitive Level:** Application; **Nursing Process:** Planning/Implementation; **Reference:** Ch 19, Manic Episode of a Bipolar Disorder, Nursing Care

256. **3** Physical activity will help use some of the excess energy without requiring the client to make decisions or forcing other clients to deal with the behavior. **1** The client needs guidance and is not able to guide others. **2** The client may greatly disrupt the unit because of the excess activity and bossiness associated with this disorder. **4** The client's extreme activity limits concentration or task completion.

Client Need: Psychosocial Integrity; **Cognitive Level:** Application; **Integrated Process:** Caring; **Nursing Process:** Planning/ Implementation; **Reference:** Ch 19, General Nursing Care of Clients With Mood Disorders

257. **2** Hyperactive clients frequently will not take the time to eat because they are overinvolved with everything in their environment. **1** This is indicative of a depressive episode. **3** The client is unable to sit long enough with the other clients to eat a meal; this is not conscious avoidance. **4** The client probably gives no thought to food because of overinvolvement with the activities in the environment.

Client Need: Psychosocial Integrity; **Cognitive Level:** Application; **Integrated Process:** Caring; **Nursing Process:** Assessment/

Analysis; **Reference:** Ch 19, Manic Episode of a Bipolar Disorder, Data Base

258. **4** Clients who are out of control need controls set for them. The staff must understand that the client is not deliberately trying to disrupt the unit. **1** Ignoring the client will not stop the disruptive behavior; the nurse has a responsibility to the other clients. **2** This may be a last resort taken to solve the problem but should not be used until other alternatives are explored. **3** This is demeaning the client in the eyes of the other clients, and does not deal with the problem directly.

Client Need: Psychosocial Integrity; **Cognitive Level:** Application; **Integrated Process:** Caring; **Nursing Process:** Planning/ Implementation; **Reference:** Ch 19, Manic Episode of a Bipolar Disorder, Nursing Care

259. **4** Hyperactive clients burn up large quantities of calories, which must be replenished. Since these clients will not take the time to sit down to eat, providing them with food they can carry with them sometimes helps. **1** The client will probably not be aware of any hunger and may go without food for a dangerously long time. **2** This is an exercise in futility for the nurse. **3** The client is not presently capable of preparing food.

Client Need: Psychosocial Integrity; **Cognitive Level:** Application; **Integrated Process:** Caring; **Nursing Process:** Planning/ Implementation; **Reference:** Ch 19, Manic Episode of a Bipolar Disorder, Data Base

260. **2** Hyperactive behavior in individuals such as this is typical of the manic flight into reality associated with mood disorders. **1** Loss of interest in usual activities and a depressed appetite are more indicative of a major depression. **3** The symptoms are more indicative of a disorder of mood than of the personality. **4** A flat affect and apathy are more indicative of a schizophrenic disorder.

Client Need: Psychosocial Integrity; **Cognitive Level:** Application; **Nursing Process:** Assessment/Analysis; **Reference:** Ch 19, Manic Episode of a Bipolar Disorder, Data Base

261. **1** This will help reduce the client's anxiety, thereby reducing hyperactivity. **2** The client is not capable of choosing activities at this time. **3** It is not possible physically to control hyperactivity. **4** The client is not capable of controlling overactive behavior; setting verbal limits will not be effective.

Client Need: Psychosocial Integrity; **Cognitive Level:** Application; **Integrated Process:** Caring; **Nursing Process:** Planning/ Implementation; **Reference:** Ch 19, Manic Episode of a Bipolar Disorder, Nursing Care

262. **4** The hyperactive client is usually rather easily distracted, so the excess energy can be redirected into constructive channels. **1** There is nothing to indicate at this time that the client is not in touch with reality. **2** The client will

talk a great deal with no encouragement. **3** The client will not be able to focus long enough on one task to finish it.

Client Need: Psychosocial Integrity; **Cognitive Level:** Application; **Nursing Process:** Planning/Implementation; **Reference:** Ch 19, Manic Episode of a Bipolar Disorder, Nursing Care

263. **4** Grandiosity is manifested by extravagant, pompous, flamboyant beliefs about the self. It frequently occurs during manic phases of bipolar disorder.

1 Passiveness is exhibited when clients turn anger inward and show little emotion. It frequently occurs during the depressive stage of bipolar disorder. **2** Dysphoria, a depressed, sad mood, is associated with the depressive stage of bipolar disorder. **3** Anhedonia, an inability to feel pleasure, is associated with the depressive stage of bipolar disorder.

Client Need: Psychosocial Integrity; **Cognitive Level:** Application; **Nursing Process:** Assessment/Analysis; **Reference:** Ch 19, Manic Episode of a Bipolar Disorder, Data Base

264. **1** The goal is 6 to 8 hours of rest at night; too much time spent sleeping in the day time will defeat the goal of adequate rest at night.

2 This intervention contributes to the client's desire for relaxation and sleep. **3** This supports the client's hypersomnia; the client already sleeps too much. **4** This will increase the metabolic rate, which is not conducive to rest.

Client Need: Psychosocial Integrity; **Cognitive Level:** Analysis; **Nursing Process:** Planning/Implementation; **Reference:** Ch 19, Depressive Episode of a Bipolar Disorder, Data Base

NURSING CARE OF CLIENTS WITH DISORDERS RELATED TO ALTERATIONS IN BEHAVIOR

265. **2** The client is too anxious to sleep in a four-bed room and should simply be moved to a private room.

1 Just talking about the problem will not improve it; quietly moving the client to a private room is a better intervention at this time. **3** This is false reassurance. **4** This probably will not help since it will not relieve the client's anxiety.

Client Need: Psychosocial Integrity; **Cognitive Level:** Application; **Integrated Process:** Caring; **Nursing Process:** Planning/Implementation; **Reference:** Ch 20, Sleep Disorders, Nursing Care

266. **2** Narcolepsy is overwhelming sleepiness that results in irresistible attacks of sleep, loss of muscle tone (cataplexy), and/or hallucinations or sleep paralysis at the beginning or end of sleep episodes; the person usually awakens from the sleep feeling refreshed.

1 Insomnia is difficulty in initiating or maintaining sleep. **3** Sleep apnea is a breathing-related sleep disorder caused by disrupted respirations or airway obstruction; the usual sleeping pattern is disrupted numerous times throughout the night. **4** Sleep terrors are recurrent episodes of abrupt awakening from sleep accompanied by intense fear, screaming, tachycardia, tachypnea, and diaphoresis with no detailed dream recall.

Client Need: Psychosocial Integrity; **Cognitive Level:** Application; **Nursing Process:** Assessment/Analysis; **Reference:** Ch 20, Sleep Disorders, Data Base

267. 1 ☐ A heavy meal places pressure against the diaphragm that may be uncomfortable and the body is expending energy to digest the food. A light, not heavy, snack may be eaten before bedtime.

2 ☐ The bed should be used exclusively for sleep so that the expectation when getting into bed is that sleep will be the outcome.

3 ☒ Lying in bed when one is unable to sleep increases frustration and anxiety, which further impede sleep; other activities, such as reading or watching television, should not be conducted in bed.

4 ☐ Although milk may promote sleep, tea contains caffeine, which is a stimulant that should be avoided after the mid-afternoon; otherwise, it may interfere with sleep.

5 ☒ Exercise during the day uses energy that promotes sleep at night; exercise too close to bedtime is stimulating and may interfere with sleep.

6 ☒ Counting backwards requires minimal concentration but it is enough to interfere with thoughts that distract a person from falling asleep.

Client Need: Basic Care and Comfort; **Cognitive Level:** Analysis; **Integrated Process:** Teaching/Learning; **Nursing Process:** Planning/Implementation; **Reference:** Ch 20, Sleep Disorders, Nursing Care

268. 1 ☒ Acute or primary insomnia is caused by emotional or physical stress not caused by the direct physiologic effects of a substance or a medical condition.

2 ☐ Severe anxiety usually is related to a psychiatric disorder and therefore causes a secondary insomnia.

3 ☐ Generalized pain usually is related to a medical or neurologic problem and therefore causes a secondary insomnia.

4 ☒ Excessive caffeine intake is an example of disruptive sleep hygiene; caffeine is a stimulant that inhibits sleep.

5 ☐ Chronic depression usually is related to a psychiatric disorder and therefore causes a secondary insomnia.

6 ☒ Environmental noise causes physical and/or emotional discomfort and therefore is related to primary insomnia.

Client Need: Psychosocial Integrity; **Cognitive Level:** Analysis; **Nursing Process:** Assessment/Analysis; **Reference:** Ch 20, Sleep Disorders, Data Base

269. 4 The problem is psychologic. Therefore the initial approach by the nurse should be directed toward establishing trust.

1 The client is convinced of being overweight; complimenting the client's lovely figure will not change the client's self-perception. **2** The client is not ready for this information. **3** This may be a nursing intervention after trust has been established.

Client Need: Psychosocial Integrity; **Cognitive Level:** Application; **Integrated Process:** Caring; **Nursing Process:** Planning/ Implementation; **Reference:** Ch 20, General Nursing Care of Clients With Eating Disorders

270. 2 A goal focuses on where the client should be after certain actions are taken; these clients need to gain weight.

1 This may set up a struggle between the client and the nurse; the focus of care should not be on the actual intake of food. **3** Behavior modification techniques work much better than group therapy; these clients lack insight and will focus on food, not eating. **4** These clients talk freely about food; this is not therapeutic.

Client Need: Psychosocial Integrity; **Cognitive Level:** Analysis; **Nursing Process:** Evaluation/Outcomes; **Reference:** Ch 20, Anorexia Nervosa, Nursing Care

271. 3 This is objective proof that eating behaviors have improved.

1 "Stashing" of food is continuing and is an eating disorder characteristic. **2** This is subjective information and may be manipulative. **4** "Marathon meals" with little actual food ingestion is a common behavior of anorexics.

Client Need: Psychosocial Integrity; **Cognitive Level:** Analysis; **Nursing Process:** Evaluation/Outcomes; **Reference:** Ch 20, Anorexia Nervosa, Nursing Care

272. 3 Electrolyte imbalances can precipitate dysrhythmias that can be life-threatening.

1 Although clients with the diagnosis of anorexia nervosa have a low self-esteem and identifying and supporting strengths promote the development of a positive self-regard, this is not the priority at this time. **2** These clients are perfectionists who usually do not display impulsivity. **4** This is difficult to accomplish initially because these clients often deny the illness and evade therapeutic treatment.

Client Need: Physiological Adaptation; **Cognitive Level:** Analysis; **Nursing Process:** Planning/Implementation; **Reference:** Ch 20, Anorexia Nervosa, Data Base

273. 3 These clients hide much of their binging and purging behaviors and, unlike clients with anorexia, may have near-ideal body weights.

1 Clients with bulimia nervosa frequently are not obese. **2, 4** This is associated with clients with both anorexia nervosa and bulimia.

Client Need: Psychosocial Integrity; **Cognitive Level:** Analysis; **Nursing Process:** Assessment/Analysis; **Reference:** Ch 20, Bulimia Nervosa, Data Base

274. 4 Realistic guidelines reduce anxiety, increase feelings of security, and increase compliance with the therapeutic regimen.

1 A controlling environment sets up a power struggle between these clients and the nurse. **2** These clients need realistic rules and regulations that they identify as helpful, not empathy. **3** This is not therapeutic; focusing on food generally results in a power struggle between these clients and the nurse.

Client Need: Psychosocial Integrity; **Cognitive Level:** Application; **Nursing Process:** Planning/Implementation; **Reference:** Ch 20, Bulimia Nervosa, Nursing Care

275. 1 ☒ Clients with borderline personality disorder often lead complex, chaotic lives because of the inability to control or limit impulses.

2 ☒ Extremes of emotions can be displayed over short periods of time and range from apathy and boredom to anger.

3 ☐ This is associated with obsessive-compulsive disorders.

4 ☒ Impulsive acts, such as reckless driving, spending money, or engaging in unsafe sex, often result in self-destructive consequences.

5 ☐ This is associated with mood disorders such as depression.

Client Need: Psychosocial Integrity; **Cognitive Level:** Analysis; **Integrated Process:** Communication/Documentation; **Nursing Process:** Assessment/Analysis; **Reference:** Ch 20, Personality Disorders, Data Base

276. 4 Clients must first become aware of their behavior before they can change it.

1, 2 Confrontation may increase anxiety, anger, and agitation. **3** This occurs after the client is aware of behavior and has a desire to change the behavior.

Client Need: Psychosocial Integrity; **Cognitive Level:** Application; **Nursing Process:** Planning/Implementation; **Reference:** Ch 20, Personality Disorders, Nursing Care

277. 1 To gain control, clients often try to split the staff apart, separating the nurse from the rest of the treatment team; confidentiality is not expected to be maintained among professionals caring for a client in a case like this, because it is detrimental to the care of the client.

2 This response reinforces the team approach to care. **3** This response both reinforces the team approach and avoids providing false assurance that the information will be kept secret. **4** This does not provide false assurance that the information will be kept secret.

Client Need: Management of Care; **Cognitive Level:** Analysis; **Integrated Process:** Communication/Documentation; **Nursing Process:** Planning/Implementation; **Reference:** Ch 20, Personality Disorders, Nursing Care

278. 4 This intervention demonstrates the nurse's caring presence, which is vital for this client.

1 Although the treatment team does need to know about the event, notification is not the immediate concern. **2** This is premature and it reinforces the client's predisposition to manipulative behavior. **3** This medication is inappropriate in this situation; vomiting is expected after the ingestion of shampoo.
Client Need: Psychosocial Integrity; **Cognitive Level:** Application; **Integrated Process:** Caring; **Nursing Process:** Planning/Implementation; **Reference:** Ch 20, Personality Disorders, Nursing Care

279. **4** Clients with borderline personality disorders frequently demonstrate a pattern of unstable interpersonal relationships, impulsiveness, affective instability, and frantic efforts to avoid abandonment; these behaviors usually create great difficulty in establishing mutual goals.
1, 2, 3 Although the client with a borderline personality disorder may have difficulty in this area, the more significant issue is addressed in answer 4.
Client Need: Psychosocial Integrity; **Cognitive Level:** Analysis; **Integrated Process:** Communication/Documentation; **Nursing Process:** Planning/Implementation; **Reference:** Ch 20, Personality Disorders, Data Base

280. **4** These clients usually display social inadequacy and lack of emotional contact with others.
1 These behaviors probably reflect an obsessive-compulsive personality disorder. **2** These behaviors probably reflect a dependent personality disorder. **3** These behaviors probably reflect a narcissistic personality disorder.
Client Need: Psychosocial Integrity; **Cognitive Level:** Application; **Nursing Process:** Assessment/Analysis; **Reference:** Ch 20, Personality Disorders, Data Base

281. **3** These clients are withdrawn, aloof, and socially distant; allowing distance and providing support may encourage the eventual development of a therapeutic alliance.
1 Manipulative behavior is typical of clients with the diagnosis of antisocial personality disorder or borderline personality disorder. **2** Group therapy will increase this client's anxiety; cognitive or behavioral therapy is more appropriate. **4** Seductive behavior is associated with clients with the diagnosis of histrionic personality disorder.
Client Need: Psychosocial Integrity; **Cognitive Level:** Analysis; **Nursing Process:** Planning/Implementation; **Reference:** Ch 20, Personality Disorders, Nursing Care

282. **1** Clients with histrionic personality disorder draw attention to themselves and demonstrate emotionality and attention-seeking behavior.
2 These are typical of clients with the diagnosis of narcissistic personality disorder. **3** These are typical of clients with the diagnosis of antisocial personality disorder. **4** These are typical of clients with the diagnosis of obsessive-compulsive personality disorder.
Client Need: Psychosocial Integrity; **Cognitive Level:** Application; **Nursing Process:** Assessment/Analysis; **Reference:** Ch 20, Personality Disorders, Data Base

283. **3** These clients interact with others through manipulation, aggressiveness, and exploitation; therefore clear limits must be set with consistently enforced consequences for crossing set boundaries.
1 These clients can be too assertive; this approach is appropriate for a client with the diagnosis of dependent personality disorder. **2** These clients need a firm, consistent approach with clear and realistic limits on inappropriate behavior; this approach should be used with clients with the diagnosis of avoidant personality disorder. **4** The nurse should provide a neutral, nonemotional approach with clear, realistic boundaries and consequences.
Client Need: Psychosocial Integrity; **Cognitive Level:** Application; **Nursing Process:** Planning/Implementation; **Reference:** Ch 20, Personality Disorders, Nursing Care

284. **3** Individuals with this personality disorder tend to be self-centered and impulsive. They lack judgment and self-control and are unable to postpone gratification.
1 Generally, the opposite is true. **2** These individuals believe that the rules do not apply to them and they do not profit from their mistakes. **4** These people are too self-centered to have a sense of responsibility to anyone.
Client Need: Psychosocial Integrity; **Cognitive Level:** Application; **Nursing Process:** Assessment/Analysis; **Reference:** Ch 20, Personality Disorders, Data Base

285. **2** The lack of superego control allows the ego and the id to control the behavior. Self-motivation and self-satisfaction are of paramount concern, and they have little or no concern for others.
1 They count on others to extricate them from their problems. **3** These people are extremely dependent on others. **4** These people are usually charming on the surface and can easily "con" people into doing what they want.
Client Need: Psychosocial Integrity; **Cognitive Level:** Application; **Nursing Process:** Assessment/Analysis; **Reference:** Ch 20, Personality Disorders, Data Base

286. **3** This accepts the client as a person of worth rather than being cold or implying rejection. However, the nurse maintains a professional rather than a social role.
1 This is shifting responsibility from the issue at hand to the institution. **2** This does not respond to the statement; the client is aware of their roles. **4** This avoids the real issue and shifts the responsibility to the ethical code.
Client Need: Management of Care; **Cognitive Level:** Analysis; **Integrated Process:** Communication/Documentation; **Nursing Process:** Planning/Implementation; **Reference:** Ch 20, Personality Disorders, Nursing Care

287. **2** When the individual consciously pretends to have an illness with no physical basis, it is called malingering.
1 People who are psychotic experience delusions, hallucinations, and disorganized thoughts, speech, or behavior. **3** A person out of contact with reality is

unable to pretend to be ill. **4** The use of conversion defenses is not a conscious act.
Client Need: Psychosocial Integrity; **Cognitive Level:** Analysis; **Nursing Process:** Assessment/Analysis; **Reference:** Ch 20, Factitious Disorders, Data Base

288. **4** This sets realistic limits on behavior without rejecting the client.
1 This will constitute a rejection of the person rather than the behavior. **2** This will encourage further manipulation of the staff by the client. **3** The other client is entitled to a special time with the nurse; this is inconsistent limit-setting on the part of the nurse.
Client Need: Psychosocial Integrity; **Cognitive Level:** Analysis; **Integrated Process:** Communication/Documentation; **Nursing Process:** Planning/Implementation; **Reference:** Ch 20, Personality Disorders, Nursing Care

289. **2** This sets limits, points out reality, and places responsibility for behavior on the client.
1 This is a punishing response and endangers the trust relationship. **3** Clients such as this need limits set; changing the time shows inconsistency. **4** The nurse using this response is showing inconsistency, endangering the trust relationship, and using a threat to gain control.
Client Need: Psychosocial Integrity; **Cognitive Level:** Application; **Integrated Process:** Communication/Documentation; **Nursing Process:** Planning/Implementation; **Reference:** Ch 20, Personality Disorders, Nursing Care

290. **2** When a client has an adjustment disorder, anxiety may be related to a disturbance in self-esteem and depression may be related to impaired social interaction.
1 Problems with memory are not specifically related to an adjustment disorder. **3** Activity intolerance, which is related to oxygenation problems, is not associated with adjustment disorders. **4** A client with an adjustment disorder does not experience a disturbance in personal identity.
Client Need: Psychosocial Integrity; **Cognitive Level:** Application; **Nursing Process:** Assessment/Analysis; **Reference:** Ch 20, Adjustment Disorders, Data Base

291. **3** Intrinsic motivation, stimulated from within the learner, is essential if rehabilitation is to be successful. Often clients are most emotionally ready for help when they have "hit bottom." Only then are clients motivationally ready to face reality and put forth the necessary energy and effort to change behavior.
1, 4 This is an important factor but not the most important one. **2** This is an important factor and a helpful one, but not the most important one.
Client Need: Psychosocial Integrity; **Cognitive Level:** Analysis; **Nursing Process:** Assessment/Analysis; **Reference:** Ch 20, Alcohol Abuse, Data Base

292. **4** Thiamine is a coenzyme necessary for the production of energy from glucose. If thiamine is not present in adequate amounts, nerve activity is diminished and damage or degeneration of myelin sheaths occurs.

1 Fats need not be restricted as long as they are tolerated. **2** These are avoided; the use of these has a higher risk for toxic side effects in older or debilitated persons. **3** Thorazine is a neuroleptic, which will not be used because it is severely toxic to the liver.
Client Need: Pharmacological and Parenteral Therapies; **Cognitive Level:** Analysis; **Nursing Process:** Planning/Implementation; **Reference:** Ch 20, Alcohol Abuse, Data Base

293. **1** This presents reality and answers the client's question.
2 This is entering into the misperception of reality. **3, 4** This intervention provides comfort and may reduce anxiety but it should follow the priority intervention of pointing out reality.
Client Need: Psychosocial Integrity; **Cognitive Level:** Analysis; **Integrated Process:** Communication/Documentation; **Nursing Process:** Planning/Implementation; **Reference:** Ch 20, Alcohol Abuse, Nursing Care

294. **2** Alcoholics Anonymous is a self-help group of individuals who meet together to attain and maintain sobriety.
1 A social group centers on building interpersonal relationships through participation in mutual activities. **3** A resocialization group centers on increasing social skills that may be diminished or lacking. **4** A psychotherapeutic group treats mental and emotional disorders by psychologic techniques and always has a member of the health care profession as its group leader.
Client Need: Psychosocial Integrity; **Cognitive Level:** Knowledge; **Nursing Process:** Assessment/Analysis; **Reference:** Ch 20, Alcohol Abuse, Data Base

295. **1** The client is using denial as a defense against feelings of guilt, which will reduce anxiety and protect the self.
2 Denial deals more with the client's own expectations. **3** Denial makes the client seem more stable to others, not independent. **4** This may be part of the reason, but the bigger motivating factor is to decrease guilt feelings.
Client Need: Psychosocial Integrity; **Cognitive Level:** Comprehension; **Nursing Process:** Assessment/Analysis; **Reference:** Ch 20, Alcohol Abuse, Data Base

296. **4** The individual is unaware of gaps in memory, so the use of stories is an unconscious attempt to deny or cover up the gaps.
1 Lying is a deliberate attempt to deceive rather than a face-saving device for loss of memory. **2** Denying is blocking out of conscious awareness rather than a cover-up for loss of memory. **3** Rationalizing is used to explain and justify the behavior rather than to cover up the loss of memory.
Client Need: Psychosocial Integrity; **Cognitive Level:** Analysis; **Nursing Process:** Assessment/Analysis; **Reference:** Ch 20, Alcohol Abuse, Data Base

297. **3** Members find empathy, patience, and understanding in the group. They are able to have their dependence needs met while helping others who are even more dependent.

1 This is helpful, but it does not have the success rate of AA. **2** This is important for the detoxification stage, not for overall therapy. **4** This does not help determine the cause of the alcohol problem.

Client Need: Psychosocial Integrity; **Cognitive Level:** Application; **Integrated Process:** Communication/Documentation; **Nursing Process:** Planning/Implementation; **Reference:** Ch 20, Alcohol Abuse, Data Base

298. **2** The CAGE screening test for alcoholism contains four questions, corresponding to the letters CAGE: **C**—Have you ever felt you ought to **C**ut down on your drinking? **A**—Have people **A**nnoyed you by criticizing your drinking? **G**—Have you ever felt bad or **G**uilty about your drinking? **E**—Have you ever had a drink first thing in the morning (as an "**E**ye-opener") to steady your nerves or get rid of a hangover?

1, 3 This question is 1 of the 26 questions that is included on the Michigan Alcohol Screening Test (MAST). **4** This question is 1 of the 10 questions that is included on the Alcohol Use Disorders Identification Test (AUDIT).

Client Need: Psychosocial Integrity; **Cognitive Level:** Analysis; **Integrated Process:** Communication/Documentation; **Nursing Process:** Assessment/Analysis; **Reference:** Ch 20, Alcohol Abuse, Nursing Care

299. **3** This focuses on the client's feelings rather than the organization itself. The organization is effective only when the client is able to discuss feelings openly.

1 This may or may not be true. **2** It may be too late by that time. **4** This is false reassurance; AA may help clients develop insight but may not be able to help them cope with their problems.

Client Need: Psychosocial Integrity; **Cognitive Level:** Analysis; **Integrated Process:** Communication/Documentation; **Nursing Process:** Planning/Implementation; **Reference:** Ch 20, Alcohol Abuse, Nursing Care

300. **1** The purpose of a self-help group is for individuals to develop their strengths and new individual patterns of coping.

2, 3, 4 This is one of the purposes of group therapy.

Client Need: Psychosocial Integrity; **Cognitive Level:** Comprehension; **Nursing Process:** Planning/Implementation; **Reference:** Ch 20, Alcohol Abuse, Data Base

301. **3** This statement reflects the underlying theme in the client's statement and nonjudgmentally encourages the client to verbalize further.

1 This is a judgmental response that may cut off further communication. **2** Although this is a true statement, it does not promote further communication nor does it promote continued attendance. **4** This is an inaccurate conclusion based on incomplete information; also, it is judgmental and may cut off further communication.

Client Need: Psychosocial Integrity; **Cognitive Level:** Analysis; **Integrated Process:** Communication/Documentation; **Nursing**

Process: Planning/Implementation; **Reference:** Ch 20, Alcohol Abuse, Nursing Care

302. **4** Referral to a community-based self-help group is an essential component of the discharge plan to provide ongoing support.

1 The client probably does not need a halfway house. **2** Referral to a family therapist can only be made at the request of the client and/or family. **3** This is not the best possible mode of therapy and may create additional anxiety.

Client Need: Psychosocial Integrity; **Cognitive Level:** Application; **Nursing Process:** Planning/Implementation; **Reference:** Ch 20, Alcohol Abuse, Data Base

303. **4** When clients with alcohol problems voice a desire for help, it usually signifies they are ready for treatment because they are admitting they have a problem.

1 Compliance with an alcohol treatment program requires abstinence. **2** This is too short a time to signal readiness for treatment. **3** Self-admission alone is often not an indication that the client is really ready for treatment because many factors can influence admission.

Client Need: Psychosocial Integrity; **Cognitive Level:** Analysis; **Nursing Process:** Assessment/Analysis; **Reference:** Ch 20, Alcohol Abuse, Nursing Care

304. **3** Attendance at AA meetings on a daily basis usually indicates an acceptance of the problem and a desire for help.

1 Attendance at inpatient group meetings is helpful but is not specific to the problem of alcoholism. **2** This drug can help maintain abstinence but may also become a crutch that fosters dependency on a pill rather than alcohol. **4** Clients with alcohol problems should not sponsor other clients until a long period of sobriety is maintained.

Client Need: Psychosocial Integrity; **Cognitive Level:** Analysis; **Nursing Process:** Assessment/Analysis; **Reference:** Ch 20, Alcohol Abuse, Nursing Care

305. **1** The client must first acknowledge that a substance abuse problem exists and is creating chaos; verbalizing that a problem exists indicates that the client is not in denial and is demonstrating the first step toward a readiness to change.

2 Once a problem is identified, then the numerous ways that drug use has controlled the client's life can be explored. **3** Once a problem is identified, then the nurse can assist the client to express and process negative feelings. **4** Once a problem is identified, then the client can explore the use of substances and the resulting lifestyle problems.

Client Need: Psychosocial Integrity; **Cognitive Level:** Application; **Nursing Process:** Evaluation/Outcomes; **Reference:** Ch 20, Drug Abuse, Nursing Care

306. 3, 2, 4, 1

   3   Of the drugs presented, codeine has the lowest potential for addiction.

   2   After codeine, alcohol has the lowest potential for addiction.

___4___   Barbiturates, which are sedatives/hypnotics, are more addicting than codeine or alcohol and are the most difficult addictions to cure.

___1___   Heroin, a semisynthetic opioid, is highly addictive.

Client Need: Psychosocial Integrity; **Cognitive Level:** Analysis; **Nursing Process:** Assessment/Analysis; **Reference:** Ch 20, Drug Abuse, Data base

307. 2 Methadone can be legally dispensed; the strength of this drug is controlled and remains constant from dose to dose, which is uncertain in illicit drugs.

1 Methadone is used in the medically supervised withdrawal period to treat physical dependence on opiates; it substitutes a legal for an illegal drug. Methadone may be administered long term to replace illegal narcotic use. If methadone treatment is abruptly stopped, there will be withdrawal symptoms. 3 Methadone is a synthetic narcotic and can cause dependence; it is mainly used in the treatment of heroin addiction but may be used with people who have chronic pain syndromes. It is not used for acute postoperative pain. 4 Methadone is not known to have this action.

Client Need: Pharmacological and Parenteral Therapies; **Cognitive Level:** Comprehension; **Nursing Process:** Planning/Implementation; **Reference:** Ch 20, Drug Abuse, Data Base

308. 2 When methadone is reduced, a craving for narcotics may occur. Without narcotics, anxiety will increase, agitation will occur, and the client may try to leave the hospital to secure drugs.

1, 3 These are not related to methadone hydrochloride reduction. 4 These may occur with methadone hydrochloride overdose.

Client Need: Pharmacological and Parenteral Therapies; **Cognitive Level:** Analysis; **Nursing Process:** Evaluation/Outcomes; **Reference:** Ch 20, Drug Abuse, Nursing Care

309. 3 Constricted pupils is a physical response to opioid intoxication; the pupils will dilate with opioid overdose.

1 Opioids cause drowsiness and psychomotor retardation; alertness is associated with the use of stimulants such as caffeine and amphetamines. 2 Opioids cause apathy or a depressed, sad mood (dysphoria); lability of mood is associated with the use of anabolic-androgenic steroids. 4 Opioids depress the respiratory center of the brain, causing slow, shallow respirations; increases in temperature, pulse, respirations, and blood pressure are associated with cocaine use.

Client Need: Pharmacological and Parenteral Therapies; **Cognitive Level:** Application; **Nursing Process:** Assessment/Analysis; **Reference:** Ch 20, Drug Abuse, Data Base

310. 4 The drug is not taken for medical reasons but for the favorable, pleasant, unusual, or desired effects it produces. It is often taken in doses that are fatal if the individual has not established a tolerance to it.

1 This is true but there is concomitant psychologic dependence on the drug. 2 This is true but there is concomitant physiologic need for the drug. 3 It is a physiologic and psychologic need to take the drug rather than a compulsion.

Client Need: Psychosocial Integrity; **Cognitive Level:** Application; **Nursing Process:** Assessment/Analysis; **Reference:** Ch 20, Drug Abuse, Data Base

311. 3 When Narcan is metabolized and its effects are diminished, the respiratory distress caused by the original drug overdose returns.

1, 4 There are no reports of these effects. 2 This combination does not cause cardiac depression.

Client Need: Pharmacological and Parenteral Therapies; **Cognitive Level:** Analysis; **Nursing Process:** Evaluation/Outcomes; **Reference:** Ch 20, Drug Abuse, Data Base

312. 1 Polydrug users abuse a variety of drugs in their search for the ultimate "high." They usually will include alcohol in their search and frequently combine their abuses.

2 This is not necessarily true. 3 This is not necessarily so; some become very happy and outgoing. 4 This has been mentioned as a possible causative factor but with no evidence to support it.

Client Need: Psychosocial Integrity; **Cognitive Level:** Application; **Nursing Process:** Assessment/Analysis; **Reference:** Ch 20, Drug Abuse, Data Base

313. 1 ☒ Cocaine is an alkaloid stimulant; euphoria or affective blunting is associated with cocaine intoxication.

2 ☒ Cocaine is an alkaloid stimulant; agitation or anger is associated with cocaine intoxication.

3 ☐ These are associated with hallucinogens.

4 ☐ This is associated with opioids.

5 ☒ Cocaine is an alkaloid stimulant; hypervigilance is associated with cocaine intoxication.

6 ☒ Cocaine is an alkaloid stimulant; impaired judgment and impaired social functioning are associated with cocaine intoxication.

Client Need: Psychosocial Integrity; **Cognitive Level:** Analysis; **Nursing Process:** Assessment/Analysis; **Reference:** Ch 20, Drug Abuse, Data Base

314. 2 If seizures were physiologically based, the client would not be able to continue to chew gum. This "attack" should be reported as a behavioral response, with the precipitating factors noted.

1 The chewing gum is not a danger when the client is not having a true seizure. 3 This is not necessary. 4 This is unsafe; it is not even used in a true seizure.

Client Need: Psychosocial Integrity; **Cognitive Level:** Application; **Integrated Process:** Communication/Documentation; **Nursing Process:** Assessment/Analysis; **Reference:** Ch 20, Factitious Disorders, Data Base

315. 2 Anger is the expected response of staff at having been duped by a client with a fictitious disorder; they feel both used and abused.

1, 3, 4 This feeling generally does not result when staff members have been involved in assessing and

caring for a client who has not had favorable outcomes from their interventions.
Client Need: Psychosocial Integrity; **Cognitive Level:** Application; **Nursing Process:** Assessment/Analysis; **Reference:** Ch 20, Factitious Disorders, Nursing Care

316. **2** Maintaining open communication is important for any therapeutic nurse-client relationship.
1 Confrontation will put the parent on the defensive and close off communication. **3** Health teaching at this time is premature; the parent is not ready for this approach. **4** Validation of the child's physical status focuses on the physical symptoms, which will reinforce the parent's behavior.
Client Need: Psychosocial Integrity; **Cognitive Level:** Application; **Integrated Process:** Communication/Documentation; **Nursing Process:** Planning/Implementation; **Reference:** Ch 20, Factitious Disorders, Nursing Care

NURSING CARE OF CLIENTS WITH SEXUAL AND GENDER IDENTITY DISORDERS

317. **1** Clients with these sexual disorders usually have many other emotional problems that may be overt or covert in nature.
2 There is no proof of a deficiency of these hormones. **3** This has no basis in fact. **4** There is normal development of sexual organs in individuals with paraphiliac sexual disorders.
Client Need: Psychosocial Integrity; **Cognitive Level:** Application; **Nursing Process:** Assessment/Analysis; **Reference:** Ch 21, Paraphilias, Data Base

318. **2** This identifies feelings and provides the client with an opportunity to talk.
1 This statement ignores feelings and does not help the client cope with the situation. **3** This may or may not be true and may be false reassurance. **4** The nurse does not know this to be a fact.
Client Need: Psychosocial Integrity; **Cognitive Level:** Analysis; **Integrated Process:** Caring, Communication/Documentation; **Nursing Process:** Planning/Implementation; **Reference:** Ch 21, Paraphilias, Nursing Care

319. **3** The nurse is legally responsible to report suspected child abuse to the appropriate child protection agency. The agency must assess the situation and intervene if necessary to protect the child.
1 Asking the child to describe the touching may cause more psychologic trauma; the nurse should listen and demonstrate concern. **2** Talking with the teacher violates the concept of confidentiality. **4** Contacting the father may result in more abuse or in the child not reporting future abuse.
Client Need: Management of Care; **Cognitive Level:** Application; **Integrated Process:** Communication/Documentation; **Nursing Process:** Planning/Implementation; **Reference:** Ch 21, Paraphilias, Nursing Care

320. 2, 1, 3, 4, 5
__2__ Because "the self" is the most important factor the nurse brings to the nurse-client therapeutic relationship, the nurse must understand personal feelings about issues surrounding this client's situation and needs; this is part of the preorientation phase of a therapeutic relationship.
__1__ In a therapeutic relationship the client is the focus of care and the relationship should be based on respect.
__3__ In an atmosphere of respect, the client will then more likely express feelings.
__4__ The client considering sex reassignment surgery should explore all alternatives. However, when the decision is made to act on this decision, the decision should be supported by the nurse.
__5__ After this important decision is made, the client may need assistance with how to inform significant others of the decision.
Client Need: Psychosocial Integrity; **Cognitive Level:** Analysis; **Integrated Process:** Caring; **Nursing Process:** Planning/Implementation; **Reference:** Ch 21, Gender Identity Disorders, Nursing Care

321. 1 ☒ Flushing is a common central nervous system response to Viagra.
2 ☒ Headache is a common central nervous system response to Viagra.
3 ☒ Diarrhea, not constipation, is a common gastrointestinal response to Viagra.
4 ☐ Dyspepsia is a common gastrointestinal response to Viagra.
5 ☐ Hypotension, not hypertension, is a cardiovascular response to Viagra. Viagra should not be taken with antihypertensives and nitrates because drug interactions can precipitate cardiovascular collapse.
Client Need: Pharmacological and Parenteral Therapies; **Cognitive Level:** Analysis; **Integrated Process:** Teaching/Learning; **Nursing Process:** Planning/Implementation; **Reference:** Ch 21, Sexual Dysfunction, Nursing Care

322. **2** Exposing the genitals and masturbating in a public place are unacceptable behaviors. Unacceptable behavior should be pointed out to the client and the client instructed to stop. Exhibitionism usually is done for shock value rather than as a preamble to sexual assault or rape. If the client wishes to masturbate, this activity can be carried out in private.
1 Unacceptable behavior should never be ignored. The client needs limits set on this type of behavior. **3** This may eventually be done. However, the client must first be given the opportunity to change his behavior. **4** Although the nurse must recognize that this behavior is related to his illness, it is not the nurse's role to seek out or prescribe medication.
Client Need: Psychosocial Integrity; **Cognitive Level:** Application; **Integrated Process:** Caring, Communication/Documentation; **Nursing Process:** Planning/Implementation; **Reference:** Ch 21,

General Nursing Care of Clients with Sexual and Gender Identity Disorders

323. 1 This response communicates to the client that the nurse is willing and able to explore this concern. It is an open-ended statement that allows the client to control the direction of the conversation. 2 With this response the nurse abdicates responsibility to the physician. The nurse is capable and legally responsible to collect information and explore client feelings and concerns. 3 Although sexual functioning changes as people age, there are many factors that influence sexual functioning (e.g., physiologic problems, interpersonal conflicts, emotional stress). 4 This response is premature; it moves immediately to a solution before adequate information has been collected. Also, the term erectile dysfunction is related to a medical diagnosis and its use at this time may increase client anxiety.

Client Need: Psychosocial Integrity; **Cognitive Level:** Analysis; **Integrated Process:** Caring; Communication/Documentation; **Nursing Process:** Planning/Implementation; **Reference:** Ch 21, General Nursing Care of Clients With Sexual and Gender Identity Disorders

324. 2 This statement is related to a sexual arousal disorder, which is a partial or complete failure to achieve a physiologic or psychologic response to sexual activity. 1 This statement may indicate a sexual desire disorder in which the individual has deficient, absent, or extreme aversion to and avoidance of sexual activity. 3, 4 This statement is related to an orgasmic disorder, which is a delay in or absence of an orgasm or premature ejaculation.

Client Need: Psychosocial Integrity; **Cognitive Level:** Analysis; **Nursing Process:** Assessment/Analysis; **Reference:** Ch 21, Sexual Dysfunction, Data Base

325. 1 During the acute phase of mania, the focus of care should be on maintaining the safety of the client and others and decreasing the client's energy expenditure. Hypersexuality is often associated with the manic episode of bipolar disorder. Obtaining sexual pleasure by exposing the genitals (exhibitionism) is a paraphilia. A private room protects the other clients and provides privacy for the client. 2 The client is too hyperactive to engage in group activities, and hypersexual behavior may precipitate anxiety in the other clients. Also, manic clients can be overly competitive, which can disturb other clients. Activities at this time should be solitary or one-on-one with the nurse or nursing assistant. 3 Manic clients have flight of ideas (rapid racing thoughts) and are easily distracted. Introspection and the development of insight cannot occur during this phase of the illness. 4 The hyperactive client will not have the self-control to sit long enough to eat a meal. The nurse should provide finger foods (sandwich, fruit, milkshake) and encourage the intake of food with short declarative statements that direct the client to eat (e.g., "finish your sandwich," "eat this banana"). Also, hypersexual behavior may precipitate anxiety in the other clients.

Client Need: Psychosocial Integrity; **Cognitive Level:** Application; **Nursing Process:** Planning/Implementation; **Reference:** Ch 21, General Nursing Care of Clients with Sexual and Identity Disorders

Nursing Care to Promote Childbearing and Women's Health

23 CHAPTER

HEALTH PROMOTION

FEMALE REPRODUCTIVE SYSTEM

Ovaries: Female Gonads

A. Location: behind and below uterine (fallopian) tubes, anchored to uterus and broad ligaments

B. Size and shape of large almonds

C. Microscopic structure: each ovary of the newborn female consists of several hundred thousand graafian follicles embedded in connective tissues; follicles are epithelial sacs in which ova develop; usually, between the years of menarche and menopause, one follicle matures each month, ruptures the surface of the ovary, and expels its ovum into the pelvic cavity; the ovum then enters a fallopian tube

D. Functions
  1. Oogenesis: formation of a mature ovum in a graafian follicle
  2. Ovulation: expulsion of the ovum from follicle into the pelvic cavity
  3. Secretion of ovarian hormones: maturing follicle secretes estrogens (estradiol, estrone, and estriol) and corpus luteum secretes progesterone and estrogens
     a. Estrogens: stimulate development of secondary sexual characteristics (e.g., breasts); thickening of endometrium, contractions of the pregnant uterus; mildly accelerate sodium and water reabsorption by kidney tubules, which increases water content of uterus; accelerate protein anabolism; stimulate long bone calcification
     b. Progesterone: prepares endometrium for implantation of fertilized ovum; inhibits uterine contractions during pregnancy; promotes development of alveoli of estrogen-primed breasts; necessary for lactation; inhibits oxytocin release by neurohypophysis; oxytocin is otherwise released in response to vaginal distention

Uterine Tubes (Fallopian Tubes, Oviducts)

A. Location: attached to upper, outer angles of uterus

B. Structure: distal ends fimbriated and open into pelvic cavity; mucosal lining of tubes and peritoneal lining of pelvis in direct contact here (permits spread of infection from tubes to peritoneum)

C. Function: serve as ducts through which ova travel from ovaries to uterus; fertilization occurs in tube

Uterus

A. Location: in pelvic cavity between the bladder and rectum

B. Structure
  1. Shape and size: pear-shaped organ approximately the size of a clenched fist
  2. Divisions
     a. Corpus (body): upper and main part of the uterus; fundus, the bulging upper surface of the body; openings include two from fallopian tubes and one into cervix
     b. Cervix: narrow, lower part of the uterus; internal os adjacent to uterus and external os adjacent to vagina
  3. Walls: composed of smooth muscle (myometrium) lined with mucosa (endometrium) and entire organ covered with perimetrium
  4. Blood supply: uterine and ovarian arteries

C. Position: flexed between body and cervix with the body portion lying over the bladder, pointing forward and slightly upward; cervix joins the vagina at right angles; ligaments hold the uterus in position (broad ligaments, uterosacral ligaments, posterior ligament, anterior ligament, round ligaments)

D. Functions: menstruation; pregnancy; labor

Vagina

A. Location: between rectum and urethra

B. Structure: collapsible, musculomembranous tube, capable of great distention; outlet to exterior covered by fold of mucous membrane called hymen

C. Functions
  1. Receives semen from the male
  2. Constitutes lower part of birth canal
  3. Acts as excretory duct for uterine secretions and menstrual flow

Vulva (Including Structures That Constitute External Genitalia)

A. Mons veneris: hairy, skin-covered pad of fat over the symphysis pubis

B. Labia majora: hairy, skin-covered folds

C. Labia minora: small inner folds covered with modified skin

D. Clitoris: small mound of erectile tissue, below junction of two labia minora

E. Urinary meatus: posterior to clitoris; opening into urethra

F. Vaginal orifice: posterior to urinary meatus; opening into vagina; hymen, fold of mucosa, partially closes orifice

G. Skene's glands: small mucous glands; ducts open on each side of the urinary meatus

H. Bartholin's glands: two small, bean-shaped glands; duct from each gland opens on side of the vaginal orifice; both Bartholin's glands and Skene's glands are prone to infection (especially by gonococci)

Breasts (Mammary Glands)

A. Location: just under skin, over the pectoralis major muscle

B. Size: depends on deposits of adipose tissue rather than on amount of glandular tissue (which is approximately same in all females)

C. Structure: divided into lobes and lobules; excretory duct leads from each lobe to opening in nipple; circular pigmented area (areola) borders nipples

D. Function: secrete milk (lactation)
1. Shedding of placenta causes marked decrease in blood levels of estrogens and progesterone, which in turn stimulates anterior pituitary to increase prolactin secretion; high blood level of prolactin stimulates alveoli of breast to secrete milk
2. Suckling controls lactation in two ways: by stimulating anterior pituitary secretion of prolactin, which stimulates milk production, and by stimulating posterior pituitary secretion of oxytocin, which stimulates release of milk from the alveoli into ducts (let-down reflex), enabling the infant to remove the milk by suckling

MALE REPRODUCTIVE SYSTEM

See Structures of the Male Reproductive System in Chapter 12: Nursing Care of Clients with Urinary/Reproductive System Disorders

PUBERTY

Period of reproductive organ maturation and preparation for reproductive function

A. Physical and physiologic changes
1. Males
   a. Occurs between 10 and 14 years of age; less dramatic than in females
   b. First sign is testicular growth and scrotal changes
   c. Growth of penis and appearance of pubic, axillary, and facial hair; deepening voice; dramatic body growth spurt
   d. Spermatogenesis occurs second year after onset; increased activity of sweat glands; periodic erections and emissions of mature sperm
   e. Ejaculation occurs early in puberty but may have few active sperm

2. Females
   a. Between 9 and 15 years of age
   b. First sign is thelarche: breast budding
   c. Acceleration of body growth
   d. Adrenarche: growth of pubic and axillary hair
   e. Menarche: onset of menses; a late pubertal event, occurring after peak of growth has passed; ovaries produce estrogen
   f. For the first year menstrual cycles are often anovulatory and irregular

B. Psychologic changes
1. Maturational changes according to age
2. Developmental task: independence versus dependence
3. Need for belonging to a peer group

MENSTRUAL CYCLE

A. Menstrual cycle refers to changes in the uterus and ovaries, which recur cyclically from the time of the menarche to the menopause

B. Length of cycle measured from the onset of a period of uterine bleeding to the onset of the next period of bleeding; mean cycle length is 28 days; range of 21 to 45 days

C. During each cycle several follicles begin the maturation process, but usually only one reaches full maturity and expels its contained ovum into the abdominal cavity and then to a fallopian tube

D. Menstrual cycle phases include ovarian and/or endometrial activity correlated with concentration fluctuations in hypothalamic, hypophyseal, and ovarian hormones
1. First phase (menstrual or ischemic stage): shedding of the spongiosum endometrium with discharge through vagina; prostaglandin content of endometrium reaches highest levels; vasoconstriction and myometrial contractions associated with menstrual events are believed to be mediated by prostaglandins; estrogen and progesterone levels are relatively low, stimulating the release of follicle-stimulating hormone (FSH); combined with a steady low level of luteinizing hormone (LH) secretion, ovarian estrogen secretion begins
2. Second phase (follicular [ovary] or proliferative [endometrium] stage): endometrium regenerates, and thickens in preparation for possible implantation; at the same time, a single dominant follicle develops from a cohort of maturing follicles and approaches full maturation under the influence of estradiol produced by ovarian follicles; rising blood levels of estradiol exert negative feedback on FSH secretion and positive feedback on LH secretion; estradiol's feedback effects are exerted on the hypothalamic secretion of FSH-releasing hormone and LH-releasing hormone, which control the hypophyseal secretion of FSH and LH; as a result of a surge in the LH level, ovulation occurs; ovulation usually

takes place 14 days before menstruation; ovum remains viable for 24 to 36 hours
3. Third phase (luteal [ovary] and secretory [endometrium] stage): begins after ovulation and is a relatively finite time period of about 12 to 14 days; under continuing LH secretion, a temporary endocrine gland is formed (corpus luteum) from the ruptured follicle; granulosa and thecal cells of the follicle enlarge, divide into and occupy the cavity of the follicle, and secrete progesterone and estrogen; progesterone stimulates the already proliferated endometrium to become glandular with a high glycogen-secreting potential (preparation for implantation); if fertilization does not occur, the corpus luteum becomes nonfunctional 10 to 12 days after ovulation; progesterone and estrogen blood levels drop, the negative feedback effect of estrogen on FSH ceases, and the first phase of the cycle begins again
E. Clinical applications
1. Family planning
  a. Synthetic preparations of estrogen-like and/or progesterone-like compounds are contained in oral, transdermal, vaginal, and parenteral contraceptive agents and on some intrauterine devices
  b. These agents prevent pregnancy by inhibiting gonadotropin (FSH and LH) secretion, affecting both pituitary and hypothalamic centers; progestational agents primarily suppress LH secretion; the estrogenic agent suppresses FSH secretion
2. Premenstrual syndrome
  a. Discomfort from ovulation to menstruation; symptoms include bloating, breast tenderness, constipation/diarrhea, acne, moodiness, fatigue, insomnia, backache, cramping
  b. Therapeutic interventions
    (1) Dietary modifications: reduction of salt, refined carbohydrates, alcohol, and caffeine
    (2) Stress management, exercise, and rest
    (3) Nonsteroidal inflammatory inhibiting agents (antiprostaglandin action) have proven effective in relieving abdominal cramping associated with the ischemic or menstrual phase of the cycle; diuretics, progesterone, oral contraceptives may also be used

PERIMENOPAUSE

A. Perimenopause: the transitional time of a gradual cessation of ovarian function and menstrual cycles, also known as the climacteric; naturally (nonsurgical) begins between 40 and 60 years of age, average age of 51; lasts 2 to 10 years
B. Menopause: the cessation of the menstrual periods for 12 consecutive months
C. Postmenopause: the time after menopause

D. Physiologic changes
1. Ovaries lose ability to respond to gonadotropic hormones with a dramatic decrease in levels of circulating estradiol and progesterone
2. Increased FSH gonadotropin blood level because ovarian production is no longer inhibited; false-positive pregnancy test may occur
E. Clinical applications
1. Atrophic changes in reproductive organs or hormonal stimulation of the sympathetic nervous system may result in dyspareunia, weight gain, facial hair growth, cardiac palpitations, hot flashes, profuse diaphoresis, constipation, pruritus, faintness, headache; long-range problems may include osteoporosis and cardiovascular disease
2. Emotional/behavioral responses may include irritability and anxiety about loss of reproductive function, sexual feelings, and feelings of womanliness; women need to understand changes and have an opportunity to discuss feelings
3. Hormonal replacement therapy (HRT) may be used to ease transition through the perimenopause (control vasomotor instability, reduce atrophic genitourinary changes), reduce the risk for cardiovascular disease, and prevent osteoporosis; used judiciously and on an individual basis because of cancer-causing potential
4. Herbal therapy, diet management, relaxation modalities, and exercise are useful in easing the transition

FAMILY PLANNING

CONTRACEPTIVE METHODS

Data Base

A. Oral contraceptives: used to prevent conception by inhibiting ovulation, causing atrophic changes in the endometrium to prevent implantation, or causing a thickening of cervical mucus to inhibit sperm travel
1. Combined form: inhibits hypothalamus, pituitary, and various hormone production
  a. Monophasic: fixed doses of estrogen and progestin in each pill that is taken for 21 days; package usually contains 28 pills, seven of which are free of estrogen; withdrawal bleeding occurs during the 7 days when the nonmedication pills are taken
  b. Biphasic: altered amounts of estrogen and progestin taken throughout the cycle; in a 21-day package, the first 10 pills contain small amounts of estrogen and the next 11 pills contain an increased amount of estrogen and progestin; this reduces the total dosage of hormones each month
  c. Triphasic: small doses of combined hormones that alter levels of estrogen and progestin throughout the cycle; this reduces the total dosage of hormones each month

d. Advantages of combined oral contraceptives: 100% effective if taken correctly; coitus independence because they are not taken in relation to intercourse; bleeding days are predictable; pills may alleviate symptoms of premenstrual syndrome (PMS), endometriosis, and dysmenorrhea

e. Examples of estrogen-progestin products (combined form): Demulen; Loestrin; Ortho-Novum

2. Minipills: a low dose of progesterone is given alone; inhibits ovulation; regimen makes uterine environment hostile to sperm; must be taken same time daily because dose is so low

a. Advantages of minipills: fewer side effects; can be used by lactating women; may be used by women older than 35 and those with a history of headaches and mild hypertension

b. Examples of progestin products (minipills): Micronor; Ovrette

3. Major side effects

a. Thrombophlebitis (increased platelets and clotting factors, intimal thickening, and vein dilation)

b. Hypertension; breast tenderness (fluid retention)

c. Libido changes (hormonal effect)

d. Hyperglycemia (decreased carbohydrate tolerance)

e. CNS disturbances (hormonal effects and fluid retention)

f. Breakthrough bleeding (estrogen effect)

4. Contraindications for the use of oral contraceptives: older than 35 years; cigarette smoking; hypertension; thrombophlebitis; breast malignancy; vascular or heart disease; less than 6 weeks of breastfeeding

B. Intrauterine devices (IUDs): device inserted into the uterus, preventing fertilization or implantation; copper IUD damages sperm and few reach ovum; progesterone IUD affects cervical mucus and endometrial maturation; may cause uterine irritability, increased bleeding, and risk for infection

C. Diaphragm: device that fits over cervix and prevents sperm from entering cervical os; used with spermicide

D. Cervical cap: a rubber thimblelike device that fits over the cervix after it is filled with a spermicide; may provide protection for up to 48 hours after insertion

E. Vaginal ring: hormonal control; worn for 3 weeks with a 1-week break; does not need to be fitted to the woman

F. Female condom: latex vaginal sheath that is an elongated pouch with a ring at each end; one ring covers the cervix and the other covers the labia; available without a prescription

G. Male condom: latex sheath that covers penis and prevents semen from entering cervical os

H. Creams, jellies, foam tablets, and vaginal suppositories: spermicidal (generally low pH) preparations inserted into vaginal canal by applicator immediately before coitus (used in conjunction with the diaphragm and condom for added protection)

I. Coitus interruptus: withdrawal during sexual intercourse before ejaculation; least effective method

J. Fertility awareness methods: the plotting of the basal body temperature to determine fertile period so that abstinence from coitus is practiced; the basal body temperature dips slightly 24 hours before ovulation, then rises sharply; stress and infection can elevate temperature, thus diminishing effectiveness of this method; used in conjunction with cervical mucus changes (Billings method)

K. Norplant system (implantable progestin): placement of six flexible rods of levonorgestrel under the skin of the upper arm; effective for 5 years; removal restores fertility; irregular periods may occur

L. Depo-Provera (injectable progestin): IM injection of medroxyprogesterone acetate that lasts 3 months; suppresses FSH and LH

M. Postcoital contraception: used after unprotected intercourse; pharmacologic management is high dose of estrogen, progesterone, or testosterone ("morning after pill"); mechanical technique is insertion of an IUD

N. Surgical sterilization

1. Bilateral vasectomy: small incision made into the scrotum and the vas deferens is ligated, producing sterilization in the male by preventing ejaculation of sperm; usually performed in ambulatory surgery center

2. Tubal ligation: interruption in the continuity of fallopian tubes by surgical transection, electric cautery, or compression with soft clamp, preventing impregnation of ovum by sperm; accomplished by laparotomy, laparoscopy, or culdoscopy; usually performed in ambulatory surgery center

Nursing Care of Clients Concerned With Family Planning

A. Assessment/Analysis

1. Medical and family history of woman

2. Couple's beliefs and feelings about sexuality, pregnancy, contraception, and abortion

3. Couple's understanding of family planning

4. Couple's readiness to learn

B. Planning/Implementation

1. Help couples to expand their knowledge about human sexuality

2. Promote optimum emotional and physical health of the family

3. Inform the couple of available methods and assist them in choosing the most appropriate method for them (e.g., barrier techniques preferred for women

with diabetes mellitus or heart disease); include both in planning if feasible

4. Provide an accepting atmosphere; offer freedom of choice
5. Review specific medication/administration schedule with client and review procedure to follow if doses are missed when oral contraceptives are being used
6. Teach side effects of oral contraceptives (e.g., vaginal bleeding) and instruct client to inform the physician if they should occur
7. Encourage periodic physical examination for all women using any contraceptive method; should include breast and pelvic examination, Papanicolaou test, and mammography
8. Teach couples electing surgical sterilization that in the female sterility is immediately achieved, whereas in the male it is not achieved until semen is free of sperm; an additional method of birth control should be used until semen is free of sperm (usually after 15 ejaculations)

C. Evaluation/Outcomes
1. Prevents conception unless desired
2. Returns for follow-up health care

INFERTILITY AND STERILITY

A. Infertility: inability on the part of a couple to conceive after consistent attempts for a 1-year period; woman has never conceived; man has never impregnated a woman
1. Primary infertility occurs when the couple has never had a child
2. Secondary infertility occurs when the couple has conceived but the woman is unable to sustain pregnancy or conceive again
B. Sterility: presence of a factor that renders a person unable to produce offspring; may be genetic, acquired, or elective
C. Male infertility and sterility
1. Coital difficulties: chordee (painful, downward-curving erection) or marked obesity
2. Spermatozoal abnormalities: small ejaculatory volume, low sperm count, increased viscosity, reduced motility of spermatozoa, and/or more than 30% abnormal sperm forms
3. Testicular abnormalities: agenesis or destruction of testes, cryptorchidism; physical injury caused by trauma, mumps, irradiation, or prolonged exposure to increased temperature; torsion of the testes
4. Varicocele: an enlarged vein in the testicle
5. Abnormalities of the penis or urethra: hypospadias or urethral stricture
6. Prostate and seminal vesicle abnormalities: chronic prostatitis or seminal vesiculitis
7. Abnormalities of the epididymis and vas deferens: inflammation or closure
8. Severe nutritional deficiencies

9. Sexually transmitted infections
10. Other factors such as radiation to testicles, excessive smoking and alcohol intake, smoking of marijuana, and (in utero) exposure to diethylstilbestrol (DES)
11. Decrease in libido and impotence; related pathologic, physiologic, and/or psychologic factors
12. Environmental factors that may influence fertility (e.g., frequent hot tub use, Agent Orange)

D. Female infertility and sterility
1. Endocrine disorders: pituitary, thyroid, or adrenal
2. Vaginal disorders: absence or stenosis of vagina, imperforate hymen, vaginitis, chronic infections
3. Cervical abnormalities: cervical obstruction by cervical polyps or tumors
4. Uterine abnormalities: hypoplasia, endometriosis, uterine neoplasms
5. Tubal disorders: obstruction (generally the result of sexually transmitted infections such as chlamydia or gonorrhea), perisalpingeal adhesions
6. Ovarian abnormalities: congenital abnormalities such as ovarian dysgenesis or agenesis, infections, tumors, multiple cysts; hormonal imbalances
7. Emotional problems: severe psychoneurosis or psychosis may cause anovulatory cycles
8. Coital factors: feminine hygiene preparations (including douches) that decrease vaginal pH may inactivate or destroy spermatozoa; sodium bicarbonate douches may be used to raise vaginal pH
9. Chronic illnesses
10. Immunologic reactions to sperm
11. Nutritional factors such as malnutrition, anorexia nervosa
12. Exposure to DES in utero
13. Environmental factors that may influence fertility (e.g., teratogenic household cleaning products)

E. Combined factors
1. Lack of coital success
2. Female antibodies to male sperm
F. Diagnostic measures
1. Genetic testing
2. Male: history, physical examination, semen analysis
3. Female: history, physical examination, CBC, sedimentation rate, serologic tests, urinalysis, triiodothyronine (T_3), thyroxine (T_4), thyroid-stimulating hormone (TSH), x-ray films of the chest, basal metabolic rate determination, postcoital (Sims-Huhner) test, ultrasonography, endometrial biopsy, tubal insufflation, hysterosalpingography, culdoscopy, use of urine luteinizing hormone predictor kits (measure the LH in the urine to predict ovulation to time intercourse or artificial insemination), laparoscopy, chlamydia test
G. Therapeutic interventions
1. Education about the menstrual cycle and timing of intercourse

2. Surgery, depending on the cause
3. Pharmacologic management
4. Intrauterine insemination (IUI) and ovulation-inducing drugs
5. In vitro fertilization (IVF)
6. IVF with intracytoplasmic sperm injection for severe male infertility
7. Stress management
8. Adoption
9. Surrogate motherhood
10. Embryo transfer

H. Drugs that affect gonadal function and fertility
   1. Androgens (testosterone derivatives)
      a. Used to replace deficient hormones in males after puberty and before the climacteric to improve development of secondary sex characteristics
      b. Adverse effects: adolescent males may have premature epiphyseal closure (decreased skeletal development, height stops increasing)
   2. Estrogens
      a. Primarily used to replace deficient hormones to control hormonal balance in menopausal or postmenopausal women or to maintain menses and fertility during reproductive years
      b. Adverse effects of estrogen: anorexia (depression of appetite center); nausea and vomiting (gastrointestinal irritation); tissue fluid accumulation (altered tissue hydrostatic pressure); growth ceases
   3. Conception enhancers
      a. Ovulatory stimulants
         (1) Clomiphene citrate (Clomid) is a follicle-maturing agent used during the fifth to tenth days of the menstrual cycle
         (2) Purified FSH (Metrodin) acts on ovarian follicles
         (3) Human menopausal gonadotropin (Pergonal) acts similarly to FSH or LH to stimulate growth and maturation of ovarian follicles
         (4) Human chorionic gonadotropin (Profasi) induces ovulation
      b. Hormone replacement therapy with conjugated estrogens and medroxyprogesterone
      c. Drugs for hyperplasia defects
         (1) Danazol (Danocrine and Cyclomen) reduces endometrial hyperplasia; acts on estrogen receptors to inhibit estrogen defects
         (2) Gonadotropin-releasing hormone (GnRH) for endometriosis and fibroid tumors
         (3) Prednisone reduces adrenal hyperplasia
      d. Adverse effects of conception enhancers
         (1) Multiple births (causes simultaneous maturation of follicles)
         (2) Visual changes (direct toxic effect)
         (3) Dizziness, lightheadedness (CNS depression)
         (4) Hyperplasia reduction drugs have an androgenic effect that can cause weight gain, hirsutism, decreased breast size, and oiliness

RELATED PROCEDURES

PELVIC EXAMINATION

A. Definition
   1. Examination of female reproductive structures
   2. Consists of
      a. Abdominal examination
      b. Inspection and palpation of external genitalia
      c. Vaginal examination bimanually and with a speculum to inspect cervix and vaginal walls; rectal examination may follow
   3. As indicated or ordered, obtain specimen for
      a. Gonorrheal culture from endocervical canal
      b. *Chlamydia trachomatis* smear from urethra and cervix
      c. Herpes simplex 1 and 2 viral culture of a smear from the lesion
      d. Cytologic examination (Papanicolaou test) of cells from endocervical canal and cervix

B. Nursing care
   1. Explain examination and collection of specimens
   2. Teach to avoid douching 24 hours before examination
   3. Request client to empty bladder before examination
   4. Help relaxation by asking client to
      a. Breathe slowly and deeply, exhaling with mouth open and lips in "O" shape
      b. Avoid squeezing eyes closed or clenching fists
   5. Instruct to bear down when speculum is introduced
   6. If client is pregnant, observe for signs of hypotension, such as pallor, dizziness, tachycardia, nausea, and diaphoresis; if symptoms occur position client on side until symptoms subside and vital signs are within acceptable limits
   7. Teach client about signs of cancer of the cervix: vaginal discharge, spotting between menstrual periods or after intercourse; discuss high cure rate if identified early in the disease

MAMMOGRAPHY

A. Definition
   1. An x-ray study of the soft tissue of the breast
   2. Technique allows detection of nonpalpable masses
   3. Women between the ages of 35 and 40 should have a baseline mammogram; after age 40, a mammogram should be performed yearly

B. Nursing care
   1. Instruct client to avoid use of deodorants or powders before test
   2. Maintain privacy
   3. Explain that stretching and compression of breast tissue may be uncomfortable

4. Stress importance of yearly clinical breast examination and regular breast self-examinations for early detection; schedule examination after menstrual period when breast density and tenderness are decreased or the same day each month if client is postmenopausal

5. Explain that reason for ultrasonography is to distinguish between cyst and tumor

BREAST BIOPSY

A. Procedure to obtain fluid or tissue
   1. Fine needle aspiration
   2. Core needle biopsy
   3. Needle localization biopsy
B. Nursing care
   1. Explain procedure to client
   2. Allow ample time to express feelings
   3. Instruct to assess site for bleeding or edema
   4. Stress importance of continued health care supervision

❋ INDUCED ABORTION
Data Base

A. Mifepristone (RU-486): administered up to 9 weeks after conception; bleeding begins within 4 days; may be combined with prostaglandin; noninvasive
B. Menstrual extraction or minisuction: vacuum of uterine contents with a 50-mL syringe; done 5 to 7 weeks after last menstrual period
C. Vacuum aspiration: done under local paracervical, epidural, or general anesthesia in first 12 weeks of pregnancy; the cervix is dilated (using mechanical means) and products of conception are suctioned through a small, hollow tube
D. Dilation and curettage: performed during the first 12 to 14 weeks of pregnancy under local paracervical or general anesthesia; the cervix is mechanically dilated and uterus is scraped and cleaned by curettage
E. Saline injection
   1. Labor is induced when a pregnancy is 14 to 24 weeks' duration by injecting a sterile saline solution into the uterus by amniocentesis; labor usually begins within 8 to 24 hours after instillation of saline; produces a macerated fetus
   2. Adverse effect: headache caused by hypernatremia
F. Prostaglandin
   1. Used during second trimester to trigger vasoconstriction and uterine contractions that interfere with endocrine function of placenta; examples: carboprost (Hemabate, Prostin/15M), dinoprostone (Prostin E2)
   2. Adverse effects: nausea, vomiting, diarrhea, pain at extrauterine sites, allergic reactions (not administered to clients with history of asthma)
G. Hysterotomy: performed after 16 weeks of pregnancy by surgically removing the fetus and placenta abdominally

H. High-dose oxytocin: first bag—50 units in 500 mL; second bag—100 units in 500 mL; if third bag is needed—150 units in 500 mL

Nursing Care of Women Undergoing Induced Abortion

A. Assessment/Analysis
   1. History and physical examination
   2. Specimens for laboratory tests
   3. Rh status
   4. Length of pregnancy
   5. Level of anxiety
   6. Understanding of procedure and postprocedure care
B. Planning/Implementation
   1. Being aware of one's own feelings about abortion is essential if the nurse is to intervene therapeutically with women having abortions; nurses with strong feelings against abortion should not counsel clients
   2. Encourage the client's expression of feelings
   3. Obtain informed consent
   4. Be objective and support the client's decision about abortion
   5. Determine that a complete history and physical examination, complete laboratory workup, pelvic examination, Papanicolaou test, and a pregnancy test are done before induced abortion
   6. Counsel concerning contraceptive methods if requested
   7. Administer RhoGAM when client is Rh-negative and negative for antibodies
   8. Teach to avoid tampons for 3 days to 3 weeks and intercourse for 1 to 2 weeks depending on practitioner's advice; report the presence of fever or bleeding that requires a new peripad every 2 hours
C. Evaluation/Outcomes
   1. Expels products of conception
   2. Remains free from complications
   3. Returns for health supervision
   4. Expresses feelings
   5. Indicates acceptance of nonpregnant state

💊 RELATED PHARMACOLOGY
Estrogens

(See Infertility and Sterility part H, Drugs that affect gonadal function and fertility)

A. Description
   1. Organic compounds secreted by ovarian follicles in females; exert effect during the proliferative phase of the menstrual cycle
   2. Used to regulate menstrual disorders, uterine bleeding, menopausal and postmenopausal problems, and as a contraceptive; also used as hormonal therapy for men with certain cancers of the reproductive/urinary system; used judiciously because of cancer-causing potential
   3. Available in oral, parenteral (IM, IV), intravaginal, and topical, including transdermal, preparations

B. Examples
1. Diethylstilbestrol (DES)
2. Estradiol preparations (Estrace, Estraderm)
3. Estrogenic substances, conjugated (Premarin)

C. Major side effects
1. Thrombophlebitis (increased clot formation)
2. Nausea (irritation of gastric mucosa)
3. Breast tenderness (promotion of sodium and water retention)
4. Hyperglycemia (decreased carbohydrate tolerance)
5. Males: gynecomastia, loss of libido, and testicular atrophy (hormonal imbalance related to estrogen antagonism)
6. Deficiency of one or more of the B complex vitamins may be induced with prolonged use

D. Nursing care
1. Obtain history to assess for medical problems that may contraindicate use
2. Assess for edema
3. Instruct client to
   a. Use correct procedure for application of topical or intravaginal preparations
   b. Report unusual vaginal bleeding immediately
   c. Avoid smoking during therapy to decrease risk for cardiovascular side effects
   d. Eat foods rich in B complex vitamins daily; B complex vitamin supplements should be considered
4. Monitor blood glucose levels of clients with diabetes for hyperglycemia
5. Reassure male clients that feminizing side effects will subside when therapy is completed

Progestins
A. Description
1. Female ovarian hormones that prepare the uterus for implantation of a fertilized ovum; essential for the maintenance of pregnancy
2. Used in the treatment of endometriosis, infertility, dysmenorrhea, secondary amenorrhea, and to suppress ovulation
3. Available in oral and parenteral (IM) preparations

B. Examples
1. Hydroxyprogesterone caproate (Hylutin)
2. Medroxyprogesterone acetate (Provera, Depo-Provera)
3. Megestrol acetate (Megace)
4. Norethindrone (Norlutin)
5. Progesterone (Progestoral)

C. Major side effects
1. Initial use may cause profuse vaginal flow (shedding of accumulation of endometrial tissue), spotting, irregular bleeding, nausea, lethargy, jaundice
2. Edema (promotion of sodium and water retention)
3. Genitourinary disturbances (renal dysfunction aggravated by fluid retention)
4. Visual disturbances (possibility of blood clots or neuro-ocular lesions)
5. Scleral jaundice (hepatic alterations)
6. Thrombophlebitis (increased clot formation)
7. Depression (CNS effect)
8. Deficiency of one or more B complex vitamins may result from prolonged use

D. Nursing care
1. Obtain client history to assess for medical problems that may contraindicate use
2. Assess client for edema during therapy
3. Inform significant others regarding potential for development of depression
4. Instruct client to eat foods rich in the B complex vitamins daily; B complex vitamin supplements should be considered

Nursing Care Related to Major Disorders Affecting Women's Health

MAJOR DISORDERS AFFECTING WOMEN'S HEALTH

CANCER OF THE CERVIX

Data Base

A. Etiology and pathophysiology
   1. Slow, malignant change in the tissue forming the neck of the uterus at the squamocolumnar junction
   2. Risk factors
      a. Multiple sexual partners
      b. Sexually transmitted infections
      c. Exposure to human papillomavirus (HPV), human immune deficiency virus (HIV), or herpes simplex virus (HSV)
      d. Erosions of cervix, often resulting from changes in pH, that can be precursors of cancer
      e. Exposure to diethylstilbestrol (DES) in utero, which increases risk for vaginal cancer
   3. High cure rate when diagnosed early
   4. Tends to spread by direct invasion of surrounding tissues and metastasizes to the lungs, bones, and liver
B. Clinical findings
   1. Subjective (when invasive): back and leg pain
   2. Objective
      a. Spotting between menstrual periods and after intercourse
      b. Vaginal discharge
      c. Lengthening of the menstrual period
      d. Papanicolaou cytologic finding of cellular changes consistent with precancerous or cancerous conditions
C. Therapeutic interventions
   1. Type of surgical intervention depends on extent of lesion and physical condition of client
      a. Stage 0—carcinoma in situ, limited to epithelial layer
      b. Stage I—confined to the cervix
      c. Stage II—extends beyond the cervix but not to the pelvic sidewall
      d. Stage III—extends to the pelvic sidewall and lower vagina
      e. Stage IV—extends beyond the pelvis to the bladder or rectum
   2. Hysterosalpingo-oophorectomy (panhysterectomy) to remove uterus, fallopian tubes, and ovaries; menstruation and ovarian function ceases; in advanced lesions parametrial tissue and lymph nodes may be removed
   3. Hysterectomy to remove uterus; menstruation ceases but ovarian function continues
   4. Internal or external radiation therapy alone or in conjunction with surgery to reduce the lesion and limit metastases
   5. Laser therapy
   6. Cryosurgery—freezing technique
   7. Conization to remove cone-shaped area of cervix while preserving reproductive functions
   8. Loop electrode excision

Nursing Care of Clients With Cancer of the Cervix

A. Assessment/Analysis
   1. Risk factors from history
   2. Description of onset and progression of signs and symptoms
   3. Cervical specimen for Papanicolaou smear
   4. Vaginal discharge following procedure; cervical interventions will produce blood-tinged discharge for 3 to 5 days
B. Planning/Implementation
   1. Assist client and family in coping with the diagnosis of cancer
   2. Allow and encourage client to express feelings and concerns about change in self-image and sexual functioning
   3. Support client's feminine image
   4. Provide care for the client receiving internal radiation
      a. Explain procedure and side effects that may occur
      b. Instruct client to maintain supine position with head of bed flat or only slightly elevated
      c. Inspect implant for proper position
      d. Provide low-residue diet and antidiarrheal agents to prevent bowel movements; insert indwelling urinary catheter to avoid displacement of radioactive substance and irradiation of adjacent tissues
      e. Explain need for isolation; explain to client and visitors that the amount of time they can spend in the room will be limited to avoid overexposure

to radiation; pregnant women and children should be restricted from visiting

    f. Use principles of time, distance, and shielding to minimize staff exposure

    g. Provide care for the client receiving chemotherapy or radiation (see Radiation under Neoplastic Disorders, especially General Nursing Care of Clients With Neoplastic Disorders in Chapter 3)

  5. Provide care following surgery

    a. Maintain patency of the urinary catheter that was inserted before surgery to decompress the bladder and reduce stress on the operative site

    b. Monitor for reestablishment of bowel sounds

    c. Maintain accurate intake and output

    d. After removal of the urinary catheter, note the amount of output and pattern of voiding; catheterize for residual urine and whenever necessary for urinary retention if ordered

    e. See Nursing Care of Clients With a Hysterectomy under Uterine Neoplasms

C. Evaluation/Outcomes

  1. Verbalizes feelings to family and health care providers

  2. Maintains satisfying sexual expression

  3. Copes with effects of treatment and potential prognosis

  4. Continues health supervision

✿ UTERINE NEOPLASMS

Data Base

A. Etiology and pathophysiology

  1. Endometrial polyps

    a. Localized overgrowths of endometrial glands and stroma that occur on the cervix and in the fundus of the uterus; usually benign

    b. Stimulated by estrogen

    c. Occur more frequently in premenopausal women who are anovulatory

  2. Uterine fibroids (leiomyomas, myomas, fibromas, and fibromyomas)

    a. Benign tumors of the uterine muscle

    b. Occur more frequently in African-American women and women who have not been pregnant

    c. Stimulated by estrogen

    d. Diminish after menopause

    e. Rarely become malignant

  3. Endometrial cancer (adenocarcinoma, adenoacanthoma, and adenosquamous carcinoma)

    a. Malignant overgrowth of the lining of the uterus

    b. Risk factors include hormone replacement therapy (HRT), unopposed estrogen therapy, pelvic radiation, obesity, and family history

    c. Most common malignancy of the female reproductive system

    d. Occurs more frequently with hormone imbalance, obesity, nulliparity, late menopause, dysfunctional bleeding, anovulation, uninterrupted estrogen stimulation, diabetes mellitus, and early menarche

    e. Occurs twice as often in Caucasian women than in African-American women

    f. Spreads by direct extension or metastasis to myometrium, vagina, and paracervical tissue

    g. Metastasizes to abdominal cavity, liver, lung, brain, and bone; progression is slow and metastasis occurs late

B. Clinical findings

  1. Endometrial polyps

    a. Frequently asymptomatic

    b. Intermenstrual bleeding (metrorrhagia)

  2. Leiomyomas

    a. Frequently asymptomatic

    b. Excessive menstrual bleeding (menorrhagia)

    c. Signs of pressure from an enlarging mass such as low abdominal discomfort, backache, visceral displacement, and constipation

    d. Painful menstruation (dysmenorrhea)

    e. Problems with pregnancy such as preterm labor, spontaneous abortion, and dystocia

  3. Endometrial cancer

    a. Premenopausal recurrent metrorrhagia

    b. Postmenopausal bleeding

    c. FIGO classification system of endometrial cancer extends from stage IA; in which tumors are limited to endometrium, to stage IVB, in which there are distant metastases to the intraabdominal area or inguinal lymph nodes

C. Therapeutic interventions

  1. Depends on the type and extent of the lesion or tumor, the physical condition of the client, and the stage of the endometrial carcinoma

  2. Dilation and curettage (D&C) for polyps

  3. Myomectomy or hysterectomy for benign neoplasms; hysterectomy results in no menstrual period; when surgery is not advisable, radiation therapy is employed

  4. Total hysterectomy with bilateral salpingo-oophorectomy (panhysterectomy) for endometrial neoplasms; results in no menstrual periods and surgical menopause

  5. Intracavitary radiation may be done before or after surgery, depending on the stage of endometrial cancer

  6. Hormonal therapy with progestins for endometrial cancer; HRT after panhysterectomy is controversial

  7. Combination chemotherapy with antineoplastic drugs such as cyclophosphamide (Cytoxan), doxorubicin (Adriamycin), and cisplatin (Platinol) for endometrial neoplasms

Nursing Care of Clients With a Hysterectomy

A. Assessment/Analysis

  1. Gynecologic and general health history

  2. Description of onset and progression of symptoms if present

  3. Feelings regarding loss of uterus

B. Planning/Implementation
1. Encourage healthy lifestyle, weight reduction if overweight, and routine pelvic examinations
2. Monitor fluid and electrolyte balance
3. Maintain patency of urinary catheter; monitor amount and characteristics of urine; blood in urine may indicate incisional tear in bladder; small voidings after catheter removal may indicate retention
4. Encourage coughing and deep breathing at frequent intervals
5. Check for bowel sounds and gas pains; insert a rectal tube or administer a Harris flush as ordered
6. Encourage frequent ambulation and elevation of extremities when sitting to prevent thrombophlebitis; apply antiembolism stockings if ordered
7. Provide emotional support; encourage ventilation of feelings
8. Teach to postpone driving for several weeks and to avoid sexual intercourse, strenuous exercise, and heavy lifting for 6 to 8 weeks
9. Provide care for the client receiving chemotherapy or radiation (see Radiation under Neoplastic Disorders, especially General Nursing Care of Clients With Neoplastic Disorders in Chapter 3)
10. Emphasize the importance of continuing health supervision
C. Evaluation/Outcomes
1. Verbalizes concerns
2. Adjusts to loss of reproductive organs
3. Establishes bowel and bladder patterns
4. Continues health supervision

CANCER OF THE OVARY

Data Base

A. Etiology and pathophysiology
1. Histologic cell types influenced by age
   a. Malignant germ cell tumors more frequent between 20 and 40 years of age
   b. Epithelial cell tumors more frequent in perimenopausal women
2. More common in Caucasian women than in African-American women; rare in Asian women
3. Incidence influenced by hormonal factors; environmental factors have been implicated but not proven
4. Risk factors: ovarian dysfunction; irregular menses; infertility; genetic predisposition (*BRCA 1* or *BRCA 2* mutations are observed in families); endometriosis; early menopause; nulliparity
5. Rarely diagnosed early because the abdominal cavity can accommodate an enlarging ovary without causing symptoms; poor prognosis because of the advanced stage at initial diagnosis, which is usually stage II to IV
6. Metastasizes to the peritoneum, omentum, and bowel surfaces

B. Clinical findings
1. Subjective: vague, lower abdominal discomfort or pain; feeling of fullness; rapid satiation; dyspepsia; nausea
2. Objective
   a. Increasing abdominal girth (ovarian enlargement or ascites)
   b. Constipation; anemia; vomiting; cachexia
   c. Change in weight
   d. Urinary frequency and urgency
   e. Enlarged ovary on palpation
   f. Elevated levels of CA-125 antigen
   g. Pleural effusion
C. Therapeutic interventions
1. Depend on the stage of disease
2. Surgical removal of the tumor via oophorectomy, salpingo-oophorectomy, panhysterectomy, and removal of any involved structures; oophorectomy causes surgical menopause
3. Cytoreductive surgery to debulk poorly vascularized large tumors; the smaller the remaining tumor, the better the response to adjuvant therapy
4. Adjuvant therapy after tumor debulking
   a. Chemotherapy with antineoplastic drugs such as cyclophosphamide (Cytoxan), cisplatin (Platinol), and doxorubicin (Adriamycin) for epithelial carcinoma
   b. Paclitaxel (Taxol) for ovarian cancer that has been unresponsive to first-line or other therapy
   c. Intraperitoneal instillation of radioactive phosphorus (^{32}P)
   d. External radiation therapy

Nursing Care of Clients With Ovarian Cancer

See Nursing Care of Clients With a Hysterectomy under Uterine Neoplasms and care for the client receiving chemotherapy or radiation (see Radiation under Neoplastic Disorders, especially General Nursing Care of Clients With Neoplastic Disorders in Chapter 3)

VAGINITIS

Data Base

A. Etiology and pathophysiology
1. Trichomoniasis: infection with *Trichomonas vaginalis,* a protozoa
2. Candidiasis (moniliasis): caused by *Candida albicans,* a fungus; incidence is high in clients with diabetes mellitus and those receiving antibiotic therapy because of the decrease in bacterial flora
3. Bacterial vaginosis: caused by overgrowth of vaginal flora
4. Atrophic vaginitis: common in the postmenopausal period
5. May occur because of oral contraceptive use, sexually transmitted infections (e.g., gonorrhea), or allergic reactions; high incidence in clients with HIV

B. Clinical findings
1. Subjective: pruritus; burning; dysuria; dyspareunia (pain with intercourse)
2. Objective
   a. Vaginal discharge
      (1) Malodorous, thin, yellow discharge (trichomoniasis)
      (2) White "cheesy" discharge (moniliasis)
      (3) Grayish-white discharge; malodorous (bacterial vaginosis)
   b. Vaginal smear can indicate *Trichomonas vaginalis, Candida albicans,* or other microorganisms
C. Therapeutic interventions
1. Antifungal preparations for candidiasis: terconazole (Terazol), OTC antifungal creams
2. Antiprotozoan preparation for trichomoniasis: metronidazole (Flagyl) tablets taken orally; clotrimazole cream inserted vaginally
3. For bacterial vaginosis clindamycin (Cleocin) cream or oral administration, metronidazole (Flagyl) cream or tablets, ceftriaxone (Rocephin)
4. Estrogen therapy prescribed for atrophic vaginitis

Nursing Care of Clients With Vaginitis
A. Assessment/Analysis
1. History of onset and progression of symptoms
2. Presence of risk factors: improper use of tampons or douches; antibiotic use; multiple sexual partners; diabetes mellitus; HIV
3. Appearance and color of vaginal discharge
4. Pelvic examination and specimen for culture
B. Planning/Implementation
1. Advise the client to have sexual partner use a condom during coitus until vaginitis is resolved; sexual partner may require treatment
2. Teach the client that douching is not recommended unless ordered by the practitioner; teach client to lie in the recumbent position on a bedpan and direct the douche nozzle toward the sacrum
3. Encourage warm sitz baths to relieve perineal discomfort (sodium bicarbonate added to the water may be ordered)
4. Teach the client the importance of wearing loose-fitting clothing and cotton underwear and to avoid wearing pantyhose, "thong" underpants, and tight pants; avoid using tampons
5. Instruct the client who is receiving antibiotics or having recurrent vaginal infections to include yogurt or food supplements containing *Lactobacillus acidophilus* in the diet to maintain the vaginal flora
C. Evaluation/Outcomes
1. Expresses relief from pruritus and pain
2. Discusses need for diagnostic screening and precautions with sexual partner
3. Achieves resolution of infection

ENDOMETRIOSIS
Data Base
A. Etiology and pathophysiology
1. Growth of endometrial tissue in areas outside the uterus, such as ovaries, ligaments, or any abdominal organ
2. May be linked to retrograde menstruation or vascular and lymphatic system dissemination of endometrial tissue relocation
3. Generally affects young, nulliparous women; unrelated to menopause
4. Endometrial cells are stimulated by the ovarian hormones; will cause bleeding during regular menstrual cycle (if located in ovary, a pseudocyst or chocolate cyst may form); endometriosis is suppressed by pregnancy and lactation
5. Adhesions are common and may result in sterility and pain
6. Adenomyosis is a similar condition affecting women 40 to 50 years old in which the endometrial cells invade the muscles of the uterus
B. Clinical findings
1. Subjective
   a. Chronic lower abdominal pain and backache beginning 2 to 7 days before menstruation, becoming progressively worse, and then diminishing as the menstrual flow decreases
   b. Dyspareunia
   c. Pain associated with defecation
2. Objective
   a. Abnormal uterine bleeding (metrorrhagia, menorrhagia)
   b. Infertility
C. Therapeutic interventions
1. Hormone therapy to suppress ovulation; young married women are advised not to delay pregnancy if children are desired; breastfeeding delays return of symptoms
   a. Oral contraceptives and/or progesterone to cause tissue to slough off
   b. Synthetic analog of gonadotropin-releasing hormone to reduce lesions, such as leuprolide (Lupron) administered IM, Sub-Q, or via implant; nafarelin (Synarel) may be administered intranasally
   c. Gonadotropin inhibitors such as danazol (Cyclomen)
2. Surgical intervention
   a. Laparoscopic evaluation to confirm diagnosis
   b. Resection of lesions; laser treatment
   c. Oophorectomy, salpingectomy, and total hysterectomy if condition is severe and childbearing is not an issue
3. Laser ablation

Nursing Care of Clients With Endometriosis
A. Assessment/Analysis
1. Description of onset and progression of symptoms
2. Pelvic examination
3. Concerns about childbearing

B. Planning/Implementation
1. Provide time for client to talk about feelings
2. Administer analgesics as ordered
3. Review administration of prescribed hormones, contraindications, and side effects (see Related Pharmacology in Chapter 23)
4. Discuss alternatives if pregnancy does not occur
5. Provide care following surgery (see Nursing Care of Clients With a Hysterectomy under Uterine Neoplasms)
6. Provide referrals to Endometriosis Society and other community-based support groups
C. Evaluation/Outcomes
1. Experiences relief from pain
2. Verbalizes concerns about altered body image and infertility

PELVIC INFLAMMATORY DISEASE (PID)

Data Base
A. Etiology and pathophysiology
1. Occurs within female pelvic cavity; can affect the uterus (endometritis), fallopian tubes (salpingitis), ovaries (oophoritis), peritoneum, surrounding connective tissue, and pelvic veins
2. May be acute, subacute, or chronic; bilateral or unilateral
3. Caused most often by the introduction of bacteria (usually through the cervical opening), such as gonococci and chlamydia, which account for 50% of causes, and a variety of other organisms
4. If untreated, can lead to adhesions, sterility, ectopic pregnancy, and peritonitis
5. Risk factors include multiple sex partners, history of sexually transmitted infections, intrauterine device (IUD) insertion, douching, sexual activity during menses, and nulliparity
B. Clinical findings
1. Subjective: pain ranging from dull aching to severe cramping in lower abdomen; nausea; malaise; dysmenorrhea; dyspareunia
2. Objective
   a. Elevated temperature; increased WBC count
   b. Foul-smelling, purulent vaginal discharge
   c. Cultures of vaginal discharge reveal causative organism
C. Therapeutic interventions
1. Medication to control pain and fever
2. Antibiotics depending on the organism
3. Identification and notification of sexual contacts and the state department of health if sexually transmitted infection is present

Nursing Care of Clients With Pelvic Inflammatory Disease
A. Assessment/Analysis
1. Description of onset and progression of symptoms
2. Potential source of infection
3. Pelvic examination and specimens for culture
4. Characteristics of discharge
5. Vital signs and WBC count for baseline data
B. Planning/Implementation
1. Monitor temperature, WBC count, and culture reports
2. Explain the importance of completing prescribed antibiotic therapy; advise client of side effects; follow-up after treatment is begun to assess response to therapy
3. Maintain on bed rest in the Fowler's or semi-Fowler's position to localize the infection and prevent the formation of abscesses within the abdominal cavity
4. Observe and record the amount and character of vaginal discharge
5. Change perineal pads frequently using gloves
6. Teach safety measures to prevent reinfection of the client or others; during the treatment phase the client should abstain from intercourse and avoid using tampons
7. Allow time for client to verbalize feelings about illness and/or possible complication of infertility
8. Explain importance of prenatal care if pregnancy occurs
9. Teach signs of ectopic pregnancy because of increased risk
C. Evaluation/Outcomes
1. Expresses relief from pain
2. Discusses need for diagnostic screening and precautions with sexual partner
3. Achieves resolution of infection
4. Verbalizes concerns
5. Verbalizes knowledge of the disease, its prevention, and its consequences

PROLAPSED UTERUS

Data Base
A. Etiology and pathophysiology
1. As a result of weakness of the pelvic floor, the uterus descends into the vagina; most often associated with childbirth injury or increased intraabdominal pressure (classified as first degree to fourth degree)
2. If severe, the entire uterus may protrude outside the vaginal orifice; in this case, the vagina is inverted; referred to as procidentia
3. Ulcerations in procidentia increase risk for cancer
B. Clinical findings
1. Subjective: heaviness within the pelvis; low back pain
2. Objective
   a. Mass in the lower vagina or outside the orifice
   b. Elongated cervix
   c. Urinary retention and/or incontinence
C. Therapeutic interventions
1. Vaginal pessary to maintain the uterus in correct position

2. Surgical intervention
  a. Suspension of the uterus and correction of retroversion
  b. Pelvic surgery to resuspend the uterus and resupport the musculature
  c. Vaginal hysterectomy (if postmenopausal or if future pregnancy is not desired)

Nursing Care of Clients With a Prolapsed Uterus
A. Assessment/Analysis
  1. Description of onset and progression of symptoms
  2. Pelvic examination; note degree (grade) of prolapse and presence of cystocele or rectocele
  3. Degree of interference with urinary and bowel elimination
  4. Presence of ulcerations on skin or mucous membranes
B. Planning/Implementation
  1. If procidentia is present, observe for ulcerations; apply warm saline compresses or protective ointment to prevent ulceration
  2. Explain that if a pessary is used, it must be taken out periodically and cleaned
  3. Monitor the color, amount, and frequency of urination; teach pelvic floor exercises (Kegel)
  4. Monitor the consistency, amount, and frequency of bowel movements
  5. Provide postoperative care (see Nursing Care of Clients With Cancer of the Cervix)
C. Evaluation/Outcomes
  1. Maintains integrity of skin and mucous membranes
  2. Establishes a regular pattern of bowel elimination
  3. Establishes a regular pattern of urinary elimination
  4. Reestablishes a satisfying sexual relationship

CYSTOCELE AND/OR RECTOCELE
Data Base
A. Etiology and pathophysiology
  1. Cystocele: herniation of the bladder into the vagina
  2. Rectocele: herniation of the rectum into the vagina
  3. Both conditions may be present at the same time and are generally associated with relaxation or injury of the pelvic muscles during childbirth
  4. Fistulas may occur
    a. Rectovaginal: opening between rectum and vagina
    b. Vesicovaginal: opening between bladder and vagina
    c. Urethravaginal: opening between urethra and vagina
B. Clinical findings
  1. Subjective: feeling of fullness in vagina, lower abdomen, and/or back; constant urge to urinate or defecate; dysuria
  2. Objective
    a. Soft, reducible mass evident during vaginal examination that increases when client is asked to bear down

  b. Stress incontinence; frequency; urgency
  c. Residual urine (60 mL or more after voiding)
  d. Constipation or diarrhea
C. Therapeutic interventions
  1. Anterior colporrhaphy to correct a cystocele
  2. Posterior colporrhaphy to correct a rectocele
  3. Insertion of a pessary for mild symptoms

Nursing Care of Clients With a Cystocele and/or Rectocele
A. Assessment/Analysis
  1. History of prolapsed uterus
  2. Description of onset and progression of symptoms
  3. Pelvic examination
  4. Presence and extent of urinary retention
  5. Impact of symptoms on client's lifestyle
B. Planning/Implementation
  1. Teach client care related to use of a pessary (e.g., cleaning, removing, or having it removed periodically)
  2. Encourage the client to perform Kegel exercises regularly to strengthen perineal muscles and use the knee-chest position for a few minutes several times a day
  3. Instruct client about preventing constipation (e.g., high-fiber diet, fluids, exercise, and stool softeners as prescribed)
  4. Provide time for client to verbalize fears and ask questions
  5. Provide postoperative care
    a. Maintain patency of urinary catheter to prevent retention; when catheter is removed assess for signs of retention
    b. Encourage voiding every 4 hours to prevent strain on the suture line from a distended bladder; perform residual urine measurements as ordered (no more than 150 mL should accumulate)
    c. After each bowel movement and voiding, cleanse perineum with warm soap and water and flush with warm water using a peri-bottle; always cleanse away from vagina and toward anus; sitz baths can be used
    d. Apply anesthetic spray, or ice packs if ordered to relieve discomfort
    e. Administer ordered stool softeners to limit straining at stool and pressure on the suture line
    f. Encourage intake of liquids on first postoperative day and a regular diet on the second day
C. Evaluation/Outcomes
  1. Establishes a regular pattern of bowel elimination
  2. Remains free from episodes of urinary incontinence

BENIGN BREAST DISEASE
Data Base
A. Etiology and pathophysiology
  1. Fibrocystic breast condition is characterized by fluid-filled cysts in the breast; linked to hormonal

imbalance and caffeine consumption; may feel soft or hard on palpation; pain is common; it is a risk factor for breast cancer

2. Fibroadenomas, the most common benign breast condition, are characterized by encapsulated, nontender tumors; increase in size during pregnancy and decrease with age

3. Papillomas are intraductal lesions within the terminal duct; occur in women between 30 and 50 years; may cause bloody nipple discharge; multiple growths may be cancerous

4. Ductal ectasia occurs in the subareolar area of aging breasts (seen in perimenopausal or postmenopausal women); duct is palpable with burning, pain, sticky nipple discharge; not generally associated with cancer

5. Lipomas are soft, fatty tumors that are mobile and nontender

B. Clinical findings
1. Subjective: painful, tender breasts (mastalgia)
2. Objective
   a. Palpable lesions that may be hard or soft, painful or nontender, fixed or mobile
   b. Nipple discharge may be bloody with papilloma or sticky with ductal ectasia
3. Mammography identifies location and shape of lesion
4. Biopsy determines pathology of lesion

C. Therapeutic interventions
1. Interventions depend on the extent of the disorder
2. Aspiration of cysts for cytology studies; biopsies with suspicious findings
3. Mammographies and breast self-examination on a regular basis
4. Dietary modification to decrease the intake of caffeine and fat

Nursing Care of Clients With Benign Breast Disease

A. Assessment/Analysis
1. Breast-oriented history that includes menstrual history, previous mammographies, biopsies, cyst aspirations, hormone therapy, and breast cancer
2. Breast examination

B. Planning/Implementation
1. Instruct client regarding importance of regular breast self-examination, yearly clinical breast examination, and mammography studies
2. Explain importance of dietary restrictions of caffeine and fat, depending on disorder
3. Listen to client's feelings and concerns regarding fear of findings; do not minimize concerns

C. Evaluation/Outcomes
1. Discusses feelings and concerns with health team members
2. Expresses decreased pain in the breasts
3. Continues planned follow-up with yearly clinical breast examination and mammography

CANCER OF THE BREAST

Data Base

A. Etiology and pathophysiology
1. Frequently begins as a hard, nontender, relatively fixed nodule; found most often in the upper, outer quadrant of the breast
2. Most breast cancers are adenocarcinomas originating in the ducts and lobes
3. Incidence increases with age; use of estrogen replacement therapy for more than 10 years; increased number of menstrual cycles (menarche before age 12, menopause after age 55); nulliparity or parity after age 35; history of benign breast disease; postmenopausal obesity; history of unrelated cancer
4. History of first-degree relative with breast cancer or presence of BRCA gene mutations increase risk
5. Most common sites of metastasis are bone, bone marrow, soft tissue, lungs, liver, and brain
6. Extent of disease reflected by staging; nodal involvement most important prognostic factor; tumors may be estrogen- or progesterone-receptor positive

B. Clinical findings
1. Subjective: lesion generally nontender; malaise in later stages
2. Objective
   a. Palpable, irregularly shaped, fixed mass; most often in upper, outer quadrant
   b. Asymmetry of breasts; inversion and discharge from nipple
   c. Dimpling and change of color of skin over lesion; in late stages, skin has orange-peel (peau d'orange) appearance
   d. Enlarged axillary lymph nodes
   e. Positive findings in following tests
      (1) Mammography: baseline between 35 and 40 years of age; every year after 40 years of age
      (2) Sonography (particularly for dense breast tissue), thermography, and transillumination for early detection; MRI
      (3) Biopsy for cytologic evaluation (see Breast Biopsy under Related Procedures in Chapter 23)
      (4) Estrogen receptor assay: if positive, indicates need for alteration of the hormonal environment by surgical or chemical means
      (5) Tumor markers: CA-15-3 and CA-125; carcinoembryonic antigen (CEA) in serum, plasma, or cerebrospinal fluid; indicative of progression of cancer, particularly of the breast, ovaries, and gastrointestinal tract

C. Therapeutic interventions
1. Intervention depends on the extent of the primary Tumor, regional lymph Node involvement, and extent of distant Metastasis (TNM classification) and the physical status of the client
2. Surgical intervention

a. Partial mastectomy (lumpectomy, wide excision, segmental resection, or quadrantectomy): removal of the lump and surrounding breast tissue

b. Simple mastectomy: removal of the breast only

c. Radical mastectomy: removal of the breast, pectoral muscles, pectoral fascia, and nodes (pectoral, subclavicular, apical, and axillary); rarely performed today

d. Modified radical mastectomy: similar to a radical mastectomy but pectoral muscles are not removed

e. Sentinel node biopsy or lymphectomy to determine the status of regional lymph node involvement and risk for metastasis

f. Breast reconstruction (tissue expanders, saline implants, muscle flaps)

g. Oophorectomy, adrenalectomy, and/or hypophysectomy to control metastases by altering endocrine environment

3. Radiation therapy through an external beam or an interstitial implant using iridium 192 (^{192}Ir)

4. Chemotherapy: regimens usually used include CMF, CAF, AC, A→CMF, AC→T, and AT; most interfere with DNA and/or RNA synthesis

a. Alkylating agent: cyclophosphamide (Cytoxan)

b. Antimetabolites: 5-fluorouracil (5-FU); methotrexate (amethopterin, MTX)

c. Antitumor antibiotic: doxorubicin (Adriamycin)

d. Taxanes: paclitaxel (Taxol), docetaxel (Taxotere); interfere with cellular microtubule function required for interphase and mitosis

e. Hormonal therapy: tamoxifen (Nolvadex), toremifene (Fareston), fulvestrant (Faslodex); reduces DNA and estrogen response

f. Corticosteroid: prednisone

5. Biologic therapy: trastuzumab (Herceptin)

6. Bone marrow/stem cell transplantation

Nursing Care of Clients With Cancer of the Breast

A. Assessment/Analysis

1. Personal and family history of breast cancer

2. Age at menarche, menopause, and birth of first child

3. Regularity of breast self-examinations, clinical breast examinations, and mammograms

4. Breast tissue, noting characteristics of lesion and skin surface

5. Enlargement of lymph nodes

6. Client's coping skills and availability of support system

7. Feelings about sexuality

8. Fears concerning consequences of cancer diagnosis and of finding another mass

B. Planning/Implementation

1. Encourage and instruct the client concerning monthly breast self-examination

a. Perform exam 7 days after the start of menstruation if premenopausal or the same time every month if postmenopausal

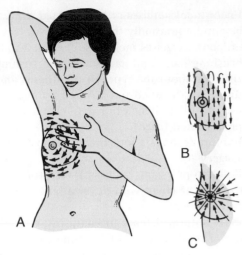

Figure 24-1 Breast self-examination. **A,** Circles; **B,** vertical lines; **C,** wedges. (From Lowdermilk DL, Perry SE: *Maternity nursing,* ed 7, St Louis, 2006, Mosby.)

b. Inspect while standing with hands at sides, overhead, and then on the hips for asymmetry, retraction of the nipple, dimpling of skin, color change

c. Palpate the axillary and supraclavicular nodes

d. Palpate the breast tissue using a systematic pattern (e.g., circles, vertical lines, wedges) when standing and lying down with the arm abducted (Figure 24-1: Breast self-examination)

e. Squeeze the nipple of each breast to check for discharge

2. Assist the client and family to cope with the diagnosis of cancer and altered body image by encouraging them to talk with staff and each other

3. Listen to and accept the client's feelings

4. Support the client's feminine image

5. Care for the client after a mastectomy

a. Observe for hemorrhage by checking all areas of the dressing underneath the client, the drainage unit, and vital signs

b. Maintain functioning of portable wound drainage system by ensuring patency of tube, emptying before half full, and supporting to avoid tension at site of insertion; drainage should not exceed 200 mL in 8 hours

c. Encourage coughing and deep breathing or use of incentive spirometer

d. Encourage correct posture and provide assistance with ambulation until the client adjusts to altered balance

e. Prevent or reduce lymphedema by elevating and supporting the client's hand above the elbow and the elbow above the shoulder; inflatable or elastic sleeve may be ordered

f. Instruct to avoid carrying heavy articles and to avoid cuts or bruises, having blood drawn, injections, or BP readings in the arm on the affected side

g. Encourage exercises of the affected arm, beginning gradually the day after surgery as ordered; exercises include squeezing a ball, brushing hair, wall hand-climbing, turning rope

h. Instruct about the types of prostheses and where to obtain them; cotton covered by gauze may be used to fill a client's bra until she is seen by a professional fitter

i. Explore feelings about breast reconstruction surgery

j. Refer to programs such as Reach for Recovery to help the client with physical and emotional readjustment

6. Support natural defense mechanisms; encourage intake of foods rich in the immune-stimulating nutrients, especially vitamins A, C, and E, and the mineral selenium; encourage low-fat diet

7. Provide care for the client receiving chemotherapy or radiation (see Radiation under Neoplastic Disorders, especially General Nursing Care of Clients With Neoplastic Disorders in Chapter 3)

C. Evaluation/Outcomes
1. Expresses improvement in body image
2. Identifies precautions necessary to prevent injury to the arm on the affected side after a mastectomy
3. Maintains strength and mobility of arm on affected side
4. Discusses feelings with health care providers, family, and sexual partner
5. Demonstrates and continues to perform monthly BSE

OSTEOPOROSIS

Data Base

A. Etiology and pathophysiology
1. Systemic skeletal disease characterized by microarchitectural deterioration of bone tissue and diminished bone mass
2. Bone fragility predisposes to pathologic fractures; most commonly affects the vertebrae, pelvis, and head of the femur
3. Risk factors include heredity (60% to 80%), low body weight (less than 127 lb), prolonged premenopausal amenorrhea, early menopause, sedentary lifestyle, prolonged immobility, inadequate intake of dietary calcium, low serum vitamin D levels, smoking, alcohol use, long-term steroid therapy

B. Clinical findings
1. Subjective: back pain that increases with activity and decreases with rest; difficulty maintaining balance
2. Objective

a. Decreased height resulting from compression of the vertebrae; kyphosis
b. Bone mass measurements (e.g., x-ray examinations, dual-energy densitometry [absorptiometry])
c. Pathologic fractures

C. Therapeutic interventions
1. Planned program of weight-bearing exercise to increase calcium deposition in bone
2. Hormone replacement therapy (HRT) with estrogen because it decreases bone reabsorption; HRT is controversial because of its relationship to increased evidence of breast cancer and cardiovascular disorders
3. Bisphosphate therapy, such as alendronate (Fosamax) and risedronate (Actonel), to inhibit osteoclasts and reduce bone resorption
4. Human recombinant parathyroid hormone, such as teriparatide (Forteo) to stimulate new bone growth
5. High-protein, high-calcium diet or calcium supplements, and vitamin D supplements
6. Support for the spine (e.g., corset, Philadelphia collar, Taylor brace)
7. Treatment of modifiable related factors

Nursing Care of Clients With Osteoporosis

A. Assessment/Analysis
1. Factors that may have contributed to development of osteoporosis
2. Usual dietary pattern and use of over-the-counter medications
3. History of loss of balance, falls, pain, fractures

B. Planning/Implementation
1. Encourage active weight-bearing and range-of-motion exercises
2. Teach effective body mechanics
3. Encourage use of assistive devices such as walker or cane to promote stability
4. Encourage diet that will supply nutrients needed for mineralization of bone (vitamins A, C, and D, and the minerals calcium, magnesium, and phosphorus); discuss calcium supplements; foods high in calcium include dairy products, turnip greens
5. Advise to lower sodium intake and to avoid caffeine and alcohol, because they increase calcium excretion
6. Encourage use of orthotic devices if ordered

C. Evaluation/Outcomes
1. Reports a reduction in pain
2. Complies with dietary and drug regimens
3. Participates in weight-bearing exercises
4. Maintains physical mobility
5. Remains free from injury

Nursing Care of Women During Uncomplicated Pregnancy, Labor, Childbirth, and the Postpartum Period

✳ PRENATAL PERIOD

Data Base

Development of the Embryo/Fetus

A. Formation of gametes
   1. The ovum and spermatozoon each have one set of 23 chromosomes; other cells of the body have two sets, or 46 chromosomes (23 pairs)
   2. The production of ova and spermatozoa requires a special type of nuclear division (meiosis) in which the chromosome number is reduced from two sets (46 chromosomes) to one set (23 chromosomes)
B. Chromosomes
   1. Humans have 23 pairs of homologous chromosomes
   2. Homologous chromosomes carry sets of matching genes (alleles); one may be dominant and the other recessive, or they may have blending expressions
C. Sex determination in humans
   1. Genetic females have two sets of autosomes (non-sex chromosomes) and two X chromosomes, whereas genetic males have two sets of autosomes and one X chromosome and one Y chromosome
   2. All ova produced by females have one set of autosomes and one X chromosome; spermatozoa produced by a male have a set of autosomes and either an X or a Y chromosome
   3. If an X-bearing spermatozoon fertilizes an ovum, a female will result; if a Y-bearing spermatozoon fertilizes an ovum, a male will result
D. Genes
   1. Sex-linked genes: genes carried on the X chromosome are always expressed in the male, even though they may be recessive; examples of such genes cause hemophilia and colorblindness
   2. Multiple genes: many different genes may combine to produce cumulative effects, such as the degree of pigmentation or height
   3. Multiple alleles: examples of human traits controlled by multiple alleles are the genes controlling blood types and eye color
E. Chromosomal alterations
   1. In rare cases additional sex chromosomes may appear and produce abnormal individuals
      a. X chromosome and no Y chromosome: Turner's syndrome
      b. Two or more X chromosomes and a Y chromosome: Klinefelter's syndrome

   2. Translocation of chromosome: a cytogenetic abnormality such as trisomy 21 (Down syndrome)
   3. Mutations
      a. Changes in DNA; chromosomal changes
      b. The frequency of mutations may be increased by certain agents such as ultraviolet radiation, x-rays, radioactive radiation, and chemical substances
F. Fertilization
   1. Spermatozoa are deposited in the vagina, and fertilization usually occurs in a fallopian tube about 24 hours after ovulation
   2. Sperm must be in the genital tract 4 to 6 hours before they can fertilize an ovum
   3. Male nucleus enters the cytoplasm of the ovum; a membrane forms around the ovum to prevent the entrance of other sperm
   4. Fertilization occurs when male pronucleus unites with female pronucleus, restoring the chromosome number to two sets (46 chromosomes)
G. Cleavage
   1. A short time after fertilization, the zygote undergoes rapid mitotic division to produce a mass of cells (morula)
   2. As the morula descends down the fallopian tube, it divides to form a hollow ball (blastocyst)
H. Implantation
   1. The blastocyst implants in the uterine wall
      a. The blastocyst is differentiated into an inner cell mass, a blastocoele; the outer covering of cells becomes the trophoderm, which forms the fetal portion of the placenta
      b. Implantation occurs 7 to 8 days after fertilization, generally in the upper fundal portion of the uterus; increased maternal hormonal action sustains implantation of the embryo
   2. Placenta and umbilical cord development
      a. Placenta
         (1) Organ of dual origin (maternal and embryonic portions) serving as the site for interchange of food, gases, and wastes between mother and embryo/fetus during pregnancy
         (2) Functions as the fetal digestive tract, lungs, and kidneys, and as a major endocrine gland

(producing estrogens, progesterone, adrenocorticotropic hormone [ACTH], growth hormone, and the gonadotropic hormones human chorionic gonadotropin [hCG] and human placental lactogen [hPL])

(3) Serves as a protective barrier against harmful effects of some drugs and microorganisms

b. Umbilical cord

(1) Inserted close to central portion of placenta and attached to fetus although there are insertion variations such as marginal (edge of the placenta) and velamentous (into amniotic sac)

(2) Cord has one vein, which transports maternal nourishment from the placenta to the fetus, and two arteries, which transport fetal wastes to the placenta

(3) Wharton's jelly, a protective covering, surrounds the entire cord

I. Embryonic period

1. During first 2 months, the conceptus is termed an embryo; after this period it is called a fetus

2. The inner cell mass differentiates into germ layers

a. Ectoderm: outer layer of skin and mouth cavity and nervous tissue

b. Mesoderm: connective tissue, including blood and muscle tissue; cardiovascular system and major organs

c. Endoderm: linings of the alimentary tract, respiratory system, and several glands

3. About 12 days after fertilization, a fetal membrane, the amnion, forms around the embryo; another membrane, the yolk sac, develops beneath the embryo

a. Amnion sac contains amniotic fluid

b. Yolk sac serves as an initial embryonic source of erythrocytes

4. Later an allantois develops that will supply the placental blood vessels

5. A chorion surrounds the embryo; this will eventually form the major part of the placenta; fingerlike projections of the chorion, called chorionic villi, grow into the decidua (endometrium); chorionic villi project into placental blood sinuses; the combination of chorionic villi, placental blood sinuses, and placental blood constitutes the placenta

6. Embryonic development—differentiation of cells occurs

a. At 14 days: heart begins to beat; brain, early spinal cord, and muscle segments present

b. At 30 days: embryo ¼ to ½ inch (0.6 to 1.2 cm) in length, definite form, umbilical cord becomes visible

c. At 31 to 36 days: both arms and legs have digits but they may be webbed

d. At 46 to 48 days: cartilage in upper arms replaced by first bone cells, amniotic fluid

surrounds the embryo (amniotic fluid is a protective cushion, equalizes pressures, maintains temperature, and facilitates fetal movements)

e. The first 8 weeks, known as the period of organogenesis, is a time of rapid growth and development; any interference with maternal physiology may cause irreparable damage (preconception counseling should include that no drugs should be taken during the first trimester without medical supervision)

f. By the end of 8 weeks every organ system and external structure that is present in the full-term newborn exists

J. Fetal development

1. Genitalia begin to differentiate at 9 weeks and are fully differentiated by 12 weeks

2. By 12 weeks: fetus moves body parts, swallows, practices breathing movements but does not inhale and exhale, weighs 28 g (1 oz); fetal heart audible with Doptone; rate range is 110 to 160 beats/min chorionic villi sampling is done between 10 and 12 weeks

3. At 16 to 20 weeks: fetal movements felt by mother (quickening), weighs 170 g (6 oz), is 20 to 25 cm (8 to 10 inches) in length; 200 mL of amniotic fluid present; amniocentesis is possible by 14 to 16 weeks; vernix and lanugo cover and protect the fetus

4. At 20 to 24 weeks: hair growth on head, eyelashes, and brow; skeleton hardens; eyelids closed; weighs 0.45 kg (1 lb); is 30.5 cm (12 inches) in length; fetal heart audible with fetoscope; respiratory movements become more regular

5. At 24 to 28 weeks: eyelids open, amniotic fluid increases to 1 quart with a daily exchange of 6 gallons, weighs 0.5 kg (1¼ lb); alveolar cells of lungs produce pulmonary surfactants that minimize surface tension

6. At 28 to 32 weeks: brown fat starts to be deposited at 28 weeks, weighs 0.5 to 0.7 kg (1 to 1½ lb)

7. At 32 to 36 weeks: stores protein for extrauterine life, gains 1.8 kg (4 lb)

8. Fetal circulation: contains mixed blood with low oxygenation (fetal oxygen saturation is 30% to 70%; the only exception is in the ductus venosus, which connects the umbilical vein to the inferior vena cava of the fetus)

a. Foramen ovale is an opening between the right and left atria during fetal life, bypassing fetal lungs

b. Ductus arteriosus is a connection between pulmonary trunk and aorta, also bypassing fetal lungs

c. Ductus venosus is a connection between umbilical vein and ascending vena cava, bypassing fetal liver

Physical, Physiologic, and Emotional Changes During Pregnancy

Pregnancy is a physiologic process that affects all body systems and results in both objective and subjective changes; it is a stressful time requiring many adaptations and may cause minor discomforts

A. Endocrine
   1. During pregnancy the chorion of the placenta secretes a hormone, hCG, that maintains the corpus luteum; the continuation of progesterone and estrogen secretion from the corpus luteum maintains the pregnancy during the first trimester; the presence of hCG hormone is an indicator of pregnancy; hCG, which plays a role in morning sickness, reaches a peak in the third month and then drops; high hCG levels are found in the presence of a hydatidiform mole
   2. Estrogen and progesterone levels increase and continue to be secreted by the placenta during the last 6 months of pregnancy; progesterone inhibits uterine contractions; the increase in these hormones leads to sodium and water retention and muscle relaxation, which results in fatigue
   3. Thyroid activity is increased; pregnancy may mimic a mild hyperthyroid state
   4. Parathyroid glands and the production of their hormone increase
   5. Human placental lactogen (hPL), sometimes called human chorionic somatomammotropin (hCS), is increased; it is a diabetogenic hormone (diminished insulin efficiency) that decreases maternal use of glucose, leaving it available for fetal use; it also affects lipid and protein metabolism
   6. Estriol levels increase; high levels in the maternal saliva may be a sign of preterm labor
   7. The posterior pituitary secretion of oxytocin, which stimulates uterine contractions, coupled with the drop in progesterone level and the increase in levels of estrogen and prostaglandins, may contribute to the initiation of labor; uterine contractions increase in frequency and intensity, culminating in fetal expulsion (birth); after birth, oxytocin contracts the uterus and stimulates the milk ejection reflex
   8. The pancreas increases the production of insulin early in pregnancy; in addition, the mother's body becomes increasingly sensitive to insulin during the first half of pregnancy

B. Reproductive
   1. Amenorrhea occurs because the corpus luteum persists, and ovulation is inhibited by the high levels of circulating estrogen and progesterone; low circulating levels of these hormones stimulate ovulation
   2. Breast changes such as fullness, tingling, soreness, and darkening of the areolae and nipples occur as a result of increased hormonal levels
   3. Leukorrhea occurs as hormonal levels rise; increased acidity in the vagina is a protection from bacterial invasion
   4. Changes in the uterus are circulatory, hormonal, and related to fetal growth
      a. Softening of the cervix: Goodell's sign
      b. Softening of the lower uterine segment: Hegar's sign
      c. Purplish hue to the cervix and vaginal mucosa: Chadwick's sign
      d. Uterus enlarges and increases in weight from 70 g to 1000 g at term
      e. Changes in position of the uterus: first trimester, uterus is in pelvic cavity; second and third trimesters, uterus is in abdominal cavity

C. Gastrointestinal
   1. Hormonal increases, especially in the first trimester, cause nausea and vomiting (morning sickness)
   2. Elevated estrogen levels cause excessive salivation (ptyalism)
   3. Hyperemia and softening of gums with accompanying hyperacidity of oral secretions result in nonspecific gingivitis; increased vitamin C intake and regular oral hygiene are indicated
   4. Decreased emptying time of gallbladder may precipitate gallstone formation
   5. Food cravings may occur; only significant if substance craving is unusual (pica); for example, clay, starch, dirt
   6. Heartburn (pyrosis) occurs because of delayed emptying time of stomach and reflux of gastric acid contents into esophagus; gastric irritants such as coffee, tea, and chocolate should be avoided; sodium antacids should be avoided
   7. Hiatal hernia is a complication that may occur in older or obese women or in those with multiple fetuses
   8. Constipation is caused by hypoperistalsis, lack of fluids, low fiber intake, pressure of the enlarged uterus on internal organs, effects of progesterone on muscle, and hemorrhoids

D. Excretory
   1. Weight of uterus on bladder in early and late pregnancy causes urinary frequency
   2. The hormonal effect on smooth muscle reduces bladder tone, which increases its capacity to 1500 mL
   3. Pressure of enlarging uterus causes dilation of renal pelves and ureters; the right ones dilate more because the uterus is displaced to the right
   4. Urine is retained in dilated urinary tract structures; flow rate decreases, leading to stasis and proneness to infection; aggressive treatment is needed to prevent preterm labor
   5. Lowered renal threshold may cause glycosuria and occasional mild proteinuria (1 +); urine must be tested at every prenatal visit to rule out gestational diabetes and preeclampsia

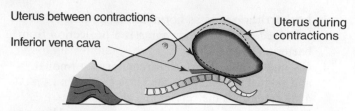

Figure 25-1 Supine hypotension. (From Lowdermilk DL, Perry SE: *Maternity nursing*, ed 7, St Louis, 2006, Mosby.)

E. Circulatory
1. Physiologic anemia occurs as a result of hemodilution of the blood; there is a 45% to 50% increase in blood volume, which is about 75% plasma and 25% RBCs; the imbalance between the plasma and RBCs leads to a reduced hematocrit; blood volume is increased to meet the needs of the mother and developing fetus
2. Cardiac output increases 30% to 50%, peaking at 28 to 32 weeks
3. Heart rate increases 10 to 15 beats/min in the latter half of pregnancy
4. Palpitations occur in early months from sympathetic nervous stimulation and in later months from increased thoracic pressure because of enlarged uterus
5. BP may drop slightly in second trimester
6. Supine hypotension syndrome (vena caval syndrome): in supine position, weight of enlarged uterus compresses vena cava, which decreases blood return to heart; decreased cardiac output ensues with hypotension, lightheadedness, faintness, and palpitations (Figure 25-1: Supine hypotension); side-lying position relieves pressure on vena cava, promoting placental perfusion
7. WBCs, fibrinogen, and other clotting factors increase; WBCs increase from 5000 to 12,000/mm^3
8. Pelvic hyperemia and pressure of the uterus on the pelvic blood vessels may cause varicose veins of legs, vulva, and perianal area
9. Edema of extremities common in the last 6 weeks of pregnancy because of stasis of blood
10. If thrombophlebitis occurs, heparin or low-molecular-weight heparin may be administered because these substances do not cross the placental barrier; bed rest with leg elevation is required

F. Respiratory
1. During the third trimester, pressure of the enlarged uterus on the diaphragm and lungs may cause dyspnea that subsides when lightening occurs at about 38 weeks
2. Oxygen consumption is increased by about 15% between the 16th and 40th weeks, although there may be only a slight increase in vital capacity during pregnancy; tidal volume increases because of an expansion of thoracic cavity up to 40%
3. Hyperventilation occurs because of mother's need to blow off increased CO_2 transferred to her from fetus
4. Nasal congestion and epistaxis may occur as a response to increased estrogen levels

G. Integumentary
1. Excretion of wastes through the skin causes diaphoresis
2. Skin changes: darkening of the areolae, darkening patches on the face (melasma, formerly chloasma), linea alba becomes nigra on the abdomen, related to increased melanin; striae on the abdomen and legs caused by skin stretching as pregnancy advances; erythematous changes on the palms and face in some women

H. Skeletal
1. Softening of all ligaments and joints, especially symphysis pubis and sacroiliac joint, caused by increased hormonal action of estrogens and relaxin
2. Leg cramps may occur from an imbalance of calcium (hypocalcemia) in the body, from pressure of the gravid uterus on nerves supplying lower extremities, or from a decrease in calcium intake

I. Emotional
1. Ambivalence about pregnancy, parenting, and impact on family
2. Acceptance of biologic fact of pregnancy and acquiring knowledge regarding physical, physiologic, and emotional changes of pregnancy; usually occurs during first trimester
3. Acceptance of growing fetus as distinct from self; usually occurs during second trimester
4. Preparation for birth; usually occurs during third trimester
5. Mood swings
6. Increase or decrease in sexual desire
7. Anxiety related to birth and adult responsibilities

J. Affirmation and confirmation of pregnancy
1. Presumptive signs: mostly subjective; may be indicative of other illnesses: amenorrhea; fatigue; nausea and vomiting; breast changes; urinary frequency; darkening of pigmentation on face, breasts, and abdomen; quickening (feeling of movement about 15 to 20 weeks)
2. Probable signs: objective but still not definite confirmations of pregnancy
   a. Uterine changes: Chadwick's sign, Hegar's sign, Goodell's sign, enlargement of the uterus
   b. Fetal outline; ballottement
   c. Pregnancy tests: urine and blood of woman tested to detect (hCG) human chorionic gonadotropin
   d. Preparatory contractions (Braxton Hicks)
3. Positive signs: confirm pregnancy
   a. Fetal heartbeat
   b. Fetal outline and movement as felt by examiner
   c. Ultrasonography revealing fetus and movement of fetal heart

4. Early determination of more than one fetus is vital; multiple gestation contributes to perinatal morbidity and mortality
5. Estimating date of birth (EDB) and duration of pregnancy
   a. Nägele's rule: count back 3 months from first day of last menstrual period and add 7 days (9 calendar months, 270 days; or 10 lunar months, 280 days) and 1 year
   b. Fundal height: measurement from symphysis pubis to top of fundus; the fundus rises about 1 cm per week up to 30 weeks; at 20 weeks it should be at the umbilicus (McDonald's rule) and at 36 weeks at the xiphoid process
   c. Ultrasonography: establishes gestational age by crown to rump measurement during first 11 weeks and then from head measurements (term pregnancy: biparietal diameter is 9.8 cm or more); when performed early in pregnancy, measurements should be made when woman has full bladder (women instructed to drink before test)

K. Nutritional needs during pregnancy
1. Consideration of preconceptional nutritional status; obesity or underweight; age and parity of mother; biologic interactions between mother, fetus, and placenta; and individual needs, such as in times of stress
2. Weight gain should be evaluated with regard to quality of gain; most of weight gain is related to size of fetus
3. Severe caloric restriction during pregnancy is contraindicated because it is a potential hazard to the mother and fetus, especially during organogenesis
4. Weight reduction should never be started as a regimen during pregnancy
5. Restriction of sodium and administration of diuretics are potentially dangerous to mother and fetus during pregnancy; they may limit interstitial fluid reserve, which may be needed if the blood volume decreases
6. Nausea and vomiting: dry crackers in morning; limited fluids with meals; small, frequent meals; restricted fat, high-carbohydrate diet; protein snacks at bedtime
7. Constipation: increased fluids and fiber; appropriate activity level
8. Consideration of demands of pregnancy related to growth and development of fetus during various trimesters; provide adequate nutrition to meet increased maternal and fetal nutrient demands
   a. Increased calories to meet increased basal metabolic needs (300 additional calories during second and third trimesters) spare protein for growth and promote weight gain to support pregnancy
   b. Average weight gain should be 14.4 to 16 kg (25 to 35 lb) but is individualized according to needs; underweight women should gain more, overweight women should gain less; women carrying multiple fetuses should gain more than the recommended weight for one fetus; body mass index may help to individualize appropriate weight gain
   c. Increased protein to provide for growth demands
   d. Increased vitamins, especially folic acid to prevent anemia and neural tube defects
   e. Increased minerals with supplement of iron to prevent anemia
   f. Iodized salt to provide needed sodium and iodine
   g. Increased calcium from milk and cheese to promote fetal bone and tooth development and prevent maternal bone mass loss
9. Dietary assessment and counseling should be an integral part of prenatal care for every pregnant woman; an adequate weight gain is about 4 lb every month after an initial 3- to 4-lb gain in the first trimester
10. Dietary assessment should consider cultural, economic, and psychologic needs
11. Food intake should be based on a balanced diet
   a. Additional calories, protein, and fluids; supplemental vitamins and minerals
   b. Daily minimum food intake during pregnancy should include 4 dairy products, which provide calcium, protein, vitamins A and D, and riboflavin; 3 (2 oz) servings of protein foods; 6 or more servings of bread and cereal; 5 servings of fruits or vegetables containing vitamin C; 1 serving of leafy, dark-green or deep-yellow vegetables; 1 serving of yellow fruit or vegetables; and 2 servings of other vegetables or fruits
   c. Minerals such as iron, calcium, phosphorus, iodine, zinc, and sodium are needed in the diet
   d. At least 6 to 8 glasses of fluid per day
12. Adolescent nutritional needs
   a. Weight gain for the pregnancy and expected weight gain for maternal growth are added together
   b. Iron needs higher to support enlarging muscle mass and increasing blood volume
   c. Calcium intake increased by 400 mg—requires a 1- to 2-g calcium diet

L. Health monitoring during pregnancy
1. History, including medical, surgical, gynecologic, and obstetric data; family history of hereditary and transmittable diseases such as diabetes, tuberculosis, heart disease; presence of domestic violence
2. Physical examination of skin, thyroid, teeth, lungs, heart, and breasts; abdominal palpation; auscultation; height of fundus; vaginal examination; and pelvic evaluation (before last 4 weeks of pregnancy)

3. Cervical smears for gonorrhea and chlamydia; Papanicolaou test for cancer; wet prep for bacterial vaginosis because this is linked to preterm labor
4. BP; weight; and urinalysis for acetone, albumin, and glucose done at all visits
5. Blood specimens taken for typing, cross-matching, Rh factor, hematocrit, hemoglobin, serologic test for syphilis (repeated at 32 weeks), and rubella titer (a titer of 1:8 is considered immune)
6. Screening tests
   a. Screening for tuberculosis
   b. Tay-Sachs screening, particularly for Jewish women
   c. Sickle cell screening, particularly for black women
   d. Alpha-fetoprotein (AFP) testing for neural tube defects, Down syndrome, and other congenital anomalies at 14 to 16 weeks
   e. Serum glucose level testing for gestational diabetes at 26 to 28 weeks
   f. Group B streptococcus culture after 36 weeks
   g. Blood type and count, assessment of Rh factor, an antibody titer test, and/or indirect Coombs' test to determine hemolytic conditions (e.g., Rh incompatibility, ABO incompatibility)
   h. Screening to determine presence of cytomegalovirus, hepatitis B, HIV, parvovirus 19, rubella, toxoplasmosis, varicella-zoster virus
   i. Herpes cultures at first visit and at 36 weeks if woman or partner has a history of genital herpes
7. Weight monitored and compared with prepregnant levels
8. Routine sonogram scheduled to confirm gestational age and assess placenta, fetus, and amniotic fluid at 18 to 20 weeks; teach client to drink 1 to 2 quarts of water 1 hour before the test and not to void
9. Chorionic villi sampling or amniocentesis for women at high risk or 35 years or older to determine chromosomal or other abnormalities

Nursing Care During the Prenatal Period

A. Assessment/Analysis
   1. Initial visit
      a. Date of last menstrual period
      b. Personal, gynecologic, and family medical history; obstetric history using GTPAL system
         (1) Gravidity: number of conceptions
         (2) Term births: number of births between 37 and 40 weeks' gestation
         (3) Preterm births: number of births between 20 and 36 weeks' gestation
         (4) Abortions and miscarriages: number of spontaneous or induced terminations of pregnancy before 20 weeks' gestation
         (5) Living children: number of children alive at the time of assessment
      c. Physical examination: including baseline vital signs and weight
      d. Current nutritional status

      e. Pelvic examination: vaginal and rectal
      f. Understanding of pregnancy and related care
      g. Presence of multiple gestation
   2. Monthly and final weekly visits
      a. Weight, BP, pulse, respirations; signs of supine hypotension
      b. Signs of facial or digital edema
      c. Fundal height and size
      d. Fetal heart rate and fetal activity
      e. Testing for glucose, albumin, and ketones in urine

B. Planning/Implementation
   1. Assist the parents in understanding the anatomy and physiology of pregnancy, labor, and birth
   2. Teach mother about changes in nutritional needs and how to meet them; consider cultural and personal preferences; obtain a dietary history
   3. Teach mother to monitor for
      a. Visual disturbances; edema of face, fingers, or feet; persistent, severe headaches; epigastric pain; seizures
      b. Persistent, severe vomiting (hyperemesis gravidarum)
      c. Signs of infection; burning on urination
      d. Any vaginal discharge, including blood
      e. Abdominal pain
      f. Absence of or decrease in fetal movements after initial presence
      g. Signs and symptoms of preterm labor
   4. Teach mother about physiologic changes and related discomforts that occur during pregnancy (nausea, vomiting, backaches, varicosities, hemorrhoids, constipation, leg pain, etc.)
   5. Respond to mother's questions about bathing, douching, work, sex, exercise, etc.
   6. Help parents discuss and explore feelings related to childbearing and rearing
   7. Prepare mother for physical work of labor through the use of relaxation and breathing exercises for the various phases of labor
   8. Identify parents' situational support systems
   9. Prepare father for a coaching and supporting role during pregnancy, labor, and birth
   10. Introduce families to health facilities available for continued health care
   11. Teach mother to avoid alcohol, tobacco, contact with second-hand smoke (causes maternal and fetal vasoconstriction and thus intrauterine growth restriction), and certain herbs
   12. Discuss various childbirth preparation techniques such as Lamaze, Read, and Bradley
   13. Refer to preparatory classes, if appropriate
   14. Teach mother to avoid OTC or prescription drugs without checking with her care provider because many drugs (e.g., NSAIDs) considered harmless may be teratogenic to the developing fetus

15. Teach mother the importance of adequate fluid intake and moderate exercise to promote circulation and prevent stasis
16. Teach mother the importance of continuing breast self-examination throughout pregnancy
17. Assess for presence of domestic violence (partner answers questions for woman, injuries to breast/abdomen, multiple health care visits); follow up on findings to prevent damage to mother and fetus
18. Teach parents to notify practitioner when the membranes rupture and/or the contractions are 5 to 8 minutes apart

C. Evaluation/Outcomes
   1. Mother
      a. Keeps weight gain within recommended limits
      b. Abstains from alcohol, drugs, and tobacco
      c. Adjusts to physiologic changes associated with pregnancy
      d. Identifies signs of complications
      e. Attends childbirth classes with partner
   2. Fetus
      a. Survives intrauterine period
      b. Maintains growth and development within acceptable parameters

✿ INTRAPARTUM PERIOD (LABOR AND BIRTH)

Data Base

A. Labor: an involuntary physiologic process whereby the contents of the gravid uterus are expelled through the birth canal into the external environment
B. Anatomy of the bony pelvis
   1. Classification of pelvis: gynecoid (female pelvis), android (male pelvis), anthropoid, and platypelloid; true pelvis is bony inner pelvis through which the infant must pass
   2. Female pelvis has an ample pubic arch, curved sacrum, curved side walls, blunt ischial spines, and a movable coccyx
   3. Diameters: at inlet: true conjugate (anterior/posterior diameter), transverse (widest diameter at inlet), right and left oblique diameters; at outlet: conjugate diagonal (anterior/posterior is widest diameter), transverse (one ischial tuberosity to the other)
C. Attitude: relationship of fetal parts to each other
D. Lie: relationship of the long axis of the fetus to the long axis of the mother
E. Presentation: body part of fetus that engages in the true pelvis
   1. Cephalic (head): vertex, brow, or face
   2. Breech: frank, complete, on single or double footling
   3. Shoulder: fetus cannot travel through birth canal
F. Position: relationship of presenting parts to four quadrants of the mother's pelvis (the letters L and R are used for left and right; A and P for anterior and posterior; O for occiput; M for mentum or face; S for sacrum)

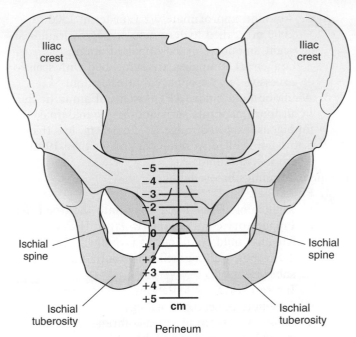

Figure 25-2 Stations of presenting part. (From Lowdermilk DL, Perry SE: *Maternity nursing*, ed 7, St Louis, 2006, Mosby.)

1. Vertex: occiput, LOA, LOP, ROA, ROP
2. Face: chin (mentum), LMA, LMP, RMA, RMP
3. Breech: sacrum, LSA, LSP, RSA, RSP
G. Station: relationship of presenting part to the false and true pelves
   1. Floating: presenting part movable above the true pelvic inlet
   2. Engaged: suboccipitobregmatic diameter fixed into the pelvic inlet
   3. Station 0: presenting part at level of the ischial spines; levels above spines −1, −2, −3; levels below spines +1, +2, +3 (Figure 25-2: Stations of presenting part)
H. Amniotic fluid: about 1000 mL of fluid in amniotic sac
   1. Spontaneous rupture of membranes (SROM or SRM): usually occurs in mid or late labor but can occur before labor begins
   2. Artificial rupture of membranes (amniotomy, AROM, or ARM): expedites labor by increasing dilation and effacement; should not be done until presenting part is engaged and against the cervix
   3. Nitrazine paper: may be used to confirm the presence of amniotic fluid; positive when pH is greater than 7.0; paper will turn color and result must be read against color code on nitrazine roll
   4. Assessment of amniotic fluid
      a. Color: strawlike and clear; may contain small particles of vernix caseosa; greenish color indicates meconium staining
      b. Odor: musky-smelling but nonoffensive; foul-smelling indicates infection (chorioamnionitis)
      c. Fern test: dried amniotic fluid on a slide examined under a microscope reveals a frondlike pattern

d. Amount: approximately 1 L at term; 1500 to 2000 mL called hydramnios or polyhydramnios; scant amount is called oligohydramnios; congenital anomalies are associated with scant or excessive (e.g., esophageal atresia) fluid

5. Amniotic fluid index (AFI): extent of amniotic fluid in all four quadrants surrounding the maternal umbilicus; expected range is 7 to 18 cm; less than 5 to 6 cm is oligohydramnios; greater than 19 to 22 cm is hydramnios

I. Clinical findings before labor
1. Physiologic
a. Lightening: fetus drops down into the true pelvis
b. Preparatory contractions (Braxton Hicks): irregular mild contractions in preparation for true labor; walking will help contractions to subside
c. Increased vaginal secretions
d. Softening of cervix (ripening)
e. Spontaneous rupture of membranes (SROM) can occur before or during labor
f. Bloody show: softening and effacement of cervix causes mucous plug to be expelled; this is accompanied by small blood loss; can occur before or during labor
2. Psychologic: mother shows signs of nesting (increased activity) caused by sudden rise in energy level (spurt of energy)

J. Clinical findings of true labor
1. Regular uterine contractions that increase in frequency, strength, and duration and do not disappear when lying down or walking around
2. Effacement (shortening or thinning of the cervix) and dilation of the cervix

K. Mechanisms of labor: rotation and descent of fetus in vertex presentation through true pelvis
1. Engagement, descent with flexion: at onset of labor, head descends and chin flexes on the chest
2. Internal rotation: as labor contractions and uterine forces move the fetus downward, the head internally rotates to pass through the ischial spines
3. Extension: occiput emerges under the symphysis pubis and the head is born by extension
4. External rotation: allows for rotation of shoulders to an anterior/posterior position
5. Expulsion: remainder of the body of the fetus is born

L. Stages of labor and maternal changes
1. First stage: from onset of true labor to complete effacement and dilation of cervix
a. Latent phase: mild, short contractions, cervix dilated 0 to 3 cm; mother excited and happy that labor has started, some apprehension; follows directions readily; walking assists labor process
b. Active phase: moderate to strong contractions about 5 minutes apart, cervix dilates from 4 to 7 cm, bloody show, membranes may rupture; slow, deep-breathing techniques help in relaxing; medication may be necessary for discomfort;

supportive measures help (e.g., encouragement, praise, reassurance, back pressure or back rubs, keeping the mother informed of progress, providing rest between contractions, presence of a supporting person); increasing difficulty in following directions
c. Transition phase: strong contractions 1 to 2 minutes apart (lasting 45 to 60 seconds or more with little rest in between); cervix dilates from 7 to 10 cm with an increased bloody show; mother becomes irritable, restless, agitated, emotional, belches, has leg tremors, perspires, pale white ring around mouth (circumoral pallor), flushed face, sudden nausea, and may vomit; feels need to have a bowel movement because of pressure on anus; may be unable to communicate or follow directions; requires emotional support
2. Second stage: beginning with full dilation of the cervix and ending with birth of the infant
a. Latent phase: may last up to 1 hour with decrease in strength and frequency of contractions and without an urge to push
b. Active phase: urge to push and stronger, closer contractions
c. Transition phase: begins with fetal head on perineum; perineum bulges, pushing with contractions, grunting sounds, behavior changes from great irritability to great involvement and work, sleep and relaxation occur between contractions, leg cramps are common
3. Third stage: after birth of the infant through expulsion of the placenta; placental separation (5 to 30 minutes) heralded by globular formation of uterus, lengthening of umbilical cord, and gush of blood; may have alteration in perineal structure either from episiotomy (prophylactic incision into perineum to allow for birth of head) or from laceration caused by rapid expulsion of presenting part
4. Fourth stage: following expulsion of placenta to 2 hours after birth; fundus firm in the midline, at or slightly above the umbilicus; bloody vaginal discharge (lochia rubra); fatigue, thirst, chills, nausea; excitement and intermittent dozing

M. Oxytocics
1. Description
a. Used to stimulate the uterus to contract
b. Used to induce labor; given slowly and in small doses during labor
c. Used to augment contractions that have already begun
d. Capable of inducing contraction of the lacteal glands, which aids in let-down reflex for breastfeeding
e. Exert vasopressor and antidiuretic effects
f. Used to control postpartum uterine atony; may be given rapidly

g. Oxytocics are available in parenteral (IM, IV), oral, and nasal preparations
2. Example: oxytocin (Pitocin, Syntocinon)
3. Major adverse side effects
  a. Maternal
    (1) Hypertension (contracture of smooth muscles of blood vessels)
    (2) Dysrhythmias; tachycardia (vasoconstriction)
    (3) Hypertonic uterus; uterine rupture
    (4) Water intoxication (antidiuretic effect)
    (5) Seizures and coma (water intoxication)
  b. Fetal
    (1) Anoxia; asphyxia (vasoconstriction)
    (2) Dysrhythmias (premature ventricular contractions [PVCs], bradycardia)
    (3) Hyperbilirubinemia (hepatic dysfunction)
4. Nursing care of clients receiving oxytocics
  a. Monitor client continuously
  b. Have O_2 and emergency resuscitative equipment available
  c. Use infusion-control device for IV administration; always given by secondary line
  d. Monitor uterine contractions; discontinue infusion if prolonged uterine contractions or inadequate uterine resting tone occur
  e. Assess BP and pulse every 30 to 60 minutes and with a dose increase
  f. Maintain fetal monitoring; assess uterine contractions and tone and fetal heart rate every 15 minutes

N. Prostaglandins
1. Description
  a. Used to stimulate the uterus to contract
  b. Used to ripen or soften the cervix
  c. Used to control postpartum uterine atony
  d. May be given orally, rectally, or vaginally
2. Examples: misoprostol (Cytotec), dinoprostone (Cervidil), carboprost (Hemabate); prostaglandin E_1 (PGE$_1$)
3. Major adverse side effects: maternal
  a. Hypertonic uterus, uterine rupture
  b. Nausea, vomiting, diarrhea, vasoconstriction; uncommon with all but PGE$_1$, and Hemabate
4. Nursing care of clients receiving prostaglandins
  a. Monitor client continuously, particularly uterine contractions
  b. Have oxygen and resuscitative equipment available
  c. Never administer Hemobate intravenously

O. Maternal analgesia and anesthesia
1. Opioid analgesics
  a. Meperidine hydrochloride (Demerol) IV, IM, epidural, or intrathecal during active labor; administration timed to allow metabolism and excretion of drug before birth to avoid respiratory depression in the newborn; naloxone (Narcan) used to counteract this respiratory depression

  b. Butorphanol (Stadol) IM; 30 to 40 times more potent than meperidine; does not interfere with labor; less neonatal depression
  c. Nalbuphine (Nubain) IV or IM; may precipitate withdrawal in clients with opioid addiction
  d. Fentanyl (Sublimaze) IV, IM, epidural, or intrathecal; 100 times more potent than meperidine; minimal respiratory depression in the newborn
2. Regional analgesia and anesthesia
  a. Epidural: may be used during labor, for anesthesia during a cesarean birth, and postcesarean anesthesia when abdomen is being closed
  b. Spinal: may be used for anesthesia during a cesarean birth; placed in the subarachnoid space; given in a single dose; may wear off before procedure is complete
  c. Combination intrathecal
  d. Pudendal: may be used during the second stage of labor
  e. Local infiltration: most frequently used to repair episiotomy
3. Nursing care of clients receiving anesthetic/analgesic agents
  a. Observe mother and newborn for respiratory depression if opioid analgesic is given; monitor mother for hypotension
  b. Epidural: monitor for maternal hypotension; if hypotension occurs, position client on left side, increase IV infusion, administer oxygen, and reassess fetal heart rate
  c. Pudendal: explain that it will eliminate discomfort of an episiotomy; assess for vaginal wall or perineal hematoma
  d. Spinal: monitor for headache that increases with head elevation; usually in first 24 to 72 hours; keep client supine

Nursing Care During the Intrapartum Period
A. Assessment/Analysis
1. Fetal heart rate and pattern
2. Age, weight, height, vital signs, allergies
3. Obstetric history; expected date of birth; intent to breastfeed or formula feed; prenatal care
4. Medical history
5. Time and type of last meal
6. Time of onset of contractions (beginning of one contraction to the beginning of the next contraction) and their frequency, duration, and intensity
7. Presence of bloody show; status of amniotic membrane
8. Leopold's maneuvers to determine fetal presentation, position, and station (see Figure 25-3: Leopold's maneuvers)
  a. A—Identifies fetal lie (longitudinal or transverse) and presentation (cephalic or breech)
  b. B—Identifies fetal presentation

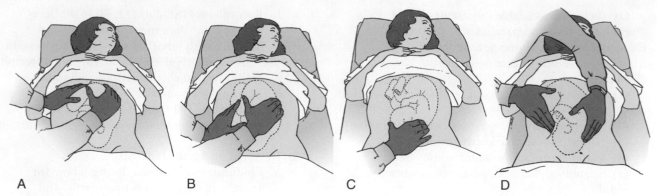

Figure 25-3 Leopold's maneuvers. (From Lowdermilk DL, Perry SE: *Maternity nursing*, ed 7, St Louis, 2006, Mosby.)

c. C—If the head is presenting and not engaged, determines attitude of the head (flexed or extended)

d. D—If the cephalic prominence is on the same side as the back, indicates that the presenting head is extended and the face is presenting

9. Factors that influence labor
   a. Power—contraction's expulsive effect
   b. Passenger—the newborn's size, position, and presentation
   c. Passageway—the maternal pelvis and soft tissue
   d. Position of the mother
   e. Psyche—the emotional energy and anxiety level of the mother side-lying, walking, sitting, semirecumbent, on hands and knee, and supine

10. Emotional response to labor; presence of support persons

B. Planning/Implementation
   1. First stage
      a. Orient to unit
      b. Time and assess contractions
      c. Assist with or perform vaginal examination
      d. Test urine for protein and glucose
      e. Assess bladder and bowel function
      f. Collect blood for CBC and cross-match
      g. Provide emotional support to mother and labor coach
      h. Monitor frequency, duration, and strength of contractions
         (1) Interpret data regarding uterine activity from fetal monitor
         (2) Observe for prolonged contractions if oxytocin is being administered
         (3) Encourage woman to limit movement to prevent interference with accurate tracings
      i. Monitor fetal heart rate (FHR) by auscultation, Doppler, internal or external fetal monitor (Figure 25-4: Areas of maximum intensity of fetal heart tones [FHTs] for different fetal positions); spiral scale electrode inserted clockwise and removed counterclockwise
      j. Interpret data of fetal monitoring (Figure 25-5: Display of FHR and uterine activity on monitor paper)

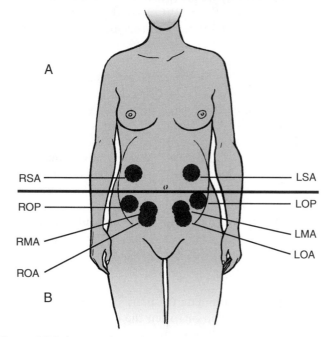

Figure 25-4 Areas of maximum intensity of fetal heart tones (FHTs) for different fetal positions. **A,** Presentation is usually breech if FHTs are heard above the umbilicus. **B,** Presentation is usually vertex if FHTs are heard below the umbilicus. *RSA,* Right sacrum anterior; *ROP,* right occipitoposterior; *RMA,* right mentum anterior; *ROA,* right occipitoanterior; *LSA,* left sacrum anterior; *LOP,* left occipitoposterior; *LMA,* left mentum anterior; *LOA,* left occipitoanterior. (From Lowdermilk DL, Perry SE: *Maternity nursing,* ed 7, St Louis, 2006, Mosby.)

(1) Baseline FHR: FHR between uterine contractions is usually 110 to 160 beats/min
(2) Periodic changes are changes that occur in relation to contractions
(3) Episodic changes do not occur in relation to contractions, including accelerations and decelerations
(4) Tachycardia: FHR above 160 beats/min lasting over 10 minutes
   (a) May result from fetal hypoxia, maternal fever or dehydration, and drugs such as atropine, Vistaril, ritodrine, and terbutaline

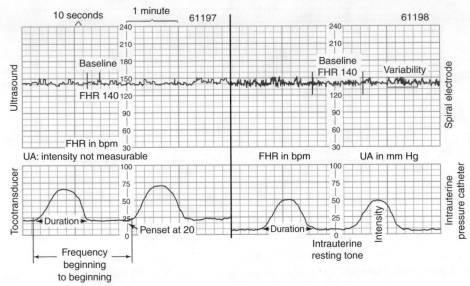

Figure 25-5 Display of fetal heart rate and uterine activity on monitor paper. (From Tucker SM, Miller LA, Miller DA: *Mosby's pocket guide to fetal monitoring*, ed 6, St. Louis, 2009, Mosby.)

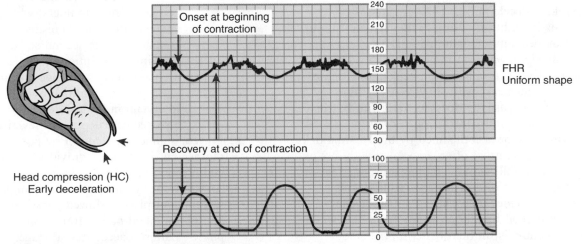

Figure 25-6 Early decelerations. (From Tucker SM, Miller LA, Miller DA: *Mosby's pocket guide to fetal monitoring*, ed 6, St. Louis, 2009, Mosby.)

 (b) Reduce underlying cause: lower maternal fever; increase maternal fluids; monitor for amnionitis

(5) Accelerations: increase in FHR of 15 beats/min lasting 15 seconds

(6) Bradycardia: FHR below 110 beats/min lasting longer than 10 minutes

 (a) May be caused by fetal hypoxia as a result of anesthetics, maternal hypotension, prolonged umbilical cord compression, or analgesics

 (b) Reduce underlying cause: reposition mother on side, assess for prolapsed cord, position mother to relieve pressure on cord, elevate mother's lower extremities, administer O_2

(7) Variability

 (a) Expected irregularity of cardiac rhythm (balance between sympathetic and parasympathetic divisions of autonomic nervous system); manifested by cyclic fluctuations of FHR; classified as absent, minimal, moderate, or marked

 (b) Absence of these fluctuations is indicative of fetal CNS depression; associated with opiates and barbiturates, fetal hypoxia, acidosis, immaturity

 (c) Reduce underlying cause: administer oxygen, reposition mother on side, increase blood volume by IV or oral fluids, turn off oxytocin

(8) Early decelerations: FHR decreases, usually not below 100 beats/min (Figure 25-6: Early decelerations)

 (a) Occur early in contraction phase, before peak, and end before uterus returns to resting tone

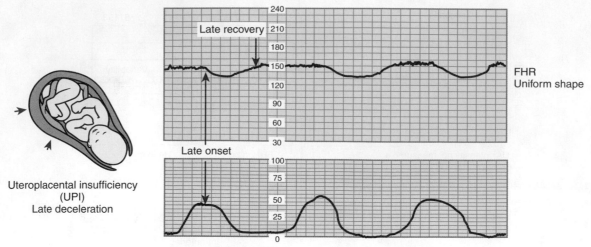

Figure 25-7 Late decelerations. (From Tucker SM, Miller LA, Miller DA: *Mosby's pocket guide to fetal monitoring*, ed 6, St. Louis, 2009, Mosby.)

(b) Indicates head compression; no nursing intervention needed

(9) Late decelerations: FHR may be very shallow, but if severe FHR may decrease to 60 beats/min (Figure 25-7: Late decelerations)

   (a) Occur as contraction peaks; lowest rate after peak; with slow recovery time; FHR usually does not return to baseline until after contraction ends

   (b) May be accompanied by bradycardia or tachycardia; often associated with loss of variability and is ominous if persistent or related to decreased variability

   (c) Indicates uteroplacental insufficiency caused by uterine tetany from oxytocin administration; postterm pregnancy; maternal supine hypotension; regional anesthesia; hypertensive disorders; diabetes mellitus; or other chronic maternal disorders; may also be associated with intrauterine growth restriction

   (d) Nursing intervention includes discontinuing oxytocin if being administered, positioning mother on left side, administering O_2 by mask at 8 to 10 L/min, increasing rate of IV fluids, assisting with fetal blood sampling, preparing for birth if there is no improvement

(10) Variable decelerations: abrupt transitory decrease in FHR that is variable in duration, intensity, and time in relation to contractions; FHR decreases at least 15 beats below baseline, lasts at least 15 seconds, and returns to baseline within 2 minutes of start (Figure 25-8: Variable decelerations)

   (a) Related to umbilical cord compression; sometimes preceded and followed by accelerations (shoulders) which are compensatory mechanisms; most common during second stage

   (b) Nursing intervention: if they occur during second stage, discourage pushing with every contraction to allow for recovery; intervention for late decelerations may also decrease depth and severity

k. Prevent supine hypotension by positioning mother on side to keep gravid uterus from compressing vena cava

l. Assist mother with breathing techniques (first stage: latent phase—slowed-paced; active phase—modified-paced; transition phase—pattern-paced; second stage: any rhythmic breathing that enhances relaxation) and rebreathing techniques to correct and prevent hyperventilation

m. Use measures to promote comfort and rest by explaining procedures and equipment, providing warmth, and administering analgesics or anesthesia; may use opioid analgesics such as butorphanol (Stadol), nalbuphine (Nubain), or fentanyl (Sublimaze); epidural or intrathecal opiate as ordered, except late in labor (less than 2 hours before birth) to prevent fetal depression

   (1) Encourage use of relaxation techniques and positions learned in childbirth classes; recognize maternal movements will be restricted with external fetal monitor; support and encourage mother and coach

   (2) Carefully monitor vital signs during administration of regional anesthesia

   (3) Have an opioid agonist such as Narcan readily available

n. Observe perineum for bloody show and appearance of amniotic fluid (indicates ruptured

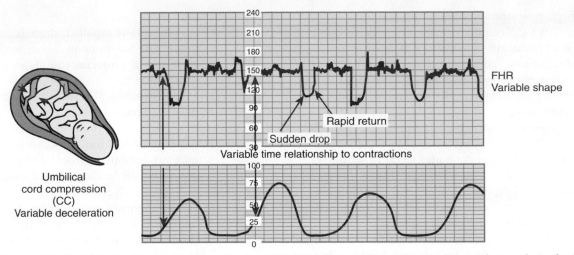

240
210
180
150
120
90
60
30

FHR
Variable shape

Rapid return
Sudden drop
Variable time relationship to contractions

100
75
50
25
0

Umbilical
cord compression
(CC)
Variable deceleration

Figure 25-8 Variable decelerations. (From Tucker SM, Miller LA, Miller DA: *Mosby's pocket guide to fetal monitoring*, ed 6, St. Louis, 2009, Mosby.)

membranes); note amount, color (if greenish, check for breech position and obtain fetal heart rate), and odor (if foul may indicate amnionitis)

o. Assess FHR following spontaneous rupture of membranes or amniotomy (AROM); assess for presence of prolapsed cord

p. Monitor for
  (1) Prolonged strong contractions; may indicate tetanic uterus
  (2) Taut, boardlike abdomen; may indicate abruptio placentae
  (3) Increase in pulse and temperature; may indicate infection
  (4) Hypertension; may indicate preeclampsia
  (5) Hypotension; may occur following epidural or spinal anesthesia
  (6) Bright red vaginal bleeding; may indicate placenta previa
  (7) Meconium-stained amniotic fluid; may indicate breech position or may be a late sign of fetal compromise
  (8) Abnormal variations in FHR patterns; may indicate a compromised fetus

q. Decrease maternal oral intake as second stage of labor approaches because vomiting often occurs

2. Second stage
a. Allow mother to choose pushing and positioning techniques, especially if she is unmedicated. Assist mother if pushing is ineffective; transfer to birthing room or prepare birthing bed when perineum bulges with contractions
b. If mother's legs are to be put in stirrups, position legs simultaneously to avoid trauma to uterine ligaments
c. Monitor FHR every 5 minutes
d. Assist with anesthesia, which could include pudendal block, saddle block, or local infiltration

3. Third stage
a. Care of newborn
  (1) Clear airway of mucus

  (2) Use Apgar scoring at 1 and 5 minutes after birth to determine respiratory effort and physical status (Table 27-1: Apgar Score)
  (3) Maintain body heat; mother-newborn skin to skin positioning is most effective; dry infant
  (4) Assess for visible anomalies
  (5) Allow parents to see newborn; place on maternal abdomen to enhance breastfeeding and begin bonding process
  (6) Administer antibiotic ophthalmic medication into each eye to prevent ophthalmia neonatorum and vitamin K injection to prevent hemorrhagic disorders
  (7) Apply identification bracelets to mother and infant (some facilities include father and significant others) before leaving birthing area according to institutional protocol
b. Assist with birth of placenta
c. Promote attachment
d. Provide support for parents if infant has an abnormality
e. Record birth and accompanying events

4. Fourth stage
a. Palpate fundus at least every 15 minutes for firmness and height in relation to umbilicus; if relaxed and bladder is not distended, massage until firm; fundus should be 2 cm below the umbilicus after third stage of labor immediately after birth; 1 hour after birth it rises to about the level of the umbilicus
b. Check for bladder distention (uterus above umbilicus and dextroverted); encourage voiding because uterus is unable to contract in the presence of a full bladder and the client may hemorrhage
c. Check perineum for vaginal and suture line bleeding; count vaginal pads; assess for concurrent uterine relaxation; massage uterus

d. Check episiotomy or laceration site for hematoma, bleeding, or edema; apply ice bag to perineum immediately after birth to reduce edema; perineal ecchymosis and perineal/rectal pressure indicate vaginal hematoma

e. Monitor temperature, BP, and pulse; report fluctuations

f. Administer oxytocic medication as ordered; after birth, an oxytocic may be administered immediately to enhance uterine contraction

g. Shivering is common after birth (exact cause unknown); keeping the client warm diminishes the sensation of chilling, which may be caused by air-conditioned birthing room

h. Provide fluid and food as tolerated

i. Encourage and teach breastfeeding within first hour of birth

C. Evaluation/Outcomes

1. Mother

a. Progresses through labor that culminates in safe birth

b. Remains free of infection

c. Maintains homeostasis

2. Newborn

a. Establishes airway, and respiratory effort sustains life without assistance

b. Achieves an Apgar score of 7 or above at 5 minutes after birth

c. Successful first breastfeeding attempt

✿ POSTPARTUM PERIOD

Data Base

A. Puerperium: 6-week period following birth in which reproductive organs undergo physical and physiologic changes, a process called involution; because of the many physiologic and psychologic stresses of the postpartum period, there is a trend to increase this period to 3 months following birth and call it the fourth trimester of pregnancy

B. Systemic changes during the puerperium

1. Reproductive system

a. Uterus: contractions bring about involution, afterpains in multiparas may cause discomfort, necessitating analgesics; oxytocin release during breastfeeding enhances involution; involution follows a one-fingerbreadth descent daily; by the seventh to ninth day, fundus cannot be felt

b. Lochia: vaginal flow following birth changes from rubra to serosa, then becomes alba

c. Vagina practically returns to its prepregnant state through healing of soft tissue and cicatrization

d. Menstruation occurs about 6 weeks after birth in nonnursing mothers and up to 24 weeks in nursing mothers but timing varies

e. Abdominal wall is soft and flabby but eventually regains tone; diastasis recti (separation of abdominal muscles) may be present

f. Breasts

(1) As placenta is expelled, there is activation of luteinizing hormone in the anterior pituitary; secretion of prolactin stimulates milk production

(2) In breastfeeding mothers, the posterior pituitary secretes oxytocin that initiates the let-down reflex with milk ejection as infant suckles

(3) Absence of suckling at breast in nonnursing mothers inhibits oxytocin and prolactin secretion; the let-down reflex diminishes, and milk production is inhibited

(4) Breast engorgement occurs in both nursing and nonnursing mothers on the second or third day because of vasodilation before lactation

2. Digestive system

a. Following birth clients are hungry and thirsty; if general anesthesia was not administered during birth, clients can be given oral nourishment

b. Proteins and calories are added to replenish those lost during labor and involution

c. Fiber, fluid, and exercise relieve constipation and distention

d. Bowel movements usually do not occur for several days, probably because of fear of pain from hemorrhoids and/or episiotomy and decreased food intake during labor; stool softeners may be prescribed and, if unsuccessful, suppositories or an enema may be ordered

3. Circulatory system

a. Blood volume usually returns to prepregnant state by the third week after birth

b. Blood fibrinogen levels and platelets increase during the first week; this may lead to thrombus formation; if deep vein thrombosis develops, heparin followed by warfarin (Coumadin) may be administered

c. Leukocytosis occurs; may be as high as $30,000/mm^3$ if labor was lengthy

d. Hemoglobin and red blood cell count decrease on fourth postpartum day

4. Excretory system

a. Urinary output increases (diuresis) from second to fifth postpartum day

b. Diminished bladder tone that occurred during pregnancy may result in small, frequent voidings indicating retention with overflow

c. Activation of lactogenic hormone may result in lactose in the urine

d. Excretion of nitrogen increases as involution occurs

5. Integumentary system

a. Profuse diaphoresis occurs as wastes are being excreted

b. Pigmentational changes such as striae, linea nigra, and darkened areolae begin to fade but do not completely return to nulliparous state

6. Vital signs
   a. Temperature elevation (not above 100.4° F) up to 24 hours after birth is a result of exertion and dehydration
   b. Blood pressure returns to baseline; drop suggests hemorrhage; elevation suggests gestational hypertension
   c. Pulse rate drops slightly because of decreased cardiac effort; blood volume decreases
7. Emotional needs
   a. Mother may experience emotional lability, exhibiting irritability, restlessness, and anxiety (postpartum blues); generally occurs on the third to tenth days after birth
   b. Mother may experience depression without psychotic features (postpartum depression); usually begins by fourth week after birth or within the first year after birth
   c. Mother may experience depression with psychotic features (postpartum psychosis); usually begins by second week after birth; often there is a history of a psychiatric disorder (e.g., bipolar disorder)

Nursing Care During the Postpartum Period

A. Assessment/Analysis (BUBBLE–HE)
   1. **B**reasts—soft, filling, engorged
   2. **U**terus—fundus firm, midline, level in relationship to umbilicus
   3. **B**owel—bowel sounds, stool
   4. **B**ladder—voiding without difficulty
   5. **L**ochia
      a. Color
         (1) Rubra: 1 to 3 days
         (2) Serosa: 4 to 10 days
         (3) Alba: 10 to 21 days
      b. Amount (pad in use less than 2 hours)
         (1) Scant: less than 1 inch
         (2) Light: less than 4 inches
         (3) Moderate: less than 6 inches
         (4) Heavy: more than 6 inches
   6. **E**pisiotomy/incision—assess for redness, edema, ecchymosis, discharge, and approximation (REEDA)
   7. **H**omans' sign/hemorrhoids
   8. **E**motional response—interaction/attachment to infant, taking-in/taking-hold, signs of postpartum blues
B. Planning/Implementation
   1. Use standard precautions and aseptic technique when giving perineal care
   2. Teach mother and assist mother with self-care
   3. Teach mother breast care; inspect breasts for tissue and nipple breakdown, palpate to rule out growths (teach breast self-examination for continued health), recommend well-fitted brassiere to support breasts, and (if ordered) apply ice compresses or cool cabbage leaves to the breasts to minimize engorgement

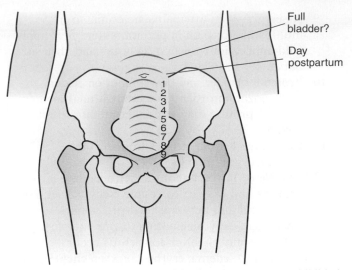

Figure 25-9 Assessment of involution of uterus after childbirth. (From Lowdermilk DL, Perry SE: *Maternity nursing*, ed 7, St Louis, 2006, Mosby.)

4. Teach the importance of handwashing when caring for self and infant
5. Observe vital signs: a temperature above 100.4° F (38° C) for 2 consecutive days (excluding first 24 hours after birth) considered sign of beginning puerperal infection, which can occur following hemorrhage or trauma; bradycardia is an expected phenomenon after birth; if infection is suspected, the practitioner will probably order a culture of lochia, antibiotics, antipyretics, and diagnostic studies
6. Palpate fundus for firmness and location (Figure 25-9: Assessment of involution of uterus after childbirth); 24 hours after birth the fundus usually is midline at the level of the umbilicus; the fundus descends (involutes) 1 fingerbreadth (1 to 2 cm) per day; a boggy fundus indicates inadequate contractile power of uterus and results in bleeding; check for full bladder, which displaces the fundus upward and to the right
7. Administer oxytocic medication as ordered to promote involution
   a. Examples
      (1) Oxytocin (Pitocin)
      (2) Methylergonovine maleate (Methergine)
      (3) Ergonovine maleate (Ergotrate)
      (4) Prostaglandin F_{2a} (Hemabate)
   b. Oxytocics maintain the uterus in a contracted state that controls bleeding from intrauterine sites and maintains tone, rate, and amplitude of rhythmic contractions required for involution; Methergine and Ergotrate may cause hypertension; withhold if blood pressure is higher than 140/90 mm Hg
8. Check lochia for color, amount, clots, odor (foul odor indicates beginning infection); observe episiotomy suture line, if present, for redness, ecchymosis, edema, discharge, and approximation (REEDA)

9. Assess for pain; afterpains are common in multiparas; for pain in perineal suture line, apply cold applications for first 24 hours and then sitz baths
10. Promote bladder and bowel function; secure catheterization order if the client is unable to void; profuse diaphoresis should not affect voiding
11. Encourage Kegel exercises to strengthen pubococcygeal muscles
12. Provide or instruct about a diet adequate in proteins and calories to restore body tissues; build on cultural and personal food preferences
13. Encourage early ambulation to prevent blood stasis; if signs of thrombophlebitis occur (discomfort, edema, erythema), keep client on bed rest and notify practitioner
14. Monitor laboratory reports for hemoglobin, hematocrit, and WBC count
15. Observe for postpartum blues, which may be caused by a drop in hormonal levels and psychologic factors; if discharged early, mother and support persons should be alerted to signs and symptoms; mothers with a history of depression are more likely to have postpartum depression

16. Meet the mother's needs to enable her to meet the infant's needs; explore feelings and concerns
17. Assist the mother with care of the infant as needed; support rooming in
18. Provide for group discussion on breastfeeding, infant care, etc.
19. Discuss resumption of intercourse and family planning; include information about when to expect menses
20. If Rh-negative mother, assess need for administration of RhoGAM and administer if ordered
21. Give rubella vaccine if indicated
22. Provide instructions to contact personnel when questions arise
23. Involve family in care and teaching

C. Evaluation/Outcomes
1. Progresses through process of involution
2. Remains free from hemorrhage, infection, and pain
3. Maintains bowel function
4. Initiates voiding and empties bladder
5. Performs perineal care after each voiding and defecation, as taught
6. Successfully feeds and cares for infant
7. Maintains emotional health

CHAPTER

26 Nursing Care of Women at Risk During Pregnancy, Labor, Childbirth, and the Postpartum Period

IDENTIFYING AND/OR MONITORING HIGH-RISK PREGNANCY

A. Alpha-fetoprotein (AFP) enzyme blood test: elevated levels may identify the pregnant woman carrying a fetus with neural tube defects (spina bifida and anencephaly); may indicate a multiple pregnancy; if AFP measurement is elevated for two samples, it is followed by ultrasonography and amniocentesis for further confirmation; done at 14 to 16 weeks' gestation

B. Ultrasonography (sonogram): high-frequency sound-wave testing; discerns multiple pregnancy, placental location, and gestational age by measurement of biparietal diameters; may be performed to assess formation of organs
   1. Visualization during first 20 weeks' gestation is improved if the bladder is full; a full bladder is not necessary after 20 weeks' gestation
   2. Nursing care: encourage fluids and teach to refrain from voiding before the test

C. Chorionic villi sampling (CVS): supplies same chromosomal data as amniocentesis but can be done earlier
   1. Aspiration of villi done during the 10th to 12th week of pregnancy
   2. Nursing care: instruct to drink fluid so that bladder is full; after test monitor for uterine contractions and vaginal discharge; teach to observe for signs of infection

D. Amniocentesis: aspiration of amniotic fluid used to detect gender, chromosomal or biochemical defects, fetal age at 12 to 15 weeks' gestation; lecithin to sphingomyelin (L/S) ratio (2:1 ratio indicates lung maturity), increased bilirubin level (associated with Rh incompatibility), and phosphatidylglycerol (PG), which appears in amniotic fluid after 35th week (indicating fetal lung maturity)
   1. Test done with sonogram
   2. Nursing care: have client void; after test monitor for uterine contractions, vaginal discharge; assess fetal heart rate; teach to observe for signs of infection; encourage rest

E. Nonstress test (NST): to observe for accelerations of fetal heart rate (FHR) in response to fetal movement over a 30- to 40-minute period

1. Classification of results
   a. A test is reactive if
      (1) Baseline FHR is 110 to 160 beats/min
      (2) There are two accelerations in 10 minutes, each increasing the FHR by 15 beats/min and lasting 15 seconds
   b. Test is nonreactive if the above criteria are not met
   c. Unsatisfactory: recording uninterpretable; repeat test in 24 hours
2. Nursing care: fasting is not necessary; observe fetal monitor; explain test to decrease anxiety; evaluate response to procedure

F. Contraction stress test (CST): to demonstrate whether a healthy fetus can withstand a decreased oxygen supply during the stress of a contraction produced by exogenous oxytocin or stimulation of nipples manually or by moist heat; if late decelerations appear, the fetus may be compromised because of uteroplacental insufficiency
   1. Classification of results
      a. Negative: no late decelerations with a minimum of three contractions in 10 minutes; indicates that the fetus should be able to survive labor
      b. Positive: repetitive late decelerations occurring with more than half the contractions; indicates consideration of early intervention
      c. Suspicious: late decelerations occurring in less than half of uterine contractions; test should be repeated in 24 hours
   2. Nursing care: void before test; monitor fetal heart rate for 30 minutes before test; monitor mother after test to observe for possible initiation of labor; evaluate response to procedure

G. Biophysical profile (BPP): assesses breathing movements, gross body movements, tone, amniotic fluid volume, and FHR reactivity during NST; a score of 2 is assigned to each finding, with a score of 8 to 10 indicating a healthy fetus (similar to Apgar scoring)
   1. Used for fetus who may be compromised
   2. Nursing care: provide emotional support; evaluate response to procedure

H. Maternal assessment of fetal activity: need to contact practitioner when there are fewer than 10 fetal movements in a 12-hour period, fewer than 3 fetal

movements in an 8-hour period, or no fetal movements in the morning
1. Used to determine vitality of fetus
2. Nursing care: teach how to record and report movements
I. Fetal scalp pH sampling: may be done during labor when fetal heart patterns begin to become nonreassuring; capillary blood samples are taken from fetal scalp in utero
1. Results: if acidosis is present, immediate birth is indicated
2. Nursing care: cleanse vaginal area to avoid contamination during test
J. Fetal acoustic stimulation test (FAST) or vibroacoustic stimulation test (VST): fetal heart baseline is measured; a buzzing (FAST) or vibration (VST) is created over the head of fetus through the maternal abdomen for 1-second and 1-minute intervals for 5 minutes
1. A reactive test occurs when an acceleration occurs
2. Test is noninvasive
K. Digital stimulation is the application of pressure to the fetal head during a vaginal examination to elicit acceleration; it is reactive if an acceleration occurs saturation of fetus
L. Fetal O_2 saturation monitoring provides continuous monitoring of O_2

PREGNANT WOMEN WITH SPECIAL NEEDS

THE PREGNANT ADOLESCENT

Data Base
A. High-risk pregnancy because
1. Physical development is not yet completed; bone growth may be incomplete and increased levels of estrogen may close epiphysis
2. Preeclampsia is a common complication because of poorly developed vascular system of placenta and possible inadequate adolescent nutrition
3. Developmental tasks of adolescence have not been fulfilled
4. Emotional maturity has not been achieved
B. Factors contributing to the incidence of adolescent pregnancy
1. Inadequate coping mechanisms
2. Need to enhance self-concept
3. Belief in own invulnerability
4. Need for immediate gratification; the present, not the future, is the focus; lack of concern for long-term consequences
5. Immature search for attention, closeness, and/or idealized or idolized love
6. Lack of knowledge about conception or contraception
7. Sexual acting out; indulgence in risk-taking behavior
8. Increase in dysfunctional families; change in morality and family life

Nursing Care of Pregnant Adolescents
A. Assessment/Analysis
1. Personal and family health; menstrual history
2. Developmental level
3. Support system; financial status
4. Potential role of infant's father
5. Attitude toward pregnancy (e.g., denial, ambivalence); understanding of responsibility of pregnancy and motherhood
B. Planning/Implementation
1. Gain trust of adolescent
2. Refer to appropriate agencies and resources
3. Promote problem-solving abilities
4. Involve father, if desired by the adolescent
5. Provide prenatal education; encourage consistent prenatal care
6. See Chapter 25: Nursing Care of Women During Uncomplicated Pregnancy, Labor, Childbirth, and the Postpartum Period
C. Evaluation/Outcomes
1. Arrives at decisions regarding the pregnancy
2. Keeps prenatal appointments and attends child-care classes
3. Involves significant others in planning concerning pregnancy and the future

THE OLDER PREGNANT WOMAN (35 YEARS OF AGE OR OLDER)

Data Base
A. High risk because
1. Increased chance of chromosomal abnormalities
2. Preexisting medical conditions
3. Increased chance of multiple gestation secondary to fertility drug use
4. Increased risk for spontaneous abortions and preterm labor
5. Emotional concerns related to changes in role, job, income, and child-care issues

Nursing Care of Older Pregnant Women
A. Assessment/Analysis
1. Personal and family health history
2. Genetic history, counseling, and testing
3. Nutritional status
4. Use of medications and drugs
5. History of fibroids
B. Planning/Implementation
1. Refer for genetic counseling
2. Provide prenatal care with an emphasis on preexisting conditions and immunizations
3. Allow for verbalization of plans regarding work, changing responsibilities, and altered lifestyle
C. Evaluation/Outcomes
1. Expresses feelings regarding expectations of body changes
2. Uses appropriate agencies for risk assessment

3. Makes appropriate plans for role change during pregnancy and after birth

THE WOMAN WITH A MULTIFETAL PREGNANCY

Data Base

A. Multiple gestation has increased 55% since 1980 in the United States, because of higher incidence of fertility drug use

B. Elective fetal reduction may be suggested when the risk for fetal death is great

C. Women with multiple gestation are at high risk for developing preterm labor, gestational hypertension, hyperemesis gravidarum, iron or folate anemia, dystocia; twin to twin transfusion, postpartum uterine atony; perinatal mortality is 2 to 3 times greater than in single gestations

D. Fetuses are at high risk for congenital anomalies and intrauterine growth restriction (IUGR)

E. Monozygotic (identical) twins develop from one fertilized ovum and are the same gender; race, heredity, parity, and maternal age have no influence on incidence

F. Dizygotic (fraternal) twins develop from separate ova that are fertilized by different sperm; they may be the same or different genders; familial; increased incidence in African-American women, women with increased parity, and women with pregnancy occurring before 35 years of age

Nursing Care of Women With a Multifetal Pregnancy

See Nursing Care of Women With Premature Rupture of Membranes and Nursing Care of Women During Preterm Labor

PREGNANT WOMEN WITH PREEXISTING HEALTH PROBLEMS

HEART DISEASE

Data Base

A. Origin: 50% had rheumatic fever (incidence expected to decrease as incidence of rheumatic fever decreases); congenital and mitral valve disorders are next most common

B. Hemodynamics of pregnancy that adversely affect the client with heart disease
1. O_2 consumption increased 10% to 20%; related to needs of growing fetus
2. Plasma level and blood volume increase; RBCs remain the same (physiologic anemia)
3. Peak cardiac output is reached around 28 weeks
4. After birth, extravascular fluid shifts into the intravascular compartment, increasing the work load of the heart

C. Functional or therapeutic classification of heart disease during pregnancy

1. Class I: no limitation of physical activity; no symptoms of cardiac insufficiency or angina
2. Class II: slight limitation of physical activity; may experience excessive fatigue, palpitation, angina, or dyspnea; slight limitations as indicated
3. Class III: moderate to marked limitation of physical activity; dyspnea, angina, and fatigue occur with slight activity, and bed rest is indicated during most of pregnancy
4. Class IV: marked limitation of physical activity; angina, dyspnea, and discomfort occur at rest; pregnancy should be avoided; indication for termination of pregnancy

Nursing Care of Pregnant Women With Heart Disease

A. Assessment/Analysis
1. Prenatal period: vital signs; weight gain; dietary patterns; emotional outlook; knowledge about self-care; signs of heart failure; stress factors such as work, household duties; drug regimen
2. Intrapartum period: vital signs (heart rate will increase); respiratory changes (dyspnea, coughing, or crackles); FHR patterns
3. Postpartum period: signs of heart failure or hemorrhage related to fluid shifts; I&O

B. Planning/Implementation
1. Prenatal period
   a. Teach importance of rest and avoidance of stress
   b. Instruct regarding use of elastic stockings and periodic elevation of legs
   c. Teach importance of continued medical supervision by cardiologist
   d. Teach appropriate dietary intake: adequate calories to ensure appropriate, but not excessive, weight gain; limited, not restricted, sodium intake (2.5 g/day)
   e. Administer medications as ordered: heparin, furosemide (Lasix), digitalis, beta blockers; antidysrhythmics
   f. Monitor for signs of heart failure, such as respiratory distress and tachycardia; may be precipitated by severe anemia; accelerated heart rate of mother in latter half of pregnancy puts extra workload on her heart
2. Intrapartum period
   a. Encourage mother to remain in semi-Fowler's or left-lateral position
   b. Provide continuous cardiac monitoring
   c. Provide electronic fetal monitoring
   d. Assist mother to cope with discomfort; regional analgesia is usually used
   e. Assist with birth (e.g., use of forceps or vacuum extraction) in second stage of labor to avoid work of pushing
   f. Monitor for signs of heart failure, such as respiratory distress and tachycardia

3. Postpartum period: most critical time because of increased circulating blood volume after birth of placenta
   a. Institute early ambulation schedule; apply elastic stockings
   b. Monitor for signs of heart failure, such as respiratory distress and tachycardia
   c. Monitor heart rate
   d. Provide for adequate rest; the increase in oxygen consumption with contractions during labor makes length of labor a significant factor
   e. Provide close supervision; sudden tachycardia during birth or sudden bradycardia along with increased cardiac output after birth may cause cardiac arrest
   f. Administer prescribed prophylactic antibiotics to mother with history of rheumatic fever
   g. Refer to various agencies for family support on discharge, if necessary
   h. Determine newborn risks, which include IUGR, preterm birth, and hypoxia

C. Evaluation/Outcomes
1. Gives birth to healthy infant
2. Maintains cardiac status within acceptable limits
3. Uses resources to obtain help in the home

DIABETES MELLITUS

Data Base

A. Physiology of pregnancy that affects woman with diabetes
1. Vomiting during pregnancy, especially in the first trimester, decreases carbohydrate intake with resulting acidosis
2. Human placental lactogen decreases insulin response; maternal sparing of glucose, and more oxidation of fats occurs to provide fetal nourishment; this leads to a greater need for insulin; although insulin production increases, resistance to insulin also increases because of the presence of placental lactogen; thus more exogenous insulin is required to maintain an acceptable serum glucose level, especially in the latter part of pregnancy
3. Elevated basal metabolic rate and decrease in CO_2 combining power increase tendency toward acidosis
4. The lower renal threshold for glucose can result in glucosuria
5. Muscular activity during labor depletes glycogen; therefore carbohydrate intake must be increased
6. During the postpartum period agonists are removed, hypoglycemia is common as involution and lactation occur and thus insulin needs decrease

B. Diabetes mellitus during pregnancy may be
1. Pregestational
   a. Type 1 diabetes: complications include retinopathy, neuropathy, and coronary artery disease
   b. Type 2 diabetes: complications may include retinopathy, neuropathy, and coronary artery disease, but women with type 1 diabetes are at greater risk
2. Gestational
   a. Controlled by diet
   b. Insulin required in 20% of women

C. Hazards of diabetes during pregnancy
1. Often a history of anomalies, stillbirths, and fetal deaths
2. Newborns are excessively large, weighing over 4000 g (macrosomia), if client does not remain euglycemic because of increased glucose utilization, increased fat synthesis and deposition, and the presence of pituitary growth hormone and somatotropin
3. Neonatal deaths occur as a result of hypoxia, hypoglycemia, congenital anomalies, and preterm labor
4. Hypertensive disorders and hydramnios are common
5. Insulin needs vary throughout pregnancy; frequent adjustments of insulin dosage required; oral hypoglycemics are contraindicated
6. Frequent hospitalization may be necessary during prenatal period
7. Cesarean birth may be necessary

Nursing Care of Pregnant Women With Diabetes Mellitus

A. Assessment/Analysis
1. Length of time client has had diabetes mellitus; type of diabetes—1 or 2
2. Dietary patterns
3. Signs of infection
4. Glucola screening test, blood glucose level, glucose tolerance test results; glycosylated hemoglobin A_{1c} level
5. Understanding of disease in relation to pregnancy
6. Presence of support persons

B. Planning/Implementation
1. Care of mother
   a. Encourage preconception counseling and early medical and prenatal supervision
   b. Teach and encourage adherence to dietary and insulin regimens
   c. Teach signs and symptoms of hyperglycemia (acidosis) and hypoglycemia (insulin reaction)
   d. Teach blood glucose testing, insulin administration, and record keeping
   e. Reinforce need for various tests for fetal well-being, such as ultrasound, stress and nonstress tests, biophysical profile, and amniocentesis for phosphatidylglycerol levels and L/S ratio
   f. Prepare client for hospitalization, induction of labor, or cesarean birth if indicated
   g. Continue monitoring for fluid and electrolyte balance and ketoacidosis during intrapartum and postpartum periods

h. Monitor glucose levels for the first 48 postpartum hours; women who were not insulin-dependent before pregnancy probably will not require it after they give birth
2. Care of neonate
   a. Admit to neonatal intensive care unit if necessary
   b. Keep warm because of inadequate temperature control mechanisms
   c. Observe respirations (stomach aspiration performed at time of birth, because hydramnios inflates stomach, which rises and interferes with diaphragm)
   d. Assess heel-stick blood specimen for glucose level because neonate continues to secrete excessive insulin and frequently becomes hypoglycemic; observe for signs of hypoglycemia and hypocalcemia such as lethargy, poor sucking reflex, cyanosis, or muscular twitching/tremors; decreased blood glucose level (30 to 45 mg/dL)
   e. Provide glucose water feeding to prevent acidosis (with poor sucking reflex, glucose should be given parenterally)
   f. Observe for congenital anomalies; there is an increased incidence in infants of diabetic mothers (IDM)
   g. Promote early mother-infant interaction
C. Evaluation/Outcomes
   1. Maintains serum glucose levels within acceptable limits
   2. Gives birth to a healthy newborn
   3. Remains free from complications

❋ RESPIRATORY DISORDERS
Data Base
A. Asthma: a lower respiratory tract disorder characterized by reversible hyperreactivity and bronchoconstriction; condition preexists and may worsen during pregnancy
   1. May experience nonproductive cough, chest tightness, wheezing, and shortness of breath
   2. Occurrence of an upper respiratory tract infection exacerbates symptoms, as does elevation of the uterus in the abdominal cavity
B. Tuberculosis: an infectious disease caused by *Mycobacterium tuberculosis;* populations at risk are those who are immunocompromised or who live under substandard conditions
   1. May experience lethargy, systemic infections, cough, night sweats, weight loss, and fever
   2. Occurrence of an upper respiratory tract infection exacerbates symptoms, as does elevation of uterus in the abdominal cavity
   3. Purified protein derivative (PPD) skin test (Mantoux) is used for screening
   4. Impaired fetal gas exchange occurs related to maternal hypoxia

C. Therapeutic interventions
   1. Asthma
      a. Identify woman's triggers for attacks and minimize exposure to respiratory tract pathogens
      b. Allergy desensitization; may be safely done during pregnancy if necessary
      c. Yearly influenza vaccination recommended by the CDC (may be administered during pregnancy because it does not contain a live organism)
      d. Inhaled bronchodilators are indicated during exacerbations; albuterol and metaproterenol are indicated
      e. When bronchodilators are ineffective, glucocorticoids may be used to decrease inflammation and mucus secretions
   2. Tuberculosis
      a. Administration of isoniazid and rifampin unless the woman demonstrates resistance to isoniazid; treatment should continue for full 9 months
      b. Ethambutol may be substituted for isoniazid
      c. Pyridoxine (vitamin B_6) 50 mg/day is indicated
      d. No other pharmacologic treatment may be substituted during pregnancy
      e. Infants of untreated mothers are at risk when cared for by the mother after birth; transmission rate is 50%
      f. Uninfected infants may receive bacille Calmette-Guérin (BCG) vaccine

Nursing Care of Pregnant Women With Respiratory Disorders
A. Assessment/Analysis
   1. Health history during initial prenatal visit to identify history of respiratory disease/exposure to tuberculosis
   2. History of symptoms of tuberculosis
   3. PPD test and follow-up sputum cultures and chest x-ray film if findings indicate possible infection
   4. Case finding to limit spread of infection to family/community
B. Planning/Implementation
   1. Refer for collaboration between pulmonary specialist and obstetric practitioners
   2. Encourage mother to follow up on therapies and tests
   3. Teach importance of adhering to pharmacologic protocols and maintaining hydration
   4. Teach importance of continued prenatal evaluations to monitor fetal heart rate and well-being
C. Evaluation/Outcomes
   1. Maintains pharmacologic regimen throughout pregnancy
   2. Modifies activities to maintain optimum oxygenation
   3. Maintains oxygenation so fetus remains optimally oxygenated and exhibits expected growth and reactivity

CANCER

Data Base

A. Cancer risks increase with age and as women postpone pregnancy

B. Cancer of the breast is most common; cervical cancer, ovarian cancer, melanoma, leukemia, lymphomas, and tubal and thyroid cancers also occur

C. Cancer during this time creates a moral dilemma for the childbearing woman, the family, and the health team

D. Laparoscopic approach may be used for node sampling; surgical procedures increase risk for preterm labor, IUGR, and fetal demise

E. Chemotherapy is contraindicated because these drugs are teratogenic, especially in the first trimester

F. Radiotherapy is contraindicated because it puts the fetus at risk for abnormalities, low birth weight, cancer later in life, possible genetic effects on future generations of that fetus

Nursing Care of Pregnant Women With Cancer

A. Assessment/Analysis

  1. Staging of cancer without exposing the fetus to radiation; ultrasound and MRI are preferred

  2. Blood studies related to organ functioning are helpful; tumor markers may be influenced by oncofetal proteins found in maternal blood

B. Planning/Implementation

  1. Explain treatment choices and plan

  2. Assess woman's understanding of her condition and its effects on her and the pregnancy

  3. Encourage woman and family to express feelings; refer to appropriate practitioners, agencies, and clergy as needed

C. Evaluation/Outcomes

  1. Maintains emotional and physiologic well-being

  2. Verbalizes fears

  3. Arrives at decisions through problem solving

  4. Uses appropriate support systems

NURSING CARE OF WOMEN WITH COMPLICATIONS DURING THE PRENATAL PEROID

HYPERTENSIVE DISORDER OF PREGNANCY

Data Base

A. Characterized by edema, hypertension, and proteinuria occurring after the 20th to 24th week of gestation and disappearing 6 weeks after birth

B. Occurs primarily in primiparas less than 17 years of age and more than 35 years of age; women who are obese or have had numerous pregnancies; women with chronic hypertension, diabetes mellitus, severe nutritional deficiencies, a multifetal pregnancy, or trophoblastic disease

C. Classification of hypertensive states of pregnancy

  1. Gestational hypertension

    a. Increased BP during pregnancy beginning in second trimester

    b. Edema and proteinuria may not be present; blood changes rarely occur in uncomplicated gestational hypertension

  2. Transient hypertension

    a. Gestational hypertension without preeclampsia

    b. Resolves by 12 weeks' postpartum

  3. Preeclampsia

    a. Mild: BP 140/90 mm Hg on two readings taken 6 hours apart; systolic BP increase of 30 mm Hg or diastolic BP increase of 15 mm Hg; proteinuria +1 (30 mg/dL) or more

    b. Severe: BP 160/110 mm Hg or higher on two readings taken 6 hours apart after bed rest; proteinuria +3 to +4; hyperreflexia; oliguria; hemoconcentration

    c. Blood chemistry: may have rise in hematocrit and hemoglobin levels; increased levels of uric acid, liver enzymes, and BUN; decrease in CO_2 combining power indicates worsening preeclampsia

    d. Qualitative urinalysis: increase in albumin output (proteinuria) and/or decreased urinary output indicates worsening preeclampsia

  4. Eclampsia

    a. Seizures and/or coma; seizure may be preceded by rolling of eyes to one side with a stare

    b. Can occur after intractable, severe preeclampsia

  5. Chronic hypertension

    a. Hypertension present before pregnancy

    b. May be diagnosed before 20 weeks' gestation

  6. Preeclampsia superimposed on chronic hypertension

    a. Proteinuria

    b. Previously controlled BP becomes elevated

    c. Blood chemistry: thrombocytopenia and elevated creatinine level with other clinical manifestations of severe preeclampsia

D. HELLP syndrome (H, hemolysis; EL, elevated liver enzymes; LP, low platelet count); preeclampsia with hepatic dysfunction

  1. Occurs with little warning and often with no previous signs of preeclampsia; occurs in 2% to 12% of women with severe preeclampsia

  2. Right upper quadrant pain occurs in 90% of affected women; proteinuria may occur

  3. Blood smear reveals broken RBCs (schistocytes or burr cells)

  4. Blood chemistry: increased uric acid, liver enzymes, and BUN concentrations and decrease in hematocrit, RBCs, and platelets

  5. Occurs after 24 weeks' gestation or after birth

E. Guidelines for prevention of hypertensive disorders of pregnancy

  1. Adherence to general pregnancy advice

2. Clinical trials of increasing vitamins C and E and exercise have shown to be beneficial, but further study is needed
3. Restriction of sodium is harmful during pregnancy and can result in electrolyte imbalance and elimination of essential nutritional components; may contribute to reduced circulatory volume
4. Diuretics are contraindicated during pregnancy because they cause hypovolemia and deplete essential nutrients for mother and fetus

F. Therapeutic interventions
   1. Gestational hypertension
      a. Frequent rest periods
      b. Dietary management with increased fluid intake
      c. Treat symptoms
   2. Mild preeclampsia
      a. High-protein diet
      b. Ambulatory care; frequent visits to practitioner
      c. Frequent rest periods with feet elevated; side-lying position to enhance renal and placental perfusion
   3. Severe preeclampsia or eclampsia
      a. Hospitalization and complete bed rest
      b. Magnesium sulfate given IV by infusion pump to prevent or limit seizures
      c. Antihypertensives: hydralazine (Apresoline), nifedipine (Adalat, Procardia), methyldopa (Aldomet), labetalol hydrochloride (Normodyne)
      d. Indwelling catheter for output assessment
      e. Labor induction or cesarean birth when condition is under control
      f. Calcium gluconate for mother and levallorphan (Lorfan) for newborn if respiratory depression occurs from magnesium sulfate
      g. If fetus is less than 34 weeks' gestation, stimulation of surfactant production with betamethasone before birth
   4. HELLP syndrome
      a. Same as for severe preeclampsia or eclampsia
      b. Blood or blood products may be administered if necessary

Nursing Care of Women With Hypertensive Disorders of Pregnancy

A. Assessment/Analysis
   1. BP elevation
   2. Albumin in urine; oliguria
   3. Hyperreflexia; persistent headache; blurred vision
   4. Epigastric pain
B. Planning/Implementation
   1. Monitor BP: every 15 minutes during critical phase; every 1 to 4 hours as condition improves
   2. Insert indwelling catheter; monitor urine for output and albumin
   3. Monitor edema: daily weights, I&O
   4. Maintain high-protein diet with adequate sodium intake
   5. Monitor hyperreflexia

6. Administer magnesium sulfate as ordered via an infusion pump (check for sufficient urinary output before starting)
7. Monitor for magnesium toxicity
   a. Assess for depressed or absent deep tendon reflexes (DTRs); patellar or brachial
   b. Observe for depressed respirations, below 12 to 14 breaths/min
   c. Assess magnesium blood levels every 6 hours; therapeutic range is 4 to 8 mg/dL
   d. Have calcium gluconate available if magnesium sulfate toxicity occurs
8. Observe for indications of a seizure; seizure may be preceded by rolling of eyes to one side with a stare; maintain seizure precautions; monitor vital signs and FHR following a seizure
9. Maintain on bed rest in side-lying position; maintain quiet, dark environment; limit visitors
10. Monitor FHR
11. Observe for signs of bleeding and labor
12. Monitor hematologic studies
13. Explore anxieties and concerns
14. Be prepared for an induced or emergency cesarean birth
15. Continue to monitor for related complications for 48 hours after birth while diuresis occurs
16. Seizures (eclampsia) may occur several weeks postpartum

C. Evaluation/Outcomes
   1. Maintains (mother and fetus) vital signs within acceptable range
   2. Remains free from seizures
   3. Maintains fluid balance

❋ SPONTANEOUS ABORTION

Data Base

A. Definition
   1. An interruption of pregnancy in which there is complete expulsion or partial expulsion (incomplete) of the products of conception before the period of viability
   2. Period of gestation is 20 weeks or less; the conceptus will weigh below 500 g and will be less than 16.5 cm long
   3. May be caused by the presence of embryonic defects, external mechanical force, or trauma
B. Types/clinical findings
   1. Threatened abortion: cervix closed, but bleeding, cramping, and backache occur; pregnancy may continue uninterrupted
   2. Imminent or inevitable abortion: bleeding and cramping become more severe, cervix dilates, and membranes may rupture
   3. Incomplete abortion: all the products of conception are not expelled after dilation of cervical os
   4. Complete abortion: all products of conception expelled within 24 to 48 hours

5. Missed abortion: fetus dies in utero but not expelled; client must be monitored for disseminated intravascular coagulopathy (DIC)
6. Habitual abortions: three consecutive pregnancies that end in abortion
C. Therapeutic interventions
   1. Complete bed rest
   2. Diagnostic/therapeutic blood studies: CBC, blood typing, Rh incompatibility, and cross-matching with availability of blood
   3. Assessment of serum progesterone or serial beta human chorionic gonadotropin (β-hCG)
   4. Dilation and curettage or vacuum aspiration performed if the products of conception are retained

Nursing Care of Women Experiencing Abortion
A. Assessment/Analysis
   1. Vital signs; amount of bleeding
   2. Pain
   3. Emotional response to loss
B. Planning/Implementation
   1. Institute measures to alleviate fear and anxiety; assist with grieving process
   2. Point out physiologic reality, but encourage client to work through feelings; grieving may last up to 24 months
   3. Encourage participation with thanatology services and bereavement groups when appropriate
   4. Monitor amount and type of bleeding: save and count number of perineal pads; distinguish between dark clotted blood and frank bleeding, which is bright red; monitor fundus for firmness after products of conception are expelled
   5. Monitor vital signs for signs of hypovolemia, shock, and infection; monitor CBC, hemoglobin, and hematocrit; prepare for administration of blood; administer O_2 if necessary
   6. Maintain fluid and electrolyte balance
   7. If appropriate, administer RhoGAM to Rh-negative client after abortion
   8. Educate about necessity for follow-up care and support groups
C. Evaluation/Outcomes
   1. Remains free from complications such as hemorrhage and infection
   2. Expresses feelings

ECTOPIC PREGNANCY (TUBAL PREGNANCY)
Data Base
A. Pregnancy in which implantation occurs outside the uterus (most frequent site is middle portion of fallopian tube; other sites are abdomen, ovaries, and cervix)
B. Early signs and symptoms are usually concealed; may be diagnosed by ultrasonography and radioimmunoassay for β-hCG

C. Pattern in tubal pregnancy: spotting after one or two missed menstrual periods; sudden, sharp, knifelike lower right or left abdominal pain radiating to shoulder; concealed bleeding from site of rupture leads to sudden shock
D. Women who have had pelvic inflammatory disease (PID), tubal surgery, or endometriosis are predisposed to ectopic pregnancies
E. Therapeutic interventions
   1. Diagnosis confirmed by ultrasound examination, laparoscopy, or culdocentesis
   2. Immediate blood replacement if blood loss is severe
   3. Removal of ruptured fallopian tube or surgical repair may be attempted
   4. Chemical therapies to salvage fallopian tube (e.g., methotrexate) or therapies to inhibit cell division if embryo is less than 4 cm by ultrasound

Nursing Care of Women With an Ectopic Pregnancy
A. Assessment/Analysis
   1. Vital signs; signs of shock
   2. Bleeding; rigid, tender abdomen
   3. Character and location of pain
   4. Level of anxiety
B. Planning/Implementation
   1. Monitor for signs of shock; administer ordered blood transfusion for excessive blood loss
   2. Administer analgesics as ordered for pain
   3. Provide emotional support
   4. Provide preoperative and postoperative care
   5. Administer RhoGAM to Rh-negative client if appropriate
C. Evaluation/Outcomes
   1. Maintains hemostasis
   2. States implications for future childbearing
   3. Expresses feelings

HYDATIDIFORM MOLE OR TROPHOBLASTIC DISEASE
Data Base
A. Definition
   1. A group of disorders in which there is an abnormal proliferation of tissues and high hGC levels
   2. These disorders include hydatidiform mole, invasive mole, and choriocarcinoma
B. Clinical findings
   1. Types include
      a. Molar pregnancy—no fetus or amnion
      b. Partial molar pregnancy—a fetus or amniotic sac present
      c. Invasive mole—locally invasive to surrounding tissues
      d. Choriocarcinoma—may occur years after a hydatidiform mole

2. Uterus is generally larger for period of gestation and fetal parts are not palpable; doughlike consistency
3. Signs and symptoms of gestational hypertension and hyperemesis are common
4. Potential for uterine perforation, hemorrhage, and infection; passing of "grapelike" substance
5. Confirmation by ultrasonography
C. Therapeutic interventions
1. If spontaneous evacuation does not occur, evacuation by dilation and curettage or hysterotomy is performed
2. Continued follow-up of serum gonadotropin levels is imperative for 1 year to rule out metastasis from choriocarcinoma (increased gonadotropin levels require chemotherapy); metastasis to lungs is common
3. Preventing a new pregnancy is essential for 1 year
4. Chemotherapy when malignant

Nursing Care of Women With Hydatidiform Mole or Trophoblastic Disease
A. Assessment/Analysis
1. Vaginal bleeding (brownish, prune juice) containing grapelike tissue
2. Uterine enlargement; fundal height greater than expected for length of pregnancy
3. Vomiting
4. Elevated BP earlier than 24 weeks' gestation
5. Absence of fetal heart tones or activity
B. Planning/Implementation
1. See Nursing Care of Women Experiencing Abortion under Spontaneous Abortion
2. Teach about importance of follow-up care
C. Evaluation/Outcomes
1. Continues follow-up care
2. Uses measures to prevent pregnancy for 1 year

INCOMPETENT CERVIX
Data Base
A. Definition
1. Cervical effacement and dilation in early second trimester, resulting in expulsion of products of conception if a cerclage procedure is not performed
2. Usually results from previous forceful dilation and curettage, difficult birth, or congenitally short cervix
B. Clinical findings
1. Painless contractions in midtrimester
2. Birth of dead or nonviable fetus
C. Therapeutic interventions
1. Cerclage procedure during 14th to 16th week of gestation; suture or ribbon placed beneath cervical mucosa to close cervix
2. At end of pregnancy, cesarean birth or cutting of suture for vaginal birth
3. Bed rest and/or activity restriction

Nursing Care of Women With an Incompetent Cervix
A. Assessment/Analysis
1. Number of weeks' gestation
2. Obstetric history
3. Knowledge of the cerclage procedure
B. Planning/Implementation
1. Maintain bed rest for 24 hours after cerclage
2. Monitor for rupture of membranes or bleeding
3. Monitor FHR
C. Evaluation/Outcomes
1. Continues pregnancy to term
2. Describes signs of labor and need to seek immediate medical care when labor begins

PLACENTA PREVIA
Data Base
A. Definition: implantation of the placenta in the lower uterine segment
B. Types
1. Type I—low-lying: placenta is in lower uterine segment next to os; as uterus stretches with gestation, placenta moves away from os
2. Type II—marginal: placental edge is at the os, but does not cover it
3. Type III—partial: placental edge partially covers the os
4. Type IV—complete: placenta is centered over the os
C. Clinical findings
1. Painless, bright-red bleeding; hemorrhage in the third trimester
2. Soft uterus in the latter part of pregnancy
3. Signs of infection may be present
D. Therapeutic interventions
1. Ultrasonography to confirm the presence of placenta previa
2. Depend on location of placenta, amount of bleeding, and status of the fetus
3. Home monitoring with repeated ultrasounds may be possible with type I—low-lying
4. Control bleeding
5. Replace blood loss if excessive
6. Cesarean birth, if necessary
7. Betamethasone before birth if indicated to increase fetal lung maturity

Nursing Care of Women With Placenta Previa
A. Assessment/Analysis
1. Presence of bright-red blood with absence of pain; assess and document amount of bleeding
2. Vital signs indicating shock (hypovolemic)
3. Changes in or absence of FHR
4. Level of anxiety (usually increases)
B. Planning/Implementation
1. No vaginal examination; if a vaginal examination must be performed, prepare double setups (vaginal and cesarean)
2. Maintain bed rest in semi-Fowler's position

3. Monitor FHR continuously; will be in expected range if placenta is functioning
4. Monitor maternal vital signs continuously; assess color for pallor or cyanosis; administer oxygen
5. Observe perineal pads to determine blood loss; monitor hemoglobin and hematocrit, prepare for cesarean birth if bleeding persists
6. Administer IV therapy and/or blood replacement

C. Evaluation/Outcomes
1. Birth of viable, stable newborn
2. Demonstrates hemodynamic stability

✼ ABRUPTIO PLACENTAE

Data Base

A. Definition: partial, marginal, or complete premature separation of the placenta in the third trimester; degree of separation may be mild, moderate, or severe (grade 1, 2, or 3, respectively)
B. Clinical findings
1. May or may not have vaginal bleeding; concealed bleeding if center of the placenta separates and margins are intact
2. Moderate to agonizing abdominal pain
3. Persistent uterine contraction; firm to boardlike abdomen
4. Hyperactivity and then cessation of fetal movements
5. Frequently associated with gestational or chronic hypertension, maternal cocaine use, previous history of abruptio placentae, trauma, and aggressive oxytocin induction
6. Predisposes client to hemorrhage, disseminated intravascular coagulopathy (DIC), and hypofibrinogenemia
C. Therapeutic interventions
1. Replacement of blood loss
2. With moderate or severe separation, maternal distress, or fetal compromise: emergency cesarean birth
3. With mild separation without fetal compromise and in the presence of some cervical effacement and dilation: induction of labor may be attempted
4. O_2 if necessary
5. Maintenance of fluid and electrolyte balance

Nursing Care of Women With Abruptio Placentae

A. Assessment/Analysis
1. Presence of pain with or without dark-red bleeding
2. Increased tonicity of abdominal wall
3. Vital signs indicating shock
4. Changes in or absence of FHR
5. Level of anxiety usually increases
B. Planning/Implementation
1. Maintain bed rest in lateral recumbent position
2. Monitor FHR continuously
3. Monitor maternal vital signs continuously; assess color for pallor or cyanosis; administer oxygen

4. Obtain blood for typing and cross-matching, coagulation studies, hemoglobin, and hematocrit
5. Prepare for a Kleihauer-Betke test to assess fetal bleeding into maternal circulation
6. Determine abdominal pain and tonicity of abdomen; observe perineal pads for bleeding; prepare for cesarean birth if abruptio is moderate or severe
7. Administer IV therapy and/or blood replacement
8. Observe for signs of DIC such as seepage of blood from IV site or incisional areas

C. Evaluation/Outcomes
1. Birth of a viable, stable newborn
2. Demonstrates hemodynamic stability

NURSING CARE OF WOMEN WITH COMPLICATIONS DURING THE INTRAPARTUM PERIOD

✼ INDUCTION OR STIMULATION OF LABOR

Data Base

A. Elective induction: initiation of labor contractions by
1. Pharmacologic means
a. Vaginal insertion of prostaglandin E_2 gel or suppository to promote cervical softening and effacement
b. Vaginal insertion of misoprostol (Cytotec) tablet to posterior fornix to promote cervical softening (ripening) and effacement
c. Approximately 8 to 12 hours after prostaglandin E_2 administration, pump infusion of oxytocin to stimulate contractions
2. Mechanical means
a. Artificial rupture of membranes (amniotomy)
b. Insertion of laminaria tent (dried seaweed that swells in presence of moisture) or other hydroscopic means to promote cervical dilation, and then induction begins
c. Nipple massage to stimulate the secretion of oxytocin from the posterior pituitary gland
B. Medical or obstetric reasons: diabetes; pyelonephritis; hypertensive disorders; Rh incompatibility; hydramnios; placental insufficiency; premature rupture of membranes at term without onset of labor; postterm gestation; history of precipitate birth; fetal jeopardy
C. Augmentation of labor: assisting client when labor process is not progressing (prolonged labor) by pharmacologic or mechanical means
D. Induction or augmentation of labor is not done with cephalopelvic disproportion, malpresentation of fetus, fetal compromise, placenta previa, or active genital herpes

Nursing Care of Women During Induction or Stimulation of Labor

A. Assessment/Analysis
1. Obstetric history, including expected date of birth
2. Maternal status: parity; contractions; status of membranes; status of cervix; ultrasonographic findings; level of anxiety
3. Fetal status: gestational age; absence of cephalopelvic disproportion or other problems; position; results of fetal monitoring and NST

B. Planning/Implementation
1. Prepare mother and labor coach for induction: explain all procedures; obtain informed consent whenever necessary
2. Obtain and record baseline information such as maternal vital signs, FHR, contractions for later comparison; continue to monitor all vital indices
3. Monitor oxytocin (Pitocin) administration
   a. Typically oxytocin is piggybacked through an infusion device; titrated at 0.5 to 2 mIU/min; titrated according to contraction pattern and fetal response
   b. Discontinue Pitocin drip if a sustained uterine contraction occurs; fetal decelerations persist; urinary flow decreases to 30 mL/hr (related to water intoxication); signs of placenta previa or abruptio placentae develop
4. Monitor effect of prostaglandin: if hypertonic contractions occur, discontinue infusion; if they persist, prepare for tocolytic therapy
5. Assist with artificial rupture of membranes (amniotomy)
   a. Maintain asepsis
   b. Immediately after rupture, monitor FHR
   c. Note color and amount of amniotic fluid
   d. Record time of rupture; prolonged time after rupture may predispose client to sepsis
6. Maintain hydration
7. Provide for blood typing, Rh compatibility, cross-matching
8. Have O_2, suction, and resuscitation equipment available
9. Prepare for emergency cesarean birth if necessary

C. Evaluation/Outcomes
1. Progresses through labor to safe birth of newborn
2. Remains free from complications

PREMATURE RUPTURE OF MEMBRANES (PROM)

Data Base
A. Definition: spontaneous rupture of membranes before onset of labor
B. Maternal implication: ascending infection
C. Fetal implications
1. Prolapsed cord
2. FHR decelerations caused by cord compression from lack of amniotic fluid

3. Sepsis from ascending infection
D. Therapeutic interventions
1. Hospitalization with bed rest after 37 weeks' gestation
2. Amnioinfusion of isotonic saline in some cases to allow for fetal movement and lessen danger of cord compression
3. Prophylactic antibiotics

Nursing Care of Women With Premature Rupture of Membranes

A. Assessment/Analysis
1. Time of rupture of membranes
2. Fetal heart rate and maternal vital signs
3. Perineum for prolapsed cord
4. Confirmation of rupture of membranes by fern test: microscopic examination reveals fernlike crystals of sodium chloride
5. Confirmation of presence of amniotic fluid by nitrazine test; paper changes color when touched by alkaline solution (7.0 to 7.5) rather than acidic vaginal secretions
6. Characteristics of leaking amniotic fluid: odor and color

B. Planning/Implementation
1. Monitor FHR and maternal vital signs; temperature and pulse every 2 hours
2. Monitor uterine activity
3. Avoid vaginal/cervical stimulation (e.g., unnecessary vaginal examinations)
4. Ensure adequate hydration
5. Educate parents: amniotic fluid is still being produced; avoid intercourse
6. Provide perineal hygiene
7. Administer antibiotics as ordered

C. Evaluation/Outcomes
1. Remains free from infection
2. Progresses through labor to safe birth of newborn

PRETERM LABOR

Data Base
A. Contractions begin after the 20th week but before the completed 37th week of gestation, causing effacement and dilation of the cervix
1. A fetus of 20 or more weeks' gestation who dies before or during birth is classified as stillborn
2. Preterm births account for 75% to 85% of neonatal morbidity and mortality
B. Contributing factors include history, risky lifestyle, multiple gestation, maternal illness with fever, opiate use, bacterial vaginitis, multiple abortions, pyelonephritis, and asymptomatic bacteriuria
C. Diagnostic studies
1. Transvaginal cervical sonography
2. Immunoassay for fetal fibronectin
3. Vaginal examinations to determine cervical changes

D. Therapeutic interventions
1. Activity restrictions; no evidence to support the effectiveness of continuous bed rest
2. Tocolytic therapy directed toward decreasing frequency and duration of contractions, postponing birth
   a. Betasympathomimetics such as ritodrine (Yutopar) and terbutaline sulfate (Brethine)
   b. Magnesium sulfate
   c. Prostaglandin inhibitors such as indomethacin (Indocin)
   d. Calcium channel blockers such as nifedipine (Procardia)
3. Glucocorticoid therapy
   a. Betamethasone (Celestone)
   b. Administered 24 to 48 hours before birth if birth appears inevitable
   c. Reduces incidence and severity of respiratory distress syndrome (RDS) in preterm infants; enhances formation of surfactant
   d. May be contraindicated if the woman has an infection
4. Home uterine monitoring has not been shown to be more effective than manual palpation and communication with an obstetric nurse
5. Treatment of etiology (e.g., antibiotics for pyelonephritis)

Nursing Care of Women During Preterm Labor

A. Assessment/Analysis
1. Number of weeks' gestation
2. Presence of live and viable fetus
3. Presence of labor: two contractions lasting 30 seconds within 15 minutes; cervical dilation less than 4 cm; effacement 50% or less
4. Signs of hemorrhage or infection
5. Presence of severe preeclampsia
6. Rupture of membranes; length of time since rupture
7. Emotional status of mother
B. Planning/Implementation
1. Prevention by decreasing risk factors when possible
   a. Discuss impact of drug use and lifestyle risks
   b. Teach the importance of early reporting of temperature elevations
   c. Check results of prenatal vaginal cultures
   d. Monitor for urinary tract infections; asymptomatic bacteriuria shows a positive culture above $100,000/mm^3$
2. Monitor vital signs, FHR, contractions, and progression of labor
3. Maintain bed rest if ordered
4. Inform client about medication; obtain consent; explain that the use of pain medications will be limited to avoid their depressive effects on the fetus
5. Provide emotional support; reduce anxiety and prepare for possible loss of infant

6. Provide special care related to the administration of tocolytic medications
   a. Use an infusion pump when IV administration of medications is indicated
   b. Obtain baseline hematologic data and electrocardiographic (ECG) readings if appropriate
   c. Monitor vital signs; hypotension can occur with all tocolytics; tachycardia can occur with terbutaline and ritodrine
   d. Maintain hydration but monitor for pulmonary edema
   e. Monitor for signs of hypokalemia and hyperglycemia
   f. Monitor I&O and neurologic reflexes
7. Prepare for use of glucocorticoid therapy for fetus
8. Prepare for preterm birth if labor continues
9. Provide home instruction for halting preterm labor
   a. Assessments by home health nurse should include vital signs, FHR, breath sounds, fetal activity, hematologic and cervical status, blood and urine glucose levels, fundal height, maternal weight, urine evaluation, presence of edema
   b. Rest periods in lateral position; avoidance of vigorous activity
   c. Increased fluid intake
   d. No sexual intercourse or sexual activity that leads to orgasm
   e. No nipple stimulation
   f. Avoidance of stressful events
   g. Empty bladder regularly and if contractions occur
C. Evaluation/Outcomes
1. Mother demonstrates cessation of labor
2. Fetus remains in utero with acceptable FHR and fetal movements
3. Mother and partner state recurring signs of preterm labor

✤ POSTTERM LABOR

Data Base

A. Extends beyond the 42nd week of gestation or 2 weeks beyond estimated date of birth (EDB); 37 to 42 weeks' gestation is considered full-term
B. Fetal risk
1. Decreased amniotic fluid may lead to cord compression during labor
2. Decreased placental function because placental aging lowers O_2 and nutritional transport; fetus becomes compromised during labor (may become asphyxic or hypoglycemic)
3. Increasing size (mainly length) and hardening of skull may contribute to cephalopelvic disproportion
C. Maternal risk present only if infant is excessively large
D. Therapeutic intervention: induction of labor

Nursing Care of Women During Postterm Labor

A. Assessment/Analysis
  1. Number of weeks' gestation; date of last menstrual period; EDB
  2. Biophysical profile, particularly amount of amniotic fluid because decreased amniotic fluid is a result of decreased kidney perfusion related to decreased fetal O_2 levels
  3. FHR; results of stress and nonstress tests
  4. Presence of meconium
  5. Level of anxiety related to delayed date of birth
  6. Newborn will have little vernix, long nails and hair, peeling wrinkled skin, reduced subcutaneous fat, meconium staining
B. Planning/Implementation
  See Planning/Implementation under Induction or Stimulation of Labor
C. Evaluation/Outcomes
  1. Progresses through labor to safe birth of neonate
  2. Remains free from complications

✽ DYSTOCIA

Data Base

A. Mechanical factors: cephalopelvic disproportion; contracted pelvis; malpresentation or position; multiple gestation
B. Faulty uterine contractions
  1. Hypertonic: increased frequency of contractions with decreased intensity; usually occurs in early labor; cervix does not dilate and mother becomes exhausted; increased fetal molding that may cause caput succedaneum or cephalohematoma; may occur in older primigravidas or very anxious women
  2. Hypotonic: slowing of rate and intensity of contractions in latter part of labor
C. Maternal complications include cervical trauma, postpartum hemorrhage, infection, and exhaustion
D. Therapeutic interventions
  1. Careful evaluation of the cause of dystocia is necessary to select an appropriate intervention; deciding factors are length of labor, condition of mother and fetus, amount of cervical effacement and dilation, and fetal presentation, position, and station
  2. Oxytocics and nonpharmacologic strategies to stimulate labor if contractions are hypotonic; analgesic and nonpharmacologic strategies to promote rest if contractions are hypertonic
  3. Cesarean birth

Nursing Care of Women With Dystocia

A. Assessment/Analysis
  1. Progress of labor with special attention to phase, fetal descent, and arrest, or prolongation of phase/descent
  2. Status of mother
  3. Status of fetus; FHR

  4. Ultrasonographic or x-ray examination to determine fetal and pelvic size
B. Planning/Implementation
  1. Relieve back pain, caused by prolonged posterior pressure from fetus in occiput posterior position, by applying sacral pressure during contractions; using the knee to apply sacral pressure may be helpful; have client avoid supine position
  2. Observe for signs of maternal exhaustion such as dehydration and acidosis/alkalosis
  3. Monitor for signs of a compromised fetus
  4. Have O_2, suction, and resuscitation equipment available
  5. Constantly monitor contractions, FHR, and vital signs when client is receiving oxytocic stimulation
  6. Provide emotional support; keep client and family informed about progress
  7. Administer fluids as ordered
  8. Administer sedatives as ordered
C. Evaluation/Outcomes
  1. Rests/sleeps between contractions and after birth
  2. Progresses through labor to safe birth of newborn
  3. Remains free from complications

✽ PRECIPITATE BIRTH

Data Base

A. Rapid labor and birth of less than 3 hours duration
B. Hazards to mother are perineal laceration and postpartum hemorrhage
C. Hazards to infant are anoxia and intracranial hemorrhage

Nursing Care of Women During Precipitate Birth

A. Assessment/Analysis
  1. Rapid cervical dilation
  2. Accelerated fetal descent
  3. History of rapid labor
  4. Rapid uterine contractions with decreased periods of relaxation between contractions
B. Planning/Implementation
  1. Remain with mother and monitor closely
  2. Keep emergency birth pack at bedside
  3. Keep mother and partner informed throughout process of labor and birth
  4. Support and guide fetal head through birth canal when birth occurs
  5. Newborn: establish airway (position head slightly lower then chest to drain mucus by gravity; rub back to precipitate crying)
C. Evaluation/Outcomes
  1. Mother remains injury-free
  2. Neonate remains injury-free

✽ BREECH BIRTH

Data Base

A. Position of fetus in which buttocks alone (frank breech), buttocks and feet (complete breech), or one or both feet (footling) descend through the birth canal first

B. Maternal implication: cesarean birth may be required, especially in primigravida
C. Fetal implications
  1. Increased mortality
  2. Occurrence of prolapsed cord, leading to asphyxia
  3. Birth trauma such as brachial palsy and fracture of the upper extremities

Nursing Care of Women During Breech Birth
A. Assessment/Analysis
  1. Recognition of breech presentation when performing Leopold's maneuvers and vaginal examination
  2. Auscultation of fetal heart tones above umbilicus
  3. Presence of meconium without signs of fetal compromise
B. Planning/Implementation
  1. Use measures to promote comfort
  2. Monitor the FHR in upper quadrants
  3. Watch for prolapsed cord; if it occurs
    a. With a sterile gloved hand, push the presenting part off the cord
    b. Place in the Trendelenburg position to keep presenting part away from the cord
    c. Keep prolapsed cord moist with sterile saline
  4. Observe for frank meconium; results from contraction of the uterus on lower colon of the fetus; not significant in breech birth
  5. Add Piper forceps to the delivery setup if vaginal birth is anticipated
  6. Prepare client for cesarean birth; usually done in primigravidas
  7. Teach mother and partner about the process of breech birth
C. Evaluation/Outcomes
  1. Mother remains free from injury
  2. Neonate remains free from injury

✿ CESAREAN BIRTH
Data Base
A. Birth of infant via transabdominal incision; transverse incision; lower uterine vertical incision
B. Indicated in cephalopelvic disproportion, dystocia, placenta previa, abruptio placentae, postmaturity, growths within the birth canal, multiple births, diabetes, hypertensive disorders, Rh incompatibility, nonreassuring fetal heart pattern, active herpes, and malpresentations such as breech or shoulder; may be indicated if there was a previous cesarean birth
C. Vaginal birth after cesarean is an alternative for a woman who has had a horizontal uterine incision for a previous cesarean birth
  1. Each pregnancy may have different variables that make this attempt possible or impossible
  2. Multiple uterine incisions may cause uterine rupture during labor
D. Informed consent must be obtained before the procedure

Nursing Care of Women After Cesarean Birth
A. Assessment/Analysis
  1. Vital signs
  2. Dressing status: intact, presence of bleeding
  3. Status of incision: REEDA (no Redness, Edema, Ecchymosis, or Discharge and well Approximated)
  4. Fundus and lochia: lochia may be less than that with vaginal birth; during the first hour after birth, the client may saturate one or two perineal pads less than after a vaginal birth
  5. Urinary output: amount; specific gravity; presence of blood
  6. Neurovascular status following regional anesthesia
  7. Presence of pain
  8. Response to neonate
B. Planning/Implementation
  1. Assist with bonding; offer emotional support; encourage touching; include father in process
  2. Encourage early ambulation to prevent circulatory stasis and promote peristalsis
  3. Check vital signs, fundus, and abdominal incision; maintain IV infusion of oxytocin if ordered; provide perineal care
  4. Encourage eating of solid foods to promote peristalsis (prevents distention) when bowel sounds have returned
  5. Administer analgesics as ordered
  6. Promote lung aeration: deep breathing and coughing; incentive spirometer
  7. Maintain fluid and electrolyte balance; monitor I&O
  8. Monitor urinary output
  9. Encourage early breastfeeding
C. Evaluation/Outcomes
  1. States relief from pain
  2. Maintains urinary and fecal elimination
  3. Remains free from complications
  4. Demonstrates bonding with newborn

✿ ASSISTED BIRTH
Data Base
A. Forceps: instrument used to shorten the second stage of labor; applied to head or presenting part to allow physician to control traction on infant's head; indicated in ineffective pushing, malposition, and large infants
B. Vacuum extraction: a cup is placed on the presenting part through which suction is applied to pull infant down; infant may develop caput succedaneum but is otherwise unharmed

Nursing Care of Women During and After Assisted Births
(See Nursing Care of Women With Complications During the Intrapartum Period and Nursing Care of Women With Complications During the Postpartum Period)

NURSING CARE OF WOMEN WITH COMPLICATIONS DURING THE POSTPARTUM PERIOD

❧ POSTPARTUM BLEEDING

Data Base

A. Definition: bleeding in excess of 500 mL within the first 24 hours following birth; usually associated with uterine atony; vaginal, cervical, and perineal lacerations; hematomas; retained placental fragments; multifetal pregnancy and numerous previous pregnancies; bleeding increases risk of infection
  1. Uterine atony may be influenced by overdistention of uterus prolonged labor, birth trauma, and high parity
  2. Lacerations are classified as
    a. First-degree: superficial, extends through skin
    b. Second-degree: extends through muscles of the perineum; episiotomies are at least second degree
    c. Third-degree: extends through the anal sphincter
    d. Fourth-degree: extends through all of these structures and the anterior rectal wall
  3. Hematomas may occur in the vagina, uterus, or perineum; they result from increased fundal pressure from fetus, forceps, or manipulation
  4. Placental abnormalities can cause life-threatening hemorrhage
    a. Placenta accreta occurs when chorionic villi adhere to the uterine myometrium
    b. Placenta increta occurs when chorionic villi invade the myometrium
    c. Placenta percreta occurs when chorionic villi invade and pass through the myometrium to the peritoneal covering
B. Clinical findings
  1. Large amount of frank, red bleeding
  2. Boggy uterus; uterus above umbilicus in postpartum period
  3. Signs of hypotension
  4. Signs of disseminated intravascular coagulopathy (DIC)
    a. Profuse, uncontrollable bleeding from uterus
    b. Oozing of blood from episiotomy, laceration, or IV site
    c. Fragmented or distorted RBCs
    d. Decreased coagulation factors (pathologic form of clotting)
C. Therapeutic interventions
  1. Maintaining an empty bladder
  2. Massaging of fundal portion of uterus
  3. Administration of oxytocics
  4. Blood replacement with severe blood loss
  5. Surgical repair of vaginal and cervical lacerations
  6. Removal of retained placental fragments
  7. Cryoprecipitate, fresh frozen plasma for DIC

Nursing Care of Women With Postpartum Bleeding

A. Assessment/Analysis
  1. Risk factors: multiparity; prolonged labor; analgesia; multiple gestation; abruptio placentae or placenta previa; hypertensive disorders, especially HELLP syndrome
  2. Vaginal bleeding and clots
  3. Uterus for lack of tone (boggy)
  4. Urinary output for decrease
  5. Vital signs for signs of shock; pallor and fatigue
  6. Level of anxiety
B. Planning/Implementation
  1. Monitor vital signs and review laboratory results of blood studies
  2. Assess fundus for height and firmness every 15 minutes; massage if boggy
  3. Keep bladder from distending so that the uterus can contract; insert indwelling catheter as ordered if voiding is insufficient; monitor intake and output
  4. Prepare for ultrasonography for retained placental fragments
  5. Monitor for bleeding: perineal pads, presence of clots; maintain standard precautions
  6. Administer an oxytocic as ordered
  7. Maintain NPO in case a surgical intervention becomes necessary
  8. Prepare for blood transfusions or emergency surgery if condition worsens
C. Evaluation/Outcomes
  1. Demonstrates hemodynamic stability
  2. Remains free from complications

❧ EPISIOTOMY

Data Base

A. Incision into perineum to facilitate birth and prevent lacerations and overstretching of the pelvic floor; it is usually made between the vaginal introitus and the rectum; may be midline or mediolateral; a restrictive episiotomy protocol to reduce perineal trauma is recommended
B. Closed surgically; usually performed under regional anesthesia
C. Tends to be more painful, more difficult to repair, and cause more perineal trauma and infection when compared to lacerations

Nursing Care of Women After an Episiotomy

A. Assessment/Analysis
  1. Assess "REEDA": no Redness, Edema, Ecchymosis, or Discharge and well Approximated edges
  2. Extent of pain
  3. Signs of hematoma

B. Planning/Implementation
   1. Apply cold to perineum to limit edema during the first 12 to 24 hours if ordered
   2. Provide and teach perineal care including when to change pads
   3. Administer analgesics as ordered; may be systemic and/or local
   4. Provide sitz baths if ordered to promote dilation of blood vessels, which increases blood to the area and facilitates healing
   5. Teach perineal exercises (Kegel)
C. Evaluation/Outcomes
   1. States relief from pain
   2. Remains free from infection

27 Nursing Care of the Newborn

FOUNDATIONS OF NURSING CARE FOR NEWBORNS

FAMILY AND PRENATAL HISTORY

A. Chronic illness in the mother's or father's family
B. Previous medical-surgical illnesses of the mother and father
C. Age and present health status of the mother and father
D. History of previous pregnancies
E. Prenatal history
   1. Medical supervision during pregnancy
   2. Nutrition during pregnancy
   3. Course of pregnancy: illnesses, medications taken, or treatments required
   4. Duration of gestation
   5. Course and amount of sedation and anesthesia required
   6. Type of birth and significant events during the immediate period after birth
   7. Immediate response of newborn (Apgar score at 1 and 5 minutes following birth)
   8. Presence of maternal infections during pregnancy
   9. History of alcohol or drug use, sexually transmitted infections, or smoking during pregnancy
   10. Group beta streptococcus (GBS) status; if positive, determine if antibiotics were administered during labor

PARENT-INFANT RELATIONSHIPS

A. Concepts basic to parent-infant relationships
   1. Early and frequent parent-infant contact is essential for survival (bonding)
   2. Childbearing is a developmental crisis; parenting abilities can be fostered and developed
   3. Biologic changes that occur at puberty and during pregnancy influence the development of nurturance
   4. Interaction between mother and infant begins from the moment of conception and can be shared with the father
   5. Love for the infant grows as the parents interact and give care
   6. As the parent gives to the infant and the infant receives, the parent in turn receives satisfaction from parenting tasks

7. Any disturbance in give-and-take cycle sets up frustrations in parents and infant
8. Parental behavior is learned and frequent parent-infant contact enhances development of parenting abilities; ambivalence is a natural phenomenon as are feelings of resentment
B. Infant's basic needs
   1. Physiologic—food, clothing, hygiene, and protection from environment
   2. Emotional—security, comfort, fondling, caressing, rocking, being spoken to, and contact with one person on a consistent basis
C. Mothering and fathering are
   1. Based on a biologic inborn desire to reproduce
   2. Based on role concepts that begin with own childhood experiences
   3. Based on primitive emotional relationships
   4. Based on level of maturity
   5. Fostered by the parent-infant interaction that constantly reinforces gratification as needs are met and security develops
   6. Abilities that are learned rather than innate
D. Parent-infant relationships are affected by
   1. Readiness for pregnancy
      a. Planned or unplanned
      b. Health status before pregnancy
      c. Determinants such as age, cultural backgrounds, number in family unit, financial status
   2. Nature of the pregnancy
      a. Health status during pregnancy
      b. Preparation for parenthood
      c. Support from family members and members of the health care team
   3. Characteristics of labor and birth
      a. Length and pattern of labor; type of birth
      b. Type and amount of analgesia/anesthesia received
      c. Support from family and health team
   4. Factors that impede bonding
      a. Impaired physical status of newborn or mother
      b. Medical therapies that interfere with bonding
      c. Disturbance of idealized image of infant
E. Reva Rubin's Significant Phases of Maternal Adjustment
   1. Taking-in phase: mother's needs have to be met before she can meet infant's needs; talks about self

rather than infant; may not touch infant; cries easily; integrates birth experience into reality

2. Taking-hold phase: characterized by mother starting to assume responsibility for her baby; lasts from day 2 to day 10; concerned about infant, interested in learning; teachable, reachable, and referable at this time
3. Letting-go phase: mother lets go of her idealized notion of childbirth; at this time there may be periods of guilt or grief over the childbirth experience

F. Supportive care to promote bonding/attachment
   1. Give parents ample time to inspect and begin to identify with infant; encourage parents to touch, fondle, and hold infant
   2. Encourage give-and-take between parents and infant; support these beginning relationships
   3. Teach parents about their newborn; showing by example helps parents to learn care necessary to meet infant's needs and their own
   4. Evaluate parents' and infant's response and revise plan as necessary; identify beginning of disturbed relationships
   5. Provide therapeutic environment for various family lifestyle types: nuclear single parent, gay, blended

ADAPTATION TO EXTRAUTERINE LIFE

A. Immediate care needed at the time of birth
   1. Aspiration of mucus to provide an open airway
   2. Evaluation by use of Apgar score 1 and 5 minutes following birth; score determined by points for heart rate (most critical), respiration, muscle tone, reflex irritability, and color (Table 27-1: Apgar Score); scores: 7 to 10, good condition; 3 to 6, moderately depressed; 0 to 2, severely depressed; the lower the score the higher the neonatal morbidity and mortality and the greater the need for resuscitative interventions
   3. Maintenance of body temperature by drying infant and placing in skin-to-skin contact with mother or under radiant warmer
   4. Promotion of interaction between parents and newborn
   5. Constant observation of physical condition
   6. Identification of infant by applying matching identification bands to infant and mother; may include father and significant others

7. Eye care: prophylactic instillation of ordered antibiotic (e.g., erythromycin) in each eye to prevent ophthalmia neonatorum
8. Heel-stick blood specimen for laboratory tests to assess adaptation to extrauterine life and the presence of congenital conditions; outer aspect of heel used to prevent lancet penetration of bone, which can cause necrotizing osteochondritis (Figure 27-1: Heel-stick sites)

B. Behavioral characteristics during transition period
   1. First stage of transition to extrauterine life (period of reactivity)
      a. Lasts 0 to 30 minutes
      b. Alert and moving
      c. Gustatory movements
      d. Heart rate increases to 160 to 180 beats/min for 15 minutes and then declines to a baseline of 100 to 120 beats/min
      e. Respirations are 40 to 60 breaths/min, abdominal, and irregular; grunting, flaring, and retractions may occur intermittently
   2. Second stage of transition to extrauterine life (period of decreased responsiveness)
      a. Lasts 30 minutes to 2 hours
      b. Relaxation and rest occur
      c. Heart rate between 100 and 120 beats/min
      d. Respirations are rapid, shallow, and synchronous; chest gradually changes shape to increase anterior-posterior diameter
      e. Bowel sounds can be heard
   3. Third stage of transition to extrauterine life (second period of reactivity)
      a. Lasts 2 to 8 hours
      b. Increased responsiveness to stimuli
      c. Cardiac and respiratory rates may increase
      d. Changes in color and muscle tone may occur

Table 27-1 Apgar Score			
	SCORE		
Sign	**0**	**1**	**2**
Heart rate (bpm)	Absent	Slow (<100)	>100
Respiratory rate	Absent	Slow, weak cry	Good cry
Muscle tone	Flaccid	Some flexion of extremities	Well flexed
Reflex irritability	No response	Grimace	Cry
Color	Blue, pale	Body pink, extremities blue	Completely pink

From Lowdermilk DL, Perry SE: *Maternity nursing*, ed 7, St Louis, 2006, Mosby.

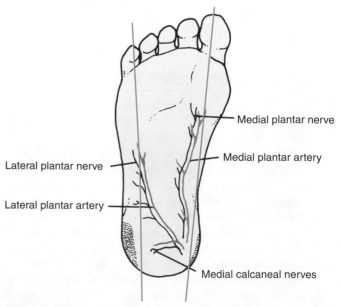

Figure 27-1 Heel-stick sites. (From Lowdermilk DL, Perry SE: *Maternity nursing*, ed 7, St Louis, 2006, Mosby.)

e. Bowel sounds become more frequent; may pass meconium

C. Characteristics of and changes in the newborn during the first week of life

1. Circulatory
   a. Clamping of cord at birth brings changes in fetal circulation: closure of foramen ovale and ductus arteriosus (after ductus arteriosus closes it is known as ligamentum arteriosum) and obliteration of umbilical arteries produce an adultlike circulation within 1 hour after birth
   b. Heart rate regular: 100 to 160 beats/min, but variable depending on infant's activity; soft heart murmur common for first month of life
   c. Clotting mechanism inadequate because intestinal bacteria are lacking that are necessary for the synthesis of prothrombin; vitamin K is given IM in the United States and orally in Canada
   d. Liver immature (although large): cannot destroy excessive red cells in newborn, resulting in physiologic jaundice by third day
   e. Hemoglobin level high: 14 to 20 g/100 mL of blood
   f. WBC count high: 6000 to 22,000/mm^3

2. Respiratory: 40 to 60 breaths/min during first 2 hours after birth, then 30 to 50 breaths/min irregular rate

3. Temperature: temperature maintained at 97.8° F or 98° F (36.6° C or 36.7° C); environmental factors may affect temperature

4. Excretory
   a. Stools: first stool is black-green and tenacious, called meconium; by third day, becomes mixed with light, yellow, milk stool, called transitional
   b. Kidneys immature: newborn should void during first 24 hours (at 2 weeks of age voids 20 times daily), albumin and urates (brick-red staining on diaper) common during first week

5. Integumentary
   a. Lanugo: fine, downy hair growth over entire body; preterm infants have more lanugo
   b. Milia: small, whitish, pinpoint spots over the nose caused by retained sebaceous secretions that resolve within a month
   c. Mongolian spots: blue-black discolorations on back, buttocks, and sacral region that disappear by first year; most common on dark-skinned infants
   d. Telangiectatic nevi or "stork bites" are pink or red areas caused by capillary dilation

6. Digestive
   a. Has stores of nutrients from intrauterine existence, therefore needs very little nourishment first few days
   b. Roots and sucks when anything is brought to mouth
   c. Digests simple carbohydrates, fats, and proteins readily

d. Cardiac sphincter of stomach not well developed; therefore regurgitates if stomach is overfull
   e. Needs to be burped frequently to remove air swallowed while suckling
   f. Gastric acidity remains low for 2 to 3 months

7. Metabolic
   a. Attempts to maintain body temperature by flexion of extremities, breaking down brown fat, and vasoconstriction
   b. Loses 5% to 10% of body weight by first week of life
   c. Needs screening for inborn errors of metabolism
      (1) Phenylketonuria (PKU) testing done 24 to 48 hours after first feeding to assess protein metabolism; some hospitals test earlier because of early discharge and repeat test at first follow-up visit; infants with excess of phenylalanine will need special diet to prevent retardation
      (2) Thyroxine (T$_4$) screening; inadequate thyroxine may lead to cretinism
      (3) Lactose intolerance; need for nonmilk formula
   d. Hypoglycemia may occur because of little glycogen reserve resulting in jitteriness, temperature and respiratory instability; higher risk in infants who are small for gestational age (SGA), large for gestational age (LGA) or have Down syndrome (e.g., infant of mother with diabetes [IDM])

8. Endocrine
   a. Enlargement of breasts in males (gynecomastia) and females is a result of hormones transmitted to infant by mother
   b. Female infants may have blood in the vagina (pseudomenstruation) because of withdrawal of maternal hormones

9. Neural
   a. CNS and brain not well developed; most responses are reflexive
   b. Breathing, sucking, and crying are early neural activities necessary for the infant's survival

10. Sleep
    a. Lowers body metabolism
    b. Helps restore energy and assimilate nutrients for growth

11. Habituation: a psychologic or physiologic phenomenon whereby the neonate's response to a repetitive stimulus decreases; promotes selectivity about the environment and promotes learning

D. Nutrition

1. Infant feeding: put to breast or give formula soon after birth; needs to ingest simple proteins, carbohydrates, fats, vitamins, and minerals for continued cell growth
   a. Fluid: 130 to 200 mL/kg or 2 to 3 oz of fluid/lb of body weight

b. Calories: 110 to 130 calories/kg or 50 to 60 calories/lb of body weight

c. Protein: 2.0 to 2.2 g per kilogram of body weight from birth to 6 months of age; 1.8 g/kg of body weight from 6 to 12 months of age

2. Self-regulation schedule
   a. Each infant born with different degree of maturity and rhythm of need
   b. Schedule is modified to meet needs of infant and parents
   c. Formula-fed infants fed on demand or about every 4 hours
   d. Breastfed infants fed on demand, approximately every 2 to 3 hours
   e. Feeding behavior and degree of satisfaction influence psychologic development
   f. Close mother-infant relationship in feeding process meets basic need of trust (Erikson's stage of trust versus mistrust)

E. Newborn immunity
   1. Passive immunity in utero: immunoglobulin G (IgG) passes from mother to fetus through the placenta
   2. Active immunity in utero: fetus produces immunoglobulin M (IgM) by the end of the first trimester
   3. Passive immunity after birth: immunoglobulin A (IgA) passes from mother to infant through colostrum, the precursor to breast milk

Nursing Care Common to All Newborns

A. Assessment/Analysis
   1. Gestational age
      a. Preterm: birth at less than 37 completed weeks' gestation
      b. Term: birth between the 37th and 42nd completed week of gestation
      c. Postterm: birth after 42 weeks' gestation
      d. Postmature: birth after 42 weeks' gestation; subjected to the effects of progressive placental insufficiency
   2. Birth weight
      a. Appropriate for gestational age (AGA): weight falls between 10th and 90th percentile (between 6 and 8.5 lb)
      b. Large for gestational age (LGA): weight is above 90th percentile
      c. Small for gestational age (SGA): weight is below 10th percentile
      d. Low birth weight (LBW): weight less than 2500 g (6 lb)
      e. Very low birth weight (VLBW): weight less than 1500 g (3.5 lb)
      f. Extremely low birth weight: weight less than 1000 g (2.2 lb)
      g. Intrauterine growth restriction (IUGR): fetal growth rate does not meet expected norms for gestational age

3. Skin
   a. Body is pink with slight cyanosis of hands and feet (acrocyanosis); jaundice is not expected during the first 24 hours of life
   b. Abrasions, rashes, crackling, turgor, and elasticity indicate the status of tissue hydration; milia (white, pinpoint spots over the nose caused by retained sebaceous secretions), birthmarks, forceps marks, ecchymosis, or papules may be present

4. Vital signs: assessment moves from least to most invasive; first monitor respirations, then heart rate, then temperature; respirations are abdominal and irregular, with a rate of 40 to 60 breaths/min during first 2 hours and then 30 to 50 breaths/min retractions with depression of the sternum are abnormal; heart rate is 100 beats/min at rest, 180 beats/min when crying; temperature range is from 97.7° F to 98.9° F

5. Head and sensory organs
   a. Head and chest circumference nearly equal with chest slightly smaller than head; if reversed, assess for microcephaly
   b. Fontanels should be flat; bulging when baby cries could indicate increased intracranial pressure; sunken fontanels indicate dehydration
   c. Symmetry of face: as infant cries, sides of the face should move equally
   d. Characteristics of head: check for molding, abrasions, or skin breakdown; observe for caput succedaneum: edema of soft tissue of scalp; cephalohematoma: edema of scalp caused by effusion of blood between the bone and periosteum; extend the head fully in all directions for adequacy in range of motion; infant's head will lag as infant is raised
   e. Eyes: observe for discharge or irritation, pupils for reaction to light, equality of eye movements (there is usually some ocular incoordination), sclerae for clarity, jaundice, or hemorrhage
   f. Nose: observe for patency of both nostrils; sneezing commonly occurs in an attempt to clear mucus from nose
   g. Mouth: observe and palpate the gums and hard and soft palates for color and continuity (white patches that bleed on rubbing indicate thrush, a monilial infection)
   h. Ears: auricles open; vernix covers tympanic membrane, making otoscopic examination useless (ring bell close to ear—infant should stir); both eyes should be at same level as ears; upper earlobes curved (flatness indicative of kidney anomaly)

6. Chest and abdomen
   a. Chest auscultation: only respiratory sounds should be audible (noisy crackling sounds are unexpected); regular heart rate

b. Nipples may have a thin discharge (witch's milk) caused by maternal oxytocin that crossed the placenta

c. Abdomen
   (1) Listen for bowel sounds over the abdomen
   (2) Palpate the spleen with fingertips under the left costal margin: tip should be palpable
   (3) Palpate liver on the right side: normally 1 cm below the costal margin
   (4) Monitor umbilical cord for redness, odor, or discharge; number of vessels present (one vein and two arteries; the presence of two vessels is associated with congenital abnormalities)
   (5) Observe for umbilical hernia when newborn cries
   (6) Palpate the femoral pulses gently at inner aspect of the groin; presence of pulses indicates intact circulation to extremities

7. Genitalia
   a. Males
      (1) Palpate the scrotum for testes: may be undescended in preterm infants, usually descend during childhood (must descend by puberty or sperm will be destroyed by high temperature within the abdominal cavity)
      (2) Enlargement of scrotum: indicates hydrocele (diagnosis confirmed by transparent appearance of the scrotum when a flashlight is held close to the scrotal sac, known as transillumination)
      (3) Observe tip of penis for the urinary meatus: epispadias, meatus on upper surface of penis; hypospadias, meatus on lower surface
      (4) Observe voiding pattern
   b. Females
      (1) Observe the genitalia for labia, urinary meatus, and vaginal opening
      (2) Edema of labia and bloody mucoid discharge are expected; these findings result from transfer of maternal hormones
      (3) Check for voiding
   c. Ambiguous genitalia
      (1) External genitalia do not allow for clear identification of gender
      (2) Further studies to determine gender are performed with surgical intervention as required

8. Extremities
   a. Hands and arms: thumbs clenched in fist; wrist angle is 0 degrees
      (1) Check for number and variation of fingers
      (2) Check the clavicles and scapulae while putting arms through range of motion; clicking or resistance indicates dislocation or fracture
      (3) Palpate for fractures; indicated by crepitation
   b. Feet and legs

      (1) Check toes: appearance and number
      (2) Adduct and abduct feet through range of motion; there should be no resistance or tightness
      (3) Flex both legs onto lower abdomen; there should be no resistance or tightness; abduct knees and listen for click (Ortolani sign—indicates developmental dysplasia of hip)
      (4) Place both feet on a flat surface and bend the knees; knees should be at the same height (when unequal, known as the Allis sign—indicates developmental dysplasia of the hip)
      (5) Observe gluteal folds for symmetry; asymmetry indicates developmental dysplasia of the hip

9. Back: turn the infant on the abdomen, run a finger along the vertebral column; any dimples, separations, or swellings are indicative of spina bifida

10. Anus: patency confirmed with passage of meconium; imperforate anus is ruled out by digital examination

11. Neuromuscular development: check reflexes
    a. Rooting: touch the infant's cheek; infant should search for finger; may persist for up to 1 year
    b. Sucking: place an object close to the infant's mouth; infant should make an attempt to suck; persists throughout infancy; presence important to prevent aspiration
    c. Gag: stimulation of posterior pharynx causes choking; persists through life
    d. Grasp: place fingers in palm of infant's hand (palmar) or on sole of foot below toes (plantar); fingers and toes flex in a grasping motion; lessen by 3 and 8 months, respectively
    e. Babinski: run thumb up middle undersurface of infant's foot; toes will separate and flare out; disappears after 1 year
    f. Moro: sudden jar or change in equilibrium causes extension and abduction of extremities followed by flexion and adduction; disappears by 3 to 4 months
    g. Startle: make a loud, sharp noise close to the infant; will result in the infant's bringing both arms and legs close to the body as if in an embrace; disappears by 4 months of age
    h. Crawl: when the infant is on a firm surface and turned on the abdomen, crawling movements will follow; disappears at about 6 weeks
    i. Step or dance: while the infant is supported under both arms, stepping movements will occur when feet are placed on a firm surface; disappears after 3 to 4 weeks
    j. Tonic neck or fencing: extension of the arm and/or leg on the side to which the head is turned quickly with flexion of the contralateral limbs; usually disappears by 3 to 4 months

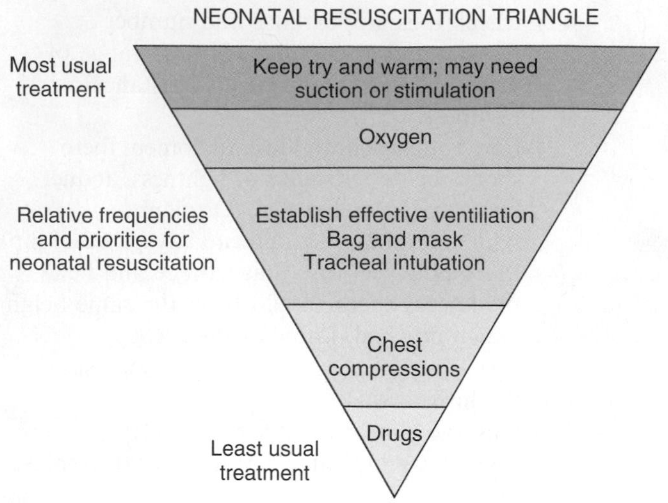

NEONATAL RESUSCITATION TRIANGLE

Figure 27-2 Neonatal resuscitation triangle. (From Hamilton P: ABCs of labor care: care of the newborn in the delivery room, *Br Med* J 318:1403-1406, 1999.)

B. Planning/Implementation
1. Monitor and maintain a patent airway (Figure 27-2: Neonatal resuscitation triangle)
   a. Suction mucus as needed to maintain an open airway
   b. Position: head in sniff position or side-lying position to facilitate drainage of mucus
   c. Observe for signs of respiratory distress: grunting, flaring of nostrils, sternal retractions
   d. Observe for signs of aspiration during first feeding (choking, cyanosis); stop feeding, suction airway, and provide O_2 before resuming feeding
2. Provide warmth
   a. Keep in radiant warmer with a surface temperature probe on until body temperature is stabilized to prevent chilling; infant is unable to shiver and breaks down brown fat to produce energy for warmth; preterm or SGA infants can be compromised by chilling because of small amount of brown fat available for breakdown
   b. Clothing should be loose, soft
   c. Environment should be warm and free from drafts
   d. Skin should be kept clean and dry
3. Monitor vital signs; weigh daily
4. Provide daily sponge bath; change diaper frequently
5. Observe umbilical cord stump for edema, redness, and drainage; provide care according to hospital protocol; clamp usually removed before discharge; keep dry; secure diaper below level of cord; sponge bathe until cord falls off
6. Administer vitamin K to prevent hemorrhagic disease of the newborn; absence of bacteria in sterile gut of newborn prevents synthesis of clotting factors
7. Administer hepatitis B vaccine
   a. Centers for Disease Control and Prevention mandate that newborns receive vaccine regardless of mother's status

   b. Vaccine may be administered in the hospital but is often administered in primary care practitioner's office
8. Administer prophylactic ophthalmic antibiotic
9. Provide for feeding (see Breastfeeding and Formula Feeding [Bottle Feeding])
10. Teach care of infant to parents; role-model acceptance of infant regardless of infant's physical characteristics or behavior
11. Care for circumcision: observe for bleeding, monitor urination, apply diaper loosely, change dressing with each diaper change or at least every 4 hours and apply petrolatum to the glans; care for uncircumcised: bathe daily, do not retract foreskin
12. Provide for human contact: touching, talking, rocking, singing
C. Evaluation/Outcomes
1. Maintains patency of the airway
2. Stabilizes body temperature within acceptable range
3. Urinates amounts commensurate with fluid intake
4. Passes stool
5. Maintains 90% of birth weight
6. Remains free from complications associated with the perinatal period

BREASTFEEDING
Data Base
A. Advantages
1. Psychologic value of closeness and satisfaction in beginning mother-infant relationship
2. Optimum nutritional value for infant
3. Economical and readily accessible
4. Infant is less likely to be allergic to mother's milk
5. Aids in the development of the infant's facial muscles, jaw, and nasal passages because stronger sucking is necessary
6. Assists in involution of uterus because it stimulates oxytocin secretion that initiates the let-down reflex
7. Reduces chances for infection because maternal antibodies are present in colostrum and milk
8. Frequent feeding stimulates evacuation of meconium, preventing reabsorption of bilirubin into circulation
B. Prerequisites
1. Psychologic readiness of mother is a major factor in successful breastfeeding
2. Adequate diet to ensure high-quality milk; increased intake of milk, protein, calories, and noncaffeinated fluids is necessary
3. Suitable rest and exercise
4. Infant's sucking at the breast stimulates the maternal posterior pituitary to produce oxytocin, the properties of which, in the blood system, constrict the lactiferous sinuses to move the milk down through the nipple ducts: known as the let-down reflex; sucking also stimulates prolactin secretion
5. Family support and absence of emotional stress in the mother, because anxiety inhibits the let-down reflex

C. Contraindications
1. In mother: active tuberculosis; acute contagious disease; HIV positive; chronic disease such as cancer, advanced nephritis, cardiac disease, hepatitis C; extensive surgery; opiate addiction
2. In infant: cleft lip or palate or any other condition that interferes with or prevents grasp of the nipple; congenital anomalies that prevent ingestion; inborn errors of metabolism that result in a negative response to breast milk
3. Many drugs are excreted in breast milk and have harmful effects on the developing infant; these drugs must be avoided or taken judiciously, if necessary; careful monitoring of the infant is required

Nursing Care of the Breastfeeding Mother and Infant

A. Assessment/Analysis
1. Condition of nipples
2. Desire to breastfeed
3. Level of anxiety and concerns regarding breastfeeding
4. Knowledge of breastfeeding and breast care
5. Family support
B. Planning/Implementation
1. Teach feeding schedule
   a. Self-demand schedule is desirable; infant usually self-regulates to a schedule, usually every 2 to 3 hours
   b. Length of feeding time is variable; about 15 to 20 minutes per breast, with greatest quantity of milk consumed in first 5 to 10 minutes
   c. Feed more often if lactation diminishes to stimulate an increase in milk production
2. Teach feeding techniques
   a. Mother and infant in comfortable position, such as semireclining or in comfortable chair
   b. Entire body of infant should be turned toward mother's breast; alternate starting breast and use both breasts at each feeding
   c. Initiate feeding by stimulating rooting reflex and direct nipple straight into infant's mouth (stroking cheek toward breast, being careful not to stroke other cheek, because this will confuse infant); as much areola as possible should be in the infant's mouth to promote latching-on (Figure 27-3: Correct attachment [latch-on] of infant at breast)
   d. Burp infant during and after feeding to allow for escape of air: sit infant on lap, flexed forward; rub or pat back (avoid jarring infant)
   e. Breast milk intake similar to formula intake: 130 to 200 mL of milk/kg (2 to 3 oz of milk/lb) of infant's weight; from one sixth to one seventh of infant's weight per day
   f. After lactation has been established, occasional formula feeding can be substituted but is not

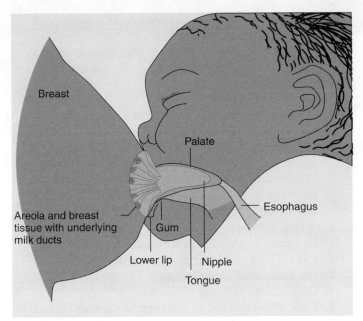

Figure 27-3 Correct attachment (latch-on) of infant at breast. (From Lowdermilk DL, Perry SE: *Maternity nursing,* ed 7, St Louis, 2006, Mosby.)

recommended; breast milk can be expelled manually or via pump, stored, and given to infant in a bottle later if the mother is not available
   g. Length of time for continuing breastfeeding is variable
3. Teach care of breasts
   a. Cleanse with plain water once daily (soap or alcohol can cause irritation and dryness)
   b. Support breasts day and night with properly fitting brassiere
   c. Nursing pads should be placed inside bra cup to absorb any milk leaking between feedings; allow nipples to air dry at intervals
   d. Plastic bra liners should be avoided because they increase heat and perspiration and decrease air circulation necessary for drying of the nipple
   e. If breasts are engorged, teach mother to take warm showers, apply icepacks between feedings, and put infant to breast more frequently
C. Evaluation/Outcomes
1. Mother demonstrates effective breastfeeding techniques
2. Mother remains free from nipple cracking and infection
3. Infant produces six or more wet diapers daily
4. Infant gains weight

FORMULA FEEDING (BOTTLE FEEDING)

Data Base

A. Advantages
1. Provides an alternative to breastfeeding
2. Less restrictive than breastfeeding; may meet needs of working mothers
3. Allows a more accurate assessment of intake

4. May be indicated in the presence of a congenital anomaly such as cleft palate
5. May be necessary for infants who require special formulas because of allergies or inborn errors of metabolism

B. Types of formulas
1. Commercial liquid or powdered formulas
2. Special formulas
3. Unmodified regular cow's milk, liquid or reconstituted; not appropriate for infants before 12 months of age; cow's milk contains more protein and calcium and less vitamin C, iron, and carbohydrate than breast milk

C. Contraindications
1. Deficient knowledge of formula preparation
2. Poor storage and refrigeration practices
3. Contaminated water supply
4. Cost of formula and equipment
5. Lack of equipment to adequately prepare bottles

Nursing Care of the Formula-Feeding Parents and Infant

A. Assessment/Analysis
1. Desire to formula feed
2. Sucking ability of infant
3. Knowledge of formulas and formula preparation

B. Planning/Implementation
1. Teach preparation of formula
   a. Calculation of formula to yield 110 to 130 calories and 130 to 200 mL of fluid/kg of body weight; caution regarding dangers of overdilution (inadequate weight gain) and underdilution (excess weight gain)
   b. Sterilization of formula by terminal heat or aseptic method
   c. Advantages and disadvantages of different commercial formulas
   d. Refrigeration of formula
2. Teach feeding techniques
   a. Always hold infant during feeding to provide warm body contact (bottle propping may contribute to aspiration of formula)
   b. Hold bottle so that nipple is always filled with milk to prevent excessive air ingestion
   c. Adjust size of nipple hole to needs of infant (a premature infant needs a larger hole that requires less sucking)
   d. Burp during and after feeding; place infant on right side to aid digestion and prevent aspiration
   e. Feeding should be offered on demand to meet the infant's needs

C. Evaluation/Outcomes
1. Mother demonstrates effective preparation of formula
2. Mother demonstrates effective formula-feeding techniques
3. Infant produces six or more wet diapers daily
4. Infant gains weight

NURSING CARE OF HIGH-RISK NEWBORNS

✿ PRETERM INFANT

Data Base

A. Prevention
1. Prevention of preterm birth is vital, because this is the cause of more than half of the neonatal deaths in the United States
2. Prevention of malnutrition and underweight in the mother because these are associated with higher preterm birth rates and IUGR
3. Education about nutrition and general hygiene before planning a family
4. Education about the hazards of drug use and smoking
5. Adequate and early prenatal health supervision
6. Referrals to community agencies to facilitate services to persons in need

B. Classification
1. Classification of newborn infants is made on the basis of gestational age as well as birth weight; full-term infant may be of low birth weight, whereas preterm infant need not be low birth weight
2. Near-term infant: 35 to 37 weeks
3. Preterm infant: born before term (36 weeks or less)
4. Low birth weight (less than 2500 g); very low birth weight (less than 1500 g); extremely low birth weight (less than 1000 g); may be both preterm and small for gestational age

C. Therapeutic interventions for the preterm neonate immediately after birth
1. Suctioning of mucus to maintain an open airway
2. Direct laryngoscopy, tracheal suctioning, intubation, and mouth-to-tube resuscitation in the absence of respirations
3. Suctioning of stomach contents at birth facilitates respirations
4. Heated isolette or radiant warmer; maintenance of body temperature is difficult because of heat loss by skin evaporation and limited subcutaneous fat
5. Readily available O_2 and resuscitation equipment at all times

D. Characteristics of preterm infant
1. Less subcutaneous fat; therefore the skin is wrinkled and blood vessels and bony structures are visible; lanugo present on face; eyebrows are absent; ears are poorly supported by cartilage; breast bud size is small with underdeveloped nipples; square window sign present
2. Circumference of the head is large in comparison with the chest; the fontanels are small and bones are soft
3. Skin color changes when infant is moved; upper half or one side of the body appears pale and lower half or one side of the body is red (harlequin sign)

4. Posture is one of complete relaxation with marked extension of the legs and abduction of the hips; random movements are common with slightest stimulus
5. Heat regulation poorly developed because of immaturity of CNS; heat loss caused by large skin surface area and lack of subcutaneous and brown fat; poorly developed respiratory center with diminished O_2 consumption causing asphyxia; weak heart action, therefore slower circulation and poor oxygenation; insufficient heat production caused by inadequate metabolism
6. Respirations are not efficient because of muscular weakness of lungs and rib cage and limited surfactant production; retraction at xiphoid is evidence of air hunger; infant should be stimulated if apnea occurs
7. Atelectasis can occur, manifested by increasing cyanosis; rapid, irregular respirations; flaring of nostrils; intercostal or suprasternal retractions; grunting on expiration
8. Greater tendency toward capillary fragility; red and WBC counts are low; anemia during first few months of life
9. Higher incidence of intracranial hemorrhage; manifested by muscle twitching, seizures, cyanosis, abnormal respirations, and a short, shrill cry
10. Weak sucking and swallowing reflexes; small capacity of stomach; low gastric acidity; slow emptying time of the stomach; the usual caloric intake of 110 to 130 calories/kg (50 to 60 calories/lb) of body weight may be increased to 200 to 220 calories/kg (100 calories/lb) for adequate growth and development
11. Reduced glomerular filtration rate results in decreased ability to concentrate urine and conserve fluid

Nursing Care of Preterm Infants
A. Assessment/Analysis
1. Respiratory rate and effort; heart rate; temperature; BP
2. O_2 concentrations via oximeter
3. Skin color and integrity
4. Daily weight; fluid and electrolyte status (radiant warmer causes dehydration)
5. Ability of infant to suck; nutritional status
6. Parents' ability to cope with preterm birth
B. Planning/Implementation
1. Maintain airway; check ventilator function if used; position with head and chest elevated to promote ventilation; suction secretions when necessary; maintain temperature of environment
2. Observe for changes in respiratory status, vital signs, and color
3. Check efficacy of isolette: maintain heat, humidity, and O_2 concentration; administer O_2 if

necessary; monitor O_2 carefully to prevent retinopathy of the newborn
4. Maintain aseptic technique to prevent infection
5. Adhere to the techniques of gavage feeding to maintain safety
6. Observe weight gain pattern
7. Determine blood gases frequently to assess for acidosis
8. Institute phototherapy should hyperbilirubinemia occur
9. Implement appropriate environmental modification: decreased or cycled light; reduced noise
10. Refer parents to support group
11. Support parents by letting them verbalize and ask questions to relieve anxiety
12. Provide liberal visiting hours for parents; encourage them to participate in care and talk to and touch infant
13. Arrange for follow-up care by a visiting nurse before and after discharge
C. Evaluation/Outcomes
1. Maintains respiratory functioning
2. Maintains body temperature within acceptable limits
3. Remains free from infection
4. Gains weight

RESPIRATORY DISTRESS SYNDROME (RDS)
Data Base
A. A deficiency in surface-active (detergent-like) lipoproteins (surfactant) results in inadequate lung inflation and ventilation
B. Can occur in preterm and low birth weight newborns, as well as in infants after cesarean birth
C. Therapeutic intervention: surfactant replacement given to preterm infants through endotracheal tube

Nursing Care of Infants With Respiratory Distress Syndrome
A. Assessment/Analysis
1. Cyanosis
2. Tachypnea; dyspnea; sternal retractions; nasal flaring; grunting
3. Respiratory and metabolic acidosis
B. Planning/Implementation
1. Admit to neonatal intensive care unit
2. Maintain patent airway
3. Keep in an isolette with O_2 and high humidity; prevent chilling
4. Administer surfactant by aerosol as ordered
5. Administer antibiotics as ordered
6. Maintain function of mechanical ventilation if employed
7. Monitor for signs of respiratory and metabolic acidosis
8. Administer feedings as ordered; prevent exhaustion

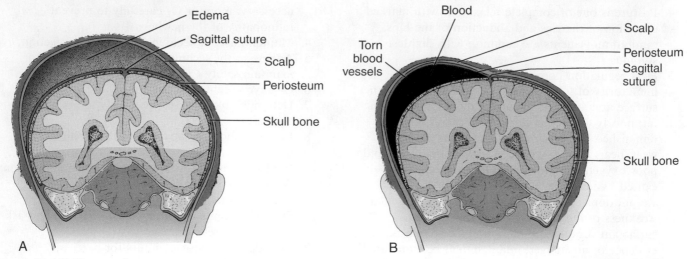

Figure 27-4 Differences between caput succedaneum and cephalohematoma. **A,** Caput succedaneum. Edema of scalp noted at birth crosses suture lines. **B,** Cephalohematoma. Bleeding between periosteum and skull bone appearing within first two hours; does not cross suture lines. (From Lowdermilk DL, Perry SE: *Maternity nursing*, ed 7, St Louis, 2006, Mosby.)

C. Evaluation/Outcomes
  1. Remains free from respiratory distress
  2. Maintains fluid and electrolyte balance
  3. Gains weight

 MECONIUM ASPIRATION SYNDROME (MAS)

Data Base

A. A hypoxic insult to fetus that causes increased intestinal peristalsis with passage of meconium into the amniotic fluid; the meconium-stained fluid is aspirated by the infant during the first few breaths after birth, causing an obstruction in the lung that results in chemical pneumonitis
B. Therapeutic interventions
  1. Amnioinfusion before birth to thin particles of meconium
  2. Suctioning after head appears outside vaginal orifice
  3. Surfactant lavages immediately after birth
  4. Oxygenation and ventilation

Nursing Care of Infants With Meconium Aspiration Syndrome

A. Assessment/Analysis
  1. Signs of fetal hypoxia and meconium-stained amniotic fluid during intrapartum
  2. Respiratory distress after birth
  3. Signs of sepsis
  4. Altered neurologic status (seizures)
B. Planning/Implementation
  1. Remove meconium and amniotic fluid from infant's nasopharynx and oropharynx immediately after birth
  2. See Planning/Implementation under Respiratory Distress Syndrome
C. Evaluation/Outcomes
  1. Maintains respiratory functioning
  2. Remains free from infection
  3. Feeds without difficulty

 CRANIAL BIRTH INJURIES (CAPUT SUCCEDANEUM, CEPHALOHEMATOMA, INTRACRANIAL HEMORRHAGE)

Data Base

A. Caput succedaneum: edema with extravasation of serum into scalp tissues caused by molding during the birth process; crosses the suture lines of the bony plates of the skull; no treatment is necessary; it subsides in a few days (Figure 27-4: Differences between caput succedaneum and cephalohematoma)
B. Cephalohematoma: edema of the scalp with effusion of blood between the bone and periosteum; stops at the suture line; no treatment is necessary; it disappears within a few weeks to a few months after birth; resolution of hematoma can lead to hyperbilirubinemia
C. Intracranial hemorrhage: bleeding into cerebellum, pons, and medulla oblongata caused by a tearing of the tentorium cerebelli; occurs in preterm infants and following prolonged labor, difficult forceps birth, precipitate birth, version, or breech extraction

Nursing Care of Infants With Intracranial Hemorrhage

A. Assessment/Analysis
  1. Abnormal respirations; cyanosis
  2. Shrill or weak cry
  3. Flaccidity or spasticity; seizures
  4. Restlessness; wakefulness
  5. Impaired sucking reflex
B. Planning/Implementation
  1. Keep in isolette with oxygen
  2. Maintain in high-Fowler's position
  3. Administer prescribed vitamins C and K to control and prevent further hemorrhage
  4. Institute ordered gavage feedings when sucking reflex is impaired

5. Support parents because of guarded prognosis

C. Evaluation/Outcomes

1. Remains free from neurologic damage

2. Gains weight

NEUROMUSCULOSKELETAL BIRTH INJURIES

Data Base

A. Facial paralysis: temporary paralysis of one side of the face caused by pressure on cranial nerve VII (facial nerve) during a difficult vaginal birth or the use of forceps; no treatment is necessary because it usually disappears in a few days

B. Erb-Duchenne paralysis (brachial palsy): paralysis of the muscles of the upper arm caused by injury to the brachial plexus during a prolonged, difficult labor or traumatic birth; treatment depends on severity of paralysis

C. Dislocations and fractures: caused by difficult birth/ extraction birth; treatment depends on the site of fracture

Nursing Care of Infants With Neuromusculoskeletal Birth Injuries

A. Assessment/Analysis

1. Facial paralysis: inability to close eye, drawing mouth to one side, and absence of forehead wrinkles when crying

2. Erb-Duchenne paralysis: flaccid arm with elbow extended, unequal Moro reflex

3. Fractures: variation in range of movement, immobility, crepitation

B. Planning/Implementation

1. Facial paralysis: continue to monitor neonate

2. Erb-Duchenne paralysis (brachial paralysis or palsy)

   a. Massage and exercise arm as ordered to prevent contractures

   b. Place in traffic cop or maitre d' position

   c. Apply ordered splints and braces, which are used when paralysis is severe

3. Dislocations and fractures: position as ordered; swaddling, splints, slings, or casts are used

4. Reassure parents and teach necessary care and positioning

C. Evaluation/Outcomes

1. Maintains correct alignment of limb

2. Achieves movement in affected part

HEMOLYTIC DISORDERS

Data Base

A. Rh incompatibility occurs when an Rh-negative woman is sensitized to Rh-positive blood from an Rh-positive fetus or other sources and develops antibodies against the Rh-positive blood

1. In subsequent pregnancies these antibodies are transferred through the placental barrier to the fetus, with a resulting agglutination and destruction of red cells (erythroblastosis fetalis); rarely a problem in first pregnancy

2. Prevention: RhoGAM, a preparation of Rh_o (D) immune globulin, is now given intramuscularly to the Rh-negative mother about the 28th week of pregnancy and within 72 hours after birth or abortion to prevent the development of antibodies in this and future pregnancies; mother must be negative for Rh antibodies to receive RhoGAM

B. The most common ABO incompatibility occurs when the fetal blood type is A, B, or AB and the mother is type O; mother's anti-A or anti-B antibodies are transferred through the placental barrier to the fetus, causing hemolysis and resulting in fetal anemia, jaundice, and kernicterus (excessively high bilirubin levels) within the first 24 hours of life (pathologic jaundice); ABO incompatibility is more common but less severe than Rh incompatibility; previous exposures to A, B, or AB blood do not increase the formation of anti-A or anti-B antibodies, so first pregnancy can be affected

C. Therapeutic interventions

1. During pregnancy, amniotic fluid determinations are done by chemical and spectrophotometric analysis; elevated readings warrant either intrauterine exchange transfusion or induction of labor, depending on the weeks of gestation

2. Phototherapy is used in an attempt to reduce mild to moderate kernicterus in the newborn

3. Exchange transfusions of Rh-negative blood are done on severely affected infants to decrease the antibody level and increase infant RBCs and hemoglobin levels

Nursing Care of Infants With Hemolytic Disorders

A. Assessment/Analysis

1. Blood incompatibility (ABO, Rh) between mother and fetus

2. Jaundice and increasing bilirubin levels during first 24 hours after birth

3. Bilirubin, hematocrit, and hemoglobin levels

4. Lethargy or irritability

5. Poor feeding pattern; vomiting

6. Enlargement of the liver and spleen

7. Signs of kernicterus; absence of Moro reflex; apnea; high-pitched cry; opisthotonos; tremors; seizures

B. Planning/Implementation

1. Monitor maternal antibody titers

2. Administer RhoGAM within 72 hours after birth if mother is Rh-negative and neonate is Rh-positive; teach why RhoGAM is necessary (not given to Rh-negative sensitized women)

3. Teach mother why intrauterine exchange transfusions may be necessary

4. Care for the neonate receiving phototherapy: protect eyes from light; monitor for signs of dehydration

C. Evaluation/Outcomes
 1. Mother, with incompatibilities other than Rh, remains free from Rh isoimmunization
 2. Neonate remains free from injury

THRUSH
Data Base
A. An oral infection caused by *Candida albicans*
B. Organism may be transmitted as the neonate passes through the vaginal canal, by unclean feeding utensils, by breasts that are improperly cleansed before breastfeeding, or by ineffective handwashing techniques

Nursing Care of Infants With Thrush
A. Assessment/Analysis
 1. White patches on tongue, palate, and inner cheeks that bleed when touched
 2. Sucking difficulties
B. Planning/Implementation
 1. Teach mother how to cleanse breasts or feeding equipment before feeding
 2. Teach mother how to apply oral topical agents such as nystatin (Mycostatin)
C. Evaluation/Outcomes
 1. Infant achieves infection-free status
 2. Infant gains weight

OPHTHALMIA NEONATORUM
Data Base
A. An eye infection caused by *Neisseria gonorrhoeae* or *Chlamydia trachomatis*
B. Organism is transmitted from the genital tract of an infected mother during birth or by infected hands
C. Chlamydial infections can also cause pneumonia
D. Prevention: ophthalmic antibiotic (0.5% erythromycin ophthalmic ointment or 1% tetracycline ointment) instilled at birth after providing for initial bonding

Nursing Care of Infants With Ophthalmia Neonatorum
A. Assessment/Analysis
 1. Perinatal history of maternal infection
 2. Purulent conjunctivitis if prophylactic treatment is not used; manifested 3 to 4 days after birth
 3. Respiratory status with chlamydial infection
B. Planning/Implementation
 1. Cleanse the eyes with normal saline by wiping from inner to outer canthus
 2. Treat with prescribed antibiotics
 3. Refer for ophthalmic evaluation
 4. Monitor vital signs and administer O_2 with chlamydial infection
C. Evaluation/Outcomes
 1. Maintains or achieves infection-free status
 2. Remains free from sequelae of infection

SYPHILIS
Data Base
A. A congenital systemic infection caused by *Treponema pallidum*
B. Prenatal syphilis transmitted to fetus by the mother
C. Incidence of fetal infection varies with stage of the disease in the mother at the time of pregnancy; newborn of infected mother should be screened for syphilis
D. Before fourth month, fetus seldom infected; Langerhans' cells in chorion are protective barrier
E. The longer the infection remains untreated the greater the damage to the fetus; pregnant women are treated with an antibiotic when diagnosed
F. Adequate treatment of pregnant woman treats the fetus

Nursing Care of Infants With Syphilis
A. Assessment/Analysis
 1. Perinatal history of maternal infection; screen neonate for signs of congenital syphilis
 2. Maculopapular lesions of the palms of the hands and soles of the feet
 3. Restlessness
 4. Rhinitis; hoarse cry
 5. Enlargement of the spleen; palpable lymph nodes
 6. Enlarged ends of long bones on x-ray examination
B. Planning/Implementation
 1. Administer ordered antibiotics, usually penicillin
 2. Teach mother the importance of continued medical supervision
C. Evaluation/Outcomes
 1. Maintains or achieves infection-free status
 2. Remains free from sequelae of infection

ACQUIRED IMMUNODEFICIENCY SYNDROME (AIDS)
Data Base
A. Generalized invasion of T cells by the human immunodeficiency virus (HIV)
B. Gynecologic manifestations occur first
 1. Recurrent vulvovaginal candidiasis
 2. Bacterial vaginosis
 3. Recurrent genital herpes simplex virus
 4. Human papillomavirus
 5. Pelvic inflammatory disease
 6. Cervical dysplasia and neoplasms
C. Transmitted by mother who is HIV positive
D. Newborn should be screened for HIV infection when either parent is at high risk for HIV or has been diagnosed as HIV positive
E. Symptoms are usually not present at birth
F. If zidovudine (AZT) is taken by pregnant woman, transmission of HIV infection to the fetus is greatly reduced

Nursing Care of Infants With Acquired Immunodeficiency Syndrome

A. Assessment/Analysis
1. Signs of prematurity or small for gestational age
2. Failure to thrive
3. Enlarged spleen and liver
4. Diarrhea; weight loss
5. Neurologic deficits
6. Frequent and debilitating infections as the child ages
B. Planning/Implementation
1. Obtain blood specimen for HIV testing
2. Institute and teach parents standard precautions
3. Inform parents that the virus may be transmitted via breast milk and that infant should be formula fed; in developing countries breastfeeding may be recommended where there are no safe alternatives
4. Stress the importance of continued medical supervision
5. Provide human contact to meet the infant's emotional needs
C. Evaluation/Outcomes
1. Infant remains free from opportunistic infections
2. Caregiver maintains standard precautions

NECROTIZING ENTEROCOLITIS (NEC)

Data Base
A. Necrotic lesions in intestines resulting from three factors: intestinal ischemia; presence of pathologic bacteria colonies; excess formula in intestines
B. More common in preterm infants and formula-fed infants; occurs several weeks after birth
C. Prevention: encouragement of breastfeeding
D. Therapeutic interventions: surgical excision often required, which may lead to short bowel syndrome; early minimal feedings may be protective against NEC

Nursing Care of Infants With Necrotizing Enterocolitis
A. Assessment/Analysis
1. Abdominal distention; diminished or absent bowel sounds
2. Impaired sucking; vomiting; loss of weight
3. Gastrointestinal bleeding
B. Planning/Implementation
1. Maintain NPO and nasogastric decompression
2. Administer IV therapy and total parenteral nutrition as ordered
3. Monitor fluid and electrolyte balance
4. Provide ileostomy or colostomy care if ostomy has been created
5. Provide nonnutritive sucking (pacifier)
C. Evaluation/Outcomes
1. Maintains fluid and electrolyte balance
2. Gains weight

SEPSIS

Data Base
A. A generalized bacterial infection
B. Precipitated by infected amniotic fluid, an infected birth canal, or a break in aseptic technique after birth while receiving care in the newborn nursery

Nursing Care of Infants With Sepsis
A. Assessment/Analysis
1. Poor feeding; vomiting
2. High temperature or inability to maintain temperature
3. Lethargy; increasing irritability
4. Signs of anemia; pallor
5. Increased number of stools
B. Planning/Implementation
1. Monitor IV fluid administration
2. Administer oxygen as ordered
3. Administer IV antibiotic therapy as ordered
4. Aid in decontaminating nursery
C. Evaluation/Outcomes
1. Maintains fluid and electrolyte status
2. Achieves infection-free status

SUBSTANCE DEPENDENCE (NEONATAL ABSTINENCE SYNDROME)

Data Base
A. Infant born with physiologic dependence on alcohol or opiates as a result of maternal drug use and/or abuse
B. Dependence: many preparations, including alcohol, methadone, heroin, cocaine
C. Perinatal mortality: 6 to 8 times higher than in control group
D. Alcohol abuse in the mother can result in fetal alcohol syndrome, producing congenital defects and retardation
E. Clinical findings
1. Infant may exhibit signs of respiratory distress, jaundice, congenital anomalies, and behavioral aberrations
2. Withdrawal symptoms appear soon after birth; severity depends on the length of maternal addiction, the type of drug used, the amount of drug taken, the concurrent use of other drugs, and the time the drug was taken before birth; may persist for up to 4 months

Nursing Care of Infants Who Are Dependent on Alcohol or Opiates
A. Assessment/Analysis
1. Maternal intake of drug, including type, time, and amount
2. Signs of withdrawal in the infant
   a. Facial scratches; hyperactivity; tremors; seizures
   b. Yawning; disturbed sleep
   c. Tachypnea; sneezing; stuffy nose
   d. Shrill cry
   e. Poor sucking; drooling; vomiting
   f. Diarrhea; excoriated buttocks

B. Planning/Implementation
1. Monitor neuromuscular status
2. Monitor vital signs; support respiratory functioning
3. Provide small, frequent feedings
4. Administer sedatives or opiates as ordered
5. Keep environmental stimuli to a minimum; maintain seizure precautions
6. Promote mother-infant bonding when possible; provide a constant caregiver
7. Hold and cuddle frequently but provide for periods of uninterrupted rest
8. Swaddle when in crib
9. Use soft nipple to reduce sucking effort; administer supplemental methods of nutritional support as ordered
10. Encourage continued medical supervision
11. Refer to appropriate community-service agencies for family support and supervision
C. Evaluation/Outcomes
1. Maintains respiratory functioning
2. Survives withdrawal from drug
3. Establishes a sleeping pattern
4. Gains weight

TORCH

Data Base
A. TORCH is an acronym for the following infections:
1. T—Toxoplasmosis *(Toxoplasma gondii):* can be acquired by eating raw or undercooked meat or contact with cat feces; organism crosses the placenta; severity of infection related to gestational age; can cause hydrocephalus, intracranial calcifications, or chorioretinitis in the infant
2. O—Others: HIV, gonorrhea *(Neisseria gonorrhoeae)*, syphilis *(Treponema pallidum)*, human papillomavirus, varicella zoster, group B streptococcus, hepatitis B, measles, mumps
3. R—Rubella (rubella virus): greatest risk to the fetus when maternal infection occurs in first 12 weeks of gestation; infant may be born with encephalitis, ocular abnormalities, cardiac maldevelopment, and other defects; these infants may have active viral infection and should be isolated until pharyngeal mucus and urine are free of virus; for mothers who have not had rubella or who are serologically negative, rubella vaccine should be given in the immediate postbirth period, not during pregnancy
4. C—Cytomegalic inclusion disease (cytomegalovirus): pregnant women usually asymptomatic; this sexually transmitted infection may cause hemolytic anemia, hydrocephalus, microcephalus, IUGR, or neonatal death
5. H—Herpes genitalis (herpesvirus): contracted by the mother during sexual relations; characterized by periods of exacerbations and remissions; first attack most severe; intercourse must be avoided during last 4 to 6 weeks of pregnancy; during an exacerbation a cesarean birth is required; a vaginal birth may cause a neonatal infection resulting in death; surviving infants suffer CNS involvement, visual impairment
B. Therapeutic interventions: care is directed toward prevention and early treatment in the pregnant woman to eliminate or reduce risk to the fetus

CONGENITAL DISORDERS

Structural or metabolic problems that may be genetically determined or a result of environmental interference during intrauterine life (see Chapter 30, Nursing Care of Infants, and Chapter 31, Nursing Care of Toddlers)

CHAPTER 28 Childbearing and Women's Health Nursing Review Questions With Answers and Rationales

QUESTIONS

NURSING CARE TO PROMOTE CHILDBEARING AND WOMEN'S HEALTH

1. A young couple attend the prenatal clinic. The wife is at 8 weeks' gestation and asks the clinic nurse for information about an abortion. The nurse expresses the opinion that abortion is immoral and that many women have long-term guilt feelings after an abortion. The couple leave the clinic in a very disturbed state. Legally, the:
   1. Client had a right to receive correct, unbiased information
   2. Nurse's statements need not be based on scientific knowledge
   3. Physician should have been notified because nurses should not discuss abortion
   4. Nurse had a right to state feelings as long as they were identified as the nurse's own

2. One day the family planning clinic is very busy, and the supervisor asks a nurse from the pediatric clinic who is strongly opposed to any chemical or mechanical method of birth control to work in the family planning clinic. What is the most professional response that this nurse could give to the supervisor?
   1. "I will go, but it is against my beliefs."
   2. "I won't do it because I do not believe in birth control."
   3. "I would prefer another assignment that is not contrary to my beliefs."
   4. "I will have to reinforce that the rhythm method is the method of choice."

3. An amniocentesis done on a client at 16 weeks' gestation reveals a fetus with Down syndrome. The client and her husband elect to have the pregnancy terminated. What should the nurse understand when caring for a client whose pregnancy is surgically terminated?
   1. The client is emotionally unstable at this time
   2. There is a high risk for a postoperative infection
   3. Contraceptive counseling should be deferred to a later time
   4. The client needs to express her feelings of guilt, anger, and frustration

4. Which research-based knowledge guides the nurse regarding the emotional factors of pregnancy?
   1. A rejected pregnancy will result in a rejected infant
   2. Ambivalence and anxiety about mothering are common
   3. Maternal love usually develops within the first week after birth
   4. An effective mother does not experience ambivalence and anxiety about mothering

5. Why is it important for the nurse to support the parents' decision to abort a fetus with a birth defect?
   1. Supporting them will eliminate feelings of guilt.
   2. The parents are legally responsible for the decision.
   3. It is essential for maintenance of the family equilibrium.
   4. The nurse's support will relieve the pressure caused by this decision.

6. During the postpartum period, a client with heart disease and type 2 diabetes asks the nurse, "Which contraceptives will I be able to use to prevent pregnancy in the near future?" The nurse should respond:
   1. "You may use oral contraceptives because they are almost 100% effective in preventing a pregnancy."
   2. "You should use foam with a condom to prevent pregnancy because they are safest for a women with your illnesses."
   3. "You will find that the intrauterine device is best for you because it prevents a fertilized ovum from implanting in the uterus."
   4. "You do not need to worry about becoming pregnant in the near future because women with heart problems usually become infertile."

7. The nurse teaches that the most frequent side effect associated with the use of an IUD is:
   1. A tubal pregnancy
   2. A rupture of the uterus
   3. An expulsion of the IUD
   4. An excessive menstrual flow

8. The nurse should explain that a common problem associated with the use of IUDs is:
   1. Perforation of the uterus
   2. Discomfort associated with coitus
   3. Development of vaginal infections
   4. Spontaneous expulsion of the device

9. A client seeking advice about contraception asks the nurse about an IUD. The nurse explains that the IUD provides contraception by:
   1. Blocking the cervical os

    2. Increasing the mobility of the uterus

    3. Preventing the sperm from reaching the vagina

    4. Interfering with either fertilization or implantation

10. In a lecture on sexual functioning, the nurse plans to include the fact that ovulation occurs when the:

    1. Oxytocin level is high

    2. Progesterone level is high

    3. Luteinizing hormone level is high

    4. Chorionic gonadotropin level is high

11. After ovulation has occurred, the nurse teaches women in the fertility clinic that the ovum is thought to remain viable for:

    1. 1 to 6 hours

    2. 12 to 18 hours

    3. 24 to 36 hours

    4. 48 to 72 hours

12. When teaching clients to determine the time of ovulation by taking the basal temperature, the nurse explains that the change in the basal temperature during ovulation:

    1. Drops slightly and then rises

    2. Rises suddenly and then falls

    3. Rises markedly and remains high

    4. Drops markedly and remains lower

13. When oral contraceptives are prescribed for a client, the nurse should teach the client about the potential of developing:

    1. Cervicitis

    2. Ovarian cysts

    3. Fibrocystic disease

    4. Breakthrough bleeding

14. Which is important for the nurse to discuss with a client who just had a vasectomy?

    1. Recanalization of the vas deferens is impossible

    2. Unprotected coitus is safe within 1 week to 10 days

    3. Some impotency is to be expected for several weeks

    4. It requires at least 15 ejaculations to clear the tract of sperm

15. Contraceptives that have estrogen-like and/or progesterone-like compounds are prepared in a variety of forms. Check all that apply.

    1. ❐ Oral agents

    2. ❐ Diaphragms

    3. ❐ Cervical caps

    4. ❐ Foam spermicides

    5. ❐ Transdermal agents

    6. ❐ Intrauterine devices

16. The nurse explains that the efficiency of the basal body temperature method of contraception depends on fluctuation of the basal body temperature. A factor that will alter its effectiveness is:

    1. Presence of stress

    2. Length of abstinence

    3. Age of those involved

    4. Frequency of intercourse

17. A biphasic antiovulatory medication of combined progestin and estrogen is prescribed for a female client. What should the nurse include when teaching about this oral contraceptive?

    1. Have bimonthly Pap smears

    2. Increase the intake of calcium

    3. Restrict sexual activity temporarily

    4. Report any irregular vaginal bleeding

18. The nurse is giving discharge instructions to a client who has had an aspiration abortion by suction curettage. What should the client be told?

    1. Avoid showering for 2 days

    2. Tampons may be used after 1 day

    3. Sexual intercourse should be delayed for 3 weeks

    4. Report bleeding that requires a pad change every 2 hours

19. A client, at 10 weeks' gestation, elects to have an induced abortion. After receiving oral mifepristone (Mifeprex), she returned to the clinic 2 days later to have misoprostol (Cytotec) inserted vaginally. The nurse should tell the client to return for a follow-up visit:

    1. 4 hours after the procedure

    2. 2 weeks after the procedure

    3. 4 to 8 days after the procedure

    4. 8 to 24 hours after the procedure

20. A couple indicate that they do not want any more children. The wife is scheduled for a laparoscopic bilateral tubal ligation. What should the nurse include in preoperative teaching?

    1. "You should stop menstruating after the surgery."

    2. "You will need to use birth control until your follow-up visit."

    3. "You will be admitted as an outpatient because you can go home the same day."

    4. "You can have the operation reversed should you decide to have more children."

21. One of the responsibilities of a nurse in a fertility specialist's office is to provide health teaching to the client in relation to timing of intercourse. Which instruction to the client addresses the best time to achieve a pregnancy?

    1. Midway between periods

    2. Immediately after menses end

    3. 14 days before the next period is expected

    4. 14 days after the beginning of the last period

22. When teaching a client about the postcoital test to evaluate fertility, the nurse should tell the client that the best time for this test is:

    1. 1 week after ovulation

    2. Immediately after menses

    3. Just before the next menstrual period

    4. Within 1 to 2 days of presumed ovulation

23. A tubal insufflation test is done to determine whether there is a tubal obstruction. The nurse knows that infertility caused by a defect in the tube is most often related to a:

    1. Tubal injury

    2. Past infection

    3. Fibroid tumor

    4. Congenital anomaly

24. When caring for a couple identified as having an infertility problem, the nurse knows that:

    1. Infertility is usually psychologic in origin

2. Infertility and sterility are essentially the same problem
3. They have been unable to have a child after trying for a year
4. One partner has a problem that makes that person unable to have children

25. A couple in the fertility clinic have become discouraged regarding their efforts to conceive. The nurse can best support them by understanding that the most stressful aspect of the process is:
   1. Obtaining the necessary specimens
   2. Visiting the fertility clinic frequently
   3. Discovering which partner is infertile
   4. Planning when intercourse should take place

26. Genetic testing is being discussed with a couple at the fertility clinic. When they express concerns, what is the nurse's best response?
   1. "You should be tested because it will be to your benefit."
   2. "Environmental factors can have an impact on genetic factors."
   3. "This type of testing will determine if you'll need in vitro fertilization."
   4. "If you carry the gene for a disease, it will probably occur in your children."

27. A client is admitted with a diagnosis of torsion of the testes. Which response by the nurse is appropriate when the client asks, "Why must I have surgery immediately?"
   1. "There is no other way to control the pain."
   2. "Irreversible damage occurs after a few hours."
   3. "Swelling is excessive, which may cause the testicle to rupture."
   4. "The reduction in testicular blood flow leads to rapid death of sperm."

28. The nurse has been asked to prepare a couple for a test to determine the number, motility, and activity of sperm. What is the name of the test?
   1. Rubin's test
   2. Postcoital test
   3. Papanicolaou test
   4. Sperm penetration test

29. Which test should the nurse schedule to evaluate the pelvic organs of reproduction in a female client?
   1. Biopsy
   2. Cystogram
   3. Culdoscopy
   4. Hysterosalpingogram

30. In response to a client's question, the nurse identifies that the chief function of progesterone is to:
   1. Develop the female reproductive organs
   2. Stimulate the follicles for ovulation to occur
   3. Prepare the uterus to receive a fertilized ovum
   4. Establish the secondary male sex characteristics

31. The pituitary hormone that stimulates the secretion of milk from the mammary glands is:
   1. Oxytocin
   2. Estrogen
   3. Prolactin
   4. Progesterone

32. A client has a history of successful treatment for papillomavirus. While preparing the client for her routine Papanicolaou smear, the nurse identifies that she appears anxious. As part of the teaching plan, the nurse should:
   1. Describe the early symptoms of cervical cancer
   2. Explain why there is a small risk for cervical cancer
   3. Offer written instructions about the Papanicolaou smear
   4. Provide the current statistics on the incidence of cervical cancer

33. What occurs in response to the large amount of progesterone secreted during the secretory phase of the menstrual cycle?
   1. Onset of ovulation
   2. Regulation of menstruation
   3. Occurrence of capillary fragility
   4. Maintenance of the thick uterine endometrium

34. The hormones responsible for the proliferation phase of the menstrual cycle are:
   1. Luteinizing hormone and estrogen
   2. Lactogenic hormone and progesterone
   3. Luteinizing hormone and progesterone
   4. Follicle-stimulating hormone and estrogen

35. The main blood supply to the uterus is directly from the:
   1. Uterine and ovarian arteries
   2. Ovarian arteries and the aorta
   3. Uterine and hypogastric arteries
   4. Aorta and the hypogastric arteries

36. A woman menstruates regularly every 30 days. Her last menses started on January 1st. She will most probably ovulate on January:
   1. 7th
   2. 17th
   3. 24th
   4. 29th

37. A nurse teaches a women's group that hot flashes are caused by the:
   1. Accumulation of acetylcholine
   2. Cessation of pituitary gonadotropins
   3. Overstimulation of the adrenal medulla
   4. Hormonal stimulation of the sympathetic system

38. Menopause is the cessation of menstrual function. The nurse understands that one of the reasons given for the cessation of menses is:
   1. A decrease in gonadotropin in the blood
   2. A decrease in the production of prostaglandins
   3. An inability of the ovary to respond to gonadotropic hormones
   4. An increase in the secretion of progesterone from the follicles in the ovary

NURSING CARE RELATED TO MAJOR DISORDERS AFFECTING WOMEN'S HEALTH

39. A client undergoing treatment for infertility is diagnosed as having endometriosis. Which of the following drugs should the nurse expect to be used for this condition?

1. Relaxin (Releasin)
2. Leuprolide (Lupron)
3. Estrogen (Premarin)
4. Ergonovine (Ergotrate)

40. At 6 weeks' gestation a client is diagnosed with gonorrhea. The nurse should anticipate that the practitioner will order:
1. Ceftriaxone (Rocephin)
2. Levofloxacin (Levaquin)
3. Sulfasalazine (Azulfidine)
4. Trimethoprim/sulfamethoxazole (Bactrim)

41. A 15-year-old client complains of persistent dysmenorrhea. The nurse should encourage her to:
1. Maintain daily activities
2. Have a gynecologic examination
3. Eat a nutritious diet containing iron
4. Practice relaxation of abdominal muscles

42. A client at the women's health clinic tells the nurse she has endometriosis. To best help this client the nurse must understand that endometriosis is characterized by:
1. Amenorrhea and insomnia
2. Ecchymoses and petechiae
3. Painful menstruation and backache
4. Early osteoporosis and pelvic inflammation

43. The nurse determines that the priority concern for a 28-year-old client who is to undergo a laparoscopic bilateral salpingo-oophorectomy is:
1. Acute pain
2. Risk for hemorrhage
3. Fear of death because of the procedure
4. Grieving for loss of childbearing potential

44. When assessing a client for a rectocele, the nurse should remember that the most common adaptation is:
1. Crampy abdominal pain
2. Bearing-down sensations
3. Urinary stress incontinence
4. Recurrent urinary tract infections

45. When taking the health history of a client who is admitted for repair of a cystocele and rectocele, the nurse should expect the client to report the occurrence of:
1. Heavy leukorrhea and pruritus
2. Sporadic bleeding and abdominal pain
3. Change in vaginal acidity and leukorrhea
4. Stress incontinence and low abdominal pressure

46. A client has an anterior and posterior surgical repair of a cystocele and rectocele (colporrhaphy) and returns from the postanesthesia care unit with an indwelling catheter in place. The primary reason for the catheter is to prevent:
1. Retention
2. Discomfort
3. Loss of bladder tone
4. Pressure on the suture line

47. After an anterior-posterior colporrhaphy in a client past menopause, the nurse should teach the client how to prevent:
1. Pregnancy
2. Constipation

3. Reflex incontinence
4. Rectovaginal fistulas

48. A client has been admitted with a diagnosis of severe procidentia (prolapse of the uterus). The nurse plans to assess the client for:
1. Edema
2. Fistulas
3. Exudate
4. Ulcerations

49. A client with a prolapsed uterus is scheduled for a vaginoplasty. Preoperatively the nurse should:
1. Encourage ambulation
2. Apply moist compresses
3. Elevate the foot of the bed
4. Support the prolapsed uterus

50. What is the most therapeutic position for a client with pelvic inflammatory disease?
1. Sims' position
2. Fowler's position
3. Supine position with knees flexed
4. Lithotomy position with head elevated

51. The nurse explains to a client with a cervical erosion that early treatment of the erosion can help prevent:
1. Metrorrhagia
2. Cancer of the cervix
3. More erosions from occurring
4. Infections in the reproductive organs

52. The nurse knows that cervical polyps are usually:
1. Precursors of uterine cancer
2. Malignant, and a curettage must be done
3. Not the cause of bleeding unless malignant
4. Benign, and curettage of the endometrium is done

53. An early manifestation of cancer of the cervix that should prompt a client to seek medical care is:
1. Abdominal heaviness
2. Pressure on the bladder
3. Foul-smelling discharge
4. Bloody spotting after intercourse

54. The most common site for cancer cell growth in the cervix is at the:
1. External os and the regional nodes
2. Internal os and the endocervical glands
3. Junction of the cervix and lower uterine segment
4. Columnosquamous junction of the internal and external ossa

55. After a client has a biopsy for suspected cervical cancer, the laboratory report reveals a stage 0 lesion. The nurse explains that according to the International Federation of Gynecology and Obstetrics, stage 0 is indicative of:
1. Carcinoma in situ
2. Early stromal invasion
3. Parametrial involvement
4. Carcinoma confined to the cervix

56. To elicit information about a client's risk for exposure to DES, the nurse, obtaining the medical history of a young woman in the prenatal clinic, should first ask:
1. "Were you born before 1963?"
2. "Have you ever taken oral contraceptives?"

3. "Have you noticed any lesions in your perineal area?"
4. "Did your mother take hormones during her pregnancy?"

57. A 35-year-old client is scheduled for a conization of the cervix to remove dysplastic cervical cells and determine the extent of involvement. The nurse can determine that the client understands the postoperative course if the client:
   1. States she will resume sexual intercourse within 48 hours
   2. Demonstrates the ability to change sterile surgical dressings
   3. Verbalizes expectations of a vaginal discharge for 3 to 5 days
   4. Makes a positive adjustment to the loss of reproductive function

58. A client who is scheduled to have an abdominal panhysterectomy asks how the surgery will affect her periods. The nurse should respond:
   1. "You will not have any more periods."
   2. "Your periods will become more regular."
   3. "Your periods will become lighter until they disappear."
   4. "You will notice that the time between periods will be longer."

59. A client is diagnosed with uterine fibroids and the practitioner advises a hysterectomy. The client expresses concern about having a hysterectomy at age 45 because she has heard from friends that she will undergo severe symptoms of menopause after surgery. The most appropriate response for the nurse is:
   1. "You are correct. This happens after this type of surgery."
   2. "This is something that does occur in older women on occasion, but you don't have to worry about it."
   3. "It's too bad you did not discuss this with your doctor. I am not allowed to give you any information about this."
   4. "Some women occasionally experience exaggerated symptoms of menopause if, in addition to their uterus, their ovaries are removed."

60. After a hysterosalpingo-oophorectomy, a client wants to know whether it would be wise for her to take hormones right away to prevent symptoms of menopause. The most appropriate response by the nurse is:
   1. "It is best to wait because you may not have any symptoms."
   2. "It is comforting to know that hormones are available if you should need them."
   3. "You have to wait until symptoms are severe; otherwise, hormones will have no effect."
   4. "You should discuss this with your doctor, because it is important to know your concerns."

61. After an abdominal hysterectomy the client returns to the unit with an indwelling catheter. The nurse notes that the urine in the client's urinary bag has become increasingly sanguineous. The nurse suspects that the client may have:
   1. An incisional nick in the bladder
   2. A urinary infection from the catheter

3. Uterine relaxation with increased lochia
4. Disseminated intravascular coagulopathy

62. A client's pathology report shows metastatic adenocarcinoma of the breast. The client is to receive doxorubicin (Adriamycin) as part of the chemotherapy protocol. This drug modifies the growth of cancer cells by:
   1. Inhibiting DNA synthesis
   2. Preventing folic acid synthesis
   3. Changing the osmotic gradient in the cell
   4. Increasing the permeability of the cell wall

63. A client who had a mastectomy asks about the term ERP-positive. The nurse explains that tumor cells are evaluated for estrogen receptor protein to determine the:
   1. Need for supplemental estrogen
   2. Feasibility of breast reconstruction
   3. Potential response to hormone therapy
   4. Degree of metastasis that has occurred

64. After a mastectomy, the nurse should position the client's arm on the affected side:
   1. In adduction supported by sandbags
   2. In abduction surrounded by sandbags
   3. On pillows with the hand higher than the arm
   4. With the arm lower than the level of the heart

65. When encouraging a client to cough and deep breathe after a bilateral mastectomy, the client says, "Leave me alone! Don't you know I'm in pain?" The nurse's most therapeutic response should be:
   1. "I'm sure you are in pain; rest now and I'll come back later."
   2. "Your pain is to be expected, but you must expand your lungs."
   3. "I'll give you something for your pain and we'll start exercising tomorrow."
   4. "If you are unable to cough, I understand, but try using the incentive spirometer."

66. When writing a teaching plan about osteoporosis, the nurse should recall that osteoporosis is best described as:
   1. Avascular necrosis
   3. Pathologic fractures
   2. Hyperplasia of osteoblasts
   4. Decrease in bone substance

67. The plan of care for a client with osteoporosis includes active and passive exercises, calcium supplements, and daily vitamins. The desired effect of therapy is identified by the nurse if the client has:
   1. Increased mobility
   2. Experienced fewer muscular spasms
   3. Developed a more regular heartbeat
   4. Had fewer bruises than before therapy

68. Which factor identified by the nurse places the client at increased risk for developing osteoporosis?
   1. Estrogen therapy
   2. Hypoparathyroidism
   3. Prolonged immobility
   4. Excess calcium intake

69. The nurse plans care for a client with osteoporosis to prevent fractures. What type of fracture is the nurse trying to prevent?
    1. Fatigue
    2. Pathologic
    3. Greenstick
    4. Compound

70. The nurse evaluates that dietary instruction for a client with osteoporosis is effective when the client's selection from the menu includes:
    1. Red meat
    2. Soft drinks
    3. Turnip greens
    4. Enriched grains

71. A thin 68-year-old female client is diagnosed with osteoporosis. What should the nurse include in the discharge plan for this client?
    1. Encouragement of gradual weight gain
    2. Monitoring for decreased urine calcium
    3. Instructions relative to diet and exercise
    4. Safety factors when using opioids and NSAIDs

72. Select all the statements by a 50-year-old obese client that indicate understanding of the strategies to prevent bone loss. "I should:
    1. Go on a strict diet."
    2. Take 1200 mg of calcium daily."
    3. Take 1000 mg of vitamin D daily."
    4. Join an aerobics class three times a week."
    5. Exercise with free weights two times a week."

73. The primary care provider prescribes teriparatide (Forteo), a parathyroid hormone (PTH) agonist, for a client with osteoporosis. What understanding about this drug does the nurse need to have when administering it to the client? Teriparatide:
    1. Requires an increase in intake of vitamin A
    2. Prevents existing bone from being destroyed
    3. Necessitates an avoidance of the use of sunscreen
    4. Stimulates osteoblastic activity more than osteoclastic activity

74. A female client is very upset with her diagnosis of gonorrhea and asks the nurse, "What can I do to prevent getting another infection in the future?" The nurse is aware that the teaching for this client has been understood when the client states, "I should:
    1. Douche after every intercourse."
    2. Avoid having sexual intercourse."
    3. Insist that my partner use a condom."
    4. Use a spermicidal cream with intercourse."

75. The nurse is caring for a client with a trichomonal infection. Which oral drug is most likely to be prescribed by the physician?
    1. Penicillin G
    2. Gentian violet
    3. Nystatin (Mycostatin)
    4. Metronidazole (Flagyl)

76. The nurse is teaching a client how to self-administer a medicated douche. In which direction should the nurse instruct the client to direct the douche nozzle? Toward the:
    1. Left
    2. Right
    3. Sacrum
    4. Umbilicus

NURSING CARE OF WOMEN DURING UNCOMPLICATED PREGNANCY, LABOR, CHILDBIRTH, AND THE POSTPARTUM PERIOD

77. A client suspects that she is pregnant, but because she is the only wage earner in her family she is ambivalent about continuing the pregnancy. The nurse recognizes that the client is in crisis and also remembers that pregnancy and birth are considered crises because:
    1. Mood changes occur during pregnancy
    2. They are periods of change and adjustment to change
    3. There are hormonal and physiologic changes in the mother
    4. Narcissism in the mother affects the husband-wife relationship

78. A pregnant woman who is at term is admitted to the birthing unit in active labor. The client is excited about the anticipated birth because she has three sons and the amniocentesis indicates that she will have a girl. Which factor in the client's history alerts the nurse that there are implications for newborn observations and care?
    1. Her membranes ruptured 2 hours ago
    2. Her first child was diagnosed with hemophilia
    3. She used NSAIDs for frequent sinus headaches
    4. There was a placenta previa in a previous pregnancy

79. A couple who recently emigrated from Israel tell the nurse in the prenatal clinic that they are concerned about a genetic disease that is prevalent among Jewish people. The nurse recommends that they have a genetic blood test to determine the possibility of any of their children being born with:
    1. Cystic fibrosis
    2. Phenylketonuria
    3. Cooley's anemia
    4. Tay-Sachs disease

80. When teaching a childbirth class, the nurse explains that during the process of gametogenesis, the male and female sex cells divide, and each mature sex cell contains:
    1. 24 pairs of autosomes in their nuclei
    2. 46 pairs of chromosomes in their nuclei
    3. A diploid number of chromosomes in their nuclei
    4. A haploid number of chromosomes in their nuclei

81. The nurse teaches that the developing cells are first called a fetus at what point in a pregnancy?
    1. When it is visualized on a sonogram

2. During the eighth week of the pregnancy
3. At the end of the second week of pregnancy
4. When the fertilized ovum becomes implanted

82. A client, at 35 weeks' gestation, tells the nurse that her breathing has become more difficult. The nurse responds that this is expected because there is:
    1. Restriction of the lower rib cage
    2. An increase in pulmonary function
    3. Upward displacement of the diaphragm
    4. An increase in the height of the rib cage

83. The nurse at the prenatal clinic examines a client and determines that her uterus has risen out of the pelvis and is now an abdominal organ. At what week during pregnancy does this occur?
    1. 8th week of pregnancy
    2. 10th week of pregnancy
    3. 12th week of pregnancy
    4. 18th week of pregnancy

84. A client has several screening tests done during pregnancy. Place the tests in the order in which they would be done during a pregnancy.
    1. _____ Sickle cell screening
    2. _____ Group B streptococcus culture
    3. _____ Serum glucose for gestational diabetes mellitus
    4. _____ Alpha-fetoprotein (AFP) testing for neural tube defects

85. At what time during prenatal development should the nurse expect the greatest fetal weight gain?
    1. First trimester
    2. Third trimester
    3. Second trimester
    4. Implantation period

86. After the first 3 months of pregnancy, the chief source of estrogen and progesterone is the:
    1. Placenta
    2. Adrenal cortex
    3. Corpus luteum
    4. Anterior pituitary gland

87. In which fetal blood vessels is the oxygen content the highest?
    1. Ductus venosus
    2. Umbilical artery
    3. Pulmonary artery
    4. Ductus arteriosus

88. A client tells the nurse that the first day of her last menstrual period was July 22, 2008. What is the estimated date of birth?
    1. May 7, 2009
    2. April 29 2009
    3. April 22, 2009
    4. March 6, 2009

89. Anticipatory guidance provided by the nurse during the first trimester of pregnancy should be primarily directed toward increasing the pregnant woman's knowledge of:
    1. Labor and birth
    2. Signs and symptoms of complications
    3. Role transition into parenthood and its acceptance

4. Physical and emotional changes resulting from pregnancy

90. When dating a pregnancy by ultrasound, what should the nurse expect to be used to determine dates?
    1. Occipital frontal diameter is used at term
    2. Biparietal diameter is 12 cm or more at term
    3. Crown to rump measurement is used until 11 weeks
    4. Diagonal conjugate is used between 26 and 37 weeks

91. The nurse recognizes that an expected change in the hematologic system that occurs during the second trimester of pregnancy is:
    1. A decrease in WBCs
    2. An increase in hematocrit
    3. An increase in blood volume
    4. A decrease in sedimentation rate

92. The nurse is aware that an adaptation of pregnancy is an increased blood supply to the pelvic region that results in a purplish discoloration of the vaginal mucosa, which is known as:
    1. Ladin's sign
    2. Hegar's sign
    3. Goodell's sign
    4. Chadwick's sign

93. The nurse should explain to the client that physiologic anemia during pregnancy is a result of:
    1. Decreased dietary intake of iron
    2. Increased plasma volume of the mother
    3. Decreased erythropoiesis after the first trimester
    4. Increased detoxification demands on the mother's liver

94. At her first prenatal visit, a client says to the nurse, "I guess I'll be having an internal examination today." What is the nurse's best response?
    1. "Yes, an internal exam is done at the mother's first visit."
    2. "Are you fearful of having an internal examination done?"
    3. "Have you ever had an internal examination done before?"
    4. "Yes, an internal will be done, but it is just slightly uncomfortable."

95. A pregnant client is making her first antepartum visit. She has a 2-year-old son born at 40 weeks, a 5-year-old daughter born at 38 weeks, and 7-year-old twin daughters born at 35 weeks. She had a spontaneous abortion 3 years ago at 10 weeks. Using the GTPAL format, the nurse should identify and document that the client is:
    1. G4 T3 P2 A1 L4
    2. G5 T2 P2 A1 L4
    3. G5 T2 P1 A1 L4
    4. G4 T3 P1 A1 L4

96. The nurse recognizes that an expected cardiopulmonary adaptation experienced by most pregnant women is:
    1. Tachycardia
    2. Dyspnea at rest
    3. Progressive dependent edema
    4. Shortness of breath on exertion

97. The nurse is aware that nausea and vomiting commonly experienced by many women during the first trimester of pregnancy is an adaptation to the increased level of which hormone?
   1. Estrogen
   2. Progesterone
   3. Luteinizing hormone
   4. Chorionic gonadotropin

98. During a client's first visit to the prenatal clinic, the nurse discusses a pregnancy diet. The client states that her mother told her she should restrict her salt intake. The nurse's best response is:
   1. "Your mother is correct. You should use less salt to prevent swelling."
   2. "Because you need salt to maintain body water balance, it is not restricted. Just eat a well-balanced diet."
   3. "Salt is an essential nutrient and is naturally reduced by the body's estrogen. There is no reason to restrict salt in your diet."
   4. "We no longer recommend that salt intake be as restricted as much as in the past. You shouldn't add any extra salt to your food."

99. A pregnant client uses a computer during her working hours. This has implications for her plan of care during pregnancy. The nurse recommends to the client that she:
   1. Try to walk about every few hours during the workday
   2. Ask for time in the morning and afternoon to elevate her legs
   3. Tell her employer she cannot work beyond the second trimester
   4. Ask for time in the morning and afternoon to obtain nourishment

100. The nurse in the prenatal clinic should provide nutritional counseling to all newly pregnant women because:
   1. Most weight gain is caused by fluid retention
   2. Dietary allowances should not increase during pregnancy
   3. Pregnant women must adhere to a specific pregnancy diet
   4. Different sources of essential nutrients are favored by different cultural groups

101. A primigravida, in her 10th week of gestation, is concerned because she has read that nutrition during pregnancy is important for the growth and development of the fetus. She wants to know something about the foods she should eat. How should the nurse respond?
   1. Instruct her to continue eating her regular diet
   2. Tell her to keep a diet history by writing down what she eats
   3. Give her a list of foods to help her plan her meals more efficiently
   4. Emphasize to her the importance of limiting highly seasoned foods

102. A client, at 8 weeks' gestation, complains of having to go to the bathroom more often to urinate. The nurse explains that urinary frequency often occurs because the capacity of the bladder during pregnancy is diminished by:
   1. Atony of the detrusor muscle
   2. Compression by the enlarging uterus
   3. Compromise of the autonomic reflexes
   4. Narrowing of the ureteral entrance at the trigone

103. While caring for a pregnant client and her partner, the nurse suspects intimate partner violence. Which assessments support this suspicion? Check all that apply.
   1. ☐ The partner refuses to come into the exam room
   2. ☐ The partner answers questions asked of the woman
   3. ☐ The woman has injuries to the breasts and abdomen
   4. ☐ The woman has been to the clinic several times in the last month

104. The nurse caring for a mother-infant dyad that just gave birth today is reviewing the mother's and infant's chart data. Using the chart data below, which nursing intervention is required?
   1. RhoGAM injection
   2. Rubella vaccination
   3. Maternal blood transfusion
   4. Neonatal 50% glucose infusion

MATERNAL: Prenatal Laboratory Tests						
Type: RH:	Rubella Titer	RPR/VDRL	HB Sag	HIV	Hgb/Hct	Sickle Prep
A Neg	1:2	Neg	Neg	Neg	11/33	Neg

INFANT: Day 2 of Life Laboratory Tests			
Blood Glucose	Total Bilirubin	Blood type	Hct
46	10 mg	O Neg	55

105. A client who is at 10 weeks' gestation calls the clinic and complains of morning sickness. What should the nurse suggest to promote relief?
   1. Eat dry crackers before arising
   2. Increase her fat intake before bedtime
   3. Have two small meals daily with a snack at noon
   4. Drink more high-carbohydrate fluids with her meals

106. Which suggestions by the nurse may help a pregnant client overcome first-trimester morning sickness?
   1. Eat protein before bedtime
   2. Take an antacid before breakfast
   3. Eat nothing until the nausea subsides
   4. Obtain a prescription for an antibiotic from the care provider

107. What should the nurse include in nutritional planning for a newly pregnant woman of average height weighing 145 lb?
   1. A decrease of 200 calories per day
   2. An increase of 300 calories per day
   3. An increase of 500 calories per day
   4. A maintenance of her present caloric intake per day

108. A client is concerned about gaining weight during pregnancy. The nurse explains that the largest part of weight gain during pregnancy is because of:
   1. Fetal growth
   2. Fluid retention
   3. Metabolic alterations
   4. Increased blood volume

109. A client at 7 weeks' gestation tells the nurse in the prenatal clinic that she is very sick every morning with nausea and vomiting and is sure that she is being punished for having initially thought of aborting the pregnancy. The nurse assures her that this is a common occurrence in early pregnancy and will probably disappear by the end of the:
   1. Fifth month
   2. Third month
   3. Fourth month
   4. Second month

110. A pregnant client is being prepared for a pelvic examination. The client complains of feeling very tired and sick to her stomach, especially in the morning. What is the nurse's best response?
   1. "Tell me about how you feel in the morning."
   2. "Perhaps you might ask the nurse-midwife about it."
   3. "There is no need to worry because these feelings are common."
   4. "Let's discuss some ways to deal with these common problems."

111. During a prenatal examination, the nurse draws blood from a young Rh-negative client and explains that an indirect Coombs' test will be performed to predict whether the fetus is at risk for developing:
   1. Acute hemolytic anemia
   2. Respiratory distress syndrome
   3. Protein metabolism deficiency
   4. Physiologic hypcrbilirubinemia

112. What is the best advice the nurse can give to a pregnant woman in her first trimester?
   1. Cut down on drugs, alcohol, and cigarettes
   2. Avoid drugs and refrain from smoking and ingesting alcohol
   3. Avoid smoking, limit alcohol consumption, and do not take any aspirin
   4. Take only prescription drugs, especially in the second and third trimesters

113. During a routine visit to the prenatal clinic, the client listens to the fetal heartbeat for the first time. The client, commenting on how rapid it is, appears frightened and asks whether this is normal. How should the nurse respond? "The heart rate is:
   1. Usually rapid and twice the mother's pulse rate."
   2. Rapid, but I'd be more concerned if it were slow."
   3. Rapid to accommodate the fetus' nutritional needs."
   4. Usually rapid, but your baby's is within the expected range."

114. When involved in prenatal teaching, the nurse should inform clients that an increase in vaginal secretions during pregnancy is called leukorrhea and is caused by an increased:
   1. Metabolic rate
   2. Production of estrogen
   3. Functioning of the Bartholin's glands
   4. Supply of sodium chloride to the vaginal cells

115. A 21-year-old client who is 26 weeks into her second pregnancy is experiencing increasing edema in the lower extremities. Besides advising rest with the legs elevated, the nurse discusses and gives instructions concerning diet. In this instance the:
   1. Nutritionist should be involved in planning a diet
   2. Foods selected do not need to have a low salt content
   3. Diet that is preferred must influence the foods that are eaten
   4. Client should be referred to the physician at the prenatal clinic

116. What advice should the nurse give to clients who have fluid retention during pregnancy?
   1. Decrease fluid intake and eat a low-sodium diet
   2. Drink adequate fluids and elevate the lower extremities
   3. Eat a low-sodium diet and elevate the lower extremities
   4. Get a prescription for a mild diuretic and drink adequate fluids

117. A 36-year-old multigravida who is at 14 weeks' gestation is scheduled for an alpha-fetoprotein test. She asks the nurse, "What does the alpha-fetoprotein test indicate?" The nurse bases a response on the knowledge that this test can detect:
   1. Kidney defects
   2. Cardiac defects
   3. Neural tube defects
   4. Urinary tract defects

118. In the 37th week of gestation, a client is scheduled for a nonstress test. The nurse explains the procedure. Which statement by the client demonstrates she understands the teaching?
   1. "I hope this test does not cause my labor to begin early."
   2. "I hope the baby doesn't get too restless after this procedure."
   3. "I hate having needles in my arm, but now I understand why it is necessary."
   4. "I know that if my baby's heart reacts well, he should do okay when I give birth."

119. A client in the 18th week of pregnancy is scheduled for ultrasonography. The nurse explains the procedure and informs the client that for this test she will have to:
   1. Be given an enema the night before the examination
   2. Refrain from voiding for at least 3 hours before the test

3. Be monitored closely afterward for signs of precipitate labor
4. Maintain NPO status for 12 hours to minimize the possibility of vomiting

120. When teaching a young primigravida about labor, the nurse should tell her to call her primary caregiver when:
1. She has a bloody show and back pressure
2. Contractions are 8 to 10 minutes apart and are getting stronger
3. Her membranes rupture or contractions are 5 to 8 minutes apart
4. Contractions are 10 to 12 minutes apart and last about 30 seconds

121. The nurse teaches a pregnant woman to avoid lying on her back during labor. What knowledge about the result of lying in the supine position is the basis of the nurse's teaching?
1. Unduly prolonged labor
2. Decreased placental perfusion
3. Transient episodes of hypertension
4. Interference with free movement of the coccyx

122. A 42-year-old client has an amniocentesis during the 16th week of gestation because of concern about Down syndrome. What additional information about the fetus will be provided by examination of the amniotic fluid at this time?
1. Lung maturity
2. Type 1 diabetes
3. A cardiac anomaly
4. A neural tube defect

123. During the postpartum period, a client tells the nurse she is having leg cramps. The nurse should suggest that the client increase her intake of:
1. Eggs and bacon
2. Liver and onions
3. Juices and water
4. Cheese and broccoli

124. When is it most important for a female client to know that a fetus is most likely to be structurally damaged by the ingestion of drugs?
1. During early adolescence
2. Throughout the entire pregnancy
3. When planning to become pregnant
4. At the beginning of the first trimester

125. A pregnant client asks the clinic nurse how smoking will affect her baby. The nurse's response reflects the knowledge that:
1. Smoking relieves tension and the fetus responds accordingly
2. Vasoconstriction affects both fetal and maternal blood vessels
3. Fetal and maternal circulation are separated by the placental barrier
4. Substances contained in smoke cross the placenta, and the fetus is affected

126. A client, at 12 weeks' gestation, arrives at the prenatal clinic complaining of severe nausea and frequent vomiting. The nurse suspects that this client has hyperemesis gravidarum and knows that this is frequently associated with:
1. A history of cholecystitis
2. A large amount of amniotic fluid
3. High levels of chorionic gonadotropin
4. Decreased secretion of free hydrochloric acid

127. The nurse caring for a pregnant woman with class I heart disease recognizes that changes in the cardiovascular system may affect her compensatory mechanisms as pregnancy progresses. Which changes should the nurse expect? Check all that apply.
1. ☐ Systemic vasodilation
2. ☐ Increased blood volume
3. ☐ Elevated blood pressure
4. ☐ Increased cardiac output
5. ☐ Enlargement of the heart
6. ☐ Decreased erythrocyte production

128. The husband of a client who is in the transitional phase of the first stage of labor becomes very tense and nervous during this period and asks the nurse, "Do you think it is best for me to leave, since I don't seem to do my wife much good?" What is the nurse's best response?
1. "This is the time your wife needs you. Don't run out on her now."
2. "This is hard for you. Let me try to help you coach her during this difficult phase."
3. "I know this is hard for you. You should go have a cup of coffee to help you relax and then come back in a little while."
4. "If you feel that way, you'd best go out and sit in the father's waiting room for a while. You may transmit your anxiety to your wife."

129. During labor a client who has been receiving epidural anesthesia has a sudden episode of severe nausea, and her skin becomes pale and clammy. What should be the immediate reaction of the nurse?
1. Notify the practitioner
2. Turn the client to her side
3. Check for vaginal bleeding
4. Monitor the FHR every 3 minutes

130. At about 5 cm dilation, a laboring client receives medication for pain. The nurse is aware that one of the medications given to women in labor that could cause respiratory depression of the newborn is:
1. Oxytocin (Pitocin)
2. Promazine (Sparine)
3. Meperidine (Demerol)
4. Promethazine (Phenergan)

131. A client in the midphase of labor becomes very uncomfortable and asks for medication. Nalbuphine (Nubain) is ordered. What effect should the nurse expect from this drug?
1. Produces amnesia
2. Acts as a preliminary anesthetic
3. Induces sleep until the time of birth
4. Decreases pain by acting on opioid receptors

132. At a prenatal visit, a client who is at 36 weeks' gestation complains of discomfort with irregularly occurring contractions. How should the nurse respond to the client?
    1. Lie down until they stop.
    2. Walk around until they subside.
    3. Time the contractions for 30 minutes.
    4. Take 1 extra-strength aspirin for relief.

133. How does the nurse identify true labor as opposed to false labor?
    1. Cervical dilation is progressive
    2. It occurs immediately after the membranes rupture
    3. The contractions stop when the client walks around
    4. The client is more comfortable in a side-lying position

134. The nurse should teach pregnant women the importance of conserving the "spurt of energy" before labor because:
    1. Energy helps to increase the progesterone level
    2. Fatigue may influence the need for pain medication
    3. Energy is needed to push during the first stage of labor
    4. Fatigue will increase the intensity of the uterine contractions

135. A client is admitted to the birthing suite in early active labor. Which admission nursing intervention takes priority?
    1. Auscultating the fetal heart
    2. Obtaining an obstetric history
    3. Determining when the last meal was eaten
    4. Ascertaining whether the membranes have ruptured

136. A client who is a gravida 1, para 0 is admitted in labor. Her cervix is 100% effaced, and she is dilated 3 cm. Her fetus is at +1 station. The nurse is aware that the head of the fetus is:
    1. Not yet engaged
    2. Below the ischial spines
    3. Entering the pelvic inlet
    4. Visible at the vaginal opening

137. After doing Leopold's maneuvers on a laboring client, the nurse determines that the fetus is in the ROP position. Where should the nurse place the Doppler to best auscultate fetal heart tones?
    1. Above the umbilicus in the midline
    2. Above the umbilicus on the left side
    3. Below the umbilicus on the right side
    4. Below the umbilicus near the left groin

138. A client in the active phase of the first stage of labor begins to tremble, becomes very tense with contractions, and is quite irritable. She frequently states, "I cannot stand this a minute longer." This behavior indicates to the nurse that she:
    1. Has not been prepared for labor
    2. Needs administration of an analgesic
    3. Is entering the transition phase of labor
    4. Is developing hypertonic uterine contractions

139. The nurse assesses the frequency of a client's contractions by timing them from the beginning of a contraction:
    1. Until the uterus starts to relax
    2. Until the uterus completely relaxes
    3. To the end of a second contraction
    4. To the beginning of the next contraction

140. The nurse observes a laboring client's amniotic fluid and decides that it is the expected color because it is:
    1. Clear, dark amber, and contains shreds of mucus
    2. Straw colored, clear, and contains little white specks
    3. Milky, greenish yellow, and contains shreds of mucus
    4. Greenish yellow, cloudy, and contains little white specks

141. A client is in active labor, and an external fetal monitor is in place. Using the monitor strip below, identify the correct assessment.
    1. Marked FHR variability
    2. FHR baseline at 145 to 150 beats/min
    3. Contractions lasting 130 to 140 seconds
    4. Contractions occurring every 3 to 4 minutes

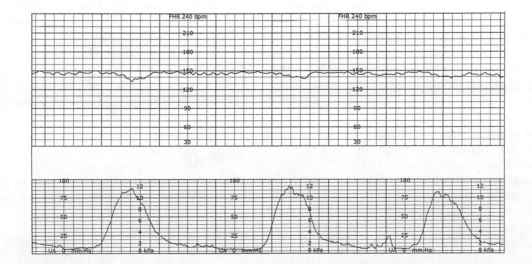

142. What is a common problem that confronts the client in labor when an external fetal monitor is being used?
    1. Intrusion on movement
    2. Inability to take sedatives
    3. Interference with breathing techniques
    4. Increased frequency of vaginal examinations

143. The nurse is examining the fetal monitor strip after rupture of the membranes in a laboring client who is having her labor augmented with an oxytocin infusion. The nurse notes variable decelerations in the fetal heart rate. What should the nurse do?
    1. Stop the oxytocin infusion
    2. Change the client's position
    3. Prepare for an immediate birth
    4. Take the client's blood pressure

144. A laboring client was given epidural anesthesia 30 minutes ago. The nurse identifies that the fetus is having late decelerations. List the following nursing actions in order of priority.
    1. _____ Increase IV fluids.
    2. _____ Reposition to side.
    3. _____ Reassess fetal heart rate pattern.
    4. _____ Document interventions and maternal/fetal response.

145. A client's membranes spontaneously rupture during active labor. What should the nurse do first?
    1. Observe the FHR
    2. Call the practitioner
    3. Time the contractions
    4. Check maternal vital signs

146. The membranes of a client who is at 39 weeks' gestation have ruptured spontaneously. She arrives at the birthing unit accompanied by her husband. Her cervix is 4 cm dilated and 75% effaced. The fetal heart rate is 136 beats/min. What should the nurse do next?
    1. Place the mother in bed and attach an external fetal monitor
    2. Let the mother undress while the nurse takes the history from the father
    3. Introduce the staff nurses to the couple and try to make them feel welcome
    4. Have them wait in the examining room while notifying the client's practitioner

147. A client is admitted to the birthing unit in active labor. What should the nurse expect if an amniotomy were done?
    1. Diminished bloody show
    2. Less discomfort with contractions
    3. Progressive dilation and effacement
    4. Increased and more variable FHR

148. A primigravida, at 40 weeks' gestation, arrives at the birthing center with abdominal cramping and a bloody show. Her membranes ruptured 30 minutes before arrival. A vaginal examination reveals 1 cm dilation and the presenting part at −1 station. After obtaining the fetal heart rate and maternal vital signs, what should the nurse do next?
    1. Teach the client how to push
    2. Encourage the client to perform pattern-paced breathing
    3. Provide the client with comfort measures used for women in labor
    4. Prepare to have the client's blood typed and cross-matched for a possible transfusion

149. When monitoring the FHR of a client in labor, the nurse identifies an elevation of 15 beats above the baseline rate of 135 beats/min lasting for 15 seconds. How should the nurse document this event?
    1. An acceleration
    2. An early elevation
    3. A sonographic motion
    4. A tachycardic heart rate

150. A client and her husband are working together during the wife's labor. The client's cervix is now dilated 7 cm, and the presenting part is low in the midpelvis. To alleviate discomfort during contractions, the nurse should instruct the husband to encourage his wife to:
    1. Deep breathe slowly
    2. Perform pelvic rocking
    3. Use the panting technique
    4. Begin pattern paced breathing

151. Why should the nurse withhold food and oral fluids as a laboring client approaches the second stage of labor?
    1. The mechanical and chemical digestive processes require energy that is needed for labor
    2. Undigested food and fluid may cause nausea and vomiting and limit the choice of anesthesia
    3. The gastric phase of digestion stimulates the release of hydrochloric acid and may cause dyspepsia
    4. Food and fluid will further aggravate gastric peristalsis, which is already increased because of the stress of labor

152. The management of a client in the transition phase of the first stage of labor is primarily directed toward:
    1. Decreasing the IV fluid intake
    2. Helping the client maintain control
    3. Reducing the client's discomfort with medications
    4. Instituting simple breathing patterns during contractions

153. Which breathing technique should the nurse instruct the client to use as the head of the fetus is crowning?
    1. Shallow
    2. Blowing
    3. Slow chest
    4. Modified paced

154. When a client's legs are placed in stirrups for birth, both legs should be positioned simultaneously to prevent:
    1. Venous stasis in the legs
    2. Pressure on the perineum
    3. Excessive pull on the fascia
    4. Trauma to the uterine ligaments

155. A laboring primipara should be prepared for birth when the nurse observes:
    1. The client becoming irritable and not following instructions
    2. That the perineum is beginning to bulge with each contraction
    3. An increase in the amount of bloody discharge from the vagina
    4. The contractions are occurring more frequently, are stronger, and last longer

156. During the period of induction of labor with an oxytocin infusion, the nurse should observe the client specifically for signs of:
    1. Severe pain
    2. Hypoglycemia
    3. Uterine tetany
    4. Umbilical cord prolapse

157. The cervix of a client in labor is fully dilated and totally effaced. The head of the fetus is at +2 station. What should the nurse encourage the client to do during contractions?
    1. Relax by closing her eyes
    2. Push with her glottis open
    3. Blow to slow the birth process
    4. Pant to prevent cervical edema

158. A laboring client is to have a pudendal block. What should the nurse teach the client about the effects of the pudendal block? She:
    1. May lose bladder sensation
    2. Will not feel the episiotomy
    3. May lose the ability to push
    4. Will no longer feel contractions

159. During the early postpartum period, when assessing a client's episiotomy, the nurse identifies edema with severe ecchymosis. Also, the client is complaining of severe perineal and rectal pressure. The fundus is firm, and there is no lochia. The client's vital signs are T 99° F, P 108 beats/min, R 20 breaths/min, BP 105/60 mm Hg. What does this assessment most likely indicate?
    1. Urinary infection
    2. Uterine infection
    3. Vaginal hematoma
    4. Postpartum hemorrhage

160. A client gives birth to a healthy baby girl. An indication to the nurse that the placenta is beginning to separate from the uterus and is about ready to be expelled is the:
    1. Relaxation of the uterus
    2. Descent of the uterus in the abdomen
    3. Appearance of a sudden gush of blood
    4. Retraction of the umbilical cord into the vagina

161. A multigravida client has a spontaneous vaginal birth of a healthy infant. Five minutes later the placenta is expelled. The nurse, assessing the fundus at this time, should expect it to be:
    1. Difficult to find
    2. Just below the xiphoid process

3. At the umbilicus and in the right quadrant
    4. Halfway between the symphysis pubis and the umbilicus

162. A client who is in labor begins to experience contractions 2 to 3 minutes apart that last about 45 seconds. Between contractions the nurse records a fetal heart rate of 100 beats/min. The nurse should:
    1. Notify the practitioner
    2. Continue to monitor the fetal heart
    3. Closely monitor the maternal vital signs
    4. Chart the rate as an expected response to contractions

163. After the birth of her infant, a woman is bleeding excessively and the practitioner orders an IV infusion containing 10 units of oxytocin (Pitocin) at 100 mL/hr and fundal massage. When evaluating the woman's response to these interventions, the BP is 135/90 mm Hg, her uterus is boggy and at 3 cm above the umbilicus and displaced to the right, and her perineal pad is saturated with bright red lochia. The nurse's next action should be to:
    1. Perform vigorous fundal massage
    2. Assess the client for a distended bladder
    3. Increase the IV infusion rate to 200 mL/hr
    4. Continue to assess the woman's vital signs

164. A primigravida, at 35 weeks' gestation, is diagnosed with hydramnios. For what should the nurse assess the newborn?
    1. Cardiac defect
    2. Kidney disorder
    3. Diabetes mellitus
    4. Esophageal atresia

165. A client who has just given birth has three young children at home. She comments to the nursery nurse that she cannot hold the baby for feedings once she gets home. She has just too much to do, and anyway, it spoils the baby. What is the nurse's best response?
    1. "You seem concerned about time. Let's talk about it."
    2. "That's up to you since you have to do what works for you."
    3. "Holding the baby when feeding is important for development."
    4. "It is not safe to prop a bottle. The baby could aspirate the fluid."

166. After giving birth at 37 weeks' gestation, a new mother is transferred to the postpartum unit. What should the nurse do to best promote the attachment process between the mother and newborn?
    1. Teach how to breastfeed the baby
    2. Allow the client extra visiting privileges in the newborn nursery
    3. Encourage the client to room-in with her infant on a 24-hour basis
    4. Arrange staffing so that one nurse is assigned to care for the client and her baby

167. A 26-year-old multigravida of Asian descent weighs 104 lb, having gained only 14 lb during this pregnancy.

On her second postpartum day, the client's temperature spikes to 102.8° F. She has a poor appetite and rarely gets out of bed. The nurse should:
1. Request the nursing supervisor to discuss this with the practitioner
2. Encourage the family to bring in special foods preferred in their culture
3. Order a high-protein milkshake as a between-meal snack to stimulate her appetite
4. Explain to the family that the dietitian plans nutritious meals that the client must eat

168. At 9 PM visiting hours are officially over, but the partner of a newly admitted postpartum client remains at the bedside. What is the most appropriate nursing intervention?
1. Remind the client and partner that visiting hours are over
2. Call the evening nursing supervisor to tactfully handle the situation
3. Encourage the partner to participate in care as much as the client wishes
4. Get written permission from the client for the partner to remain

169. Three weeks after giving birth a client develops thrombophlebitis of the left leg and is admitted to the hospital for bed rest and anticoagulant therapy. Which anticoagulant should the nurse expect to administer?
1. Clopidogrel (Plavix)
2. Warfarin (Coumadin)
3. Continuous infusion of heparin
4. Intermittent doses of a low molecular weight heparin

170. During the postpartum period, the nurse teaches a client to cleanse her episiotomy to prevent infection. The nurse determines that the teaching was effective when the client:
1. Changes her perineal pad twice daily
2. Rinses with water after applying an analgesic spray
3. Washes her hands whenever she changes her perineal pads
4. Cleanses her perineum from the anus toward the symphysis pubis

171. The nurse identifies that a client is voiding frequently in small amounts 8 hours after giving birth. Intake and output measurements are important in the early postpartum period because small amounts of output:
1. May indicate retention of urine with overflow
2. May be indicative of beginning glomerulonephritis
3. Are common because less fluid is excreted after birth
4. Are commonly voided because fluid intake diminishes

172. When checking a client's fundus on the second postpartum day, the nurse observes that the fundus is above the umbilicus and displaced to the right. The nurse evaluates that the client probably has:
1. A slow rate of involution
2. Retained placental fragments

3. An overdistended bladder
4. Overstretched uterine ligaments

173. The nurse examines a client who had a cesarean birth. It is 3 days since the birth and she is about to be discharged. Where should the nurse expect the fundus to be located?
1. 1 fingerbreadth below the umbilicus
2. 2 fingerbreadths below the umbilicus
3. 3 fingerbreadths below the umbilicus
4. 4 fingerbreadths below the umbilicus

174. The nurse working on the postpartum unit should teach clients to ambulate early. This is done to:
1. Enhance respirations
2. Increase bladder tonicity
3. Strengthen abdominal muscles
4. Promote peripheral vasomotor activity

175. When performing discharge teaching for a postpartum client, the nurse should inform her that:
1. The episiotomy sutures will be removed at the first postpartum visit
2. She may not have a bowel movement for up to a week after the birth
3. She should schedule a postpartum checkup as soon as her menses returns
4. The perineal tightening exercises she started during pregnancy should be continued indefinitely

176. The nurse should plan to teach a client who is formula-feeding her infant to minimize breast discomfort by:
1. Applying covered ice packs to her breasts
2. Gently applying cocoa butter to her nipples
3. Placing warm, wet washcloths on her nipples
4. Manually expressing colostrum from her breasts

177. Two days after having had a cesarean birth, a client complains of pain in the right leg. What should be the nurse's initial response?
1. Apply warm soaks
2. Massage the affected area
3. Encourage ambulation and exercise
4. Maintain bed rest and notify the practitioner

178. The nurse teaches a multipara who has just given birth to a large baby how she can maintain a contracted uterus. The nurse recognizes that teaching has been effective when the client states:
1. "If I start to bleed, I will call for help."
2. "I will massage my uterus regularly to keep it firm."
3. "If I urinate frequently, my uterus will stay contracted."
4. "I will call you every 15 minutes to massage my uterus."

179. Two days after giving birth, a woman has a temperature of 101° F. The nurse calls the practitioner and receives the following orders. Place them in the order that they should be implemented.
1. _____ Culture the lochia
2. _____ Begin IV antibiotics
3. _____ Obtain a chest x-ray film
4. _____ Give Tylenol PRN fever >100° F

NURSING CARE OF WOMEN AT RISK DURING PREGNANCY, LABOR, CHILDBIRTH, AND THE POSTPARTUM PERIOD

180. A 16 year old visits the prenatal clinic because she has missed three menstrual periods. Before her physical examination, the client says, "I don't know what the problem is, but I can't be pregnant." What is the most therapeutic response by the nurse?
    1. "Should I ask the doctor to talk to you?"
    2. "What brought you to the prenatal clinic then?"
    3. "Many young women are irregular at your age."
    4. "If you had intercourse, you are probably pregnant."

181. A client visiting the prenatal clinic for the first time asks the nurse about the probability of having twins because her husband is one of a pair of fraternal twins. What should the nurse tell the client?
    1. The probability of having twins is 25%
    2. She will be monitored closely for the presence of twins
    3. There is no greater probability of having twins than in the general population
    4. The husband's history of being a twin increases the probability of having twins

182. A pregnant client with severe abdominal pain and heavy bleeding is prepared for a cesarean birth. What care should the nurse include?
    1. Teaching coughing and deep-breathing techniques
    2. An abdominal prep and administration of a Fleet enema
    3. Obtaining an informed consent and assessment for drug allergies
    4. Inserting an indwelling catheter and administering a tap-water enema

183. When caring for a client who is having a prolonged labor, the nurse must be aware that the client is very concerned when her labor deviates from what she sees as the norm. A response conveying acceptance of the client's expressions of frustration and hostility would be:
    1. "I'll leave so you can talk to your husband."
    2. "I'll rub your back and you tell me if it helps."
    3. "Women usually get weary and frustrated during labor."
    4. "Perhaps you will feel better if we talk about what's bothering you."

184. A client at 26 weeks' gestation is admitted with an influenza infection. She is in labor. Which of these physician orders should the nurse question?
    1. Betamethasone 12 mg IV every 12 hours
    2. I&O and IV Ringer's lactate at 500 mL/24 hr
    3. Vital signs and fetal heart tones every 30 minutes
    4. IV loading dose of magnesium sulfate per protocol

185. A client who was admitted in active labor has only progressed from 2 to 3 cm in 8 hours. She is diagnosed as having hypotonic dystocia and is given oxytocin (Pitocin) to augment her contractions. What is the most important nursing action at this time?
    1. Checking the perineum for bulging
    2. Preparing for an emergency cesarean birth
    3. Documenting the fetal heart rate and its variations
    4. Monitoring the duration and intensity of the contractions

186. A client, at 38 weeks' gestation, is admitted for induction of labor. She has a history of ruptured membranes for the past 12 hours. She has no other signs of labor. Which medication should the nurse expect to be prescribed?
    1. Oxytocin (Pitocin)
    2. Estrogen (Premarin)
    3. Ergonovine (Ergotrate)
    4. Progesterone (Prometrium)

187. A pregnant client's labor is to be induced at 39 weeks' gestation. The nurse is aware that several drugs are currently utilized for inducing labor. Check all that apply.
    1. ☐ Oxytocin (Pitocin)
    2. ☐ Misoprostol (Cytotec)
    3. ☐ Ergonovine (Ergotrate)
    4. ☐ Carboprost (Hemabate)
    5. ☐ Dinoprostone (Prepidil)

188. A client begins preterm labor and the physician orders terbutaline sulfate (Brethine). After its administration, which therapeutic effect should the nurse expect?
    1. Reduction of pain in the perineal area
    2. Lowering the blood pressure and pulse
    3. Decrease in frequency and duration of contractions
    4. Dilation of the cervix by 0.5 cm every hour of labor

189. A client is receiving magnesium sulfate therapy for severe preeclampsia. The nurse must be alert for the first sign of an excessive blood magnesium level, which is:
    1. Increase in respiratory rate
    2. Stimulation of the sensorium
    3. Disappearance of the knee-jerk reflex
    4. Development of a cardiac dysrhythmia

190. The nurse admits a woman with preterm labor. A loading dose of 6 g of magnesium sulfate over 20 minutes is ordered to be followed by 2 g/hr. Premixed stock is available with 40 g of magnesium sulfate in 1000 mL of D_5W. At how many milliliters should the nurse set the infusion pump to complete the loading dose?
    Answer: _____ mL

191. Despite medication, a client's preterm labor continues, her cervix dilates, and birth appears to be inevitable. Which medication should the nurse expect to be prescribed that increases the chance of extrauterine survival?
    1. Ritodrine (Yutopar)
    2. Ampicillin by piggyback
    3. Betamethasone by IM injection
    4. An intrauterine exchange transfusion

192. A client at the prenatal clinic, who is at 9 weeks' gestation, asks the nurse if she can have her chorionic villi sampling (CVS) done at this visit. The nurse should respond that the best time for this test is at:
1. 8 weeks and less than 10 weeks
2. 10 weeks and less than 12 weeks
3. 12 weeks and less than 14 weeks
4. 14 weeks and less than 16 weeks

193. When assessing a client with a tentative diagnosis of hydatidiform mole, the nurse should be alert for:
1. Hypotension
2. Decreased fetal heart rate
3. Unusual uterine enlargement
4. Painless, heavy vaginal bleeding

194. When obtaining the nursing history from a client with a diagnosis of a ruptured tubal pregnancy, when should the nurse expect the client to indicate that her symptoms of pain in the lower abdomen and vaginal bleeding started?
1. About the sixth week of pregnancy
2. At the beginning of the last trimester
3. Midway through the second trimester
4. Immediately after implantation occurred

195. Which complaint leads the nurse to suspect that a client has a tubal pregnancy?
1. An adherent painful ovarian mass
2. Lower abdominal cramping for a long period of time
3. Sharp lower right or left abdominal pain radiating to the shoulder
4. Leukorrhea or dysuria a few days after the first missed menstrual period

196. The nurse is caring for a client who had a spontaneous abortion. The nurse's priority should be assessing the client for:
1. Hemorrhage
2. Dehydration
3. Hypertension
4. Subinvolution

197. The nurse is caring for a client who has had a spontaneous abortion. The client asks why spontaneous abortions occur. Before responding, the nurse recalls that the most common cause is:
1. Physical trauma
2. Unresolved stress
3. Embryonic defects
4. Congenital defects

198. A client is admitted to the hospital with vaginal staining but no pain. The client's history reveals amenorrhea for the last 2 months and pregnancy confirmation after her first missed period. She is admitted for observation. Which is the most likely tentative diagnosis?
1. Missed abortion
2. Inevitable abortion
3. Threatened abortion
4. Incomplete abortion

199. A few hours after being admitted with a diagnosis of inevitable abortion, a client begins to experience bearing-down sensations and suddenly expels the products of conception in bed. What should the nurse do first?
1. Notify the practitioner
2. Give her the sedation ordered
3. Check the fundus for firmness
4. Take her to the operating room

200. After an incomplete abortion, a client tells the nurse that although her doctor explained what an incomplete abortion was, she did not understand. What is the nurse's best response?
1. "I don't think you should focus on this any more."
2. "This is when the fetus dies but is retained in the uterus for 8 weeks or more."
3. "I think it would be best if you asked your doctor for the answer to that question."
4. "This is when the fetus is expelled but part of the placenta and membranes are not."

201. A client asks the nurse at the prenatal clinic whether she can continue to have sexual relations. The nurse's response is based on the knowledge that coitus during pregnancy is contraindicated if there is:
1. Leukorrhea
2. Fetal tachycardia
3. Gestation past 32 weeks
4. Premature rupture of membranes

202. An expectant couple asks the nurse about the cause of low back pain in labor. The nurse replies that this pain occurs most when the position of the fetus is:
1. Breech
2. Transverse
3. Occiput anterior
4. Occiput posterior

203. A laboring client complains of low back pain. To increase the client's comfort, the nurse recommends that the client's coach:
1. Instruct her to flex her knees
2. Place her in the supine position
3. Apply pressure to her back during contractions
4. Perform neuromuscular control exercises with her

204. To promote comfort caused by back pain during labor, the nurse teaches the client to avoid the:
1. Sims' position
2. Supine position
3. Sitting position
4. Side-lying position

205. A client arrives at the hospital in the second stage of labor. The head of the fetus is crowning, the client is bearing down, and birth appears imminent. What should the nurse do?
1. Show her how to pant while pushing gently
2. Transfer her by stretcher to the birthing unit
3. Tell her to breathe through her mouth so as not to bear down
4. Instruct her to pant while supporting her perineum with the hand

206. A client requests that she not have an episiotomy and would rather tear naturally. The nurse responds based on the knowledge that:
1. Lacerations are more painful than an episiotomy
2. Lacerations are easier to repair than an episiotomy
3. An episiotomy causes less posterior trauma than lacerations
4. An episiotomy is preferred over lacerations according to evidence-based practice

207. A client who had a postpartum hemorrhage is to receive 1 unit of packed RBCs. The nurse manager observes the staff nurse administering the packed RBCs without wearing gloves. The nurse manager concludes that the:
1. Client does not have an infection
2. Donor blood is free of blood-borne pathogens
3. Nurse should have worn gloves for self-protection
4. Nurse was skilled enough to prevent exposure to the blood

208. When caring for a client with an episiotomy during the postpartum period, the practitioner orders sitz baths. The nurse encourages her to take the sitz baths because they primarily aid the healing process by:
1. Promoting vasodilation
2. Softening the incision site
3. Cleansing the perineal area
4. Tightening the rectal sphincter

209. An infant is born precipitously in the emergency department. What should be the nurse's initial action?
1. Tie and cut the umbilical cord
2. Establish an airway for the newborn
3. Ascertain the condition of the fundus
4. Move mother and newborn to the birthing unit

210. Women who become pregnant for the first time at a later reproductive age (35 years of age or older) are at risk for complications. Check all that apply.
1. ☐ Preterm labor
2. ☐ Multiple gestation
3. ☐ Development of seizures
4. ☐ Chromosomal anomalies
5. ☐ Bleeding in the first trimester

211. What is the cause of more than half the neonatal deaths in the United States?
1. Atelectasis
2. Preterm births
3. Congenital heart disease
4. Respiratory distress syndrome

212. What complication is a contraindication for a contraction stress test?
1. Hypertension
2. Fetal activity
3. Preterm labor
4. Drug addiction

213. When caring for a woman with a positive contraction stress test, what complication should the nurse suspect?
1. Preeclampsia
2. Placenta previa

3. Imminent preterm birth
4. Uteroplacental insufficiency

214. What is the initial responsibility of the nurse when teaching the pregnant adolescent?
1. Informing her of the benefits of breastfeeding
2. Advising her about the proper care of an infant
3. Instructing her to watch for danger signs of preeclampsia
4. Impressing her with the importance of consistent prenatal care

215. The major concern about pregnant, unmarried teenagers is that they often are:
1. Diabetogenic
2. Socially ostracized
3. Financially dependent
4. Prone to gestational hypertension

216. Why should the presence of multiple gestation be detected as early as possible and the pregnancy managed as high risk?
1. Postpartum hemorrhage is an expected complication
2. Perinatal mortality is 2 to 3 times greater in multiple than in single births
3. Maternal mortality is higher during the prenatal period with a multiple gestation
4. Optimum adjustment following a multiple birth requires 6 months to 1 year of time

217. The nurse knows that a client is at risk for hypotonic uterine dystocia if she has:
1. A twin gestation
2. Gestational anemia
3. A pelvic contracture
4. Gestational hypertension

218. At 28 weeks' gestation the ultrasonography results indicate that the fetus is small for gestational age and there is evidence of a low-lying placenta. The nurse should use this information in the last trimester of pregnancy by assessing the client for signs of:
1. Preterm labor
2. Placenta previa
3. Precipitate birth
4. Premature placental separation

219. A client who is at 26 weeks' gestation arrives at the prenatal clinic complaining of painful urination, flank tenderness, and pink-tinged urine. A diagnosis of pyelonephritis is made. What is the most important nursing intervention at this time?
1. Limiting fluid intake
2. Examining her urine for protein
3. Observing for signs of preterm labor
4. Maintaining her on a 2-g sodium diet

220. Why does the nurse encourage continued health care supervision for the pregnant woman with pyelonephritis?
1. Preeclampsia frequently occurs after pyelonephritis
2. A low-protein diet is needed until the pregnancy is terminated

3. Antibiotic therapy should be administered until the urine is sterile
4. Pelvic inflammatory disease can occur with untreated pyelonephritis

221. A 25-year-old primigravida, at 15 weeks' gestation, is diagnosed as having a twin gestation. After having the risks of a multifetal pregnancy explained, the nurse determines that further instruction is needed when the client states that multiple gestation is associated with:
1. A preterm birth
2. Twin to twin transfusion
3. Gestational hypertension
4. A higher incidence of Down syndrome

222. A client comes to the clinic for a sonogram at 36 weeks' gestation. Before the test begins, the client complains of severe abdominal pain. Heavy vaginal bleeding is noted, the client's BP drops, and her pulse rate increases. What complication should the nurse suspect when the client develops these signs and symptoms?
1. Hydatidiform mole
2. Vena caval syndrome
3. Marginal placenta previa
4. Complete abruptio placentae

223. The nurse realizes the abdominal pain associated with abruptio placentae initially may be caused by:
1. Hemorrhagic shock
2. Concealed hemorrhage
3. Blood in the myometrium
4. Disseminated intravascular coagulation

224. The nurse is aware that the bleeding following severe abruptio placentae is usually caused by:
1. Polycythemia
2. Thrombocytopenia
3. Hyperglobulinemia
4. Hypofibrinogenemia

225. What maternal condition is associated with abruptio placentae?
1. Cardiac disease
2. Hyperthyroidism
3. Gestational hypertension
4. Cephalopelvic disproportion

226. A client who is at 38 weeks' gestation arrives at the hospital with profuse vaginal bleeding. What is the most likely cause of the bleeding?
1. Placenta previa
2. Placenta accreta
3. Ruptured uterus
4. Concealed abruptio

227. What nursing care should be included in the care of a client with placenta previa?
1. Vital signs at least once per shift
2. A tap-water enema before the birth
3. Documentation of the amount of bleeding
4. Limited ambulation until the bleeding stops

228. A client who is in the third trimester arrives at the hospital with vaginal bleeding. She states that she snorted cocaine approximately 2 hours ago. Which complication is most likely causing the client's vaginal bleeding?
1. Placenta previa
2. Ectopic pregnancy
3. Abruptio placentae
4. Spontaneous abortion

229. The nurse should explain to a client who is experiencing preterm contractions in the 35th week of gestation and whose cervix is dilated 2 cm that sexual intercourse:
1. Need not be restricted
2. Is prohibited because it may stimulate labor
3. Should be restricted to the side-lying position
4. Is permitted as long as penile penetration is shallow

230. After the birth of twins, a client may be predisposed to experiencing a postpartum hemorrhage. What is the most likely cause of hemorrhage for this client?
1. Atony of the uterus
2. Mediolateral episiotomy
3. Lacerations of the cervix
4. Retained placental fragments

231. A client who is at 39 weeks' gestation is now in labor. She has been told that she will have to have a cesarean birth. What in relation to the client's physical status is the most likely reason for the cesarean birth?
1. Gonorrhea
2. Chlamydia
3. Chronic hepatitis
4. Active genital herpes

232. The nurse notifies the practitioner that a client has been admitted in her 36th week of gestation. The client is bleeding, has severe abdominal pain and a hard fundus, and is demonstrating signs of shock. The nurse should prepare for:
1. A high-forceps birth
2. An immediate cesarean birth
3. The administration of oxytocin
4. The insertion of a fetal monitor

233. The nurse in the birthing suite has just admitted four clients. Which one should the nurse prepare for a cesarean birth?
1. Multipara with a shoulder presentation
2. Multipara with a documented station of "floating"
3. Primigravida with a fetus presenting in the occiput posterior position
4. Primigravida with a twin gestation with the lower-most in vertex presentation

234. During the first hour after a cesarean birth, the nurse notes that the client's lochia has saturated one perineal pad. Based on the knowledge of expected lochial flow, what should the nurse conclude that this indicates?
1. Scant lochial flow
2. Postpartum hemorrhage
3. Retained placental fragments
4. Lochial flow within normal limits

235. Which client should the nurse identify as at risk for developing a hypertensive disorder of pregnancy? A woman who:
    1. Is 31 years old
    2. Is an obese primigravida
    3. Has had six previous pregnancies
    4. Took oral contraceptives within 3 months of conception

236. When examining a pregnant client, a diagnosis of preeclampsia is made when the client's BP is:
    1. Elevated and accompanied by a headache
    2. 150/100 mm Hg while standing and sitting
    3. Above the baseline and fluctuating at each reading
    4. Greater than 140 mm Hg systolic and the client has proteinuria

237. When a client is admitted to the birthing suite with a BP of 150/90 mm Hg, 3+ proteinuria, and edema of the hands and face, the nurse should ask the client about the presence of:
    1. Constipation, edema, visual problems, headache
    2. Visual disturbances, headaches, constipation, bleeding
    3. Leakage of fluid, bleeding, edema, pain in the abdomen
    4. Headache, visual disturbances, edema, pain in the abdomen

238. The first assessable objective sign of a seizure in a client with eclampsia is frequently:
    1. Epigastric pain, nausea, and vomiting
    2. Persistent headache and blurred vision
    3. Spots with flashes of light before the eyes
    4. Rolling of the eyes to one side with a fixed stare

239. The nurse evaluates that the danger of a seizure in a woman with eclampsia subsides:
    1. After labor begins
    2. After birth occurs
    3. 48 hours postpartum
    4. 24 hours postpartum

240. During an emergency birth, the nurse notes the infant's head crowning on the perineum. The nurse's priority action is to support the head by:
    1. Applying suprapubic pressure over it
    2. Distributing the fingers evenly around it
    3. Placing a hand firmly against the perineum
    4. Maintaining pressure against the anterior fontanel

241. What is the safest position for a woman in labor when the nurse notes a prolapsed cord?
    1. Prone
    2. Fowler's
    3. Lithotomy
    4. Trendelenburg

242. The hemodynamics of pregnancy that affect the pregnant client with heart disease include the:
    1. Decrease in the number of RBCs
    2. Gradually increasing size of the uterus
    3. Rise in cardiac output after the 34th week
    4. Heart rate acceleration in the last half of pregnancy

243. A pregnant client with a class II heart disease is concerned that her pregnancy will be an added burden on her already compromised heart. The nurse explains that during pregnancy the cardiac system is most compromised during the:
    1. First trimester
    2. Third trimester
    3. Transitional phase of labor
    4. First 48 hours after the birth

244. A pregnant client with a history of rheumatic heart disease since childhood is concerned about the birth of her baby and asks what to expect. The nurse should mention that at term her care will probably include:
    1. An elective cesarean birth
    2. General anesthesia and forceps-assisted birth
    3. Regional anesthesia and forceps-assisted birth
    4. Induction of labor to reduce the stress of the birth

245. A client with class I heart disease is admitted to the birthing suite in active labor. How should the client be positioned?
    1. Supine, high-Fowler's
    2. Supine, semi-Fowler's
    3. Left lateral, semi-Fowler's
    4. Right lateral, low Fowler's

246. A nursing intervention that is specific for clients with cardiac problems who are in active labor is:
    1. Monitoring blood pressure hourly
    2. Encouraging the client to void frequently
    3. Auscultating the lungs for crackles every 30 minutes
    4. Having the client turn from side to side at 15-minute intervals

247. The nurse is aware that in the second half of pregnancy, women who have type 1 diabetes require increased dosages of:
    1. Insulin
    2. Antihypertensives
    3. Pancreatic enzymes
    4. Estrogenic hormones

248. The nurse should anticipate that on the first postpartum day, the insulin requirements of a client with diabetes will:
    1. Rapidly increase
    2. Remain unchanged
    3. Decrease sharply and suddenly
    4. Demonstrate a slow and steady decrease

249. A client has given birth to a healthy girl. During the second postpartum hour, the nurse notes heavy vaginal bleeding that does not diminish after fundal massage. The client states, "I am so thirsty after my long labor. Can I have some ginger ale?" The nurse should reply:
    1. "It is good to regain your fluids. I will bring some for you right now."
    2. "I can imagine how thirsty you are. However, I must get an order before giving you any fluid."

3. "As difficult as it is, it is best for you to wait for the bleeding to slow. I can give you a moisturizer for your lips to relieve the dryness."

4. "Your fluid level should return to normal as quickly as possible. The blood loss can begin to balance if you drink enough fluids."

250. A client who has six living children has just given birth. After the expulsion of the placenta an infusion of lactated Ringer's solution with 10 units of oxytocin is ordered. The nurse understands that this infusion is indicated for this client because:
1. She had a precipitate birth
2. This was an extramural birth
3. Retained placental fragments must be expelled
4. Multigravidas are at increased risk for uterine atony

251. When assessing clients who have given birth, the nurse should be aware that postpartum hemorrhage rarely occurs as a result of:
1. Twin births
2. Retained placenta
3. Overdistended bladder
4. Uncomplicated hypertension

252. When reviewing a client's history, the nurse should know that the two most important predisposing causes of puerperal (postpartum) infection are:
1. Hemorrhage and trauma during labor
2. Preeclampsia and retention of placenta
3. Malnutrition and anemia during pregnancy
4. Organisms in the birth canal and trauma during labor

253. During the postpartum period it is not uncommon for a new mother to have an increased cardiac output with tachycardia. This knowledge should motivate the nurse who is caring for a client with cardiac problems to vigilantly observe for signs of:
1. Irregular pulse
2. Hypovolemic shock
3. Respiratory distress
4. Increased vaginal bleeding

254. The nurse screens the newborn of a diabetic mother for hypoglycemia by:
1. Drawing blood for serum glucose
2. Beginning a glucose tolerance test
3. Scheduling a fasting blood glucose
4. Using a glucose-oxidase strip on heelstick blood

255. In the nursery, the newborn of a mother with a history of long-standing diabetes should be provided with:
1. Fast-acting insulin
2. Special high-risk care
3. Routine newborn care
4. Limited glucose intake

256. The nurse understands that after birth infants of diabetic mothers often have tremors, periods of apnea, cyanosis, and poor sucking ability. These signs are associated with:
1. Hypoglycemia
2. Hypercalcemia
3. Central nervous system edema
4. Congenital depression of the islets of Langerhans

257. The nurse is aware that infants of diabetic mothers are usually larger than other newborns because of:
1. Increased somatotropin and lowered glucose utilization
2. Increased somatotropin and increased glucose utilization
3. Decreased somatotropin and increased glucose utilization
4. Decreased somatotropin and decreased glucose utilization

NURSING CARE OF THE NEWBORN

258. An infant is born with a bilateral cleft palate. Plans are made to begin reconstruction immediately. What nursing intervention should be included to promote parent-infant bonding?
1. Demonstrating a positive acceptance of the infant
2. Placing the baby in a nursery away from view of the general public
3. Explaining to the parents that the infant will look normal after the surgery
4. Encouraging the parents to limit contact with the infant until after the surgery

259. After an 8-hour, uneventful labor a client gives birth to a boy spontaneously under epidural block anesthesia. As the nurse places the newborn in the mother's arms, the mother asks, "Is he normal?" What is the best response by the nurse?
1. "Most babies are normal; of course he is."
2. "He must be all right; he has such a good strong cry."
3. "Yes; because your entire pregnancy has been so normal."
4. "We will unwrap him now; you can look him over for yourself."

260. Supportive nursing care in the beginning mother-infant relationship should include:
1. Requiring the mother to assist with simple aspects of her infant's care
2. Encouraging the mother to decide between breast-feeding and formula feeding
3. Observing the mother and her infant unobtrusively to watch for a disturbed relationship
4. Allowing the mother time to undress her infant so that she can proceed with an inspection

261. Which behavior indicates to the nurse that a new mother is in the taking-hold phase?
1. Talking about the baby
2. Calling the baby by name
3. Touching the baby with her fingertips
4. Involving herself passively with the baby

262. When selecting nursing measures to help parent-child relationships during the postpartum period, what is the most important factor for the nurse to consider?
1. Anesthesia during labor
2. Duration and difficulty of labor

3. Physical condition of the infant
4. Health and emotional status during pregnancy

263. When caring for a family on a postpartum unit, the nurse must be aware that all the tasks, responsibilities, and attitudes that make up child care can be called parenting and that either parent can exhibit these qualities. Which factor most importantly influences parenting ability?
1. Marriage with flexible roles
2. Inborn ability based on instinct
3. Positive childhood roles and concepts
4. Education about growth and development

264. What type of immunity is transferred to the fetus through the placenta?
1. Active natural immunity
2. Passive natural immunity
3. Active artificial immunity
4. Passive artificial immunity

265. Closure of the newborn's foramen ovale is caused by:
1. A decrease in the aortic blood flow
2. A decrease in pressure in the left atrium
3. An increase in the pulmonary blood flow
4. An increase in the pressure in the right atrium

266. After the birth of a healthy neonate, the ductus arteriosus becomes the:
1. Vesical ligament
2. Venous ligament
3. Ligamentum teres
4. Ligamentum arteriosum

267. A client gives birth to a 6-lb baby girl. The client is rooming-in with her baby. The nurse observes the infant lying quietly in the bassinet with her eyes wide open. In response to the infant's behavior, the nurse:
1. Begins the physical assessment
2. Turns up the lights in the room
3. Encourages the mother to talk to her baby
4. Wraps the infant and then turns her to the side

268. What is the primary critical observation for Apgar scoring?
1. Heart rate
2. Respiratory rate
3. Presence of meconium
4. Evaluation of Moro reflex

269. When performing a newborn assessment, the nurse should measure the vital signs in the following sequence:
1. Pulse, respirations, temperature
2. Temperature, pulse, respirations
3. Respirations, temperature, pulse
4. Respirations, pulse, temperature

270. Within 3 minutes after birth the heart rate of a healthy, alert neonate may range between:
1. 120 and 180 beats/min
2. 130 and 170 beats/min
3. 110 and 160 beats/min
4. 100 and 130 beats/min

271. In a noisy room a newborn initially startles and has rapid movements initially to the noise but soon goes to sleep. The most appropriate nursing action in response to this behavior is to:
1. Test the infant's hearing
2. Accept the infant's behavior
3. Assess the infant's vital signs
4. Stimulate the infant's respirations

272. The nurse knows that neonates have difficulty maintaining their body temperature. However, they have several mechanisms to help them maintain it. Check all that apply.
1. ☐ Flexed fetal position
2. ☐ Hepatic insulin stores
3. ☐ Brown fat metabolism
4. ☐ Peripheral vasoconstriction
5. ☐ Parasympathetic nervous system

273. The nurse is aware that a healthy newborn's respirations are:
1. Irregular, thoracic, 30 to 60/min, deep
2. Regular, abdominal, 40 to 50/min, deep
3. Regular, thoracic, 40 to 60/min, shallow
4. Irregular, abdominal, 30 to 60/min, shallow

274. Just after beginning the first feeding, a newborn begins to cough and choke, and the lips turn cyanotic. What should be the immediate nursing action?
1. Stimulate crying
2. Suction and then provide oxygen
3. Change the feeding to sterile water
4. Stop the feeding momentarily and then restart

275. At 10 hours of age an infant has a large amount of mucus and becomes cyanotic. What should the nurse do first?
1. Suction
2. Administer oxygen
3. Record the incident
4. Insert a nasogastric tube

276. Which behavior should the nurse recognize as the Moro reflex response?
1. Extension of the arms
2. Adduction of the arms
3. Abduction and then adduction of the arms
4. Extension of the legs and fanning of the toes

277. A newborn has small, whitish, pinpoint spots over the nose, which the nurse knows are caused by retained sebaceous secretions. When charting this observation, the nurse identifies it as:
1. Milia
2. Lanugo
3. Whiteheads
4. Mongolian spots

278. The nurse observes a healthy newborn lying in a supine position with the head turned to the side, legs and arms extended on the same side and flexed on the opposite side. Which reflex does this posture represent?
1. Moro reflex
2. Grasp reflex

3. Babinski reflex

4. Tonic neck reflex

279. An infant's intestines are sterile at birth, therefore lacking the bacteria necessary for the synthesis of:
1. Bilirubin
2. Bile salts
3. Prothrombin
4. Intrinsic factor

280. The nurse explains to a new mother why there must be a delay of 36 to 48 hours before her newborn can have a:
1. Screening for PKU
2. Vitamin K injection
3. Heelstick for blood glucose level
4. Test for necrotizing enterocolitis

281. The nurse teaches a group of postpartum clients that all their newborns will be screened for PKU to:
1. Detect possible retardation
2. Measure protein metabolism
3. Detect chromosomal damage
4. Identify thyroid insufficiency

282. When assessing a 9-lb neonate 2 hours after birth, the nurse identifies jitteriness, irregular respirations, and temperature instability. The nurse knows that these are indications that the neonate probably has:
1. Hyponatremia
2. Hypoglycemia
3. A cardiac defect
4. An immature CNS

283. The practice of separating the parents and the newborn immediately after birth and limiting their time with the infant in the first few days contradicts studies based on:
1. Bonding
2. Rooming-in
3. Taking-in behaviors
4. Taking-hold behaviors

284. After birth, when inspecting her newborn girl, the mother notices a discharge from the nipples of both of her infant's breasts. The nurse should explain that this is evidence of:
1. Monilia contracted during birth
2. An infection contracted in utero
3. Congenital hormonal imbalance
4. An effect from maternal hormones

285. The nurse decides on a teaching plan for a new mother and her infant. The plan should include:
1. Discussing the topic with her in a nonthreatening manner
2. Showing by example and explanation how to care for the infant
3. Setting up a schedule for teaching her how to care for her infant
4. Supplying emotional support and encouraging her dependence on the nurse's expertise

286. A client asks the nurse what advantage breastfeeding has over formula feeding. The nurse replies that one major group of substances in human milk is of special importance to the newborn and cannot be reproduced in a bottle formula. This group of substances is:
1. Amino acids
2. Gamma globulins
3. Essential electrolytes
4. Complex carbohydrates

287. The nurse knows that certain newborns are at risk to develop hypoglycemia. Check all that apply.
1. ☐ Preterm infants
2. ☐ Infants with Down syndrome
3. ☐ Infants of mothers with diabetes
4. ☐ Small-for-gestational-age infants
5. ☐ Large-for-gestational-age infants
6. ☐ Appropriate-for-gestational-age infants

288. Which assessment, observed immediately after birth, will probably necessitate prolonged follow-up care of a newborn?
1. Apgar score of 5
2. Weight of 3500 g
3. Umbilical cord that contains 2 blood vessels
4. Aspiration of 20 mL of milky-colored gastric fluid

289. A neonate at 1 minute of age has a weak cry, a heart rate of 90 beats/min, some flexion of the extremities, grimacing, and acrocyanosis. What is the Apgar score for this neonate?
1. 5
2. 6
3. 7
4. 8

290. A low Apgar score at 5 minutes after birth correlates with the occurrence of:
1. Cerebral palsy
2. Genetic defects
3. Mental retardation
4. Neonatal morbidity

291. An infant born in the 36th week of gestation weighs 4 lb 3 oz (2062 g) and has Apgar scores of 7/9. On admission to the nursery, it is not necessary for the nurse to:
1. Record vital signs
2. Administer oxygen
3. Evaluate the neonate's health status
4. Support the neonate's body temperature

292. The nurse understands that one of the factors influencing the availability of milk in the lactating woman is the:
1. Distribution of erectile tissue in nipples
2. Age of the woman at the time of the birth
3. Amount of milk products consumed during the pregnancy
4. Viewpoint of the woman's family toward breastfeeding

293. While teaching a prenatal class about infant feeding, the nurse is asked a question about the relationship between the size of breasts and breastfeeding. How should the nurse respond?
1. "You should be successful at breastfeeding."
2. "You seem to have some concern about breastfeeding."

3. "The size of your breasts has nothing to do with the production of milk."
4. "The amount of glandular tissue in the breasts determines the amount of milk produced."

294. A woman learning about infant feedings asks how anyone who is breastfeeding gets anything done with a baby on demand feedings. How should the nurse respond?
    1. "Most mothers find that feeding the baby whenever the baby cries works out fine."
    2. "Perhaps a schedule might be better because the baby is already accustomed to the hospital routine."
    3. "Babies on demand feedings eventually set a schedule, so there will be time for you to do other things."
    4. "Most breastfeeding mothers find that their babies do better on demand because the amount of milk ingested may vary at each feeding."

295. The nurse should explain to a client that breastfeeding is always contraindicated with:
    1. Mastitis
    2. Hepatitis C
    3. Inverted nipples
    4. Herpes genitalis

296. The client response that indicates understanding of teaching regarding breast care for the mother who is breastfeeding is, "I will:
    1. Use a mild soap for washing."
    2. Remove my brassiere at night."
    3. Air dry my nipples after feeding."
    4. Line my breast pads with plastic."

297. A client who is breastfeeding is being discharged. The client tells the nurse that she is worried because her neighbor's breasts "dried up" when she got home and had to discontinue breastfeeding. What should the nurse reply?
    1. "Once lactation is established, this rarely happens."
    2. "You have little to worry about because you already have a good milk supply."
    3. "This can happen with the excitement of going home, but putting the baby to breast more often should reestablish lactation."
    4. "This commonly happens, so we will give you a bottle of formula to take home so the baby won't go hungry until your milk supply returns."

298. When teaching breastfeeding, the nurse should recognize the client needs further instructions when she states, "I will:
    1. Try to empty my breasts at each feeding."
    2. Start with an alternate breast at each feeding."
    3. Wash my breasts with water before each feeding."
    4. Use soap and water to wash my breasts before each feeding."

299. To limit the development of hyperbilirubinemia in the breastfed neonate, the plan of care should include:
    1. Instituting phototherapy for 30 minutes every 6 hours
    2. Substituting breastfeeding for formula during the second day after birth

3. Supplementing breastfeeding with glucose-water during the first 24 hours
4. Encouraging more frequent breastfeeding during the first 2 days after birth

300. A new mother is breastfeeding her 2-day-old infant and tells the home health nurse that she cannot believe her newborn wants to breastfeed again, since she just fed him 2½ hours ago. The nurse should plan to teach the client that a newborn usually should be nursed:
    1. Every hour
    2. On demand
    3. Every 4 hours
    4. At 5-hour intervals

301. The nurse identifies that a woman needs further teaching about breastfeeding her newborn when she:
    1. Leans forward to put her breast into the infant's mouth
    2. Holds the infant level with her breast and in a side-lying position
    3. Touches her nipple to the infant's lips when beginning the feeding
    4. Puts her finger in the infant's mouth to break the suction when switching breasts

302. A 2-day-old infant who weighs 2722 g (6 lb) is fed formula every 4 hours. Newborns need about 73 mL of fluid per pound of body weight each day. Based on this information, approximately how much formula should the infant receive at each feeding?
    1. 1 to 2 oz
    2. 2 to 3 oz
    3. 3 to 4 oz
    4. 4 to 5 oz

303. A client asks about the difference between cow's milk and the milk from her breasts. The nurse should respond that cow's milk differs from human milk in that it contains:
    1. Less protein, less calcium, and more carbohydrates
    2. Less protein, more calcium, and more carbohydrates
    3. More protein, less calcium, and fewer carbohydrates
    4. More protein, more calcium, and fewer carbohydrates

304. While performing bag and mask ventilation on a newborn, the nurse does not see the newborn's chest rise. Place the following interventions in order of their priority.
    1. _____ Reposition the head
    2. _____ Open the mouth slightly and reventilate
    3. _____ Check for secretions and suction if necessary
    4. _____ Reapply the mask for a better seal and reventilate

305. At 12 weeks' gestation, a client who is Rh-negative completely expels the products of conception. After determining that she has not been previously sensitized, the nurse should:
    1. Administer RhoGAM within 72 hours
    2. Make certain the client receives RhoGAM at her first clinic visit
    3. Withhold the RhoGAM, because it is not used after the birth of a stillborn

4. Withhold administration of the RhoGAM, because the gestation lasted only 12 weeks

306. A client who has type O Rh-positive blood gives birth. The neonate has type B Rh-negative blood. When the nurse assesses the neonate 11 hours after birth, the infant's skin appears yellow. This is most likely caused by:
1. Neonatal sepsis
2. Rh incompatibility
3. Physiologic jaundice
4. ABO incompatibility

307. The nurse in the newborn nursery observes a yellowish skin color of an infant whose mother had a cesarean birth. The immediate nursing action should be to:
1. Notify the practitioner
2. Ascertain the age of the neonate
3. Take a heel blood sample and send it to the laboratory
4. Cover the eyes and place the infant under the ultraviolet light

308. A primigravida has just given birth. The nurse notes that she has type AB negative blood. Her newborn's blood type is B positive. The nurse is aware that the mother's plan of care should include:
1. Obtaining an order for RhoGAM
2. Observing for ABO incompatibility
3. Determining the father's blood type
4. Preparing for a maternal blood transfusion

309. When observing a newborn for signs of pathologic jaundice, the nurse should be alert for:
1. Muscular irritability at birth
2. Neurologic signs during the first 24 hours
3. Jaundice developing between 48 and 72 hours after birth
4. Jaundice developing between the first 12 and 24 hours

310. The nurse is differentiating between cephalohematoma and caput succedaneum. What adaptation is unique to caput succedaneum?
1. Scalp over the area is tender
2. Edema crosses the suture line
3. Edema increases during the first day
4. Scalp over the area becomes ecchymosed

311. The nurse should be aware that the major hazard to a newborn during a precipitate birth is:
1. Brachial palsy
2. Dislocated hip
3. Fractured clavicle
4. Intracranial hemorrhage

312. A preterm neonate admitted to the neonatal intensive care nursery has muscle twitching, seizures, cyanosis, abnormal respirations, and a short, shrill cry. The nurse suspects that this infant may have:
1. Tetany
2. Spina bifida
3. Hyperkalemia
4. Intracranial hemorrhage

313. An infant is born in the breech position. Because Erb's palsy may occur as the result of a difficult vaginal breech birth, the nurse should assess the infant for:
1. An absent grasp reflex on the affected side
2. A negative Moro reflex on the unaffected side
3. An inability to turn the head to the affected side
4. A flaccid arm with the elbow extended on the affected side

314. Nursing care for the affected arm of an infant born with Erb's palsy should include:
1. Constant immobilization of the affected arm
2. Teaching the parents to manipulate the muscle
3. Daily measurement of the length of the affected arm
4. Immediate passive ROM exercises to the affected arm

315. A newborn is diagnosed as having Erb's palsy. The nurse is aware that this problem is caused by:
1. A disease acquired in utero
2. An X-linked inheritance pattern
3. A tumor arising from muscle tissue
4. An injury to the brachial plexus during birth

316. The nurse should know that an asymmetric Moro reflex is frequently associated with:
1. Down syndrome
2. Cranial nerve damage
3. Cerebral or cerebellar injuries
4. Brachial plexus, clavicular, or humeral injuries

317. The nurse suspects that a newborn is exhibiting signs of opiate withdrawal when assessment demonstrates:
1. Lethargy and constipation
2. Grunting and a low-pitched cry
3. Irritability and nasal congestion
4. Watery eyes and rapid respirations

318. Typical signs of withdrawal in opiate-dependent newborns usually begin within 24 hours after birth. The nurse should observe newborns of suspected or known drug users for:
1. Dehydration
2. Hyperactivity
3. Hypotonicity of muscles
4. Prolonged periods of sleep

319. On a home visit the visiting nurse assesses that the 4-day-old infant who was born at home has a purulent discharge from the eyes. The nurse suspects that the infant has:
1. Signs of *Chlamydia trachomatis* infection
2. Acquired immunodeficiency syndrome (AIDS)
3. Retinopathy of prematurity (retrolental fibroplasia)
4. A reaction to the ophthalmic antibiotic instilled after birth

320. An infant develops purulent conjunctivitis on the fourth day of life and is brought to the emergency department. The nurse first should:
1. Teach the mother about handwashing
2. Assess the infant for signs of pneumonia

3. Secure an order for allergy testing of the infant
4. Bathe the infant's eyes with tepid boric acid solution

321. The care of a newborn infant whose mother has had untreated syphilis since the second trimester of the pregnancy includes:
   1. Assessing for cleft palate
   2. Eliciting hypotonicity of skeletal muscles
   3. Screening immediately for congenital syphilis
   4. Observing for maculopapular lesions of the soles

322. The nurse must continuously monitor a preterm infant's temperature and provide appropriate nursing care because the preterm infant, unlike the full-term infant, has:
   1. An inability to use shivering to produce heat
   2. An inability to break down glycogen to glucose
   3. A limited supply of brown fat available to provide heat
   4. A limited amount of pituitary hormones to control internal heat

323. When meeting a preterm infant's hydration needs, the nurse should know that the preterm infant's urinary function:
   1. Is the same as in a full-term newborn
   2. Results in the loss of large amounts of urine
   3. Leads to urine with an elevated specific gravity
   4. Adequately maintains an acid-base and electrolyte balance

324. The nurse must continuously monitor preterm infants for the most common preterm complication, which is:
   1. Hemorrhage
   2. Brain damage
   3. Respiratory distress
   4. Aspiration of mucus

325. When caring for preterm infants with respiratory distress, the nurse should keep:
   1. Them prone to prevent aspiration
   2. Them in a high-humidity environment
   3. Their caloric intake low to decrease metabolic rate
   4. Their oxygen concentration low to prevent eye damage

ANSWERS AND RATIONALES

NURSING CARE TO PROMOTE CHILDBEARING AND WOMEN'S HEALTH

1. **1** Nurses with positive attitudes toward abortion should counsel women who are thinking of undergoing the procedure; they should know what services are available and the various methods that are used to induce abortion.

   2 Nursing practice necessitates scientific knowledge; statements must be based on fact, not personal feelings or beliefs. **3** The nurse is capable of giving information about abortion and need not defer to the physician. **4** The nurse should give the client only the information requested and should not state personal feelings.

   Client Need: Management of Care; **Cognitive Level:** Application; **Nursing Process:** Evaluation/Outcomes; **Reference:** Ch 23, Induced Abortion, Nursing Care

2. **3** This response is a positive negotiation to be reassigned to an area where the nurse's personal values will not pose a problem.

   1 This is an ineffective way to resolve value conflict; undoubtedly, any client would sense this conflict. **2** The nurse may not have the legal, ethical, or professional right to refuse this assignment if employed by the facility. **4** Imposing this kind of advice would be unethical and unprofessional.

   Client Need: Management of Care; **Cognitive Level:** Analysis; **Nursing Process:** Planning/Implementation; **Reference:** Ch 23, Contraceptive Methods, Nursing Care

3. **4** The client must feel comfortable enough to verbalize her feelings; this helps to complete the grieving process.

   1 This is a false assumption. **2** Induced abortion is a sterile procedure and should not predispose the client to postoperative infection. **3** Studies show that contraceptive counseling at this time is most important, because the client may not return after the abortion.

   Client Need: Psychosocial Integrity; **Cognitive Level:** Application; **Integrated Process:** Caring, Communication/Documentation; **Nursing Process:** Assessment/Analysis; **Reference:** Ch 23, Induced Abortion, Nursing Care

4. **2** Because mothering is not an inborn instinct, almost all mothers, including multiparas, report some ambivalence and anxiety about their ability to be good mothers.

   1 Frequently maternal feelings are nurtured by the sight of the infant. **3** It may take a much longer time. **4** Ambivalent feelings are universal in response to a neonate.

   Client Need: Psychosocial Integrity; **Cognitive Level:** Comprehension; **Nursing Process:** Assessment/Analysis; **Reference:** Ch 25, Prenatal Period: Physical, Physiologic, and Emotional Changes During Pregnancy

5. **3** Although support may help minimize guilt, it will not eliminate it; however, support will sustain family cohesion and unity.

   1 Support may help, but it does not completely alleviate guilt feelings. **2** Support does not affect the legal responsibility of the parents. **4** This may help, but it cannot completely relieve pressure.

   Client Need: Psychosocial Integrity; **Cognitive Level:** Application; **Integrated Process:** Caring; **Nursing Process:** Planning/Implementation; **Reference:** Ch 23, Induced Abortion, Nursing Care

6. **2** Some type of a barrier contraceptive (condom with foam or jelly or a diaphragm) is usually recommended for the client with diabetes mellitus and heart disease.

   1 Oral contraceptives are not recommended for this client because of their tendency to alter glucose tolerance. **3** An IUD is not recommended because it may predispose this client to infection. **4** Clients with heart disease can become pregnant again in the future.

   Client Need: Health Promotion and Maintenance; **Cognitive Level:** Application; **Integrated Process:** Teaching/Learning; **Nursing Process:** Planning/Implementation; **Reference:** Ch 23, Contraceptive Methods, Nursing Care

7. **4** Subsequent to IUD insertion, there may be an excessive menstrual flow for several cycles; because the IUD is a foreign body, there is an increase in the blood supply as a result of the inflammatory process.

   1 There is no documentation of this. **2** This may occur on insertion but is uncommon. **3** This may occur but it is not classified as a side effect.

   Client Need: Health Promotion and Maintenance; **Cognitive Level:** Application; **Integrated Process:** Teaching/Learning; **Nursing Process:** Planning/Implementation; **Reference:** Ch 23, Contraceptive Methods, Data Base

8. **4** The IUD may cause irritability of the myometrium, inducing contraction of the uterus and expulsion of the device.

   1 This is a rare, rather than a common, occurrence. **2** Clients do not complain of discomfort during coitus when an IUD is in place. **3** Increased vaginal infections are not reported with the use of an IUD.

   Client Need: Health Promotion and Maintenance; **Cognitive Level:** Application; **Integrated Process:** Teaching/Learning; **Nursing Process:** Planning/Implementation; **Reference:** Ch 23, Contraceptive Methods, Data Base

9. **4** Sperm are damaged by copper IUDs, whereas progesterone IUDs interfere with endometrial maturation.

   1 A diaphragm blocks the cervical os. **2** Mobility of the uterus is not related to contraception. **3** This is the function of a condom.

   Client Need: Health Promotion and Maintenance; **Cognitive Level:** Application; **Integrated Process:** Teaching/Learning; **Nursing Process:** Planning/Implementation; **Reference:** Ch 23, Contraceptive Methods, Data Base

10. **3** It is the surge of LH (luteinizing hormone) secretion in midcycle that is responsible for ovulation.

    1 Oxytocin stimulates ejection of milk into the mammary ducts. **2** Ovulation occurs when the

progesterone level is low. **4** Human chorionic gonadotropin is secreted after pregnancy occurs.
Client Need: Health Promotion and Maintenance; **Cognitive Level:** Comprehension; **Integrated Process:** Teaching/Learning; **Nursing Process:** Planning/Implementation; **Reference:** Ch 23, Menstrual Cycle

11. **3** The ovum is capable of being fertilized for 24 to 36 hours following ovulation; after this time it travels a variable distance between the fallopian tube and uterus, and, if not fertilized, disintegrates and is phagocytized by leukocytes.
1 The ovum is viable for 24 to 36 hours. **2** The ovum is viable a longer time. **4** The ovum is not fertilizable after 36 hours.
Client Need: Health Promotion and Maintenance; **Cognitive Level:** Knowledge; **Integrated Process:** Teaching/Learning; **Nursing Process:** Planning/Implementation; **Reference:** Ch 23, Menstrual Cycle

12. **1** As ovulation approaches, there may be a drop in the basal temperature because of an increased production of estrogen; when ovulation occurs, there will be a rise in the basal temperature because of an increased production of progesterone.
2 At ovulation the temperature rises after a slight drop. **3** At ovulation the temperature drop is slight, not marked. **4** At ovulation the temperature drops slightly and then rises.
Client Need: Health Promotion and Maintenance; **Cognitive Level:** Comprehension; **Integrated Process:** Teaching/Learning; **Nursing Process:** Planning/Implementation; **Reference:** Ch 23, Contraceptive Methods, Data Base

13. **4** This commonly occurs when clients begin taking oral contraceptives; it is midcycle bleeding, and if it persists, the dosage is changed.
1 Cervicitis is unrelated to oral contraceptive use.
2 At this time there is no evidence that ovarian cysts are related to oral contraceptive use.
3 Fibrocystic breast disease is unrelated to oral contraceptive use.
Client Need: Pharmacological and Parenteral Therapies; **Cognitive Level:** Application; **Integrated Process:** Teaching/Learning; **Nursing Process:** Planning/Implementation; **Reference:** Ch 23, Contraceptive Methods, Data Base

14. **4** Some spermatozoa will remain viable in the vas deferens for a variable time after vasectomy.
1 There has been some success in reversing this procedure. **2** Precautions must be taken to prevent fertilization until absence of sperm in the semen has been verified. **3** The procedure does not affect sexual functioning.
Client Need: Health Promotion and Maintenance; **Cognitive Level:** Application; **Integrated Process:** Teaching/Learning; **Nursing Process:** Planning/Implementation; **Reference:** Ch 23, Contraceptive Methods, Nursing Care

15. 1 ☒ Oral agents have a hormonal component.
2 ☐ Diaphragms act as a barrier.
3 ☐ Cervical caps act as a barrier.
4 ☐ Foam spermicides kill the sperm; there is no hormonal effect.

5 ☒ Transdermal agents have a hormonal component.
6 ☒ Some intrauterine devices (IUDs) have a hormonal component as well as the ability to interfere with implantation.
Client Need: Pharmacological and Parenteral Therapies; **Cognitive Level:** Analysis; **Nursing Process:** Assessment/Analysis; **Reference:** Ch 23, Contraceptive Methods, Data Base

16. **1** Stress or infection can alter the body's metabolism, causing an elevation in temperature; a rise in temperature from these causes may be misinterpreted as ovulation.
2 This may increase sperm volume but does not affect the female's basal temperature. **3** Age is not a factor concerning efficiency of the basal body temperature method of contraception. **4** Frequency of intercourse may affect the volume of sperm but does not alter the female's basal temperature.
Client Need: Health Promotion and Maintenance; **Cognitive Level:** Application; **Integrated Process:** Teaching/Learning; **Nursing Process:** Planning/Implementation; **Reference:** Ch 23, Contraceptive Methods, Data Base

17. **4** Antiovulatory drugs suppress menstruation. Breakthrough bleeding is not expected with biphasic drugs. The drug is given for 21 days, and a menstrual flow does not occur during this time.
1 There is no indication for increased Papanicolaou smears; once a year is sufficient. **2** Increasing calcium intake is not relevant to the administration of oral contraceptives. **3** No restriction of sexual activity is indicated when one is taking oral contraceptives.
Client Need: Pharmacological and Parenteral Therapies; **Cognitive Level:** Application; **Integrated Process:** Teaching/ Learning; **Nursing Process:** Planning/Implementation; **Reference:** Ch 23, Contraceptive Methods, Nursing Care

18. **4** Excessive bleeding should be reported because it is an indication that all of the products of conception have not been evacuated.
1 The client may shower daily. **2** Tampons should be avoided for at least 3 days, although some protocols stress avoidance of tampons for 3 weeks. **3** Depending on the protocol, sexual intercourse should be avoided for at least 1 week and up to 2 weeks.
Client Need: Health Promotion and Maintenance; **Cognitive Level:** Analysis; **Integrated Process:** Teaching/Learning; **Nursing Process:** Planning/Implementation; **Reference:** Ch 23, Induced Abortion, Nursing Care

19. **3** A follow-up visit 4 to 8 days later should confirm that the abortion has occurred.
1 This is too soon. **2** This is too late. **4** This is too early.
Client Need: Pharmacological and Parenteral Therapies; **Cognitive Level:** Application; **Integrated Process:** Teaching/ Learning; **Nursing Process:** Planning/Implementation; **Reference:** Ch 23, Induced Abortion, Data Base

20. **3** A laparoscopic tubal ligation takes about 20 minutes to perform. The client is admitted as an outpatient and goes home the same day after she recovers from the anesthesia.

1 Menstruation will continue because there is no trauma to the ovaries or the endocrine glands involved with reproduction. **2** Sterility is immediate; a waiting period is not required as with a vasectomy. **4** Microsurgery to reverse the procedure is not guaranteed or easily accomplished.
Client Need: Reduction of Risk Potential; **Cognitive Level:** Application; **Integrated Process:** Teaching/Learning; **Nursing Process:** Planning/Implementation; **Reference:** Ch 23, Contraceptive Methods, Data Base

21. **3** Ovulation occurs 14 days before the onset of menses.
1 Midway between her cycles would be appropriate only if the client had a 28-day cycle. **2** This would mean that ovulation would occur on approximately day 5 of the menstrual cycle. **4** Variations in the cycle occur in the preovulation period; it is not as accurate as counting 14 days before the next expected menses.
Client Need: Health Promotion and Maintenance; **Cognitive Level:** Application; **Integrated Process:** Teaching/Learning; **Nursing Process:** Planning/Implementation; **Reference:** Ch 23, Menstrual Cycle

22. **4** At this time, because of increased estrogen levels, the cervical mucus is abundant, and its quality changes in such a way as to optimize sperm survival time.
1 Cervical mucus at this time is no longer receptive to spermatozoa. **2** Cervical mucus is destructive to spermatozoa and sperm penetration at this time. **3** The cervical mucus at this time is not yet receptive to spermatozoa.
Client Need: Health Promotion and Maintenance; **Cognitive Level:** Application; **Integrated Process:** Teaching/Learning; **Nursing Process:** Planning/Implementation; **Reference:** Ch 23, Menstrual Cycle

23. **2** Past infections may cause tubal occlusions, most of which are caused by postinfection adhesions.
1 This is possible, but infections in the tube are more common. **3** This is a tumor of the uterus and does not affect the tube. **4** This is rare; anomalies of the uterus are more common than those of a tube.
Client Need: Physiological Adaptation; **Cognitive Level:** Analysis; **Nursing Process:** Assessment/Analysis; **Reference:** Ch 23, Infertility and Sterility

24. **3** Infertility is the inability of a couple to conceive after at least 1 year of adequate exposure to the possibility of pregnancy.
1 Infertility may be psychogenic; however, statistics show that physiologic problems are more often the cause. **2** Infertility may be corrected, but sterility is irreversible. **4** Although this may be true, it is not the definition of the existence of infertility.
Client Need: Health Promotion and Maintenance; **Cognitive Level:** Comprehension; **Nursing Process:** Assessment/Analysis; **Reference:** Ch 23, Infertility and Sterility

25. **4** A strategy for increasing the chances of conceiving requires the couple to plan intercourse only while the woman is ovulating; this removes spontaneity and is often stressful.
1 Obtaining and delivering the necessary specimens may be inconvenient but should not be stressful. **2** The number of office visits and examinations that are required may be cumbersome but should not be stressful. **3** The couple probably knows that one of them has a fertility problem; it may be helpful knowing what the problem is so that measures can be taken to correct it, which usually reduces stress.
Client Need: Health Promotion and Maintenance; **Cognitive Level:** Application; **Nursing Process:** Planning/Implementation; **Reference:** Ch 23, Infertility and Sterility

26. **2** This is an accurate, objective statement that should be included in a discussion of genetic factors that influence fertility.
1 This is not the role of the nurse; based on the objective data imparted by the nurse, the couple should make the decision whether or not to be tested. **3, 4** This information is not relevant at this time and might cause unnecessary concern.
Client Need: Physiological Adaptation; **Cognitive Level:** Application; **Integrated Process:** Teaching/Learning; **Nursing Process:** Planning/Implementation; **Reference:** Ch 23, Infertility and Sterility

27. **2** When the testes are twisted, a decrease in their blood supply occurs. This can result in gangrene.
1 Medication can be given to relieve pain. **3** The testes do not rupture if edema occurs. **4** Sperm are continually produced, so their destruction is not the concern.
Client Need: Physiological Adaptation; **Cognitive Level:** Comprehension; **Integrated Process:** Teaching/Learning; **Nursing Process:** Planning/Implementation; **Reference:** Ch 23, Infertility and Sterility

28. **2** This test determines the number and condition of sperm aspirated from the cervix within 2 hours after coitus.
1 Rubin's test determines the patency of the fallopian tubes. **3** The Papanicolaou test is used for the early diagnosis of cervical cancer. **4** The sperm penetration assay determines the sperm's ability to enter an egg
Client Need: Reduction of Risk Potential; **Cognitive Level:** Analysis; **Nursing Process:** Assessment/Analysis; **Reference:** Ch 23, Infertility and Sterility

29. **4** This test enables the examiner to visualize the uterus and fallopian tubes and the pelvic organs of reproduction.
1 A biopsy is the surgical excision of tissue for diagnostic purposes. **2** A cystogram is used to visualize the urinary bladder. **3** A culdoscopy is the direct examination of female pelvic viscera using an endoscope introduced through a perforation in the vagina.
Client Need: Reduction of Risk Potential; **Cognitive Level:** Analysis; **Nursing Process:** Planning/Implementation; **Reference:** Ch 23, Infertility and Sterility

30. **3** Progesterone stimulates the differentiation of the endometrium into a secretory type of tissue, which makes it receptive to the fertilized ovum.
1 This is influenced by estrogen. **2** This is influenced by high levels of luteinizing hormone. **4** Secondary male characteristics are influenced by testosterone.
Client Need: Health Promotion and Maintenance; **Cognitive Level:** Comprehension; **Integrated Process:** Teaching/Learning; **Nursing Process:** Planning/Implementation; **Reference:** Ch 23, Female Reproductive System, Ovaries: Female Gonads

31. **3** Prolactin is the hormone secreted by the anterior pituitary gland that stimulates mammary gland secretion.
1 Oxytocin, a posterior pituitary hormone, stimulates the uterine musculature to contract and causes the let-down reflex. **2** Estrogen is not a pituitary hormone; it is secreted by the ovaries and placenta and is not involved with lactation. **4** Progesterone is not a pituitary hormone; it is secreted by thc corpus luteum of the ovary and is not involved with lactation.
Client Need: Health Promotion and Maintenance; **Cognitive Level:** Knowledge; **Nursing Process:** Assessment/Analysis; **Reference:** Ch 23, Female Reproductive System, Breasts

32. **4** Providing factual information decreases fear and fosters further communication.
1 Cervical cancer is asymptomatic in the early stages. **2** This offers false reassurance. **3** At this time the client may not be able to focus on written instructions; also, the anxiety may be related to the potential implications of the results of the test rather than the actual procedure.
Client Need: Reduction of Risk Potential; **Cognitive Level:** Application; **Integrated Process:** Teaching/Learning; **Nursing Process:** Planning/Implementation; **Reference:** Ch 23, Related Procedures, Pelvic Examination

33. **4** The function of progesterone is to relax the uterus and maintain a succulent endometrium to foster implantation of the fertilized ovum.
1 Ovulation is stimulated by increases in the levels of luteinizing hormone (LH) and estrogcn. **2** Menstruation is controlled by regulating factors from the hypothalamus and pituitary: the hormones they produce stimulate the production of ovarian follicles, as well as estrogen and progesterone by the ovarian cells. **3** Capillary fragility is often associated with deficiency of vitamin C (ascorbic acid); progesterone is not responsible.
Client Need: Health Promotion and Maintenance; **Cognitive Level:** Comprehension; **Nursing Process:** Assessment/Analysis; **Reference:** Ch 23, Menstrual Cycle

34. **4** Estrogen is found in the follicular fluid of the ovaries and aids in the growth of the endometrium.
1 The luteinizing hormone promotes the development of ovarian follicles and also stimulates ovulation and the production of estrogen and progesterone by the ovarian cells. **2** These hormones prepare the breasts for milk secretion (lactation). **3** The luteinizing hormone promotes the development of ovarian follicles and also stimulates ovulation and the production of estrogen and progesterone; progesterone prepares the endometrium for implantation and the breasts for lactation.
Client Need: Health Promotion and Maintenance; **Cognitive Level:** Knowledge; **Nursing Process:** Assessment/Analysis; **Reference:** Ch 23, Menstrual Cycle

35. **1** A generous supply of blood is carried by the uterine arteries (branches of the internal iliac arteries). The vaginal and ovarian arteries also supply the uterus with blood by anastomosing with the uterine vessels.
2 The aorta does not supply the uterus directly. **3** The hypogastric or internal iliac arteries supply the pelvic wall and viscera. **4** The hypogastric arteries (internal iliac) supply the pelvic wall and gluteal area, and the external branches (called uterine arteries) supply the uterus and genitalia; the aorta does not supply the uterus directly.
Client Need: Health Promotion and Maintenance; **Cognitive Level:** Knowledge; **Nursing Process:** Assessment/Analysis; **Reference:** Ch 23, Female Reproductive System, Uterus

36. **2** January 17. The time between ovulation and the next menstruation is relatively constant. Within a 30-day cycle the first 15 days are preovulatory, ovulation occurs on day 16, and the next 14 days are postovulatory.
1, 3, 4 This answer reflects an inaccurate calculation of the date of ovulation.
Client Need: Health Promotion and Maintenance; **Cognitive Level:** Application; **Nursing Process:** Assessment/Analysis; **Reference:** Ch 23, Menstrual Cycle

37. **4** Alteration of ovarian hormones causes vasomotor instability; periodic systemic vasodilation is triggered by the sympathetic nervous system, causing the feeling of warmth.
1 Acetylcholine does not cause hot flashes; it is the chemical mediator of cholinergic nerve impulses. **2** Gonadotropins do not cause hot flashes; they stimulate the function of the testes and ovaries. **3** Hot flashes may be associated with understimulation of the adrenals.
Client Need: Health Promotion and Maintenance; **Cognitive Level:** Application; **Integrated Process:** Teaching/Learning; **Nursing Process:** Planning/Implementation; **Reference:** Ch 23, Perimenopause

38. **3** The lack of utilization of gonadotropin by the ovaries causes an elevation of gonadotropin level in the blood; ovarian function is diminished; there is little or no follicular activity.
1 There would be an increase in gonadotropin level in the blood, because it is not used by the ovaries. **2** There would be an increase in prostaglandins. **4** There would be a decrease in secretion of progesterone.

Client Need: Health Promotion and Maintenance; **Cognitive Level:** Comprehension; **Nursing Process:** Assessment/Analysis; **Reference:** Ch 23, Perimenopause

NURSING CARE RELATED TO MAJOR DISORDERS AFFECTING WOMEN'S HEALTH

39. 2 Continuous administration of Lupron decreases LH and FSH levels, as well as hormone-dependent tissue.

1 Relaxin is used for dysmenorrhea; it causes relaxation of the symphysis pubis. 3 Estrogen affects the release of pituitary gonadotropins and inhibits ovulation. 4 Ergotrate is used to contract the uterus.

Client Need: Pharmacological and Parenteral Therapies; **Cognitive Level:** Analysis; **Nursing Process:** Assessment/Analysis; **Reference:** Ch 24, Endometriosis, Data Base

40. 1 Rocephin is a broad-spectrum antibiotic and is preferred during pregnancy.

2 Levaquin, although effective for urinary tract infections, is not the drug of choice during pregnancy. 3 Sulfonamides may cause hemolysis in the fetus. 4 Bactrim contains a sulfonamide and is contraindicated during pregnancy.

Client Need: Pharmacological and Parenteral Therapies; **Cognitive Level:** Analysis; **Nursing Process:** Planning/Implementation; **Reference:** Ch 24, Vaginitis, Data Base

41. 2 Persistent pain of any kind usually indicates a problem, and the client should seek medical attention.

1 Although diversion is a method to alter pain perception, the presence of pain requires investigation of possible causes. 3 Although a nutritious diet is beneficial, iron does not prevent the pain of dysmenorrhea. 4 Voluntary relaxation of the abdominal muscles does not cause cessation of dysmenorrhea.

Client Need: Management of Care; **Cognitive Level:** Application; **Integrated Process:** Communication/Documentation; **Nursing Process:** Planning/Implementation; **Reference:** Ch 24, Endometriosis, Data Base

42. 3 Endometriosis is the presence of aberrant endometrial tissue outside the uterus. The tissue responds to ovarian stimulation, bleeds during menstruation, and causes pain.

1, 2 These are not related to endometriosis. 4 Osteoporosis may be a complication of menopause because of decreased estrogen levels; pelvic inflammation usually results from infection.

Client Need: Physiological Adaptation; **Cognitive Level:** Application; **Nursing Process:** Assessment/Analysis; **Reference:** Ch 24, Endometriosis, Data Base

43. 4 The nurse must determine the client's feelings concerning loss of fertility; if she is childless, the client must cope with the knowledge that unless ova are removed and frozen before the surgery,

her genes will not be passed to the next generation, even with in vitro fertilization.

1 Laparoscopic surgery is relatively painless. 2 Since the abdominal cavity is not entered, there is minimal risk of hemorrhage. 3 Although the client may be fearful, the death rate for people undergoing laparoscopic surgery is significantly lower than for those undergoing abdominal surgery.

Client Need: Psychosocial Integrity; **Cognitive Level:** Application; **Integrated Process:** Caring; **Nursing Process:** Assessment/Analysis; **Reference:** Ch 24, Endometriosis, Nursing Care

44. 2 The posterior vaginal wall is pushed forward by the herniation of the rectum; this protrusion increases rectal pressure and causes the bearing-down sensation.

1 A rectocele is not accompanied by abdominal pain. 3 This is the primary symptom of a cystocele. 4 A cystocele is associated with urinary tract infections.

Client Need: Physiological Adaptation; **Cognitive Level:** Application; **Nursing Process:** Assessment/Analysis; **Reference:** Ch 24, Cystocele and/or Rectocele, Data Base

45. 4 As the uterus drops, the vaginal wall relaxes. When the bladder herniates into the vagina (cystocele) and the rectal wall herniates into the vagina (rectocele), the individual feels pressure or pain in the lower back and/or pelvis. When there is an increase in intraabdominal pressure in the presence of a cystocele, incontinence results.

1 These do not indicate cystocele and rectocele; they are common with infection. 2 Sporadic bleeding is not expected with cystocele and rectocele. 3 These are not expected with cystocele and rectocele.

Client Need: Physiological Adaptation; **Cognitive Level:** Application; **Nursing Process:** Assessment/Analysis; **Reference:** Ch 24, Cystocele and/or Rectocele, Data Base

46. 1 The effects of anesthesia and the inflammatory process may impede voiding, leading to urinary retention; an indwelling catheter empties the bladder continuously, preventing retention.

2 Distention causes discomfort; this is avoided by preventing retention. 3 Because the bladder is continually empty when an indwelling catheter is in place, it loses tone; this is an expected side effect. 4 Distention places pressure on the suture line; this is avoided by preventing retention.

Client Need: Reduction of Risk Potential; **Cognitive Level:** Application; **Nursing Process:** Planning/Implementation; **Reference:** Ch 24, Cystocele and/or Rectocele, Nursing Care

47. 2 Immediately after this type of surgery, pain is associated with bearing down; to prevent constipation, the client should be instructed to increase fluid, fiber, and activity.

1 The client is past childbearing age. 3 The anterior colporrhaphy is expected to reduce incontinence. 4 The colporrhaphy involves only the vaginal wall; the rectum should not be involved.

Client Need: Basic Care and Comfort; **Cognitive Level:** Application; **Integrated Process:** Teaching/Learning; **Nursing Process:** Planning/Implementation; **Reference:** Ch 24, Cystocele and/or Rectocele, Nursing Care because of the potential for drying and trauma

48. **4** Ulcerations may occur when the vagina and uterus are displaced and exposed.

1 Edema is not usually the problem. **2** Fistulas are not associated with procidentia. **3** Exudate is not present with procidentia.

Client Need: Physiological Adaptation; **Cognitive Level:** Application; **Nursing Process:** Assessment/Analysis; **Reference:** Ch 24, Prolapsed Uterus, Nursing Care

49. **2** Moist compresses may be indicated to prevent ulcerations.

1 Ambulation would encourage the development of ulcerations. **3** This would be ineffective; gravity alone does not correct the prolapse. **4** This could cause irritation and should be avoided.

Client Need: Reduction of Risk Potential; **Cognitive Level:** Application; **Nursing Process:** Planning/Implementation; **Reference:** Ch 24, Prolapsed Uterus, Nursing Care

50. **2** The Fowler's position facilitates localization of the infection by pooling exudate in the lower pelvis.

1, 3 This position does not use gravity to promote pooling of exudate in the lower pelvis. **4** This position does not use gravity to promote pelvic drainage despite an elevated head.

Client Need: Reduction of Risk Potential; **Cognitive Level:** Application; **Nursing Process:** Planning/Implementation; **Reference:** Ch 24, Pelvic Inflammatory Disease, Nursing Care

51. **2** Erosion of the cervix frequently occurs at the columnosquamous junction, the most common site for carcinoma of the cervix.

1 Metrorrhagia, abnormal bleeding from the uterus, may be present as erosion develops into carcinoma; however, spotting may be the earliest sign and will be eliminated when the cancer is treated. **3** The goal of treatment of the erosion is to prevent cancer. **4** Infection may occur in the cancerous area accompanied by profuse, malodorous discharge; treatment of the erosion is done to prevent cancer, not the secondary infection.

Client Need: Reduction of Risk Potential; **Cognitive Level:** Application; **Integrated Process:** Teaching/Learning; **Nursing Process:** Planning/Implementation; **Reference:** Ch 24, Cancer of the Cervix, Data Base

52. **4** Polyps are usually benign, but a biopsy should be done because epidermoid cancer occasionally arises from cervical polyps.

1 Polyps rarely are the precursors of uterine cancer. **2** Polyps usually are benign. **3** Bleeding may occur whether they are benign or malignant.

Client Need: Physiological Adaptation; **Cognitive Level:** Application; **Nursing Process:** Assessment/Analysis; **Reference:** Ch 24, Uterine Neoplasms, Data Base

53. **4** Any sign of abnormal vaginal bleeding may indicate cervical cancer and must be investigated.

1 Discomfort is a late sign because there are few nerve endings in this area. **2** The cancer must be extensive to cause pressure. **3** Discharge becomes foul-smelling after there is necrosis and infection; it is not an early sign.

Client Need: Reduction of Risk Potential; **Cognitive Level:** Application; **Nursing Process:** Assessment/Analysis; **Reference:** Ch 24, Cancer of the Cervix, Data Base

54. **4** This area, called the transitional zone, frequently is altered by metaplasia or covered by a variant of squamous epithelium. Also, this area often is distorted by eversion and laceration, especially during pregnancy.

1 Extension to lymph nodes is a later stage. **2** Adenocarcinoma, accounting for only 5% of cervical cancers, may be found in the endocervical glands. **3** The cervix is the lower portion of the uterus; the juncture of the uterine body with the cervical canal is called the internal os; erosion most frequently occurs distal to this point, between the external and internal ossa, closer to the external os.

Client Need: Physiological Adaptation; **Cognitive Level:** Comprehension; **Nursing Process:** Assessment/Analysis; **Reference:** Ch 24, Cancer of the Cervix, Data Base

55. **1** When the cancerous cells are completely confined within the epithelium of the cervix without stromal invasion, it is stage 0 and called carcinoma in situ or preinvasive carcinoma.

2 This is Stage IA; there is minimal stromal invasion. **3** This is Stage II and involves the area around the broad ligaments but not the pelvic wall; there is extension to the corpus of the uterus. **4** This is Stage I.

Client Need: Reduction of Risk Potential; **Cognitive Level:** Application; **Integrated Process:** Teaching/Learning; **Nursing Process:** Planning/Implementation; **Reference:** Ch 24, Cancer of the Cervix, Data Base

56. **4** Rare cell adenoma of daughters is associated with mothers who took DES or DES-type drugs during pregnancy.

1 Although DES was prescribed between 1941 and 1971 to reduce the risk for spontaneous abortion in high-risk women; this question will not elicit this information. **2** Use of oral contraceptives is not associated with DES exposure. **3** The client with DES-related problems may exhibit abnormal bleeding or a heavy mucoid vaginal discharge, not lesions on the perineum.

Client Need: Health Promotion and Maintenance; **Cognitive Level:** Application; **Integrated Process:** Communication/Documentation; **Nursing Process:** Assessment/Analysis; **Reference:** Ch 24, Cancer of the Cervix, Data Base

57. **3** The physical trauma of the intervention will result in a blood-tinged vaginal discharge for several days.

1 Vaginal packing will be in place for 2 to 3 days; intercourse and tampon use should be delayed until total healing occurs. **2** Conization does not involve an external incision or dressing. **4** Conization affects only the cervix and does not alter reproductive ability.

Client Need: Physiological Adaptation; **Cognitive Level:** Application; **Integrated Process:** Teaching/Learning; **Nursing Process:** Evaluation/Outcomes; **Reference:** Ch 24, Cancer of the Cervix, Nursing Care

58. **1** An abdominal panhysterectomy in the premenopausal woman produces artificial onset of menopause.

2, 3, 4 Because the uterus was removed, there will be no uterine endometrial proliferation and no desquamation.

Client Need: Reduction of Risk Potential; **Cognitive Level:** Application; **Integrated Process:** Teaching/Learning; **Nursing Process:** Planning/Implementation; **Reference:** Ch 24, Uterine Neoplasms, Data Base

59. **4** A hysterectomy involves only removal of the uterus. The ovaries, which secrete estrogen and progesterone, are not removed. Therefore menopause will not be precipitated but will occur naturally.

1 Surgical menopause is precipitated by the removal of the ovaries, not the uterus. **2** When the ovaries are removed, older women might have less severe symptoms than younger women; however, in this instance the ovaries are not removed. **3** This does not answer the question. The nurse should serve as a resource person.

Client Need: Reduction of Risk Potential; **Cognitive Level:** Application; **Integrated Process:** Teaching/Learning; **Nursing Process:** Planning/Implementation; **Reference:** Ch 24, Uterine Neoplasms, Data Base

60. **4** The nurse cannot prescribe medication. In addition, the use of hormones is controversial and depends on the practitioner's beliefs and the client's needs.

1, 3 This is advice the nurse is not legally licensed to provide. **2** This is an evasive response; it does not answer the client's question.

Client Need: Management of Care; **Cognitive Level:** Application; **Integrated Process:** Communication/Documentation; **Nursing Process:** Planning/Implementation; **Reference:** Ch 24, Uterine Neoplasms, Data Base

61. **1** During an abdominal hysterectomy, the urinary bladder may be nicked.

2 The client is not likely to develop an infection with bleeding so soon. **3** The uterus is removed with a hysterectomy; therefore there would be no lochia. **4** Bleeding would be present from other sites, such as the incision, as well as in the urinary bag.

Client Need: Physiological Adaptation; **Cognitive Level:** Application; **Integrated Process:** Teaching/Learning; **Nursing Process:** Evaluation/Outcomes; **Reference:** Ch 24, Uterine Neoplasms, Nursing Care

62. **1** Doxorubicin (Adriamycin) is a chemotherapeutic agent classified as an antibiotic and antineoplastic. It achieves its therapeutic effect by inhibiting the synthesis of DNA, thus blocking protein synthesis and cell division.

2, 3, 4 This is not a physiologic action of Adriamycin.

Client Need: Pharmacological and Parenteral Therapies; **Cognitive Level:** Comprehension; **Nursing Process:** Planning/Implementation; **Reference:** Ch 24, Cancer of the Breast, Data Base

63. **3** Estrogen receptor protein–positive tumors have a more dramatic response to hormonal therapies that reduce estrogen.

1 Estrogen contributes to tumor growth; supplements are not indicated. **2** This does not influence breast reconstruction. **4** ERP-positive is unrelated to metastasis.

Client Need: Pharmacological and Parenteral Therapies; **Cognitive Level:** Application; **Integrated Process:** Teaching/Learning; **Nursing Process:** Planning/Implementation; **Reference:** Ch 24, Cancer of the Breast, Data Base

64. **3** Postoperatively the arm on the operated side is elevated on pillows, with the hand higher than the arm to prevent muscle strain and edema.

1 Total immobilization should be avoided, and adduction may put undue pressure on the operative site. **2** Although the arm is slightly abducted, sandbags are not used because complete immobility should be prevented. **4** This would impair venous return and increase edema.

Client Need: Reduction of Risk Potential; **Cognitive Level:** Application; **Nursing Process:** Planning/Implementation; **Reference:** Ch 24, Cancer of the Breast, Nursing Care

65. **4** Deep breathing aids in expanding lung tissue and prevents stasis of pulmonary secretions.

1 This may result in atelectasis and retained respiratory secretions. **2** This only states a fact and provides no option to meet the need to limit pain or the need to prevent atelectasis. **3** Although empathetic, delay could compromise the client's respiratory status.

Client Need: Reduction of Risk Potential; **Cognitive Level:** Application; **Integrated Process:** Caring; **Nursing Process:** Planning/Implementation; **Reference:** Ch 24, Cancer of the Breast, Nursing Care

66. **4** This defect in bone matrix formation weakens the bones, making them unable to withstand usual functional stresses.

1 Avascular necrosis is death of bone tissue that results from reduced circulation to bone. **2** Pathologic fractures can result from osteoporosis. **3** Hyperplasia of osteoblasts is not related to osteoporosis. This occurs during bone healing.

Client Need: Physiological Adaptation; **Cognitive Level:** Comprehension; **Integrated Process:** Teaching/Learning; **Nursing Process:** Planning/Implementation; **Reference:** Ch 24, Osteoporosis, Data Base

67. **1** This regimen limits bone demineralization and reduces bone pain, which promote increased activity.

2 This is unrelated to osteoporosis; it would be an expected outcome if the client were receiving calcium for hypocalcemia. **3** This is unrelated to osteoporosis or its therapy. **4** This is unrelated to osteoporosis; it would be expected if the client were receiving vitamin C for capillary fragility.

Client Need: Physiological Adaptation; **Cognitive Level:** Application; **Nursing Process:** Evaluation/Outcomes; **Reference:** Ch 24, Osteoporosis, Nursing Care

68. 3 Prolonged immobility results in bone demineralization because there is decreased bone production by osteoblasts and increased resorption by osteoclasts.
1 Estrogen helps prevent bone demineralization.
2 Hypoparathyroidism decreases mobilization of calcium from the bones, and thus serum calcium level is lowered. 4 Decreased calcium intake or absorption may precipitate osteoporosis.
Client Need: Physiological Adaptation; Cognitive Level: Application; Nursing Process: Assessment/Analysis; Reference: Ch 24, Osteoporosis, Data Base

69. 2 Pathologic fractures occur as a result of minimal injury to an already weakened bone; osteoporosis is one cause of this weakening.
1 Fatigue fractures occur when muscles are so fatigued that they no longer act as shock absorbers to protect the bone, a condition not related to osteoporosis. 3 Greenstick fractures occur in young children whose long bones are not yet completely mineralized. 4 Compound fractures refer to the protrusion of the bone fragments through the skin; this is not related to osteoporosis.
Client Need: Reduction of Risk Potential; Cognitive Level: Application; Nursing Process: Planning/Implementation; Reference: Ch 24, Osteoporosis, Data Base

70. 3 Turnip greens are high in calcium and vitamins.
1 High levels of nitrogen from protein breakdown may increase the release of calcium from bone to serve as a buffer of the nitrogen. 2 Soft drinks that are high in phosphorus may interfere with calcium absorption from the GI tract. 4 Enriched grains that are high in phosphorus may interfere with calcium absorption from the GI tract.
Client Need: Basic Care and Comfort; Cognitive Level: Analysis; Integrated Process: Teaching/Learning; Nursing Process: Evaluation/Outcomes; Reference: Ch 24, Osteoporosis, Nursing Care

71. 3 A diet high in calcium and exercise, which helps deposit calcium into bone, are the most important factors in limiting the extent of osteoporosis.
1 Weight gain should be discouraged to limit stress on the client's bones. 2 Increased, not decreased, urine calcium should be monitored because it reflects demineralization of bone. 4 Opioids usually are not prescribed; other analgesics are used for pain.
Client Need: Health Promotion and Maintenance; Cognitive Level: Application; Integrated Process: Teaching/Learning; Nursing Process: Planning/Implementation; Reference: Ch 24, Osteoporosis, Nursing Care

72. 1 ☐ Weight loss should be slow and reasonable; restricting calories promotes production of the hormone leptin, which stimulates bone loss.
2 ☒ This is the recommended daily intake of calcium for a 50-year-old adult.
3 ☐ 800 international units, not 1000 mg, of vitamin D are the recommended daily intake for a 50-year-old adult.
4 ☒ High-impact exercises (such as tennis, running, aerobics, and dancing) are best for building bone mass.
5 ☐ This may promote overall health and vigor; it will not increase the strength or mass of bone.
Client Need: Health Promotion and Maintenance; Cognitive Level: Analysis; Integrated Process: Teaching/Learning; Nursing Process: Evaluation/Outcomes; Reference: Ch 24, Osteoporosis, Nursing Care

73. 4 Teriparatide is a 34–amino acid polypeptide that represents the biologically active part of human parathyroid hormone; it enhances bone microarchitecture and increases bone mass and strength.
1 Supplemental intake of vitamin A should not exceed normal recommended daily requirements; too much vitamin A has been associated with bone loss and an elevated rate of fractures. 2 Alendronate sodium (Fosamax), a regulator of bone metabolism, not teriparatide (Forteo), inhibits osteoclast-mediated bone resorption, minimizing loss of bone density. 3 Sunscreen may be used but only after exposure to the sun for 5 to 20 minutes so that vitamin D can be converted in the skin; vitamin D helps the body absorb calcium.
Client Need: Pharmacological and Parenteral Therapies; Cognitive Level: Comprehension; Nursing Process: Assessment/Analysis; Reference: Ch 24, Osteoporosis, Data Base

74. 3 Although not 100% effective, a condom is the best protection against gonorrhea in a sexually active person.
1 Douching has no proven protective effect against sexually transmitted infections; excessive douching can alter the natural environment of the vagina and may even promote an ascending infection. 2 Although this is the best way to prevent a sexually transmitted infection, it is not the most realistic response for a sexually active person. Once people become sexually active, they usually remain sexually active.
4 Spermicidal creams do not have a protective effect against sexually transmitted infections; spermicides kill sperm and limit the risk for pregnancy.
Client Need: Health Promotion and Maintenance; Cognitive Level: Application; Integrated Process: Teaching/Learning; Nursing Process: Evaluation/Outcomes; Reference: Ch 24, Vaginitis, Nursing Care

75. 4 Metronidazole (Flagyl) is a potent amebicide. It is extremely effective in eradicating the protozoan *Trichomonas vaginalis*.
1 Penicillin is administered for its effect on bacterial, not protozoal, infections. 2 This is a local antiinfective that is applied topically; it may cause discoloration of the skin; it is particularly effective against *Candida albicans*. 3 This is an antifungal for infections caused by *Candida albicans*.
Client Need: Pharmacological and Parenteral Therapies; Cognitive Level: Analysis; Nursing Process: Planning/Implementation; Reference: Ch 24, Vaginitis, Data Base

76. 3 This is the anatomic direction of the vaginal tract in the back-lying position.

1, 2, 4 The vaginal tract may be injured when the douche nozzle is not directed with consideration of normal anatomy.

Client Need: Pharmacological and Parenteral Therapies; **Cognitive Level:** Application; **Integrated Process:** Teaching/Learning; **Nursing Process:** Planning/Implementation; **Reference:** Ch 24, Vaginitis, Nursing Care

NURSING CARE OF WOMEN DURING UNCOMPLICATED PREGNANCY, LABOR, CHILDBIRTH, AND THE POSTPARTUM PERIOD

77. 2 Expected periods of marked change and adjustment are called developmental crises and predispose the woman to a situational crisis.

1 These are transient; they are similar to previous mood changes and should not affect the mother's ability to cope. **3** These occur throughout the life cycle of a mature woman and should not now be classified as a crisis. **4** It becomes a crisis only if the husband withdraws support.

Client Need: Psychosocial Integrity; **Cognitive Level:** Comprehension; **Nursing Process:** Assessment/Analysis; **Reference:** Ch 25, Prenatal Period: Physical, Physiologic, and Emotional Changes During Pregnancy

78. 3 NSAIDs, as well as other OCT drugs taken during pregnancy, may cause problems in the newborn during the neonatal period.

1 This is not a cause for concern; if membranes ruptured more than 24 hours before birth, infection may ensue. **2** Hemophilia affects males; this fetus is known to be a female; the female may be a carrier but would not have hemophilia. **4** A history of a placenta previa in an earlier pregnancy would not have implications for this newborn.

Client Need: Pharmacological and Parenteral Therapies; **Cognitive Level:** Analysis; **Nursing Process:** Assessment/Analysis; **Reference:** Ch 25, Prenatal Period, Nursing Care

79. 4 This is a genetic disorder transmitted as an autosomal recessive trait that occurs primarily among Ashkenazi Jews.

1, 2, 3 This disease does not have a higher prevalence in the Jewish population.

Client Need: Reduction of Risk Potential; **Cognitive Level:** Analysis; **Integrated Process:** Teaching/Learning; **Nursing Process:** Planning/Implementation; **Reference:** Ch 25, Prenatal Period: Physical, Physiologic, and Emotional Changes During Pregnancy

80. 4 This is the result of a reduced chromosome number, from 46 to 23, readying the sex cells for fertilization.

1 They each have one set of chromosomes (23). **2** There are 23 pairs of chromosomes in the nuclei. **3** The diploid number (46 chromosomes) is reached when fertilization occurs.

Client Need: Health Promotion and Maintenance; **Cognitive Level:** Knowledge; **Integrated Process:** Teaching/Learning; **Nursing Process:** Planning/Implementation; **Reference:** Ch 25, Prenatal Period, Development of the Embryo/Fetus

81. 2 During the eighth week of pregnancy the organ systems and other structures are developed to the extent that they take the human form; at this time the embryo becomes a fetus and remains so until birth.

1 The embryo can be visualized on a sonogram before it becomes a fetus. **3** At this time the developing cells are called an embryo. **4** At the time of implantation the group of developing cells is called a blastocyst.

Client Need: Health Promotion and Maintenance; **Cognitive Level:** Comprehension; **Integrated Process:** Teaching/Learning; **Nursing Process:** Planning/Implementation; **Reference:** Ch 25, Prenatal Period, Development of the Embryo/Fetus

82. 3 The pressure of the enlarging fetus causes the upward displacement of the diaphragm, which results in thoracic breathing; this limits the descent of the diaphragm on inspiration.

1 The lower rib cage expands. **2** There is no change in pulmonary function during pregnancy unless there is a preexisting problem. **4** The thoracic cage enlarges; it does not rise.

Client Need: Health Promotion and Maintenance; **Cognitive Level:** Application; **Integrated Process:** Teaching/Learning; **Nursing Process:** Planning/Implementation; **Reference:** Ch 25, Prenatal Period: Physical, Physiologic, and Emotional Changes During Pregnancy

83. 3 By this time the fetus and placenta have grown, expanding the size of the uterus. The extended uterus expands into the abdominal cavity.

1 The uterus is still within the pelvic area. **2** The uterus is still within the pelvic area. **4** The uterus has already risen out of the pelvis and is expanding further into the abdominal area.

Client Need: Health Promotion and Maintenance; **Cognitive Level:** Knowledge; **Nursing Process:** Assessment/Analysis; **Reference:** Ch 25, Prenatal Period: Physical, Physiologic, and Emotional Changes During Pregnancy

84. 1, 4, 3, 2

____1____ Sickle cell screening, particularly for black women, should be done on the initial visit.

____4____ Alpha-fetoprotein (AFP) testing for neural tube defects should be done between 14 and 16 weeks.

____3____ Serum glucose testing for gestational diabetes mellitus should be done between 26 and 28 weeks.

____2____ Group beta streptococcus culture should be done between 36 and 38 weeks.

Client Need: Reduction of Risk Potential; **Cognitive Level:** Analysis; **Nursing Process:** Assessment/Analysis; **Reference:** Ch 25, Prenatal Period: Physical, Physiologic, and Emotional Changes During Pregnancy

85. 2 This is the period in which the fetus stores deposits of fat.

1 The first trimester is the period of organogenesis, when cells differentiate into major organ systems. **3** Growth is occurring, but fat deposition does not

occur in this period. **4** This is the period of the blastocyst, when initial cell division takes place.
Client Need: Health Promotion and Maintenance; **Cognitive Level:** Knowledge; **Nursing Process:** Assessment/Analysis; **Reference:** Ch 25, Prenatal Period, Development of the Embryo/Fetus

86. **1** When placental formation is complete, around the 12th week of pregnancy, it produces progesterone and estrogen.
2 This is not the chief source of progesterone and estrogen; only small amounts are secreted. **3** The corpus luteum supplies the estrogen and progesterone needed to sustain the pregnancy until the placenta is ready to take over. **4** Neither estrogen nor progesterone is secreted by the anterior pituitary gland.
Client Need: Health Promotion and Maintenance; **Cognitive Level:** Comprehension; **Nursing Process:** Assessment/Analysis; **Reference:** Ch 25, Prenatal Period: Physical, Physiologic, and Emotional Changes During Pregnancy

87. **1** The umbilical vein carries blood high in O_2 concentration from the placenta and empties it into the fetal vena cava by way of the ductus venosus.
2 The blood in the umbilical artery is deoxygenated fetal blood that flows back to the placenta. **3** The pulmonary artery carries only a small amount of oxygenated blood, since the lungs are not functioning. **4** This contains a mixture of arterial and venous blood.
Client Need: Health Promotion and Maintenance; **Cognitive Level:** Comprehension; **Nursing Process:** Assessment/Analysis; **Reference:** Ch 25, Prenatal Period, Development of the Embryo/Fetus

88. **2** April 29, 2009. Nägele's rule is an indirect, noninvasive method for estimating the date of birth: EDB = (LMP + 1 year) − 3 months + 7 days.
1 This is beyond the expected date of birth. **3, 4** This is before the expected date of birth.
Client Need: Health Promotion and Maintenance; **Cognitive Level:** Application; **Nursing Process:** Assessment/Analysis; **Reference:** Ch 25, Prenatal Period: Physical, Physiologic, and Emotional Changes During Pregnancy

89. **4** Increasing the client's knowledge of physical and psychologic changes resulting from pregnancy prepares the client for expected changes as pregnancy continues; it is most effective when taught during the first trimester.
1 This is too early; this should be done in the last trimester. **2** The client should be alerted to danger signs and symptoms; however, primary teaching is directed toward increasing her knowledge of expected physiologic changes. **3** Concerns about role transition to parenthood should be addressed in the third trimester.
Client Need: Health Promotion and Maintenance; **Cognitive Level:** Application; **Integrated Process:** Teaching/Learning; **Nursing Process:** Assessment/Analysis; **Reference:** Ch 25,

Prenatal Period: Physical, Physiologic, and Emotional Changes During Pregnancy

90. **3** Crown to rump measurement is used to determine the age of the embryo until 11 weeks.
1 Occipital frontal diameter is not an ultrasound measurement used at term. **2** Biparietal diameter at term would be approximately 9.8 cm. **4** Diagonal conjugate is not used as an ultrasound measurement; it is the estimated size of the maternal pelvic outlet; the actual size, as it relates to fetal size, is best determined with ultrasonography.
Client Need: Health Promotion and Maintenance; **Cognitive Level:** Application; **Nursing Process:** Assessment/Analysis; **Reference:** Ch 25, Prenatal Period: Physical, Physiologic, and Emotional Changes During Pregnancy

91. **3** The blood volume increases by approximately 50% during pregnancy. Peak blood volume occurs between 30 and 34 weeks' gestation.
1 WBC values remain stable during the antepartum period. **2** The hematocrit decreases as a result of hemodilution. **4** The sedimentation rate increases because of a decrease in plasma proteins.
Client Need: Health Promotion and Maintenance; **Cognitive Level:** Comprehension; **Nursing Process:** Assessment/Analysis; **Reference:** Ch 25, Prenatal Period: Physical, Physiologic, and Emotional Changes During Pregnancy

92. **4** A purplish color results from the increased vascularity and blood vessel engorgement of the vagina.
1 This is increased vascularity and cervical softening. **2** This is softening of the lower uterine segment. **3** This is softening of the cervix.
Client Need: Health Promotion and Maintenance; **Cognitive Level:** Analysis; **Nursing Process:** Assessment/Analysis; **Reference:** Ch 25, Prenatal Period: Physical, Physiologic, and Emotional Changes During Pregnancy

93. **2** There is a 30% to 50% increase in maternal plasma volume at the end of the first trimester, leading to a decrease in the concentrations of hemoglobin and erythrocytes.
1 Dietary intake of iron is unrelated to the development of physiologic anemia of pregnancy. **3** Erythropoiesis is increased after the first trimester. **4** Detoxification demands are unchanged during pregnancy.
Client Need: Health Promotion and Maintenance; **Cognitive Level:** Comprehension; **Integrated Process:** Teaching/Learning; **Nursing Process:** Planning/Implementation; **Reference:** Ch 25, Prenatal Period: Physical, Physiologic, and Emotional Changes During Pregnancy

94. **3** Before health teaching is instituted, the nurse should ascertain the client's past experiences; they will influence the teaching plan.
1 This answer does not give the client a chance to discuss her feelings about the examination. **2** This response presupposes that the client is fearful and does not address the client's question. **4** This answer does not give the client a chance to discuss her feelings about the examination; the nurse is assuming that the client's concerns are related to discomfort.

Client Need: Health Promotion and Maintenance; **Cognitive Level:** Analysis; **Integrated Process:** Caring; **Nursing Process:** Planning/Implementation; **Reference:** Ch 25, Prenatal Period, Nursing Care

95. 3 The acronym GTPAL reflects **G,** gravidity; **T, term** birth; **P, p**reterm births; **A, a**bortions; and **L, l**iving children; G5 T2 P1 A1 L4 indicates that there were 5 pregnancies; 2 term births; twins count as 1 preterm birth; 1 abortion; 4 living children.

1 G4 T3 P2 A1 L4: this indicates that there were 4, not 5, pregnancies; 3, not 2, term births; twins count as 1, not 2, preterm birth; 1 abortion; 4 living children. 2 G5 T2 P2 A1 L4: this indicates that there were 5 pregnancies; 2 term births; twins count as 1, not 2, preterm birth; 1 abortion; 4 living children. 4 G4 T3 P1 A1 L4: this indicates that there were 4, not 5, pregnancies; 3, not 2, term births; twins count as 1 preterm birth; 1 abortion; 4 living children.

Client Need: Health Promotion and Maintenance; **Cognitive Level:** Analysis; **Integrated Process:** Communication/Documentation; **Nursing Process:** Assessment/Analysis; **Reference:** Ch 25, Prenatal Period, Nursing Care

96. 4 This is an expected cardiopulmonary adaptation during pregnancy caused by an increased ventricular rate and elevated diaphragm.

1, 2, 3 This is pathologic, a sign of impending cardiac decompensation.

Client Need: Health Promotion and Maintenance; **Cognitive Level:** Application; **Nursing Process:** Assessment/Analysis; **Reference:** Ch 25, Prenatal Period: Physical, Physiologic, and Emotional Changes During Pregnancy

97. 4 Chorionic gonadotropin, secreted in large amounts by the placenta during gestation, and the metabolic changes associated with pregnancy can precipitate nausea and vomiting in early pregnancy.

1 Estrogen is elevated throughout pregnancy; usually the symptoms of morning sickness disappear after the first trimester. 2 Progesterone is elevated throughout pregnancy; usually the symptoms of morning sickness disappear after the first trimester. 3 The luteinizing hormone is present only during ovulation.

Client Need: Health Promotion and Maintenance; **Cognitive Level:** Analysis; **Nursing Process:** Assessment/Analysis; **Reference:** Ch 25, Prenatal Period: Physical, Physiologic, and Emotional Changes During Pregnancy

98. 2 Sodium is needed to maintain body water balance; sodium requirements increase slightly during pregnancy to accommodate the increased blood volume; a healthy pregnant woman should not limit her sodium intake.

1 This could be detrimental to the client's health. 3 Sodium, although essential, is not a nutrient; it is a mineral. 4 Although this statement is correct, it does not explain why sodium intake is not restricted during pregnancy.

Client Need: Basic Care and Comfort; **Cognitive Level:** Application; **Integrated Process:** Teaching/Learning; **Nursing Process:** Planning/Implementation; **Reference:** Ch 25, Prenatal Period: Physical, Physiologic, and Emotional Changes During Pregnancy

99. 1 Maintaining the sitting position for prolonged periods may constrict the vessels of the legs, particularly in the popliteal spaces, as well as diminish venous return. Walking contracts the muscles of the legs, which applies gentle pressure to the veins in the legs, thus promoting venous return.

2 A better means of improving circulation would be to walk about several times each morning and afternoon; she could also keep her legs elevated while sitting at her desk. **3** If the client is feeling well, there are no contraindications to working throughout her pregnancy. **4** Adequate nourishment can be obtained during mealtimes; the client does not require extra nutrition breaks.

Client Need: Health Promotion and Maintenance; **Cognitive Level:** Application; **Integrated Process:** Teaching/Learning; **Nursing Process:** Planning/Implementation; **Reference:** Ch 25, Prenatal Period, Nursing Care

100. 4 The nurse should become informed about the cultural eating patterns of clients so that foods containing the essential nutrients that are part of these dietary patterns will be included in the diet.

1 Fluid retention is only one component of weight gain; growth of the fetus, placenta, breasts, etc. also contribute to weight gain. 2 Calories and nutrients are increased during pregnancy. 3 Pregnancy diets are not specific; they are composed of the essential nutrients.

Client Need: Basic Care and Comfort; **Cognitive Level:** Analysis; **Integrated Process:** Teaching/Learning; **Nursing Process:** Planning/Implementation; **Reference:** Ch 25, Prenatal Period, Nursing Care

101. 2 By taking a diet history, the nurse can assess the woman's level of nutritional knowledge and gain clues for appropriate methods of counseling.

1 A "regular" diet does not indicate that the client is eating a nutritious diet; also, the client will need increased protein and calories. 3 These foods may be too expensive and different from her usual choices, leading to noncompliance. 4 If the client's diet includes highly seasoned foods and they are well tolerated, they need not be excluded.

Client Need: Basic Care and Comfort; **Cognitive Level:** Application; **Integrated Process:** Teaching/Learning; **Nursing Process:** Planning/Implementation; **Reference:** Ch 25, Prenatal Period, Nursing Care

102. 2 The uterus and bladder occupy the pelvic cavity and lie closely together; as the uterus enlarges with the growing fetus, it impinges on the space occupied by the bladder and thereby diminishes bladder capacity.

1 Atony would not cause frequency; more likely, it would lead to retention. 3 This would lead to incontinence rather than frequency. 4 This is an unlikely occurrence; the uterus would not impinge on that area.

Client Need: Basic Care and Comfort; **Cognitive Level:** Application; **Integrated Process:** Teaching/Learning;

Nursing Process: Planning/Implementation; **Reference:** Ch 25, Prenatal Period: Physical, Physiologic, and Emotional Changes During Pregnancy

103. 1 ☐ Control is a primary concern of the batterer, so it would be highly unlikely for a batterer to leave the battered woman alone with the care provider.

    2 ☒ It is common for the batterer to control the conversation by answering for the woman.

    3 ☒ During pregnancy, batterers may focus their anger at the pregnancy itself and focus their assaults on the breasts, buttocks, and abdomen.

    4 ☒ Women who are battered are at risk for stress illness such as gastrointestinal distress and chest pain. They are also more likely to suffer from frequent headaches and depression.

Client Need: Health Promotion and Maintenance; **Cognitive Level:** Analysis; **Nursing Process:** Assessment/Analysis; **Reference:** Ch 25, Prenatal Period, Nursing Care

104. 2 A titer of 1:2 is inadequate immunization. A titer of 1:8 is considered immune. Rubella immunization protects the fetuses of future pregnancies from significant birth defects caused by a rubella infection.

    1 A RhoGAM injection is not needed because the infant also has negative Rh factor. 3 There is no evidence the mother is in need of a transfusion. These laboratory results are borderline for pregnancy but were taken during the prenatal period and do not represent the woman's current status. 4 This is an expected glucose level for a neonate.

Client Need: Safety and Infection Control; **Cognitive Level:** Analysis; **Nursing Process:** Planning/Implementation; **Reference:** Ch 25, Prenatal Period: Physical, Physiologic, and Emotional Changes During Pregnancy

105. 1 Nausea and vomiting in the morning occur in almost 50% of all pregnancies. Eating dry crackers before getting out of bed in the morning is a simple remedy that may provide relief.

    2 Increasing fat intake does not relieve the nausea. 3 Two small meals and a snack at noon would not meet the nutritional needs of a pregnant woman, nor would it relieve nausea. Some women find that eating five or six small meals daily instead of three large ones is helpful. 4 This is not helpful; separating fluids from solids at mealtime is more advisable.

Client Need: Basic Care and Comfort; **Cognitive Level:** Application; **Integrated Process:** Teaching/Learning; **Nursing Process:** Planning/Implementation; **Reference:** Ch 25, Prenatal Period: Physical, Physiologic, and Emotional Changes During Pregnancy

106. 1 Nausea and vomiting of pregnancy can be relieved with small snacks of protein before bedtime to slow digestion.

    2 An antacid may affect electrolyte balance; also this will not help morning sickness. 3 This is contraindicated, because both fetus and mother need nourishment. 4 Medications in the first trimester are contraindicated because this is the period of organogenesis, and congenital anomalies could result.

Client Need: Basic Care and Comfort; **Cognitive Level:** Application; **Integrated Process:** Teaching/Learning; **Nursing Process:** Planning/Implementation; **Reference:** Ch 25, Prenatal Period: Physical, Physiologic, and Emotional Changes During Pregnancy

107. 2 This is the recommended caloric increase for adult women to meet the increased metabolic demands of pregnancy.

    1, 4 This would not meet the metabolic demands of pregnancy and may result in weight reduction. 3 This is the recommended caloric increase for breastfeeding mothers.

Client Need: Basic Care and Comfort; **Cognitive Level:** Knowledge; **Integrated Process:** Teaching/Learning; **Nursing Process:** Planning/Implementation; **Reference:** Ch 25, Prenatal Period: Physical, Physiologic, and Emotional Changes During Pregnancy

108. 1 The average weight gain during pregnancy is 25 to 35 lb (11.9 to 15.8 kg); of this, the fetus accounts for 7 to 8 lb (3.18 to 3.6 kg), or approximately 30% of weight gain.

    2 Fluid retention accounts for about 20% to 25% of weight gain. 3 Metabolic alterations do not cause a weight gain. 4 Increased blood volume accounts for about 12% to 16% of weight gain.

Client Need: Health Promotion and Maintenance; **Cognitive Level:** Application; **Integrated Process:** Teaching/Learning; **Nursing Process:** Planning/Implementation; **Reference:** Ch 25, Prenatal Period: Physical, Physiologic, and Emotional Changes During Pregnancy

109. 2 Because of changes in the hormone levels, morning sickness seldom persists beyond the first trimester.

    1, 3 It usually ends at the end of the third month, when the chorionic gonadotropin level falls. 4 It is still present at this time; it is related to the high level of chorionic gonadotropin.

Client Need: Basic Care and Comfort; **Cognitive Level:** Application; **Integrated Process:** Teaching/Learning; **Nursing Process:** Planning/Implementation; **Reference:** Ch 25, Prenatal Period: Physical, Physiologic, and Emotional Changes During Pregnancy

110. 4 This allows the client to discuss her feelings and participate in her care.

    1 The client has already told the nurse how she feels. 2 This cuts off communication; this also may cause the client to worry that something is seriously wrong. 3 This statement cuts off communication and does not address the totality of the client's concern.

Client Need: Basic Care and Comfort; **Cognitive Level:** Analysis; **Integrated Process:** Caring; Communication/Documentation; **Nursing Process:** Planning/Implementation; **Reference:** Ch 25, Prenatal Period: Physical, Physiologic, and Emotional Changes During Pregnancy

111. 1 When an Rh-negative mother carries an Rh-positive fetus there is a risk for maternal antibodies against Rh-positive blood; antibodies cross the placenta and destroy the fetal RBCs.

    2 Determination of the lecithin/sphingomyelin ratio, not the Rh factor, may provide information about

the risk for developing RDS. An indirect Coombs' test will determine whether the mother has antibodies against Rh-positive blood. **3** Testing for the Rh factor will not provide information about protein metabolism deficiency. **4** Physiologic bilirubinemia is a common occurrence in newborns; it is not associated with the Rh factor.
Client Need: Reduction of Risk Potential; **Cognitive Level:** Analysis; **Integrated Process:** Teaching/Learning; **Nursing Process:** Planning/Implementation; **Reference:** Ch 25, Prenatal Period: Physical, Physiologic, and Emotional Changes During Pregnancy

112. **2** The first trimester is the period when all major embryonic organs are forming; drugs, alcohol, and tobacco may cause major defects.
1 Cutting down is insufficient; these teratogens should be eliminated. **3** Even 1 oz of alcohol is considered harmful; baby aspirin is now given to some women who are considered at risk for pregnancy-induced hypertension. **4** Drugs, unless absolutely necessary, should be avoided throughout pregnancy; but the first trimester is most significant.
Client Need: Health Promotion and Maintenance; **Cognitive Level:** Application; **Integrated Process:** Teaching/Learning; **Nursing Process:** Planning/Implementation; **Reference:** Ch 25, Prenatal Period, Nursing Care

113. **4** With spontaneous or stimulated activity, the FHR is usually between 110 and 160 beats/min. This is to be expected, and the mother should be made aware of this.
1 The heart rate for a fetus is 110 to 160 beats/min, not twice the mother's heart rate. **2** This implies that the heart rate is too rapid; this is misinformation that may cause more concerns. **3** The heart rate is rapid to accommodate the metabolic, not nutritional, needs of the fetus.
Client Need: Reduction of Risk Potential; **Cognitive Level:** Application; **Integrated Process:** Teaching/Learning; **Nursing Process:** Planning/Implementation; **Reference:** Ch 25, Prenatal Period, Development of the Embryo/Fetus

114. **2** Increased estrogen production during pregnancy causes hyperplasia of the vaginal mucosa, which leads to increased production of mucus by the endocervical glands. The mucus contains exfoliated epithelial cells.
1 Increased metabolism leads to systemic changes but does not increase vaginal discharge. **3** The functioning of the Bartholin glands, which lubricate the vagina during intercourse, remains unchanged during pregnancy. **4** There is no additional supply of sodium chloride to the vaginal cells during pregnancy.
Client Need: Health Promotion and Maintenance; **Cognitive Level:** Application; **Integrated Process:** Teaching/Learning; **Nursing Process:** Planning/Implementation; **Reference:** Ch 25, Prenatal Period: Physical, Physiologic, and Emotional Changes During Pregnancy

115. **2** Dependent edema is common during the last trimester; there is no need to lower the salt

content of the client's diet. Teaching should be based on optimum nutrition as well as the caloric content of the diet.
1 Immediate planning based on the nurse's knowledge of dietary needs is sufficient. **3** Not all preferences can be included; the diet should contain normal sodium, high protein, and sufficient calories. **4** Unless the nurse thought there was a need for medical intervention, the nurse could supervise prenatal care.
Client Need: Basic Care and Comfort; **Cognitive Level:** Application; **Integrated Process:** Teaching/Learning; **Nursing Process:** Planning/Implementation; **Reference:** Ch 25, Prenatal Period: Physical, Physiologic, and Emotional Changes During Pregnancy

116. **2** Fluids, proteins, and sodium should not be restricted, for they are necessary to the well-being of the mother and fetus; elevation of the extremities several times daily is recommended to decrease the edema.
1 Sodium and fluid intake should not be limited. **3** Sodium intake should not be limited. **4** Diuretics can be harmful and are not used during a healthy pregnancy.
Client Need: Basic Care and Comfort; **Cognitive Level:** Application; **Integrated Process:** Teaching/Learning; **Nursing Process:** Planning/Implementation; **Reference:** Ch 25, Prenatal Period: Physical, Physiologic, and Emotional Changes During Pregnancy

117. **3** The alpha-fetoprotein test can detect neural tube defects, Down syndrome, and other congenital anomalies. It is a screening test that affords a tentative diagnosis; confirmation requires more definitive testing.
1, 2, 4 These are not detected by the alpha-fetoprotein test.
Client Need: Reduction of Risk Potential; **Cognitive Level:** Comprehension; **Integrated Process:** Teaching/Learning; **Nursing Process:** Planning/Implementation; **Reference:** Ch 25, Prenatal Period: Physical, Physiologic, and Emotional Changes During Pregnancy

118. **4** The nonstress test evaluates the response of the fetus to movement and activity. A reactive test indicates that the fetus is healthy.
1 This is unlikely because it is a noninvasive test. **2** This test will not influence the activity of the fetus because no exogenous stimulus is used. **3** No injections of any kind are used during a nonstress test; this test involves only the use of a fetal monitor to record the fetal heart rate during periods of activity.
Client Need: Reduction of Risk Potential; **Cognitive Level:** Application; **Integrated Process:** Teaching/Learning; **Nursing Process:** Evaluation/Outcomes; **Reference:** Ch 25, Prenatal Period, Nursing Care

119. **2** A full bladder is required for effective visualization of the uterus in early pregnancy.
1 The procedure is not done via the colon and will not cause fecal contamination. **3** This procedure is noninvasive; it cannot irritate the uterus and initiate

labor. **4** For this noninvasive procedure the GI tract is not involved.

Client Need: Reduction of Risk Potential; **Cognitive Level:** Application; **Integrated Process:** Teaching/Learning; **Nursing Process:** Planning/Implementation; **Reference:** Ch 25, Prenatal Period: Physical, Physiologic, and Emotional Changes During Pregnancy

120. **3** When the membranes rupture, the potential for infection is increased, and when the contractions are 5 to 8 minutes apart, they are usually of sufficient force to warrant professional supervision.

1 These may be early signs of labor or signs of posterior fetal position; it is too early to notify the primary caregiver. **2, 4** This is too early; the client should be with her family and moving about at home.

Client Need: Health Promotion and Maintenance; **Cognitive Level:** Analysis; **Integrated Process:** Teaching/Learning; **Nursing Process:** Planning/Implementation; **Reference:** Ch 25, Prenatal Period, Nursing Care

121. **2** The supine position results in pressure on the vena cava by the gravid uterus; this impedes venous return, causing hypotension and decreased systemic perfusion.

1 This may be partially true, but more significantly, it may cause hypotension. **3** It can lead to hypotension, not hypertension. **4** Even if true, this is not the reason for discouraging the supine position.

Client Need: Physiological Adaptation; **Cognitive Level:** Application; **Integrated Process:** Teaching/Learning; **Nursing Process:** Planning/Implementation; **Reference:** Ch 25, Prenatal Period: Physical, Physiologic, and Emotional Changes During Pregnancy

122. **4** Alpha-fetoprotein in amniotic fluid is elevated in the presence of a neural tube defect.

1 Lung maturity cannot be determined until after 35 weeks' gestation. **2** Diabetes cannot be detected. **3** Cardiac disorders cannot be detected via an amniocentesis.

Client Need: Reduction of Risk Potential; **Cognitive Level:** Knowledge; **Nursing Process:** Assessment/Analysis; **Reference:** Ch 25, Prenatal Period: Physical, Physiologic, and Emotional Changes During Pregnancy

123. **4** The leg cramps may be related to low calcium intake; cheese and broccoli both have high calcium content.

1, 2, 3 These are inadequate sources of calcium.

Client Need: Basic Care and Comfort; **Cognitive Level:** Analysis; **Integrated Process:** Teaching/Learning; **Nursing Process:** Planning/Implementation; **Reference:** Ch 25, Prenatal Period: Physical, Physiologic, and Emotional Changes During Pregnancy

124. **3** The greatest danger of drug-induced malformations is in the first trimester of pregnancy during the period of organogenesis; because a woman may not know she is pregnant, she should be aware of this before becoming pregnant.

1 Although adolescent girls may be aware of this, it is not a priority concern for them. **2** Drugs should

be avoided throughout pregnancy, but the first trimester (period of organogenesis) is the most critical. **4** If the client is not aware of her pregnancy, it may be too late to start discontinuing drugs.

Client Need: Health Promotion and Maintenance; **Cognitive Level:** Application; **Integrated Process:** Teaching/Learning; **Nursing Process:** Assessment/Analysis; **Reference:** Ch 25, Prenatal Period, Development of the Embryo/Fetus

125. **2** Cigarette smoking or continued exposure to secondary smoke causes both maternal and fetal vasoconstriction, resulting in fetal growth retardation and increased fetal and infant mortality.

1 There is no concrete evidence that smoking relieves tension or that the fetus is more relaxed. **3** Although the fetal and maternal circulations are separate, vasoconstriction occurs in both mother and fetus. **4** Smoking causes vasoconstriction; permeability of the placenta to smoke is irrelevant.

Client Need: Health Promotion and Maintenance; **Cognitive Level:** Application; **Integrated Process:** Teaching/Learning; **Nursing Process:** Planning/Implementation; **Reference:** Ch 25, Prenatal Period, Nursing Care

126. **3** High levels of chorionic gonadotropin frequently are associated with severe vomiting of pregnancy, especially in the presence of hydatidiform mole and often in a twin pregnancy.

1 Cholecystitis is unrelated to this problem. **2** Hydramnios (excessive amniotic fluid) is associated with a multiple gestation; maternal dehydration generally is associated with hyperemesis gravidarum. **4** When undigested food remains in the stomach, it leads to a reflexive action and vomiting; this is common but not severe in early pregnancy.

Client Need: Physiological Adaptation; **Cognitive Level:** Application; **Nursing Process:** Assessment/Analysis; **Reference:** Ch 25, Prenatal Period, Nursing Care

127. 1 ☐ Systemic vasodilation is not expected during pregnancy.

2 ☒ Blood volume is increased during pregnancy to meet the metabolic demands of pregnancy.

3 ☐ There is little variation in BP during pregnancy with a slight decrease during the second trimester.

4 ☒ Increased cardiac output is necessary to accommodate the increased blood volume needed to meet the demands of the growing fetus.

5 ☒ Cardiac hypertrophy is a result of the demands made by the increased blood volume and cardiac output.

6 ☐ Erythrocyte production increases during pregnancy; because the plasma volume increases more than the RBCs, the hematocrit is lower.

Client Need: Health Promotion and Maintenance; **Cognitive Level:** Analysis; **Nursing Process:** Assessment/Analysis; **Reference:** Ch 25, Prenatal Period: Physical, Physiologic, and Emotional Changes During Pregnancy

128. **2** Both the father and the mother need additional support during the transitional phase of the first stage of labor.
1 This statement is judgmental; this approach suggests that the father will be failing his wife. **3** The husband should be present throughout labor to support his wife; he should be assisted in this role. **4** This does not encourage the husband to fulfill his role of supporting his wife during labor.
Client Need: Psychosocial Integrity; **Cognitive Level:** Application; **Integrated Process:** Caring; **Nursing Process:** Planning/Implementation; **Reference:** Ch 25, Intrapartum Period, Data Base

129. **2** Maternal hypotension is a common complication of this anesthesia during labor, and nausea is one of the first clues that this has occurred. Turning the client onto her side will deflect the uterus from putting pressure on the inferior vena cava, which causes a decrease in blood flow.
1 If signs and symptoms do not abate after turning on the side, the practitioner should be notified. **3** This is not a specific observation after epidural anesthesia; it is part of the general nursing care during labor. **4** If the FHR is being monitored, it is a constant process; if not, the FHR should be monitored every 15 minutes.
Client Need: Pharmacological and Parenteral Therapies; **Cognitive Level:** Analysis; **Nursing Process:** Planning/Implementation; **Reference:** Ch 25, Intrapartum Period, Data Base

130. **3** Respiratory depression occurs with the use of meperidine (Demerol) and produces significant depression of the infant at birth if circulating levels are high at the time of birth.
1 Oxytocin is not used for pain; it is used to stimulate contractions; used judiciously, it will not harm the fetus. **2** Promazine (Sparine), an anxiolytic, augments the effects of Demerol, thereby lessening the amount of drug needed. **4** Promethazine (Phenergan), an antihistamine, does not cause respiratory depression.
Client Need: Pharmacological and Parenteral Therapies; **Cognitive Level:** Analysis; **Nursing Process:** Evaluation/Outcomes; **Reference:** Ch 25, Intrapartum Period, Data Base

131. **4** Nalbuphine is classified as an opioid analgesic and is effective for the relief of pain, causing little or no respiratory depression in the newborn.
1 Nalbuphine does not induce amnesia. **2** Nalbuphine acts as an analgesic, not an anesthetic. **3** Nalbuphine does not induce sleep, but can cause more sedation than meperidine.
Client Need: Pharmacological and Parenteral Therapies; **Cognitive Level:** Comprehension; **Nursing Process:** Evaluation/Outcomes; **Reference:** Ch 25, Intrapartum Period, Data Base

132. **2** Ambulation relieves preparatory (Braxton Hicks) contractions.
1 These contractions increase when the client is resting. **3** These contractions are not indicative of true labor and need not be timed. **4** Aspirin may be harmful to the fetus because it can hemolyze RBCs.

133. **1** Progressive dilation of the cervix is the most accurate indication of true labor.
2 Contractions may not begin until 24 to 48 hours later. **3** With true labor contractions will increase with activity. **4** Contractions of true labor persist in any position.
Client Need: Health Promotion and Maintenance; **Cognitive Level:** Analysis; **Nursing Process:** Assessment/Analysis; **Reference:** Ch 25, Intrapartum Period, Data Base

134. **2** Fatigue will influence other coping strategies, such as distraction.
1 Progesterone level is decreased at this time. **3** The client does not push during the first stage of labor; pushing is done during the second stage. **4** This may decrease the quality of the contractions.
Client Need: Basic Care and Comfort; **Cognitive Level:** Application; **Integrated Process:** Teaching/Learning; **Nursing Process:** Planning/Implementation; **Reference:** Ch 25, Intrapartum Period, Data Base

135. **1** Determining fetal well-being takes priority over all other measures. If the FHR is absent or persistently decelerating, immediate intervention is required.
2, 3, 4 Although this is important, the determination of fetal well-being is the priority.
Client Need: Reduction of Risk Potential; **Cognitive Level:** Application; **Integrated Process:** Teaching/Learning; **Nursing Process:** Assessment/Analysis; **Reference:** Ch 25, Intrapartum Period, Nursing Care

136. **2** A station of +1 indicates that the fetal head is 1 cm below the ischial spines.
1 The head is now past the points of engagement, which are the ischial spines. **3** This is designated as 0 station. **4** The head must be at +3 to +4 station to be visible at the vaginal opening.
Client Need: Health Promotion and Maintenance; **Cognitive Level:** Comprehension; **Nursing Process:** Assessment/Analysis; **Reference:** Ch 25, Intrapartum Period, Data Base

137. **3** Fetal heart tones are best auscultated through the fetal back; because the position is ROP (right occiput presenting), the back would be below the umbilicus and on the right side.
1 This could be used when the fetus is lying in the midline in a breech position. **2** This would be appropriate for an LSA position. **4** This would be appropriate for LOA or LOP position.
Client Need: Reduction of Risk Potential; **Cognitive Level:** Application; **Nursing Process:** Assessment/Analysis; **Reference:** Ch 25, Intrapartum Period, Nursing Care

138. **3** The contractions become stronger, last longer, and are erratic during this stage; the intervals during the contractions are shorter than the contractions themselves; much concentration and effort are needed by the mother to pace herself with each contraction.

1 Even clients who have been adequately prepared will experience these behaviors during the transition phase of the first stage of labor. **2** Administration of an analgesic at this point could reduce the effectiveness of labor and depress the fetus. **4** There is no indication that the contractions are hypertonic.

Client Need: Health Promotion and Maintenance; **Cognitive Level:** Application; **Nursing Process:** Assessment/Analysis; **Reference:** Ch 25, Intrapartum Period, Data Base

139. **4** This is the accepted way to determine the frequency of the contractions.

1 This does not determine the length of a contraction. **2** This identifies the end of a contraction, but it is not the accepted way of timing the frequency of contractions. **3** This does not indicate the frequency of contractions.

Client Need: Health Promotion and Maintenance; **Cognitive Level:** Application; **Nursing Process:** Assessment/Analysis; **Reference:** Ch 25, Intrapartum Period, Nursing Care

140. **2** By 36 weeks' gestation, amniotic fluid should be straw colored with small particles of vernix caseosa present.

1 Dark amber-colored fluid suggests the presence of bilirubin, an ominous sign. **3** Greenish yellow fluid may indicate the presence of meconium and suggests fetal compromise. **4** Cloudy fluid suggests the presence of purulent material, and greenish yellow may indicate the presence of meconium.

Client Need: Health Promotion and Maintenance; **Cognitive Level:** Application; **Nursing Process:** Assessment/Analysis; **Reference:** Ch 25, Intrapartum Period, Data Base

141. **2** Electronic fetal monitoring provides a continuous graphic printout of rate patterns and periodic changes; on this FHR strip the heart rate is 145 to 150 beats/min.

1 Long-term, not short-term, variability is present. **3** Contractions are lasting 100 seconds. **4** Contractions are occurring every 2½ to 3 minutes.

Client Need: Reduction of Risk Potential; **Cognitive Level:** Analysis; **Nursing Process:** Assessment/Analysis; **Reference:** Ch 25, Intrapartum Period, Nursing Care

142. **1** Because the client is attached to a machine and movement may alter the tracings, movement is discouraged.

2 Placement of the monitor leads does not interfere with the administration of sedatives. **3** Breathing techniques do not interfere with the use of a monitor. **4** An external monitor does not necessitate more frequent vaginal examinations.

Client Need: Reduction of Risk Potential; **Cognitive Level:** Application; **Nursing Process:** Evaluation/Outcomes; **Reference:** Ch 25, Intrapartum Period, Nursing Care

143. **2** Variable decelerations usually are seen as a result of cord compression; a change of position will relieve the pressure on the cord.

1 Variable decelerations are not oxytocin related. **3** This is premature; other nursing measures should

be tried first. **4** Variable decelerations are not related to the mother's BP.

Client Need: Health Promotion and Maintenance; **Cognitive Level:** Application; **Nursing Process:** Planning/Implementation; **Reference:** Ch 25, Intrapartum Period, Nursing Care

144. 2, 1, 3, 4

_____ 2 _____ Repositioning to the side increases uterine blood flow, improves cardiac output, and moves pressure of the uterus off of the vena cava.

_____ 1 _____ Increasing IV fluids increases uterine blood flow and improves cardiac output.

_____ 3 _____ Reassessing the FHR pattern enables the nurse to determine if the FHR has returned to a safe level without reflex late decelerations.

_____ 4 _____ Documentation of the response to interventions provides communication to other care providers and documents interventions.

Client Need: Health Promotion and Maintenance; **Cognitive Level:** Analysis; **Integrated Process:** Communication/Documentation; **Nursing Process:** Planning/Implementation; **Reference:** Ch 25, Intrapartum Period, Nursing Care

145. **1** When the membranes rupture, there is always the possibility of a prolapsed cord leading to fetal compromise, which would manifest itself in a slow FHR.

2 This is unnecessary unless there is a marked change in the FHR. **3** This is regularly done before and after the membranes rupture; however, fetal status takes priority. **4** This is done routinely throughout the entire labor process; at this point, fetal status takes priority.

Client Need: Reduction of Risk Potential; **Cognitive Level:** Application; **Nursing Process:** Planning/Implementation; **Reference:** Ch 25, Intrapartum Period, Nursing Care

146. **3** The client is in the first stage of labor, and the priority of care is to establish a trusting relationship with her and her husband. This will help to allay their anxiety.

1 This may be necessary later; however, it is not the priority. **2** The history should be taken from the client as long as she is capable of providing it. **4** This is not an initial priority; the practitioner may have been notified already.

Client Need: Psychosocial Integrity; **Cognitive Level:** Application; **Integrated Process:** Caring; **Nursing Process:** Planning/Implementation; **Reference:** Ch 25, Intrapartum Period, Nursing Care

147. **3** Artificial rupture of the membranes (amniotomy) allows for more effective pressure of the fetal head on the cervix, enhancing dilation and effacement.

1 Vaginal bleeding may increase because of the progression of labor. **2** Discomfort may become greater because contractions usually increase after an amniotomy. **4** This does not directly affect the fetal heart rate.

Client Need: Health Promotion and Maintenance; **Cognitive Level:** Application; **Nursing Process:** Evaluation/Outcomes; **Reference:** Ch 25, Intrapartum Period, Data Base

148. **3** The client is experiencing the expected discomforts of labor; the nurse should initiate measures that will promote relaxation.

1 The client is in early first-stage labor; pushing commences during the second stage. **2** This breathing technique should be used in the transition phase, not the early phase of the first stage of labor **4** There is no evidence at this time that the client's bleeding is excessive.

Client Need: Health Promotion and Maintenance; **Cognitive Level:** Application; **Integrated Process:** Caring; **Nursing Process:** Planning/Implementation; **Reference:** Ch 25, Intrapartum Period, Nursing Care

149. **1** An acceleration is an abrupt elevation above the baseline of 15 beats/min for 15 seconds; if the acceleration persists for more than 10 minutes, it is considered a change in baseline rate.

2 Early decelerations, not elevations, occur. An early deceleration generally starts before the peak of the uterine contraction and returns to the baseline when the uterine contraction ends. **3** A sonographic motion is not a fetal monitoring descriptive term. **4** A tachycardic FHR is above 160 beats/min.

Client Need: Reduction of Risk Potential; **Cognitive Level:** Analysis; **Integrated Process:** Communication/Documentation; **Nursing Process:** Assessment/Analysis; **Reference:** Ch 25, Intrapartum Period, Nursing Care

150. **1** This slow, deep breathing expands the spaces between the ribs and raises the abdominal muscles, allowing room for the uterus to expand and preventing painful pressure of the uterus against the abdominal wall.

2 Pelvic rocking is used to relieve pressure from back labor. **3** Panting is used to halt or delay the expulsion of the infant's head before complete dilation. **4** This breathing technique is used during the transition phase of the first stage; the client has not yet reached this phase.

Client Need: Health Promotion and Maintenance; **Cognitive Level:** Application; **Integrated Process:** Teaching/Learning; **Nursing Process:** Planning/Implementation; **Reference:** Ch 25, Intrapartum Period, Nursing Care

151. **2** Gastric peristalsis often ceases during periods of stress. Abdominal contractions put pressure on the stomach and can cause nausea and vomiting, increasing the risk for aspiration.

1 Although this is a true statement, it is not the reason for withholding/limiting food or fluid during labor. **3** Although food may cause dyspepsia, the primary reason for withholding it is to prevent aspiration. **4** Gastric peristalsis is decreased, not increased, during the stress of labor and birth.

Client Need: Health Promotion and Maintenance; **Cognitive Level:** Application; **Nursing Process:** Planning/Implementation; **Reference:** Ch 25, Intrapartum Period, Nursing Care

152. **2** This is the most difficult part of labor, and the client needs encouragement and support to cope.

1 IV fluids may need to be increased because of the increase in metabolism. **3** Medication at this time

will depress the newborn and is contraindicated. **4** Breathing patterns should be complex and require a high level of concentration to distract the client.

Client Need: Health Promotion and Maintenance; **Cognitive Level:** Application; **Integrated Process:** Caring; **Nursing Process:** Planning/Implementation; **Reference:** Ch 25, Intrapartum Period, Data Base

153. **2** Blowing forcefully through the mouth controls the strong urge to push and allows for a more controlled birth of the head.

1 This breathing pattern does not help to control expulsion. **3** This is used during the latent phase of the first stage of labor; it is not helpful in overcoming the urge to push. **4** This is used during active labor when the cervix is 3 to 7 cm dilated; it is not helpful in overcoming the urge to push.

Client Need: Health Promotion and Maintenance; **Cognitive Level:** Application; **Nursing Process:** Planning/Implementation; **Reference:** Ch 25, Intrapartum Period, Nursing Care

154. **4** As the uterus rises into the abdominal cavity, the uterine ligaments become elongated and hypertrophied; raising both legs at the same time limits the tension placed on these ligaments.

1 Lifting the legs simultaneously does not affect circulation in the legs. **2** There is already pressure on the perineum from the head of the fetus; this maneuver eases tension on the uterine ligaments. **3** There is no effect on the fascia with this maneuver.

Client Need: Health Promotion and Maintenance; **Cognitive Level:** Application; **Nursing Process:** Planning/Implementation; **Reference:** Ch 25, Intrapartum Period, Nursing Care

155. **2** The bulging perineum indicates that the fetal head is on the pelvic floor and birth is imminent.

1, 3 This occurs during the transition phase or at the beginning of the second stage. **4** This describes the progress of labor; it is not a sign that birth is imminent.

Client Need: Health Promotion and Maintenance; **Cognitive Level:** Application; **Nursing Process:** Assessment/Analysis; **Reference:** Ch 25, Intrapartum Period, Nursing Care

156. **3** Uterine tetany could result from the use of oxytocin to induce labor. Because oxytocin promotes powerful uterine contractions, uterine tetany may occur. The oxytocin infusion must be stopped to prevent uterine rupture and fetal compromise.

1 Severe pain is associated with intense contractions. **2** This is unrelated to uterine contractions. **4** This is not likely to occur.

Client Need: Pharmacological and Parenteral Therapies; **Cognitive Level:** Application; **Nursing Process:** Evaluation/Outcomes; **Reference:** Ch 25, Intrapartum Period, Data Base

157. **2** The contractions in this stage of labor are expulsive in nature; having the client push or bear down with the glottis open will hasten expulsion.

1 Contractions are now very intense and the client will be unable to relax; relaxation occurs between contractions. **3** Blowing is encouraged to slow down

pushing; she should be encouraged to push. **4** The client should be pushing; panting will prevent this.
Client Need: Health Promotion and Maintenance; **Cognitive Level:** Application; **Integrated Process:** Teaching/Learning; **Nursing Process:** Planning/Implementation; **Reference:** Ch 25, Intrapartum Period, Nursing Care

158. **2** A pudendal block provides anesthesia to the perineum.
1 This affects only the perineum, not the bladder. **3** This does not affect muscle control. **4** This anesthetizes only the perineum, not the cervix or body of the uterus.
Client Need: Pharmacological and Parenteral Therapies; **Cognitive Level:** Application; **Integrated Process:** Teaching/Learning; **Nursing Process:** Planning/Implementation; **Reference:** Ch 25, Intrapartum Period, Data Base

159. **3** These are the classic signs and symptoms of a vaginal hematoma.
1, 2 The signs and symptoms do not indicate this infection; the temperature would be elevated in the presence of infection. **4** This condition would reveal persistent vaginal bleeding with a dropping BP.
Client Need: Physiological Adaptation; **Cognitive Level:** Analysis; **Nursing Process:** Assessment/Analysis; **Reference:** Ch 25, Intrapartum Period, Nursing Care

160. **3** When the placenta separates from the uterine wall, it tears blood vessels and results in a gush of blood from the vagina.
1 This is not a desired outcome; the uterus should become tense and firm. **2** When the placenta separates, the fundus rises in the abdomen. **4** The reverse occurs; as the placenta separates it descends into the vaginal introitus and the umbilical cord appears longer and protrudes from the vagina.
Client Need: Health Promotion and Maintenance; **Cognitive Level:** Application; **Nursing Process:** Assessment/Analysis; **Reference:** Ch 25, Intrapartum Period, Data Base

161. **4** Immediately after birth the fundus is found midway between the symphysis pubis and the umbilicus.
1 The fundus is easily palpable midway between the symphysis pubis and the umbilicus. **2** The fundus is never elevated this high. **3** The fundus is not this high until 1 hour after birth; if the uterus is deviated to the right, it usually indicates bladder distention.
Client Need: Health Promotion and Maintenance; **Cognitive Level:** Application; **Nursing Process:** Assessment/Analysis; **Reference:** Ch 25, Intrapartum Period, Data Base

162. **1** Bradycardia (baseline FHR below 110 beats/min) indicates the fetus may be compromised, requiring medical intervention.
2 This may be dangerous; the fetus may be compromised, and time should not be spent on monitoring. **3** There is no indication of maternal distress. **4** The expected FHR is 110 to 160 beats/min.
Client Need: Management of Care; **Cognitive Level:** Application; **Nursing Process:** Planning/Implementation; **Reference:** Ch 25, Intrapartum Period, Nursing Care

163. **2** The displaced and boggy uterus is mostly caused by a full bladder; if the bladder is distended, the nurse should have the client void and then reassess the fundus, and if still boggy, massage gently until firm.
1 This is necessary if the fundus remains boggy after the client has voided and more gentle massage has been ineffective. **3** The oxytocin infusion may need to be increased if voiding and fundal massage are ineffective. **4** This is unsafe; the nurse must intervene.
Client Need: Health Promotion and Maintenance; **Cognitive Level:** Analysis; **Nursing Process:** Evaluation/Outcomes; **Reference:** Ch 25, Intrapartum Period, Nursing Care

164. **4** Esophageal atresia is associated with hydramnios.
1 Cardiac defects are not associated with hydramnios. **2** Kidney disorders are associated with oligohydramnios, not hydramnios. **3** Diabetes in the newborn is not associated with hydramnios.
Client Need: Physiological Adaptation; **Cognitive Level:** Application; **Nursing Process:** Assessment/Analysis; **Reference:** Ch 25, Intrapartum Period, Data Base

165. **1** This opens up an area of communication to determine what really is troubling the mother about feeding her baby.
2 The nurse is aware that this is not the best method; the problem of time should be explored with the mother. **3** Holding can be accomplished at times other than feeding periods; it does not explore the client's feelings. **4** Although this is true, the mother should not be frightened; a more gentle explanation should be offered.
Client Need: Health Promotion and Maintenance; **Cognitive Level:** Application; **Integrated Process:** Communication/Documentation; **Nursing Process:** Planning/Implementation; **Reference:** Ch 25, Postpartum Period, Nursing Care

166. **3** Rooming-in provides time for the mother and newborn to be together; the mother can become acquainted with the infant more quickly.
1 It is possible that the client does not want to breastfeed; attachment can be furthered by rooming-in. **2** Rooming-in is far more preferable. **4** This will not promote bonding and attachment.
Client Need: Health Promotion and Maintenance; **Cognitive Level:** Application; **Integrated Process:** Caring; **Nursing Process:** Planning/Implementation; **Reference:** Ch 25, Postpartum Period, Nursing Care

167. **2** Family-centered childbearing should adapt needs to the cultural system whenever possible.
1 This is the nurse's responsibility. **3** This may be useful, but the primary intervention is to address the client's cultural needs. **4** Forcing the issue does not address the underlying problem.
Client Need: Health Promotion and Maintenance; **Cognitive Level:** Application; **Nursing Process:** Planning/Implementation; **Reference:** Ch 25, Postpartum Period, Nursing Care

168. 3 Family-centered maternity care focuses on the whole family, including the relatives, in the care that will be most therapeutic for the client.

1 This is an inappropriate intervention; family-centered care focuses on the whole family, and the relative should be permitted to take part in the care of the client. 2 The nurse should be able to handle this situation. 4 Written permission is not required.

Client Need: Health Promotion and Maintenance; Cognitive Level: Application; Integrated Process: Caring; Nursing Process: Planning/Implementation; Reference: Ch 25, Postpartum Period, Nursing Care

169. 3 Heparin is the drug of choice during the acute phase of a deep vein thrombosis; it prevents conversion of fibrinogen to fibrin and of prothrombin to thrombin.

1, 4 A low molecular weight heparin is not administered during the acute stage of a deep vein thrombosis; it may be administered later to prevent future deep vein thromboses. 2 IV heparin is given for 3 to 5 days; Coumadin is started toward the end of this time and continued for 2 to 3 months.

Client Need: Pharmacological and Parenteral Therapies; Cognitive Level: Analysis; Nursing Process: Planning/Implementation; Reference: Ch 25, Postpartum Period, Data Base

170. 3 This action prevents the transfer of microorganisms from the hands to the genital tract or from the genital tract to the hands.

1 This is an inadequate number of changes; soiled pads promote the growth of microorganisms because they are warm and moist and provide a medium for growth. 2 This action interferes with analgesic action and does not prevent infection. 4 This action promotes contamination of the vagina and urethra by organisms from the perianal area.

Client Need: Safety and Infection Control; Cognitive Level: Application; Integrated Process: Teaching/Learning; Nursing Process: Evaluation/Outcomes; Reference: Ch 25, Postpartum Period, Nursing Care

171. 1 Retention of urine with overflow will be manifested in small, frequent voidings. The bladder should be palpated for distention.

2 An elevated temperature with urinary symptoms would indicate impending infection. 3 More circulating fluid is present, causing an increased output. 4 The client is usually thirsty and fluid intake increases.

Client Need: Health Promotion and Maintenance; Cognitive Level: Comprehension; Nursing Process: Assessment/Analysis; Reference: Ch 25, Postpartum Period, Data Base

172. 3 A distended bladder will displace the fundus upward and laterally.

1 This would be manifested by a slow contraction and uterine descent into the pelvis. 2 If this were true, in addition to being displaced the uterus would be boggy and vaginal bleeding would be heavy.

4 From this assessment the nurse cannot make a judgment about overstretched uterine ligaments.

Client Need: Health Promotion and Maintenance; Cognitive Level: Application; Nursing Process: Assessment/Analysis; Reference: Ch 25, Postpartum Period, Nursing Care

173. 3 The fundus descends one fingerbreadth per day from the first postpartum day.

1, 2 If the fundus were at this level, the nurse should suspect that involution has been delayed and further investigation is required. 4 Although this is not expected, it is a benign occurrence.

Client Need: Health Promotion and Maintenance; Cognitive Level: Comprehension; Nursing Process: Assessment/Analysis; Reference: Ch 25, Postpartum Period, Nursing Care

174. 4 There is extensive activation of the blood clotting factors after a birth; this, together with immobility, trauma, or sepsis, encourages thromboembolization, which can be limited through activity.

1 This can be accomplished by encouraging the client to turn from side to side and to deep breathe and cough. 2 Bladder tone would be improved by the regular emptying and filling of the bladder. 3 Exercise during the next 6 weeks can strengthen the abdominal muscles.

Client Need: Health Promotion and Maintenance; Cognitive Level: Comprehension; Integrated Process: Teaching/Learning; Nursing Process: Planning/Implementation; Reference: Ch 25, Postpartum Period, Nursing Care

175. 4 Kegel exercises can be resumed immediately and should be done for the rest of the client's life because they help strengthen muscles needed for urinary continence and may enhance sexual intercourse.

1 Episiotomy sutures do not have to be removed. 2 Bowel movements should spontaneously return in 2 to 3 days after giving birth; a delay of bowel movements promotes constipation, perineal discomfort, and trauma. 3 The usual postpartum examination is 6 weeks after birth; menses can return earlier or later than this and should not be a factor when scheduling a postpartum examination.

Client Need: Health Promotion and Maintenance; Cognitive Level: Application; Integrated Process: Teaching/Learning; Nursing Process: Planning/Implementation; Reference: Ch 25, Postpartum Period, Nursing Care

176. 1 Covered ice packs promote comfort by decreasing vasocongestion.

2, 3 Nipple stimulation precipitates the release of prolactin, which leads to more milk production and further engorgement and discomfort. 4 Emptying the breasts stimulates lactation, leading to further engorgement and discomfort.

Client Need: Basic Care and Comfort; Cognitive Level: Application; Integrated Process: Teaching/Learning; Nursing Process: Planning/Implementation; Reference: Ch 25, Postpartum Period, Nursing Care

177. 4 Although thrombophlebitis is suspected, before a definitive diagnosis the client should be

confined to bed so that further complications may be avoided.
1 This may cause vasodilation, which would allow a thrombus to dislodge and circulate freely.
2, 3 If a thrombus is present, this may dislodge it and lead to a pulmonary embolism.
Client Need: Management of Care; **Cognitive Level:** Application; **Integrated Process:** Communication/Documentation; **Nursing Process:** Planning/Implementation; **Reference:** Ch 25, Postpartum Period, Nursing Care

178. **2** The uterus responds rapidly to touch and this involves the mother in her care.
1 The uterus must be massaged before there are signs of bleeding. **3** Although this would be beneficial, the client should be taught to massage the uterus to cause it to contract. **4** This does not actively involve the mother in her own care and could be unsafe if the uterus becomes boggy between the 15-minute time periods.
Client Need: Health Promotion and Maintenance; **Cognitive Level:** Application; **Integrated Process:** Teaching/Learning; **Nursing Process:** Evaluation/Outcomes; **Reference:** Ch 25, Postpartum Period, Nursing Care

179. 1, 2, 4, 3
___1___ The culture should be obtained before antibiotics are given to ensure that the antibiotic does not interfere with accurate culture results.
___2___ Antibiotics are the most important of these orders and should be given as soon as possible to counteract any infective processes, but should not be given before obtaining the specimen for the culture.
___4___ The Tylenol is a comfort measure that can be done at any time but does not take precedence over the antibiotics.
___3___ A chest radiograph will not interfere with any of the other orders but is not as important as starting the antibiotics right away and providing comfort; it may take time to arrange for a radiograph and the other interventions should be implemented.
Client Need: Management of Care; **Cognitive Level:** Analysis; **Nursing Process:** Planning/Implementation; **Reference:** Ch 25, Postpartum Period, Nursing Care

NURSING CARE OF WOMEN AT RISK DURING PREGNANCY, LABOR, CHILDBIRTH, AND THE POSTPARTUM PERIOD

180. **2** This response points out reality and allows the client to elaborate.
1 This response would close off any future communication with the client. **3** This may be a true statement, but it does not allow for much discussion to follow. **4** This response implies that the nurse does not believe the client; it would probably cut off further communication.

Client Need: Management of Care; **Cognitive Level:** Analysis; **Integrated Process:** Communication/Documentation; **Nursing Process:** Assessment/Analysis; **Reference:** Ch 26, The Pregnant Adolescent, Nursing Care

181. **3** Fraternal twins may occur as a result of a hereditary trait, but it is related to the ovaries releasing two eggs during one ovulation; the fact that the father is a fraternal twin would not influence the female to release two eggs during one ovulation.
1, 4 If there is no maternal family history of twin pregnancies, it would be a chance occurrence that is equal to the probability found in the general population. **2** Pregnant women are routinely monitored for multiple pregnancies; this client needs information about her risk for having twins.
Client Need: Health Promotion and Maintenance; **Cognitive Level:** Comprehension; **Integrated Process:** Teaching/Learning; **Nursing Process:** Planning/Implementation; **Reference:** Ch 26, The Woman With a Multifetal Pregnancy, Data Base

182. **3** In an emergency surgical situation when invasive techniques are necessary, it is important to have a consent signed as well as a history of the client's known allergies.
1 This is not a priority in an emergency such as this.
2, 4 An enema is not given to a bleeding client; it may stimulate contractions and further bleeding.
Client Need: Management of Care; **Cognitive Level:** Analysis; **Nursing Process:** Planning/Implementation; **Reference:** Ch 26, Cesarean Birth, Data Base

183. **2** This response provides the client with a comfort measure while giving her an opportunity to verbalize her concerns.
1 This closes off communication with the client. **3** The nurse should focus on the client, not on how other women may feel; this may close off communication. **4** The client's concerns are obvious; talking about them might cause more frustration.
Client Need: Psychosocial Integrity; **Cognitive Level:** Analysis; **Integrated Process:** Caring, Communication/Documentation; **Nursing Process:** Planning/Implementation; **Reference:** Ch 26, Dystocia, Nursing Care

184. **1** Antenatal glucocorticoid therapy is contraindicated when the client has an infection because the antiinflammatory effect may exacerbate the infection.
2 An available IV line should be maintained. **3** This is the usual monitoring for preterm labor. **4** Measures to halt labor should be started.
Client Need: Pharmacological and Parenteral Therapies; **Cognitive Level:** Analysis; **Integrated Process:** Communication/Documentation; **Nursing Process:** Planning/Implementation; **Reference:** Ch 26, Preterm Labor, Data Base

185. **4** Oxytocin increases the intensity and duration of contractions; prolonged (tetanic) contractions will jeopardize the safety of the fetus and necessitate discontinuing the drug.
1 Because she is dilated only 2 to 3 cm, there will be no bulging. **2** There is no indication at this time that

a cesarean birth is necessary. **3** This is important throughout labor.
Client Need: Pharmacological and Parenteral Therapies; **Cognitive Level:** Application; **Nursing Process:** Planning/Implementation; **Reference:** Ch 26, Dystocia, Nursing Care

186. **1** Oxytocin is a small polypeptide hormone synthesized in the hypothalamus and secreted from the neurohypophysis during parturition or suckling; it promotes powerful uterine (smooth muscle) contractions and thus is used to induce labor.
2 Estrogen suppresses the follicle-stimulating and luteinizing hormones, thus helping to maintain the pregnancy. **3** Ergonovine can lead to sustained contractions, which would be undesirable in labor. **4** Progesterone causes hyperplasia of the endometrium in preparation for implantation of the fertilized ovum; later it helps to maintain the pregnancy.
Client Need: Pharmacological and Parenteral Therapies; **Cognitive Level:** Analysis; **Nursing Process:** Planning/Implementation; **Reference:** Ch 26, Induction or Stimulation of Labor, Data Base

187. **1** ☒ Pitocin is an oxytocic used for labor induction.
2 ☒ Cytotec is a prostaglandin used for cervical ripening and labor induction.
3 ☐ Ergotrate is an oxytocic used for postpartum or postabortion hemorrhage.
4 ☐ Hemabate is a prostaglandin used for postpartum hemorrhage.
5 ☐ Prepidil is used for cervical ripening to induce abortion.
Client Need: Pharmacological and Parenteral Therapies; **Cognitive Level:** Analysis; **Nursing Process:** Planning/Implementation; **Reference:** Ch 26, Induction or Stimulation of Labor, Data Base

188. **3** Terbutaline sulfate (Brethine) is a beta-mimetic drug that acts on the smooth muscles of the uterus to reduce contractility, which in turn inhibits dilation and contractions.
1 Terbutaline sulfate (Brethine) has no analgesic effects. **2** Terbutaline sulfate (Brethine) does not decrease BP; it may increase the pulse rate. **4** Terbutaline sulfate (Brethine) should stop cervical dilation, rather than increase it.
Client Need: Pharmacological and Parenteral Therapies; **Cognitive Level:** Application; **Nursing Process:** Evaluation/Outcomes; **Reference:** Ch 26, Preterm Labor, Data Base

189. **3** Magnesium sulfate has a CNS depressant effect; therefore toxic levels will be reflected by the loss of the knee-jerk reflex.
1 There is a deceleration of the respiratory rate with excessive magnesium sulfate. **2** The level of consciousness is decreased with excessive magnesium sulfate. **4** This may be caused by increased potassium, not magnesium sulfate.
Client Need: Pharmacological and Parenteral Therapies; **Cognitive Level:** Application; **Nursing Process:** Evaluation/Outcomes; **Reference:** Ch 26, Preterm Labor, Nursing Care

190. Answer: 450 mL
Solve the problem by using ratio and proportion.

$$\frac{\text{Desired}}{\text{Have}} \frac{6 \text{ grams}}{40 \text{ grams}} \times \frac{x \text{ mL}}{1000 \text{ mL}}$$

An infusion pump is set at milliliters per hour. 150 mL is needed in 20 minutes. There are 60 minutes in an hour; therefore, $3 \times 150 = 450$ mL/hr.
Client Need: Pharmacological and Parenteral Therapies; **Cognitive Level:** Application; **Nursing Process:** Planning/Implementation; **Reference:** Ch 26, Preterm Labor, Nursing Care

191. **3** This steroid, when administered before a preterm birth, enhances fetal lung maturity.
1 Ritodrine is a tocolytic agent used to prevent preterm birth; this birth is inevitable. **2** Antibiotics would not be indicated if there were no signs of infection. **4** This would be indicated if an Rh incompatibility were present in the fetus.
Client Need: Pharmacological and Parenteral Therapies; **Cognitive Level:** Analysis; **Nursing Process:** Planning/Implementation; **Reference:** Ch 26, Preterm Labor, Data Base

192. **2** This is the ideal time for CVS; this allows the client time to consider other options if a problem is discovered.
1 CVS is no longer done at this time because it has been associated with digit reduction. **3** This is late for CVS. **4** This is when a genetic amniocentesis is done.
Client Need: Reduction of Risk Potential; **Cognitive Level:** Application; **Integrated Process:** Teaching/Learning; **Nursing Process:** Planning/Implementation; **Reference:** Ch 26, Identifying and/or Monitoring High-Risk Pregnancy

193. **3** The proliferation of trophoblastic tissue filled with fluid causes the uterus to enlarge more quickly than it would with a fetus without a health problem.
1 Hypertension, not hypotension, often occurs with a molar pregnancy. **2** There is no living fetus with a hydatidiform mole. **4** There may be slight vaginal bleeding without pain.
Client Need: Physiological Adaptation; **Cognitive Level:** Application; **Nursing Process:** Assessment/Analysis; **Reference:** Ch 26, Hydatidiform Mole or Trophoblastic Disease, Data Base

194. **1** At this time the products of conception are too large for the tube to accommodate and rupture occurs.
2 Tubal pregnancies cannot advance to this stage because of the tube's inability to expand to accommodate a pregnancy of this size. **3** Tubal pregnancies cannot advance to this stage because the tube cannot expand to accommodate a pregnancy of this size. **4** The size of the fertilized egg at this time is miniscule and will cause no problem.
Client Need: Physiological Adaptation; **Cognitive Level:** Comprehension; **Nursing Process:** Assessment/Analysis; **Reference:** Ch 26, Ectopic Pregnancy, Data Base

195. **3** A fallopian tube is unable to contain and sustain a pregnancy to term; as the fertilized ovum grows, there is excessive stretching or rupture of the fallopian tube, causing pain. **1** This would be difficult for the client to identify correctly. **2** The pain is sudden, intense, knifelike, and is usually located on one side. **4** Leukorrhea and dysuria may be indicative of a vaginal or bladder infection.

Client Need: Physiological Adaptation; **Cognitive Level:** Application; **Nursing Process:** Assessment/Analysis; **Reference:** Ch 26, Ectopic Pregnancy, Data Base

196. **1** Hemorrhage may result from retained placental tissue or uterine atony.

2 There is no indication at this time that the client has been deprived of fluids. **3** Hypotension, not hypertension, may occur with postabortion hemorrhage. **4** Subinvolution usually occurs after a full-term birth.

Client Need: Health Promotion and Maintenance; **Cognitive Level:** Application; **Nursing Process:** Assessment/Analysis; **Reference:** Ch 26, Spontaneous Abortion, Nursing Care

197. **3** About 75% of all spontaneous abortions take place between 8 and 12 weeks' gestation and show embryonic defects.

1 Though possible, physical trauma rarely causes an abortion. **2** Unresolved stress is rarely associated with abortion; 50% to 60% result from chromosomal abnormalities. **4** Congenital defects are asymptomatic during pregnancy and do not usually cause an abortion.

Client Need: Physiological Adaptation; **Cognitive Level:** Application; **Integrated Process:** Teaching/Learning; **Nursing Process:** Planning/Implementation; **Reference:** Ch 26, Spontaneous Abortion, Data Base

198. **3** Spotting in the first trimester may indicate that the client is having a threatened abortion; any client with the possibility of hemorrhage should not be left alone; therefore admitting this client for observation is safe medical practice.

1 This may not cause any outward symptoms, only the signs of pregnancy disappearing. **2** This can be confirmed only if vaginal examination reveals cervical dilation. **4** This indicates that some, but not all, of the products of conception have been expelled.

Client Need: Health Promotion and Maintenance; **Cognitive Level:** Analysis; **Nursing Process:** Assessment/Analysis; **Reference:** Ch 26, Spontaneous Abortion, Data Base

199. **3** After a spontaneous abortion the fundus should be checked for firmness, which indicates effective uterine tone; if the uterus is not firm or appears to be hypotonic, hemorrhage may occur; a soft or boggy uterus may also indicate retained placental tissue.

1 The nurse would do this if necessary after checking for fundal firmness. **2** The priority action is to check for firmness of the fundus and possible bleeding. **4** This is unnecessary; fetal and placental contents are small and expelled easily.

Client Need: Health Promotion and Maintenance; **Cognitive Level:** Application; **Nursing Process:** Planning/Implementation; **Reference:** Ch 26, Spontaneous Abortion, Nursing Care

200. **4** A correct and simple definition answers the question and fulfills the client's need to know.

1 This denies the client's right to know. **2** This is the definition of a missed abortion. **3** The nurse can independently reinforce information and correct misconceptions.

Client Need: Health Promotion and Maintenance; **Cognitive Level:** Application; **Integrated Process:** Teaching/Learning; **Nursing Process:** Planning/Implementation; **Reference:** Ch 26, Spontaneous Abortion, Data Base

201. **4** Intact membranes act as a barrier against organisms that may cause an intrauterine infection.

1 This is common because of increased production of mucus containing exfoliated vaginal epithelial cells; intercourse is not contraindicated. **2** This may occur during sex but there is no literature indicating that it is harmful for the fetus. **3** Intercourse is not contraindicated if membranes are intact; modification of sexual positions may be needed because of the enlarged abdomen.

Client Need: Health Promotion and Maintenance; **Cognitive Level:** Application; **Integrated Process:** Teaching/Learning; **Nursing Process:** Planning/Implementation; **Reference:** Ch 26, Premature Rupture of Membranes, Nursing Care

202. **4** A persistent occiput posterior position causes intense back pain because of fetal compression of the maternal sacral nerves.

1 Breech positions are not associated with back pain. **2** The transverse position usually does not cause back pain. **3** This is the most common fetal position and does not cause back pain.

Client Need: Health Promotion and Maintenance; **Cognitive Level:** Application; **Integrated Process:** Teaching/Learning; **Nursing Process:** Planning/Implementation; **Reference:** Ch 26, Dystocia, Nursing Care

203. **3** The application of back pressure combined with frequent positional changes will help alleviate the discomfort.

1 Although this may be comfortable for some individuals, rubbing the back and alternating positions are more universally effective. **2** The supine position places increased pressure on the back and often aggravates the pain. **4** Neuromuscular control exercises are used to teach selective relaxation in childbirth classes; they will not relieve back pain.

Client Need: Health Promotion and Maintenance; **Cognitive Level:** Application; **Integrated Process:** Caring; **Nursing Process:** Planning/Implementation; **Reference:** Ch 26, Dystocia, Nursing Care

204. **2** Low back pain is aggravated when the mother is in the supine position because of increased pressure from the fetus.

1, 3, 4 This position helps relieve back pain.

Client Need: Health Promotion and Maintenance; **Cognitive Level:** Application; **Integrated Process:** Teaching/Learning; **Nursing Process:** Planning/Implementation; **Reference:** Ch 26, Dystocia, Nursing Care

205. 4 Gentle pressure is applied against the head of the fetus as it emerges so it is not born too rapidly. The head should be supported as it emerges to avoid vaginal lacerations.

1 It is impossible to pant and push at the same time. 2 Birth is imminent and there is no time to transfer the client. 3 Unless she is in a pant-blow breathing pattern, she will push involuntarily.

Client Need: Health Promotion and Maintenance; **Cognitive Level:** Analysis; **Nursing Process:** Planning/Implementation; **Reference:** Ch 26, Precipitate Birth, Nursing Care

206. 2 Lacerations require less suture time and cause less perineal trauma, which can have lifelong implications such as rectal-vaginal fistulas.

1 Lacerations are less painful than an episiotomy and tend to heal more quickly. 3 An episiotomy causes more posterior trauma than lacerations. 4 Evidence indicates that a routine episiotomy policy results in more perineal trauma, more suturing time, and more complications than lacerations.

Client Need: Health Promotion and Maintenance; **Cognitive Level:** Comprehension; **Integrated Process:** Teaching/Learning; **Nursing Process:** Planning/Implementation; **Reference:** Ch 26, Episiotomy, Data Base

207. 3 According to the Centers for Disease Control and Prevention (CDC) recommendations for isolation precautions, gloves should be worn when there is potential contact with blood or other body fluids.

1 Even if the client does not have an infection, gloves are always worn when exposure to blood or other body fluids is a possibility. 2 All blood is considered to be potentially infectious. 4 Nurses are required to take precautions that limit exposure; gloves must be worn.

Client Need: Safety and Infection Control; **Cognitive Level:** Application; **Nursing Process:** Evaluation/Outcomes; **Reference:** Ch 26, Postpartum Bleeding, Nursing Care

208. 1 Heat causes vasodilation and an increased blood supply to the area.

2 Sitz baths do not soften the incision site. 3 Cleansing is done with a perineal bottle and cleansing solution immediately after voiding and defecating. 4 Neither relaxation nor tightening of the rectal sphincter will increase healing of an episiotomy.

Client Need: Basic Care and Comfort; **Cognitive Level:** Comprehension; **Integrated Process:** Caring; **Nursing Process:** Planning/Implementation; **Reference:** Ch 26, Episiotomy, Nursing Care

209. 2 The nurse should position the infant with head slightly lower than the chest to allow mucus to flow by gravity and rub the back to stimulate crying, which promotes oxygenation.

1 This is not the priority; there is no need for haste in cutting the cord. 3 This is not the priority; the uterus still contains the placenta and will not contract. 4 This is not the priority; the well-being of the newborn and mother must be confirmed before moving them.

Client Need: Health Promotion and Maintenance; **Cognitive Level:** Application; **Nursing Process:** Planning/Implementation; **Reference:** Ch 26, Precipitate Birth, Nursing Care

210. 1 ☒ Increased risk for developing preterm labor is age associated; it occurs more commonly in older primigravidas and adolescents.

2 ☒ Mature gravidas have an increased incidence of multiple gestation secondary to fertility drug use and in vitro fertilization.

3 ☐ This is not seen more frequently in mature gravidas.

4 ☒ After 35 years of age, mature gravidas have an increasing incidence of chromosomal abnormalities.

5 ☒ Bleeding in the first trimester as a result of spontaneous abortion is seen more frequently in mature gravidas.

Client Need: Physiological Adaptation; **Cognitive Level:** Analysis; **Nursing Process:** Assessment/Analysis; **Reference:** Ch 26, The Older Pregnant Woman, Data Base

211. 2 About two thirds of neonatal deaths are associated with preterm births; there appears to be a correlation with teenage pregnancy, lack of prenatal care, nonwhite mothers, and chronic health problems.

1 Atelectasis may occur from respiratory distress, which in turn is associated with preterm births, the leading cause of death. 3 Most infants who die from congenital heart disease die after the neonatal period. 4 This is just one complication of a preterm birth.

Client Need: Physiological Adaptation; **Cognitive Level:** Comprehension; **Nursing Process:** Assessment/Analysis; **Reference:** Ch 26, Preterm Labor, Data Base

212. 3 Preterm labor, a history of preterm births, nipple stimulation, or administration of oxytocin too early in pregnancy can cause uterine contractions and a preterm birth.

1 The contraction stress test is indicated to assess the influence of hypertension on the placental circulation. 2, 4 The contraction stress test is indicated to determine the response of the fetus to labor.

Client Need: Reduction of Risk Potential; **Cognitive Level:** Analysis; **Nursing Process:** Assessment/Analysis; **Reference:** Ch 26, Identifying and Monitoring High-Risk Pregnancy

213. 4 A positive contraction stress test (CST) indicates a compromised FHR during contractions, which is associated with uteroplacental insufficiency.

1 Preeclampsia does not cause a positive CST. 2 Ultrasonography would show placenta previa and a contraction stress test is contraindicated, because oxytocin may stimulate contractions. 3 A contraction stress test is contraindicated for a woman with a suspected preterm birth or a pregnancy of less than 33 weeks' gestation because oxytocin may induce labor.

Client Need: Reduction of Risk Potential; **Cognitive Level:** Application; **Nursing Process:** Evaluation/Outcomes; **Reference:** Ch 26, Identifying and Monitoring High-Risk Pregnancy

214. 4 It is not uncommon for adolescents to avoid prenatal care; many do not recognize the deleterious effect that lack of prenatal care can have on them and their infants.
1 This should come later in pregnancy, but not before ascertaining the client's feelings about breastfeeding. 2 This can be done in the later part of pregnancy and reinforced during the postpartum period. 3 This will have to be done, but it is not the priority intervention at this time.

Client Need: Health Promotion and Maintenance; **Cognitive Level:** Application; **Integrated Process:** Teaching/Learning; **Nursing Process:** Planning/Implementation; **Reference:** Ch 26, The Pregnant Adolescent, Nursing Care

215. 4 The pregnant teenager generally is more prone to gestational hypertension because of age, inadequate diet, and lack of prenatal care.
1 There is no proof that teenagers are more diabetogenic than are other pregnant women. 2 This is a false assumption; societal mores vary, and the pregnancy of an unmarried adolescent may be acceptable. 3 This may or may not be true.

Client Need: Physiological Adaptation; **Cognitive Level:** Application; **Nursing Process:** Assessment/Analysis; **Reference:** Ch 26, The Pregnant Adolescent, Data Base

216. 2 Perinatal morbidity and mortality are greatly increased with a multiple gestation because the high metabolic demands and the possibility of malpositioning of one or more fetuses may increase the potential for medical and obstetric complications.
1 Although postpartum hemorrhage does occur more frequently after multiple births, it is not a routine occurrence. 3 Maternal mortality during the prenatal period is not increased in the presence of a multiple gestation. 4 Adjustment to a multiple gestation and birth is individual; the time needed for adjustment does not place the pregnancy at high risk.

Client Need: Physiological Adaptation; **Cognitive Level:** Application; **Nursing Process:** Assessment/Analysis; **Reference:** Ch 26, The Woman With a Multifetal Pregnancy, Data Base

217. 1 A multiple gestation thins the uterine wall by overstretching; thus the efficiency of contractions is reduced.
2 Gestational anemia is physiologic anemia that is benign; although anemia may cause fatigue during labor; it does not affect uterine contractility. 3 A pelvic contracture may lead to a difficult birth because of cephalopelvic disproportion; it does not affect uterine contractions. 4 Gestational hypertension may trigger preterm labor; it does not cause hypotonic uterine dysfunction.

Client Need: Physiological Adaptation; **Cognitive Level:** Application; **Nursing Process:** Assessment/Analysis; **Reference:** Ch 26, The Woman With a Multifetal Pregnancy, Data Base

218. 2 Placenta previa is defined as an abnormally implanted placenta in the thin, lower uterine segment (i.e., low-lying or covering the cervical os).
1 This can occur at any time; it is not specific to a low-lying placenta. 3 This can occur without a low-lying placenta; factors such as poor muscular tone of the uterus and excessive oxytocin during induction may cause this to occur. 4 Premature separation of the placenta can occur with a normally implanted placenta.

Client Need: Physiological Adaptation; **Cognitive Level:** Analysis; **Nursing Process:** Planning/Implementation; **Reference:** Ch 26, Placenta Previa, Data Base

219. 3 Pyelonephritis often causes preterm labor, leading to increased neonatal morbidity and mortality.
1 Fluids should be increased; the inflammatory process may lead to fever, dehydration, and an accumulation of toxins. 2 Proteinuria occurs with preeclampsia; the client's signs and symptoms are indicative of a kidney infection. 4 This is not necessary.

Client Need: Physiological Adaptation; **Cognitive Level:** Application; **Nursing Process:** Assessment/Analysis; **Reference:** Ch 26, Preterm Labor, Data Base

220. 3 Health care supervision requires treatment with an appropriate antibiotic until two negative cultures are obtained; recurring pyelonephritis often leads to preterm birth.
1 Preeclampsia is not preceded by specific infections. 2 A low-protein diet inhibits fetal development and is contraindicated during pregnancy. 4 Pelvic inflammatory disease is associated with infections of the genital, not the urinary, tract.

Client Need: Safety and Infection Control; **Cognitive Level:** Application; **Nursing Process:** Planning/Implementation; **Reference:** Ch 26, Preterm Labor, Data Base

221. 4 This is not associated with multiple gestation and therefore the client needs further instruction.
1 Preterm birth with multiple gestation occurs for a variety of reasons such as spontaneous rupture of the membranes, abruptio placentae, and marked uterine distention. 2 Shunting of blood between placentas can occur only with multiple gestations because of the presence of multiple placentas. 3 The increased blood volume and metabolism necessary to sustain a multiple gestation predisposes the mother to hypertension.

Client Need: Health Promotion and Maintenance; **Cognitive Level:** Analysis; **Integrated Process:** Teaching/Learning; **Nursing Process:** Evaluation/Outcomes; **Reference:** Ch 26, The Woman With a Multifetal Pregnancy, Data Base

222. 4 Severe pain accompanied by bleeding at term or close to it is symptomatic of complete premature detachment of the placenta (abruptio placentae).
1 A hydatidiform mole is diagnosed before 36 weeks' gestation; it is not accompanied by severe pain. 2 There is no bleeding with vena caval syndrome. 3 Bleeding caused by marginal placenta previa should not be painful.

Client Need: Physiological Adaptation; **Cognitive Level:** Analysis; **Nursing Process:** Assessment/Analysis; **Reference:** Ch 26, Abruptio Placentae, Data Base

223. 2 The blood cannot escape from behind the placenta; thus the abdomen becomes boardlike and painful because of the entrapment.

1 Symptoms of hemorrhagic shock do not include pain. 3 This is not related to the initial pain of abruptio placentae; eventually blood at the site of placental separation may seep into the uterine muscle (Couvelaire uterus). 4 This is not related to the initial pain of abruptio placentae; it is a life-threatening complication.

Client Need: Physiological Adaptation; **Cognitive Level:** Application; **Nursing Process:** Assessment/Analysis; **Reference:** Ch 26, Abruptio Placentae, Data Base

224. 4 Clotting defects are common in moderate and severe abruptio placentae because of the loss of fibrinogen caused by severe internal bleeding.

1 An excessive amount of RBCs is not related to the depletion of fibrinogen. 2 The bleeding with abruptio placentae is caused by depletion of fibrinogen, not thrombocytes (platelets). 3 Excessive globulin in the blood is unrelated to clotting.

Client Need: Physiological Adaptation; **Cognitive Level:** Analysis; **Nursing Process:** Assessment/Analysis; **Reference:** Ch 26, Abruptio Placentae, Data Base

225. 3 Hypertension during pregnancy leads to vasospasms; this in turn causes the placenta to tear away from the uterine wall (abruptio placentae).

1 Generally cardiac disease does not cause abruptio placentae. 2 This may cause endocrine disturbance in the infant but does not affect the blood supply to the uterus. 4 This may affect the birth of the fetus but does not affect the placenta.

Client Need: Physiological Adaptation; **Cognitive Level:** Application; **Nursing Process:** Assessment/Analysis; **Reference:** Ch 26, Abruptio Placentae, Data Base

226. 1 Placenta previa is classically painless bleeding; the placenta partially or completely covers the cervical os and as the cervix dilates the placenta separates and bleeds.

2 Placenta accreta is an abnormally adherent placenta; the placenta attaches through the endometrium to the myometrium. 3 A ruptured uterus is a painful occurrence; the fetus may be expelled from the uterus into the abdomen. 4 If the abruptio were concealed, there would be no visible bleeding; abruptio placentae is painful as the blood accumulates between the placenta and the uterine muscle.

Client Need: Physiological Adaptation; **Cognitive Level:** Application; **Nursing Process:** Assessment/Analysis; **Reference:** Ch 26, Placenta Previa, Data Base

227. 3 Observation and documentation of bleeding are necessary for implementing safe care, because hemorrhage and shock can be life-threatening.

1 Vital signs should be checked more often while there is bleeding. 2 This is contraindicated, because it may cause further separation of the placenta. 4 The client should be restricted to complete bed rest until bleeding stops.

Client Need: Physiological Adaptation; **Cognitive Level:** Application; **Integrated Process:** Communication/ Documentation; **Nursing Process:** Planning/Implementation; **Reference:** Ch 26, Placenta Previa, Nursing Care

228. 3 Abruptio placentae is associated with cocaine use and seen in the third trimester.

1 Placenta previa is seen in the third trimester but is not associated with cocaine use. 2 Ectopic pregnancy occurs in the first trimester, not the third trimester. 4 Spontaneous abortion is seen in the first trimester, not the third trimester.

Client Need: Physiological Adaptation; **Cognitive Level:** Application; **Nursing Process:** Assessment/Analysis; **Reference:** Ch 26, Abruptio Placentae, Data Base

229. 2 Prostaglandins in semen may stimulate labor, and penile contact with the cervix may increase myometrial contractility.

1 Sexual intercourse may cause labor to progress; it is contraindicated. 3 The position is irrelevant; sexual intercourse is not advised in week 35 of pregnancy with 2-cm cervical dilation. 4 Regardless of the penile penetration, sexual intercourse may precipitate labor.

Client Need: Reduction of Risk Potential; **Cognitive Level:** Application; **Integrated Process:** Teaching/Learning; **Nursing Process:** Planning/Implementation; **Reference:** Ch 26, Preterm Labor, Nursing Care

230. 1 Atony often results from an overdistended uterus; uterine contractions do not occur readily and the uterus fills with blood.

2 This might cause a hematoma to form, but not a hemorrhage. 3 This is unusual; it may cause some bleeding, but not a hemorrhage. 4 This can occur in single, not just multiple, births if careful inspection of the placenta is not done.

Client Need: Health Promotion and Maintenance; **Cognitive Level:** Application; **Nursing Process:** Evaluation/Outcomes; **Reference:** Ch 26, The Woman With a Multifetal Pregnancy, Data Base

231. 4 Once the membranes have ruptured, the active herpes infection ascends and can infect the fetus; since herpes does not cross the placenta, a cesarean birth can prevent transfer of the virus to the fetus.

1, 2, 3 This is not an indication for cesarean birth; pharmacologic therapy will be administered.

Client Need: Reduction of Risk Potential; **Cognitive Level:** Application; **Nursing Process:** Assessment/Analysis; **Reference:** Ch 26, Cesarean Birth, Data Base

232. 2 This is the treatment of choice for complete placental separation (abruptio placentae). The risk for fetal death is too high to delay.

1 A high-forceps birth rarely is used because the forceps may further complicate the situation by tearing the cervix. 3, 4 The fetus would probably expire if this course of action were taken.

Client Need: Physiological Adaptation; **Cognitive Level:** Application; **Nursing Process:** Planning/Implementation; **Reference:** Ch 26, Abruptio Placentae, Data Base

233. 1 A multipara with a shoulder presentation is indicative of a transverse lie; this necessitates a cesarean birth.

2 It is not uncommon for the fetus of a multipara to be high at the beginning of labor; early engagement occurs more often with a primigravida. 3 With an occiput posterior presentation, the labor may be longer but usually the mother can give birth vaginally. 4 If the first twin is in the vertex presentation, a vaginal birth will be attempted with a double setup; if possible, the birth of the second twin also will be attempted vaginally.

Client Need: Management of Care; **Cognitive Level:** Analysis; **Nursing Process:** Planning/Implementation; **Reference:** Ch 26, Cesarean Birth, Data Base

234. 4 It is expected that up to two perineal pads can be saturated in the first hour.

1 A scant flow would be less and probably would not even saturate one pad. 2 Hemorrhage would saturate more than two pads in 1 hour. 3 This would be accompanied by heavy bleeding and require more than two pads during the first hour.

Client Need: Health Promotion and Maintenance; **Cognitive Level:** Application; **Nursing Process:** Evaluation/Outcomes; **Reference:** Ch 26, Cesarean Birth, Nursing Care

235. 2 First pregnancy and obesity are both documented risk factors.

1 The risk age for a hypertensive disorder of pregnancy is under 20 and over 35 years. 3, 4 This is not a documented risk factor.

Client Need: Health Promotion and Maintenance; **Cognitive Level:** Application; **Nursing Process:** Assessment/Analysis; **Reference:** Ch 26, Hypertensive Disorders of Pregnancy, Data Base

236. 4 A BP greater than 140 mm Hg systolic and 90 mm Hg diastolic is diagnostic of preeclampsia; assessments should be done twice 4 to 6 hours apart.

1 Hypertension is not always accompanied by headaches. 2 The data are incomplete; many women have low baseline BPs and could be hypertensive at 120/75 mm Hg. 3 This can occur at any time, not specifically in clients with pregnancy-induced hypertension.

Client Need: Physiological Adaptation; **Cognitive Level:** Application; **Nursing Process:** Assessment/Analysis; **Reference:** Ch 26, Hypertensive Disorders of Pregnancy, Data Base

237. 4 To ascertain the severity of preeclampsia, these are the signs that must be assessed.

1 Constipation is not related to preeclampsia. 2 Constipation and bleeding are not associated with preeclampsia. 3 Leakage of fluid and bleeding are not related to preeclampsia.

Client Need: Physiological Adaptation; **Cognitive Level:** Analysis; **Nursing Process:** Assessment/Analysis; **Reference:** Ch 26, Hypertensive Disorders of Pregnancy, Data Base

238. 4 This is a sign of CNS involvement that the nurse can observe without obtaining subjective data from the client.

1 Pain and nausea are subjective symptoms and are not directly observable. 2 These are subjective symptoms; the client must indicate their presence. 3 These are subjective symptoms that are not obvious to the nurse.

Client Need: Physiological Adaptation; **Cognitive Level:** Application; **Nursing Process:** Assessment/Analysis; **Reference:** Ch 26, Hypertensive Disorders of Pregnancy, Nursing Care

239. 3 The danger of a seizure in a woman with eclampsia subsides when postpartum diuresis has occurred, usually 48 hours after birth; however, the risk for seizures may remain for up to 2 weeks postpartum.

1, 2, 4 This is too soon.

Client Need: Physiological Adaptation; **Cognitive Level:** Comprehension; **Nursing Process:** Evaluation/Outcomes; **Reference:** Ch 26, Hypertensive Disorders of Pregnancy, Nursing Care

240. 2 Distribution of the fingers around the head will prevent a rapid change in intracranial pressure while the head is being born and keeps the head from "popping out," causing maternal perineal trauma.

1 This will not assist with the birth of the head. 3 This may interfere with the birth and harm the neonate. 4 This may injure the neonate.

Client Need: Safety and Infection Control; **Cognitive Level:** Application; **Nursing Process:** Planning/Implementation; **Reference:** Ch 26, Precipitate Birth, Nursing Care

241. 4 A position in which the mother's head is below the level of the hips helps decrease compression of the cord and therefore maintains the blood supply to the fetus.

1 This position is impossible to maintain and will not relieve the pressure of the oncoming head on the cord. 2 This will increase the pressure of the presenting part on the cord. 3 The pressure of the presenting part on the cord is not relieved in this position.

Client Need: Physiological Adaptation; **Cognitive Level:** Application; **Nursing Process:** Planning/Implementation; **Reference:** Ch 26, Breech Birth, Nursing Care

242. 4 The heart rate increases by about 10 beats/min in the last half of pregnancy; this increase plus the increase in total blood volume can strain a damaged heart beyond the point at which it can efficiently compensate.

1 The number of RBCs does not decrease during pregnancy. 2 The increased size of the uterus is related to the growth of the fetus, not to any hemodynamic change. 3 Cardiac output begins to decrease by the 34th week of gestation.

Client Need: Physiological Adaptation; **Cognitive Level:** Application; **Nursing Process:** Assessment/Analysis; **Reference:** Ch 26, Heart Disease, Data Base

243. 4 This is the most critical period because of the rapid fluid shift as extravascular fluid returns to the bloodstream; this mobilization of fluid can place a strain on the heart and lead to cardiac decompensation.

1 During the first trimester the increased amount of circulating blood volume is minimal and occurs gradually; thus usually it does not place a large burden on the heart. **2** The risk for cardiac decompensation increases as pregnancy progresses; however, the increase in blood volume occurs gradually and the mother is monitored closely. **3** There is an increased risk for stress on the heart during labor; however, close monitoring and the use of agents to provide rest and pain relief have decreased these risks.

Client Need: Physiological Adaptation; **Cognitive Level:** Application; **Integrated Process:** Teaching/Learning; **Nursing Process:** Evaluation/Outcomes; **Reference:** Ch 26, Heart Disease, Nursing Care

244. **3** Forceps reduces the mother's need to push, conserving energy; regional anesthesia will relieve the stress of pain, and it does not compromise cardiovascular function.

1 Abdominal surgery is performed on clients with cardiac problems only when absolutely necessary. **2** Forceps reduces the mother's need to push, conserving energy; however, general anesthesia would compromise cardiovascular function. **4** Induced labor is often more stressful and painful than spontaneous labor.

Client Need: Physiological Adaptation; **Cognitive Level:** Application; **Integrated Process:** Teaching/Learning; **Nursing Process:** Planning/Implementation; **Reference:** Ch 26, Heart Disease, Nursing Care

245. **3** The semi-Fowler's position facilitates easier oxygen exchange, and the side-lying position promotes venous return.

1 This is too uncomfortable; the gravid uterus will impede venous return from the legs. **2** In the supine position the gravid uterus may inhibit venous return and result in placental congestion and supine hypotension. **4** At full term, the left side-lying position is preferred to the right side-lying position to enhance venous return.

Client Need: Physiological Adaptation; **Cognitive Level:** Application; **Nursing Process:** Planning/Implementation; **Reference:** Ch 26, Heart Disease, Nursing Care

246. **3** Clients with cardiac problems are prone to heart failure in this stage of labor; crackles indicate the presence of pulmonary edema.

1, 2 This is done for all clients who are in labor. **4** This is not necessary; clients who are in labor are maintained on the side to facilitate venous return.

Client Need: Reduction of Risk Potential; **Cognitive Level:** Application; **Nursing Process:** Planning/Implementation; **Reference:** Ch 26, Heart Disease, Nursing Care

247. **1** Usually as pregnancy progresses, there are alterations in glucose tolerance and in the metabolism and utilization of insulin. The result is an increased need for exogenous insulin.

2 Antihypertensives are administered only to clients with severe hypertensive preeclampsia. **3** Pancreatic enzymes or hormones other than insulin are not taken by pregnant women with diabetes. **4** Estrogenic hormones are not administered during pregnancy.

Client Need: Physiological Adaptation; **Cognitive Level:** Analysis; **Nursing Process:** Planning/Implementation; **Reference:** Ch 26, Diabetes Mellitus, Data Base

248. **3** Insulin requirements may fall suddenly during the first 24 to 48 postpartum hours because the endocrine changes of pregnancy are reversed.

1 Insulin requirements do not suddenly rise at this time. **2** Insulin requirements do not remain unchanged at this time. **4** Insulin requirements do not slowly, steadily decrease at this time.

Client Need: Physiological Adaptation; **Cognitive Level:** Application; **Nursing Process:** Evaluation/Outcomes; **Reference:** Ch 26, Diabetes Mellitus, Data Base

249. **3** The client should receive nothing by mouth while heavy bleeding continues because surgical intervention may become necessary.

1 Providing oral fluids at this time is inappropriate and could result in aspiration if surgery becomes necessary in the near future. **2** The nurse does not need an order to give fluids to a postpartum client; the nurse must make an independent judgment regarding the withholding of fluids. **4** Although oral fluids can increase the blood volume, it would be inappropriate to provide fluids at this time.

Client Need: Physiological Adaptation; **Cognitive Level:** Analysis; **Nursing Process:** Planning/Implementation; **Reference:** Ch 26, Postpartum Bleeding, Nursing Care

250. **4** Previous multiple full-term pregnancies and births result in overstretched uterine muscles that do not contract efficiently, and bleeding may ensue; oxytocin promotes uterine contractions.

1 A precipitate birth does not predispose to uterine atony unless there is a complication. **2** Giving birth outside the birthing area does not predispose the client to uterine atony. **3** Multiparity does not predispose to retained placental fragments.

Client Need: Pharmacological and Parenteral Therapies; **Cognitive Level:** Analysis; **Nursing Process:** Planning/Implementation; **Reference:** Ch 26, Postpartum Bleeding, Data Base

251. **4** Uncomplicated hypertension does not interfere with uterine involution, return of uterine tone, or constriction of vessels at the placental site.

1 Overdistention of the uterus may lead to delayed or inadequate uterine myometrial contractions at the placental site. **2** Retained placenta inhibits uterine myometrial contractions; also, manual removal of the placenta may cause uterine trauma. **3** This may inhibit myometrial contraction of the uterus at the placental site.

Client Need: Health Promotion and Maintenance; **Cognitive Level:** Application; **Nursing Process:** Evaluation/Outcomes; **Reference:** Ch 26, Postpartum Bleeding, Data Base

252. 1 Blood loss depletes the cellular response to infection; trauma provides an excellent avenue for bacteria to enter.

2 Preeclampsia is not a predisposing cause of postpartum infection. 3 These may create problems if hemorrhage occurs because the hemoglobin and hematocrit are already low. 4 Endogenous infection is rare; infection is usually caused by outside contamination; trauma and the denuded placental site contribute to the development of infection.

Client Need: Health Promotion and Maintenance; **Cognitive Level:** Application; **Nursing Process:** Assessment/Analysis; **Reference:** Ch 26, Postpartum Bleeding, Data Base

253. 3 As the heart fails, the respiratory rate and effort increase in an attempt to maintain O_2 to all body cells.

1 Although pulse rate is important, the primary observation should be for respiratory distress. 2 Signs of heart failure, not hypovolemic shock, might develop. 4 Increased vaginal bleeding is not caused by alterations in cardiac status.

Client Need: Physiological Adaptation; **Cognitive Level:** Analysis; **Nursing Process:** Evaluation/Outcomes; **Reference:** Ch 26, Heart Disease, Nursing Care

254. 4 Glucose-oxidase strips are used by nurses to screen infants for hypoglycemia.

1 This test is not used to screen for hypoglycemia. 2 This test is not used as a screening tool. 3 Fasting blood glucose levels are not used routinely to screen newborns for hypoglycemia; fasting may reduce glucose levels further.

Client Need: Reduction of Risk Potential; **Cognitive Level:** Application; **Nursing Process:** Planning/Implementation; **Reference:** Ch 26, Diabetes Mellitus, Nursing Care

255. 2 The infant of a diabetic mother (IDM) is a newborn at risk because of the interplay between the maternal disease and the developing fetus.

1 A newborn of a diabetic mother is generally hypoglycemic because of oversecretion of insulin by the infant's hypertrophied pancreas. 3 Infants of diabetic mothers are at high risk and require intensive monitoring. 4 The IDM may be prone to hypoglycemia and will need increased glucose.

Client Need: Management of Care; **Cognitive Level:** Application; **Nursing Process:** Planning/Implementation; **Reference:** Ch 26, Diabetes Mellitus, Nursing Care

256. 1 The pancreas of a fetus of a diabetic mother responds to the mother's hyperglycemia by secreting large amounts of insulin; this leads to infant hypoglycemia after birth.

2 Hypocalcemia, not hypercalcemia, occurs. 3 Edema may be generalized, not specific to the central nervous system. 4 In response to the increased glucose received from the mother, the islets of Langerhans in the fetus may have become hypertrophied; they are not congenitally depressed.

Client Need: Physiological Adaptation; **Cognitive Level:** Application; **Nursing Process:** Assessment/Analysis; **Reference:** Ch 26, Diabetes Mellitus, Nursing Care

257. 2 The higher-than-normal glucose level in a fetus of a diabetic mother leads to increased fat synthesis and deposition; increased glucose utilization is also promoted by the combined presence of the pituitary growth hormone and placental somatotropin.

1 Glucose utilization is increased, with resultant macrosomia. 3 Somatotropin concentration is increased during pregnancy. 4 Somatotropin concentration and glucose utilization are increased.

Client Need: Physiological Adaptation; **Cognitive Level:** Application; **Nursing Process:** Assessment/Analysis; **Reference:** Ch 26, Diabetes Mellitus, Data Base

NURSING CARE OF THE NEWBORN

258. 1 By demonstrating acceptance of the infant, without regard for the defect, the nurse acts as a role model for the parents, thus enhancing their acceptance.

2 Infants with cleft palates can remain in the newborn nursery; they should not be hidden. 3 This is false reassurance; it does not promote parent-infant bonding. 4 The parents should be encouraged to have frequent contact with their infant to promote bonding.

Client Need: Psychosocial Integrity; **Cognitive Level:** Application; **Integrated Process:** Caring; **Nursing Process:** Planning/Implementation; **Reference:** Ch 27, Nursing Care Common to All Newborns

259. 4 Mothers need to explore their infants visually and tactilely to assure themselves that the infants are normal in all respects.

1 This is false reassurance; this comment closes off communication with the mother at a very opportune moment. 2 Crying is not indicative of congenital defects; a strong cry does not ensure "normalcy." 3 The "normalcy" of the mother's pregnancy does not always have a relationship to the "normalcy" of the infant.

Client Need: Health Promotion and Maintenance; **Cognitive Level:** Application; **Nursing Process:** Planning/Implementation; **Reference:** Ch 27, Parent-Infant Relationships

260. 4 Allowing the mother time to inspect the child permits viewing, touching, and holding, promoting bonding.

1 The client will proceed at her own rate; requiring her to do things is not supportive. 2 The mother usually makes this decision before the birth. 3 Early observation is not adequate; this can be done only by allowing the mother ample time to interact with her baby.

Client Need: Health Promotion and Maintenance; **Cognitive Level:** Application; **Integrated Process:** Caring; **Nursing Process:** Planning/Implementation; **Reference:** Ch 27, Parent-Infant Relationships

261. **2** The mother has completed the taking-in phase (the mother's needs predominate) and has moved into the taking-hold phase (active maternal involvement with self and infant) when she calls her infant by name.

1 This may occur in either phase. **3** This is the initial early action of the taking-in phase. **4** This is part of the taking-in phase.

Client Need: Health Promotion and Maintenance; **Cognitive Level:** Analysis; **Nursing Process:** Assessment/Analysis; **Reference:** Ch 27, Parent-Infant Relationships

262. **3** Bonding between parent and infant is most successful when interaction is possible immediately after birth; if the infant is ill, contact is limited.

1 Though the effect of anesthesia is a factor, the most important factor is the physical condition of the infant. **2** Though the duration and difficulty of labor is a factor, the most important factor is the physical condition of the infant. **4** Health and emotional status during pregnancy may be factors, but the most important factor after the birth is the physical condition of the infant.

Client Need: Health Promotion and Maintenance; **Cognitive Level:** Analysis; **Nursing Process:** Planning/Implementation; **Reference:** Ch 27, Parent-Infant Relationships

263. **3** Parenting is a learned behavior based on past experiences or current instruction.

1 Marriage is not essential for good parenting. **2** Parenting is learned, not inborn. **4** This knowledge does not ensure the ability to parent.

Client Need: Health Promotion and Maintenance; **Cognitive Level:** Analysis; **Nursing Process:** Assessment/Analysis; **Reference:** Ch 27, Parent-Infant Relationships

264. **2** This immunity is developed from an antigen-antibody response in the mother that is passed to the fetus.

1 This is acquired by an individual in response to a disease or an infection. **3** This is acquired by an individual in response to small amounts of antigenic material (e.g., vaccination). **4** This is conferred by the injection of antibodies already prepared in another host.

Client Need: Health Promotion and Maintenance; **Cognitive Level:** Comprehension; **Nursing Process:** Assessment/Analysis; **Reference:** Ch 27, Adaptation to Extrauterine Life

265. **3** The increased pulmonary blood flow raises the pressure in the left atrium, functionally forcing the septum to close the foramen ovale.

1 There is an increased aortic blood flow. **2** This is caused by increased pressure in the left atrium. **4** There is decreased pressure in the right atrium.

Client Need: Health Promotion and Maintenance; **Cognitive Level:** Application; **Nursing Process:** Assessment/Analysis; **Reference:** Ch 27, Adaptation to Extrauterine Life

266. **4** There is anatomic obliteration of the lumen by fibrous proliferation, leading to the term ligamentum arteriosum.

1 There is no such ligament. **2** This refers to the ductus venosus after it closes. **3** This is a descriptive term meaning a long and round ligament.

Client Need: Health Promotion and Maintenance; **Cognitive Level:** Application; **Nursing Process:** Assessment/Analysis; **Reference:** Ch 27, Adaptation to Extrauterine Life

267. **3** A quiet, alert state is an optimum time for infant stimulation.

1 Physical assessment is not the priority and can be delayed. **2** Bright lights are disturbing to newborns and may impede mother-child interaction. **4** This position is used for the sleeping infant; increased stimulation and interaction are appropriate when the infant is alert.

Client Need: Psychosocial Integrity; **Cognitive Level:** Application; **Integrated Process:** Teaching/Learning; **Nursing Process:** Planning/Implementation; **Reference:** Ch 27, Parent-Infant Relationships

268. **1** The heart rate is vital for life and is the most critical observation in Apgar scoring.

2 Respiratory effort rather than rate is included in the Apgar score; the rate is very erratic. **3** This may or may not be present at this time and is not a part of Apgar scoring. **4** This is not a part of Apgar scoring, but should be assessed later.

Client Need: Reduction of Risk Potential; **Cognitive Level:** Analysis; **Nursing Process:** Assessment/Analysis; **Reference:** Ch 27, Adaptation to Extrauterine Life

269. **4** This sequence is least disturbing. Touching with the stethoscope and inserting the thermometer increase anxiety and elevate vital signs.

1 Measuring the respirations should precede heart rate measurement because the vital signs will change when the baby is touched. **2** Temperature should be measured last. **3** Respirations should be measured first, but temperature should be measured after the heart rate.

Client Need: Health Promotion and Maintenance; **Cognitive Level:** Application; **Nursing Process:** Assessment/Analysis; **Reference:** Ch 27, Nursing Care Common to Newborns

270. **3** The newborn's heart rate varies with activity; crying can increase it to 180 beats/min, whereas deep sleep may lower it to 80 to 100 beats/min; a rate between 110 and 160 beats/min is average.

1, 2 The heart rate of an alert, noncrying newborn that is above 160 beats/min indicates tachycardia. **4** The heart rate of an alert newborn that is below 110 beats/min indicates bradycardia.

Client Need: Health Promotion and Maintenance; **Cognitive Level:** Comprehension; **Nursing Process:** Assessment/Analysis; **Reference:** Ch 27, Adaptation to Extrauterine Life

271. **2** The initial response is a reflection of the startle reflex; when the stimulus is repetitive, the response to the stimulus decreases; this decrease in response by the neonate is called habituation and is expected.

1 The infant is responding to noise and therefore hears. **3, 4** This is not necessary because the neonate's response is expected.

Client Need: Health Promotion and Maintenance; **Cognitive Level:** Application; **Nursing Process:** Planning/Implementation; **Reference:** Ch 27, Adaptation to Extrauterine Life

272. 1 ☒ Full-term neonates have a flexed fetal position, which provides heat conservation.
2 ☐ Insulin is not stored in the liver and is not involved with maintaining neonatal body temperature.
3 ☒ Brown fat starts being deposited at 28 weeks' gestation and is innervated by the sympathetic nervous system; when the body becomes cool, the sympathetic nervous system stimulates the breakdown of brown fat, which releases heat as a byproduct.
4 ☒ Peripheral vasoconstriction helps conserve heat by keeping the central core warm and not allowing heat to dissipate.
5 ☐ The sympathetic, not parasympathetic, nervous system is involved in thermoregulation.

Client Need: Health Promotion and Maintenance; **Cognitive Level:** Analysis; **Nursing Process:** Assessment/Analysis; **Reference:** Ch 27, Adaptation to Extrauterine Life

273. 4 The healthy newborn's breathing is abdominal and irregular in rhythm and depth (alternates between shallow and deep); the rate ranges from 30 to 60 breaths/min.
1 Newborns' respirations are abdominal.
2 Newborns' respirations usually are irregular.
3 Newborns' respirations are irregular and abdominal in origin.

Client Need: Health Promotion and Maintenance; **Cognitive Level:** Application; **Nursing Process:** Assessment/Analysis; **Reference:** Ch 27, Adaptation to Extrauterine Life

274. 2 Cyanosis, choking, and coughing denote aspiration and hypoxia, for which suctioning and oxygenation are needed.
1 Crying could add to the infant's distress. 3 The water could be aspirated and intensify the infant's problems. 4 The infant is showing signs of a blocked airway; the priority action is to stop the feeding, suction the airway, and then oxygenate the infant before trying to restart the feeding.

Client Need: Physiological Adaptation; **Cognitive Level:** Application; **Nursing Process:** Planning/Implementation; **Reference:** Ch 27, Adaptation to Extrauterine Life

275. 1 To maintain a patent airway and promote respiration and gaseous exchange, mucus must be removed.
2 If the airway is obstructed, O_2 will be of no use.
3 Documentation is important, but secondary to clearing a passageway for air. 4 This is for aspirating the stomach contents, not for airway clearance.

Client Need: Physiological Adaptation; **Cognitive Level:** Application; **Nursing Process:** Planning/Implementation; **Reference:** Ch 27, Nursing Care Common to Newborns

276. 3 The Moro reflex is a sudden extension and abduction of the arms at the shoulders and spreading of the fingers, with the index finger and thumb forming the letter "C"; this is followed by flexion and adduction; the infant may cry vigorously.
1 This is only part of the normal Moro response; it should be accompanied by abduction and spreading of the fingers, followed by flexion.
2 The reflex is abduction, followed by adduction.
4 The legs generally flex weakly.

Client Need: Health Promotion and Maintenance; **Cognitive Level:** Comprehension; **Nursing Process:** Assessment/Analysis; **Reference:** Ch 27, Nursing Care Common to Newborns

277. 1 Milia occur commonly, are not indicative of any illness, and eventually disappear.
2 Lanugo is fine, downy hair. 3 This is a lay term for milia; it would not be used when documenting. 4 These are bluish-black areas on the buttocks that may be present on darkly pigmented infants.

Client Need: Health Promotion and Maintenance; **Cognitive Level:** Application; **Nursing Process:** Assessment/Analysis; **Reference:** Ch 27, Nursing Care Common to Newborns

278. 4 The tonic neck reflex (fencing position) is a spontaneous postural reflex of the newborn; it persists until the third month.
1 The Moro reflex is exhibited when a sudden change in equilibrium causes extension and abduction of the extremities followed by flexion and adduction. 2 The grasp reflex is exhibited when an infant's fingers flex around another person's finger when it is placed in the infant's palm.
3 The Babinski reflex is exhibited when the infant's toes separate and flare out when the examiner runs a finger up the middle undersurface of the infant's foot.

Client Need: Health Promotion and Maintenance; **Cognitive Level:** Application; **Nursing Process:** Assessment/Analysis; **Reference:** Ch 27, Nursing Care Common to Newborns

279. 3 Bacteria, especially *Escherichia coli*, produce substances necessary to synthesize prothrombin.
1 This is an orange bile pigment produced by the breakdown of hemoglobin. 2 Bile salts are manufactured in the liver, not synthesized by bacteria. 4 This is secreted by the gastric glands, not synthesized by bacteria.

Client Need: Health Promotion and Maintenance; **Cognitive Level:** Application; **Nursing Process:** Assessment/Analysis; **Reference:** Ch 27, Adaptations to Extrauterine Life

280. 1 In 36 to 48 hours the newborn will have ingested an ample amount of the amino acid phenylalanine, which, if not metabolized because of a lack of a specific liver enzyme, can result in excess levels of phenylalanine in the bloodstream and brain, resulting in mental retardation; early detection is essential to prevent this.
2 The infant will have a vitamin K injection soon after birth to prevent bleeding problems.
3 Heelsticks are done soon after birth to rule out hypoglycemia; heelsticks are not related to a 36- to 48-hour delay after birth. 4 The infant will

demonstrate clinical signs that suggest necrotizing enterocolitis at any time and are not related to a 36-hour intake of formula.
Client Need: Reduction of Risk Potential; **Cognitive Level:** Application; **Integrated Process:** Teaching/Learning; **Nursing Process:** Planning/Implementation; **Reference:** Ch 27, Adaptation to Extrauterine Life

281. **2** Phenylalanine is an essential amino acid necessary for growth that may be absent in infants with PKU; testing is done on all newborns.
1 Untreated PKU can lead to retardation; the test will not identify retardation. **3** PKU is a genetic, not a chromosomal, disorder. **4** This is done at the same time as PKU testing, but thyroid deficiency does not lead to PKU.
Client Need: Reduction of Risk Potential; **Cognitive Level:** Application; **Integrated Process:** Teaching/Learning; **Nursing Process:** Planning/Implementation; **Reference:** Ch 27, Adaptation to Extrauterine Life

282. **2** Hypoglycemia causes central nervous system and sympathetic nervous symptom responses.
1, 3, 4 These are not signs of this problem.
Client Need: Physiological Adaptation; **Cognitive Level:** Application; **Nursing Process:** Assessment/Analysis; **Reference:** Ch 27, Adaptation to Extrauterine Life

283. **1** There is a sensitive period in the first minutes or hours after birth during which it is important, for later interpersonal development, that the mother and father have close contact with their new infant.
2 Rooming-in may not be instituted immediately after birth. **3** Taking-in is a maternal psychologic behavior described by Reva Rubin that occurs during the first 2 postpartum days. **4** Taking-hold is a maternal psychologic behavior described by Reva Rubin that occurs after the third postpartum day.
Client Need: Psychosocial Integrity; **Cognitive Level:** Comprehension; **Nursing Process:** Assessment/Analysis; **Reference:** Ch 27, Parent-Infant Relationships

284. **4** Some maternal oxytocin crosses the placenta and induces the secretion of fluids that have accumulated in the fetal breasts (sometimes called "witch's milk").
1 This usually is manifested in the oral mucosa as thrush (white, adherent patches). **2** Evidence of infection would not appear so rapidly after birth. **3** This is uncommon and usually undetectable in the newborn period.
Client Need: Health Promotion and Maintenance; **Cognitive Level:** Application; **Integrated Process:** Teaching/Learning; **Nursing Process:** Planning/Implementation; **Reference:** Ch 27, Nursing Care Common to Newborns

285. **2** Teaching the mother by example is a nonthreatening approach that allows her to proceed at her own pace.
1 Mothers need demonstration of appropriate mothering skills, not just a discussion. **3** Learning does not occur by schedule; questions must be answered as they arise. **4** Although emotional

support is required, the plan should encourage independent caregiving.
Client Need: Health Promotion and Maintenance; **Cognitive Level:** Application; **Integrated Process:** Teaching/Learning; **Nursing Process:** Planning/Implementation; **Reference:** Ch 27, Nursing Care Common to Newborns

286. **2** The antibodies in human milk provide the infant with immunity against all or most of the pathogens that the mother has encountered.
1, 3 These are present in commercial formulas. **4** Complex carbohydrates are not required by the infant.
Client Need: Health Promotion and Maintenance; **Cognitive Level:** Application; **Integrated Process:** Teaching/Learning; **Nursing Process:** Planning/Implementation; **Reference:** Ch 27, Adaptation to Extrauterine Life

287. **1** ☒ These infants have low glycogen stores.
2 ☐ These infants usually have no problem with hypoglycemia.
3 ☒ After prolonged exposure to high circulating glucose levels while in utero, hyperplasia of the pancreas occurs, resulting in hyperinsulinemia.
4 ☒ Same as answer 1.
5 ☒ These infants are prone to hyperinsulinemia; often they have mothers who have diabetes, which exposes them to high circulating glucose levels while in utero.
6 ☐ These infants are not at risk for developing hypoglycemia.
Client Need: Physiological Adaptation; **Cognitive Level:** Analysis; **Nursing Process:** Assessment/Analysis; **Reference:** Ch 27, Adaptation to Extrauterine Life

288. **3** The congenital absence of a blood vessel in the umbilical cord is often associated with life-threatening congenital anomalies.
1 If the Apgar score 5 minutes later showed marked improvement, there would be no need for placing the infant in the ICU. **2** This is the average weight for a full-term newborn. **4** The fetus may have swallowed some amniotic fluid; this is not unusual or dangerous.
Client Need: Physiological Adaptation; **Cognitive Level:** Analysis; **Nursing Process:** Assessment/Analysis; **Reference:** Ch 27, Nursing Care Common to Newborns

289. **1** The Apgar score is 5. Weak cry = 1; heart rate of 90 bpm = 1; some flexion of extremities = 1; grimacing = 1; and acrocyanosis = 1.
2, 3, 4 This score is too high.
Client Need: Reduction of Risk Potential; **Cognitive Level:** Analysis; **Nursing Process:** Assessment/Analysis; **Reference:** Ch 27, Adaptation to Extrauterine Life

290. **4** This is related to neonatal morbidity and mortality; by 5 minutes the healthy neonate is relatively stable and requires routine care.
1 The diagnosis of cerebral palsy is not related to the Apgar score. **2** Genetic defects may or may not be apparent at this time. They are not related to the Apgar score. **3** This has not been proven, although research continues in this area.

Client Need: Reduction of Risk Potential; **Cognitive Level:** Application; **Nursing Process:** Evaluation/Outcomes; **Reference:** Ch 27, Adaptation to Extrauterine Life

291. 2 The baby's Apgar score (7/9) does not indicate a need for O_2.

1 This is an important part of record keeping for all newborns. 3 All newborns are evaluated immediately. 4 Poor thermoregulation necessitates keeping the baby warm to stabilize body temperature.

Client Need: Reduction of Risk Potential; **Cognitive Level:** Application; **Nursing Process:** Planning/Implementation; **Reference:** Ch 27, Nursing Care Common to Newborns

292. 4 If the woman perceives a negative viewpoint about breastfeeding from significant others, she may be tense and the let-down may not occur; a positive attitude from significant others toward breastfeeding promotes relaxation and the let-down reflex.

1, 2 This has no influence on lactation. 3 Milk or milk product intake during pregnancy has little influence on lactation.

Client Need: Psychosocial Integrity; **Cognitive Level:** Application; **Nursing Process:** Assessment/Analysis; **Reference:** Ch 27, Breastfeeding, Data Base

293. 2 Some mothers will respond to mores and pressures by trying to breastfeed in spite of the fact that they would prefer to formula-feed. The nurse should elicit more information before responding.

1 This is false reassurance; successful breastfeeding requires mastery, and some women have great difficulty. 3 Although this is true, the mother's statement indicates some concerns about breastfeeding that should be explored further. 4 The baby's suckling and emptying the breasts will determine the amount of milk produced.

Client Need: Psychosocial Integrity; **Cognitive Level:** Application; **Integrated Process:** Caring, Teaching/Learning; **Nursing Process:** Planning/Implementation; **Reference:** Ch 27, Breastfeeding, Nursing Care

294. 3 Most average-sized babies regulate themselves on an approximate 3- to 4-hour schedule. However, wide variations do exist.

1 Some of the episodes of crying do not indicate that the baby is hungry; the mother will learn the difference. 2 It is best to allow the baby to set the schedule. 4 Although this is true, this does not answer the mother's question concerning when she will have free time.

Client Need: Health Promotion and Maintenance; **Cognitive Level:** Application; **Integrated Process:** Teaching/Learning; **Nursing Process:** Planning/Implementation; **Reference:** Ch 27, Breastfeeding, Nursing Care

295. 2 Breastfeeding by a mother with hepatitis C is contraindicated to limit the transmission of infection.

1 Breastfeeding by a mother with mastitis is not always contraindicated; the baby already has the organism in the mouth. 3 Breastfeeding is not contraindicated with inverted nipples, because a breast shield can provide mild suction to help evert a nipple. 4 Breastfeeding is not always contraindicated with this disorder.

Client Need: Safety and Infection Control; **Cognitive Level:** Application; **Integrated Process:** Teaching/Learning; **Nursing Process:** Planning/Implementation; **Reference:** Ch 27, Breastfeeding, Data Base

296. 3 Air-drying nipples after feedings limits irritation and disruption of skin integrity.

1 Application of soap to breast tissue may result in drying and cracking. 2 Wearing a brassiere continuously, except for bathing, is recommended for 2 to 3 weeks postpartum to provide support to breast tissue structures. 4 Plastic liners trap moisture against tissue and may cause skin breakdown.

Client Need: Health Promotion and Maintenance; **Cognitive Level:** Application; **Integrated Process:** Teaching/Learning; **Nursing Process:** Evaluation/Outcomes; **Reference:** Ch 27, Breastfeeding, Nursing Care

297. 3 Frequently the emotional excitement of going home will diminish lactation and/or the let-down reflex for a brief period. When the mother is aware that this may happen and knows how to cope with it, the problem is apt to be a minor one and easily overcome.

1 This is false reassurance. Many factors (stresses) inhibit lactation, and the client should be aware of this. 2 This is false reassurance. This supply may diminish or stop under stress. 4 This response lacks an explanation of why it happens as well as concrete instructions for remedying the situation.

Client Need: Health Promotion and Maintenance; **Cognitive Level:** Application; **Integrated Process:** Teaching/Learning; **Nursing Process:** Planning/Implementation; **Reference:** Ch 27, Breastfeeding, Nursing Care

298. 4 Soap irritates, cracks, and dries breasts and nipples, making it painful for the mother when the baby sucks.

1 The client should empty the breasts at each feeding to keep milk flowing. 2 This is a permissible and often-used technique of breastfeeding. 3 The breasts should be washed with water before feeding to remove encrustations and microorganisms.

Client Need: Safety and Infection Control; **Cognitive Level:** Application; **Integrated Process:** Teaching/Learning; **Nursing Process:** Evaluation/Outcomes; **Reference:** Ch 27, Breastfeeding, Nursing Care

299. 4 More frequent breastfeeding stimulates more frequent evacuation of meconium, thus preventing resorption of bilirubin into the circulatory system.

1 Phototherapy is the treatment for hyperbilirubinemia and it is maintained continuously; it does not prevent the development of hyperbilirubinemia. 2 Early feeding tends to keep the bilirubin level low by stimulating GI activity.

3 Increasing water intake does not limit the development of hyperbilirubinemia because only small amounts of bilirubin are excreted by the kidneys.
Client Need: Basic Care and Comfort; **Cognitive Level:** Application; **Nursing Process:** Planning/Implementation; **Reference:** Ch 27, Breastfeeding, Data Base

300. **2** Breast milk is digested faster than formula; therefore breastfed newborns become hungry sooner.
1 A newborn may want to nurse hourly if irritable, but this is not a usual feeding pattern. **3** A breastfed newborn must be fed more often than this. **4** All newborns must be fed more often than this.
Client Need: Basic Care and Comfort; **Cognitive Level:** Application; **Integrated Process:** Teaching/Learning; **Nursing Process:** Planning/Implementation; **Reference:** Ch 27, Breastfeeding, Nursing Care

301. **1** When the breast is pushed into the infant's mouth, a typical response is for the mouth to close too soon, resulting in inadequate latching-on.
2 This facilitates latching-on and maintains the infant's head in correct alignment, which promotes sucking and swallowing. **3** This will stimulate the rooting reflex and promote latching-on. **4** This prevents trauma to the nipple when removing the infant from the breast.
Client Need: Basic Care and Comfort; **Cognitive Level:** Application; **Integrated Process:** Teaching/Learning; **Nursing Process:** Evaluation/Outcomes; **Reference:** Ch 27, Breastfeeding, Nursing Care

302. **2** Infants require about 73 mL of fluid per pound and 60 calories a day per pound for growth. The infant's weight of 6 lb × 73 mL of fluid = 438 mL. If fed every 4 hours the infant will have 6 feedings; 438 ÷ 6 = 73 mL; 73 ÷ 30 (30 mL/oz) = 2.4 oz. Therefore the infant should be given 2 to 3 oz per feeding.
1 This amount of formula is inadequate for this newborn. **3, 4** This amount of formula is excessive for this newborn.
Client Need: Basic Care and Comfort; **Cognitive Level:** Analysis; **Nursing Process:** Planning/Implementation; **Reference:** Ch 27, Formula Feeding, Nursing Care

303. **4** Cow's milk is more difficult to digest because it is meant to meet the calf's, not the infant's, nutritional needs. It is not recommended until after the infant is 1 year old.
1 Cow's milk contains more protein and more calcium. **2** Cow's milk contains more protein and fewer carbohydrates. **3** Cow's milk contains more calcium.
Client Need: Health Promotion and Maintenance; **Cognitive Level:** Application; **Integrated Process:** Teaching/Learning; **Nursing Process:** Planning/Implementation; **Reference:** Ch 27, Formula Feeding; Data Base

304. 1, 4, 3, 2,
_____1_____ Repositioning the newborn's head may open the airway.
_____4_____ Reapplying the mask may create a better seal when the bag is compressed again.

_____3_____ Checking for secretions and suctioning, if necessary, will clear the airway of obstructions.
_____2_____ Opening the mouth slightly reduces resistance to the positive pressure of the air being ventilated; newborns breathe through the nose, and if an obstruction is present, they do not know how to breathe through the mouth.
Client Need: Physiological Adaptation; **Cognitive Level:** Analysis; **Nursing Process:** Planning/Implementation; **Reference:** Ch 27, Respiratory Distress Syndrome, Nursing Care

305. **1** RhoGAM must be given within 72 hours postpartum if the client has not been sensitized previously, irrespective of the length of the gestation.
2 It would be useless at this time because antibodies have been produced already. **3** RhoGAM is always indicated at the termination of a pregnancy, even with fetal demise. **4** RhoGAM is always indicated at the termination of a pregnancy, even with a short-term pregnancy.
Client Need: Pharmacological and Parenteral Therapies; **Cognitive Level:** Application; **Nursing Process:** Planning/Implementation; **Reference:** Ch 27, Hemolytic Disorders, Data Base

306. **4** ABO incompatibility is the issue because the mother is O and the infant is B; incompatibility can cause jaundice within the first 24 hours.
1 The information provided does not indicate neonatal sepsis. **2** Rh incompatibility is not a factor because the mother is Rh-positive. **3** Jaundice in the first 24 hours is not physiologic; it is pathologic.
Client Need: Physiological Adaptation; **Cognitive Level:** Analysis; **Nursing Process:** Assessment/Analysis; **Reference:** Ch 27, Hemolytic Disorders, Data Base

307. **2** The infant's age is critical because the development of jaundice before 24 to 48 hours after birth may indicate a blood dyscrasia requiring immediate investigation. Jaundice occurring between 48 and 72 hours after birth (physiologic jaundice) is a consequence of the expected breakdown of fetal red cells and immaturity of the liver.
1 Unless the jaundice was pathologic (occurring in the first 24 hours of life), this is not necessary. **3** First, the age of the infant must be ascertained to determine if this is physiologic or pathologic jaundice; then, the nurse should perform a heelstick to determine the amount of bilirubin in the blood. **4** Bilirubin studies would be done first to determine whether the amount of bilirubin present warranted phototherapy.
Client Need: Health Promotion and Maintenance; **Cognitive Level:** Application; **Nursing Process:** Assessment/Analysis; **Reference:** Ch 27, Hemolytic Disorders, Data Base

308. **1** RhoGAM will prevent sensitization from Rh incompatibility that may arise between an Rh-negative mother and an Rh-positive infant.
2 There is no incompatibility; incompatibility might occur if the mother was O positive and the infant

had type A, B, or AB blood. **3** This is unnecessary because only the mother's and infant's Rh factors are relevant. **4** This is unnecessary.
Client Need: Pharmacological and Parenteral Therapies; **Cognitive Level:** Application; **Nursing Process:** Planning/ Implementation; **Reference:** Ch 27, Hemolytic Disorders, Nursing Care

309. **4** Development of jaundice in the first 24 hours indicates hemolytic disease of the newborn.
1 This may or may not be present during the first 24 hours; usually it develops later. **2** These may or may not be present during the first 24 hours; they are dependent on the bilirubin level. **3** Serum bilirubin normally accumulates in the neonatal period because of the short life span of fetal erythrocytes, reaching levels of 7 mg/ 100 mL the second to third day, when jaundice appears.
Client Need: Health Promotion and Maintenance; **Cognitive Level:** Application; **Nursing Process:** Assessment/Analysis; **Reference:** Ch 27, Hemolytic Disorders, Data Base

310. **2** This is the sign that differentiates between these two conditions; cephalohematoma does not extend beyond the suture line.
1 Pain usually is not associated with either condition. **3** This is unusual; it usually decreases in size. **4** Bruising can occur with either condition.
Client Need: Health Promotion and Maintenance; **Cognitive Level:** Analysis; **Nursing Process:** Assessment/Analysis; **Reference:** Ch 27, Cranial Birth Injuries, Data Base

311. **4** A rapid birth does not give the fetal head adequate time for molding, so pressure against the head is increased.
1, 3 This results from excessive pulling on the head and shoulders during birth. **2** This is more likely to occur in a footling breech delivery.
Client Need: Physiological Adaptation; **Cognitive Level:** Analysis; **Nursing Process:** Evaluation/Outcomes; **Reference:** Ch 27, Cranial Birth Injuries, Data Base

312. **4** Intracranial bleeding may occur in the subdural, subarachnoid, or intraventricular spaces of the brain, causing pressure on vital centers; clinical signs are related to the area and degree of cerebral involvement.
1 This is caused by hypocalcemia; it is manifested by exaggerated muscular twitching. **2** This is an obvious defect of the spinal column; it is easily recognized. **3** Elevated potassium level causes cardiac irregularities.
Client Need: Physiological Adaptation; **Cognitive Level:** Application; **Nursing Process:** Assessment/Analysis; **Reference:** Ch 27, Cranial Birth Injuries, Nursing Care

313. **4** With Erb-Duchenne paralysis there is damage to spinal nerves C5 and C6, which causes paralysis of the arm.
1 The grasp reflex is intact because the fingers usually are not affected; if C8 is injured, paralysis of the hand results (Klumpke's paralysis).
2 There would be a negative Moro reflex only

on the affected side. **3** There is no interference with turning of the head; usually injury results from excessive lateral flexion of the head as the shoulder is born.
Client Need: Physiological Adaptation; **Cognitive Level:** Application; **Nursing Process:** Evaluation/Outcomes; **Reference:** Ch 27, Neuromusculoskeletal Birth Injuries, Data Base

314. **2** Gentle massage and manipulation of the muscles help prevent contractures.
1 This would be dangerous because it would lead to permanent contractures. **3** The length of the arm will not change on a daily basis. **4** Passive range-of-motion exercises should be delayed for 10 days to prevent additional injury to the brachial plexus.
Client Need: Reduction of Risk Potential; **Cognitive Level:** Application; **Integrated Process:** Teaching/Learning; **Nursing Process:** Planning/Implementation; **Reference:** Ch 27, Neuromusculoskeletal Birth Injuries, Nursing Care

315. **4** The brachial plexus is injured by excessive pressure during a difficult birth or during a vaginal breech birth.
1 Erb's palsy is an injury that occurs during the process of birth; it is not acquired before or after birth. **2** Erb's palsy is a birth injury, not a genetic problem. **3** Erb's palsy is a birth injury to nervous tissue, not a tumor arising from muscle tissue.
Client Need: Physiological Adaptation; **Cognitive Level:** Application; **Nursing Process:** Assessment/Analysis; **Reference:** Ch 27, Neuromusculoskeletal Birth Injuries, Data Base

316. **4** Injury to the brachial plexus, clavicle, or humerus prevents abduction and adduction movements of an upper extremity.
1 Children with Down syndrome exhibit a normal Moro reflex. **2** This frequently is not associated; however, if the cochlea were undeveloped or the eighth cranial (vestibulocochlear) nerve were injured, it would affect equilibrium and response to the test. **3** These injuries usually cause a symmetric loss of the Moro reflex.
Client Need: Physiological Adaptation; **Cognitive Level:** Application; **Nursing Process:** Assessment/Analysis; **Reference:** Ch 27, Neuromusculoskeletal Birth Injuries, Nursing Care

317. **3** Opiate withdrawal affects the CNS and respiratory system.
1 These may occur in a newborn with thyroid deficiency. **2** These may indicate that the newborn is experiencing cold or respiratory distress. **4** These may occur in a newborn affected with syphilis.
Client Need: Physiological Adaptation; **Cognitive Level:** Application; **Nursing Process:** Assessment/Analysis; **Reference:** Ch 27, Substance Dependence, Nursing Care

318. **2** As the opioid is cleared from the body, signs of withdrawal become evident. Tremors, irritability, difficulty sleeping, twitching, and convulsions result.
1 Dehydration is secondary to poor feeding; it is not a direct result of withdrawal. **3** Hypertonicity of muscles occurs. **4** Drug withdrawal involves signs of excessive stimulation.

Client Need: Physiological Adaptation; **Cognitive Level:** Application; **Nursing Process:** Assessment/Analysis; **Reference:** Ch 27, Substance Dependence, Nursing Care

319. 1 This conjunctivitis occurs about 3 to 4 days after birth; if it is not treated with an antibiotic, chronic follicular conjunctivitis with conjunctival scarring will occur.

2 AIDS in the newborn does not manifest itself with conjunctivitis. 3 High O_2 concentrations given to severely compromised preterm infants cause vasoconstriction of retinal capillaries, which can lead to blindness; there are no data to indicate that this infant was preterm or severely compromised. 4 This chemical conjunctivitis occurs within the first 48 hours and is not purulent.

Client Need: Physiological Adaptation; **Cognitive Level:** Analysis; **Nursing Process:** Assessment/Analysis; **Reference:** Ch 27, Ophthalmia Neonatorum, Data Base

320. 2 *Chlamydia trachomatis* is associated with the development of pneumonia in the newborn.

1 This would be done eventually; the priority is to monitor for signs of pneumonia. 3 Purulent conjunctivitis at this time suggests a *Chlamydia* infection, not an allergic response. 4 This requires an order; bathing the eyes with a solution will not stop the infection; the infant should receive antibiotic therapy.

Client Need: Physiological Adaptation; **Cognitive Level:** Analysis; **Nursing Process:** Assessment/Analysis; **Reference:** Ch 27, Ophthalmia Neonatorum, Data Base

321. 3 Because physical signs of congenital syphilis are difficult to detect at birth, the infant should be screened immediately to determine if treatment is necessary.

1 This defect occurs in the first trimester; *Treponema pallidum* does not affect a fetus before the 16th week of gestation. 2 This is found in children with Down syndrome, not congenital syphilis. 4 This does not manifest in the infant with congenital syphilis until about 3 months of age.

Client Need: Reduction of Risk Potential; **Cognitive Level:** Application; **Nursing Process:** Planning/Implementation; **Reference:** Ch 27, Syphilis, Nursing Care

322. 3 Because neonates are unable to shiver, they use the breakdown of brown fat to supply body heat; the preterm infant has a limited supply of brown fat available for this breakdown.

1 This is not specific to preterm neonates; all newborns are unable to use shivering to supply body heat. 2 The breakdown of glycogen into glucose does not supply body heat. 4 Pituitary hormones do not regulate body heat.

Client Need: Health Promotion and Maintenance; **Cognitive Level:** Application; **Nursing Process:** Assessment/Analysis; **Reference:** Ch 27, Preterm Infant, Data Base

323. 2 The preterm infant has a reduced glomerular filtration rate and reduced ability to concentrate urine or conserve water.

1 All systems of the preterm neonate are less developed than in the full-term neonate. 3 The opposite occurs; urine is very dilute. 4 The fluid and electrolyte balance of preterm infants is easily upset.

Client Need: Health Promotion and Maintenance; **Cognitive Level:** Application; **Nursing Process:** Assessment/Analysis; **Reference:** Ch 27, Preterm Infant, Data Base

324. 3 Immaturity of the respiratory tract in preterm infants can be evidenced by a lack of functional alveoli, smaller lumina with increased possibility of collapse of the respiratory passages, weakness of respiratory musculature, and insufficient calcification of the bony thorax, leading to respiratory distress.

1 This is not a common occurrence at the time of birth unless trauma has occurred. 2 This is not a primary concern unless severe hypoxia occurred during labor; it is difficult to diagnose at this time. 4 This may be a problem, but generally the air passageway is well suctioned at birth.

Client Need: Physiological Adaptation; **Cognitive Level:** Application; **Nursing Process:** Planning/Implementation; **Reference:** Ch 27, Preterm Infant, Data Base

325. 2 The moisture provided by the humidity liquefies the tenacious secretions, making gas exchange possible.

1 They should be positioned side-lying rather than prone; the prone position is associated with apnea and SIDS. 3 Actually the caloric intake is increased; the amount, number, and type of feedings are related to the metabolic rate. 4 This is not a routine action; the concentration of oxygen that is administered depends on the O_2 concentration of the blood gases.

Client Need: Physiological Adaptation; **Cognitive Level:** Application; **Nursing Process:** Planning/Implementation; **Reference:** Ch 27, Preterm Infant, Nursing Care

CHAPTER 29

Foundations of Child Health Nursing

HUMAN GROWTH AND DEVELOPMENT

PRINCIPLES OF GROWTH

A. Children are individuals, not little adults, who must be seen as part of a family
B. Children are influenced by genetic factors, home and environment, parental attitudes, and culture
C. Chronologic and developmental ages of children are the most important contributing factors influencing their care
D. Play is a natural medium for expression, communication, and growth in children
E. Growth is complex, with all aspects closely related
F. Growth is measured both quantitatively and qualitatively over a period of time
G. Although the rate is uneven, growth is a continuous and orderly process
   1. Infancy: most rapid period of growth
   2. Preschool to puberty: slow and uniform rate of growth
   3. Puberty: second most rapid growth period (growth spurt)
   4. After puberty: decline in growth rate until death
H. There are specific principles regarding developmental direction, including the cephalocaudal principle (from head to toe) and the proximodistal principle (from center of body to periphery)
I. Different parts of the body grow at different rates
   1. Prenatally: head grows fastest
   2. During the first year: elongation of trunk dominates
J. Both rate and pattern of growth can be modified, most obviously by nutrition
K. There are critical or sensitive periods in growth and development, such as brain growth during uterine life and infancy
L. Although there are specified sequences for achieving growth and development, each individual proceeds at own rate
M. Development is closely related to the maturation of the nervous system; as primitive reflexes disappear, they are replaced by voluntary activity

CHARACTERISTICS OF GROWTH

Circulatory System
A. Heart rate decreases with increasing age
   1. Infancy: 100 to 180 beats/min
   2. One year: 80 to 150 beats/min
   3. Childhood: 70 to 110 beats/min
   4. Adolescence to adulthood: 55 to 90 beats/min
   5. Specific sites for heart rate assessment include apical, femoral, brachial
B. Blood pressure increases with age
   1. The 50th percentile ranges from 55 to 70 mm Hg diastolic to 100 to 110 mm Hg systolic
   2. These levels increase about 2 to 3 mm Hg per year starting at age 7 years
   3. Systolic pressure in adolescence: higher in males than in females
   4. Appropriate size cuff should be used
C. Hemoglobin
   1. Highest at birth, 17 g/100 mL of blood; then decreases to 10 to 15 g per 100 mL by 1 year
   2. Fetal hemoglobin (60% to 90% of total hemoglobin) gradually decreases during first year to less than 5%
   3. Gradual increase in hemoglobin level to 14.5 g/100 mL between 1 and 12 years of age
   4. Level is higher in males than in females
D. The extracellular body fluid represents 45% at birth, 25% at 2 years of age, and 20% at maturity

Respiratory System
A. Respiratory rate decreases as age increases
   1. Infancy: 30 to 40 breaths beats/min
   2. Childhood: 20 to 24 breaths beats/min
   3. Adolescence and adulthood: 16 to 18 breaths/min
B. Vital capacity
   1. Gradual increase throughout childhood and adolescence, with a decrease in later life
   2. Capacity in males exceeds that in females
C. Basal metabolism
   1. Highest metabolic rate is found in the newborn
   2. Rate declines with increase in age; higher in males than in females

Urinary System
A. Preterm and full-term newborns cannot concentrate urine effectively
   1. Specific gravity (newborn): 1.001 to 1.02
   2. Specific gravity (other age-groups): 1.002 to 1.03
B. Glomerular filtration rate increases rapidly in first 6 months; reaches adult values between 1 and 2 years; gradually decreases after 20 years

Digestive System

A. Stomach size is small at birth; rapidly increases during infancy and childhood

B. Peristaltic activity decreases with advancing age

C. Blood glucose levels gradually rise from 75 to 80 mg/100 mL of blood in infancy to 95 to 100 mg/100 mL during adolescence

D. Preterm infants have lower blood glucose levels than do full-term infants

E. Enzymes are present at birth to digest proteins and a moderate amount of fat but only simple sugars can be digested (amylase is produced as starch is introduced)

F. Secretion of hydrochloric acid and salivary enzymes increases with age until adolescence; then decreases with advancing age

Nervous System

A. Brain reaches 90% of total size by 2 years of age

B. All brain cells are present by end of the first year, although their size and complexity will increase

C. Maturation of brainstem and spinal cord follows cephalocaudal and proximodistal principles

PLAY

FUNCTIONS OF PLAY

A. Educational: teaches about physical world and helps to associate names with objects

B. Recreational: helps to release surplus energy

C. Sensorimotor: stimulates muscle development and tactile, auditory, visual, and kinesthetic senses

D. Social and emotional adjustment: aids in learning moral values; helps to develop the idea of sharing

E. Therapeutic: releases tension and stress; encourages the manipulation of syringes and other equipment, thus allowing control over threatening events

TYPES OF PLAY

A. Type of play is characteristic of developmental level
   1. Infancy: solitary play is one-sided
      a. They explore using their senses; choose with whom to interact
      b. Play provides interpersonal contact; provides recreational and educational stimulation
   2. Toddler: parallel play is characteristic of developmental level
      a. Plays alongside, not with, other children
      b. Less emphasis on exploration of senses
      c. Imitation is a distinguishing characteristic
   3. Preschooler: associative play is characteristic of developmental level
      a. Play occurs in groups; consists of similar or identical activities without rigid organization or rules
      b. Play becomes cooperative and imitative of life in their environment

   4. School age: characterized by increased physical skills, intellectual ability, and fantasy; groups are formed, which help evolve a sense of belonging

B. Active and physical: push-and-pull toys; riding toys; sports and gym equipment

C. Manipulative, constructive, creative, or scientific: blocks; construction toys such as erector sets; drawing sets; microscope and chemistry sets; books; computer programs

D. Imitative, imaginative, and dramatic: dolls; dress-up costumes; puppets

E. Competitive and social: games; role playing

SUITABILITY OF TOYS

Criteria for Judging the Suitability of Toys

A. Safety
   1. Infants, toddlers and all children who put objects in their mouths should not be given toys with small parts that may present choking hazards
   2. Infants should not be given toys with strings or cords that are 18 cm or longer
   3. Safety labels should designate flame retardant/flame resistant, nontoxic
   4. Toys should not be given to children under the recommended age

B. Compatibility: child's age; level of development; experience

C. Usefulness
   1. Challenge to child's development; assist child to achieve mastery
   2. Support social and personality development; increase motor and sensory skills; develop creativity; help express emotions
   3. Implement therapeutic procedures

Criteria for Judging the Unsuitability of Toys

A. Unsafe

B. Beyond the child's level of growth and development; overstimulating; frustrating

C. Foster isolation from peer group

THE FAMILY

STRUCTURE OF THE FAMILY

A. The basic unit of a society

B. Composition varies, although one member is usually recognized as head

C. Usually share common goals and beliefs

D. Roles change within the family and reflect both individual's and family's needs

E. Status of members determined by position in family in conjunction with views of society

FUNCTIONS OF THE FAMILY

A. Reproduction

B. Maintenance to provide

1. Clothing, housing, food, and medical care
2. Social, psychologic, and emotional support for family members
3. Protection: immaturity of young children necessitates that care be given by adults
4. Status: child is member of a family that is also a part of the larger community

C. Socialization
   1. Child is acculturated by introduction to social situations and instruction in appropriate social behaviors
   2. Self-identity develops through relationships with other family members
   3. Child learns appropriate sex roles and responsibilities

D. Growth and development of individual members toward maturity and independence

Nursing Care Related to Meeting the Needs of the Family of a Child With Special Needs

A. Recognize that members of the family will exhibit a variety of responses, such as acute grief and mourning, chronic grief, and excessive use of defense mechanisms

B. Understand the stages of chronic grief
   1. Shock and denial—parents tend to
      a. Learn about the problem but deny the facts
      b. Feel inadequate and guilty
      c. Feel insecure in their ability to care for the child
      d. "Shop for doctors" in hope of finding solutions
   2. Adjustment to special needs—parents tend to
      a. Feel guilty and self-accuse
      b. Envy well children: closely related to bitterness and anger
      c. Search for clues or reasons why this happened to them
      d. Have special feelings toward child: overprotectiveness, rejection, denial; can lead to gradual acceptance
   3. Reintegration and acknowledgment—parents tend to
      a. See the child's special needs in perspective
      b. Function more effectively and realistically
      c. Socially and emotionally accept the child
      d. Reintegrate family life without centering it around the child

C. Help parents and siblings gain awareness of the child's special needs
   1. Learning cannot take place until awareness of the problem exists
   2. Support parents as they develop an awareness through their own realization of the problem, rather than identifying the problem for them

D. Help parents understand their child's potential ability and assist them in setting realistic goals
   1. Enhance the parents' ability to achieve a sense of adequacy in parenting by emphasizing appropriate care, identifying small steps in child's learning progress

   2. Teach family how to stimulate the child's learning of new skills (e.g., sitting, walking, talking, toileting)
   3. Teach parents how to help the child deal with frustration

E. Encourage the parents to treat the child equal to other children within the family
   1. Encourage them to avoid overprotection, to set limits, and to be consistent
   2. Help them become aware of the effects of this child on siblings, who may resent the excessive attention given to this child

F. Provide the family with an outlet for their emotional tensions and needs
   1. Be a listener, not a preacher; explore parental concerns by using interviewing techniques (e.g., reflection, paraphrasing, clarification)
   2. Acquaint the family with organizations, especially groups of parents who have children with similar problems
   3. Assist siblings, who may fear having children with similar problems

G. Teach parents the importance of continued health supervision; provide follow-up nursing care in the home; ensure home visits are convenient for the family

H. Support parents' decisions about extent of health care interventions

I. Evaluate the family's responses and revise plan as necessary

AGE-RELATED REPONSES TO PAIN

INFANT

A. Total body response; arms and legs may tremor
B. Facial expressions: grimaces, surprise, frowns, facial flinching
C. Tense, harsh cry
D. Increase in blood pressure and heart rate, decrease in oxygen saturation

TODDLER

A. Generalized restlessness; guards or rubs painful area
B. Loud crying; uses words to describe pain (e.g., boo-boo, ouch)
C. Tries to delay painful situations

PRESCHOOLER

A. Crying; can describe pain location
B. Regression to earlier stage of development; withdrawal
C. May believe pain is punishment for bad behavior
D. May have been told to be brave and deny pain; fear of injections may contribute to denial of pain
E. May hit or kick caregiver

SCHOOL-AGE CHILD

A. Stiff body posture; withdrawal
B. Able to describe pain
C. Afraid of bodily harm; may delay or bargain to avoid painful situations
D. Recognizes that death exists

ADOLESCENT

A. Increased muscle tension; decreased activity; withdrawal
B. Describes location and intensity of pain
C. Understands cause and effect
D. Perceives pain at physical, emotional, and mental levels

Nursing Care Related to Pain Assessment

A. Use pain rating scales: children's pain is real and must be addressed
   1. Behavioral scales are used for infants, toddlers, and nonverbal children; assess facial expression, leg movement, activity, cry, and consolability (Table 29-1: FLACC Scale)
   2. Face scales can be used for children ages 3 and older; pictures representing facial response to pain progress from "no hurt" to "hurts worst" (Figure 29-1: Faces Pain Rating Scale)
   3. Numerical scales (0 to 5, 0 to 10) should be used for older children and adolescents
B. Address parental concerns about treatment of pain in children
   1. Explore with the parents their perceptions of the child's behavioral responses and their concerns

2. Fear of addiction: clarify differences between physical dependence, tolerance, and addiction in relation to acute pain
3. Fear of respiratory depression: explain that pain is natural antidote to respiratory depressant effects of opiates
4. Fear of adverse effects of opiates such as constipation: explain that side effects are treatable
5. Help parents to understand that physiologic responses do not distinguish between physical responses to pain and other sources of stress to the body

RELATED PHARMACOLOGY—CHILD HEALTH NURSING

Overview

A. Pediatric dosages differ from adult medication dosages as a result of differences in physiology
   1. Immature liver and kidney function
   2. More rapid metabolic rate
   3. Lower plasma protein concentration
   4. Different body composition: less fat; more fluid
B. Most reliable method of calculating dosage is based on body surface area (m^2); ensures that child receives correct dose within a safe therapeutic range
C. Dosage prescribed by practitioner is frequently ordered based on kg of body weight; guideline is manufacturer's recommended daily dose (mg/kg of body weight)
D. IV solutions administered via volume control devices; hourly rate, determined by dividing total volume to be infused by the total number of hours infusion is to run

Table 29-1 FLACC Scale			
	0	1	2
Face	No particular expression or smile	Occasional grimace or frown, withdrawn, disinterested	Frequent to constant frown, clenched jaw, quivering chin
Legs	Normal position or relaxed	Uneasy, restless, tense	Kicking, or legs drawn up
Activity	Lying quietly, normal position, moves easily	Squirming, shifting back and forth, tense	Arched, rigid, or jerking
Cry	No cry (awake or asleep)	Moans or whimpers, occasional complaint	Crying steadily, screams or sobs, frequent complaints
Consolability	Content, relaxed	Reassured by occasional touching, hugging, or talking to; distractible	Difficult to console or comfort

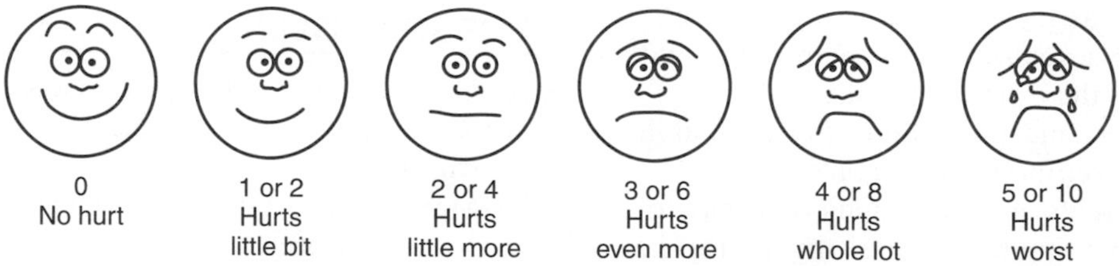

0	1 or 2	2 or 4	3 or 6	4 or 8	5 or 10
No hurt	Hurts little bit	Hurts little more	Hurts even more	Hurts whole lot	Hurts worst

Figure 29-1 Faces Pain Rating Scale. (From Hockenberry M, Wilson D: *Wong's essentials of pediatric nursing*, ed 8, St Louis, 2009, Mosby.)

Nursing Care Related to Administration of Medication to Children

A. Determine amount child should receive (child's weight in kilograms multiplied by the ordered dose per kilogram); assess whether amount ordered is within safe limits for this medication; use ratio and proportion to calculate ordered dose in relation to the amount supplied by the pharmacy

B. Assess child's developmental level to determine whether suspension or pill form can be used; tablets that are not time released or enteric coated may be crushed and mixed with a half teaspoon of pureed fruit

C. Use administration tools to ensure accurate dosage and to minimize loss of medication (e.g., dropper, nipple); infusion pumps should be set at milliliters per hour; secure IV site to prevent dislodgment

D. Give medications as prescribed to maintain therapeutic drug levels

E. Closely monitor child for signs and symptoms of effectiveness, side effects, hypersensitivity reactions, and toxicity

F. Administer ear drops by placing child in side-lying position with affected ear up; pull pinna down and back for child 3 years old or younger because eustachian tube is shorter, wider, and straighter than in adult and this facilitates passage of fluid to the eardrum; pull pinna up and back for children older than 3 years

G. Allow child to manipulate equipment (e.g., syringe, multidose inhaler); demonstrate use of equipment and assess return demonstration

H. Follow procedures for safe administration of medications (e.g., standard precautions, 7 rights, 3 checks, verification of placement of central line before administering medications)

Nursing Care of Infants 30

GROWTH AND DEVELOPMENT

DEVELOPMENTAL TIMETABLE

One Month
A. Physical
 1. Weight: gains about 150 to 210 g (5 to 7 oz) weekly during first 6 months of life
 2. Height: grows about 2.5 cm (1 inch) a month for first 6 months of life
 3. Head circumference: grows about 1.5 cm (½ inch) a month for first 6 months
B. Motor
 1. Assumes flexed position with pelvis high, but knees not under abdomen, when prone
 2. Holds head parallel with body when suspended in prone position
 3. Can turn head from side to side when prone; lifts head momentarily from flat surface
 4. Asymmetric posture dominates, such as tonic neck reflex
 5. Primitive reflexes still present
C. Sensory
 1. Eye movements coordinated most of the time; follows a light to midline
 2. Visual acuity 20/100
D. Socialization and vocalization
 1. Watches face intently while being spoken to
 2. Utters small, throaty sounds

Two to Three Months
A. Physical: posterior fontanel closed
B. Motor
 1. Holds head erect for a short time; can raise chest supported on forearms
 2. Bears some weight on legs when held in standing position
 3. Actively holds rattle but will not reach for it
 4. Grasp, tonic neck, and Moro reflexes are fading; step or dance reflex disappears
 5. Plays with fingers and hands
C. Sensory
 1. Follows a light to the periphery
 2. Has binocular coordination (vertical and horizontal vision)
 3. Listens to sounds
D. Socialization and vocalization
 1. Smiles in response to a person or object; cries less

2. Laughs aloud and shows pleasure in making sounds

Four to Five Months
A. Physical
 1. Birth weight doubles
 2. Drools because salivary glands are functioning; does not have sufficient coordination to swallow saliva
B. Motor
 1. Can sit when back is supported; knees will be flexed and back rounded; can balance head
 2. Symmetric body position predominates
 3. Can sustain a portion of own weight when held in a standing position
 4. Reaches for and grasps an object with the whole hand but misjudges distances
 5. Can move own hand or an object to mouth at will
 6. Can roll over from abdomen to back
 7. Lifts head and shoulders at a 90-degree angle when prone
 8. Primitive reflexes (e.g., grasp, tonic neck, and Moro) have disappeared
C. Sensory
 1. Recognizes familiar objects and people
 2. Has coupled eye movements; accommodation is developing
D. Socialization and vocalization
 1. Coos and gurgles when talked to; enjoys social interaction
 2. Vocalizes displeasure when an object is removed

Six to Seven Months
A. Physical
 1. Weight: gains about 90 to 150 g (3 to 5 oz) weekly during second 6 months of life
 2. Height: grows about 1.25 cm (½ inch) a month
 3. Head circumference: grows about 0.5 cm (⅕ inch) a month
 4. Teething may begin with eruption of two lower central incisors, followed by upper incisors
B. Motor
 1. Can turn over equally from stomach or back
 2. Sits unsupported, especially if placed in a forward-leaning position
 3. Lifts head off table when supine; when lying down, lifts head as if trying to sit up
 4. Can approach a toy and grasp it with one hand; can transfer a toy from one hand to the other and from hand to mouth

5. Plays with feet and puts them in mouth
6. Neurologic reflexes
   a. Landau (from 6 to 8 months to 12 to 24 months): when suspended in a horizontal prone position, the head is raised, legs and spine are extended
   b. Parachute (7 to 9 months, persists indefinitely): when infant is suspended in a horizontal prone position and suddenly thrust forward, hands and fingers extend forward as if to protect from falling
C. Sensory
   1. Has taste preferences; will spit out disliked food
   2. Begins to recognize that things are still present even though they cannot be seen
D. Socialization and vocalization
   1. Begins to differentiate between strange and familiar faces and shows "stranger anxiety"
   2. Makes polysyllabic vowel sounds
   3. Vocalizes "m-m-m-m" when crying; cries easily on slightest provocation but laughs just as quickly

Eight to Nine Months
A. Motor
   1. Sits steadily alone; pulls self to standing position; stands holding onto furniture
   2. Has developed hand-to-mouth coordination
   3. Developing pincer grasp, with preference for use of one hand over the other
   4. Crawls; may go backward at first
B. Sensory
   1. Depth perception is improving
   2. Displays interest in small objects
C. Socialization and vocalization
   1. Definite social attachment is evident (e.g., stretches out arms to loved ones); shows anxiety with strangers (e.g., turns or pushes away and cries)
   2. Responds to own name; is separating self from mother by desire to act on own
   3. Reacts to adult anger; cries when scolded
   4. Has imitative and repetitive speech, using vowels and consonants such as "Dada"; no true words as yet, but comprehends words such as "bye-bye"

Ten to Twelve Months
A. Physical
   1. Weight: birth weight triples
   2. Height: birth length increases by 50%
   3. Head and chest circumference are equal
   4. Upper and lower lateral incisors usually have erupted, for total of 6 to 8 teeth
   5. Hematocrit: 29% to 41%
B. Motor
   1. Creeps (creeping is more advanced than crawling because abdomen is supported off floor)
   2. Stands alone for short times; walks with help; moves around by holding onto furniture ("cruising")
   3. Can sit down from a standing position without help
   4. Can eat from a spoon and a cup but needs help; prefers using fingers

5. Can play pat-a-cake and peek-a-boo; holds a crayon to make a mark on paper
6. Helps in dressing, such as putting arm through sleeve
C. Sensory
   1. Visual acuity 20/50; amblyopia (lazy eye) may develop with lack of binocularity
   2. Discriminates simple geometric forms
D. Socialization and vocalization
   1. Shows emotions such as jealousy, affection, anger
   2. Enjoys familiar surroundings and will explore away from mother
   3. Fearful in strange situations or with strangers; clings to mother
   4. May develop habit of "security" object
   5. Can say two words besides Dada or Mama with meaning; understands simple verbal requests, such as, "Give it to me"

HEALTH PROMOTION OF INFANTS
PLAY DURING INFANCY

A. Primarily narcissistic and revolves around their own body
B. Initially responses are global, largely undifferentiated
C. Initially dependent; then progresses to interdependent and then independent
D. Directed toward physical, motor, sensory, language, cognitive, and personal-social development; peek-a-boo uses the developing ability to understand object permanence
E. Safety is chief determinant in choosing toys (aspirating small objects is one cause of accidental death, no strings or pulls longer than 18 cm)
F. Toys
   1. Mostly used for physical development
   2. Should be simple because of short attention span
   3. Should provide visual, auditory, tactile, and kinetic stimulation
G. Suggested toys: rattles; soft, stuffed toys; mobiles; push-pull toys; simple musical toys; unbreakable mirrors; weighted or suction toys; squeeze toys; teething toys; books with textures; activity boxes; nested boxes and fitting forms

NUTRITION DURING INFANCY

Nutrition in Relation to Growth and Development
A. Nutrition as it affects growth
   1. Birth weight usually doubled by 5 months of age and tripled by 1 year
   2. Growth during the first year should be charted to observe for comparable gain in length, weight, and head circumference
   3. Growth charts demonstrate percentile of child's growth (below 5th and above 95th percentile are outside the norm)

4. Growth curves are observed in relation to deviation from a steady rate of growth, hereditary factors (size and body shape), and height as it compares to weight
5. Satisfactory rate of growth judged by
   a. Weight and length (overweight and underweight constitute malnutrition)
   b. General appearance; muscular development; tissue tone and turgor
   c. Activity level; amount of crying and needed sleep
   d. Mental status and behavior in relation to norms for the age
   e. Presence or absence of illness
B. Optimum feeding essential to growth and development
   1. Diet should promote growth, prevent overweight, and avoid nutritional deficiencies
   2. Gastrointestinal disturbances such as vomiting, diarrhea, or constipation interfere with optimum nutrition despite adequate diet
   3. Appropriate eating habits should be established
   4. Consistency of foods should progress from liquid to semisoft to soft to solids as dentition and the jaw develop

Feeding Milestones

A. At birth the full-term infant has sucking, rooting, and swallowing reflexes
B. Newborn feels hunger and indicates desire for food by crying; expresses satiety by contentedly falling asleep
C. At 1 month has strong extrusion reflex
D. By 5 to 6 months can use fingers to eat teething cracker or toast
E. By 6 to 7 months is developmentally ready to chew solids
F. By 8 to 9 months can hold a spoon and play with it during feeding
G. By 9 months can hold own bottle
H. By 12 months usually can drink from a cup, although fluid may spill and bottle may be preferred at times

Guidelines for Infant Nutrition

A. Breast milk is most complete diet for first 6 months
   1. Requires supplements of iron by 4 to 6 months
   2. Requires fluoride if mother's water supply is not fluoridated
   3. The American Academy of Pediatrics recommends vitamin D supplementation beginning in the first 2 months to prevent rickets
B. Iron-fortified commercial formula is an acceptable alternative to breastfeeding; requires fluoride supplements in areas where fluoride content of drinking water is below 0.3 ppm
C. Breast milk or iron-fortified commercial formula is recommended for the first year of life
D. Whole cow's milk should not be introduced to infants until after 1 year of age; inadequate in iron and vitamin C
E. Solids can be introduced by about 6 months; the first food can be commercially prepared iron-fortified infant cereals; rice cereal is usually introduced first because of its low allergenic potential; infant cereals should be continued until 18 months of age
F. With the exception of infant cereals, the order of introducing other foods is variable; recommended sequence is approximately weekly introduction of one food; vegetables and/or fruits, and then meats
G. First solid foods are strained, puréed, or mashed
H. Finger foods such as toast, teething cracker, or raw fruit are introduced at 6 to 7 months
I. Chopped table food or commercially prepared junior foods can be started by 9 to 12 months
J. Fruit juices should be offered from a cup as early as possible to reduce development of dental caries; juice can be substituted for milk for one feeding each day
K. Method for introducing foods
   1. Feed when infant is hungry, after a few sucks of breast milk or formula
   2. Introduce one food at a time, usually at intervals of 4 to 7 days, to allow for identification of food allergies
   3. Begin spoon feeding by placing food on back of tongue because of infant's natural tendency to thrust tongue forward (extrusion reflex, which begins to fade by 3 to 4 months)
   4. Small spoon with a straight handle should be used; begin with 1 or 2 teaspoons of food; gradually increase to several tablespoons per feeding
   5. As amount of solid food increases, milk should be decreased to approximately 900 mL (30 oz) daily to prevent overfeeding
   6. Foods should not be introduced by mixing them with formula in the bottle
L. Weaning
   1. Giving up bottle or breast for a cup is psychologically significant because it requires the relinquishing of a major source of pleasure
   2. Usually, readiness develops during second half of first year because of pleasure from receiving food by a spoon and desire for more freedom and control over body and the environment
   3. One bottle at a time is gradually replaced with a cup; nighttime bottle is last to be relinquished
   4. If breastfeeding must be terminated before 5 or 6 months of age, a bottle should be used to allow for continued sucking needs; after about 6 months, infant can be weaned directly to a cup

IMMUNIZATIONS

A. Types of immunizations that provide active immunity
   1. Hepatitis B vaccine (Hep B)
      a. Infants receive 3 doses (given at birth to 1 month, 2 months, and 6 months); should be considered for all adolescents not immunized; advised for health care providers because of risk of transmission via needle sticks or exposure to blood
      b. Vaccine is given by IM injection; can be given at same time as diphtheria, tetanus, acellular pertussis (DTaP) but separate sites must be used; vastus lateralis or deltoid muscles are used in

older infants; dorsogluteal site is not used because of low seroconversion rate

2. Hepatitis A vaccine
   a. Recommended for children 1 year of age and older
   b. Two doses administered at least 6 months apart

3. Diphtheria, tetanus, pertussis (DTP)
   a. Diphtheria, tetanus, and acellular pertussis (DTaP): given at 2, 4, and 6 months; fourth dose may be administered as early as 12 months if there is concern that child may not return at 15 months and 6 months have elapsed since previous dose; next dose should be given at ≥4 years of age
   b. Diphtheria toxoid: effective for about 10 years; febrile reaction more commonly seen in older children, so adult type tetanus and diphtheria (Td) toxoid is recommended every 10 years after last booster at 5 years of age; Td is used for any child over the age of 7 who has not been previously immunized
   c. Tetanus toxoid: nearly 100% effective; induces immunity for about 10 years; given at 5-year intervals if there is a possibility of a contaminated wound; tetanus is characterized by severe muscle spasms and is potentially fatal
   d. Pertussis vaccine: started early because there is no passive immunity from mother, as with diphtheria and tetanus; not given after seventh birthday because risk for disease is less than vaccine's side effects

4. Measles (rubeola), mumps, and rubella (German measles) vaccine (MMR)
   a. MMR vaccine (live attenuated vaccine): generally given at 12 months of age because of the presence of natural immunity from mother; a second dose should be administered at 4 to 6 years of age
   b. Not given to any nonimmunized pregnant woman or if pregnancy is suspected because of potential infection of the fetus; pregnancy must be prevented until 3 months after immunization to eliminate danger to fetus
   c. Rubella vaccine: given to prevent its occurrence in women during the first trimester; causes a maculopapular rash
   d. Mumps vaccine: given because mumps may cause sterility in postpubescent males; causes swelling of the parotid glands
   e. Measles causes Koplik's spots on the buccal mucosa; vaccine at this time is ineffective

5. Inactivated polio vaccine (IPV)
   a. Recommended for all children younger than 18 years of age
   b. Infants receive 3 doses (given at 2, 4, and 6 months); fourth dose given at 4 to 6 years of age

   c. Intramuscular polio vaccine preferred because oral polio vaccine is associated with the danger of acquiring vaccine-associated paralysis (VAPP)
   d. Infants/children who are asymptomatic HIV-positive or those with immune deficiencies and their siblings should receive IPV

6. *Haemophilus influenzae* type B vaccine (Hib)
   a. Polysaccharide vaccine given at 2, 4, 6, and 15 months of age; can be given sooner if child is in high-risk category (e.g., child who attends daycare center, is asplenic, or has sickle cell anemia)
   b. DTP can be given at same visit, but a different site should be used

7. Chickenpox vaccine (Varivax)
   a. Children under 12 receive 1 dose; teenagers and adults need 2 doses 4 to 8 weeks apart; given to children at risk and those who will require steroid therapy
   b. Vaccine is 70% to 90% effective in preventing chickenpox and its sequelae, such as encephalitis and thrombocytopenia
   c. Causes malaise and a pruritic rash that begins on the abdomen and progresses to the face and proximal extremities

B. Factors influencing administration of immunizations
   1. The benefit from being protected by the immunization is thought to greatly outweigh the risk from the disease
   2. Presence of maternal antibodies; antibodies received in utero through the placenta and via breast milk if the mother is breastfeeding provide the infant with passive immunity against most viral, bacterial, and fungal infections during the first several weeks of life
   3. Administration of blood transfusion or immune serum globulin within 3 months
   4. High fever, serious illness (common cold is not a contraindication)
   5. Impaired immune system or immunosuppressive therapy in child or family member
   6. Generalized malignancy such as leukemia
   7. Neurologic problems such as seizures after administration of pertussis vaccine
   8. Allergic reaction to a previously administered vaccine or anaphylactic reaction to egg protein

INJURY PREVENTION DURING INFANCY

A. Accidents are one of the leading causes of death during infancy
   1. Mechanical suffocation causes most accidental deaths in children less than 1 year of age
   2. Aspiration of small objects and ingestion of poisonous substances occur most often during second half of the first year and into early childhood

3. Trauma from rolling off a bed or falling down stairs can occur at any time

B. Teaching is an essential aspect of prevention

1. Birth to 4 months
   a. Sudden infant death: place infant to sleep on back; do not use soft, moldable bedding such as pillows and quilts
   b. Aspiration: not as great a danger to this age-group but should begin practicing safeguards early (see 4 to 7 months) (e.g., danger inherent in use of baby powder)
   c. Suffocation
      (1) Keep plastic bags away; do not cover mattress or pillows with soft plastic
      (2) Use a firm mattress; do not use pillows and loose blankets
      (3) Be sure crib design follows regulations and mattress fits snugly
      (4) Keep crib away from other furniture and cords from window blinds
      (5) Do not tie pacifier on string around infant's neck; remove bibs after use
      (6) Never leave infant alone in bath; danger of drowning
   d. Falls
      (1) Always raise crib rails
      (2) Never leave infant on a raised, unguarded surface; when in doubt, use the floor
      (3) Restrain in an infant seat and never leave infant unattended while seat is resting on a raised surface
      (4) Avoid using a high chair until infant is old enough to sit
   e. Poisoning: not as great a danger to this age-group but should begin practicing safeguards early (see 4 to 7 months)
   f. Burns
      (1) Set hot water heater at temperature no greater than 120° F
      (2) Check temperature of bath water and warmed formula and food
      (3) Do not pour hot liquids when infant is nearby, such as sitting on lap
      (4) Keep cigarettes and their ashes away from infant; do not allow smoking in infant's presence
      (5) Do not leave infant in the sun for more than a few minutes; use hats and sunscreens
      (6) Wash flame-retardant clothes according to label directions
      (7) Check surface heat of car restraint; do not leave infant unattended in parked car
   g. Motor vehicles
      (1) Transport infant in a specially constructed rear-facing car seat with appropriate restraints (infants should face the rear from birth to 9070 g [20 lb] or 1 year of age); car seat should always be on rear seat of car,

never in front passenger seat; infant should always be secured in car seat, never on the seat of the car or in an adult's lap
      (2) Do not place a carriage or stroller behind a parked car
   h. Bodily damage: keep sharp, jagged-edged objects away from infant's environment

2. 4 to 7 months
   a. Aspiration
      (1) Keep buttons, beads, and other small objects out of infant's reach; keep floor free of small objects; inspect toys for removable parts
      (2) Obtain pacifier with one-piece construction and loop handle
      (3) Do not feed infant hard candy, nuts, food with pits or seeds, or whole hot dogs; cut foods, such as hot dogs, into small irregularly shaped pieces
      (4) Do not offer balloons as playthings
   b. Suffocation: begin to teach swimming as part of water safety
   c. Falls: restrain in high chair; keep crib rails raised to full height
   d. Poisoning
      (1) Verify that paint for furniture or toys does not contain lead
      (2) Place toxic substances on a high shelf and/or locked cabinet; do not store toxic substances in food containers; avoid storing large quantities of cleaning fluids, paints, pesticides, and other toxic substances; discard used containers of poisonous substances
      (3) Place purses/backpacks on tables or counters where infant cannot reach
      (4) Hang plants or place on a high surface rather than on floor
      (5) Know national toll free telephone number of Poison Control Center (800-222-1222)
   e. Burns
      (1) Always check temperature of bath water and adjust household hot-water temperature to 120° F (49° C) or lower
      (2) Place hot objects (cigarettes, candles, incense) on high surfaces
   f. Motor vehicles: see Birth to 4 months
   g. Bodily damage: avoid long, pointed objects as toys; give toys that are smooth and rounded, made of wood or plastic

3. 8 to 12 months
   a. Aspiration: see 4 to 7 months
   b. Suffocation/drowning
      (1) Keep doors of bathrooms, ovens, dishwashers, refrigerators, and front-loading clothes washers and dryers closed at all times
      (2) If storing or discarding an appliance, such as a refrigerator, remove door

(3) Fence swimming pools; always supervise when near any source of water, including toilets, filled bathtubs, and cleaning buckets

c. Falls: fence stairways at top and bottom if infant has access to either end

d. Poisoning

(1) Administer medications as a drug, not as a candy

(2) Do not administer adult medications unless prescribed by a practitioner

(3) Replace caps to medications and poisons immediately after use; use child protector caps

e. Burns

(1) Place guards in front of any heating appliance, fireplace, or furnace

(2) Keep electrical wires hidden or out of reach; do not allow infant to play with electrical appliances

(3) Use plastic guards in electrical outlets; place furniture in front of outlets

(4) Avoid use of overhanging tablecloths

f. Motor vehicles

(1) Do not use adult seat or shoulder belt without infant car seat

(2) Do not allow infant to crawl behind a parked car

(3) If infant plays in a yard, have yard fenced; use a playpen and provide supervision

g. Bodily damage

(1) Do not allow infant to use a fork for self-feeding; use plastic cups or dishes

(2) Check safety of toys and toy box

(3) Protect from animals, especially dogs

HOSPITALIZATION OF INFANTS

DATA BASE

A. Reactions to parental separation begin later in infancy (see Hospitalization of Toddlers in Chapter 31)

B. Infant recognizes pain but is not emotionally traumatized by intrusive procedures

C. Procedures, such as urinary catheterization, that may have a sexual connotation to older children usually are not emotionally traumatic for infants

D. Appropriate analgesia and sedation should be used for painful procedures to minimize effects of pain

GENERAL NURSING CARE OF INFANTS

A. Assess infant's physical, physiologic, and behavioral responses because infant cannot communicate needs verbally

B. Meet physical and emotional needs immediately to support development of trust

C. Provide nonnutritive sucking to meet oral needs

D. Allow significant others to stay with infant to provide support, particularly when separation anxiety occurs

E. Provide consistent caregivers

HEALTH PROBLEMS PRESENT IN THE INFANT AT BIRTH

FETAL ALCOHOL SYNDROME (FAS)

Data Base

A. Predictable abnormal patterns of fetal and neonatal morphogenesis attributed to severe, chronic alcoholism in women who continue to drink heavily during pregnancy; exact amount of alcohol needed to produce teratogenic effect is unknown

1. Infants may not initially display the dysmorphic facial features; these features become more pronounced with increasing age

2. Syndrome describes full spectrum disorder from mild effects (fetal alcohol effects [FAE]) to more severe neurodevelopmental defects

B. Leading cause of preventable mental retardation

1. Occurs in approximately 0.2 to 1.5 per 1000 live births

2. Women with history of heavy drinking should be informed of risks

3. Women who drink should be made aware of treatment sources to decrease or eliminate alcohol ingestion

C. Clinical findings

1. CDC criteria: growth restriction (prenatal and postnatal); midfacial dysmorphic features; central nervous system (CNS) involvement (structural, neurologic, or functional abnormality)

2. Growth: prenatal growth restriction; persistent postnatal growth lag

3. Neurologic: includes mental retardation, motor retardation, microcephaly, hypotonia; hearing disorders

4. Facial features: includes hypoplastic maxilla, micrognathia, hypoplastic philtrum, short palpebral features

5. Behavior: includes irritability, sleeplessness, inconsolable crying, and feeding difficulties in infants; hyperactivity in children

D. Therapeutic interventions

1. Pharmacologic management depending on severity of CNS dysfunction and withdrawal symptoms

2. Reduction of noxious environmental stimuli

3. Encouragement of infant to achieve self-regulation

4. Provision of IV fluids and nutrients until able to maintain feedings

5. Therapy specific to individualized needs of infant; may be similar to needs of preterm infants

Nursing Care of Alcohol-Exposed Infants

A. Assessment/Analysis

1. Mother's prenatal record indicating alcohol use

2. Growth deficiencies
3. Central nervous system adaptations associated with fetal alcohol syndrome (FAS)
4. Distinctive craniofacial characteristics related to FAS
5. Behaviors related to neonatal abstinence syndrome

B. Planning/Implementation
   1. Monitor vital signs
   2. Be alert for signs of withdrawal
      a. Usually within 6 to 12 hours after birth and persist for about 3 days
      b. Include CNS, GI, respiratory, and autonomic nervous system manifestations
      c. Monitor for seizure activity; protect from injury during a seizure; seizures after the newborn period are rare
   3. Maintain a protective environment
      a. Limit environmental stimuli; keep in quiet, dimly lit room
      b. Provide a warm physical environment
      c. Touch gently and avoid sudden postural changes
      d. Position on side
      e. Have suctioning equipment available to maintain patent airway
   4. Console infant
      a. Encourage parent to engage in "skin-to-skin care"
      b. Use containment devices or swaddle with extremities in a flexed position
      c. Allow hand to mouth activity to promote self-soothing
      d. Provide opportunities for nonnutritive sucking with a pacifier
      e. Provide safe objects for infant to grasp
   5. Provide fluid and nutrients as ordered; breastfeeding is not contraindicated, but excessive alcohol consumption may intoxicate the newborn and inhibit the let-down reflex
      a. Provide time for feedings
      b. Provide frequent, small feedings
      c. Burp infant often during feedings
      d. Elevate head of mattress after feedings
      e. Reinforce positive parenting activities

C. Evaluation/Outcomes
   1. Remains free from injury
   2. Exhibits resolution of withdrawal
   3. Demonstrates ingestion and retention of adequate nutrients
   4. Has consistent weight gain
   5. Parents demonstrate effective infant care

CHROMOSOMAL ABERRATIONS

General Nursing Care of Children With Chromosomal Aberrations

A. Assessment/Analysis
   1. Presence of chromosomal abnormality
   2. Parental perceptions of child

3. Infant's health status; functional limitations; and presence of other congenital abnormalities such as cardiac malformation

B. Planning/Implementation
   1. Provide emotional support to parents
   2. Encourage genetic counseling appropriate for type of problem
   3. Assist parents in setting realistic expectations and goals for their child
   4. Refer for testing of intellectual functioning for guidance to parents
   5. Identify necessary interventions specific to associated congenital malformations
   6. See Planning/Implementation under Nursing Care of Children Who Are Cognitively Impaired in Chapter 31

C. Evaluation/Outcomes
   1. Breathes without difficulty
   2. Maximizes growth and development potential
   3. Communicates needs, feelings, and concerns
   4. Demonstrates behavior indicative of positive self-esteem

TRISOMY 21 (DOWN SYNDROME)

Data Base

A. Types
   1. Free trisomy 21: frequently associated with advanced maternal age (older than 40 years of age); can occur in all age-groups
   2. Translocation 15/21: translocated chromosome transmitted most often by mother, who is a carrier; age not a factor
   3. Mosaicism: mixture of healthy cells and cells that are trisomic for 21; do not necessarily have a better developmental outcome than those with trisomy 21
   4. Often associated with congenital heart defects and respiratory problems

B. Clinical findings
   1. Brachycephaly, flat occiput, broad nose with a depressed bridge (saddle nose)
   2. Inner epicanthic folds and oblique palpebral fissures; speckling of the iris (Brushfield's spots)
   3. Small, sometimes low-set, ears; short, thick neck
   4. Protruding, sometimes fissured, tongue; respiratory problems
   5. Hypotonic musculature (protruding abdomen, umbilical hernia); hyperflexible and lax joints
   6. Broad, short, and stubby hands and feet; one transverse palmar crease
   7. Delayed or incomplete sexual development (men with Down syndrome usually are infertile)
   8. May have a cardiac malformation, respiratory problems, and/or obesity

Nursing Care of Children With Trisomy 21

A. Prevent infection, especially respiratory
B. Assess and monitor cardiac status if cardiac defect is present

C. Provide activity consistent with abilities and limits
D. Provide physical supervision and habilitation
E. See General Nursing Care of Children With Chromosomal Aberrations

TRISOMY 18 (EDWARDS' SYNDROME)

Data Base

A. Types: trisomy; translocation; mosaicism
B. Clinical findings
   1. Deformed and low-set ears; abnormal smallness of the jaws, especially lower jaw (micrognathia); rocker-bottom feet; prominent occiput; webbed neck; short digits
   2. Failure to thrive and short survival; if surviving, severe mental retardation

Nursing Care of Children With Trisomy 18

A. Because of short survival, prepare parents for loss of their child
B. See General Nursing Care of Children With Chromosomal Aberrations

TURNER'S SYNDROME (GONADAL DYSGENESIS)

Data Base

A. Chromosome monosomy (XO karyotype) in females
B. Clinical findings
   1. Congenital malformations such as short stature, webbed neck, coarctation of the aorta, ovarian dysgenesis, and developmental failure of secondary sex characteristics at puberty
   2. Usually average intelligence; problems in directional sense and space-form recognition

Nursing Care of Children With Turner's Syndrome

A. Prepare child for lack of pubertal changes and need for hormonal replacement
B. Counsel with emphasis on adoption rather than on person's inability to conceive
C. See General Nursing Care of Children With Chromosomal Aberrations

KLINEFELTER'S SYNDROME

Data Base

A. Sex-chromosomal abnormality of XXY in males

B. Clinical findings
   1. Physical characteristics: slightly taller than average; long legs and arms; small, firm testes; gynecomastia; and inadequately developed secondary sex characteristics
   2. Average to borderline intelligence

Nursing Care of Children With Klinefelter's Syndrome

A. Counsel with emphasis on positive aspects such as adoption or donor insemination of mate
B. Recognize that emotional problems may require life-long counseling
C. See General Nursing Care of Children With Chromosomal Aberrations

GASTROINTESTINAL MALFORMATIONS

CLEFT LIP (CL) AND CLEFT PALATE (CP)

Data Base

A. Results from incomplete fusion of embryonic structures surrounding the primitive oral cavity (cleft lip) or failure of the primary and secondary palatine plates to fuse (cleft palate) (Figure 30-1: Variations in clefts of lip and palate at birth)
   1. CL: incomplete fusion of maxillary and premaxillary processes; fusion should be completed between 5 and 8 weeks of fetal life
   2. CP: incomplete fusion of palatal structures; may involve soft or hard palate and may extend into nose, forming an oronasal passageway; fusion should be completed between 9 and 12 weeks of fetal life
B. Cause unknown; evidence of hereditary influence
   1. Multifactorial inheritance; increased frequency in relatives; higher incidence in monozygotic twins than in dizygotic twins
   2. CL more common in males; CP more common in females
   3. Linked to maternal nutrition including folic acid deficiency
   4. Linked to prenatal exposure to substances such as phenytoin, valproic acid, thalidomide, and maternal smoking and alcohol ingestion
   5. Occurs with other congenital anomalies

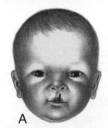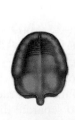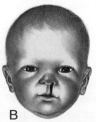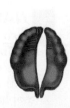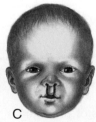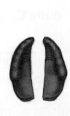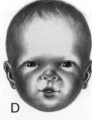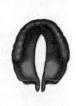

Figure 30-1 Variations in clefts of lip and palate at birth. **A,** Notch in vermillion border. B, Unilateral cleft lip and cleft palate. C, Bilateral cleft lip and cleft palate. D, Cleft palate. (From Hockenberry MJ, Wilson D: *Wong's nursing care of infants and children*, ed 8, St Louis, 2007, Mosby.)

C. Classification
  1. Bilateral or unilateral; if unilateral, more common on left side
  2. Cleft lip can be several degrees; complete cleft usually continuous with cleft palate
D. Related difficulties
  1. Cleft lip
    a. Difficult feeding: infant cannot form vacuum with mouth to suck; may be able to breastfeed (breast may fill cleft, making sucking easier)
    b. Special feeding devices include Cleft Lip/ Cleft Palate Nurser (squeezable plastic bottle and cross-cut nipple) and Haberman Feeder (bottle with valve and nipple; adjusts flow of formula)
    c. Mouth breathing dries mucous membranes, predisposing infant to infection
  2. Cleft palate
    a. Prone to infection, especially otitis media
    b. Altered speech; complete palate needed to trap air in the mouth
    c. Malposition of teeth and maxillary arch; extensive orthodontic and prosthodontics needed to correct
    d. Hearing problems caused by recurrent otitis media (eustachian tube connects nasopharynx and middle ear and transports pathogens to ear)
    e. Requires special feeding devices similar to those used with cleft lip
E. Therapeutic intervention
  1. Surgical repair
    a. Cleft lip: repaired in first few weeks after birth; further modification may be necessary; aids infant's ability to suck; helps parents with visible aspects of the defect
    b. Cleft palate: surgical intervention and repair may occur as early as the neonatal period but not later than between 12 and 18 months; done before speech is fully developed
  2. Multidisciplinary team approach, including pediatric plastic surgeons, orthodontists, otolaryngologists, speech and language therapists, audiologists, nurses, and social workers
  3. Cleft palate: temporary or permanent dental prostheses needed to replace missing teeth; other dental appliances used to mechanically close clefts until surgical closure can be performed

Nursing Care of Children With Cleft Lip/Cleft Palate

A. Assessment/Analysis
  1. Feeding behaviors; consumption of adequate calories for growth without excessive energy expenditure; oral hygiene
  2. Mucous membranes for dryness, signs of infection
  3. Parent/infant interaction and effect of facial defect on bonding
  4. Cleft palate: respiratory status and hearing ability

B. Planning/Implementation
  1. Preoperative care
    a. Feed in upright position to prevent aspiration; encourage breastfeeding or use of adaptive feeding device
    b. Feed slowly, burp frequently because of swallowed air
    c. Prevent infection from irritation of the lip
    d. Teach parents the need for oral/dental hygiene and regular dental supervision
  2. Postoperative nursing care for CL
    a. Maintain patent airway because of edema and infant's habit of mouth breathing; keep laryngoscope, endotracheal tube, and suction equipment nearby
    b. Cleanse suture line to prevent crust formation and eventual scarring
    c. Minimize crying, because of pressure on suture line; encourage a parent to stay with child
    d. Use pain rating scale and medicate infant appropriately
    e. Place infant in supine position with arm or elbow restraints; change position to side or sitting up to prevent hypostatic pneumonia; remove restraints only when infant is supervised
    f. Feed (see preoperative care)
    g. Support parents during healing process
  3. Postoperative nursing care for CP
    a. Avoid traumatizing operative site; tell child who can follow directions not to rub tongue on roof of mouth; avoid using straw, spoon, toothbrush
    b. Use pain rating scale and medicate appropriately
    c. Provide liquid or blenderized diet
    d. Provide emotional support for parents; recovery is prolonged and prognosis is uncertain
  4. See Meeting the Needs of the Family of a Child With Special Needs
C. Evaluation/Outcomes
  1. Maintains integrity of suture line
  2. Experiences no trauma to operative site
  3. Experiences minimal or no pain
  4. Consumes adequate calories for growth and development
  5. Demonstrates ability to be comforted by means other than sucking
  6. Family members accept infant despite altered appearance

NASOPHARYNGEAL AND TRACHEOESOPHAGEAL ANOMALIES

Data Base

A. Result from failure of esophagus to develop a continuous passage and failure of trachea and esophagus to develop into separate distinct structures
B. Associated with low birth weight; approximately 50% associated with other anomalies including vertebral anomalies, imperforate anus, radial

and renal dysplasia, limb anomalies, and cardiac malformations

C. Chalasia: an incompetent cardiac sphincter

D. Choanal atresia: a nasopharyngeal anomaly (lack of an opening between one or both of the nasal passages and nasopharynx)

E. Tracheopharyngeal anomalies
   1. Absence of esophagus
   2. Atresia of esophagus without a tracheal fistula
   3. Tracheoesophageal fistula
   4. Most common type of anomaly: proximal esophageal atresia combined with distal tracheoesophageal fistula

F. Clinical findings
   1. Excessive salivation and drooling
   2. Choking, sneezing, and coughing during feeding, with regurgitation of formula through mouth and nose
   3. Catheter cannot be passed into the stomach (depending on type)
   4. Abdominal distention (depending on type)

G. Therapeutic intervention: surgical repair, which can be done in one procedure or several, depending on infant's condition and severity of defect

---

Nursing Care of Children With Nasopharyngeal and Tracheoesophageal Anomalies

A. Assessment/Analysis
   1. Three Cs of tracheoesophageal fistula: coughing; choking; cyanosis
   2. Signs of respiratory distress
   3. Nutrition/weight
   4. Fluid and electrolyte balance
   5. Parent/infant interaction

B. Planning/Implementation
   1. Preoperative nursing care
      a. Keep NPO; monitor intake and output; change position to prevent pneumonia
      b. Maintain position with head elevated on inclined plane of at least 30 degrees
      c. Observe for signs of respiratory distress; suction oropharynx to remove accumulated secretions
      d. Maintain patency of nasogastric tube if used to decompress stomach
   2. Postoperative nursing care
      a. Maintain body temperature
      b. Maintain nasogastric/gastrostomy tube to drainage
      c. Change position to prevent pneumonia
      d. Maintain functions of chest tubes if used
      e. Maintain nutrition by oral, parenteral, or gastrostomy route
      f. Use pain rating scale and medicate appropriately
      g. Provide comfort and physical contact; provide a pacifier for nonnutritive sucking until oral feedings are resumed

C. Evaluation/Outcomes
   1. Maintains patent airway

2. Receives adequate calories for growth and development

✸ INTESTINAL OBSTRUCTION
Data Base
A. Congenital life-threatening obstruction of lower gastrointestinal tract
   1. Mechanical: constricted or occluded lumen
   2. Muscular: interference with regular muscular contractions
   3. May be caused by inguinal hernia that is irreducible (incarcerated) progressing to interruption of blood supply (strangulated)

B. Clinical findings
   1. Abdominal distention; paroxysmal pain
   2. Absence of stools, especially meconium in the newborn (meconium ileus)
   3. Vomiting of bile-stained material; may be projectile
   4. Weak, thready pulse; cyanosis; and weak, grunting respirations from abdominal distention, causing the diaphragm to compress the lungs

C. Therapeutic interventions
   1. Surgical repair: either by single-staged or by multistaged procedures if defect is severe
   2. Prevention of pneumonia
   3. Supportive nutritional therapy

Nursing Care of Children With an Intestinal Obstruction

A. Assessment/Analysis
   1. Abdomen for distention and visible peristaltic waves
   2. Absence of bowel movements
   3. Bowel sounds

B. Planning/Implementation
   1. Preoperative nursing care
      a. Keep NPO; provide a pacifier; observe for signs of dehydration and shock
      b. Maintain nasogastric suction; monitor intake and output
   2. Postoperative nursing care: depends on type of surgery performed
      a. Keep operative site clean and dry, especially after passage of stool
      b. Use pain rating scale and medicate appropriately
      c. Position on side to prevent pulling legs up under chest
      d. Provide colostomy care; prevent excoriation of skin by frequent cleansing and use of skin protective agent, diaper, or ostomy appliance
      e. Instruct parents about colostomy care (include avoidance of tight diapers and clothes around abdomen)

C. Evaluation/Outcomes
   1. Establishes a regular pattern of bowel elimination
   2. Maintains fluid and electrolyte balance
   3. Rests comfortably

ANORECTAL ANOMALIES (IMPERFORATE ANUS)

Data Base

A. Failure of membrane separating rectum from anus to absorb during eighth week of fetal life; anomalies range from simple (imperforate anus only) to complex (genitourinary and pelvic organs involved); one of the most common congenital malformations

B. Imperforate anus: may include fistula from distal rectum to perineum, urinary system, or reproductive system

C. Rectal atresia and stenosis: anal opening present, but midline intergluteal groove without fistula limits or prevents defecation

D. Persistent cloaca: rectum, vagina, urethra open into common lumen in the perineum, emptying through the urethral opening

E. Classification according to gender
   1. Male: perineal, rectourethral, and bladder neck fistulas; simple imperforate anus; rectal atresia and stenosis
   2. Female: perineal and vestibular fistulas; simple imperforate anus; rectal atresia and stenosis; cloaca

F. Clinical findings: absence of an anal opening; failure to pass meconium stool; abdominal distention; meconium on perineum via fistula

G. Therapeutic interventions: immediate surgical correction unless fistula is present; possible colostomy with multistaged surgical repair; breastfeeding recommended to prevent constipation

Nursing Care of Children With Anorectal Anomalies

A. Assessment/Analysis
   1. Rectum for opening, passage of meconium
   2. Abdomen for distention, bowel sounds

B. Planning/Implementation
   1. See Planning/Implementation under Intestinal Obstruction

C. Evaluation/Outcomes
   1. Rests comfortably
   2. Achieves pattern of regular bowel elimination
   3. Family demonstrates ability to care for child

HYPERTROPHIC PYLORIC STENOSIS (HPS)

Data Base

A. Circular muscle of the pylorus thickens as a result of hypertrophy, usually within the first weeks of life
   1. Narrowed opening between stomach and duodenum
   2. Inflammation and edema can cause total obstruction
   3. Compensatory dilation, hypertrophy, and hyperperistalsis of the stomach result

4. Not a congenital disorder; usually an isolated problem, but can be associated with intestinal malrotation, esophageal and duodenal atresia, and anorectal anomalies

B. Five times more common in males than females
   1. Inheritance is polygenic
   2. Increased incidence in first-born children and in offspring of affected persons

C. Clinical findings
   1. Palpable olive-shaped mass in right upper quadrant
   2. Vomiting, progressively projectile; non–bile-stained vomitus
   3. Dehydration; weight loss; failure to thrive; electrolyte and acid-base imbalances
   4. Constipation; distention of the epigastrium
   5. Complete obstruction within 4 to 6 weeks: visible peristaltic waves across abdomen; discomfort; colicky pain

D. Therapeutic intervention: surgical repair

Nursing Care of Children With Hypertrophic Pyloric Stenosis

A. Assessment/Analysis
   1. Feeding history and type of vomiting; failure to gain weight, dehydration
   2. Upper abdomen for distention; epigastrium just to right of umbilicus for palpable olive-shaped mass
   3. Visible peristaltic waves
   4. Evidence of pain or discomfort

B. Planning/Implementation
   1. Preoperative nursing care
      a. Keep NPO
      b. Assess vital signs for indications of fluid and electrolyte imbalance
      c. Monitor intake and output
      d. Monitor for signs of dehydration and metabolic alkalosis
   2. Weigh daily
   3. Postoperative nursing care
      a. Keep NPO as ordered
      b. Monitor IV fluid/electrolytes; administered until infant is consuming sufficient oral feedings
      c. Administer ordered liquid electrolyte solution for first feeding and, if tolerated, breast milk or formula for subsequent feedings; usually within 24 hours
   4. Teach parents specific feeding method
      a. Give small, frequent feedings; feed slowly
      b. Hold infant in an upright position during feeding; after feeding place in infant seat or on right side with head of bed elevated
      c. Burp frequently during feeding; avoid handling afterward

C. Evaluation/Outcomes
   1. Maintains fluid and electrolyte balance
   2. Rests comfortably
   3. Consumes adequate calories for growth and development

HIRSCHSPRUNG'S DISEASE (MEGACOLON)

Data Base

A. Absence of parasympathetic ganglion cells in a portion of the bowel, which causes enlargement of the bowel proximal to the defect
  1. Length of involved bowel varies from only internal sphincter to entire colon
  2. Rectosigmoid colon is the most commonly affected site
B. Four times more common in males than females
C. Clinical findings
  1. Symptoms may occur gradually
  2. Constipation or passage of ribbonlike or pelletlike, foul-smelling stool; intestinal obstruction
  3. Rectum is empty of feces with leakage of liquid stool and gas
  4. Refusal of food; vomiting; abdominal distention
  5. Biopsy of intestine identifies absence of ganglion cells
D. Therapeutic intervention
  1. Surgical intervention usually in two stages: removal of aganglionic portion of bowel and temporary colostomy followed later by anastomosis
  2. Management with isotonic enemas for some children; tap water contraindicated because it can cause fluid and electrolyte imbalances; fluid amount depends on age (100 to 150 mL for small infant; 155 to 250 mL for older/larger infant; 255 to 360 mL for young child; 365 to 500 mL for older child)

Nursing Care of Children With Megacolon

A. Assessment/Analysis
  1. Elimination history; characteristics of stools; onset of constipation
  2. Abdomen for distention
  3. Bowel sounds
  4. Nutrition and hydration status; poor feeding
  5. Behavior for fussiness; irritability
B. Planning/Implementation
  1. Teach parents about disorder and preparation for surgery
  2. Postoperative nursing care depends on type of surgery performed (see Planning/Implementation under Intestinal Obstruction)
C. Evaluation/Outcomes
  1. Rests comfortably
  2. Achieves pattern of regular bowel evacuation
  3. Family demonstrates ability to care for child

CARDIAC MALFORMATIONS

Data Base

A. Circulatory changes that occur at or shortly after birth are disrupted, including the rapid increase in pulmonary circulation and the closure of the foramen ovale, ductus arteriosus, and ductus venosus, resulting from decreased oxygen concentration
B. Classification of cardiac defects
  1. Defects with increased pulmonary blood flow: occur with atrial and ventricular septal defects and patent ductus arteriosus
    a. Intracardiac communication along the septum or an abnormal connection between the great arteries allows blood to flow from high-pressure left side to lower-pressure right side (left to right shunt)
    b. The shunting of blood from left to right results in increased BP on right side of heart
    c. The increased pulmonary blood flow decreases systemic circulation
    d. Clinical findings: signs and symptoms of heart failure
  2. Defects with decreased pulmonary blood flow: occur with tetralogy of Fallot, transposition of great vessels, truncus arteriosus, and tricuspid atresia
    a. An obstruction of pulmonary blood flow exists and there is an anatomic defect (atrial septal defect or ventricular septal defect) between the right and left sides of the heart
    b. Blood cannot exit the right side of the heart because of the obstruction, which raises the pressure on the right side of the heart, exceeding the pressure on the left side of the heart
    c. Desaturated, O_2-poor blood flows from right to left, causing desaturation in the left side of the heart and in the systemic circulation (right to left shunt)
    d. Clinical findings: hypoxemia; apparent cyanosis; polycythemia
  3. Obstructive defects: occur with coarctation of the aorta, aortic stenosis, and pulmonic stenosis
    a. Blood exiting the heart meets an area of anatomic narrowing or stenosis, causing an obstruction to blood flow
    b. The pressures in the ventricle and in the great artery before the obstruction are increased
    c. The pressure beyond the obstruction is decreased
    d. Usually located near a valve
    e. There is an increased pressure load on the ventricle and decreased cardiac output
    f. Clinical findings: heart failure occurs with significant obstruction
C. General clinical findings
  1. Dyspnea, especially on exertion
  2. Feeding difficulty and failure to thrive, often first signs noted by the parent
  3. Stridor or choking spells
  4. During infancy: heart rate over 200 beats/min; respiratory rate about 60 breaths/min
  5. In older child: restricted physical development; delayed milestones; and decreased exercise tolerance
  6. Recurrent respiratory tract infections
  7. Heart murmurs

8. Squatting or knee-chest position: helps decrease venous return to the heart, resulting in lowered cardiac workload
9. Signs of heart failure
   a. Tachycardia and hypotension progressing to extreme pallor or duskiness
   b. Tachypnea, dyspnea, and costal retractions progressing to grunting respirations
   c. Weight gain, ascites, and pleural effusions progressing to peripheral edema
D. General therapeutic interventions
   1. Surgical intervention
      a. Prophylactic antibiotic therapy may be necessary before surgery, before invasive procedures, and throughout life
      b. Postoperative prevention of constipation to prevent straining and the Valsalva maneuver, which increases intrathoracic pressure and places stress on heart sutures
   2. Pharmacologic approach: cardiac glycosides to increase efficiency of heart action
      a. Positive inotropic effect is achieved by increasing the permeability of muscle membranes to the calcium and sodium ions required for contraction of muscle fibrils
         (1) Forceful contraction during systole improves peripheral tissue perfusion
         (2) Chamber emptying allows additional venous blood to enter the cardiac chambers during diastole
      b. Negative chronotropic effect is achieved through an action mediated by the vagus nerve that slows firing of the sinoatrial (SA) node and impulse transmission through the atrioventricular (AV) node
      c. Variety of medications have same qualitative effect on heart action but differ in potency, rate of absorption, amount absorbed, onset of action, and speed of elimination
         (1) Digitalis: longer onset, peak action, and half-life
         (2) Digoxin (Lanoxin): rapid onset and peak action with a short half-life; drug of choice in children, especially because risk for toxicity is lessened by the shorter half-life
      d. Digitalization
         (1) Provides an initial loading dose for acute effect on the enlarged heart
         (2) After desired effect is achieved, dosage is lowered to maintenance level, replacing the drug metabolized and excreted each day
      e. Adverse effects
         (1) Most frequent are nausea, vomiting, headache, drowsiness, insomnia, vertigo, confusion; all attributable to drug action at CNS sites; oral forms also cause nausea and vomiting by irritation of the gastric mucosa

      (2) Bradycardia attributable to drug-induced slowing of SA node firing
      (3) Dysrhythmias are first evidence of toxicity in one third of children; premature nodal or ventricular impulses; varying degrees of heart block caused by drug action that slows transmission of impulses through the AV node
      (4) Xanthopsia (yellow vision) caused by drug effect on visual cones
      (5) Gynecomastia (mammary enlargement) in males resulting from the estrogen-like steroid portion of digitalis glycosides
   f. Considerations during therapy
      (1) Premature contractions elevate the audible apical rate and mask the pacemaker conduction rate; apical pulse is taken before administration and drug is withheld when pulse rate drops to 110 to 90 beats/min in infants and below 70 beats/min in older children
      (2) Immaturity of hepatic and renal systems in preterm and newborn infants or depressed hepatic or renal function in children may result in accumulation
      (3) Because potassium ions are required for interaction of digitalis glycosides with sodium-potassium–dependent membranes, lowering of serum potassium ions may foster digitalis toxicity
      (4) Because calcium ions act synergistically with digitalis on myocardial membranes, an elevation of serum calcium ion levels may increase sensitivity of cardiac muscle to digitalis action
   g. Drug interactions
      (1) Phenobarbital, phenytoin, and phenylbutazone accelerate metabolism of digitalis glycosides by induction of hepatic microsomal enzymes; serum levels are lower when drugs are used concomitantly
      (2) Diuretics that cause hypokalemia may contribute to incidence of serious dysrhythmias when administered concurrently with digitalis glycosides; supplemental potassium may be used for replacement of losses, or potassium-sparing diuretics may be prescribed to prevent potassium ion losses

General Nursing Care of Children With Cardiac Malformations

A. Assessment/Analysis
   1. Color: cyanosis, pallor
   2. Apical pulse rate, peripheral pulse rates, presence of murmurs
   3. Respirations, dyspnea, frequency of colds
   4. BP
   5. Chest abnormalities

B. Planning/Implementation
   1. Calculate dosage of digoxin; usually prescribed in micrograms (1000 mcg = 1 mg)
   2. Take apical pulse before administering drug; withhold if below age norm
   3. Observe for signs of digitalis toxicity
   4. Teach parents home administration of digoxin
      a. Give digoxin at regular intervals, usually every 12 hours
      b. Plan times so that drug is given 1 hour before or 2 hours after feedings
      c. Use a calendar to mark off each dose that is given or post a reminder, such as a sign on the refrigerator
      d. Have prescription refilled before medication is completely used
      e. Administer the drug carefully by slowly squirting it in the side and back of the mouth
      f. Do not mix it with other foods or fluids because refusal to consume these results in inaccurate intake of the drug
      g. If child has teeth, give water after administering drug; whenever possible, brush teeth to prevent tooth decay from the sweetened liquid
      h. If a dose is missed and more than 4 hours have elapsed, withhold the dose and give next dose at the regular time; if less than 4 hours have elapsed, give the missed dose
      i. If child vomits within 15 minutes of receiving the digoxin, repeat dose once; if more than 15 minutes have elapsed, do not give a second dose
      j. If more than two consecutive doses have been missed, notify the practitioner
      k. Do not increase or double the dose for missed doses
      l. If child becomes ill, notify practitioner immediately
      m. Keep digoxin in a safe place, preferably in a locked cabinet
      n. If accidental overdose of digoxin, call nearest poison control center immediately
   5. Help parents cope with symptoms of the illness
      a. During dyspneic/cyanotic spell, place child in a side-lying knee-chest position, with head and chest elevated
      b. Keep child warm; encourage rest and sleep
      c. Decrease child's anxiety by remaining calm
      d. Feed child slowly; allow frequent burping; gavage feedings may be ordered
      e. Administer small, frequent meals
      f. Introduce solids and spoon-feeding early
      g. Encourage anorectic child to eat
      h. Encourage parents to include others in child's care to prevent parental exhaustion
   6. Foster growth-promoting family relationships
      a. Encourage family members to discuss their feelings about each other and the child's defect
      b. Encourage family members to maintain expectations from all siblings as equally as possible
      c. Encourage parents to provide consistent discipline, especially from infancy, to prevent behavioral problems
      d. Encourage acceptable pursuits for the child
      e. Discuss school entry with teacher and school nurse
      f. Guide parents to the eventual hazards of fostering overdependency
      g. Help parents feel adequate in their maternal-paternal roles by emphasizing growth and developmental progress of the child
      h. Help parents foster their child's development by formulating age-appropriate goals consistent with the child's activity tolerance
      i. Encourage parents to provide social experiences for the child
   7. Preoperative assessment areas necessary for planning postoperative care
      a. Keep a sleep record so that care can be organized around the child's usual rest pattern
      b. Avoid constipation and straining after surgery: assess child's elimination pattern; know words child uses; have child practice using a bedpan
      c. Record the level of activity and list favorite toys or games that require gradually increased exertion
      d. Determine child's fluid preferences for postoperative maintenance
      e. Identify and document child's activity at the time of vital sign measurement
      f. Observe the child's verbal and nonverbal responses to pain
   8. Prepare child physically and emotionally for surgery
      a. Priority assessment factor in preparation of child is developmental and chronologic age
         (1) Explanation of the heart differs according to age of the child
         (2) Children 4 to 6 years of age know that the heart is in the chest; they describe it as valentine-shaped and characterize its function by the sound of "tick tock"
         (3) Children 7 to 10 years of age do not see the heart as valentine-shaped; they know it has veins and have an idea of its function (e.g., "It makes you live"), but they do not understand the concept of pumping
         (4) Children more than 10 years of age have a concept of veins, valves, circulation, and why death occurs when the heart stops
      b. Preparation is based on the principle that fear of the unknown increases anxiety
      c. The same nurse should participate in preoperative and postoperative preparation as a source of support for both child and parents

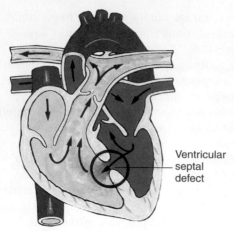

Figure 30-2 Ventricular septal defect. (From Hockenberry MJ, Wilson D: *Wong's nursing care of infants and children*, ed 8, St Louis, 2007, Mosby.)

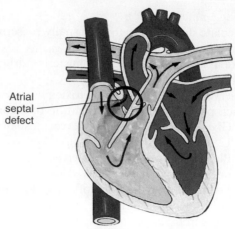

Figure 30-3 Atrial septal defect. (From Hockenberry MJ, Wilson D: *Wong's nursing care of infants and children*, ed 8, St Louis, 2007, Mosby.)

d. Know what equipment is usual after open or closed heart surgery

e. Let child play with equipment such as stethoscope, BP machine, oxygen mask, suction, and syringes without needles

f. For the young child, especially the preschooler, use dolls and puppets to describe procedures

g. Prepare child for cardiac catheterization before surgery

  (1) Frequent assessments (e.g., vital signs, assessment of catheter insertion site)

  (2) Immobility of extremity used for catheter insertion site for several hours

h. For the young child, talk about size of the bandage; for the older child, discuss the actual incision

i. Familiarize child with postoperative environment, such as the postanesthesia and intensive care units, stressing the strange noises

j. Have child practice coughing and breathing with an incentive spirometer

k. Explain to child why coughing and moving are necessary even though there is discomfort

l. Explain to child what tubes may be used and what they will look like; explain to parents that chest tubes may be used to drain air and fluid from pleural cavity

9. Specifics of postoperative care are similar to those for any major surgery

10. Help child and family adjust to correction of the cardiac defect

a. Improved physical status is often difficult for the child who has become accustomed to the sick role and its secondary gains

b. Improved physical status of the child may also be difficult for parents, because it reduces child's dependency on them

c. The child may have difficulty learning to relate to peers and siblings on a competitive basis

d. The child can no longer use the disability as a crutch for educational and social shortcomings

e. Parental expectations must be adjusted to accommodate the child's new physical vigor and search for independence

C. Evaluation/Outcomes

1. Chooses and participates in appropriate activities for age, energy, and developmental level

2. Consumes sufficient nutrients for growth and development

3. Family and child discuss fears and feelings about disorder and limitations

4. Family demonstrates home care for child

DEFECTS WITH INCREASED PULMONARY BLOOD FLOW

Ventricular Septal Defect (VSD)

(Figure 30-2: Ventricular septal defect)

A. Abnormal opening between the two ventricles

B. Severity of defect depends on size of the opening

C. Higher pressure in right ventricle causes hypertrophy, with development of pulmonary hypertension

D. Low, harsh murmur heard throughout systole

E. Specific therapeutic intervention: surgical closure of the opening at the septum

F. Prognosis: a single membranous defect has less than a 5% death rate; multiple muscular defects can have a mortality risk of 20%

Atrial Septal Defect (ASD)

(Figure 30-3: Atrial septal defect)

A. Types

1. Ostium primum defect (ASD1): opening at lower end of septum; may be associated with mitral valve abnormalities

2. Ostium secundum defect (ASD2): opening is near the center of the septum

3. Sinus venosus defect: superior portion of the atrial septum fails to form near the junction of the atrial wall with the superior vena cava

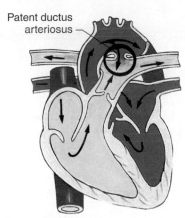

Figure 30-4 Patent ductus arteriosus. (From Hockenberry MJ, Wilson D: *Wong's nursing care of infants and children*, ed 8, St Louis, 2007, Mosby.)

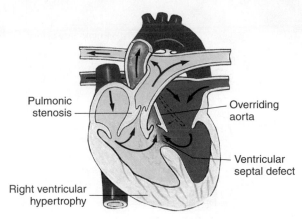

Figure 30-5 Tetralogy of Fallot. (From Hockenberry MJ, Wilson D: *Wong's nursing care of infants and children*, ed 8, St Louis, 2007, Mosby.)

B. Murmur heard high on the chest, with fixed splitting of second heart sound
C. Specific therapeutic intervention: surgical closure of the opening at the septum
D. Prognosis: has less than a 1% operative mortality

Patent Ductus Arteriosus (PDA)
(Figure 30-4: Patent ductus arteriosus)
A. Failure of the fetal connection between the aorta and pulmonary artery to close
B. Blood shunted from aorta back to the pulmonary artery; may progress to pulmonary hypertension and cardiomegaly
C. Machinery-type murmur; heartbeat heard in left second or third intercostal site
D. Specific therapeutic intervention: closure of the opening between the aorta and the pulmonary artery; in critically ill newborns, pharmacologic closure may be attempted with a prostaglandin inhibitor (e.g., indomethacin)
E. Prognosis: has less than a 1% mortality

DEFECTS WITH DECREASED PULMONARY BLOOD FLOW
Tetralogy of Fallot
(Figure 30-5: Tetralogy of Fallot)
A. Four associated defects
 1. Pulmonary valve stenosis
 2. Ventricular septal defect, usually high on the septum
 3. Overriding aorta, receiving blood from both ventricles, or an aorta arising from the right ventricle
 4. Right ventricular hypertrophy
B. Specific therapeutic interventions
 1. Palliative treatment: surgery performed to increase pulmonary blood flow; anastomosis of subclavian and pulmonary artery (Blalock-Taussig procedure)
 2. Complete repair: closure of the ventricular septal defect and resection of the infundibular stenosis,

possibly with a pericardial patch to enlarge the right ventricular outflow tract
C. Prognosis: has less than a 5% surgical repair mortality

Transposition of the Great Vessels (Arteries)
(Figure 30-6: Transposition of the great vessels [arteries])
A. Aorta exits from right ventricle and pulmonary artery leaves the left ventricle
B. Incompatible with life unless there is a communication between both sides of the heart, such as an atrial septal defect, ventricular septal defect, or patent ductus arteriosus
C. Specific therapeutic interventions
 1. Palliative procedures performed to prevent pulmonary vascular resistance and heart failure until child is able to tolerate complete repair
  a. Rashkind procedure: enlargement of an existing atrial septal defect by pulling a balloon through the defect (balloon septostomy) during a cardiac catheterization
  b. Pulmonary artery banding if a ventricular septal defect (VSD) is present to decrease blood flow to the lungs and increase shunting of oxygenated blood intraventricularly to the aorta
  c. Pharmacologic dilation of patent ductus arteriosus with use of prostaglandins (e.g., Prostin VR)
  d. Blalock-Hanlon operation: surgical creation of an atrial septal defect
 2. Complete repair
  a. Arterial switch procedure: transposing the great vessels to their correct anatomic placement with reimplantation of the coronary arteries
  b. Rastelli's procedure: closure of VSD (directing left ventricular blood through VSD into aorta, pulmonic valve closed, and conduit made from right ventricle to pulmonary artery) results in usual physiologic circulation but requires revision as child grows; procedure of choice for infants with transposition of the great vessels, VSD, and severe pulmonic stenosis
D. Prognosis: has a 5% to 10% surgical mortality

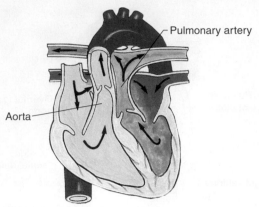

Figure 30-6 Transposition of the great vessels (arteries). (From Hockenberry MJ, Wilson D: *Wong's nursing care of infants and children*, ed 8, St Louis, 2007, Mosby.)

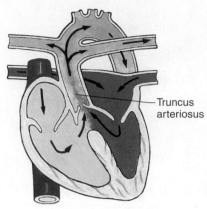

Figure 30-8 Truncus arteriosus. (From Hockenberry MJ, Wilson D: *Wong's nursing care of infants and children*, ed 8, St Louis, 2007, Mosby.)

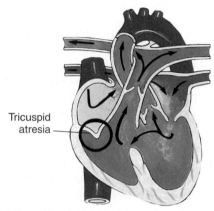

Figure 30-7 Tricuspid atresia. (From Hockenberry MJ, Wilson D: *Wong's nursing care of infants and children*, ed 8, St Louis, 2007, Mosby.)

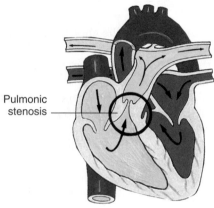

Figure 30-9 Pulmonary (pulmonic) stenosis. (From Hockenberry MJ, Wilson D: *Wong's nursing care of infants and children*, ed 8, St Louis, 2007, Mosby.)

Tricuspid Atresia
(Figure 30-7: Tricuspid atresia)
A. Absence of the tricuspid valve
B. Incompatible with life unless there is a communication between the right and left sides of the heart, such as atrial septal defect, ventricular septal defect, or patent ductus arteriosus
C. Specific therapeutic interventions
  1. Palliative treatment procedures: same as for tetralogy of Fallot
  2. Complete repair: modified Fontan procedure—conversion of the right atrium into an outlet for the pulmonary artery, which involves placing a tubular conduit with a valve between the two and closing the atrial septal defect; physiologically corrects tricuspid atresia by preventing any mixing of systemic blood in the left atrium and shunting the entire venous blood to the lungs for oxygenation
D. Prognosis: has a surgical mortality greater than 10%

Truncus Arteriosus
(Figure 30-8: Truncus arteriosus)
A. Single great vessel arising from the base of the heart, serving as a pulmonary artery and aorta

B. Systolic murmur is heard, and a single semilunar valve produces a loud second heart sound that is not split
C. Specific therapeutic intervention: complete repair (Rastelli's operation) excising pulmonary arteries from aorta and attaching them to the right ventricle by means of a prosthetic valve conduit; septal defects also repaired)
D. Prognosis: requires complex repair and has a mortality of 10%

✿ OBSTRUCTIVE DEFECTS
Pulmonary (Pulmonic) Stenosis
(Figure 30-9: Pulmonary [pulmonic] stenosis)
A. Narrowing of the pulmonary valve
B. Causes decreased blood flow to lungs and increased pressure to right ventricle
C. Specific therapeutic intervention: valvotomy or balloon angioplasty
D. Prognosis: has less than a 2% mortality
Aortic Stenosis
(Figure 30-10: Aortic stenosis)
A. Narrowing of the aortic valve

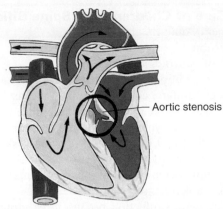

Figure 30-10 Aortic stenosis. (From Hockenberry MJ, Wilson D: *Wong's nursing care of infants and children*, ed 8, St Louis, 2007, Mosby.)

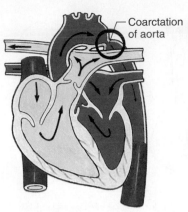

Figure 30-11 Coarctation of the aorta. (From Hockenberry MJ, Wilson D: *Wong's nursing care of infants and children*, ed 8, St Louis, 2007, Mosby.)

B. Causes increased workload on left ventricle, and lowered pressure in the aorta reduces coronary artery blood flow
C. Specific therapeutic intervention: division of the stenotic valves of the aorta
D. Prognosis: has a significant (greater than 20%) mortality in critically ill newborns; older children have a lower mortality risk

Coarctation of the Aorta

(Figure 30-11: Coarctation of the aorta)
A. Localized narrowing of aorta near the insertion of the ductus arteriosus
B. Increased systemic circulation above stricture: bounding radial and carotid pulses; headache; dizziness; epistaxis
C. Decreased systemic circulation below stricture: absent femoral pulses; cool lower extremities
D. Increased pressure in aorta above defect causes left ventricular hypertrophy
E. Murmur may or may not be heard
F. Specific therapeutic intervention: angioplasty; resection of the defect and anastomosis of ends of the aorta
G. Prognosis: has less than a 5% mortality in children with isolated coarctation

NEUROLOGIC MALFORMATIONS

DEFECTS OF NEURAL TUBE CLOSURE (SPINA BIFIDA)

Data Base
A. Abnormalities that are derived from the embryonic neural tube constitute the largest group of congenital anomalies with multifactorial inheritance
B. Malformation of the spine in which the posterior portion of the laminae of the vertebrae fails to close; may involve the entire length of the spinal column or be restricted to a small area; most common site is the lumbosacral area

C. Associated defects include weakness or paralysis below the defect, bowel and bladder dysfunction, clubfeet, dislocated hip, and hydrocephalus
D. Defect of the occipitocervical region with swelling and displacement of the medulla into the spinal cord (Arnold-Chiari malformation) is associated with hydrocephalus
E. Incidence of spina bifida is higher in females than males
F. Rates of neural tube disorders (NTDs) have decreased from 1.3 per 1000 in 1990 to 0.3 per 1000 after the introduction of mandatory food fortification with folic acid
G. Classifications (Figure 30-12: Midline defects of osseous spine with varying degrees of neural herniation)
   1. Spina bifida occulta: defect only of the vertebrae; spinal cord and meninges are intact
   2. Spina bifida cystica
      a. Meningocele: meninges, but no neural elements, protrude through the defect; spinal fluid exits through the defect
      b. Myelomeningocele: meninges and a portion of the spinal cord with its nerves protrude through the defect, usually in lumbosacral area spinal fluid exits through the defect
   3. Anencephaly
      a. Brain degenerated to a spongiform mass with no bony covering
      b. Absence of both cerebral hemispheres
      c. Incompatible with life; intact brainstem maintains vital functions from several hours to several weeks
H. Clinical findings
   1. Defect readily apparent on inspection
   2. Degree of neurologic dysfunction directly related to anatomic level of defect and nerves involved
   3. Sensory disturbances usually parallel motor dysfunction
   4. Defective nerve supply to bladder affects sphincter and muscle tone

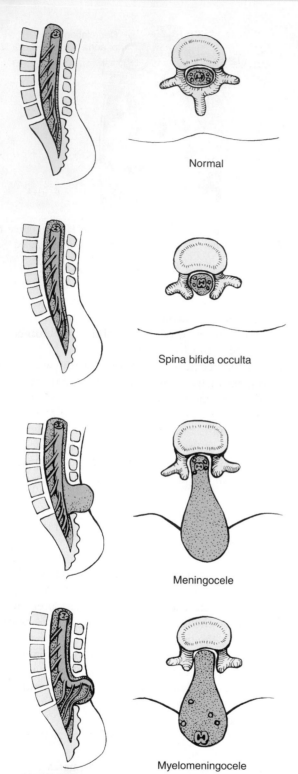

Normal

Spina bifida occulta

Meningocele

Myelomeningocele

Figure 30-12 Midline defects of osseous spine with varying degrees of neural herniation. (From Hockenberry MJ, Wilson D: *Wong's nursing care of infants and children*, ed 8, St Louis, 2007, Mosby.)

   5. Ineffective anal sphincter control
I. Therapeutic interventions
   1. Multidisciplinary approach including rehabilitation
   2. Surgical repair of sac as soon as possible to maintain neurologic function and prevent infection

Nursing Care of Children With Spina Bifida

A. Assessment/Analysis
   1. Condition of the myelomeningocele sac
   2. Level of neurologic involvement
   3. Neurologic impairment of elimination
   4. Head circumference and fontanels at least daily; head measured at greatest circumference (usually slightly above eyebrows and pinna of ears and around occipital prominence at back of skull); marks may be placed on both sides of child's head to facilitate accurate serial measurements
B. Planning/Implementation
   1. Protect against infection because breakdown of sac exposes spinal cord to the environment
     a. Keep area clean of urine and feces
     b. Apply sterile, moist, nonadherent dressing over sac to prevent drying; moistening solution is usually sterile normal saline; diapers are not used
     c. Change dressing every 2 to 4 hours to maintain moistness; inspect sac for leaks, abrasions, irritation, or signs of infection
     d. Avoid pressure on sac
   2. Place in prone position before and after surgical correction; after surgery prone position may aggravate coexisting hip dysplasia or may permit undesirable hip flexion; provide passive range-of-motion exercises to extremities when permitted
   3. Provide meticulous skin care because areas of sensory and motor impairment are susceptible to skin breakdown
   4. Foster elimination in the infant with a neurogenic bladder
     a. When urinary retention is detected, intermittent straight catheterization is used
     b. When bowel sphincter is affected, there may a continual passage of stool that may be misinterpreted as diarrhea
   5. Postoperative nursing care
     a. Measure head circumference because increase may indicate that hydrocephalus is developing
     b. Monitor for signs of increased intracranial pressure
     c. Use pain rating scale and medicate appropriately
     d. With skin grafts covering a large defect, maintain prone position indefinitely; restrict movement to minimize tension on operative site
C. Evaluation/Outcomes
   1. Remains free of infection
   2. Maintains skin integrity
   3. Family demonstrates ability to care for child

✿ HYDROCEPHALUS

Data Base

A. Abnormal accumulation of cerebrospinal fluid within the ventricular system
B. Classifications
   1. May be classified according to the cause, either congenital or acquired hydrocephalus; also may be classified according to the presence or absence of an

obstruction, either noncommunicating or communicating hydrocephalus

   a. Noncommunicating: obstruction within the ventricles such as congenital malformation, neoplasm, or hematoma

   b. Communicating: inadequate absorption of cerebrospinal fluid (CSF), resulting from infection, trauma, or obstruction by thick arachnoid membrane or meninges

C. Clinical findings

  1. Increasing head size because of open sutures and bulging fontanels

  2. Prominent scalp veins and taut, shiny skin

  3. "Sunset" eyes (sclera visible above iris), bulging eyes, and papilledema of retina

  4. Head lag, especially important after 4 to 6 months

  5. Increased intracranial pressure: projectile vomiting not associated with feeding; irritability; anorexia; high; shrill cry; seizures; tense fontanels in infant

  6. Brain damage because increased pressure compresses brain against unyielding skull, decreasing blood flow to brain cells and causing necrosis

D. Therapeutic interventions

  1. Relief of hydrocephalus

   a. Removal of obstruction if noncommunicating hydrocephalus

   b. Mechanical shunting of fluid to another area of body; with ventricular peritoneal shunt, catheter is passed subcutaneously to peritoneal cavity and placement is revised as necessary

  2. Treatment of complications

  3. Management of complications that cause psychomotor problems

Nursing Care of Children With Hydrocephalus

A. Assessment/Analysis

  1. Head circumference measured at least daily (see Assessment/Analysis under Nursing Care of Children with Spina Bifida for procedure)

  2. Fontanels and suture lines are palpated for size, signs of bulging, tenseness, and separation.

  3. Signs of increased intracranial pressure

  4. Status of neurologic reflexes

B. Planning/Implementation

  1. Prevent breakdown of scalp, infection, and damage to spinal cord

   a. Position with head elevated to facilitate draining of fluid; after shunt placement, position flat with head resting on side without the shunt

   b. Support neck and head when holding infant

   c. Observe shunt site (abdominal site in peritoneal procedure) for infection

  2. Monitor for increasing intracranial pressure

   a. Monitor neurologic signs

   b. Measure head circumference

   c. Control pain with acetaminophen with or without codeine for mild to moderate pain and opioids for severe pain as ordered

  3. Promote adequate nutrition

   a. Monitor for vomiting, irritability, lethargy, and anorexia because these will decrease the intake of nutrients

   b. Provide small, frequent feedings

   c. Perform all care before feeding to minimize vomiting; hold infant if possible

   d. Observe for signs of dehydration

  4. Keep eyes moist and free of irritation if eyelids incompletely cover corneas

  5. Place on bed rest after surgery, with minimal handling to prevent damage to shunt

  6. Support parents (shunt revisions are necessary as growth occurs)

  7. Provide anticipatory guidance to parents about observing for and recording developmental milestones; perform range-of-motion exercises to lower extremities when medically permitted

  8. Teach parents

   a. To pump the shunt, if indicated to maintain patency

   b. Signs of increasing intracranial pressure, infection, and dehydration

C. Evaluation/Outcomes

  1. Remains free of increased intracranial pressure

  2. Remains free from infection

  3. Maintains skin integrity

  4. Family demonstrates ability to care for child

GENITOURINARY MALFORMATIONS

✿ EXSTROPHY OF THE BLADDER

Data Base

A. Absence of portion of abdominal wall and bladder wall, causing bladder to appear to be turned inside-out and outside the abdominal cavity

B. May be accompanied by defects such as pubic bone malformations, inguinal hernia, epispadias, undescended testes, or short penis in boys and a cleft clitoris or absent vagina in girls

C. Occurs two times more frequently in males than females

D. Clinical findings

  1. Bladder is exposed and appears to be turned inside-out

  2. Constant seepage of urine leading to skin breakdown and infection

  3. Progressive renal failure may result from infection and obstruction

E. Therapeutic interventions

  1. Plastic surgery

  2. Closure of the bladder within 48 hours if possible; final repair attempted before school age

  3. Ileal conduit (also called ureteroileal cutaneous ureterostomy); child wears ileostomy appliance over stoma, which collects the continuously flowing urine

4. Cutaneous ureterostomy; ureters are attached directly to the abdominal wall, usually at a site proximal to the level of kidneys; two collecting appliances are worn over bilateral openings

Nursing Care of Children With Exstrophy of the Bladder

A. Assessment/Analysis
1. Condition of skin
2. Renal function; urine output
3. Parental interaction with child
B. Planning/Implementation
1. Help parents to accept disorder and long-term sequelae
2. Scrupulously clean area around bladder and apply sterile, nonadherent, moist dressing over exposed bladder tissue to prevent infection
3. Monitor and maintain fluid balance because of large insensible water losses from exposed viscera
4. Dress with loose clothing to avoid pressure over area
5. Change clothing frequently because of odor
6. Care for the urine-collecting appliance; change frequently
C. Evaluation/Outcomes
1. Maintains skin integrity
2. Remains free from infection
3. Maintains renal function within acceptable limits
4. Family demonstrates ability to care for child

DISPLACED URETHRAL OPENINGS

Data Base
A. Urethral opening is abnormally located
B. In males severity varies, depending on distance from tip of penis and presence of other penile anomalies
C. Classification
1. Hypospadias
   a. In males urethra opens on lower surface of penis from just behind the glans to the perineum (placement varies)
   b. In females urethra opens into the vagina
2. Epispadias
   a. Occurs only in males
   b. Urethra opens on dorsal surface of penis; often associated with exstrophy of the bladder
3. Defect can be a sign of ambiguous genitalia
D. Clinical findings
1. Interference with procreation if severely affected
2. Increased risk for urinary tract infection
E. Therapeutic interventions
1. Surgical repair of defect; circumcision, if desired, is delayed until after surgical repair
2. Surgical repair may be performed in several stages

Nursing Care of Children With a Displaced Urethral Opening

A. Assessment/Analysis
1. Parental knowledge of defect
2. Origin of urinary stream

B. Planning/Implementation
1. Provide parents with an explanation of child's future functioning
2. Help boy to cope with anatomic difference from peers and adjustment to voiding in sitting position
3. Prepare child for surgery
C. Evaluation/Outcomes
1. Remains free from pain
2. Maintains peer interactions
3. Child and parents verbalize feelings/concerns effects of the defect
4. Surgical repair corrects voiding pattern

SKELETAL MALFORMATIONS

CLUBFOOT

Data Base
A. Congenital clubfoot involves bone deformity and malposition with soft tissue contracture; foot is twisted out of usual shape or position
B. Talipes equinovarus is most common type; foot is fixed in plantar flexion (downward) and deviated medially (inward)
C. Clinical findings
1. Deformity is apparent at birth
2. Classification
   a. Deformity is rigid or flexible
   b. Mild or positional deformity may correct spontaneously or require passive exercise and serial casting
   c. Syndromic clubfoot: associated with other congenital anomalies
   d. Congenital clubfoot: wide range of rigidity and prognosis; usually requires surgical intervention
D. Therapeutic interventions
1. Treatment is most successful when started during newborn period because delay causes leg muscles and bones to develop abnormally, with shortening of tendons
2. Nonsurgical treatment: gentle, repeated manipulation of foot with casting; done every few days for 1 to 2 weeks, then at 1- to 2-week intervals
3. Surgical treatment: done if nonsurgical treatment not effective
   a. Tight ligaments released
   b. Tendons lengthened or transplanted
4. Follow-up care
   a. Extended medical supervision is required because there is a tendency for this deformity to recur (considered cured when the child is able to wear regular shoes and walk properly)
   b. Care emphasizes muscle reeducation (by manipulation) and proper walking
   c. Heels and soles of shoes prescribed following correction must be kept in repair
   d. Corrective shoes may have sole and heel lifts on lateral border to maintain proper position

Nursing Care of Children With Clubfoot

A. Assessment/Analysis
   1. Parental understanding of treatment regimen
   2. Skin and circulation of affected limb
B. Planning/Implementation
   1. After casting
      a. Observe toes for signs of circulatory impairment (toes should be visible at end of cast)
      b. Check cast for weakness and wear, especially if child is allowed to walk on it
      c. For other areas of cast care, see Developmental Dysplasia of the Hip
   2. Teach parents necessary care and emphasize need for follow-up, which may be prolonged
C. Evaluation/Outcomes
   1. Remains free from complications
   2. Parents demonstrate ability to care for child

❖ DEVELOPMENTAL DYSPLASIA OF THE HIP

Data Base

A. Imperfect development of hip—can affect femoral head, acetabulum, or both
B. Head of the femur does not lie deep enough within the acetabulum and slips out on movement
C. Sixty percent of affected children are females
D. Classification
   1. Acetabular dysplasia: mildest form; femoral head remains in acetabulum
   2. Subluxation: most common form; femoral head partially displaced
   3. Dislocation: femoral head not in contact with acetabulum; displaced posteriorly and superiorly
E. Clinical findings
   1. Limitation in abduction of leg on affected side
   2. Asymmetry of gluteal, popliteal, and thigh folds
   3. Audible click when abducting and externally rotating hip on affected side (Ortolani's sign)
   4. Apparent shortening of femur on affected side (Galeazzi's sign)
   5. Waddling gait and lordosis when child begins to walk
F. Therapeutic interventions
   1. Directed toward enlarging and deepening acetabulum by placing head of femur within acetabulum and applying constant pressure
   2. Positioned with legs slightly flexed and abducted: Pavlik harness; spica cast; brace
   3. Surgical intervention (e.g., open reduction with casting)

Nursing Care of Children With Developmental Dysplasia of the Hip

A. Assessment/Analysis
   1. Limb shorter on affected side
   2. Positive Ortolani's test (hip click)
   3. Restricted abduction of hip on affected side

B. Planning/Implementation
   1. Support child experiencing respiratory problems such as hypostatic pneumonia caused by immobility
      a. Change position frequently; raise head of mattress/crib rather than just the head to prevent flexion of the neck
      b. Teach parents postural drainage and exercises for child, such as blowing bubbles to increase lung expansion
      c. Encourage parents to seek immediate medical care if child develops congestion or cough
   2. Maintain skin integrity
      a. Assess circulation to toes: pedal pulses and signs of blanching
      b. Do not let child put small toys or food inside cast
      c. Teach parents to recognize signs of infection, such as odor
      d. Protect cast edges with adhesive tape or waterproof material, especially around perineum
      e. Use diapers and plastic lining to minimize soiling of cast by feces and urine
   3. Prevent constipation
      a. Teach parents to observe child for straining on defecation and constipation
      b. Increase fluids and fiber
   4. Encourage intake of nutritious foods appropriate for activity level
      a. Provide small, frequent meals because of inflexibility of cast around waist (a window may be made over abdominal area to allow for expansion with meals)
      b. Teach parents to adjust calorie intake, because less energy expenditure can lead to obesity
   5. Move and position child safely when in a spica cast
      a. Use wagon or stroller with back flat or mechanic's creeper for transportation
      b. Protect child from falling when positioned
      c. Never lift child by using bar between legs of cast (two people needed to provide adequate body support if necessary)
      d. Use specially designed car restraint system for transportation in motor vehicle
   6. Meet emotional needs
      a. Use touch as much as possible; small children can be picked up and cuddled
      b. Stimulate and provide for play activities appropriate to age
   7. Provide parents with help and support
      a. Give written instructions
      b. Schedule routine home visits with telephone or e-mail counseling available
      c. Stress need for follow-up care because treatment may be prolonged
      d. Prepare parents for possible use of an abduction brace after cast is removed
   8. For additional care for the child with a spica cast, see Chapter 11 in Medical-Surgical Nursing for Care of the Client With a Cast

C. Evaluation/Outcomes
1. Moves about and controls environment
2. Remains free of injury
3. Regains earlier movement (crawling/walking) when device is removed
4. Parents demonstrate ability to care for child

INBORN ERRORS OF METABOLISM

Inherited autosomal recessive trait disorders are caused by absence of substances essential to cellular metabolism. They are characterized by abnormal fat, protein, or carbohydrate metabolism

General Nursing Care of Children With Inborn Errors of Metabolism

A. Assessment/Analysis
1. Verification of test results
2. Parents' understanding of disorder
3. Growth and development
B. Planning/Implementation
1. Help parents to understand disorder and the role of diet (see Therapeutic interventions under Phenylketonuria [PKU] and Galactosemia for specific diets)
2. Refer parents for genetic counseling
3. Specific nursing care for children with hypothyroidism
   a. Instruct parents regarding administration of thyroid replacement medications and signs of overdose (rapid pulse rate, dyspnea, insomnia, irritability, sweating, fever, and weight loss)
   b. Teach parents to take child's pulse
C. Evaluation/Outcomes
1. Achieves satisfactory growth and development
2. Consumes adequate nutrients for growth
3. Child and family verbalize feelings about necessity of dietary modifications
4. Child and family verbalize and demonstrate ability to follow medical regimen (prescribed diet/ medications)

PHENYLKETONURIA (PKU)

Data Base

A. Lack of the enzyme phenylalanine hydroxylase, which changes phenylalanine (essential amino acid) into tyrosine
B. Clinical findings
1. Growth failure
   a. Frequent vomiting
   b. Irritability
2. Mental retardation from damage to nervous system by buildup of phenylalanine if untreated
   a. Altered mental processes apparent by 4 months of age
   b. IQ: usually below 50 and most frequently under 20
3. Strong musty odor in urine from phenylacetic acid

4. Absence of tyrosine reduces production of melanin and results in blond hair and blue eyes
5. Fair skin is susceptible to eczema
C. Therapeutic interventions
1. Early detection is essential; newborn testing is mandatory in all 50 states
2. Guthrie blood test: testing is done after protein ingestion; if testing is done during initial 24 hours, it is repeated by 2 weeks of age
3. Dietary: low-phenylalanine diet is calculated to allow 20 to 30 mg of phenylalanine per kg of body weight
   a. Breastfeeding: highly recommended or use of Lofenalac or Phenex-1 as breast milk substitute
   b. Phenylalanine-free formulas such as Phenex-2 or Phenyl-Free for children more than 3 years of age
   c. Dietary restrictions of phenylalanine through adolescence and possibly life
   d. Low-phenylalanine diet required for pregnant women with phenylketonuria
   e. Artificial sweetener aspartame is prohibited
4. Treatment for eczema—see Atopic Dermatitis (Eczema)

GALACTOSEMIA

Data Base

A. Missing enzyme that converts galactose to glucose
B. Clinical findings
1. Weight loss/vomiting
2. Hepatosplenomegaly; jaundice
3. Cataracts
C. Therapeutic interventions
1. Early detection: test for galactosemia at birth; Beutler test (method similar to Guthrie test for PKU) mandatory in many states
2. Dietary reduction of lactose: soy-based formula as milk substitute and restriction of foods to those low in lactose (usually continued until child is 7 to 8 years of age), followed by dietary modifications throughout life

HYPOTHYROIDISM

Data Base

A. Types
1. Congenital hypothyroidism: failure of embryonic development of the thyroid gland or inborn enzyme defect in the formation of thyroxine
2. Lymphocytic thyroiditis (Hashimoto's disease): genetic predisposition to the development of autoimmune thyroiditis; most common thyroid disease in children; may be transient and regress spontaneously within 1 to 2 years
B. Clinical findings
1. Congenital hypothyroidism
   a. Prolonged physiologic jaundice, feeding difficulties, inactivity (excessive sleeping, little crying), anemia, problems resulting from

hypotonic abdominal muscles (constipation, protruding abdomen, and umbilical hernia)

b. Apparent at 3 to 6 months of age in formula-fed infants; may be delayed in breastfed infants

c. Impaired development of nervous system leads to mental retardation; level depends on degree of hypothyroidism and interval before therapy is begun

d. Decreased growth and decreased metabolic rate, resulting in increased weight

e. Characteristic infant facies: short forehead; wide, puffy eyes; wrinkled eyelids; broad, short, upturned nose; large, protruding tongue; dry, brittle, and lusterless hair with low hairline

f. Mottled skin because of decreased heart rate and circulation

g. Yellowish skin color from carotenemia resulting from decreased conversion of carotene to vitamin A

2. Lymphocytic thyroiditis

a. Enlarged thyroid gland

b. Tracheal compression: hoarseness; dysphagia

c. Some have signs of hyperthyroidism: nervousness; hyperactivity; irritability; increased perspiration

C. Therapeutic interventions

1. Congenital hypothyroidism

a. Detection: neonatal screening for thyroxine (T_4) and thyroid-stimulating hormone (TSH)

(1) Newborn testing is mandatory in all 50 states

(2) Performed by heelstick blood test at same time as other neonatal metabolic tests

b. Replacement therapy with thyroid hormone; if therapy is begun before 3 months of age, chances for adquate growth and normal IQ are increased

2. Lymphocytic thyroiditis: thyroid replacement to depress thyroid-stimulating hormone, thus reducing the size of the thyroid gland

HEALTH PROBLEMS THAT DEVELOP DURING INFANCY

(Some problems may continue past infancy)

✽ INTUSSUSCEPTION

Data Base

A. Telescoping of a proximal section of intestine into a more distal segment; most common site is at the ileocecal valve where the ileum invaginates into another section of the ileum (Figure 30-13: Ileocecal valve [ileocolic] intussusception)

B. Males affected two times more frequently than females

C. Usually occurs between 5 and 9 months of age

D. Clinical findings

1. Healthy, well-nourished infant who awakens with severe paroxysmal abdominal pain, evidenced by kicking and drawing legs up to abdomen

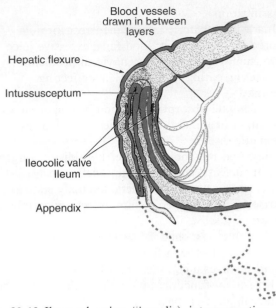

Figure 30-13 Ileocecal valve (ileocolic) intussusception. (From Hockenberry MJ, Wilson D: *Wong's nursing care of infants and children*, ed 8, St Louis, 2007, Mosby.)

2. One or two regular stools, then bloody mucus in stool ("currant jelly" stool)

3. Palpation of sausage-shaped mass in abdomen

4. Other signs of intestinal obstruction usually present

E. Therapeutic interventions

1. Medical reduction by hydrostatic pressure (water-soluble contrast material given as enema or air pressure; barium enemas used less frequently)

2. Surgical reduction; sometimes with intestinal resection

Nursing Care of Children With Intussusception

A. Assessment/Analysis

1. Presence and extent of abdominal pain, vomiting

2. Stools for color and consistency

3. Abdomen for presence of sausage-shaped mass

B. Planning/Implementation

1. Same as for any abdominal surgery

2. Make provisions for parental rooming-in/visits because problem usually occurs when infant is 6 to 8 months of age and separation anxiety is acute

C. Evaluation/Outcomes

1. Remains free from pain

2. Consumes sufficient nutrients for growth

3. Maintains fluid balance

4. Family can verbalize feelings about illness

✽ FAILURE TO THRIVE (FTT)

Data Base

A. The term used to describe infants and children whose weight and sometimes height fall below the 5th percentile for their age

B. Persistent deviation from established growth curve

C. Classification
1. Inadequate caloric intake: incorrect formula preparation; neglect; food fads; excessive juice consumption; poverty; behavioral problems affecting eating; CNS problems affecting intake
2. Inadequate absorption: cystic fibrosis; celiac disease; vitamin or mineral deficiencies; biliary atresia; or hepatic disease
3. Increased metabolism: hyperthyroidism; congenital heart defects; chronic immunodeficiency
4. Defective utilization: genetic anomaly such as trisomy 21 or 18; congenital infection; metabolic storage disease

D. Clinical findings: child
1. Etiology of growth failure is often multifactorial and involves a combination of infant organic disease, dysfunctional parenting behaviors, subtle neurologic or behavioral problems, and disturbed parent-child interactions
2. Growth failure: below 5th percentile in weight only or height and weight
3. Developmental: social, motor, adaptive, and language deficit; hearing not affected
4. Apathy; difficulty forming meaningful relationships; withdrawn behavior
5. Feeding or eating disorders, such as vomiting, anorexia, voracious appetite, pica, rumination
6. Stiff and unyielding or flaccid and unresponsive; minimal smiling; not comforted by touch
7. Prone to development of illnesses

E. Clinical findings: caregiver
1. Difficulty perceiving and assessing infant's needs
2. Inadequate support systems
3. Frequently under stress and in crisis, with emotional, social, and financial problems

F. Therapeutic interventions
1. Nutritional
a. Correction of nutritional deficiencies and achievement of appropriate weight for height
b. Allowance for catch-up growth
c. Restoration of optimum body composition
d. Education of parents or primary caregivers regarding child's nutritional needs and appropriate feeding methods
2. Treatment of underlying cause: coexisting medical problems; parent-child relationship

Nursing Care of Children With Failure to Thrive

A. Assessment/Analysis
1. Accurate baseline height and weight
2. Feeding behavior
3. Parent-child behavior/interactions
4. Developmental level

B. Planning/Implementation
1. Provide a consistent caregiver who can begin to satisfy routine needs

2. Provide optimum nutrients
a. Make feeding a priority intervention
b. Keep accurate record of intake to determine daily calories
c. Weigh daily and record to ascertain weight gain
3. Introduce a positive feeding environment
a. Establish a structured routine and follow it consistently; assign one nurse for feeding; follow child's rhythm of feeding; be persistent
b. Hold young child for feeding; maintain eye-to-eye contact; maintain a calm, even temperament; provide a quiet, nonstimulating environment
c. Talk to child by giving appropriate directions and praise for eating
4. Increase stimulation appropriate to child's present developmental level
5. Provide parent with opportunities to talk
6. When necessary, relieve parent of childrearing responsibilities until able and ready emotionally to support the child
7. Demonstrate proper infant care by example, not lecturing (allow parent to proceed at own pace)
8. Supply parent with emotional support without fostering dependency
9. Promote parent's self-respect and confidence by praising achievements with child's behavior, growth, and development

C. Evaluation/Outcomes
1. Demonstrates a positive response to interventions
2. Gains weight steadily
3. Parents demonstrate ability to care for child

SHAKEN BABY SYNDROME

Data Base
A. Injuries caused by vigorously shaking while infant is held by the shoulders or upper extremities
B. Can cause fatal intracranial trauma without external signs of abuse
C. Clinical findings
1. Retinal hemorrhages
2. Central nervous system
a. Intracranial bleeding
b. Seizures; coma
3. Bruising
4. Skull fractures
5. Tense or bulging fontanel
6. Respiratory irregularities without stridor or adventitious breath sounds; apnea

Nursing Care of Children With Shaken Baby Syndrome

Nursing care depends on the type of injuries sustained. Most frequently injuries involve the CNS, fractures of the skull and long bones, and trauma to the organs in the thoracic and abdominal cavities

SUDDEN INFANT DEATH SYNDROME (SIDS)

Data Base

A. The third leading cause of death in infants between 1 month and 1 year of age; incidence of 0.7 in every 1000 live births
B. Peak age of occurrence: healthy infants 2 to 4 months of age—95% occur by 6 months
C. Prevention: infants should be placed on their backs on a firm surface for sleep; breastfeeding
D. Risk factors
   1. Sleeping on abdomen or on soft bedding, pillows, comforters, quilts, and sheepskin
   2. Males
   3. Low birth weight
   4. Low Apgar scores
   5. CNS disturbances
   6. Respiratory disorders such as bronchopulmonary dysplasia
   7. Mothers who are very young, smoked during pregnancy, or abused drugs
   8. Exposure to environmental tobacco smoke
E. Lower incidence in breastfed infants
F. May be greater incidence in siblings of children with SIDS
G. Clinical findings
   1. Sudden, unexplained death of an infant under 1 year of age
   2. Frothy, blood-tinged fluid fills mouth and nose
   3. Diaper wet and full of stool, which is consistent with cataclysmic type of death
   4. Disheveled bedding
   5. Pulmonary edema and intrathoracic hemorrhages found on autopsy
H. Therapeutic interventions
   1. Avoidance of implying wrongdoing, abuse, or neglect
   2. Provision of support to parents
   3. Nonjudgmental attitude toward parents' attempts at resuscitation

Nursing Care of Families of Children With Sudden Infant Death Syndrome

A. Assessment/Analysis
   1. Parental knowledge of SIDS
   2. Parental support system
B. Planning/Implementation
   1. Know signs of SIDS to distinguish them from child neglect or abuse; do or say nothing that instills guilt in parents
   2. Reassure parents that they could not have prevented the death or predicted its occurrence
   3. Reinforce that an autopsy by experienced practitioners should be done on every infant to confirm diagnosis
   4. Arrange a home visit to discuss the cause of death and help the parents with their guilt and grief
   5. Refer parents to a national SIDS parent group

C. Evaluation/Outcomes
   1. Family exhibits positive coping behavior
   2. Family uses support services
   3. Family exhibits effective bereavement behaviors
   4. Parents maintain supportive relationship with other children

APNEA OF INFANCY (AOI)

Data Base

A. Apnea of 15 seconds or less is expected at any age
B. Pathologic apnea lasts at least 20 seconds
C. May be symptomatic of sepsis, seizures, upper airway abnormalities, gastroesophageal reflux, hypoglycemia, or impaired regulation of sleep or feeding
D. No cause identified in 50% of infants with apnea
E. At risk for SIDS but account for only 7% to 12% of SIDS cases
F. Clinical findings
   1. Usually presents as an apparent life-threatening event
   2. Is associated with cyanosis, marked pallor, hypotonia, or bradycardia
G. Therapeutic interventions
   1. Continuous home monitoring of cardiorespiratory rhythm
   2. Respiratory stimulant medication such as caffeine
   3. Treatment discontinued when child has gone 2 to 3 months without a significant number of alarms or with apneic episodes that did not require intervention

Nursing Care of Children with Apnea

A. Assessment/Analysis
   1. Parental fears and concerns
   2. Knowledge about cardiopulmonary resuscitation (CPR) and home monitoring
   3. Description of apparent life-threatening event
B. Planning/Implementation
   1. Monitor type and quality of apneic episodes
   2. Teach parents about home monitoring and how to stimulate/resuscitate infant
   3. Assist parents to identify support system
C. Evaluation/Outcomes
   1. Maintains respiratory functioning
   2. Parents demonstrate effective use of equipment for home monitoring
   3. Parents demonstrate CPR
   4. Parents verbalize fears
   5. Parents identify support system

DIARRHEA

Data Base

A. Frequent, watery stools caused by increased peristalsis resulting from a variety of causes, local or systemic
B. Classification
   1. Acute: sudden increase in frequency and a change in consistency of stools; leading cause of illness in children younger than 5 years throughout the world
   2. Chronic: often caused by chronic conditions such as malabsorption syndromes, inflammatory bowel

disease, food allergy, lactose intolerance, or chronic nonspecific diarrhea
  3. May cause diaper dermatitis as a result of exposure of skin to enzymes and other substances in feces and the warm, moist environment
C. Clinical findings
  1. Frequent, watery stools
  2. If fluid loss is severe
    a. Weight loss greater than 10% (moderate dehydration)
    b. Diminished skin turgor and dry mucous membranes
    c. Depressed fontanels and sunken eyeballs
    d. Decreased urine output, increased specific gravity, and increased hematocrit
    e. Irritability, stupor, and seizures from loss of intracellular water and decreased plasma volume
    f. Metabolic acidosis, which decreases available bicarbonate
D. Therapeutic interventions
  1. Severe diarrhea: correction of fluid and electrolyte imbalance (oral rehydration therapy or intravenous fluids)
  2. Identification of causative agent and institution of appropriate therapy (antibiotics are used if a bacterial agent is identified)

Nursing Care of Children With Diarrhea
A. Assessment/Analysis
  1. Assess diarrhea: onset; duration; presence of fever; frequency of vomiting; frequency and character of stools
  2. State of hydration
    a. Mucous membranes
    b. Skin turgor
  3. Electrolyte and acid-base balance
  4. Characteristics of bowel sounds
  5. Perianal area for redness and skin breakdown
  6. Possible source of infection
B. Planning/Implementation
  1. Explain to parents why antibiotics and an increase in food are ineffective in treating viral diarrhea
  2. Offer oral rehydration fluids or administer IV fluids/electrolytes to correct dehydration if present
  3. Record and monitor intake and output; assess for fluid overload if receiving IV fluids
  4. Continue regular diet
C. Evaluation/Outcomes
  1. Consumes sufficient calories and fluids
  2. Maintains skin integrity
  3. Child and family do not transmit infection to others
  4. Episodes of diarrhea cease

✿ VOMITING
Data Base
A. Forcible ejection of stomach contents: usually associated with nausea
  1. Under control of CNS

  2. Response to stress
  3. Protective mechanism to remove toxins from body (gastric acidity not effective to protect infant)
B. Associated hazard: aspiration with risk for asphyxiation, atelectasis, or pneumonia
C. Common in childhood, usually minor and of short duration
D. Causes
  1. Most commonly caused by infection
  2. Response to allergen, drug ingestion
  3. Recurrent or prolonged vomiting may be caused by increased intracranial pressure
E. Clinical findings
  1. One or more episodes of regurgitation or emesis
  2. If vomiting is severe
    a. Dehydration
    b. Tetany and seizures in severe alkalosis resulting from hypokalemia and hypocalcemia
    c. Metabolic alkalosis from loss of hydrogen ions
F. Therapeutic intervention: correction of underlying disorder

Nursing Care of Children With Vomiting
A. Assessment/Analysis
  1. Amount and character of vomitus
  2. Circumstances preceding vomiting
  3. Child's behavior
  4. Bowel sounds
  5. Associated signs and symptoms are fever, diarrhea, constipation, localized abdominal pain, and fluid and electrolyte imbalances
B. Planning/Implementation
  1. Maintain in side-lying position with body inclined at 30 degrees at all times
  2. Do not disturb infant after feeding
  3. If associated with gastroesophageal reflux or cardiac sphincter problems: thicken consistency of foods and provide small-volume feedings every 2 to 3 hours
  4. Rinse mouth after each episode of vomiting
C. Evaluation/Outcomes
  1. Demonstrates evidence of rehydration
  2. Consumes adequate nutrients for growth and development
  3. Episodes of vomiting cease

✿ COLIC
Data Base
A. Paroxsymal abdominal pain or cramping reported in 5% to 30% of infants
B. More common in infants less than 3 months old
C. Less than 5% of infants with colic have an identified etiology
D. Infants with cow's milk allergy are more prone to colic (44%)
E. Associated with excessive swallowing of air, size of nipple opening or shape of nipple, too rapid feeding or overfeeding, tenseness or anxiety in caregiver,

maternal diet, CNS immaturity, and neurochemical dysregulation

F. Clinical findings
1. Pulling up of arms and legs
2. Red-faced crying over long periods of time
3. Presence of excessive gas

G. Therapeutic intervention: correction of underlying cause when identified

Nursing Care of Children With Colic

A. Assessment/Analysis
1. Characteristics of cry (duration and intensity)
2. Diet of breastfeeding mother
3. When attacks occur in relationship to feeding
4. Activity of caregiver around time of attack
5. Mother's habits, such as smoking
6. Measures to relieve crying and their effectiveness

B. Planning/Implementation
1. Watch parent feed infant before attempting to counsel
2. Instruct parents to offer smaller, more frequent feedings
3. Teach parents to burp infant frequently and to position on side after feeding
4. Encourage caregiver to spend time without infant
5. Reassure parents that condition is not life-threatening; infant will gain weight, and the colic will eventually subside

C. Evaluation/Outcomes
1. Decreased pain episodes
2. Parents and infant are rested and able to continue activities of daily living
3. Parents demonstrate effective feeding practices
4. Family can discuss impact of infant's colic

CONSTIPATION

Data Base

A. Hard, dry stools that are difficult to pass or are infrequent
B. Usually result of diet, although may have a psychologic component
C. May be indicative of Hirschsprung's disease
D. Classification
1. Obstipation: long periods between defecations
2. Encopresis: constipation with fecal soiling
E. Clinical findings
1. "Stool withholding" behavior
2. Pain on defecation
F. Therapeutic interventions
1. Dietary: increased fiber and fluid
2. If mineral oil is administered, it is not given with foods because it decreases absorption of nutrients
3. Avoidance of enemas; institution of bowel retraining

Nursing Care of Children With Constipation

A. Assessment/Analysis
1. History of bowel habits, diet
2. Stool characteristics, frequency
3. Parent/child knowledge of elimination

B. Planning/Implementation
1. Teach parents to provide foods high in fiber and ways to promote healthy food choices for their children
2. Teach parents to increase amount of fluid offered
3. Place infant in knee-chest position if distention or cramping is present
4. Cuddle infant to provide comfort as necessary

C. Evaluation/Outcomes
1. Consumes appropriate amount of fiber and fluid
2. Establishes a regular pattern of bowel elimination

RESPIRATORY TRACT INFECTIONS

Data Base

A. Frequent cause of morbidity
B. Young children have four to five infections per year
C. Children between 3 months and 3 years react more severely
D. Acute infection may be bacterial or viral
E. Respiratory syncytial virus (RSV) is single most important respiratory pathogen; causes 50% of pediatric hospitalizations for bronchiolitis in children under 1 year of age
F. Classification: acute nasopharyngitis (common cold); pneumonia; bronchitis; bronchiolitis; tonsillitis; epiglottitis; croup; acute laryngotracheobronchitis
G. Clinical findings
1. Infection: elevated temperature; purulent discharge from nose, ears, lungs; enlarged cervical lymph nodes
2. Cough; wheeze
3. Adventitious breath sounds; tachypnea
4. Cyanosis
5. Grunting respirations
H. Therapeutic interventions
1. Interruption of spasms and bronchial dilation
2. Antibiotics based on culture and sensitivity results

Nursing Care of Children With Respiratory Tract Infections

A. Assessment/Analysis
1. Respirations: rate; depth; ease; and rhythm
2. Color: cyanosis
3. Adventitious breath sounds
4. Nasal discharge; presence of sputum
5. Cough; occurrence of laryngeal spasms
6. Inflammation of the pharynx

B. Planning/Implementation
1. Airborne, droplet, or contact precautions as indicated by CDC
2. Increase fluid intake to prevent dehydration from fever and perspiration, and to prevent secretions from becoming more tenacious
3. Increase humidity and environmental coolness
   a. Decreases febrile state and limits inflammation of mucous membrane
   b. Causes vasoconstriction and bronchiolar dilation
4. Promote nasal and pulmonary drainage
   a. Clean nares with a bulb syringe

b. Suction oronasal pharynx
c. Perform postural drainage and chest physiotherapy
5. Decrease stimulation to promote rest
6. Elevate head of bed
7. Monitor O_2 saturation
8. Administer oxygen as indicated
9. Avoid use of a tongue blade to visualize the posterior pharynx in children with epiglottitis
10. Keep a tracheostomy set at bedside; if a tracheostomy is necessary, see Tracheostomy Care in Chapter 7 under Medical-Surgical Nursing
11. Assess for presence of a mucous plug if a tracheostomy is present and child is exhibiting restlessness, pallor, and/or tachycardia
C. Evaluation/Outcomes
1. Rests and sleeps with unlabored respirations within norms for age range
2. Maintains patent airway

OTITIS MEDIA

Data Base

A. Acute infection of the middle ear; causative bacterial organisms usually *Streptococcus pneumoniae* or *Haemophilus influenzae;* incidence is decreasing secondary to immunization; causative viral organisms usually RSV and influenza
B. One of most common illnesses of early childhood
C. Highest incidence between ages 6 months and 2 years
D. Breastfed infants have lower incidence
E. Classification
1. Otitis media: inflammation of middle ear without reference to cause or pathogenesis
2. Acute otitis media: inflammation of middle ear space with rapid onset of signs and symptoms, mainly fever and ear pain
3. Otitis media with effusion: middle ear inflammation with fluid present
4. Chronic otitis media with effusion: fluid in middle ear space without signs of acute infection
F. Clinical findings
1. Acute otitis media
a. Pain: infant frets and rubs ear or rolls head from side to side; may also hit head against hard surface
b. Drum bulging, red, may rupture; no light reflex
2. Otitis media with effusion
a. No pain or fever, but "fullness" in the ear
b. Drum appears gray, bulging
c. Possible loss of hearing from scarring of eardrum
G. Therapeutic interventions
1. Antibiotic therapy
2. Topical analgesics for ear pain
3. Surgery, including myringotomy with insertion of tympanotomy tubes

Nursing Care of Children With Otitis Media

A. Assessment/Analysis
1. Pain

2. Signs and symptoms of infection
3. Allergies
B. Planning/Implementation
1. Teach parents administration of antibiotics if ordered; stress importance of full course of therapy
2. Teach parents how to instill ear drops: for children under 3 years, pull auricle down and back; for older child, pull auricle up and back
3. Minimize recurrence: eliminate environmental allergens and tobacco smoke; feed in upright position; keep water out of ears
4. Encourage follow-up care to check for complications such as chronic hearing loss, mastoiditis, or possible meningitis
C. Evaluation/Outcomes
1. Sleeps and rests without signs of discomfort
2. Remains free from infection
3. Parents verbalize techniques to minimize otitis media
4. Parents verbalize importance of antibiotic therapy

MENINGITIS

Data Base

A. Most common CNS infection of infants and children
B. Acute inflammation of meninges; cerebral spinal fluid affected
C. Classification: culture of cerebrospinal fluid used to identify organism
1. Bacterial: caused by variety of bacteria, especially *H. influenzae* type b, *S. pneumoniae*, and *Neisseria meningitidis* (meningococcus); account for 95% of meningitis in children older than 2 months
2. Tuberculous: caused by tubercle bacillus
3. Viral or aseptic: caused by wide variety of viral agents
4. Causative organism enters cranial apertures or sinuses; may be caused by an infection of a ventriculoperitoneal shunt used to prevent or treat hydrocephalus
D. Clinical findings
1. Infants
a. Opisthotonos: rigidity and hyperextension of neck
b. Irritability; high-pitched cry
c. Fever
d. Poor feeding
e. Bulging or tense fontanels
f. Meningococcal meningitis: vomiting; petechiae and purpuric skin rash; peripheral circulatory collapse and shock
2. Children and adolescents
a. Signs of increased intracranial pressure: headache; bradycardia; irritability; vomiting
b. Fever; nausea and vomiting
c. Irritability and agitation
d. Photophobia

e. Meningococcal meningitis: petechiae and purpuric skin rash; peripheral circulatory collapse and shock

E. Therapeutic intervention: intravenous antibiotics

Nursing Care of Children With Meningitis

A. Assessment/Analysis
1. Fever
2. Headache; irritability; vomiting
3. Seizures; nuchal rigidity
4. Bulging fontanels
5. Lumbar puncture result indicates causative organism

B. Planning/Implementation
1. Provide for rest; decrease environmental stimuli (control light and noise)
2. Position on side with head gently supported in extension
3. Maintain droplet precautions for at least 48 hours (usually no longer contagious 48 hours after start of antibiotic therapy)
4. Maintain fluid balance because of meningeal edema: monitor I&O, IV fluids, and daily weights; correct deficits
5. Administer antibiotic therapy as prescribed
6. Provide emotional support for parents, because onset of illness is sudden
7. Monitor for complications such as septic shock and circulatory collapse

C. Evaluation/Outcomes
1. Demonstrates a positive response to interventions
2. Parents verbalize fears regarding child's prognosis

FEBRILE SEIZURES

Data Base

A. A seizure in association with a febrile illness in the absence of a CNS infection or an acute electrolyte imbalance

B. Usually occurs in children between 3 months and 5 years of age; most occur between 6 months and 3 years

C. Affects 3% to 4% of children in this age-group

D. Clinical findings
1. Associated with disease outside CNS
2. Temperature usually exceeds 102° F (38.8° C)
3. 30% to 40% of children have a recurrence

E. Therapeutic interventions
1. Control of seizures with medication
2. Reduction of fever
3. Treatment of underlying cause

Nursing Care of Children With Febrile Seizures

A. Assessment/Analysis
1. Description of seizure
2. History of present illness

B. Planning/Implementation
1. Reduce fever with antipyretic drugs; monitor tympanic or axillary temperature
2. General seizure precautions
   a. Protect from injury: do not restrain; pad crib rails; do not use tongue blade
   b. Place on flat surface in side-lying position to prevent aspiration
   c. Observe and record time of seizure, duration, and body parts involved
   d. Suction nasopharynx and administer oxygen after seizure as required
   e. Observe degree of consciousness and behavior after seizure
   f. Provide rest after seizure
3. Teach parents to give antipyretics at first sign of elevated temperature
4. Prevent shivering because it raises the metabolic rate, further raising the body temperature
5. For further discussion of seizures, see Epilepsy (Seizure Disorders) in Chapter 11 under Medical-Surgical Nursing

C. Evaluation/Outcomes
1. Maintains patent airway
2. Remains free from injury during and after seizure
3. Episodes of febrile seizures cease

ATOPIC DERMATITIS (ECZEMA)

Data Base

A. A type of pruritic eczema that usually begins during infancy and is associated with allergy and a hereditary component

B. Most common during first 2 years of life

C. Involves periods of remissions and exacerbations

D. Majority of children with infantile form have a family history of eczema, asthma, food allergies, or allergic rhinitis

E. Classification
1. Infantile: begins between 2 and 6 months of age; spontaneous remission by 3 years
2. Childhood: occurs at 2 to 3 years of age; 90% manifest disorder by 5 years
3. Preadolescent/adolescent: begins at about 12 years and continues into adulthood

F. Clinical findings
1. Erythema and edema from dilation of capillaries
2. Papules, vesicles, and crusts
3. Occurs mostly on cheeks, scalp, neck, and flexor surfaces of arms and legs
4. Itching that may precipitate infection from scratching

G. Therapeutic interventions
1. Relief of pruritus using systemic (e.g., diphenhydramine [Benadryl]) and topical medications
2. Provision of tepid baths and within 3 minutes application of an emollient
3. Increased fluid intake to promote skin hydration
4. Reduction of inflammation
5. Prevention or control of secondary infections

Nursing Care of Children With Atopic Dermatitis

A. Assessment/Analysis
1. Family history of allergies
2. Environmental or dietary factors associated with previous exacerbations

3. Skin lesions: distribution; type; presence of secondary infection
4. Parent/child attitude toward lesions

B. Planning/Implementation
1. Support parents—this long-term problem is often discouraging because infant is difficult to comfort
2. Restrain infant's hands when unsupervised to prevent scratching; keep nails short; provide supervised, unrestrained play periods
3. Pick up frequently because infant is irritable, fretful, and anorectic
4. Keep skin hydrated
5. Provide parents with list of foods permitted or omitted on an elimination or restricted diet
6. Instruct parents how to apply prescribed topical ointments

C. Evaluation/Outcomes
1. Remains free from injury and infection in affected areas
2. Child and parents rest/sleep adequate amounts for age
3. Parents demonstrate ability to follow medical regimen

 HUMAN IMMUNODEFICIENCY VIRUS (HIV) AND ACQUIRED IMMUNODEFICIENCY SYNDROME (AIDS)

Data Base

A. Infection with human immunodeficiency virus (HIV)
B. Viral infection occurs either
1. Vertically from an HIV-infected mother to child (breastfeeding has been identified as a source of the virus); accounts for 91% of AIDS in children
2. Horizontally by sexual contact or parenteral exposure to blood
C. Immunosuppression results from decreased number of CD4 T cells, as well as functional defects in B cells
D. Populations of affected children
1. Children exposed during perinatal period
2. Adolescents who are infected after engaging in high-risk behaviors
E. Clinical findings
1. Failure to thrive
2. Hepatosplenomegaly
3. Diffuse lymphadenopathy
4. Chronic or recurrent diarrhea
5. Oral candidiasis
6. Parotitis
7. *Pneumocystis* pneumonia (PCP) caused by *Pneumocystis jiroveci*
8. Neurologic involvement

F. Therapeutic interventions
1. Combination antiviral medication to suppress viral replication; nucleoside reverse transcriptase inhibitors (zidovudine [AZT, Retrovir], didanosine [ddl, Videx]); nonnucleoside reverse transcriptase inhibitors (nevirapine [Viramune]); and protease inhibitors (indinavir [Crixavan], saquinavir [Fortavase, Invirase])
2. Immunizations
   a. HIV asymptomatic: DTP; inactivated polio virus (Salk vaccine); measles, mumps, and rubella (MMR) vaccine; pneumococcal and influenza immunizations; child monitored to observe results; no varicella vaccine
   b. Children with suppressed immune systems: may not be able to mount active immunity against the immunizations
   c. HIV symptomatic: usually no immunizations
3. Prevention and management of secondary infections
4. Treatment of pain
5. Nutritional support

Nursing Care of Children With AIDS

A. Assessment/Analysis
1. Family support; determine who is able to care for child
2. History to determine source of infection
3. Health status
B. Planning/Implementation
1. Prevent transmission of virus
   a. Standard and transmission-based precautions
   b. Education of child and parent about modes of transmission
2. Provide emotional support to child and family
3. Monitor child for signs and symptoms of sepsis and other complications
C. Evaluation/Outcomes
1. Does not transmit the HIV virus
2. Remains free of opportunistic infections and other complications
3. Child and family maintain positive interpersonal relationships
4. Family members demonstrate appropriate care of child
5. Family members demonstrate effective bereavement behaviors

EMOTIONAL DISORDERS

For common emotional disorders of infancy, see Chapter 17: Nursing Care of Clients With Disorders Usually First Evident in Infancy, Childhood, or Adolescence under Mental Health/Psychiatric Nursing

31 Nursing Care of Toddlers

GROWTH AND DEVELOPMENT

DEVELOPMENTAL TIMETABLE

Fifteen Months

A. Physical
1. Growth rate begins to decrease
2. Capacity of urinary bladder increases

B. Motor
1. Walks alone by 14 months with a wide-based gait; creeps up stairs
2. Builds tower of two blocks; enjoys throwing objects and picking them up
3. Drinks from a cup and can use a spoon

C. Vocalization and socialization
1. Can use four to six words, including name
2. Has learned "No," which may be said while complying with a request

Eighteen Months

A. Physical
1. Growth has decreased and appetite lessened ("physiologic anorexia")
2. Anterior fontanel is usually closed
3. Abdomen protrudes, larger than chest circumference

B. Motor
1. Runs clumsily; climbs stairs or up on furniture
2. Imitates strokes in drawing
3. Drinks from a cup; manages a spoon
4. Builds tower of three to four cubes

C. Vocalization and socialization
1. Says 10 or more words
2. Has new awareness of strangers
3. Begins to have temper tantrums
4. Ritualistic, has favorite toy or blanket, thumb-sucking may be at peak

Two Years

A. Physical
1. Weight—about 11 to 12 kg (26 to 28 lb)
2. Height—about 80 to 82 cm (32 to 33 inches)
3. Teeth—16 temporary; should begin visits to dentist

B. Motor
1. Gross motor skills refined
2. Can walk up and down stairs, both feet on one step at a time, holding onto rail
3. Builds tower of six to seven cubes or will make cubes into a train

C. Sensory
1. Eye accommodation has developed
2. Visual acuity 20/40

D. Vocalization and socialization
1. Vocabulary of about 300 words; uses short, 2- to 3-word phrases, also pronouns
2. Obeys simple commands; shows signs of increasing autonomy and individuality; makes simple choices when possible
3. Still ritualistic, especially at bedtime
4. Can help undress self and pull on simple clothes
5. Does not share possessions, everything is "mine"

Thirty Months

A. Physical
1. Full set of 20 temporary teeth; dentist visits should begin between 2 to 3 years of age
2. Decreased need for naps

B. Motor
1. Walks on tiptoe; stands on one foot momentarily
2. Builds tower of eight blocks
3. Copies horizontal or vertical line
4. May attend to own toilet needs during the day
5. Increasing ability to use a spoon

C. Vocalization and socialization
1. Beginning to see self as a separate individual from reflected appraisal of significant others
2. Still sees other children as objects
3. Increasingly independent, ritualistic, and negativistic

Major Learning Events

A. Toilet training: most important physiologic task of the toddler
1. Physical maturation must be reached before training is possible; approach and attitude of parents play vital role
   a. Sphincter control adequate when child can walk
   b. Able to retain urine for at least 2 hours
   c. Usual age for bowel training is 22 to 30 months
   d. Daytime bowel and bladder control: during second year
   e. Night control takes several months to years after daytime control is achieved; if night wetting persists to 6 years of age, investigation into cause is indicated
2. Psychologic readiness
   a. Aware of the act of elimination

b. Able to inform caregiver of need to urinate or defecate

c. Desire to please parents

3. Process of training

a. Usually begins with bowel, then bladder; uses potty chair

b. Accidents and regressions frequently occur

4. Parental response

a. Choose a specific word for the act

b. Have a specific time and place

c. Do not punish for accidents

B. Need for independence without overprotection; parents should

1. Be consistent; set realistic limits; provide choices

2. Reinforce desired behavior

3. Be constructive, geared to teach self-control

4. Punish immediately after a wrongdoing; punish appropriately

HEALTH PROMOTION OF TODDLERS

PLAY DURING TODDLERHOOD (PARALLEL PLAY)

A. Plays alongside other children but not with them

B. Mostly free and spontaneous, no rules or regulations

C. Short attention span requires frequent change of toys

D. Safety is important; there is danger of

1. Breaking a toy through exploration and ingesting small pieces

2. Ingesting lead from lead-based paint on toys

3. Being burned by potentially flammable toys

E. Imitation and make-believe play begins by end of second year

F. Suggested toys

1. Play furniture, dishes, cooking utensils, telephone

2. Puzzles with a few large pieces

3. Pedal-propelled toys, such as tricycle; straddle toys such as rocking horse

4. Play-Doh, clay, sandbox toys, crayons, finger paints

5. Pounding toys; blocks; push-pull toys

CHILDHOOD NUTRITION

A. Nutritional objectives include provision of

1. Adequate nutrient intake to meet continuing growth and development needs

2. A basis for support of psychosocial development in relation to food patterns, eating behavior, and attitudes

3. Sufficient calories for increasing physical activity and energy needs

4. Fresh fruits and vegetables rather than processed foods

B. Diet

1. Reflects patterns and preferences of culture, parents, and siblings

2. Calorie and nutrient requirements increase with age, despite slower growth

3. Increased variety in types and textures of foods; provision of choices to address growing independence

4. Increased involvement in the feeding process; stimulation of curiosity about food environment; language learning

5. Consideration for child's appetite, choices, motor skills

C. Possible nutritional problem areas

1. Anemia: increased need for foods containing iron (e.g., enriched cereals, meat, eggs, green vegetables); iron supplements should be diluted and administered through a straw

2. Obesity or underweight: increased or decreased caloric intake; maintenance of core foods

3. Low intake of calcium, iron, vitamins A and C; usually caused by dietary fads

4. Breakfast often omitted

5. Influence of commercialism on selection of foods and emphasis on fast foods, "empty-calorie" snacks, and high-carbohydrate convenience foods

INJURY PREVENTION DURING TODDLERHOOD

A. Leading cause of death in children between 1 and 4 years of age

B. Children under 5 years of age account for over half of all accidental deaths during childhood

C. More than half of accidental child deaths are related to automobiles and fire

D. Accidents can be viewed in terms of child's growth and development, especially curiosity about the environment

1. Motor vehicle

a. Walking or running, especially chasing after objects thrown into the street

b. Inability to determine speed; lack of experience to foresee danger

c. Child often unseen because of small size; can be hit by car backing out of driveway, or when playing in leaves or snow

d. Failure to restrain in car (sitting in a person's lap; incorrect use of seat belts rather than appropriate car restraint)

2. Burns

a. Investigating: pulls a pot off stove; plays with matches; inserts an object into wall socket

b. Climbing: reaches stove, oven, ironing board and iron, cigarettes on a table

3. Poisons

a. Learning new tastes and textures; uses oral exploration

b. Developing fine motor skills: able to open bottles, cabinets, jars

c. Climbing to previously unreachable shelves and cabinets

4. Drowning
   a. Child and parents do not recognize danger of playing in or near water
   b. Child is unaware of inability to breathe under water
5. Aspirating small objects and putting foreign objects in ear or nose
   a. Puts everything in mouth
   b. Very interested in body and newly found openings
6. Fractures
   a. Climbing, running, and jumping
   b. Still developing sense of balance

HOSPITALIZATION OF TODDLERS

DATA BASE

A. Toddler experiences basic fear of loss of love, fear of unknown, fear of punishment
B. Immobilization and isolation represent additional crises; may influence physical (particularly neurologic) and psychosocial development; rarely affects hearing ability
C. Regression to earlier behaviors may occur
D. Stages of separation anxiety
   1. Protest
      a. Prolonged loud crying, consoled by no one but the parent or usual caregiver
      b. Continually asks to go home
      c. Rejection of nurse or any other stranger
   2. Despair
      a. Alteration in sleep pattern
      b. Decreased appetite and weight loss
      c. Diminished interest in environment and play
      d. Relative immobility and listlessness
      e. No facial expression or smile
      f. Unresponsive to stimuli
   3. Detachment or denial
      a. Cheerful, undiscriminating friendliness
      b. Lack of preference for parents

GENERAL NURSING CARE OF TODDLERS

A. Prepare parents and child for hospitalization
   1. Give primary consideration to maintaining parent-child relationship by limiting separation
   2. Recognize that only minimal advance preparation for hospitalization is possible, because the toddler's cognitive ability to grasp verbal explanation is limited
   3. Determine child's routines and rituals in the areas of toilet training, feeding, bathing, sleep pattern so that they can be continued during hospitalization
   4. Ask parents to bring child's favorite items from home (e.g., a blanket, a toy, a bottle, or a pacifier)
   5. Prepare parents for child's reaction to separation; pounding toys helps release anger associated with temper tantrums or separation; limit temper tantrums by preventing unreasonable demands on child
   6. Prepare parents for child's regression to previous modes of behavior and loss of newly learned skills
B. Minimize separation anxiety and other emotional traumas during hospitalization
   1. Encourage parents to stay with child in hospital; if possible, have one parent room-in with child throughout hospitalization
   2. If parent is not rooming-in, encourage frequent visits; explain that frequent visits for short periods of time are more therapeutic than one long visit
   3. Associate parents' visits with familiar events, such as "Mommy is coming after lunch"
   4. Involve parents in child's care as much as possible; however, understand that parental anxiety may be transmitted to child and involve parents appropriately
   5. When parents are unable to visit, establish phone contact
   6. Provide a consistent caregiver who can offer individual attention, physical touch, sensory stimulation, and affection
   7. Avoid teaching new skills during hospitalization
   8. Encourage release of tension, especially aggression, through play (knocking blocks over, scribbling on paper, peg and pounding board)
   9. Establish a routine similar to the home routine by continuing rituals and providing favorite items from home
   10. Maintain familiarity with home by talking about parents, having child listen to a tape recording of family members' voices, and showing photographs of family members
   11. When family members leave, stay with child for comfort and to reassure parents
   12. Understand that regression may occur; accept regression and support child emotionally
   13. Understand that sedation may be necessary during procedures that require the child to remain still (e.g., CT scan, MRI)

HEALTH PROBLEMS MOST COMMON IN TODDLERS

❁ BURNS

(See Burns in Chapter 10 under Medical-Surgical Nursing for additional information)

Data Base

A. Burn injuries are the third leading cause of unintentional injury and related death among children 14 years of age and under
B. Children under 5 years of age are at greatest risk because of their limited control of their

environment and limited ability to act promptly and appropriately

C. Causative agents: thermal (flame, hot water); chemical; electrical; radiation

D. Classification
1. Depth of injury
   a. Superficial (first-degree): tissue damage minimal; pain predominant symptom
   b. Partial-thickness (second-degree): involves epithelium and part of dermis; severity and rate of healing depend on amount of damaged dermis; very painful
   c. Full-thickness (third and fourth degree): all layers of skin destroyed; systemic effects can be life-threatening; requires skin grafting
2. Extent of injury
   a. Described as a percentage of total body surface area (TBSA) injured
   b. Standard adult rule of nines cannot be used in children under 15 years of age; modifications exist for newborn, infant, 5 year old, 10 year old, 15 year old

E. Clinical findings
1. Local response
   a. Edema formation
   b. Fluid loss from nonprotected skin
   c. Occurrence of circulatory stasis; usually restored within 24 to 48 hours in partial-thickness burns
2. Systemic response
   a. "Burn shock" causes precipitous drop in cardiac output; returns to normal in 24 to 36 hours
   b. Metabolic rate greatly increased
   c. Physiologic stress response
   d. Anemia and metabolic acidosis: initially hematocrit is elevated because of fluid shifts from the intravascular space; increased red cell fragility contributes to a decreased RBC life span, resulting in anemia
   e. Post-burn growth retardation: severe growth delays in height and weight seen in children who sustain greater than 40% TBSA burn; growth lag may last for up to 3 years without catch-up growth

F. Therapeutic interventions
1. Burning process is stopped
   a. Source of danger removed
   b. Smoldering clothes removed
   c. For superficial burns, affected area is immersed in cool water
2. First aid administered promptly
   a. Patent airway maintained
   b. For superficial burns, area is cleansed, application of sterile dressing soaked in sterile saline if possible
   c. Avoidance of creams, butter, or any household remedies
   d. Oral fluids not offered for severe burns (more than 10% of body)

3. Transportation of child to an appropriate health care facility as quickly as possible because
   a. Child's large body surface area in proportion to weight results in greater potential for fluid loss
   b. Shock: primary cause of death in first 24 to 48 hours
   c. Infection: primary cause of death after initial period
4. Treatment of fluid and electrolyte loss
   a. Greatest in first 24 to 48 hours because of tissue damage
   b. Immediate replacement of both fluids and electrolytes is essential
   c. Determination of hematocrit, hemoglobin, and blood chemistry levels should be done daily to provide a guide for replacement
5. Tetanus prophylaxis as needed

Nursing Care of Children With Burns

A. Assessment/Analysis
1. Wound assessment/classification; presence and extent of pain
2. Vital signs; respiratory status
3. Fluid balance; nutritional needs
4. Pain rating

B. Planning/Implementation
1. Monitor fluids and electrolytes
   a. Administer prescribed fluids accurately, both in time and in volume
   b. Accurately measure intake and output (daily weights, weigh diapers)
2. Maintain precautions (standard, protective, and/or contact)
   a. Understand that child has feelings of guilt and punishment
   b. Recognize that children under 5 years of age rarely understand the reason for isolation or the use of personal protective equipment, which further separates child from others
   c. Encourage child to express feelings
3. Compensate for touch deprivation
   a. Recognize that touch, a child's main means of comfort and security, is now painful
   b. Reestablish pleasurable touch (apply lotion to unaffected areas)
   c. Maximize use of other senses to promote security and comfort
4. Provide for adequate nutrition
   a. Understand that children with burns initially experience a hypometabolic state followed by a hypermetabolic state, that usually begins on the fifth day post injury, which causes erosion of lean body mass, muscle weakness, immunodepression, and inadequate wound healing
   b. Diet high in protein, vitamins, and calories should be started as soon as paralytic ileus resolves
   c. Encourage eating; child is frequently anorectic because of discomfort, isolation, emotional depression

d. Provide child's food preferences when feasible; do not force eating or use it as a weapon; encourage parent participation

e. If child is unable to consume the necessary calories, provide care related to tube feeding; assess for gastric return and residual before feeding; flush with normal saline before and after feeding

f. Alter diet as needs change, especially when high-calorie foods are no longer needed and can cause obesity

5. Prevent contractures

a. Make moving a game; use play that uses the affected part, such as throwing a ball for arm movement

b. Provide for functional body alignment; place child so attention is focused on an object that will keep the body in a specific position

c. Do passive exercises during bath or whirlpool treatments

d. Give analgesics before exercise

6. Meet child's emotional needs

a. Allow child to play with gown, mask, gloves, and bandages so that they are less strange

b. Prepare child for baths and whirlpool treatments, which can be frightening and painful

c. Allow child to reenact treatments and care on a doll to work through feelings

d. Help child deal with changes in body

(1) For younger child: support parents whose reactions are communicated to their child

(2) For older child, especially the adolescent: body appearance is of great concern; devise ways to conceal affected areas, especially when peers visit; emphasize what can be done to improve looks (e.g., plastic surgery, wigs, cosmetics, clothing)

7. Help limit pain

a. Assess extent of pain by observing behavior of the young child, as well as verbal complaints

b. Distinguish pain from fear of dark, being left alone, or being in strange surroundings

c. Use pain rating scale and medicate child appropriately

d. Medicate before procedures; anesthetic agents such as nitrous oxide, propofol (Disoprofol, Diprivan), and ketamine are used

e. Opioids may be required for burn pain; IV is the preferred route because of impaired peripheral absorption

8. Teach prevention of burn injuries

a. Educate children regarding fire safety

(1) Tell children to leave the house as soon as smoke is smelled or flames are seen, without stopping to retrieve a pet or toy

(2) Involve all members of the family in fire drills

(3) Demonstrate and practice "stop, drop, and roll" rather than running, if clothes are on fire

b. Educate parents especially in regard to their child's growth and development and specific dangers at each age level

c. Teach parents how to prevent fires in the home

(1) Supervise children at all times; maintain escape route

(2) Cautiously use heaters, barbecue grill, and fireplace; place shield in front of heating unit

(3) Maintain integrity of electrical system

(4) Regulate water heater to no higher than 120° F (mandated in several states)

(5) Use and maintain smoke detectors

C. Evaluation/Outcomes

1. Remains comfortable

2. Maintains fluid and nutritional balance

3. Heals with minimal scarring

4. Remains free from infection

5. Regains flexibility and functional capacity of joints

6. Child and family members verbalize feelings and concerns about appearance

POISONING

Data Base

A. Ingestion of a toxic substance or an excessive amount of a substance

B. More than 90% of poisonings occur in the home

C. Highest incidence occurs in children under 4 years

D. Most commonly ingested substances

1. Cosmetics and personal care products—13% (e.g., perfume, aftershave)

2. Cleaning products—10.7% (e.g., household bleach, pine oil disinfectant)

3. Analgesics—7.6% (e.g., acetaminophen, ibuprofen)

4. Plants—6.9% (e.g., nontoxic gastrointestinal irritants, oxalates)

5. Foreign bodies, toys, miscellaneous—6.6% (e.g., desiccants, thermometer, bubble blowing solution)

E. Improper storage is major contributing factor to poisonings

General Nursing Care of Children With Poisoning

A. Assessment/Analysis

1. Child's general response

2. Vital signs

3. Need for respiratory or cardiac support

4. See Clinical findings under specific type of poisoning

B. Planning/Implementation

1. Terminate the exposure

a. Empty mouth of pills, plant parts, or other material

b. Thoroughly flush eyes with tap water if they were involved

c. Flush skin and wash with soap and soft cloth

d. Remove clothing, especially if pesticide, acid, alkali, or hydrocarbon involved

e. Bring child into fresh air if an inhalation poisoning

2. Communicate that a poisoning has occurred
   a. Call the poison control center, emergency facility, or physician for immediate advice regarding treatment
   b. Save all evidence of poison (e.g., container, vomitus, urine)

3. Do not induce vomiting because
   a. If a low-viscosity hydrocarbon (e.g., gasoline, lighter fluid, mineral seal oil [found in furniture polishes]) is aspirated, it can cause severe chemical pneumonitis
   b. If poison is a strong corrosive (e.g., acid or alkali, such as drain cleaners, bleach, electric dishwasher detergent, batteries), emesis of the corrosive redamages the mucosa of the esophagus and pharynx

4. Remove the poison
   a. Administer activated charcoal (1 g per kilogram body weight) if possible within 1 hour of ingestion; can be effective within 4 hours of ingestion of injurious substance
   b. Prepare equipment for gastric lavage if can be initiated within 1 hour of ingestion

5. Prevent aspiration if child is vomiting
   a. Keep head lower than the chest
   b. When alert, place head between the child's legs
   c. When unconscious, position on the side

6. Observe for latent symptoms and complications of poisoning
   a. Monitor vital signs
   b. Treat as appropriate (e.g., institute seizure precautions, keep warm, and position correctly in case of shock; reduce temperature if hyperpyretic)

7. Support child and parent
   a. Keep calm and quiet
   b. Do not admonish or accuse child or parent of wrongdoing

8. Teach prevention of poisoning
   a. Assess possible contributing factors in the occurrence of an accident, such as lack of discipline, parent-child relationship, developmental ability, environmental factors, and behavior problems
   b. Institute anticipatory guidance for possible future accidents based on child's age and developmental level
   c. Refer to an appropriate agency for evaluation of the home environment and need for safety measures
   d. Provide assistance with environmental manipulation when necessary

e. Educate parents regarding safe storage of all substances

f. Teach children the hazards of ingesting nonfood items

g. Caution against keeping large amounts of medicines on hand, especially children's varieties

h. Discourage transferring medications to containers without safety caps

i. Discuss problems of discipline and children's noncompliance

C. Evaluation/Outcomes
   1. Recuperates free from complications
   2. Parents and child demonstrate knowledge concerning prevention of future poisoning

ACETAMINOPHEN POISONING

Data Base

A. One of the most common drugs taken by children
   1. Toxic dose: 150 mg/kg body weight
   2. Therapeutic dose of 150 mg/kg/day for several days has resulted in toxicity

B. Clinical findings: signs and symptoms of overdose
   1. First 2 to 4 hours after ingestion: nausea; vomiting; profuse diaphoresis; pallor
   2. Latent period (24 to 36 hours): symptoms subside; slow, weak pulse
   3. Hepatic involvement (may last up to 7 days or be permanent): pain in right upper quadrant; jaundice; confusion; stupor; coagulation abnormality
   4. Gradual recovery for children who do not die during hepatic coma

C. Therapeutic interventions
   1. IV fluids
   2. Administration of oral antidote (acetylcysteine)

Nursing Care of Children With Acetaminophen Poisoning

A. Determine amount ingested
B. Monitor the electrocardiograph
C. Measure I&O
D. Measure and record vital signs frequently
E. Obtain blood for hepatic and renal function tests
F. Support child and family
G. See General Nursing Care of Children With Poisoning

SALICYLATE POISONING AND TOXICITY

Data Base

A. Toxic dose: 300 to 500 mg/kg body weight or 7 adult aspirins (28 baby aspirin) for a 9-kg (20-lb) child

B. Clinical findings
   1. Acute poisoning
      a. Nausea, vomiting, disorientation, dehydration, diaphoresis, oliguria
      b. Hyperpyrexia; hyperpnea
      c. Ringing in the ears, dizziness, disturbances of hearing and vision
      d. Delirium, confusion, coma

2. Chronic poisoning
   a. Can occur from chronic ingestion: more than 100 mg/kg/day for 2 or more days
   b. Same as acute poisoning but subtle onset; dehydration, coma, and seizures more severe
   c. Bleeding, especially if chronic ingestion
C. Therapeutic interventions
   1. Emesis, gastric lavage, activated charcoal, and saline cathartics if life-threatening
   2. IV fluids with sodium bicarbonate for correction of acidosis
   3. Vitamin K if bleeding
   4. Peritoneal dialysis if severe complication
   5. Hypothermia blanket when hyperthermia is present

Nursing Care of Children With Salicylate Poisoning

A. Identify salicylate overdose
B. Assess blood gases and serum electrolyte concentration frequently
C. Administer sodium bicarbonate, elcctrolytes, and vitamin K as indicated
D. Continue use of hypothermia blanket if hyperthermia is present
E. See General Nursing Care of Children With Poisoning

❧ PETROLEUM DISTILLATE POISONING

Data Base

A. Distillates include kerosene, turpentine, gasoline, lighter fluid, furniture polish, metal polish, benzene, naphthalene, some insecticides, and cleaning fluid
B. Clinical findings
   1. Gagging; choking; and coughing
   2. Nausea; vomiting
   3. Weakness; alterations in sensorium, such as lethargy
   4. Signs of pulmonary involvement: tachypnea; cyanosis; substernal retractions; grunting
C. Therapeutic interventions
   1. Vomiting not induced: aspiration is a particular danger because of risk for chemical pneumonia
   2. Gastric decontamination and emptying are questionable: if gastric lavage must be performed because of a life-threatening situation, a cuffed endotracheal tube is in place before lavage because of high risk of aspiration

Nursing Care of Children With Petroleum Distillate Poisoning

A. Identify distillate ingested and amount
B. Prevent further irritation
   1. Avoid causing emesis
   2. Implement gastric lavage only if ordered
C. See General Nursing Care of Children With Poisoning

❧ CORROSIVE CHEMICAL POISONING

Data Base

A. Corrosive chemicals include oven and drain cleaners, electric dishwasher granules, and strong detergents
B. Clinical findings
   1. Severe burning pain in mouth, throat, and stomach
   2. White, edematous mucous membranes; edema of lips, tongue, and pharynx (respiratory obstruction)
   3. Violent vomiting; hemoptysis; hematemesis
   4. Signs of shock
   5. Anxiety and agitation
C. Therapeutic intervention: vomiting is never induced because regurgitation of the substance will further damage mucous membranes

Nursing Care of Children With Corrosive Chemical Poisoning

A. Identify ingested substance and amount
B. Maintain a patent airway
   1. Examine pharynx for burns; monitor for respiratory difficulty
   2. Have emergency equipment available; provide an airway if necessary
   3. Administer steroids if prescribed
C. Prevent further irritation
   1. Avoid causing emesis
   2. Give nothing by mouth except as ordered and tolerated; dilute with water or milk (no more than 120 mL)
   3. Do not neutralize substance; neutralization can cause an exothermic reaction, which produces heat and causes increased symptoms or produces a thermal burn in addition to the chemical burn
D. Provide comfort and support to child and family
   1. Use pain rating scale and medicate appropriately
   2. Remain with child
   3. Keep parents informed of their child's progress
E. See General Nursing Care of Children with Poisoning

❧ LEAD POISONING (PLUMBISM)

Data Base

A. A prevalent, significant, preventable health problem that causes neurologic, intellectual, and developmental problems from even low levels of lead
B. Blood lead concentration should be less than 10 mg per 100 mL of blood
C. Associated with increased levels of lead in the environment and pica: lead-based paint (most common source); other sources include soil, dust, drinking water with lead, parental occupations, and hobbies involving lead
D. Child does not have to eat loose paint chips to be exposed to the toxin; typical hand to mouth behavior coupled with presence of lead dust in the environment is the usual method of poisoning
E. Clinical findings (chronic ingestion)
   1. Anemia; pallor; listlessness; fatigue
   2. Lead line on teeth and long bones; joint pain
   3. Protein in urine as a result of proximal tubular damage
   4. Behavioral changes: impulsiveness; irritability; hyperactivity; lethargy

5. Headache; insomnia; brain damage; convulsions; death

F. Therapeutic interventions
1. Reduction of lead concentration in blood and soft tissue using chelation therapy (removal of lead from circulating blood and, theoretically, some lead from organs in tissues)
    a. Calcium disodium edetate (calcium disodium versenate, calcium EDTA)
        (1) Administered through IV or IM route
        (2) Urine lead content monitored; peak excretion in 24 to 48 hours
        (3) Adverse effects: acute tubular necrosis; malaise; fatigue; numbness of extremities; GI disturbances; fever; pain in muscles and joints
    b. Succimer (Chemet)
        (1) Oral chelating agent
        (2) Adverse effects: nausea; vomiting; diarrhea; loss of appetite; rash; liver damage; and neutropenia
        (3) Adequate hydration to facilitate clearance of chelates through kidney
    c. Dimercaprol (BAL)
        (1) Administered by deep IM injection
        (2) Generally used in conjunction with calcium disodium edetate
        (3) Adverse effects: local pain at site of injection; may cause persistent fever; rise in BP accompanied by tachycardia after injection
        (4) Cannot be used in children with peanut allergy
2. Prevention of further ingestion

Nursing Care of Children With Lead Poisoning

A. Determine environmental exposure and oral ingestion
B. Screen children at risk by recognizing clinical findings, especially behavior changes
C. Plan preparation of child and rotation of injection sites if therapeutic intervention includes IM chelating agents; warm, moist applications may relieve discomfort of injections
D. Use therapeutic play including a syringe and doll to help child express feelings
E. Monitor for side effects of chelation therapy
F. Monitor urinary output; keep well hydrated
G. Prevent future lead poisoning with parental and child education, appropriate environment, and supervision of child and siblings

❁ FRACTURES

(See Fractures of the Extremities in Chapter 11 under Medical-Surgical Nursing for additional information)
Data Base
A. An interruption in the integrity of a bone
B. In children, bones are more easily injured; fractures can result without major injury to surrounding tissue

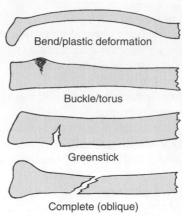

Figure 31-1 Common types of fractures in children. (From Hockenberry MJ, Wilson D: *Wong's nursing care of infants and children*, ed 8, St Louis, 2007, Mosby.)

C. Fractures of the forearm (most often the radius) are common bone injuries in children; usually caused when child extends the palm of the hand to break a fall
D. Healing occurs rapidly in children; rapidity of healing is inversely related to age of child
E. Types of fractures (Figure 31-1: Common types of fractures in children)
1. Bend: bone is bent, not broken
2. Buckle: bone is compressed; appears as a bulge
3. Greenstick: incomplete break and bending of a long bone, occurs in young children because bones are soft and not fully mineralized
4. Complete: bone fragments are divided; may be connected by a periosteal hinge; subtypes include transverse, oblique, spiral
F. Clinical findings
1. Generalized swelling
2. Pain or tenderness
3. Diminished function or use of part
G. Therapeutic interventions
1. Splints
2. Casts: hard or soft to promote bone alignment and prevent further damage
3. Internal or external fixation

Nursing Care of Children With Fractures

A. Assessment/Analysis
1. The five P's associated with neurovascular assessment
    a. Pain and point of tenderness
    b. Pulselessness distal to fracture site (late and ominous sign)
    c. Pallor
    d. Paresthesia: sensation distal to fracture site
    e. Paralysis: lack of movement distal to fracture site
2. Cause of injury
B. Planning/Implementation
1. Use pain rating scale and medicate appropriately
2. Monitor neurovascular status of distal extremity
3. Allow cast to dry by exposing casted extremity to air
4. Provide activity to keep child occupied and entertained

5. Maintain functional alignment
   a. Keep child positioned by using supportive devices
   b. Jacket restraint may be necessary to prevent twisting or turning
C. Evaluation/Outcomes
   1. Maintains neurovascular status in affected extremity
   2. Experiences minimal discomfort
   3. Maintains skin integrity
   4. Regains tone and flexibility in muscles and joints, respectively
   5. Plays and interacts with others

ASPIRATION OF FOREIGN OBJECTS
Data Base
A. Obstruction of the airway by a foreign object; can occur anywhere from larynx to bronchi
B. Most common in children 1 to 3 years of age; leading cause of accidental death in children less than 1 year of age
C. Foods that cause asphyxiation include hot dogs, round candy, peanuts, grapes, and popcorn
D. Classification
   1. Partial obstruction has time interval (hours to days) without symptoms
   2. Complete obstruction is an emergency
E. Clinical findings
   1. Complete obstruction: substernal retractions; inability to cough or speak; increased pulse and respiratory rates; cyanosis
   2. Partial obstruction: persistent respiratory tract infection; hoarseness or garbled speech; wheeze; stridor
F. Therapeutic interventions
   1. Incomplete obstruction: no intervention; child is allowed to continue coughing until object is dislodged
   2. Complete obstruction: immediate first aid
      a. Small child is turned upside down (head lower than chest) and given up to five quick, sharp back blows with the heel of the hand; child is turned over and given up to five quick chest thrusts using the technique for CPR
      b. Abdominal thrust for children ages 1 year and older (formerly called the Heimlich maneuver): child is grasped from behind around the upper abdomen and squeezed, forcing the diaphragm up
   3. Medical removal by bronchoscopy
   4. Surgical relief by a tracheotomy below level of the object

Nursing Care of Children Who Aspirate Foreign Objects
A. Assessment/Analysis
   1. Breathing pattern
   2. Absence of speech
   3. Color
B. Planning/Implementation
   1. Keep small objects such as balloons, buttons, and batteries out of child's reach; inspect larger toys for removable parts

2. Avoid giving young children foods easily aspirated, such as nuts or hot dogs
3. Teach child not to run or laugh with food or fluid in the mouth and to chew food well before swallowing
C. Evaluation/Outcomes
   1. Regains a patent airway
   2. Child and parents verbalize ways to prevent future airway obstruction

CHILD MALTREATMENT
Data Base
A. One of the most significant social problems affecting children
B. Intentional physical abuse or neglect, emotional abuse or neglect, and sexual abuse of children
C. The Child Abuse Prevention and Treatment Act (CAPTA) defines child abuse and neglect as any recent act or failure to act that results in imminent risk of death, serious physical or emotional harm, sexual abuse, or exploitation of a child by a parent or caretaker who is responsible for the child's welfare
D. Sexual abuse is defined as employment, use, persuasion, inducement, enticement, or coercion of any child to engage in, or assist any other person to engage in, any sexually explicit conduct or any simulation of such conduct for the purpose of producing any visual depiction of such conduct; definition includes rape, statutory rape, molestation, prostitution, or other forms of sexual exploitation of children or incest with children
E. Family characteristics
   1. Parental history of abuse or neglect
   2. Parental report of severe punishment as a child, which makes them more likely to injure their own children
   3. Difficulty controlling aggressive impulses
   4. Use of violence to resolve conflict
   5. Unpredictable, unstable family environment
   6. Inability to deal with serial crises
   7. Lack of trust for outsiders and family members
   8. Isolation from community and social supports
F. Child characteristics
   1. Difficult temperament; difficult interaction between parent and child; hyperactive
   2. Position in family
   3. Additional physical needs: physical or mental disability; preterm birth
   4. Lack of sensitivity to parental needs
G. Environmental characteristics
   1. Atmosphere of chronic stress; crowded living conditions
   2. Presence of alcohol or substance abuse
   3. Divorce; unemployment; and frequent change of location
H. Classification
   1. Physical abuse: minor physical abuse responsible for more reported cases than major physical abuse, which results in increased mortality

2. Neglect: most common form of maltreatment; includes emotional neglect, physical neglect, and emotional abuse
3. Sexual abuse: incest; molestation; exhibitionism; pedophilia; child pornography or prostitution
4. Rate of sexual abuse of females approximately 4 times that of males
5. Emotional abuse includes acts or omissions by parents or other caregivers that have caused, or could cause, serious behavioral, cognitive, emotional, or mental disorders
I. Clinical findings
   1. Physical evidence of abuse/previous injuries
   2. Conflicting stories about injury; injury blamed on sibling or another party
   3. Inappropriate parental response; exaggerated or absent emotional response; rarely looks at or touches child; failure to sign consent for additional tests; delay in seeking treatment
   4. Inappropriate response of child: little or no response to pain; fear of being touched; excessive or lack of separation anxiety; indiscriminate friendliness to strangers
J. Therapeutic interventions
   1. Treatment of injury
   2. Suspected abuse reported to local authorities; all states and provinces in North America have laws for mandatory reporting
   3. Protection of child from further abuse

Nursing Care of Children Who Are Maltreated

A. Assessment/Analysis
   1. History of injury: objective data from examination of child does not match story told by parents ("Toddler fell off of chair" while examination shows a spiral fracture of femur, which would not be a likely result of this report)
   2. Physical status; evidence of past injuries (skeletal and soft tissue injuries); failure to thrive
   3. Parent-child interaction
   4. Developmental level of child
B. Planning/Implementation
   1. Be alert for clues that indicate child neglect or abuse
      a. Child has many unexplained injuries, scars, bruises
      b. Parents offer inconsistent stories explaining child's injuries when questioned
      c. Emotional response of parents is inconsistent with the degree of child's injury
      d. Parents may resist or fail to be present for questioning
      e. Child exhibits physical signs of neglect: malnourished; dehydrated; unkempt
      f. Child cringes when physically approached and appears unduly afraid
      g. Child responds in a manner that indicates avoiding punishment rather than gaining reward

h. Child has excessive interest in sexual matters
      i. Child has a sexually transmitted infection
   2. Be aware of child abuse laws
   3. Recognize that the main objective is to protect the child from further abuse
   4. Place child in a room near the nurses' station; provide a consistent caregiver
   5. Focus on helping parents with their own dependency needs; use group therapy, home visiting, and foster grandparents
   6. Help parents learn to control frustration through other outlets
   7. Educate parents about the child's needs and development, new modes of discipline, and realistic expectations
   8. Use therapeutic play to help child express feelings
   9. Provide emotional support and therapy for the child because abused children may grow up to be abusing parents
C. Evaluation/Outcomes
   1. Child remains free from injury or neglect
   2. Parents demonstrate effective parenting activities

COGNITIVE IMPAIRMENT (MENTAL RETARDATION)

Data Base

A. Causes
   1. Infection and intoxication: congenital rubella; syphilis; maternal alcohol or drug consumption; chronic lead ingestion; kernicterus (high bilirubin level)
   2. Injury to the brain suffered during the prenatal, perinatal, or postnatal periods; intracranial hemorrhage; anoxia; physical injury
   3. Inadequate nutrition and metabolic or endocrine disorders such as PKU or hypothyroidism
   4. Associated with cerebrospinal and craniofacial malformations, such as microcephaly, hydrocephalus, myelomeningocele, and craniostenosis
   5. Gestational disorders including low birth weight, prematurity, or postmaturity
   6. Chromosomal abnormalities resulting from radiation, viral infection, chemical exposure, parental age, and genetic mutations, such as Down syndrome and fragile X syndrome
   7. Environmental influences including deprived environment associated with parents and siblings with mental retardation
B. Conditions that may lead to a false diagnosis of mental retardation
   1. Emotional disturbance (e.g., maternal deprivation)
   2. Sensory problems (e.g., deafness, blindness)
   3. Cerebral dysfunctions (e.g., cerebral palsy, learning disorders, hyperkinesia, seizure disorders)
C. Classification
   1. Normal: 90 to 110 IQ
   2. Borderline: 71 to 89 IQ
   3. Mild: 50/55 to 70 IQ

a. Can achieve a mental age of 8 to 12 years

b. Educable: can learn to read, write, do arithmetic, achieve a vocational skill, and function in society

4. Moderate: 35/40 to 50/55 IQ

a. Can achieve a mental age of 3 to 7 years

b. Trainable: can learn the activities of daily living and social skills; can be trained to work in a sheltered workshop

5. Severe: below 20/25 to 35/40 IQ

a. Can achieve a mental age of birth to 2 years

b. Barely trainable; totally dependent on others and in need of custodial care

6. Profound: below 20/25 IQ

a. May attain mental age of young infant

b. Requires total care

D. Clinical findings

1. Delayed milestones: infant fails to suck; head lag after 4 to 6 months of age; slow in learning self-help; slow to respond to new stimuli; slow or absent speech development

2. Mental abilities are concrete; abstract ability is limited; may repeat words (echolalia)

3. Lacks power of self-appraisal; does not learn from errors

4. Cannot carry out complex instructions; learns rote responses and socially acceptable behavior

5. Does not relate to peers; more secure with adults; comforted by physical touch

6. Short attention span, but usually attracted to music

E. Therapeutic interventions

1. Prevention of causes that damage brain cells such as hypoxia, untreated PKU

2. Early identification of condition

3. Effort to minimize long-term consequences: treatment of associated problems; infant stimulation; parental education

Nursing Care of Children Who Are Cognitively Impaired

A. Assessment/Analysis

1. Developmental screening

2. Associated illnesses/risk factors

3. Parental perception of developmental delays

B. Planning/Implementation

1. Consider child's developmental, not chronologic, age

a. Educate the parents regarding developmental age

b. Near adolescence, sexual feelings accompany maturation and need to be explained according to the child's mental capacity

2. Set realistic goals; teach by simple steps for habit formation rather than for understanding or transference of learning

a. Break down the process of skills' learning into simple steps that can be easily achieved; ensure each step is learned completely before teaching child the next step

b. Recognize that behavior modification is a very effective method of teaching these children; praise accomplishments to develop child's self-esteem

c. Keep discipline simple, geared toward learning acceptable behavior rather than developing judgment

d. Recognize that routines and simple repetetive tasks are the foundation of the child's lifestyle; hospital activities should be based on the child's routine schedule

C. Evaluation/Outcomes

1. Performs activities of daily living at optimum level

2. Family members make realistic decisions based on their needs and capabilities

CEREBRAL PALSY (CP)

Data Base

A. Nonspecific term for a neuromuscular disability or difficulty in controlling voluntary muscles (caused by damage to some portion of the brain, with associated sensory, intellectual, emotional, or seizure disorders)

B. Characteristics of CP

1. Affects young children, usually becoming evident before 3 years of age

2. Nonprogressive, but persists throughout life

3. Some motor dysfunction always present

4. Mental deficiency may be present; language deficit may be present

C. Major causes

1. Prenatal brain abnormalities: estimated that these account for as many as 80% of cases

2. Prematurity: prevalence of CP in infants born before 36 weeks' gestation and weighing less than 2000 g is 12%

3. Anoxia of the brain caused by a variety of insults at or near time of birth

4. Trauma; brain attack (cerebral vascular accident)

5. No identified cause in some children

D. Classification (based on predominant clinical manifestations)

1. Spastic type: hypertonicity with poor control of posture, balance, and coordinated movements; impairment of gross and fine motor skills

2. Dyskinetic type: abnormal involuntary movements

a. Athetosis; characterized by slow, wormlike, writhing movements

b. Involvement of mouth and throat that results in drooling

3. Ataxic type: wide-based gait; rapid repetitive movements performed inadequately

4. Mixed type: combination of spasticity and athetosis

E. Clinical findings

1. Difficulty in feeding, especially sucking and swallowing; many children have gastroesophageal reflux

2. Delayed motor development; abnormal motor performance; asymmetry of motion or contour of body

3. Alteration in muscle tone
4. Abnormal posture
5. Delayed speech development
6. Reflex abnormalities (e.g., hyperreflexia)
7. Any of the muscular abnormalities listed under classification

F. Therapeutic interventions
1. Multidisciplinary approach
2. Mobility devices
3. Surgery to correct spastic muscle imbalance
4. Medications, such as skeletal muscle relaxants and anticonvulsants; implanted pump for intrathecal baclofen administration
5. Medications to treat pain that may occur with muscle spasms
6. Physiotherapy, occupational and speech therapy

Nursing Care of Children With Cerebral Palsy

A. Assessment/Analysis
1. Presence of prenatal/perinatal risk factors
2. Ineffective feeding
3. Muscles for rigidity, tenseness, hypotonia
4. Delayed developmental milestones

B. Planning/Implementation
1. Feeding
   a. Recognize drooling results from difficulty in swallowing
   b. Use a spoon and blunt fork, with plate attached to the table, for easier self-feeding
   c. Provide increased calories because of excessive energy expenditure, increased protein for muscle activity, and increased vitamins (especially B_6) for amino acid metabolism
2. Relaxation: provide rest periods in an area with few stimuli; set limits and control activity level
3. Safety
   a. Protect from accidents resulting from altered sensation, impaired balance, and lack of muscle control
   b. Provide helmet for protection against head injuries
   c. Evaluate need for restraint
4. Play
   a. Keep safety as main objective; do not overstimulate
   b. Provide play that has educational value, appropriate to developmental level and ability
5. Elimination
   a. Teach parents that difficulty in toilet training results from poor muscle control
   b. Provide special bowel and bladder training
6. Speech
   a. Teach parents that incoordination of lips, tongue, cheeks, and larynx and impaired control of diaphragm make formation of words difficult
   b. Refer for speech therapy

7. Respirations
   a. Recognize impaired control of the intercostal muscles and diaphragm makes child prone to respiratory tract infection
   b. Protect child from exposure to infection as much as possible; be alert for symptoms of aspiration pneumonia
8. Dental problems
   a. Recognize problems in muscular control affect development and alignment of teeth
   b. Explain that frequent dental caries occur and that there is continued need for dental supervision and care
   c. Teach parents to brush child's teeth if muscular dysfunction is present
9. Vision
   a. Recognize that common ocular problems such as strabismus and refractive errors may be related to impaired muscular control
   b. Observe and report visual disorders to prevent further problems, such as amblyopia
10. Hearing
    a. Understand that hearing problems may be present, depending on the area of brain damage
    b. Encourage parents to have child's hearing checked periodically
11. Mobility
    a. Perform passive and encourage active range-of-motion exercises to prevent contractures and stretch ligaments and muscles
    b. Encourage use of leg braces, if prescribed, to maintain functional alignment and prevent deformities
    c. Encourage use of assistive devices such as a wheeled walker to promote stability

C. Evaluation/Outcomes
1. Remains safe from injury
2. Consumes adequate nutrients for growth
3. Communicates needs to caregivers
4. Performs self-care activities within capabilities
5. Exhibits behavior indicative of positive self-image
6. Family verbalizes effect of child's disability on family

❈ HEARING IMPAIRMENT

Data Base

A. Causes
1. Family history of childhood hearing impairment
2. Anatomic malformations; Down syndrome; cerebral palsy
3. Perinatal factors: low birth weight; severe perinatal asphyxia; infection (cytomegalovirus, rubella, herpes, syphilis, toxoplasmosis, bacterial meningitis)
4. Chronic ear infections
5. Ototoxic drugs such as gentamicin
6. Environmental factors: continuous exposure to noises made by equipment in a neonatal intensive

care unit; loud noises such as gunfire or continuous exposure to less intense noises such as music

B. Types of hearing loss by location of defect
  1. Conductive: loss results from interference of transmission of sound to middle ear
     a. Interferes mainly with loudness of sound
     b. Most frequent cause is recurrent otitis media
     c. Most common of all types of hearing loss
  2. Sensorineural: damage to inner ear structures and to the auditory nerve
     a. Distortion in clarity of words
     b. Problem in discrimination of sounds
     c. Common causes: kernicterus; ototoxic drugs; excessive noise exposure
  3. Mixed conductive-sensorineural
  4. Central auditory imperception
     a. Not explained by other three causes
     b. Child hears but does not understand

C. Classification of hearing loss
  1. Slight (16 to 25 decibels): has difficulty hearing faint or distant speech; usually unaware of problem; may have some problems in school; no speech defects
  2. Mild to moderate (26 to 55 decibels): may have some speech difficulties; understands face-to-face conversational speech at 3 to 5 feet
  3. Moderately severe (56 to 70 decibels): unable to understand conversational speech unless loud; considerable difficulty with group or classroom discussion
  4. Severe (71 to 90 decibels): may hear loud noises if nearby; may be able to identify loud environmental noises; requires speech training
  5. Profound (>90 decibels): may hear only loud noises; requires extensive speech training

D. Clinical findings
  1. Lack of Moro reflex in response to a sharp clap; failure to respond to loud noise
  2. Failure to locate a source of sound at 2 to 3 feet after 6 months of age
  3. Absence of babble by 7 months of age
  4. Inability to understand words or phrases by 12 months of age
  5. Use of gestures rather than verbalization to establish wants, especially after 15 months of age
  6. History of frequent respiratory tract infections and otitis media
  7. Older children: monotone quality to and unintelligible speech; inattentive; shy; withdrawn; tinnitus

E. Therapeutic interventions
  1. Conductive loss: tympanostomy tubes for chronic otitis media; hearing aids to amplify sounds
  2. Sensorineural: cochlear implants; hearing aids of less value
  3. Central auditory imperception: may not respond to any therapy
  4. Speech therapy

Nursing Care of Children With Impaired Hearing

A. Assessment/Analysis
  1. Prenatal or family history that places child at risk
  2. Response to auditory stimuli
  3. Failure to develop intelligible speech by 24 months

B. Planning/Implementation
  1. Observe for manifestations beginning at birth
  2. Face child to facilitate lip reading; have adequate light on speaker's face
  3. Educate others concerning how best to communicate with child
  4. Be level with the child's face and speak toward the unaffected ear; do not walk back and forth while talking
  5. Enunciate and articulate carefully; do not talk too loudly, especially if the loss is sensorineural
  6. Use facial expressions, since verbal intonations are not communicated
  7. Encourage active play to express feelings and build self-confidence

C. Evaluation/Outcomes
  1. Remains safe
  2. Uses a hearing aid
  3. Engages in activities appropriate to developmental level
  4. Child/family communicates effectively

✼ VISUAL IMPAIRMENT

Data Base

A. Definition: visual impairment is a general term referring to visual loss that cannot be corrected with regular prescription glasses
  1. School vision (partially sighted): visual acuity is between 20/70 and 20/200; able to participate in school with usual size print
  2. Legal blindness: visual acuity 20/200 or less or a visual field of 20 degrees or less in the better eye; child is eligible for special services

B. Strabismus: imbalance of the extraocular muscles causing a physiologic incoordination of the eye
  1. Amblyopia develops in the weak eye from disuse; must be corrected before 4 years of age to prevent blindness
  2. Treatment: patch on unaffected eye to force the weak eye to fixate; surgery to lengthen or shorten the extraocular muscles

C. Causes other than strabismus
  1. Perinatal infections: herpes, rubella, gonococci
  2. Congenital cataracts
  3. Retinopathy of prematurity
  4. Postnatal infections: meningitis
  5. Postnatal: trauma; tumor; diabetes mellitus

D. Clinical findings
  1. Delayed motor development
  2. Rocking for sensory stimulation

3. Squinting; rubbing eyes; sitting close to television; holding book close to face
4. Clumsiness (e.g., bumping into objects)

E. Therapeutic interventions
1. Surgical intervention for strabismus and cataracts
2. Corrective lenses

Nursing Care of Children With Impaired Vision

A. Assessment/Analysis
1. Factors that indicate children at risk
2. Behavior indicative of vision loss
3. Visual acuity and signs of ocular disorders

B. Planning/Implementation
1. Assess for early signs of visual problems
2. Explain to and encourage parents to follow treatments for strabismus and other visual problems
3. Talk clearly; use noise so child can locate your position
4. Help child learn through other senses, especially touch, with play activities
5. Facilitate eating
   a. Arrange food on the plate at clock hours and teach child its location
   b. Provide finger foods when possible
   c. Provide a light spoon and deep bowl so that the child can feel weight of food on spoon

C. Evaluation/Outcomes
1. Remains free from injury
2. Engages in appropriate activities for level of development
3. Child and other family members demonstrate a positive relationship

❊ CELIAC DISEASE

Data Base

A. Also known as gluten-sensitive enteropathy; an immunologically mediated small intestine enteropathy; mucosal lesions show features suggestive of both humoral and cell-mediated immunologic stimulation

B. Chronic intestinal malabsorption and inability to digest gluten, a protein found mostly in wheat, rye, oats, and barley

C. Malabsorption syndrome: characterized by chronic diarrhea and malabsorption of fluid and nutrients, resulting in failure to thrive

D. Diagnosis based on finding of villous atrophy with hyperplasia of the crypts and abnormal epithelium; full remission of symptoms occurs after gluten is withdrawn from diet

E. Identified several months after introduction of gluten-containing grain into the diet; usually between 1 and 5 years of age

F. Progression of illness
1. Fat absorption affected in early stage of disease
2. Protein, carbohydrate, mineral, and electrolyte absorption then affected
3. Growth failure and muscle wasting finally occur

G. Clinical findings
1. Progressive malnutrition: anorexia; muscle wasting; distended abdomen
2. Secondary deficiencies: anemia and rickets
3. Behavioral changes: irritability; fretfulness; apathy
4. Stool: watery; pale; foul-smelling
5. Celiac crisis: severe episode of dehydration and acidosis from diarrhea

H. Therapeutic intervention: dietary
1. Low in glutens; no wheat, rye, oats, or barley
2. High in calories and protein
3. Low fat
4. Small, frequent feedings; adequate fluids
5. Vitamin supplements, all in water-miscible form; supplemental iron

Nursing Care of Children With Celiac Disease

A. Assessment/Analysis
1. Nutritional status
2. Parent/child knowledge of dietary regimen

B. Planning/Implementation
1. Teach parents and child about dietary modifications; restrict foods containing wheat, rye, oats, and barley; permit foods containing corn, rice, and millet
2. Explain need for frequent health supervision
3. Provide support to facilitate adherence to dietary regimen

C. Evaluation/Outcomes
1. Parent/child verbalizes correct dietary information
2. Consumes adequate calories for growth and development

❊ CYSTIC FIBROSIS

Data Base

A. Autosomal recessive disorder affecting the exocrine (mucus-producing) glands

B. Most common lethal genetic disease of children; estimated that 1 in 29 Caucasian children are symptom-free carriers

C. Basic defect reduces ability of the epithelial cells in the airways and pancreas to transport chloride; abnormal transport of sodium and chloride across the epithelium leads to increased viscosity of airway mucus, abnormal mucociliary clearance, and lung disease

D. Elevation in sweat electrolytes: sodium and chloride levels are 3 to 5 times higher than expected; chloride levels more than 60 mEq/L are diagnostic

E. Increased viscosity of mucous gland secretions is responsible for clinical findings
1. Pancreas: becomes fibrotic, with a decreased production of pancreatic enzymes (lipase, trypsin, chymotrypsin, amylase)
2. Respiratory system: increased viscous mucus in trachea, bronchi, and bronchioles interferes with expiration (emphysema) and increases incidence of infection
3. Liver: possible cirrhosis from biliary obstruction, malnutrition, or infection; portal hypertension leads to esophageal varices

4. Rectal prolapse
5. A late complication is cystic fibrosis related diabetes mellitus
6. Sexual organs: infertility may occur

F. Clinical findings
1. Early manifestations during infancy
   a. Meconium ileus at birth (about 15%); abdominal distention
   b. Failure to regain expected 10% weight loss at birth
   c. Presence of cough or wheezing during first 6 months of age
2. Respiratory involvement evidenced by increased frequency of pulmonary infection; hyperaeration of functioning alveoli contributes to barrel-shaped chest, cyanosis, clubbing of fingers
3. GI involvement evidenced by decreased pancreatic enzymes (lipase, trypsin, chymotrypsin, and amylase), which prevent conversion of foods into substances that can be absorbed by the intestinal mucosa; consequently, undigested food (unabsorbed fats and proteins) is excreted, increasing the bulk of feces to 2 or 3 times the normal amount; as solid foods are added to the diet, the excessively large stools become frothy and extremely foul-smelling
4. Cardiac involvement evidenced by enlargement of the heart, particularly right ventricular hypertrophy (cor pulmonale)

G. Therapeutic interventions
1. Pulmonary problems: chest physiotherapy; bronchodilators; antibiotic therapy as indicated
2. Gastrointestinal problems: pancreatic enzyme supplements; water-miscible forms of fat-soluble vitamins (A, D, E, K); balanced nutritional intake; caloric intake should be 150% to 200% more than that of child who does not have cystic fibrosis

---

Nursing Care of Children With Cystic Fibrosis

A. Assessment/Analysis
1. Respiratory status
2. GI status
3. Failure to thrive
4. Cognitive level
5. Effect of chronic illness on social status

B. Planning/Implementation
1. Prevent respiratory tract infections
   a. Postural drainage, percussion, and vibration between feedings
   b. Use of expectorants, antibiotics, aerosol therapy; avoid antitussives and antihistamines
2. Promote optimal nutrition
   a. Administer pancreatic enzymes with cold food in middle of meal
   b. Administer fat-soluble vitamins in water-miscible form
   c. Encourage high-protein, moderate-fat, high-calorie diet of easily digested food

3. Promote mobility and activity
   a. Encourage activity and regular exercise
   b. Help child regulate activity to own tolerance
4. Promote a positive body image
   a. Help child cope with barrel-shaped chest, low weight, thin extremities, bluish coloring, smell of stools
   b. Encourage hygiene and selection of clothes that compensate for protuberant abdomen and emaciated extremities
5. Provide for emotional support and counseling for child and family
   a. Recognize that CF is a long-term problem that causes financial and emotional stresses
   b. Understand that this chronic illness can become a major controlling factor in the family
      (1) The child begins to recognize that wheezing brings attention and uses this knowledge
      (2) Parents can deal with such behavior by recognizing false attacks and using consistent discipline
   c. Encourage family to join a support group
   d. Refer family for genetic counseling

C. Evaluation/Outcomes
1. Engages in activities that maintain a balance between oxygen supply and demand
2. Maintains a patent airway
3. Consumes adequate calories for growth and development
4. Family members demonstrate ability to care for child

IRON DEFICIENCY ANEMIA

Data Base

A. Most prevalent nutritional disorder among children in the United States; caused by lack of adequate sources of dietary iron
1. Infant usually has iron reserve for 6 months
2. Preterm infant lacks sufficient reserves; usually depleted by 2 to 3 months of age
3. Children receiving only milk have no source of iron ("milk babies")

B. Insidious onset: usually diagnosed because of an infection or chronic GI problems

C. Causes
1. Decreased intake
2. Increased loss

D. Clinical findings
1. Pallor; weakness; tachycardia; dizziness; cardiac decompensation if severe
2. Slow motor development; poor muscle tone
3. Hemoglobin level below average for age

E. Therapeutic interventions
1. Food sources rich in iron
   a. Iron-fortified formula
   b. Iron-fortified infant cereal

2. Iron replacement
   a. Oral iron sources
      (1) Ferrous sulfate—most absorbable form of iron
      (2) Adverse effects: nausea and vomiting; fatalities in children who ingest enteric-coated tablets, thinking they are candy
   b. Parenteral iron sources for children with iron malabsorption or chronic hemoglobinuria
      (1) Parenteral iron-dextran (Imferon)
      (2) Adverse effects: tissue staining; fever; lymphadenopathy; nausea; vomiting; arthralgia; urticaria; severe peripheral vascular failure; anaphylaxis; secondary hematochromatosis

Nursing Care of Children With Iron Deficiency Anemia

A. Assessment/Analysis
   1. Nutritional history and status
   2. History of chronic infection
   3. Family history of hematologic disorder
   4. Eating habits: pica; ingestion of lead
   5. Bowel habits; blood in stools
B. Planning/Implementation
   1. Prevent development of anemia
      a. Teach pregnant women the importance of iron intake
      b. Encourage feeding of iron-fortified infant formula or breastfeeding
      c. Encourage feeding of iron-fortified infant cereal and chopped meat
      d. Teach parents which foods are high in iron
      e. Teach parents about other nutrients essential for RBC production (e.g., protein, vitamin B_{12}, folic acid, ascorbic acid)
   2. Teach parents about administration of supplemental iron
      a. Vitamin C aids absorption
      b. Folic acid acts as a coenzyme in the formation of heme; proteins are necessary for synthesis of hemoglobin; ascorbic acid promotes conversion of folic acid to folinic acid
      c. Oxalates, phosphate, and caffeine decrease absorption
      d. Some liquid preparations stain teeth; straw should be used during administration
      e. Color of stools is blackish green
      f. Gastric irritation or constipation may occur
C. Evaluation/Outcomes
   1. Engages in appropriate activities without fatigue
   2. Consumes adequate nutrients for correction of anemia
   3. Parents can verbalize dietary requirements of child

SICKLE CELL ANEMIA
Data Base
A. Autosomal disorder affecting hemoglobin
B. Substitution of the amino acid valine for glutamic acid in the beta chain of the hemoglobin; defective hemoglobin causes RBCs to become sickle-shaped and clump together under reduced O_2 tension; during the newborn period, high levels of fetal hemoglobin prevent sickling; as this form of hemoglobin decreases during the first year of life, increased episodes of sickling can occur
C. Classification
   1. Sickle cell anemia: homozygous for sickle cell gene
   2. Sickle cell trait: heterozygous for sickle cell gene; have same basic defect, but only 35% to 45% of total hemoglobin is sickle hemoglobin (HbS)
D. Clinical findings
   1. Sickle turbidity test (Sickledex) determines presence of HbS
   2. Vasoocclusive crisis (preferably called "painful episode"): most common and not life-threatening
      a. Results from sickled cells obstructing blood vessels, causing occlusion, ischemia, and potential necrosis
      b. Signs and symptoms include fever, acute abdominal pain (visceral hypoxia), hand-foot syndrome, priapism, and arthralgia without an exacerbation of anemia
   3. Sequestration crisis
      a. Results from the spleen pooling large quantities of blood, which causes a precipitous drop in BP and ultimately shock
      b. Acute episode occurs most commonly in children between 8 months and 5 years of age; can result in death from anemia and cardiovascular collapse
   4. Multiple splenic infarctions result in functional asplenia
   5. Aplastic crisis: diminished RBC production
      a. May be triggered by a viral or other infection
      b. Profound anemia results from rapid destruction of RBCs combined with decreased production
   6. Hyperhemolytic crisis: increased rate of RBC destruction
      a. Characterized by anemia, jaundice, and reticulocytosis
      b. Rare complication that frequently suggests a coexisting abnormality such as glucose-6-phosphate dehydrogenase deficiency
   7. Cerebral vascular accident (brain attack)
      a. Sickled cells block major blood vessels in the brain
      b. Repeat brain attacks in 60% of children who have experienced previous one
   8. Chest syndrome: clinically similar to pneumonia
   9. Overwhelming infection: *Streptococcus pneumoniae; Haemophilus influenzae* type B; major cause of death in children under 5 years of age.

E. Therapeutic interventions
1. Prevention of sickling phenomenon
   a. Adequate oxygenation
   b. Adequate hydration
   c. Administration of hydroxyurea to increase fetal hemoglobin
   d. Blood transfusions to decrease production of cells with sickle hemoglobin
2. Treatment of crisis
   a. Pain management; rest
   b. Hydration/electrolyte replacement
   c. Antibiotic therapy
   d. Blood products

Nursing Care of Children With Sickle Cell Anemia

A. Assessment/Analysis
1. Vital signs; neurologic signs
2. Vision/hearing
3. Location and intensity of pain
4. Fluid balance
5. Spleen size

B. Planning/Implementation
1. Avoid dehydration
   a. May cause rapid thrombus formation and crisis
   b. Daily fluid intake should be calculated according to body weight (130 to 200 mL/kg)
   c. During crisis, fluid needs to be increased, especially if child is febrile
2. Prevent crisis
   a. Avoid infection, dehydration, and other conditions causing stress on body, which precipitate a crisis; prophylactic use of pneumococcal, meningococcal, and *Haemophilus* flu vaccines; hepatitis B for those children who did not receive it with routine immunizations
   b. Avoid hypoxia; treat respiratory tract infections immediately
3. During crisis provide for
   a. Adequate hydration (may need IV therapy)
   b. Effective positioning (head of bed elevated; joints supported); careful handling
   c. Exercise as tolerated (immobility promotes thrombus formation and respiratory problems)
   d. Adequate ventilation
   e. Control of pain; use comfort measures; administer ordered opioids; schedule medication administration to prevent onset of pain; warm soaks to joints as ordered
   f. Blood transfusions for severe anemia
4. Provide for genetic counseling
   a. Disorder mostly of blacks; can be found in individuals of Mediterranean descent
   b. Parents need to know the risk for having other children with trait or disease
   c. If both parents are carriers, each pregnancy has 25% chance of producing a child with the disease

d. Screen infants for the disorder because clinical manifestations usually do not appear before 6 months of age
5. Support parents

C. Evaluation/Outcomes
1. Reports minimal pain
2. Verbalizes feelings about disease process
3. Demonstrates behaviors reflective of a positive body image
4. Remains free from crisis

β-THALASSEMIA (COOLEY's ANEMIA)

Data Base
A. Autosomal disorder with varied expressivity
B. Basic defect is a deficiency in the synthesis of β-chain polypeptides, which results in a decreased rate of production of the globin molecule
C. Classification
1. Thalassemia trait: heterozygous; mild anemia
2. Thalassemia intermedia: splenomegaly; severe anemia
3. Thalassemia major: severe anemia; incompatible with life without transfusions
D. Clinical findings
1. Severe anemia
2. Unexplained fever; headache
3. Anorexia; impaired feeding
4. Enlarged abdomen; splenomegaly; hepatomegaly
5. Impaired physical growth
6. Listlessness; exercise intolerance
E. Therapeutic interventions
1. Blood transfusions to maintain adequate hemoglobin levels
2. Iron-chelating agents such as deferoxamine (Desferal) are given to reduce iron storage; transfusions greatly increase risk for hemosiderosis (excessive iron storage in various tissues of the body, especially the spleen, liver, lymph glands, heart, and pancreas), hemochromatosis (excessive iron storage with resultant cellular damage), and pulmonary edema
3. Bone marrow transplantation

Nursing Care of Children With β-Thalassemia
A. Assessment/Analysis
1. Family history
2. RBCs for significant anemia
3. Cardiovascular status
B. Planning/Implementation
1. Be alert for signs and symptoms in older infants or young children who are black or of Mediterranean descent (Italian, Greek, Syrian)
2. Prevent infection: child should avoid contact with persons who have infections
3. Ensure immunizations are current
4. Prevent complications
   a. Monitor during transfusions; stop infusion if signs of a transfusion reaction occur

b. Administer chelating agents and folic acid as ordered
c. Teach to avoid activities that increase risk for fractures
d. Observe for signs of cholecystitis in the adolescent
5. Prepare child and family for bone marrow transplantation
   a. Encourage participation in support group
   b. Identify family support
   c. Provide education on the preprocedure and postprocedure periods
6. Assist child in coping with the disorder and its effects
   a. Explore child's feelings about being different from other children
   b. Emphasize child's abilities and focus on realistic endeavors
   c. Encourage quiet activities, creative efforts, and "thinking" games
   d. Encourage interaction with peers; introduce child to other children who have adjusted to this or a similar disorder
   e. Help plan therapies and medical care so they do not interfere with child's regular activities and social interactions
   f. Assist child with vocational planning
7. Support parents
   a. Explore feelings regarding the hereditary nature of the disease
   b. Emphasize need for their child to lead as active a life as possible
   c. Help family deal with the potentially fatal nature of the disease
8. Refer for genetic counseling; reinforce and clarify counseling information
C. Evaluation/Outcomes
   1. Participates in appropriate activities for energy level
   2. Verbalizes feelings about disease/hospitalization
   3. Demonstrates behaviors reflective of a positive body image
   4. Parents demonstrate ability to care for child
   5. Parents verbalize feelings and concerns about seriousness of illness

✿ PINWORMS

Data Base
A. Most common intestinal parasite in United States
B. Children reinfest themselves by fingers-to-anus-to-mouth route; can also be infested by breathing airborne ova

C. Crowded conditions such as classrooms and day-care centers increase risk for transmission
D. Clinical findings
   1. Severe pruritus of the anal area; pinworm eggs isolated from the perianal area; cellophane-tape test done early in the morning before first bowel movement
   2. Irritability and insomnia
   3. Anorexia; weight loss
   4. Eosinophilia
   5. Signs of complications: vaginitis; appendicitis
E. Therapeutic interventions: mebendazole (Vermox) is drug of choice
   1. Selectively and irreversibly inhibits uptake of glucose and other nutrients of pinworms
   2. Adverse effects: occasional, transient abdominal pain and diarrhea

Nursing Care of Children With Pinworms
A. Assessment/Analysis
   1. Perianal area for signs of inflammation
   2. Cellophane-tape test in morning before a bowel movement
B. Planning/Implementation
   1. Prevent reinfestation
      a. Wash anal area thoroughly at least once a day
      b. Place a tight diaper or underpants on child; change child's clothes and bedding daily and wash in hot water
      c. Do not allow child to scratch the anus; keep fingernails short; child may need to wear mittens
      d. Air out bedroom; dust and vacuum house thoroughly
   2. Teach parents about administration of medication
      a. Increasing dose will not produce a quicker recovery
      b. Stools contain worms; may turn bright red from medication
      c. Additional series of medication may be used, frequently 2 weeks after initial dose; all family members are usually treated
C. Evaluation/Outcomes
   1. Maintains intact perianal skin
   2. Produces stool that is free of infestation

✿ EMOTIONAL DISORDERS

For common emotional disorders of the toddler, see Chapter 17: Nursing Care of Clients With Disorders Usually First Evident in Infancy, Childhood, or Adolescence under Mental Health/Psychiatric Nursing

32 Nursing Care of Preschoolers

GROWTH AND DEVELOPMENT
DEVELOPMENTAL TIMETABLE

Three Years
A. Physical
1. Usual weight gain 1.8 to 2.7 kg (4 to 6 lb)
2. Usual height gain 7.5 cm (3 inches)
B. Motor
1. Jumps off bottom step; walks upstairs alternating feet; stands on one foot
2. Rides a tricycle using pedals
3. Constructs three-block bridge; builds tower of 9 or 10 cubes
4. Can unbutton front or side button; uses a spoon
5. Usually toilet trained at night
C. Sensory: visual acuity 20/30
D. Vocalization and socialization
1. Vocabulary of about 900 words; uses 3- to 4-word sentences; uses plurals; may have hesitation in speech pattern
2. Begins to understand ideas of sharing and taking turns
E. Mental abilities
1. Beginning understanding of the past, present, future, or any aspect of time
2. Stage of magical thinking

Four Years
A. Physical
1. Height and weight increases are similar to previous year
2. Length at birth is doubled
B. Motor
1. Skips and hops on one foot; walks up and down stairs like an adult
2. Can button buttons and lace shoes
3. Throws ball overhand; uses scissors to cut outline
C. Vocalization and socialization
1. Vocabulary of 1500 words or more
2. May have an imaginary companion
3. Tends to be selfish and impatient but takes pride in accomplishments; exaggerates, boasts, and tattles on others
D. Mental abilities
1. Unable to conserve matter
2. Can repeat 4 numbers and is learning number concept

3. Knows which is the longer of two lines; has poor space perception

Five Years
A. Physical: height and weight increases are similar to previous year
B. Motor
1. Gross motor abilities well developed; can balance on one foot for about 10 seconds; can jump rope, skip, and roller skate
2. Can draw a picture of a person; prints first name and other words as learned
3. Dresses and washes self; may be able to tie shoelaces
C. Sensory
1. Color recognition is well established
2. Minimal potential for amblyopia to develop
D. Vocalization and socialization
1. Vocabulary of about 2100 words; talks constantly; asks meaning of new words
2. Generally cooperative and sympathetic toward others
3. Basic personality structure is well established
E. Mental abilities (Piaget's phase of intuitive thought)
1. Beginning understanding of time in terms of days as part of a week
2. Beginning understanding of conversion of numbers
3. Has not mastered concept that parts equal a whole regardless of their appearance; difficulty with abstract thought

HEALTH PROMOTION OF PRESCHOOLERS
PLAY (COOPERATIVE PLAY)

A. Loosely organized group play where membership changes readily, as do rules
B. Through play, child deals with reality, learns control of feelings, and expresses emotions more through action than through words
C. Play is still physically oriented but is also imitative and imaginary; imaginary playmates are common because of a blurred line between reality and fantasy
D. Tend to exaggerate, and be impatient, noisy, and selfish
E. Increased sharing and cooperation among preschool children, especially 5-year-old children

F. Suggested toys
   1. Dress-up clothes; dolls; doll house; small trucks; animals; puppets
   2. Painting sets; coloring books; paste; and cutout sets
   3. Illustrated books; puzzles with large pieces and varied shapes
   4. Tricycle; swing; slide; other playground equipment

NUTRITION AND INJURY PREVENTION DURING THE PRESCHOOL YEARS

See Chapter 31: Health Promotion of Toddlers: Childhood Nutrition and Injury Prevention During Toddlerhood

HOSPITALIZATION OF PRESCHOOLERS

DATA BASE

A. Child's reaction
   1. Fears about body image and bodily harm are now greater than fear of separation
   2. Fears include
      a. Intrusive experiences: needles; thermometer; otoscope
      b. Punishment and rejection
      c. Pain
      d. Castration and mutilation
   3. May regress and exhibit earlier developmental behaviors
   4. Views death as temporary
   5. Cries when parents arrive/leave but usually is calm
   6. Physical assessment of preschoolers (as well as toddlers) is challenging and may require modification of procedures (e.g., handling equipment, allowing child to guide hand during assessment of the abdomen)
B. If possible, parents can be helped to prepare the child beforehand because increased cognitive and verbal ability makes explanations possible

✿ GENERAL NURSING CARE OF PRESCHOOLERS

A. Begin preparing for elective hospitalization a few days before but not too early because of the child's vague concept of time; encourage child to bring a security article or appropriate special toy to the hospital
B. Clarify cause and effect because of the child's phenomenalistic thinking (in the child's mind, proximity of two events relates them to each other)
C. Explain routines of hospital admission but not all procedures at one time, because this may be overwhelming
D. Understand play is an excellent medium for preparation (use dolls, puppets, make-believe equipment, dress-up doctor and nurse clothes, story books)
E. Provide time for play as an outlet for fear, anger, and hostility, as well as a temporary escape from reality

F. Keep verbal explanation as simple as possible and always honest
G. Add details about procedures, drugs, surgery, as the child's cognitive level and personal experiences increase
H. Encourage parents to stay or visit as often as possible
I. Facilitate therapeutic play for emergent hospitalization

HEALTH PROBLEMS MOST COMMON IN PRESCHOOLERS

✿ LEUKEMIA

Data Base

A. Cancer of the blood-forming organs; overproduction of immature, nonfunctioning leukocytes
B. The most common type of childhood cancer; peak incidence between 2 and 6 years of age; more common in males than females after the age of 1; prognosis is improving
C. Classification
   1. Acute lymphoblastic (also called lymphoid, lymphatic, lymphocytic) leukemia (ALL); subdivided into 3 subtypes (L1, L2, and L3); L1 is most common; 84% long-term disease-free survival
   2. Acute myelogenous leukemia (AML) (also called acute nonlymphoblastic leukemia); subdivided into 8 subtypes; constitutes 20% of leukemias in children; prognosis depends on several factors but has less favorable survival rates than ALL
D. Clinical findings
   1. Anemia: pallor; weakness; irritability; result of decreased erythrocytes
   2. Infection: fever; result of neutropenia
   3. Bleeding: petechiae; result of decreased platelets
   4. Bone pain and fractures; bones weakened by invasion of bone marrow by leukemic cells
   5. Enlargement of spleen, liver, and lymph glands
   6. Anorexia and vague abdominal pain caused by areas of intestinal inflammation
   7. Necrosis and bleeding of gums and other mucous membranes
   8. Later signs and symptoms: CNS involvement and frank hemorrhage
E. Therapeutic interventions
   1. Remission induced with chemotherapy; protocols for AML and ALL are significantly different; each protocol is modified based on child and disease factors (see Related Pharmacology under Neoplastic Disorders in Chapter 3)
      a. Induction therapy for ALL: 4 to 6 weeks
         (1) Corticosteroids: prednisone (Metacortin) or dexamethasone (Decadron)
         (2) Plant alkaloid: vincristine (Oncovin)
         (3) Asparaginase (Elspar)
         (4) Cytotoxic antibiotic: doxorubicin (Adriamycin)
      b. Consolidation therapy for ALL: further decreases number of leukemic cells; combination of two or more drugs given in routine periodic stretches of administration (pulses) during the first 6 months

(1) Asparaginase
(2) Methotrexate (Rheumatrex); high
    or intermediate dose
(3) Vincristine
(4) Doxorubicin
(5) Corticosteroids
(6) Cytarabine (Cytosar)
(7) Mercaptopurine (6-MP)
c. CNS prophylactic therapy: irradiation and triple intrathecal medications (methotrexate, cytarabine, and hydrocortisone) because leukemic cells invade the brain; most antileukemic drugs do not pass the blood-brain barrier
d. Maintenance therapy: preserves remission and further reduces number of leukemic cells
(1) Oral 6-mercaptopurine
(2) Weekly doses of methotrexate
(3) Vincristine and steroid pulses
2. Transfusions to replace and provide needed blood factors such as RBCs, platelets, and WBCs

Nursing Care of Children With Leukemia

A. Assessment/Analysis
1. Hematologic status: anemia (pallor, fatigue); thrombocytopenia (hematuria, bleeding gums); neutropenia (signs of infection)
2. Activity level
3. Complications of therapy/disease process
4. Family/child knowledge of disease process
5. Family support systems and coping strategies
B. Planning/Implementation
1. Encourage adjustment to chronic illness; stress need for maintaining regular lifestyle
2. Identify child's perception of illness and death; discussion should be appropriate to level of understanding
    a. Preschoolers: concept that death is reversible; greatest fear is separation
    b. Children 6 to 9 years of age: concept that death is personified; a person actually comes and removes the child
    c. Children over 9 years of age: adult concept of death as irreversible and inevitable
3. Support child experiencing side effects of drugs
    a. Prophylactic use of antinausea agents such as ondansetron (Zofran) before chemotherapy
    b. Cyclophosphamide (Cytoxan): bone marrow depression (10 to 14 days); severe nausea; vomiting; hemorrhagic cystitis; and alopecia
    c. Vincristine: neurotoxicity; fever; constipation; alopecia
    d. Methotrexate: nausea; vomiting; immunosuppression; photosensitivity; oral and rectal ulcers
    e. Corticosteroids: mood swings; fluid retention
4. Teach prevention of infection: handwashing; avoiding contact with people who have active infections; avoiding crowded places

5. Handle child carefully because of pain and risk for hemorrhage
6. Use pain rating scale and medicate appropriately
7. Provide gentle oral hygiene using soft-tipped applicator; saline mouth rinses; soft, bland foods; cool liquids/food rather than cold or hot liquids/food
8. Provide for frequent rest periods; quiet play
C. Evaluation/Outcomes
1. Participates in developmental, age-appropriate activities
2. Remains comfortable
3. Consumes adequate calories for growth
4. Remains free from complications (infection, bleeding, anemia, impaired skin)
5. Expresses feelings about altered body image
6. Family and child discuss fears, concerns, and needs

✿ WILMS' TUMOR (NEPHROBLASTOMA)

Data Base

A. Most common malignant neoplasm of the kidney in children
B. Estimated frequency is 9 cases per 1 million Caucasian children less than 15 years old
C. Peak age at diagnosis between 3 and 4 years of age; 80% are diagnosed by 5 years of age
D. Increased incidence among siblings; mode of familial inheritance (less than 2% of diagnoses) is autosomal dominant
E. May be associated with congenital anomalies: aniridia (congenital absence of iris); hemihypertrophy; hypospadias; cryptorchidism
F. Prognosis
1. Stages I and II with localized tumor: 90% cure with multimodal therapy
2. Factors that favorably affect the success of further therapy
    a. Favorable histology of tumor
    b. Relapse more than 12 months after first remission
G. Clinical findings
1. Swelling or nontender mass in abdomen; confined to one side of midline
2. Weight loss; fever; fatigue; malaise if there is compression of abdominal organs
3. Hematuria, caused by intrarenal hemorrhage, occurs in less than 25% of affected children
4. Hypertension occasionally occurs
5. Other symptoms associated with compression of neighboring organs or metastasis (e.g., lungs: cough, dyspnea, shortness of breath)
H. Therapeutic interventions
1. Abdominal palpation and renal biopsy contraindicated to prevent rupture of encapsulated tumor
2. Surgery: should be scheduled soon after confirmation of renal mass
    a. Tumor, kidney, and associated adrenal gland removed; precautions taken not to rupture the capsule of the tumor

b. Contralateral kidney is inspected; when other kidney is involved, partial nephrectomy is done on the less affected side

c. Regional lymph nodes and organs inspected and biopsied; when indicated, they are removed

3. Chemotherapy
   a. Indicated for all stages; continued for 6 to 15 months varying by the tumor stage
   b. Drugs used include dactinomycin (Cosmegen), vincristine (Oncovin), and doxorubicin (Adriamycin)

4. Radiation therapy: indicated for children with large tumors, metastasis, residual disease after surgery, and unfavorable cell type

Nursing Care of Children With Wilms' Tumor

A. Assessment/Analysis
1. Manifestations of Wilms' tumor
   a. Abdomen for mass or swelling; firm, nontender; does not cross midline
   b. RBCs for anemia; weight loss
2. Symptoms of compression
3. Signs of metastasis: dyspnea; cough; shortness of breath

B. Planning/Implementation
1. Preoperative
   a. Handle and bathe carefully to prevent trauma to the abdomen, which may result in rupture of the tumor capsule; place sign over bed, stating "Do not palpate abdomen"
   b. Monitor BP and I&O
   c. Prepare parents and child for large size of incision and drainage
   d. Begin teaching family about chemotherapy and radiation therapy
2. Postoperative
   a. Monitor BP and intake and output
   b. Use pain rating scale and medicate appropriately
   c. Encourage child to turn, cough, and deep breathe to prevent pulmonary complications
   d. Teach parents to identify untoward reactions from chemotherapy and radiation therapy
3. See Nursing Care of Children With Leukemia

C. Evaluation/Outcomes
1. Remains free from complications (infection, rupture of encapsulated tumor)
2. Maintains BP within acceptable range
3. Consumes adequate calories for growth
4. Child and family members discuss feelings and concerns

❋ NEPHROTIC SYNDROME (MINIMAL CHANGE NEPHROTIC SYNDROME)

Data Base

A. Abnormal, increased permeability of the glomerular basement membrane to plasma albumin; cause unknown

B. Peak incidence: 2 to 7 years of age; in North America approximately 100,000 children are affected each year

C. Males outnumber females 2:1

D. Classification
1. Minimal change nephrotic syndrome (MCN) has greatest incidence (80%)
   a. Glomerular membrane becomes permeable to protein, especially albumin, which leaks through membrane
   b. Serum albumin level is decreased
   c. Capillary oncotic pressure is decreased
   d. Hydrostatic pressure of tissues exceeds pull of capillary oncotic pressure and fluid accumulates in body cavities, especially the abdomen (ascites)
2. Secondary nephrotic syndrome
3. Congenital nephrotic syndrome (children usually die by second year of life without kidney transplant)

E. Clinical findings
1. Weight gain from fluid retention
2. Puffiness of face; periorbital edema on arising
3. Abdominal swelling (ascites)
4. Generalized edema
5. Scrotal edema in males
6. Irritability
7. Easily fatigued
8. BP average for age or slightly decreased
9. Decreased urinary volume, may be frothy
10. Proteinuria
11. Impending chronic renal failure: pale; muddy appearance; malaise; headache; muscle cramps; nausea; anorexia

F. Therapeutic interventions
1. Supportive therapy
2. Nutrition
   a. Sodium-restricted diet during periods of massive edema; edema does not resolve with low-sodium diet but rate of increase may be limited
   b. Diet adjusted to child's appetite, which must not interfere with nutrient intake
   c. Protein restriction if renal failure and azotemia are present
3. Children with MCN are usually categorized by their response to steroid therapy
   a. Steroid sensitive (20% to 40%): responds to a single short course of steroids without evidence of relapse after cessation of therapy
   b. Steroid dependent (60% to 80%): responds to steroids and can be tapered off completely; has remission when placed on steroids but tends to relapse on lower dosage; has three or more relapses in a 6- to 12-month period
   c. Steroid unresponsive or steroid resistant: never responds to steroids, or becomes resistant to steroids at some point during course of the illness
4. Corticosteroid therapy; prednisone drug of choice
   a. Response to therapy usually within 7 to 21 days or promotes diuresis
   b. Lower dose or gradual discontinuation when satisfactory response noted
5. Immunosuppressant therapy for children who do not respond to steroids or those who have frequent

relapses; cyclophosphamide (Cytoxan) is drug of choice

6. Diuretics; edema of nephrotic syndrome is usually unresponsive to diuretic agents

Nursing Care of Children With Nephrotic Syndrome

A. Assessment/Analysis
1. Vital signs, particularly BP
2. Fluid balance: daily weight; edema; abdominal girth
3. Urine studies: specific gravity; albumin
4. Skin monitoring when edema is present
5. Side effects of steroids are edema, lability of mood, thin extremities, truncal obesity, signs of infection

B. Planning/Implementation
1. Prevent infection: both illness and drug therapy increase susceptibility
   a. Protect child from others who are ill
   b. Teach parents signs of impending infection and encourage them to seek medical care
2. Prevent malnutrition: caused by loss of protein and anorexia
   a. Provide regular diet; encourage nutritious selection of foods
   b. Restrict fluids if ordered; when indicated, teach child and parents about sodium-restricted diet
3. Promote respirations: respiratory difficulty caused by ascites
   a. Place in a seated position to decrease pressure against the diaphragm
   b. Monitor vital signs and respiratory status
4. Promote comfort: discomfort caused by edema, pressure areas
   a. Provide some relief by positioning and giving skin care
   b. Support the genitalia if edematous
5. Promote a positive body image: altered body image as a result of edema and steroids
   a. Recognize that this becomes a greater problem as the child gets older
   b. Emphasize clothes, hairdo, etc. that make the child attractive
   c. Stress that "diets" will not help weight loss
6. Provide emotional support: irritability and depression commonly occur
   a. Help parents understand that mood swings are influenced by illness
   b. Encourage child to participate in own care
   c. Encourage diversionary activities that provide satisfaction

C. Evaluation/Outcomes
1. Engages in activities appropriate to capabilities
2. Maintains fluid balance
3. Adheres to dietary regimen
4. Remains free from infection
5. Maintains skin integrity
6. Child and family members discuss feelings and concerns

✿ URINARY TRACT INFECTION (UTI)

Data Base

A. More common in females because of anatomy of the lower urinary tract: urethra is short and meatus is close to anus; after neonatal period females have 10 to 30 times greater likelihood of UTI
B. Peak incidence occurs at 2 to 6 years of age
C. Classification
1. Bacteriuria: asymptomatic; symptomatic
2. Recurrent UTI
3. Persistent UTI
4. Febrile UTI
5. Cystitis
6. Urethritis
7. Pyelonephritis
8. Urosepsis
D. Clinical findings
1. In children under 2 years of age symptoms mimic GI disorders, failure to thrive, feeding problems, vomiting, and diarrhea
2. Children more than 2 years of age have more characteristic symptoms
   a. Enuresis; daytime incontinence
   b. Dysuria
   c. Urgency; frequency of urination
E. Therapeutic interventions
1. Antibiotics to eliminate infection
2. Identification and correction of structural anomalies if present
3. Prevention of recurrence; preservation of renal function

Nursing Care of Children With Urinary Tract Infection

A. Assessment/Analysis
1. Discomfort on urination
2. Pattern of urinary elimination
3. Pattern of bowel elimination
4. Dietary recall for fluid intake
5. Urine sample

B. Planning/Implementation
1. Develop voiding schedule to limit holding urine in bladder
2. Encourage to increase fluids to enhance urine production and need for voiding
3. Encourage routine health care supervision
4. Encourage increase in dietary fiber to minimize constipation, which contributes to UTI

C. Evaluation/Outcomes
1. Resolves infection
2. Receives follow-up health care supervision

✿ ASTHMA

Data Base

A. Chronic inflammatory disorder of airways characterized by increased responsiveness and inflammation of the airway, spasms of bronchi and bronchioles, edema of mucous membranes, increased secretions; respiratory acidosis results from buildup of CO_2

B. Results from immunologic exposure to an antigen that is deposited on the respiratory mucosa; and/or nonimmunologic stimuli such as viral infections, physical and chemical substances

C. Incidence, severity, and mortality associated with asthma are increasing; it is the most common chronic disease of childhood; primary cause of school absences; and a leading cause of pediatric hospitalizations

D. Classification
   1. Mild intermittent: symptoms 2 or fewer times each week; brief exacerbations; nighttime symptoms 2 or fewer times each month
   2. Mild persistent: symptoms more than 2 times per week but no more than 1 per day; exacerbations affect activity; nighttime symptoms more than twice per month
   3. Moderate persistent asthma: daily symptoms; daily use of inhaled short-acting beta agonists; frequent nighttime symptoms; limited physical activity
   4. Severe persistent asthma: continual symptoms; frequent exacerbations; frequent nighttime symptoms; limited physical activity

E. Clinical findings
   1. Wheezing, especially on expiration
   2. Labored breathing; flaring nares
   3. Cough; increased secretions
   4. Tachycardia
   5. Restlessness; apprehension
   6. Upright sitting position with shoulders forward
   7. Diminished peak expiratory flow rate (PEFR)

F. Therapeutic interventions
   1. Long-term control medications (preventive medicines) achieve and maintain control of inflammation
   2. Quick-relief medications (rescue medications) treat symptoms and exacerbations
   3. Current recommendations include addition of a long-acting beta-adrenergic medication to inhaled steroid; combination therapy has allowed reduction in steroid dosing
   4. Corticosteroids
      a. Action: antiinflammatory effect diminishes the inflammatory component of asthma and reduces airway obstruction; first-line therapy for children more than 5 years of age; oral steroids given initially to gain control of moderately persistent asthma
      b. Inhaled corticosteroids have few side effects and are associated with decreased risk of death; child must rinse mouth after inhalation to reduce risk of oral thrush
      c. If oral steroids are indicated, lowest dose and alternate day administration minimize adverse effects
   5. NSAID: cromolyn sodium (Intal)

a. Action: prevents release of mediators of type I allergic reactions (histamine, slow-reacting substance of anaphylaxis) from sensitized mast cells; prophylactic use lessens bronchoconstriction
      b. Adverse effects: similar to bronchodilator group; anxiety, nervousness, tremors, nausea, vomiting, headache, and dizziness can occur
   6. Beta-adrenergic agonists: albuterol (Proventil); metaproterenol (Alupent); terbutaline (Brethine)
      a. Action: act on beta-adrenergic receptors in the bronchi to relax smooth muscle and increase respiratory volume; used for quick relief in rescue situations
      b. Adverse effects: cardiac palpitation, hyperactivity, insomnia, and tremor can occur; overuse of inhalants may cause "congestive rebound"
   7. Status asthmaticus: beta-adrenergic agents such as epinephrine and albuterol are given when the child continues to experience respiratory distress despite usual interventions; a medical emergency

Nursing Care of Children With Asthma

A. Assessment/Analysis
   1. Respiratory status
   2. History of current and previous attacks
   3. Precipitating events/environmental factors
   4. Knowledge of drug therapy

B. Planning/Implementation
   1. Administer parenteral drugs per procedures to minimize adverse effects
   2. Teach parents how to give controller and rescue medications and explain why control medications must be given even if child does not have an attack
   3. Teach parents chest physiotherapy, need for increased fluids, and use of a cool mist humidifier to provide high humidity in the home
   4. Improve ventilating capacity
      a. Position in a high-Fowler's or the orthopneic position
      b. Teach breathing exercises and controlled breathing
      c. Have child return demonstrate how to use peak expiratory flow meter (PEFM) to monitor airflow
   5. Teach parents that a controlled environment can limit attacks
      a. Allergy-proof home (e.g., damp dust, no carpets)
      b. Manage exertion, exposure to cold air, and people with infections

C. Evaluation/Outcomes
   1. Breathes without dyspnea when at rest or engaging in activities
   2. Manages respiratory secretions
   3. Obtains sufficient sleep to feel rested
   4. Maintains family and peer-group relationships
   5. Child and family members cope with impact of chronic illness

MUCOCUTANEOUS LYMPH NODE SYNDROME (KAWASAKI DISEASE)

Data Base

A. Acute febrile illness of unknown cause; principally involving the cardiovascular system, with extensive perivasculitis of arterioles, venules, capillaries, including the coronary arteries; panvasculitis and perivasculitis of main coronary arteries may cause stenosis or obstruction with aneurysm formation, pericarditis, interstitial myocarditis and endocarditis, and phlebitis of the larger veins

B. Geographic and seasonal outbreaks

C. Clinical findings
   1. Fever for 5 or more days; cervical lymphadenopathy
   2. Bilateral congestion of the ocular conjunctiva without exudation
   3. Changes in mucous membranes of the oral cavity, such as erythema, dryness and fissuring of lips, oropharyngeal reddening, or "strawberry tongue"
   4. Changes in the extremities, such as peripheral edema, peripheral erythema, and desquamation of the palms and soles, particularly periungual peeling; polymorphous rash, primarily of the trunk
   5. Extreme irritability
   6. Joint stiffness and pain

D. Therapeutic interventions
   1. Primarily supportive and directed toward preventing dehydration, and minimizing possible cardiac complications; cardiac monitoring
   2. Intravenous gamma globulin
   3. Large doses of aspirin initially, then low-dose therapy

Nursing Care of Children With Kawasaki Disease

A. Assessment/Analysis
   1. Cardiac status; signs of heart failure
   2. Fluid balance
   3. Symptoms associated with syndrome

B. Planning/Implementation
   1. Administer aspirin; assess for early signs of toxicity
   2. Monitor for signs of cardiac complications, especially dysrhythmias
   3. Observe for allergic reaction to and side effects of IV gamma globulin
   4. Use pain rating scale and medicate appropriately for joint pain
   5. Minimize skin discomfort: cool baths; nonscented lotions; soft, loose clothing
   6. Provide emotional support to child and parents; child is often inconsolable

C. Evaluation/Outcomes
   1. Regains skin integrity
   2. Remains free from complications (cardiac problems, aspirin toxicity)
   3. Remains comfortable
   4. Child and parents discuss feelings

 TONSILLECTOMY AND ADENOIDECTOMY

Data Base

A. Not done routinely, because lymphoid tissue helps prevent invasion of organisms

B. Indications for surgical removal
   1. Recurrent tonsillitis or otitis media
   2. Enlargement that interferes with breathing or swallowing

C. Contraindications for removal
   1. Occasional infections that resolve rapidly
   2. Cleft palate, hemophilia, or debilitating disease such as leukemia

D. Clinical findings: postoperative
   1. Postsurgical hemorrhage: first 24 hours after surgery because of trauma; 5 to 10 days after surgery because of sloughing of tissue
   2. Signs of hemorrhage: frequent swallowing; bright-red blood in vomitus; restlessness; increased pulse rate; pallor

Nursing Care of Children Having a Tonsillectomy and/or Adenoidectomy

A. Assessment/Analysis
   1. Presence of bleeding; frequent swallowing
   2. Presence and extent of pain
   3. Swallowing ability

B. Planning/Implementation
   1. Keep positioned on the side to allow secretions to drain from mouth
   2. Give cool liquids that are not red in color, or thick
   3. Ask child to talk; provide assurance that it is possible
   4. Apply an ice collar to decrease edema
   5. Use pain rating scale and medicate appropriately; avoid use of salicylates
   6. During initial postoperative days: provide only soft food; nothing with sharp edges such as crisp bacon, pretzels, or chips, which could interrupt suture line

C. Evaluation/Outcomes
   1. Maintains patent airway
   2. Manages respiratory secretions
   3. Reports minimal pain
   4. Maintains fluid and nutritional status

 EMOTIONAL DISORDERS

For common emotional disorders of the preschooler, see Chapter 17: Nursing Care of Clients with Disorders Usually First Evident in Infancy, Childhood, or Adolescence in Unit 3 Mental Health/Psychiatric Nursing

Nursing Care of School-Age Children

GROWTH AND DEVELOPMENT

DEVELOPMENTAL TIMETABLE

A. Physical growth
  1. Permanent dentition, beginning with 6-year molars and central incisors at 7 or 8 years of age
  2. Tends to look lanky because bone development precedes muscular development
     a. 6 years: height and weight gain slower; 2 inches and 2 to 3 kg (4½ to 6½ lb) a year
     b. 7 years: continues to grow, 5 cm (2 inches) and 2.5 kg (5½ lb) a year
     c. 8 to 9 years: continues to grow, 5 cm (2 inches) and 3 kg (6½ lb) a year
     d. 10 to 12 years: slow growth in height compared to rapid weight gain, 6.25 cm (2½ inches) and 4.5 kg (10 lb) a year; pubescent changes may begin to appear, earlier in females than males
B. Motor
  1. Refinement of coordination, balance, and control
  2. Motor development becomes important; necessary for competitive activity
C. Sensory: visual acuity should be 20/20
D. Mental abilities
  1. Readiness for learning, especially in perceptual organization: names months of year; knows right from left; can tell time; can follow several directions at once
  2. Acquires use of reason and understanding of rules; needs consistency
  3. Trial-and-error problem solving becomes conceptual rather than action oriented
  4. Reasoning ability allows greater understanding and use of language
  5. Concrete operations (Piaget): knows that quantity remains the same even though appearance differs

HEALTH PROMOTION OF SCHOOL-AGE CHILDREN

PLAY

A. Play activities vary with age; number of play activities decreases, whereas amount of time spent in one particular activity increases
B. Prefers games with rules because of increased mental abilities

C. Prefers games of athletic competition because of increased motor ability
D. Learns how to work as well as play, with a beginning appreciation for economics and finances
E. In beginning of school years, boys and girls play together but gradually separate into sex-oriented types of activities; socialization should be supported
F. Suggested play for 6 to 9 year olds
  1. Housekeeping toys that work; doll accessories; paper-doll sets; simple sewing machine; needlework; building toys
  2. Simple word, number, and card games that require increased skills
  3. Physically active games such as hopscotch, jump rope, tree climbing, bicycle riding
  4. Collections and hobbies such as stamp collecting and building simple models
G. Suggested play for 9 to 12 year olds
  1. Handicrafts of all kinds; model kits; pottery clay; hobbies; collections
  2. Skilled and intellectual play: archery; dart games; chess; puzzles; sports; science toys; magic sets

HOSPITALIZATION OF SCHOOL-AGE CHILDREN

DATA BASE

A. Typical reactions
  1. Usually handles separation well but prefers parents to be near
  2. Fears the unknown, especially when dependency or loss of control is expected
  3. Fears bodily harm, especially disfigurement
  4. Young school-age children personify death as a "bogeyman"; possesses realistic concept of death by 9 to 10 years of age, which may add to other fears
  5. Concerned about self-image when reacting to pain; may use avoidance to deal with physical discomfort
  6. Wants to know scientific rationale for treatments and procedures; willing to participate in self-care
B. If possible parents can be helped to prepare child, since increased cognitive and verbal ability makes explanations possible

GENERAL NURSING CARE OF SCHOOL-AGE CHILDREN

A. Begin preparing child for hospitalization before admission, if possible
B. Provide explanations that are simple and honest and at child's level of understanding; add details about procedures, drugs, surgery, and related issues based on child's cognitive level and personal experiences
C. Involve child and parents in planning care
D. Provide time for play as an outlet for fear, anger, and hostility, as well as a temporary escape from reality
E. Provide diversional play activities that support/ challenge child's mental and motor skills as indicated
F. Encourage and allow child to express feelings, emotions, and fears; expect and accept regression
G. Check child for the presence of loose teeth, especially before surgery
H. Provide for tutoring if absence from school is prolonged
I. Encourage visits from siblings and peers and the formation of new peer relationships; assign age-appropriate roomates who do not have a negative effect on physical status
J. Allow dependency, but foster independence as much as possible

HEALTH PROBLEMS MOST COMMON IN SCHOOL-AGE CHILDREN

DIABETES MELLITUS

Data Base

A. Peak incidence in school-age group
B. Differences in diabetes in children and adults
1. Children are usually diagnosed with type 1 diabetes and adults with type 2 diabetes
2. Onset of type 1 diabetes: rapid in children; insidious in adults
3. Dietary treatment: rarely adequate for children; may be beneficial for some children and adults with type 2 diabetes
4. Oral hypoglycemics: not used for type 1 diabetes
5. Insulin: almost universally necessary in children with type 1 diabetes; may be necessary for type 2
6. Hypoglycemia and ketoacidosis: frequent in children; less common in adults
7. Obesity: not a factor in type 1 diabetes; becoming an increasing factor in both children and adults with type 2 diabetes
8. Degenerative vascular changes: develop after adolescence in children; may be present at time of diagnosis in adults
C. Classification
1. Type 1 diabetes: onset usually in childhood but can be at any age; both genetic and immunologic factors are associated with onset
2. Type 2 diabetes: involves resistance to insulin action and defective glucose-mediated insulin secretion; 100% concordance in identical twins
3. Other types caused by pancreatic defects

a. Maturity-onset diabetes of the young: associated with defects in pancreatic beta cell function; characterized by impaired insulin secretion with minimum or no defect in insulin action; occurs as an autosomal dominant inheritance with onset before age 25
b. Cystic fibrosis–related diabetes
D. Clinical findings: type 1 diabetes
1. Onset: rapid and obvious
2. Child usually thin, underweight
3. Three Ps: polydipsia; polyphagia; polyuria
4. Hyperglycemia: ketoacidosis or diabetic coma
a. Causes
(1) Inadequate amount of insulin
(2) Emotional stress
(3) Physical stress such as fever, infection
(4) Increased food intake
b. Signs and symptoms
(1) Onset: gradual (days)
(2) Mood: lethargic
(3) Mental status: dulled sensorium; confused
(4) Symptoms: thirst; weakness; nausea/ vomiting; abdominal pain
(5) Skin: flushed; signs of dehydration
(6) Mucous membranes: dry and crusty
(7) Vital signs: respirations deep and rapid (Kussmaul); pulse less rapid and weaker than baseline
(8) Breath odor: fruity; acetone
(9) Blood glucose level: high, 250 mg/dL or higher
(10) Urine output: polyuria (early); oliguria (late); enuresis; nocturia
(11) Vision: diplopia
(12) Neurologic: diminished reflexes and paresthesia
(13) Ominous signs: acidosis and coma
5. Hypoglycemia: related to insulin therapy
a. Causes
(1) Overdose of insulin
(2) Decreased food intake
(3) Increased physical exercise: increases muscle activity and movement of glucose into muscle cells
b. Signs and symptoms
(1) Onset: rapid
(2) Mood: labile; irritable; and anxious
(3) Mental status: difficulty concentrating; speaking; focusing
(4) Symptoms: shaky feeling; hunger; headache; dizziness
(5) Skin: pallid and sweating
(6) Mucous membranes: moist
(7) Vital signs: respirations shallow; pulse rapid; palpitations
(8) Breath odor: normal
(9) Blood glucose level: below 60 mg/dL
(10) Urine output: within usual range

(11) Vision: diplopia

(12) Neurologic: tremors; hyperreflexia; dilated pupils

(13) Ominous signs: shock and coma

E. Therapeutic interventions

1. Calories, carbohydrate, fat, and protein intake balanced with physical activity and metabolic needs

2. Insulin (see Related Pharmacology in Chapter 9: Nursing Care of Clients With Endocrine System Disorders [Medical-Surgical Nursing])

3. Exercise to reduce need for insulin

4. Hyperglycemia: hospitalization with administration of fluids, electrolytes, and insulin

5. Hypoglycemia: immediate supply of readily available glucose followed by a complex carbohydrate and protein

Nursing Care of Children With Diabetes Mellitus

A. Assessment/Analysis

1. Knowledge and attitudes about the disease and its management

2. Blood glucose monitoring; expected values: child, 50 to 85 mg/dL; adolescent, 60 to 110 mg/dL

3. Insulin administration

4. Signs of hypoglycemia/hyperglycemia

5. Early signs of complications

B. Planning/Implementation

1. Explain differences between type 1 and type 2 diabetes to parents

2. Teach factors that affect insulin requirements and signs of insulin overdose and diabetic coma

a. Teach onset of action and peak action of insulin being taken

b. Provide a written list explaining signs and symptoms and appropriate interventions

c. Emphasize that a glucose source and skim milk can be given if insulin reaction is suspected but that insulin should not be increased if diabetic ketoacidosis is developing; practitioner should be notified

d. Explain orders for insulin coverage

3. Teach need for prevention of infection: skin care; frequent baths; properly fitting shoes; prompt treatment of any small cut; protection from undue exposure to illness

4. Encourage well-balanced diet, with fairly equal quantities of food to be eaten frequently and regularly; usually unrestricted within reason; regularly scheduled snacks particularly before bed time if taking intermediate-acting insulin

5. Help plan exercise and adjust food intake and insulin dosage to meet child's requirements; food intake should increase before exercising

6. Teach child how to do blood glucose testing to increase independence

7. Teach child how to administer insulin (by injection or pump)

a. Child should be taught as early as motor and mental abilities allow, usually by 7 to 9 years of age

b. Explanations should be simple; diagrams for administration sites should be used

c. Periodic observation by an adult to ensure proper technique

8. Allow child to make choices when possible for sense of control

9. Encourage continued health care supervision

C. Evaluation/Outcomes

1. Maintains blood glucose levels within acceptable range

2. Consumes adequate calories for growth and development

3. Remains free from complications (insulin coma; ketoacidosis)

4. Demonstrates behaviors reflective of a positive self-image

5. Child and parents demonstrate the ability to follow health care regimen

HEMOPHILIA

Data Base

A. Defect in clotting mechanism of blood

B. Genetic disorder; X-linked recessive transmission

C. Occurs in males; females are carriers but do not have the illness

D. Classification

1. Factor VIII deficiency (hemophilia A, classic hemophilia); 80% to 85% of cases

2. Factor IX deficiency (hemophilia B, Christmas disease)

E. Clinical findings

1. Expression of gene varies markedly in relation to degree and severity of bleeding

2. Bleeding into the joints (hemarthrosis), resulting in pain, deformity, and impaired growth

3. Intracranial hemorrhage

4. Severity of bleeding depending on factor VIII activity

a. Mild: bleeding with severe trauma or surgery; factor VIII activity 5% to 40%

b. Moderate: bleeding with trauma; factor VIII activity 2% to 4.9%

c. Severe: spontaneous bleeding without trauma; factor VIII activity less than 2%

F. Therapeutic interventions

1. Control of bleeding when it occurs

2. Prevention of bleeding with use of factor replacement

a. Drugs that replace deficient coagulation factors

(1) Factor VIII concentrate from recombinant DNA

(2) Factor IX concentrate from recombinant DNA; complex contains factors II, VII, IX, X

b. Adjunctive measures

(1) DDAVP (l-deamino-8-D-arginine vasopressin) treatment of choice in mild

hemophilia and von Willebrand's disease; vigorous treatment to prevent joint bleeding is done if child responds to this drug therapy

(2) NSAIDs such as ibuprofen are effective in relieving pain caused by synovitis; must be used with caution because of potential effect on platelet function

(3) Corticosteroids used for hematuria, acute hemarthrosis, and chronic synovitis

(4) Aminocaproic acid (Amicar) oral administration or local application prevents clot destruction; use limited to mouth or trauma surgery

(5) Regular program of exercise and physical therapy to strengthen muscles around joints and minimize bleeding

Nursing Care of Children With Hemophilia

A. Assessment/Analysis
1. Parent/child knowledge of disease process
2. Knowledge of injury prevention and protective attire
3. Location and extent of bleeding
4. Mobility of joints

B. Planning/Implementation
1. Teach child and parents about the treatment for bleeding, especially when it occurs in joints
   a. Resting the area
   b. Application of cool/ice compresses
   c. Compression of the area
   d. Elevation of the affected body part
2. Provide for appropriate activity that lessens the chance of trauma, which is often difficult because boys are physically active
3. Select safe toys and inform parents to safe-proof house to minimize injuries; secure throw rugs
4. Explain reason for avoiding use of aspirin and for using ibuprofen sparingly
5. Use pain rating scale and medicate to control joint pain
6. Plan physical activity program that encourages use of extremities to prevent muscle atrophy
7. Provide for genetic counseling
8. Encourage parents to avoid overprotection or overpermissiveness
9. Administer ordered blood products in the morning so that the child benefits the most from the therapeutic effects

C. Evaluation/Outcomes
1. Reports minimal pain
2. Remains free from injury (hemorrhage)
3. Maintains range of motion of joints
4. Participates in desired activities
5. Child and parents discuss feelings and concerns

RHEUMATIC FEVER (RF)

Data Base
A. Inflammatory disease affecting heart, joints, CNS, and subcutaneous tissue; most significant sequela is

rheumatic heart disease with damage and scarring of the mitral valve

B. Strong relationship between upper respiratory tract infection with group A beta-hemolytic streptococci and RF

C. Most common among children in developing countries because of inadequate health care and limited access to antibiotics

D. Clinical findings
1. Heart: endocarditis and mitral and aortic stenosis may occur
2. Joints: edema, inflammation, and effusion, especially in knees, elbows, hips, shoulders, and wrists
3. Skin: erythematous macules with a clear center and wavy demarcated border usually on trunk and proximal extremities
4. Neurologic: chorea
5. Low-grade fever, epistaxis, abdominal pain, arthralgia, weakness, fatigue, pallor, anorexia, and weight loss

E. Therapeutic interventions
1. Antibiotic therapy to eradicate organism and prevent recurrence; life-long prophylactic therapy before dental work or invasive procedures
2. Prevention of permanent cardiac damage
3. Palliation of other symptoms
4. Salicylates to control inflammatory process
5. Prevention of recurrences

Nursing Care of Children With Rheumatic Fever

A. Assessment/Analysis
1. Presence of symptoms
2. Activity level
3. Pain
4. Compliance with drug regimen

B. Planning/Implementation
1. Encourage bed rest to reduce workload of the heart during acute phase of illness; gradually increase activities as child recovers
2. Handle painful joints carefully; maintain functional alignment to prevent deformities
3. Use pain rating scale and medicate appropriately
4. Provide small, frequent meals; encourage intake of nutritious fluids
5. Emphasize abilities rather than limitations; stimulate development of quiet hobbies and collections
6. Maintain child's status in home and school by keeping communication channels open; obtain tutor as necessary; encourage child to do schoolwork and keep up with class

C. Evaluation/Outcomes
1. Maintains cardiac output within acceptable limits
2. Consumes adequate calories for growth
3. Reports minimal pain
4. Maintains mobility of joints

ACUTE POSTSTREPTOCOCCAL GLOMERULONEPHRITIS (APSGN)

Data Base

A. Most common form of postinfectious glomerulonephritis
B. Peak age of onset is during early school-age years (6 to 7)
C. Terminates with full recovery in 1 to 3 weeks; illness confers immunity; recurrence is rare
D. Clinical Findings
  1. Manifested about 10 days after an infection; infection may range from mild to severe
  2. Signs and symptoms during acute phase
    a. Urine: analysis reveals hematuria; proteinuria; elevated specific gravity
    b. Blood: studies show azotemia from elevated BUN and creatinine
    c. Serology: tests show post streptococcal infection (e.g., antistreptolysin O [ASO])
    d. Edema: periorbital in morning; spreads to rest of body during day
    e. General malaise: irritable; anorexic; lethargic
    f. Hypertension: mild to moderate
E. Therapeutic interventions
  1. No specific treatment; supportive measures as needed
  2. Monitoring course of illness to prevent complications

Nursing Care of Children With Acute Post Streptococcal Glomerulonephritis

A. Assessment/Analysis
  1. Extent of edema
  2. Extent of kidney involvement; results of urinalysis
  3. Changes in vital signs
  4. Blood and serologic findings
  5. Behavior: irritability; lethargy
  6. Complaints of headache; discomfort; signs of impending seizures
B. Planning/Implementation
  1. Maintain fluid balance: monitor daily weights, vital signs I&O; restrict fluids as ordered
  2. Provide nutritious diet based on child's preferences; implement moderate sodium restriction when edematous and/or hypertensive
  3. Document and report signs of complications: severe hypertension; gross hematuria; gross edema; behavioral changes that may signify cerebral involvement
  4. Administer prescribed medications: diuretics; antihypertensives; antibiotics; all based on child's response to illness
  5. Instruct parents about supportive care if child is treated at home (e.g., balancing rest and activity; nutritious diet; dietary restrictions; prevention of infection)
  6. Emphasize importance of follow-up care: weekly and then monthly visits for health supervision and evaluation of the progress and resolution of the illness
C. Evaluation/Outcomes
  1. Child will be free from illness within 3 weeks
  2. There are no complications or recurrences
  3. Health supervision and follow-up care continue until discharged by practitioner

JUVENILE IDIOPATHIC ARTHRITIS (JUVENILE RHEUMATOID ARTHRITIS)

Data Base

A. Group of inflammatory diseases affecting joints and other tissues; incidence is approximately 1 in 1000 children
B. Two peak ages of onset: 1 to 3 and 8 to 10 years of age; female predominance of 2:1
C. Classification
  1. Systemic onset
  2. Monoarticular or pauciarticular: involves a few joints; usually fewer than five
  3. Polyarticular: simultaneous involvement of five or more joints
D. Clinical findings
  1. Differences from adult RA: onset before age 16; 90% of children negative for rheumatoid factor (RF); only 30% will have RA that persists to adulthood
  2. Stiffness, swelling, and loss of motion in affected joints; most common in morning and after inactivity
  3. Joint enlargement results from edema, joint effusion, and synovial thickening
E. Therapeutic interventions
  1. Medications
    a. First-line drugs: nonsteroidal antiinflammatory drugs (NSAIDs)
    b. Second-line drugs: slow-acting antirheumatic drugs (SAARDs), such as methotrexate (Rheumatrex), sulfasalazine (Azulfidine)
    c. Tumor necrosis factor inhibitor: etanercept (Enbrel)
    d. Corticosteroids: used when other drugs fail; affects growth and development
  2. Physical and occupational therapy

Nursing Care of Children With Juvenile Idiopathic Arthritis

A. Assessment/Analysis
  1. Status of involved joints
  2. Physical restrictions
  3. Location and extent of pain
  4. Child's response to disease process
B. Planning/Implementation
  1. Emphasize that medication must be taken regularly, even in periods of remission, to decrease inflammation and pain; NSAIDs should be taken with food to prevent GI irritation
  2. Promote functional alignment; provide passive range of motion

3. Have physical therapist design activity program to provide exercise with limited impact on joints
4. Encourage a warm bath or moist heat compresses to joints in the morning to decrease stiffness and increase mobility; discourage prolonged sitting
5. Encourage parents to accept their child's illness but to avoid using the disease as a means of fostering dependency or controlling relationships
6. Encourage verbalization of feelings; emphasize abilities rather than limitations

C. Evaluation/Outcomes
1. Reports minimal pain
2. Maintains mobility of joints
3. Participates in activities with minimal discomfort and sufficient energy
4. Participates in self-care to fullest extent of abilities
5. Child and family maintain health care regimen

❀ SKIN INFECTIONS AND INFESTATIONS

General Nursing Care of Children With Skin Infections and infestation

A. Assessment/Analysis
1. Type of skin lesion
2. Location and extent of discomfort or itching
3. Knowledge of cause, prevention, and treatment
4. Self-concept and social isolation as a result of change in appearance

B. Planning/Implementation
1. Prevent secondary infection: keep nails short; administer medications to limit pruritus
2. Encourage daily bathing with tepid water; dry thoroughly; expose area to light and air
3. Encourage completion of full regimen of antimicrobial medication
4. Prevent spread of infection to other members of the family: prevent direct contact between children; keep oozing lesions covered; prevent athlete's foot by not walking barefooted, drying feet carefully, wearing lightweight shoes to decrease heat, disinfecting shoes and socks, and not sharing towels
5. Teach proper hygiene: hair care; frequent bathing; clean clothes; avoidance of strong alkalis or bleach when washing clothes
6. Encourage screening in schools to identify source of infection

C. Evaluation/Outcomes
1. Confines skin lesions to primary site and infection/infestation to self
2. Remains free from secondary infection
3. Remains free from discomfort
4. Child and parents verbalize how to prevent future infection/infestation

❀ PEDICULOSIS (LICE)

Data Base
A. Infestation of head, body, or pubic hair; nits (grayish white, oval eggs) attach to hair

B. Severe itching may lead to secondary infection
C. Therapeutic interventions
1. Special shampoo; use of fine-toothed comb to remove nits
2. All bed linens and clothes must be washed in hot water and detergent
3. Return to school as soon as possible per policy; many schools allow child to return after treatment

❀ SCABIES

Data Base
A. Produced by itch mite; female burrows under skin to lay eggs (usually in folds)
B. Intensely pruritic; scratching can lead to secondary infection with development of papules and vesicles
C. Therapeutic interventions: all members of the family must be treated because it is highly contagious; wash with sulfur or other special soap; wear clean clothes

❀ RINGWORM (FUNGAL DISEASE)

Data Base
A. Scalp (tinea capitis)
1. Reddened oval or round areas of alopecia
2. Pruritus
B. Feet (athlete's foot, tinea pedis)
1. Scaly fissures between toes, vesicles on sides of feet, pruritus
2. Particularly common in summer; contracted in swimming areas and gymnasium locker rooms
C. Therapeutic interventions
1. Griseofulvin, micronized (Fulvicin-U/F, Grifulvin V, Grisactin); topical or oral
2. Terbinafine (Lamisil); topical cream

❀ INTERTRIGO

Data Base
A. Excoriation of any adjacent body surfaces
B. Caused by moisture and chafing

❀ IMPETIGO

Data Base
A. Bacterial infection of skin by streptococci or staphylococci
B. Highly contagious; other areas of body frequently become infected
C. Therapeutic interventions: antibiotics systemically and locally; isolation of child; prevention from scratching other areas of the body

❀ REYE'S SYNDROME

Data Base
A. Acute toxic encephalopathy associated with characteristic organ involvement
B. Usually follows viral illness, influenza, or varicella; associated with aspirin administration
C. Use of aspirin and NSAIDs, such as ibuprofen, is not recommended for children with varicella or influenza

D. Clinical findings
1. Fever
2. Profound impaired consciousness
3. Disordered hepatic function
E. Therapeutic interventions
1. Early diagnosis with aggressive therapy
2. Treatment: determined by clinical stage of the disease

Nursing Care of Children With Reye's Syndrome
A. Assessment/Analysis
1. Vital signs and neurologic status
2. Fluid balance
3. Level of consciousness
4. Signs of impaired coagulation (related to hepatic dysfunction)
B. Planning/Implementation
1. Maintain a patent airway
2. Monitor vital signs; neurologic status; hemodynamics
3. Monitor fluid balance
4. Assist with invasive procedures
5. Keep parents informed of child's progress; include parents in child's care whenever possible; provide emotional support
6. Foster dissemination of information concerning role of aspirin in relation to viral disease and development of Reye's syndrome
C. Evaluation/Outcomes
1. Maintains a patent airway and appropriate breathing pattern
2. Remains free from injury
3. Maintains fluid balance
4. Parents can verbalize questions and concerns about child's status

LEGG-CALVÉ-PERTHES DISEASE (COXA PLANA)
Data Base
A. A disturbance of circulation to the femoral capital epiphysis that produces an ischemic aseptic necrosis of the femoral head, epiphysis, and acetabulum; cause unknown
B. Occurs between 2 to 12 years of age; most common in males 4 to 8 years of age; male to female ratio 4:1; more common in Caucasians than in African Americans (10:1)
C. In 10% to 15% of incidences, both hips are involved; most children have skeletal ages below chronologic age
D. Stages: stage I—avascular; stage II—fragmentation or revascularization; stage III—reparative; stage IV—regenerative

E. Clinical findings
1. Insidious onset
2. Persistent pain in affected hip(s)
3. Limitation of movement in affected hip(s); limp
F. Therapeutic interventions
1. Maintenance of head of the femur in the acetabulum and full range of motion
2. Conservative therapy is continued for 2 to 4 years, whereas surgical correction returns the child to usual activities in 3 to 4 months
3. Non–weight-bearing devices such as an abduction brace, leg casts, or a leather harness sling that prevent weight-bearing on the affected limb
4. Abduction-ambulation braces or casts after a period of bed rest and traction
5. Surgical reconstructive and containment procedures

Nursing Care of Children With Legg-Calvé-Perthes Disease
A. Assessment/Analysis
1. Extent of pain
2. Extent of joint dysfunction
B. Planning/Implementation
1. Educate child and parents regarding correct use of appliances, including skin care at brace edges
2. Instruct child and parents regarding what constitutes non–weight-bearing (e.g., no standing or kneeling on affected leg)
3. Assist child and family in selecting activities according to child's age, interests, and physical limitations (e.g., quiet games, hobbies, collections, model building, crafts, indoor gardening)
4. Encourage peer interaction; help child determine alternatives to weight-bearing activity (e.g., scorekeeping, acting as sideline "coach")
5. Help child devise explanations for appliances
C. Evaluation/Outcomes
1. Reports minimal pain
2. Remains free from injury
3. Participates in activities with immobilizing device
4. Discusses feelings and concerns

EMOTIONAL DISORDERS
For common emotional disorders of the school-age child, see Chapter 17: Nursing Care of Clients With Disorders Usually First Evident in Infancy, Childhood, or Adolescence in Unit 3 (Mental Health/Psychiatric Nursing)

34 Nursing Care of Adolescents

GROWTH AND DEVELOPMENT
DEVELOPMENTAL TIMETABLE

A. Physical growth: includes physical changes associated with puberty such as secondary sexual characteristics
B. Pubertal growth spurt
  1. Females between 10 and 14 years
     a. Weight gain 7 to 25 kg (15 to 55 lb), mean 17.5 kg (38 lb)
     b. Approximately 95% of mature height achieved by onset of menarche or by skeletal age of 13 years; height gain 5 to 25 cm (2 to 10 inches), mean 20.5 cm (8¼ inches)
     c. Secondary sexual characteristics: usually breasts begin to develop first, then pubic and axillary hair appear, followed by pigmentation of genital skin and menarche
  2. Males between 12 and 16 years
     a. Weight gain 7 to 30 kg (15 to 65 lb), mean 23.7 kg (52 lb)
     b. Approximately 95% of mature height achieved by skeletal age of 15 years; height gain 10 to 30 cm (4 to 12 inches), mean 27.5 cm (11 inches)
     c. Secondary sexual characteristics: usually deepening of the voice, testicular enlargement, and pubic, facial, and body hair growth occur first; then a lengthening and thickening of the penis occurs followed by the initiation of ejaculation of semen; gynecomastia occurs in one third of adolescent boys during midpuberty but usually disappears within 2 years
C. Mental abilities
  1. Abstract thinking
     a. New level of social communication and understanding; can comprehend satire and double meanings; can say one thing and mean another
     b. Can conceptualize thought; more interested in exploring ideas than facts
     c. Can appreciate scientific thinking, problem solve, and theoretically explore alternatives
  2. Perception
     a. Can appreciate nonrepresentational art
     b. Can understand that the whole is more than the sum of its parts
  3. Learning
     a. Long attention span

     b. Learns through inference, intuition, and theorizing, rather than repetition and imitation
     c. Enjoys experimenting with language by using jargon to suit changing moods
D. Social patterns
  1. Peer-group identity
     a. One of the strongest motivating forces of behavior
     b. Extremely important to be part of the group and be like everyone else
     c. Clique formation; usually based on common denominators such as race, social class, ethnic group, or special interests
  2. Interpersonal relationships
     a. Major goal is learning to form a close intimate relationship with the opposite sex
     b. May develop crushes and worship idols
     c. Time of sexual exploration and questioning of one's sexual role
     d. Concerned more with the present than the future
  3. Independence
     a. By 15 or 16 years of age, feel they should be treated as adults
     b. Ambivalence: wants freedom but has difficulty accepting corresponding responsibilities; frequently yearns for more carefree days of childhood
     c. Parental ambivalence and discipline problems are common as parents try to allow for increasing independence but continue to offer constructive guidance and enforce discipline

HEALTH PROMOTION DURING ADOLESCENCE
NUTRITION DURING ADOLESCENCE

A. Nutritional objectives
  1. Provide optimum nutritional support for demands of rapid growth and high energy expenditure
  2. Support development of appropriate eating habits through variety of foods, regular food pattern, quality snacks (high in protein; low in refined carbohydrate, primarily sugar)
B. Range of nutrient requirements increases, so adequate intake of all nutrients should form basis of diet

C. Nutritional problems
  1. Inadequate intake of calcium, vitamins A and C, and iron in females
  2. Anemia
  3. Obesity or underweight
D. Possible causes of nutritional deficiencies
  1. Psychologic factors: food aversions; emotional problems
  2. Fear of overweight: crash diets, mainly in girls; cultural pressure
  3. Fad diets: caused by misinformation; need for effective counseling
  4. Choice of junk foods for snacks: usually high in sugar and fat
  5. Irregular eating pattern
  6. Pregnancy: requires higher intake of protein, calcium, and calories
E. Nutrition education may be provided through association with teenagers' concerns about physical appearance, figure control, complexion, physical fitness, athletic ability

INJURY PREVENTION DURING ADOLESCENCE

A. Appropriate education regarding sexual maturity, reproduction, and sexual behavior
B. Driver education
C. Education regarding use and abuse of drugs, especially alcohol
D. Education about health hazards associated with smoking

Topics for Health Guidance During Adolescence

A. Accidents: leading cause of death, with motor vehicle accidents causing most fatalities; homicide and suicide: next two leading causes of death
B. Substance abuse
C. Sexually transmitted infections
D. Pregnancy
E. Anorexia nervosa and bulimia nervosa; obesity
F. Delinquency
G. Acne
H. Orthopedic problems
I. Cancer

HOSPITALIZATION OF ADOLESCENTS

Data Base

A. Reactions
  1. Need for privacy, sense of control, and independence
  2. Concern for mutilation, disfigurement, and loss of function; body image changes
  3. Concern about separation from peers and possible loss of status in group
B. Parents and health team members can help prepare adolescent for hospitalization by providing full explanations and answering questions completely and honestly

General Nursing Care of Adolescents

A. Understand that problems are magnified by illness during this period of development
B. Involve adolescent in planning care
C. Be open concerning feelings, care, and prognosis; answer questions honestly and directly to help develop a trusting relationship
D. Foster independence as much as possible
E. Provide for contact with peers
F. Encourage compliance with health program
G. Arrange for continuity in schoolwork
H. Encourage involvement of positive support systems
I. Accept self-appraisal but point out reality
J. Encourage use of clothing or makeup to minimize perceived shortcomings

HEALTH PROBLEMS MOST COMMON IN ADOLESCENTS

SCOLIOSIS
Data Base

A. Lateral curvature of spine usually associated with a rotary deformity that eventually causes cosmetic and physiologic alterations in spine, chest, and pelvis
B. Usually unknown cause (idiopathic); possible genetic etiology
C. Most common spinal deformity; more frequent in girls during growth spurt
D. Classification
  1. Nonstructural scoliosis: curve is flexible and corrects by bending
  2. Structural scoliosis: curve fails to straighten on side-bending; characterized by changes in spine and its supporting structures
E. Clinical findings
  1. Curve in vertebral spinous process alignment
  2. Prominence of one hip
  3. Prominence of one scapula; difference in shoulder or scapular height
  4. Deformity of rib cage; breasts appear unequal in size
  5. Other signs: clothes do not fit; skirt or pant hems are uneven
F. Therapeutic interventions
  1. Screening for scoliosis beginning at age 10; diagnosis confirmed by x-ray examination
  2. Exercise for nonstructural scoliosis
  3. Mild to moderate curvature
    a. Bracing
      (1) Boston or Wilmington brace: worn 16 to 23 hours/day; gradually weaned over 1- to 2-year period; then worn only at night until spine is mature
      (2) Charleston nighttime bending brace: worn only for sleeping because it prevents walking
      (3) Not entirely effective; retrospective studies show only slight variation in outcome with different types of braces

4. More severe curves usually require surgery: techniques consist of spinal realignment and straightening by way of external or internal fixation and instrumentation combined with bony fusion (arthrodesis) of realigned spine (Harrington rods); L-rod segmental instrumentation
5. Most severe scoliotic curvatures require traction devices and exercises before spinal fusion to provide partial correction and more flexibility

Nursing Care of Adolescents With Scoliosis

A. Assessment/Analysis
   1. Symmetry of shoulders and hips while child stands erect, clothed only in underpants (and bra if older girl); observation occurs from behind
   2. Symmetry or prominence of ribs while child bends forward so that back is parallel with floor; observation occurs from the side
B. Planning/Implementation
   1. Maintain spinal alignment
   2. Examine skin surfaces in contact with brace for signs of irritation; implement corrective action to treat or prevent skin breakdown
   3. Reinforce instructions about plan of care, use of appliance, activities permitted or restricted (encourage activities that do not require twisting of the spinal column), and adolescent's and parents' responsibilities in therapy
   4. Help in selection of appropriate wearing apparel to be worn over brace to minimize altered appearance and low-heeled footwear to maintain balance
   5. Prepare for surgery if required
C. Evaluation/Outcomes
   1. Demonstrates correct use of brace
   2. Reports minimal pain
   3. Maintains skin integrity
   4. Verbalizes feelings and concerns
   5. Engages in activities appropriate to limitations and developmental level

✿ BONE TUMORS

Data Base

A. Neoplastic disease that can arise from any tissues involved in bone growth
B. Less than 5% of all malignant neoplasms; more common in children than adults; peak ages 15 to 19 years
C. Classification
   1. Osteosarcoma
      a. Most frequent bone tumor in children
      b. Primary tumor site: metaphysis (wider part of shaft) of a long bone, especially the femur
      c. Arises from osteoid tissue
   2. Ewing's sarcoma
      a. Most frequent sites: shaft of long and trunk bones, especially the femur, tibia, fibula, humerus, ulna, vertebra, scapula, ribs, pelvic bones, and skull
      b. Arises from medullary tissue (marrow)

D. Clinical findings
   1. Signs and symptoms
      a. Localized pain in affected site
      b. Limp; voluntary curtailment of activity
      c. Inability to hold heavy objects
      d. Weight loss; frequent infections
   2. Diagnosis
      a. Radiographic examination; CT (bone); MRI; bone scan
      b. Bone marrow aspiration
      c. Surgical biopsy (Ewing's sarcoma)
E. Therapeutic interventions
   1. Osteogenic sarcoma
      a. Preoperative and postoperative use of chemotherapy with en bloc resection of primary tumor followed by a prosthetic replacement
      b. Amputation of affected bone followed by high-dose methotrexate with citrovorum factor rescue
      c. Administration of doxorubicin (Adriamycin), bleomycin (Blenoxane), dactinomycin (Cosmegen), cyclophosphamide (Cytoxan), ifosfamide (Ifex), and cisplatin (Platinol) singly or in combination both before and after surgery
      d. Currently approximately 85% of those treated can expect long-term survival
   2. Ewing's sarcoma
      a. Intensive irradiation of involved bone and chemotherapy including vincristine (Oncovin), dactinomycin, cyclophosphamide, or ifosfamide, etoposide (VePesid), and doxorubicin
      b. Prognosis is best when no metastasis is present at diagnosis
      c. Current 3-year survival is 80%

Nursing Care of Adolescents With Bone Tumors

A. Assessment/Analysis
   1. Location and extent of pain
   2. Functional status of involved area
   3. Inflammation at site; lymph node involvement
   4. Systemic involvement
B. Planning/Implementation
   1. Preoperative and postoperative intervention
      a. Employ straightforward honesty; avoid disguising diagnosis with terms such as "infection"
      b. Answer questions regarding information presented by surgeon and clarify any misconceptions; avoid overwhelming adolescent or parents with too much information
      c. Emphasize lack of alternatives if amputation is planned
      d. Use pain rating scale and medicate appropriately during postoperative period
      e. Assist adolescent in becoming adept at using prosthesis
      f. Help adolescent select clothing to camouflage prosthesis

2. Radiotherapy used for Ewing's sarcoma
   a. Explain procedure; explain side effects
   b. Suggest and/or implement measures to reduce physical effects of radiotherapy: select loose-fitting cotton clothing over irradiated areas to decrease additional irritation; protect area from sunlight and sudden changes in temperature; avoid use of ice packs, heating pads
   c. Help adolescent cope with side effects of radiotherapy
3. Chemotherapy
   a. Explain procedure, stressing importance of chemotherapy
   b. Explain probable side effects of antimetabolites (e.g., nausea, hair loss, stomatitis)
   c. Use preventative therapies including ondansetron (Zofran) to minimize associated nausea
   d. Help adolescent cope with side effects of chemotherapy; discuss supportive therapies (e.g., antiemetics, nutrition, soft-tipped applicator for oral hygiene)
   e. Encourage hygiene, grooming, and items to enhance appearance such as a wig
4. Emotional support to child and family members
   a. Clarify misconceptions and provide technical information as needed
   b. Allow time and opportunity to go through the grieving process
   c. Allow for expression of feelings regarding losses and undesirable effects of therapy

   d. Allow dependence but encourage independence
   e. Emphasize need for continuing regular activities, interactions, and behaviors
C. Evaluation/Outcomes
   1. Reports minimal pain
   2. Adolescent and parents express feelings and concerns
   3. Adolescent and parents demonstrate positive coping skills
   4. Adolescent and parents verbalize understanding of therapies and side effects
   5. Adolescent and parents adjust to alterations in adolescent's appearance
   6. Resumes peer relationships and activities commensurate with abilities

EMOTIONAL DISORDERS

For common emotional disorders of the adolescent, see Chapter 17: Nursing Care of Clients With Disorders Usually First Evident in Infancy, Childhood, or Adolescence, Unit 3: Mental Health/Psychiatric Nursing

OTHER HEALTH PROBLEMS

Many problems of adolescence are similar to those of adults; see specific areas in Unit 4: Childbearing and Women's Health Nursing, and in Unit 2: Medical-Surgical Nursing, for further discussions

35 Child Health Nursing Review Questions With Answers and Rationales

QUESTIONS

FOUNDATIONS OF CHILD HEALTH NURSING

1. The mother of a 2-year-old child tells the nurse she is having difficulty disciplining her child. What is the nurse's most appropriate response to this comment?
   1. "This is a difficult age that your child is going through right now."
   2. "Tell me more about your difficulty. I'm not sure what you mean by this."
   3. "It's important to be consistent with toddlers when they need disciplining."
   4. "I can understand what you mean. That's why this age is called the terrible twos."

2. Which nursing intervention provides the most support to the parents of a newborn with an obvious physical defect?
   1. Encourage them to express their concerns
   2. Discourage them from talking about their baby
   3. Tell them not to worry because the defect can be repaired
   4. Show them postoperative photographs of infants who had similar defects

3. A child who is known to have the human immunodeficiency virus (HIV) is admitted with the diagnosis of *Pneumocystis jiroveci* pneumonia. The practitioner orders trimethoprim/sulfamethoxazole (Bactrim) and pentamidine (Pentam). When administering Bactrim to a child with AIDS, for which common side effect should the nurse monitor?
   1. Jaundice
   2. Headache
   3. Toxic nephrosis
   4. Hypersensitivity reactions

4. The nurse practitioner orders amoxicillin 145 mg po three times daily for a 28-lb toddler. It is supplied as a suspension of 250 mg/5 mL. The safe dosage is 35 mg/kg/24 hours. How many milligrams within the safe dosage limit is the ordered dose?
   Answer: _____ mg

5. A 7-year-old girl develops a urinary tract infection. The practitioner orders a sulfonamide preparation. What is a major nursing responsibility when administering this drug?
   1. Weigh the child daily
   2. Give milk with the medication
   3. Monitor the child's temperature frequently
   4. Administer the drug at the prescribed times

6. Based on developmental norms for a 5-year-old child, the nurse should withhold a scheduled dose of digoxin (Lanoxin) elixir and notify the practitioner when the child's apical pulse rate first drops below:
   1. 60 beats/min
   2. 70 beats/min
   3. 90 beats/min
   4. 100 beats/min

7. A father calls the clinic and tells the nurse that his child is irritable and has a 102° F temperature after having had a routine immunization. The clinic protocol indicates acetaminophen 15 mg/kg is to be administered every 4 to 6 hours. The child's last weight was 9.6 kg. The father states he has a bottle of acetaminophen that indicates 160 mg/5 mL. How much should the nurse tell the father to administer for each dose?
   Answer: _____ mL

8. A father calls the outpatient clinic requesting information about the appropriate dose of acetaminophen for his 16-month-old child who has symptoms of an upper respiratory tract infection and fever. The box of acetaminophen says to give 120 mg every 4 hours when needed. At the child's 15-month visit, the nurse practitioner prescribed 150 mg. What is the nurse's best response to the parent?
   1. "The doses are close enough and it doesn't really matter which one is given."
   2. "From your description, medications are not necessary. They should be avoided at this age."
   3. "It is appropriate to use dosages based on age. Children have a wide range of weights at different ages."
   4. "The nurse practitioner ordered the drug based on weight, and this is a more accurate way of determining a therapeutic dose."

9. When planning to provide teaching about self-administration of insulin to a school-age child newly diagnosed with diabetes mellitus, the nurse should first:
   1. Assess the child's developmental level
   2. Determine family's understanding of the procedure
   3. Discuss community resources for the child in the future
   4. Collaborate with the school nurse for ensuring continuity of care in school

10. When teaching the correct way to administer ear drops to a 2-year-old child, the nurse should instruct the parent to position the child on the side and instill the drops while pulling the auricle:
    1. Forward
    2. Up and back
    3. Straight back
    4. Down and back

11. The nurse teaches a 5-year-old girl with cystic fibrosis how to use an inhaler. What is the most appropriate way to evaluate her understanding?
    1. Showing the nurse how to use the inhaler
    2. Asking questions about using the inhaler
    3. Explaining how the inhaler will be used at home
    4. Telling the nurse about the things that have been learned

12. A 7-year-old child with cystic fibrosis is receiving an intravenous antibiotic. The medication is supplied in a 125-mL bag of normal saline. It is to be infused over 30 minutes. At what rate should the infusion pump be set to deliver the medication at the prescribed time?
    Answer: _____ mL/hour

13. When picked up by the mother or the nurse, an 8-month-old infant screams and seems to be in pain. The nurse notes the behavior and talks to the mother about:
    1. Accidents and the importance of their prevention
    2. Limiting play time with other children in the family
    3. Food and specific vitamins that should be given to infants
    4. Any other behaviors that the mother may have noticed

14. A 1-week-old infant has been in the pediatric unit for 18 hours following placement of a spica cast. The nurse notes that the respiratory rate is less than 24 breaths/min. No other changes are observed, and because the infant is apparently well, there is no report or documentation of the slow respiratory rate. Several hours later, the infant experiences severe respiratory distress and emergency care is necessary. Legal responsibility in this instance should take into consideration that:
    1. Most infants' respirations are slow when they are uncomfortable
    2. The respirations of young infants are irregular so a drop in rate is unimportant
    3. Vital signs that are outside the expected parameters are significant and should be documented

    4. The respiratory tract of young infants is underdeveloped and their respiratory rate is not significant

15. After orthopedic surgery, a 15 year old reports a pain rating of 5 on a 0 to 10 scale. The adolescent is given 5 mg of oxycodone as ordered every 3 hours PRN. Two hours after having been given this medication, the adolescent reports a pain rating of 10 out of 10. What action should the nurse take?
    1. Administer another dose of oxycodone within 30 minutes
    2. Report that the adolescent has an apparent idiosyncrasy to oxycodone
    3. Tell the adolescent that additional medication cannot be given for 1 more hour
    4. Request that the practitioner evaluate the adolescent's need for additional medication

16. An adolescent is hospitalized for dehydration. The practitioner orders an IV of 1000 mL of 0.9% sodium chloride with 20 mEq/L of potassium chloride. A 500-mL bag of 0.9% sodium chloride is available. The potassium chloride label reads 2 mEq/mL. How many milliliters of potassium chloride should the nurse add to the 500-mL bag?
    Answer: _____ mL

17. The maintenance of fluid and electrolyte balance is more critical in infants and toddlers than in adults because:
    1. Cellular metabolism is less stable than in adults
    2. The proportion of water in the body is less than in adults
    3. Renal function is immature in children until they reach school age
    4. The extracellular fluid requirement per unit of body weight is greater than in adults

18. An infant is receiving parenteral therapy. The IV orders are 400 mL of $D_5 0.45$ NS to run in 8 hours. At what rate should the nurse maintain the hourly rate?
    1. 20 mL/hr
    2. 30 mL/hr
    3. 40 mL/hr
    4. 50 mL/hr

19. The nurse plans specific care for infants based on the knowledge that infants are at greater risk for a fluid volume deficit and hyperosmolar imbalance than adults because:
    1. Their metabolic processes are slower
    2. They have a slower glomerular filtration rate
    3. Their body fluid loss is proportionately greater per kilogram of weight
    4. They have not yet developed a generalized response to insensible fluid loss

20. It is suspected that an infant has a congenital heart defect. When monitoring the infant's vital signs, the nurse also assesses the presence and strength of the femoral pulses. Identify the site on the illustration on the next page that should be palpated to evaluate the femoral pulse.
    Answer: _____

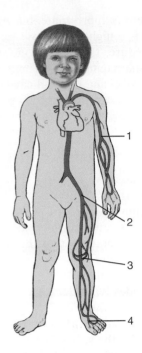

21. During a vaccination drive at a well-child clinic, a nurse observes that a recently hired nurse is not wearing gloves. The nurse should advise the newly hired nurse to:
   1. Speak with the nurse manager regarding techniques
   2. Put on gloves because standard precautions are required
   3. Continue with the immunizations since gloves are not needed
   4. Evaluate the child's appearance to determine whether gloves are needed

22. A peripheral central venous catheter has just been inserted in the arm of a 7-year-old child on the pediatric unit. A peripheral IV line is still in place. An antibiotic is to be administered immediately. Which intravenous access line should the nurse use for the antibiotic infusion and why?
   1. Central venous catheter, because this will help determine its patency
   2. Peripheral line, because the central venous catheter is reserved for fluids
   3. Central venous catheter, because the antibiotic must be given systemically as quickly as possible
   4. Peripheral line, because the central venous catheter placement has not been confirmed by radiograph

23. An order for prednisone reads 10 mg four times per day. The dose for children is 2 mg/kg/day. How many pounds does the child weigh?
   Answer: _____ pounds

24. A family has decided to withhold "extraordinary care" for a newborn with severe abnormalities. How should the nurse interpret this decision?
   1. The newborn has no rights
   2. It is the same as euthanasia
   3. It is illegal professional practice
   4. The newborn is being allowed to die

25. A nurse, planning an initial home care visit to a mother who gave birth to a high-risk infant, understands that the visit will be more productive if scheduled when the:
   1. Husband is out of the home
   2. Mother is feeding the infant
   3. Time is convenient for the family
   4. Nurse has time to spend with the family

NURSING CARE OF INFANTS

26. What should the nurse do before administering a tube feeding to an infant?
   1. Irrigate the tube with water
   2. Slowly instill 10 mL of formula
   3. Provide the infant with a pacifier
   4. Place the infant in the Trendelenburg position

27. What suggestion should the nurse give to the mother who is having difficulty coping with her 2-month-old son who has colic?
   1. Give him a warm bath to calm him down
   2. Arrange for some time away from your son each day to rest
   3. Provide him with warm, sweetened tea when he begins to cry
   4. Sit comfortably in a quiet, darkened room while holding your son when he cries

28. Before surgery to relieve an intestinal obstruction, a 3-month-old infant is kept NPO and has a nasogastric tube in place. Which nursing intervention will help to calm the infant, as well as meet developmental needs?
   1. Allow the infant to suck on a pacifier
   2. Offer the infant a favorite toy to hold
   3. Hang a brightly colored mobile in the infant's crib
   4. Place the infant on the abdomen to permit crawling

29. A child with eczema complains of itching. Which drug can be ordered by the practitioner to relieve this symptom?
   1. Nitrofurazone (Furacin)
   2. Hyaluronidase (Wydase)
   3. Acetylsalicylic acid (Ecotrin)
   4. Diphenhydramine (Benadryl)

30. The parents of an infant ask the nurse why their baby is scheduled to receive the intramuscular polio vaccine rather than the oral vaccine. What is the nurse's best response?
   1. "The American Academy of Pediatrics recommends the intramuscular vaccine because it is safer."
   2. "The consensus is that either can be used since both produce the same results and are equally safe."
   3. "The oral vaccine is more expensive, so the intramuscular vaccine is preferred unless it is contraindicated."
   4. "The U.S. Center for Infectious Disease Control and Prevention recommends intramuscular vaccine unless the infant or a family member is immunocompromised."

31. At a well-child clinic visit, a 1-year-old boy's length is assessed by the nurse to be below what is expected. His current height is 28 inches, and his birth length was 20 inches. What should his current length be?
    1. 27 inches
    2. 30 inches
    3. 32 inches
    4. 35 inches

32. What nursing intervention best meets a major developmental need of a newborn in the immediate postoperative period?
    1. Give a pacifier to the infant
    2. Put a mobile over the infant's crib
    3. Provide the infant with a soft cuddly toy
    4. Warm the infant's formula before feeding

33. The nurse is aware that children born with a missing chromosome are most likely to have:
    1. Cretinism
    2. Phenylketonuria
    3. Down syndrome
    4. Turner's syndrome

34. Play during infancy is important because it enhances:
    1. Social development
    2. Physical development
    3. Cognitive development
    4. Emotional development

35. The nurse caring for infants and young children who have experienced maternal deprivation expects them to be:
    1. Overweight
    2. Hyperactive
    3. Prone to illness
    4. Responsive to stimuli

36. A mother and her 3-month-old infant visit the well-baby clinic for a routine examination. What should the nurse include in the accident prevention teaching plan?
    1. Remove small objects from the floor
    2. Cover electric outlets with safety plugs
    3. Keep crib rails up to the highest position
    4. Remove poisonous substances from low areas

37. When teaching a mother how to prevent accidents while caring for her 6-month-old infant, the nurse should emphasize that at this age, the infant can usually:
    1. Sit up
    2. Roll over
    3. Crawl short distances
    4. Stand while holding on to furniture

38. A 7-month-old girl is to be catheterized to obtain a sterile urine specimen. The infant's mother expresses fear that this procedure may traumatize her baby psychologically. The nurse reassures the mother that:
    1. Her fear is justified and the nurse will obtain a "clean catch" specimen
    2. She has every right to refuse the catheterization, and her concerns are realistic

    3. Her concern is appropriate, but the need for a sterile specimen is a higher priority
    4. The procedure, though uncomfortable, should not have any damaging long-term effect

39. The nurse is assessing the oral cavity of a 6-month-old child. The nurse can predict the appearance of incoming teeth by understanding that the teeth that bud first tend to be the:
    1. Canines
    2. Incisors
    3. Upper molars
    4. Lower molars

40. When teaching a class of mothers about how to position their infants during the first few weeks of life, the nurse tells them that the safest position is on their:
    1. Stomachs lying flat
    2. Backs or sides lying flat
    3. Stomachs with their heads slightly elevated
    4. Right or left sides with their heads slightly elevated

41. What should be the school nurse's first action when a child complains of a sore throat?
    1. Examine the throat
    2. Have the child sent home
    3. Take the child's temperature
    4. Secure an order for an oral analgesic

42. A 17-year-old female arrives in the emergency clinic with her 3-month-old son who she says stopped breathing for "a while." The infant continues to have difficulty breathing. Which assessment data should alert the nurse to suspect shaken baby syndrome (SBS)?
    1. Birth occurred before 32 weeks' gestation
    2. Lack of stridor and adventitious breath sounds
    3. Previous episodes of apnea lasting 10 to 15 seconds
    4. Retractions and use of accessory respiratory muscles

43. A mother talks to the nurse about her sick infant. She is concerned that she did not realize her baby was ill. The nurse explains that a major indication of illness in an infant is:
    1. Profuse perspiration
    2. Longer periods of sleep
    3. Rapid grunting respirations
    4. Crying immediately after feedings

44. A newborn is admitted to the neonatal intensive care unit (NICU) with the diagnosis of choanal atresia. The nurse is aware that choanal atresia is an anomaly located in the:
    1. Anal area
    2. Nasopharynx
    3. Intestinal tract
    4. Laryngopharynx

45. While feeding a newborn with the diagnosis of choanal atresia, the nurse observes that the newborn:
    1. Chokes on the feeding
    2. Lacks a swallowing reflex
    3. Does not appear to be hungry
    4. Takes about half of the feeding

46. An infant is admitted to the pediatric intensive care unit after open-heart surgery for the repair of a ventricular septal defect. A nursing priority is to:
    1. Monitor the infant's urinary output
    2. Ascertain the infant's pulmonary status
    3. Determine the status of the operative site
    4. Check the patency of the intravenous catheter

47. The most critical factor in the immediate care of an infant after repair of a cleft lip is the:
    1. Preventing vomiting
    2. Maintaining a patent airway
    3. Monitoring parenteral fluid infusions
    4. Administering medications that reduce oral secretions

48. When preparing for the admission of a child with acute laryngotracheobronchitis (croup), what should be the nurse's priority intervention?
    1. Pad the side rails of the crib
    2. Arrange for a quiet, cool room
    3. Obtain a cot so that a parent can stay
    4. Place a tracheotomy set at the bedside

49. When caring for a child with croup, what should be the nurse's priority action?
    1. Initiate measures to reduce fever
    2. Ensure delivery of humidified O_2
    3. Continually assess respiratory status
    4. Provide support to reduce apprehension

50. A child with cystic fibrosis has been hospitalized with bacterial pneumonia. The nurse determines that the child has no known allergies. Selection of the antibiotic to treat the pneumonia depends primarily on the:
    1. Tolerance of the child
    2. Selectivity of the bacteria
    3. Sensitivity of the bacteria
    4. Preference of the practitioner

51. A 3-month-old infant has been hospitalized with respiratory syncytial virus (RSV). What is the priority nursing intervention?
    1. Administering an antiviral agent
    2. Clustering care to conserve energy
    3. Providing an antitussive agent PRN
    4. Offering oral fluids to promote hydration

52. A 6-year-old child is admitted to the hospital with pneumonia. What is the priority need that must be included in the nursing care plan for this child?
    1. Rest
    2. Exercise
    3. Nutrition
    4. Elimination

53. A 6-month-old infant is brought to the emergency department in severe respiratory distress. A diagnosis of respiratory syncytial virus (RSV) is made and the infant is admitted to the pediatric unit. What instruction should be included in the nursing plan of care?
    1. Place in a warm, dry environment
    2. Allow parents and siblings to visit
    3. Maintain standard and contact precautions
    4. Administer prescribed antibiotic immediately

54. An infant is admitted to the neonatal intensive care unit (NICU) with exstrophy of the bladder. What covering should the nurse use to protect the exposed area?
    1. Loose diaper
    2. Moist dressing
    3. Dry gauze dressing
    4. Petroleum jelly gauze pad

55. The nurse is aware that an additional defect associated with exstrophy of the bladder is:
    1. Imperforate anus
    2. Absence of one kidney
    3. Congenital heart disease
    4. Pubic bone malformation

56. When caring for an infant born with exstrophy of the bladder, the nurse understands that the infant is at the greatest risk for:
    1. Infection
    2. Dehydration
    3. Urinary retention
    4. Intestinal obstruction

57. A child born with exstrophy of the bladder is admitted to the pediatric unit for urinary diversion surgery wherein the ureters are transplanted to a resected section of the colon with one end attached to the abdominal wall as an ileostomy. The nurse explains the procedure to the parents and states that it is called:
    1. A cystostomy
    2. An ileal conduit
    3. An ureterosigmoidostomy
    4. A cutaneous ureterostomy

58. The nurse explains to a parent group that immunizations are important because a complication of mumps in postpubertal males is:
    1. Sterility
    2. Hypopituitarism
    3. Decrease in libido
    4. Decrease in androgens

59. When performing a physical assessment of a newborn with Down syndrome, the nurse suspects that the infant may have:
    1. Bulging fontanels
    2. Stiff lower extremities
    3. Abnormal heart sounds
    4. Unusual pupillary reactions

60. A mother expresses concerns about her 9-month-old child's development, noting that her infant no longer has the same strong grasp that was present shortly after birth, nor does the infant have a startle response to loud noise. How should the nurse explain these changes in behavior?
    1. "I will check these responses before deciding how to proceed."
    2. "Failure of these responses may be related to a developmental delay."
    3. "These responses are replaced by voluntary activity at 5 to 6 months of age."
    4. "Additional sensory stimulation is needed to aid in the return of these responses."

61. The nurse is teaching a group of parents about the side effects of the immunization vaccines. Which side effect is expected when an infant receives the *Haemophilus influenzae* (Hib) vaccine?
    1. Lethargy
    2. Urticaria
    3. Low-grade fever
    4. Generalized rash

62. When explaining the occurrence of febrile seizures to a parents' class, what information should the nurse include?
    1. They may occur in minor illnesses
    2. The cause is usually readily identified
    3. They usually do not occur during the toddler years
    4. The frequency of occurrence is greater in females than males

63. A mother tells the nurse in the emergency department that her 3 year old has had a fever for several days and has been vomiting. While instituting nursing measures to reduce the child's fever, the nurse should also:
    1. Prevent shivering
    2. Restrict oral fluids
    3. Measure output hourly
    4. Take vital signs hourly

64. The nurse notes that a 3-year-old child in a crib has a clamped jaw and is having a tonic-clonic seizure. What is the priority nursing responsibility at this time?
    1. Start O_2 by mask
    2. Insert a plastic airway
    3. Protect the child from self-injury
    4. Prevent injury by applying restraints

65. A child sitting on a chair in a playroom starts to have a tonic-clonic seizure with a clenched jaw. What is the nurse's best initial action?
    1. Call for assistance
    2. Attempt to open the jaw
    3. Lower the child to the floor
    4. Place a large pillow under the head

66. The nurse is caring for a child with the diagnosis of meningitis. What sign or symptom indicates an increase in intracranial pressure?
    1. Bradycardia
    2. Hyperalertness
    3. A decreased pulse pressure
    4. A decreased systolic blood pressure

67. An infant is diagnosed as having communicating hydrocephalus. When helping the parents understand the practitioner's explanation of their baby's problem, the nurse should respond:
    1. "Too much CSF is produced within the ventricles of the brain."
    2. "The flow of CSF through the brain cells does not empty effectively into the spinal cord."
    3. "The CSF is prevented from adequate absorption by a blockage in the ventricles of the brain."
    4. "There is a part of the brain surface that usually absorbs CSF after its production that is not functioning adequately."

68. The nurse understands that hydrocephalus, if it is untreated, can cause mental retardation because the:
    1. CSF dilutes blood supply, causing cells to atrophy
    2. Hypertonic CSF disturbs normal plasma concentration, depriving nerve cells of vital nutrients
    3. Increasing head size necessitates more oxygen and nutrients than normal blood flow can supply
    4. Gradually increasing size of the ventricles presses the brain against the bony cranium; anoxia and decreased blood supply result

69. What should be included in the nursing care of an infant with increased intracranial pressure?
    1. Weigh the infant daily before feeding
    2. Elevate the infant's head higher than hips
    3. Check the infant's reflexes at regular intervals
    4. Monitor the infant's level of consciousness by stimulating frequently

70. The parents of an infant who has just had a ventriculoperitoneal shunt inserted for hydrocephalus are concerned about the prognosis. What information should the nurse give the parents?
    1. The shunt may need to be revised as the child grows older
    2. The prognosis is excellent and the valve is permanent
    3. If any brain damage has occurred, it is reversible during the first year of life
    4. Hydrocephalus usually is self-limiting by 2 years of age and then the shunt is removed

71. An infant who was born with a meningomyelocele develops hydrocephalus. A ventriculoperitoneal shunt is inserted. What nursing intervention is essential in the care of the infant during the first postoperative 24 hours?
    1. Sedating the infant
    2. Placing the infant in a high-Fowler's position
    3. Positioning the infant on the side that has the shunt
    4. Monitoring the infant for increasing intracranial pressure

72. The discharge of a newborn with a surgically repaired myelomeningocele is anticipated at about 2 weeks of age. What teaching should the nurse include when preparing the parents for the discharge?
    1. Demonstration of restrictive positions to prevent the infant from turning
    2. Discussion about the need to limit the infant's fluid intake to formula only
    3. Instructions on how to do passive range-of-motion exercises to the infant's lower extremities
    4. Explanation of the need to provide the infant with a quiet environment to reduce external stimuli

73. A 4-year-old child who has had a revision of a ventriculoperitoneal shunt is visiting the clinic for follow-up care. What observation might alert the nurse that the child has an infected shunt?
    1. Lethargy
    2. Decreased pulse rate

3. Complaint of a headache
4. Complaint of a stiff neck

74. The nurse in the clinic is assessing an infant who had a revision of a ventriculoperitoneal shunt. What observation alerts the nurse that the intracranial pressure has increased?
1. Hypoactive reflexes
2. A lower blood pressure
3. A more rapid pulse rate
4. Tension of the anterior fontanel

75. What is the primary nursing intervention for an infant with a myelomeningocele before surgical correction?
1. Minimize infection
2. Prevent trauma to the sac
3. Observe for increasing paralysis
4. Assess the degree of bowel and bladder control

76. A newborn with a meningomyelocele is admitted to the high-risk nursery. The Apgar scores were 9/10. While the newborn is awaiting surgical correction of the defect, what is the most appropriate nursing intervention?
1. Use disposable diapers
2. Place in the prone position
3. Perform neurologic checks above the site of the lesion
4. Wash the area below the defect with a nontoxic antiseptic

77. After closure of a newborn's meningomyelocele, what essential nursing intervention must be included in the plan of care?
1. Strict limitation of leg movement
2. Decrease of environmental stimuli
3. Measurement in head circumference daily
4. Observation for serous drainage from the nares

78. The nurse is caring for an infant with meningitis. By which route does the nurse understand that the bacteria responsible for meningitis may have entered the infant's CNS?
1. Genitourinary tract
2. Gastrointestinal tract
3. Skin or mucous membranes
4. Cranial apertures or sinuses

79. The nurse should maintain isolation of a child with a diagnosis of bacterial meningitis:
1. For 12 hours after admission
2. Until the cultures are negative
3. Until antibiotic therapy is completed
4. For 48 hours after antibiotic therapy begins

80. A 2 year old has been admitted with a tentative diagnosis of bacterial meningitis. A lumbar puncture is performed to confirm the diagnosis. The diagnosis is confirmed because the spinal fluid has
1. A decreased cell count
2. An elevated protein level
3. An increased glucose level
4. A low spinal fluid pressure

81. When caring for a child with meningococcal meningitis, the nurse should observe for the:
1. Presence of severe glossitis
2. Identifying purpuric skin rash

3. Low-grade nature of the fever
4. Constant tremors of the extremities

82. The nurse is caring for a 2-year-old child with meningitis. What signs and symptoms should alert the nurse to possible increasing intracranial pressure?
1. Restlessness, anorectic, rapid respirations
2. Vomiting, seizures, complaints of head pain
3. Anorectic, irritability, subnormal temperature
4. Bulging fontanels, decreased blood pressure, elevated temperature

83. What is the most serious complication of meningitis in young children?
1. Epilepsy
2. Blindness
3. Peripheral circulatory collapse
4. Communicating hydrocephalus

84. After many episodes of otitis media, a child is to have a myringotomy with tubes implanted surgically. What should the nurse include in the discharge preparation for this family?
1. Apply an ointment to the ear canal daily
2. Use cotton swabs to clean the inner ears
3. Keep the child out of daycare for 1 week
4. Have the child use ear plugs when bathing

85. The nurse identifies that a newborn has asymmetric gluteal folds. For which disorder should the nurse perform a focused assessment?
1. Congenital inguinal hernia
2. Central nervous system damage
3. Peripheral nervous system damage
4. Developmental dysplasia of the hip

86. A 3-month-old infant with severe developmental dysplasia of the hip has a hip spica cast applied. To prevent a serious complication that can occur in infants in a spica cast, the nurse should teach the parents to:
1. Change diapers frequently
2. Decrease the number of feedings per day
3. Call the practitioner if a foul smell develops
4. Avoid turning from prone to supine positions

87. A 4-month-old infant is in a spica cast. What should the nurse include in the discharge instructions?
1. Obtain a specially designed car seat
2. Change infant's position every 8 hours
3. Diapers alone should be used to reduce soiling of the cast
4. Use the abduction bar between the infant's legs for position changes

88. When elevating the head of an infant in a spica cast, the nurse should:
1. Place 2 pillows under the shoulders
2. Limit this position to 1 hour at a time
3. Pad the edge of the cast with folded diapers
4. Raise the entire mattress at the head of the crib

89. A 3-month-old infant has been diagnosed with congenital hypothyroidism. What is the probable effect on the child's future if treatment is not begun in early infancy?
1. Lifelong myxedema
2. More severe mental retardation

3. Development of spastic paralysis

4. Repeated episodes of thyrotoxicosis

90. A 10 year old is diagnosed with lymphocytic thyroiditis (Hashimoto's disease). The nurse should explain to the parents and child that this condition is:

1. Chronic

2. Inherited

3. Difficult to treat

4. Probably temporary

91. At a visit to the well-baby clinic, a mother is upset because her 9-month-old son has a severe diaper rash; the mother wants to know how to treat it and prevent it from recurring. What explanation should the nurse give the mother about the etiology of diaper dermatitis?

1. Use of disposable diapers

2. Prolonged contact with an irritant

3. Too early introduction of solid foods

4. Decreased pH of the infant's urine output

92. When teaching parents of school-age children about communicable diseases, the nurse reminds them that these diseases are serious, and that encephalitis can be a complication of:

1. Pertussis

2. Varicella

3. Scarlet fever

4. Poliomyelitis

93. A mother asks the nurse how to tell the difference between measles (rubeola) and German measles (rubella). The nurse should tell the mother that rubeola is characterized by:

1. A high fever and Koplik spots

2. A rash on the trunk with pruritus

3. Nausea, vomiting, and abdominal cramps

4. Signs that are similar to those of a cold, followed by a rash

94. The nurse should recommend to parents the varicella (chickenpox) vaccination for children at risk for contracting it and who are about to receive:

1. Insulin

2. Steroids

3. Antibiotics

4. Anticonvulsants

95. A viral disease that begins with malaise and a highly pruritic rash that begins on the abdomen, spreads to the face and proximal extremities, and possibly results in grave complications is:

1. Rubella

2. Rubeola

3. Chickenpox

4. Yellow fever

96. A mother brings her 1-week-old infant to the clinic because the infant continually regurgitates. Chalasia is suspected. What instructions should the nurse give the mother?

1. Keep the infant prone following feedings

2. Prevent the infant from crying for prolonged periods

3. Be sure the infant drinks a full bottle of formula at each feeding

4. Keep the infant in a semi-sitting position, particularly after feedings

97. A mother brings her 9-month-old son to the pediatric clinic and asks about the introduction of new foods. What should the nurse suggest?

1. "Introduce a new food after he has had his regular feeding."

2. "Offer a new food every day until he likes one and then offer it again."

3. "Offer a new food after he has had some milk when he is still hungry."

4. "Mix the pureed food with formula and have him drink it from the bottle."

98. What should nursing care for an infant after the surgical repair of a cleft lip include?

1. Preventing the infant from crying

2. Placing the infant in a semi-sitting position

3. Keeping the infant NPO for 1 day after surgery

4. Feeding the infant with a spoon for 2 days after surgery

99. A cleft lip predisposes an infant to infections primarily because of:

1. Deficient nutrition from ineffective feeding

2. Inadequate circulation in the defective area

3. Waste products that accumulate along the defect

4. Mouth breathing that dries the oropharyngeal mucous membranes

100. For an infant born with a unilateral cleft lip and palate, feeding will probably be:

1. Limited to IV fluids

2. Accomplished with a cross-cut nipple

3. Achieved with a rubber-tipped syringe or medicine dropper

4. Different from feeding an infant with a bilateral cleft lip or palate

101. The mother of an 18-month-old boy with a cleft palate asks the nurse why the pediatrician recommended that closure of the palate should be done before he is 2 years old. The nurse responds:

1. "As he gets older the palate gets wider and more difficult to repair"

2. "After age 2 surgery is very frightening and should be avoided if possible"

3. "The eruption of the 2-year molars often complicates the surgical procedure"

4. "Surgery should be performed before the child starts to use faulty speech patterns"

102. An infant with hypertrophic pyloric stenosis (HPS) is admitted to the pediatric unit. When palpating this infant's abdomen, the nurse expects:

1. A distended colon

2. Marked tenderness around the umbilicus

3. An olive-sized mass in the right upper quadrant

4. Rhythmic peristaltic waves in the lower abdomen

103. The nurse should carefully observe the infant with a tentative diagnosis of hypertrophic pyloric stenosis for:

1. Signs of dehydration

2. The quality of the cry

3. Coughing after feeding

4. The character of the stool

104. Surgery to correct hypertrophic pyloric stenosis is performed on a 2-week-old infant who had been formula-fed. Which postoperative feeding order is appropriate?
1. Thickened formula 24 hours after surgery
2. Withholding feedings for the first 24 hours
3. Regular formula feeding within 24 hours after surgery
4. Additional glucose feedings as desired after the first 24 hours

105. Corrective surgery for hypertrophic pyloric stenosis is completed, and the infant is returned to the pediatric unit with an IV infusion in place. What is the priority nursing action?
1. Apply adequate restraints
2. Administer a mild sedative
3. Assess the IV site for infiltration
4. Attach the nasogastric tube to wall suction

106. An infant has had corrective surgery for hypertrophic pyloric stenosis. To reduce vomiting, the nurse should teach the mother that immediately after feeding the infant, she should:
1. Rock the infant
2. Place the infant in an infant seat
3. Place the infant flat on the right side
4. Keep the infant awake with sensory stimulation

107. Which type of hernia involves an impaired blood supply?
1. Hiatal
2. Incarcerated
3. Omphalocele
4. Strangulated

108. A newborn with an anorectal anomaly had an anoplasty performed. At the 2-week follow-up visit, a series of anal dilations are begun. What should the nurse recommend to the parents to help prevent the infant from becoming constipated?
1. Use a soy formula
2. Breastfeed if possible
3. Administer a suppository nightly
4. Offer glucose water between feedings

109. Exposure to hepatitis B may occur on pediatric units because of:
1. Careless handling of feces by staff
2. Increasing use of ventilating systems
3. Needle sticks and mucous membrane exposure
4. Early diagnosis and improved treatment of hepatitis A

110. Dietary treatment of children with PKU includes a:
1. Protein-free diet
2. Protein-enriched diet
3. Phenylalanine-free diet
4. Low-phenylalanine diet

111. What should the nurse include in the teaching plan for parents of an infant diagnosed with PKU?
1. Mental retardation occurs if PKU is untreated
2. Testing for PKU is done immediately after birth

3. Treatment for PKU includes lifelong medications
4. PKU is transmitted by an autosomal dominant gene

112. The parents of a newborn with PKU need help and support in adhering to specific dietary restrictions. A frequent question asked by parents is, "How long will my child have to be on this diet?" How should the nurse respond?
1. "We still are not sure, but you should discuss this with your practitioner."
2. "If your baby does well, foods containing protein can gradually be introduced."
3. "Unfortunately, this is a lifelong problem and dietary restrictions must be continued."
4. "As of now, research shows that a child needs to be on this diet at least through adolescence and into adulthood."

113. The nurse plans to discuss childhood nutrition with a group of parents whose children have Down syndrome in an attempt to minimize a common nutritional problem, which is:
1. Obesity
2. Rickets
3. Anemia
4. Rumination

114. The nurse is caring for a 3-month-old infant whose abdomen is distended and whose vomitus is bile stained. The nurse, suspecting an intestinal obstruction, should observe the infant for:
1. High-pitched cry and weak pulse
2. Constant pain and absence of stools
3. Irregular heart rate and hypotonicity
4. Paroxysmal pain and grunting respirations

115. The nurse explains to the parents of an infant with colic that the typical behavior is caused by:
1. Inadequate peristalsis
2. Paroxysmal abdominal pain
3. An allergic response to certain proteins in milk
4. A protective mechanism designed to eliminate foreign proteins

116. A 1-month-old infant is admitted to the pediatric unit with a tentative diagnosis of Hirschsprung's disease (congenital aganglionic megacolon). What procedure will probably be ordered to confirm the diagnosis?
1. Rectal tube
2. Suction biopsy
3. Multiple saline enemas
4. Fiberoptic nasoenteric tube

117. The practitioner orders a tap-water enema for a 6-month-old infant with suspected Hirschsprung's disease. What rationale would cause the nurse to question the order?
1. The result could be loss of necessary nutrients
2. It could cause a fluid and electrolyte imbalance
3. It could increase the fear of intrusive procedures
4. The result could cause shock from a sudden drop in temperature

118. An order is written for an isotonic enema for a 2-year-old child. What is the maximum amount of fluid the nurse should give to this child without a practitioner's specific order?
    1. 100 to 150 mL
    2. 155 to 250 mL
    3. 255 to 360 mL
    4. 365 to 500 mL

119. A 5 month old develops severe diarrhea and is given IV fluids. What is the rationale for frequent observation of the IV flow rate?
    1. Restriction of output
    2. Replacement of lost fluids
    3. Avoidance of IV infiltration
    4. Prevention of cardiac overload

120. What is an essential nursing action when caring for a young child with severe diarrhea?
    1. Maintain the IV
    2. Take daily weights
    3. Replace lost calories
    4. Promote perianal skin integrity

121. When an infant's vomiting is uncontrolled, it is most important for the nurse to assess for which complication?
    1. Acidosis
    2. Alkalosis
    3. Hyperkalemia
    4. Hypernatremia

122. The nurse is administering IV fluids to a dehydrated infant. Which intervention is necessary?
    1. Ensuring the sterility of equipment
    2. Calculating the total necessary intake
    3. Continuing the prescribed rate of flow
    4. Maintaining the fluid at body temperature

123. A 5-month-old infant is brought to the pediatric clinic for a routine monthly examination. The nurse should seek immediate medical attention if the infant:
    1. Has tachycardia
    2. Exhibits mild hypotonia
    3. Appears to have strabismus
    4. Cannot sit without support

124. When assessing infants and children with cardiac disorders, the nurse understands that one of the last signs of heart failure in infants and children is:
    1. Tachypnea
    2. Tachycardia
    3. Peripheral edema
    4. Periorbital edema

125. What is a common finding that the nurse can identify in most children with symptomatic cardiac malformations?
    1. Mental retardation
    2. Inherited genetic factors
    3. Delayed physical growth
    4. Clubbing of the fingertips

126. A 2-year-old child has a congenital cardiac malformation that causes right-to-left shunting of blood through the heart. What clinical finding should the nurse expect?
    1. Proteinuria
    2. Peripheral edema
    3. Elevated hematocrit
    4. Absence of pedal pulses

127. The nurse explains to the mother of a child who is awaiting surgery to correct a congenital cardiac malformation that the child will be given prophylactic long-term antibiotic therapy to prevent:
    1. Pericarditis
    2. Myocarditis
    3. Subacute bacterial endocarditis
    4. Upper respiratory tract infections

128. Anticipating that a 4-year-old child, scheduled for open-heart surgery, will have chest tubes in place postoperatively the nurse informs the parents that the chest tubes will:
    1. Increase tidal volumes
    2. Promote drainage of air and fluid
    3. Maintain positive intrapleural pressure
    4. Regulate pressure on the pericardium and chest wall

129. After a discussion with the pediatric cardiologist, the parents of an infant with patent ductus arteriosus (PDA) ask the nurse to explain once again what PDA is. The nurse explains that it is:
    1. An enlarged diameter of the aorta
    2. A narrowing of the entrance to the pulmonary artery
    3. A connection between the pulmonary artery and the aorta
    4. An opening in the wall between the right and left ventricles

130. The nurse caring for a child with a cardiac malformation associated with left-to-right shunting should be aware that the major characteristic of this type of congenital disorder is:
    1. Severe growth retardation
    2. Clubbing of the fingers and toes
    3. Increased blood flow to the lungs
    4. Polycythemia and elevated hematocrit

131. A young child has coarctation of the aorta. What should the nurse expect to identify when taking the child's vital signs?
    1. A weak radial pulse
    2. An irregular heartbeat
    3. A bounding femoral pulse
    4. An elevated blood pressure in the arm

132. A 2-week-old boy is admitted with a tentative diagnosis of a ventricular septal defect. The parents report that their baby has had difficulty feeding since he has been home. The nurse explains that:
    1. Feeding problems are common in neonates
    2. Inadequate sucking is not significant in the absence of cyanosis
    3. Ineffective sucking and swallowing may be early indications of a heart defect
    4. Many neonates retain mucus and this may interfere with feeding for several weeks

133. A 3 year old is scheduled for a cardiac catheterization. What is the priority nursing care after this procedure?
    1. Encouraging early ambulation
    2. Monitoring the site for bleeding
    3. Restricting fluids until blood pressure is stabilized
    4. Comparing the blood pressure of both lower extremities

134. A newborn has been diagnosed with Down syndrome. The nurse recognizes that these infants usually have several problems in conjunction with Down syndrome. On what should the nurse focus when doing the initial assessment?
    1. Reflex responses for hypotonicity
    2. Eye examination for congenital cataracts
    3. Sensory stimulation for muscle flaccidity
    4. Cardiac irregularities for congenital heart disease

135. Which cardiac defects are associated with tetralogy of Fallot?
    1. Right ventricular hypertrophy, atrial and ventricular defects, and mitral valve stenosis
    2. Origin of the aorta from the right ventricle and of the pulmonary artery from the left ventricle
    3. Right ventricular hypertrophy, ventricular septal defect, pulmonic stenosis, and overriding aorta
    4. Altered connection between the pulmonary artery and the aorta, right ventricular hypertrophy, and an atrial septal defect

136. The laboratory analysis for a 5-year-old child admitted for repair of tetralogy of Fallot indicates an elevated RBC count. This polycythemia is a compensatory mechanism for:
    1. Tissue O_2 need
    2. Low blood pressure
    3. Diminished iron level
    4. Hypertrophic cardiac muscle

137. What common adaptation of children with tetralogy of Fallot should the nurse expect?
    1. Slow respirations
    2. Clubbing of fingers
    3. Subcutaneous hemorrhages
    4. Decreased RBC counts

138. A child undergoes heart surgery to repair the defects associated with tetralogy of Fallot. Postoperatively, it is essential that the nurse prevent:
    1. Crying
    2. Coughing
    3. Hard stools
    4. Unnecessary movement

139. An infant who has had cardiac surgery for a congenital defect is to be discharged. What should the nurse emphasize to the parents regarding the infant's prophylactic antibiotic?
    1. Give the antibiotic to the infant between feedings
    2. Ensure the infant receives the antibiotic as prescribed
    3. Shake the bottle thoroughly before giving the antibiotic to the infant

    4. Keep the antibiotic in the refrigerator after the bottle has been opened

140. The nurse explains to the parents of an infant with a congenital heart defect why gavage feedings have been instituted. It is because:
    1. Vomiting is prevented
    2. Gavage feedings can be given quickly
    3. The amount of food can be regulated
    4. It conserves energy that would be expended on sucking

141. Occasionally infants are born without an immune system. They can live with no apparent problems during their first months after birth because:
    1. Exposure to pathogens during this time can be limited
    2. Limited antibodies are produced by the infant's colonic bacteria
    3. Antibodies are passively received from the mother through the placenta and breast milk
    4. Fewer antibodies are produced by the fetal thymus during the eighth and ninth months of gestation

142. When evaluating the laboratory report of a 1-year-old infant's hematocrit, the nurse compares it with the expected hematocrit range for this age-group, which is:
    1. 19% to 32%
    2. 29% to 41%
    3. 37% to 47%
    4. 42% to 69%

143. What explanation should the nurse give a mother about the purpose of a tetanus toxoid injection for her child?
    1. Passive immunity is conferred for life
    2. Long-lasting active immunity is conferred
    3. Lifelong active natural immunity is conferred
    4. Passive natural immunity is conferred temporarily

144. Using live virus vaccines is contraindicated for children receiving corticosteroid, antineoplastic, or irradiation therapy because they may:
    1. Be susceptible to infection as a result of a depressed immunity
    2. Have had the disease or have been immunized previously
    3. Be unlikely to need this protection during their shortened life span
    4. Have an allergy to rabbit serum, which may have been used as a basis for these vaccines

145. The mother of a child who has received all of the primary immunizations asks the nurse which ones her child should receive before starting kindergarten. The nurse tells the mother that her child should receive boosters of:
    1. IPV, HepB, Td
    2. DTaP, HepB, Td
    3. MMR, DTaP, Hib
    4. DTaP, IPV, MMR

146. When reviewing the immunization schedule for an 11 month old, the nurse should expect that the infant had been previously immunized against:
    1. Pertussis, tetanus, polio, and measles
    2. Polio, pertussis, tetanus, and diphtheria

3. Rubella, polio, tuberculosis, and pertussis
4. Measles, mumps, rubella, and tuberculosis

147. A mother asks the nurse how the DTaP immunization works. The nurse should base an answer on the information that:
1. Lipid agents are formed by the body against antigens
2. Antigens are formed in the blood to fight invading antibodies
3. Protein substances are formed by the body to destroy or neutralize antigens
4. Blood antigens are aided by phagocytes in defending the body against pathogens

148. An infant has become immunosuppressed after chemotherapy. When preparing the parents for the infant's discharge, what information should the nurse give concerning the measles, mumps, and rubella (MMR) immunization?
1. It should not be given until the infant reaches 2 years of age
2. The infant is still receiving chemotherapy so it should not be given
3. The parents should discuss this with the pediatrician at the next visit
4. It should be given to protect the infant from contracting any of these diseases

149. The mother of a 4-year-old boy, whose family recently emigrated from Columbia, arrives at the pediatric clinic with her son who has a temperature of 102° F. He is irritable and has a runny nose, a rash, and several small, red, irregularly shaped spots with blue-white centers in his mouth. The nurse identifies that the child has:
1. Measles
2. Chickenpox
3. Fifth disease
4. Scarlet fever

NURSING CARE OF TODDLERS

150. The nurse in the emergency department observes large welts and scars on the back of a child who has been admitted for an asthma attack. What additional information must be included in the nurse's assessment?
1. Signs of child abuse
2. History of an injury
3. Presence of food allergies
4. Recent recovery from chickenpox

151. A 13-year-old girl tells the nurse at the pediatric clinic that she took a pregnancy test and it was positive. She tells the nurse that her grandfather, with whom she, her younger siblings, and her mother live, has repeatedly molested her for the past 3 years. When the nurse asks the girl if she has told this to anyone, she replies, "Yes, but my mother doesn't believe me." The nurse's legal responsibility is to notify the:
1. Police concerning a possible sex crime
2. Child Protective Services for immediate intervention

3. Girl's mother about the pregnancy test's positive result
4. Physician to do a vaginal examination to confirm the pregnancy

152. The nurse manager should place a 5 year old admitted with injuries that may be related to abuse:
1. In a private room
2. With another 5 year old
3. With an older friendly child
4. In a room near the nurses' desk

153. What is one of the most important factors that the nurse must consider when parents of a toddler request to be present at a procedure occurring on the hospital unit?
1. Type of procedure to be performed
2. Individual assessment of the parents
3. Whether the child wants the parents present
4. Presence of the parents on the unit if the procedure is painful

154. The response that would be unusual in toddlers subjected to prolonged hospitalization is:
1. Slowness of weight gain
2. Limited emotional response to stimuli
3. Excessive crying and clinging when approached
4. Looking at ceiling lights rather than at persons caring for them

155. At 2 years of age, a child is readmitted to the hospital for additional surgery. What is the most important factor in preparing the child for this experience?
1. Gratification of the child's wishes
2. The child's previous hospital visits
3. Avoiding leaving the child with strangers
4. The assurance of continuation of affection

156. On the third day of hospitalization, a 2-year-old child who had been screaming and crying inconsolably begins to regress and is now lying quietly in the crib with a blanket. The nurse recognizes that the child is in the stage of:
1. Denial
2. Despair
3. Mistrust
4. Rejection

157. During the second week of hospitalization for intravenous antibiotic therapy, a 2-year-old girl whose family is unable to visit often smiles easily, goes to all the nurses happily, and does not express interest in her mother when she does visit. The mother tells the nurse she is pleased about the adjustment but somewhat concerned about her child's reaction to her. The nurse explains to the mother that her child:
1. Has established a routine and feels safe
2. Is repressing her feelings for her mother
3. Has given up fighting and accepts the separation
4. Is feeling better physically so her behavior has improved

158. The nurse accompanies a 3-year-old child to the playroom. The toddler seems afraid to select a toy or activity. The nurse should offer a:
1. Mold and clay
2. Stuffed animal

3. Pencil and paper
4. Simple video game

159. The practitioner prescribes mebendazole (Vermox) for a 4-year-old child with pinworms. When preparing to teach the parents about this medication, the nurse should recall that the medication will cause:
1. Constipation
2. Hypertension
3. Blood in the stool
4. Passage of worms in the stool

160. A child with a high blood level of lead is started on a regimen of chelation therapy that consists of calcium disodium edetate (EDTA) and dimercaprol (BAL) q4h for 5 days. The nurse understands that this combination of drugs:
1. Removes lead from the bone marrow more efficiently
2. Eliminates lead from the body more rapidly through the urine
3. Decreases blood lead levels and increases deposition in the bones
4. Has fewer side effects and removes lead from the brain more effectively

161. A 15 month old is playing in the child life center. The nurse evaluates that the child's ability to perform physical tasks is at the age-related norm when the child:
1. Builds a tower of six blocks
2. Walks with a wide-based gait
3. Throws the toys around the room
4. Stands in the playpen holding onto the sides

162. A father brings his 18-month-old son to the clinic. He asks the nurse why his son is so difficult to please, has temper tantrums, and annoys him by throwing food from the table. How can the nurse best address the father's concern?
1. He needs discipline to prevent the development of antisocial behaviors
2. Toddlers are learning to assert independence, and his behavior is expected for his age
3. This is the usual way that a toddler expresses his needs during the initiative stage of development
4. It is best to leave the toddler alone in his crib after calmly telling him why his behavior is unacceptable

163. A mother tells the nurse that each morning she offers her 24-month-old son juice and he always shakes his head and says, "No." She asks the nurse what to do, because she knows the child needs fluids. What strategy should the nurse suggest to the mother?
1. Distract him with some food
2. Hand him the glass in a firm manner
3. Let him see that he is making her angry
4. Offer him a choice of two juices to drink

164. A 2-year-old boy, admitted to the hospital for further surgical repair of a clubfoot, is standing in his crib crying. The child refuses to be comforted and calls for his mother. As the nurse approaches the crib to provide morning care, the child screams louder.

Recognizing that this behavior is typical of the stage of protest, what is the most appropriate nursing intervention?
1. Fill the basin with water and proceed to bathe him
2. Try to comfort him while carrying him around the room
3. Sit by his crib and bathe him later when his anxiety decreases
4. Skip the bath because a child this upset does not really need a bath

165. A major developmental milestone of the toddler is the achievement of autonomy. The nurse should teach the parents the importance of helping their toddler to:
1. Share with others
2. Learn society's roles
3. Accept external limits
4. Develop superego control

166. The nurse observes a 2-year-old child at play and identifies that the child is engaging in age-appropriate behavior for a toddler. Check all that apply.
1. ☐ Is possessive of toys
2. ☐ Follows simple directions
3. ☐ Can play simple card games
4. ☐ Enjoys playing with other children
5. ☐ Attempts to stay within the lines when coloring.

167. After the nurse has completed an oral examination of a healthy 2 year old, the mother asks when she should start taking her child to the dentist. When is the most appropriate time for the nurse to suggest?
1. Before starting school
2. Within the next few months
3. When the first deciduous teeth are lost
4. At the same time a family member goes to the dentist

168. The nurse explains to the mother of a 2-year-old girl that the child's negativism is expected at her age and that it is helping her meet her need for:
1. Trust
2. Attention
3. Discipline
4. Independence

169. The mother of a 2-year-old girl tells the nurse that whenever she takes her toddler to a store the child has a screaming tantrum demanding a toy or candy on the shelves. The mother asks the nurse how best to cope with this situation without further embarrassment. The nurse's best response is to advise the mother to:
1. Take the child to another part of the store
2. Say nothing and allow the tantrum to continue until it ends
3. Hire a baby sitter when she shops until the child outgrows this typical toddler behavior
4. Give the child the item while in the store and when the child loses interest return the item to the shelf

170. When ordering a regular diet for a young toddler, the nurse should choose foods such as:
1. Hamburger with bun and grapes
2. Chicken fingers and french fries

3. Hot dog with bun and potato chips

4. Macaroni and cheese and Cheerios

171. During a nap, a 3-year-old hospitalized boy wets the bed. The nurse should:
    1. Ask him to help with remaking the bed
    2. Put clean sheets on his bed over a rubber sheet
    3. Change his clothes without discussing the incident
    4. Explain that big boys should call the nurse when they need to void

172. When evaluating a 3-year-old child's developmental progress, the nurse should identify that there is a developmental delay when the child is unable to:
    1. Copy a square
    2. Hop on one foot
    3. Catch a ball reliably
    4. Use a spoon effectively

173. Which healthy snack should the nurse teach the parents to give their 2-year-old child who has the diagnosis of acute asthma is:
    1. Grapes
    2. Apple slices
    3. Oatmeal cookies
    4. Cold glass of milk

174. When observing a toddler and other children in the playroom, the nurse should expect the toddler to engage in:
    1. Parallel play
    2. Solitary play
    3. Competitive play
    4. Cooperative play

175. While assessing an 18 month old, the nurse observes that the toddler can crawl upstairs, but needs assistance when climbing the stairs upright. The nurse recognizes that this:
    1. Indicates evidence of neurologic damage
    2. Signifies the presence of talipes equinovarus
    3. Reflects expected behavior in a toddler of this age
    4. Verifies the existance of developmental dysplasia of the hip

176. The nurse is aware that an appropriate toy for a young toddler during hospitalization is a:
    1. Mobile
    2. Tricycle
    3. Ten-piece puzzle
    4. Carton of Play-Doh

177. A mother tells the nurse that the pediatrician is concerned that her 4-year-old child exhibits developmental delays. The mother expresses readiness to place her child in a preschool program for cognitively impaired children. What is the nurse's most appropriate response?
    1. Praise the mother for her acceptance and encourage her plan
    2. Advise the mother to have the pediatrician help choose an appropriate program
    3. Ask the mother for more specific information related to the developmental delays
    4. Tell the mother that this is probably a premature action because developmental delays often disappear

178. A nurse on the pediatric unit is observing the developmental skills of several 2 year olds in the playroom. The nurse should continue to evaluate the child who:
    1. Cannot stand on 1 foot
    2. Builds a tower of 7 blocks
    3. Uses echolalia when speaking
    4. Colors outside the lines of a picture

179. The nurse plans to talk to a mother about toilet-training her toddler, knowing that the most important factor in the process of toilet-training is the:
    1. Child's desire to be dry
    2. Child's ability to sit still
    3. Parents' attitude concerning it
    4. Parents' willingness to work at it

180. A mother asks the nurse what to do when her toddler has temper tantrums. What play materials should the nurse suggest for the mother to offer the child as another way of expressing anger?
    1. Ball and bat
    2. Wad of clay
    3. Punching bag
    4. Pegs and pounding board

181. When the working mother of a toddler is preparing to take her child home after a prolonged hospitalization, she asks the nurse what type of behavior she should expect to be displayed. What is the nurse's most appropriate description of her child's probable behavior?
    1. Excessively demanding behavior
    2. Hostile attitude toward the mother
    3. Cheerful, with shallow attachment behaviors
    4. Withdrawn, without emotional ties to the mother

182. The nurse is aware that the primary pathology that produces the clinical manifestations of cystic fibrosis is:
    1. Hyperactivity of the eccrine (sweat) glands
    2. Hypoactivity of the autonomic nervous system
    3. Mechanical obstruction of mucus-secreting glands
    4. Atrophic changes in the mucosal lining of the intestines

183. Although there is no history of cystic fibrosis in a 5-year-old child's family, the nurse understands that cystic fibrosis is inherited through genes that are:
    1. X-linked
    2. Mutant in nature
    3. Autosomal recessive
    4. Autosomal dominant

184. What assessment by the nurse in the newborn nursery is suggestive of cystic fibrosis?
    1. Excessive crying
    2. Rapid heart rate
    3. Sternal retractions
    4. Abdominal distention

185. When is the most appropriate time for the nurse to plan for chest percussion and postural drainage for a toddler with cystic fibrosis?
    1. After suctioning
    2. One hour before meals
    3. Before aerosol therapy
    4. Fifteen minutes after meals

186. When caring for the hospitalized child with cystic fibrosis, the nurse should:
    1. Discourage coughing
    2. Perform postural drainage
    3. Encourage active exercise
    4. Provide small, frequent feedings

187. A child with cystic fibrosis is predisposed to bronchitis mainly because of:
    1. Associated heart defects that cause heart failure and respiratory depression
    2. Neuromuscular irritability that causes spasm and constriction of the bronchi
    3. Tenacious secretions that obstruct the respiratory tract and provide a favorable medium for growth of bacteria
    4. Elevated salt content in saliva that irritates the mucous membranes and causes inflammation of the nasopharynx

188. The nurse teaches the parents of a toddler newly diagnosed with cystic fibrosis that vitamins A, D, E, and K should be:
    1. Given in a water-miscible form
    2. Taken during meals and snack time
    3. Calibrated based on height and weight
    4. Offered with fruit juice rather than milk

189. Studies of young children who have had a prolonged hospitalization indicate that they show signs of developmental delay. Least affected by this type of delay is the child's:
    1. Sense of hearing
    2. Ability to understand
    3. Capacity for self-expression
    4. Neuromuscular development

190. A 15-month-old child with the diagnosis of hydrocephalus is to have a CT scan. What should the nurse include when preparing the toddler for the CT scan?
    1. Shaving the head
    2. Starting the prescribed IV infusion
    3. Administering the prescribed sedative
    4. Giving a simple explanation of the procedure

191. At the age of 7 years, a child with cerebral palsy is admitted to the hospital for a tendon-lengthening procedure. After the surgery, the parents ask the nurse why their child must wear braces and shoes for at least 8 hours a day even while in bed. The nurse responds that this is to:
    1. Encourage ambulation as soon as possible
    2. Maintain body alignment and help prevent footdrop
    3. Stretch the child's ligaments and strengthen muscle tone
    4. Continue the child's acceptance of physical restraints

192. A child with diminished sensation in the legs because of cerebral palsy should be taught special safety precautions, including:
    1. Tightening brace straps securely before ambulating
    2. Setting the clock twice during the night to change position

    3. Testing the temperature of the water before starting water-related activities
    4. Looking down at the legs when crutch walking to determine if they are appropriately positioned

193. When planning long-term care for a child with cerebral palsy, it is important for the nurse to understand that the:
    1. Illness is not progressively degenerative
    2. Effects of cerebral palsy are unpredictable
    3. Child probably has some degree of mental retardation
    4. Child should have genetic counseling before planning a family

194. The exact sociocultural reason for lead poisoning in children is:
    1. Understood to be caused by the ingestion of foods that are high in fat
    2. Environmental, because there is lead available for ingestion and inhalation
    3. Attributed to an indigent and passive mother who fails to supervise her children
    4. Socioeconomic, because inadequately maintained old buildings have more lead-based paint

195. Although lead poisoning affects various organ systems, its irreversible side effects are exerted mainly on the:
    1. Urinary system
    2. Skeletal system
    3. Hematologic system
    4. Central nervous system

196. For a child with the diagnosis of lead poisoning, the most damaging adverse effect is:
    1. Inadequate nutrition
    2. Delayed development
    3. Anemia and constipation
    4. Renal and skeletal damage

197. If a child cannot be given oral chelating agents, parenteral medication must be used. To effectively prepare a child to cope with this painful treatment, the nurse should give priority to:
    1. Rotating the injection sites and adding procaine to the chelating agents to lessen the discomfort
    2. Role-playing with puppets dressed as hospital personnel to minimize the child's fear of unfamiliar adults
    3. Therapeutic play using a needleless syringe and a doll before therapy is initiated and after receiving each injection
    4. Explaining the rationale for the injections so that the child does not view them as a punishment for bad behavior

198. The nurse should encourage parents to have their young children's eyes tested because if monocular strabismus is not corrected early enough:
    1. Dyslexia will develop
    2. Peripheral vision will disappear
    3. Amblyopia develops in the weak eye
    4. Vision in both eyes will be diminished

199. The nurse explains to parents of a toddler with strabismus that if this condition is not corrected in early childhood, it can lead to:
    1. Cataracts
    2. Glaucoma
    3. Refractive errors
    4. Partial loss of sight

200. The nurse observes that a 6-month-old infant is startled by a loud noise but does not turn in the direction of the sound. How should the nurse interpret this response?
    1. Risk for vision deficits
    2. Evidence of hearing loss
    3. Low-normal hearing range
    4. Developmentally appropriate

201. An adolescent has arrived at the clinic complaining of buzzing in the ears. What assessment data are essential for the nurse to obtain?
    1. Emotional upsets
    2. Music preferences
    3. Childhood ear infections
    4. Familial history of deafness

202. During a well-child visit parents tell the nurse that their 3-year-old daughter does not listen to them when they speak to her and ignores them. After an auditory screening, the nurse determines that the child has a mild hearing loss. The nurse explains to the parents why a mild hearing loss:
    1. Will not require immediate follow-up
    2. May progress to a severe hearing deficit
    3. Will not interfere with progress in school
    4. May require hearing aids along with speech therapy

203. A young child with a leg fracture of suspicious origin is brought into the emergency department by the mother and the mother's boyfriend. It is the child's first visit to this hospital. After assessing the child, the nurse suggests that the practitioner order a skeletal survey because it:
    1. Will pinpoint the exact location and extent of the fracture
    2. Is more cost-effective than ordering three separate x-ray films of the leg and hip
    3. Is the first step toward a complete assessment before a CT scan and an MRI is done
    4. Will provide a skeletal history of the current fracture and any previous healing or healed fractures

204. A 9-year-old child has a fractured tibia, and a full leg cast has been applied. Which assessment should the nurse immediately report to the practitioner?
    1. ☐ An increased urinary output
    2. ☐ An inability to move the toes
    3. ☐ A pedal pulse of 90 beats/min
    4. ☐ A tingling sensation in the foot
    5. ☐ A fiberglass cast that is damp after 4 hours

205. An infant has a plaster cast applied for clubfoot correction. What nursing intervention will hasten the drying of the cast?
    1. Using a blow dryer
    2. Exposing the casted extremity
    3. Covering the cast with a light sheet
    4. Promote circulation of air by opening the window

206. An 11-year-old child has just received a cast for a fractured wrist. The wrist and elbow are immobilized. What information should the nurse include in the home care instructions before discharge? Check all that apply.
    1. ☐ Resume usual activities
    2. ☐ Report swelling of fingers
    3. ☐ Elevate casted arm when standing
    4. ☐ Keep affected shoulder immobilized

207. A 3-year-old child is admitted with partial- and full-thickness burns over 30% of the body. What significant adverse outcome during the first 48 hours should the nurse try to prevent?
    1. Shock
    2. Pneumonia
    3. Contractures
    4. Hypertension

208. A 6-year-old child has partial-thickness burns of the face and upper chest. What is the priority nursing assessment for the first 24 hours?
    1. Wound sepsis
    2. Pulmonary distress
    3. Fear and separation anxiety
    4. Fluid and electrolyte imbalance

209. A 15-year-old male is admitted with partial- and full-thickness burns of the arms and upper torso. The nurse plans for the administration of pain medication intravenously rather than intramuscularly because this method of administration:
    1. Decreases risk for tissue irritation
    2. Reduces severe pain more effectively
    3. Bypasses impaired peripheral circulation
    4. Provides for more prolonged relief of pain

210. Nurses understand that the major influence on eating habits of the early school-age child is the:
    1. Smell and appearance of food
    2. Availability of food selections
    3. Food preferences of the peer group
    4. Example of parents and siblings at mealtime

211. A child receives a gastrostomy tube feeding every 4 hours. What is the priority nursing intervention for this child?
    1. Open the tube 1 hour before feeding
    2. Flush the tube with normal saline after feeding
    3. Position the child on the right side after feeding
    4. Keep the child's head flat before raising the tube 12 inches above the head

212. An unconscious child requires intermittent nasogastric feeding. When should the nurse check placement of the tube?
    1. Once a day
    2. At every shift change
    3. Before administering each feeding
    4. During the night shift for the morning report

213. A nurse can assist in confirming a suspected diagnosis of intestinal infestation with pinworms in a 6-year-old child by:
    1. Teaching the mother the procedure for an anal cellophane-tape test

2. Asking the mother to collect stools for 3 consecutive days for culture
3. Having the mother bring in the child's stools for visual examination for 3 days
4. Assisting the mother to schedule a hypersensitivity test of the child's blood serum

214. The stools of children with celiac disease are:
1. Small, pale, mucoid
2. Large, frothy, green
3. Large, pale, foul-smelling
4. Moderate, green, foul-smelling

215. The mother of a 6-year-old girl with celiac disease tells the school nurse that her daughter becomes dejected because she cannot have "snack" food like her playmates. The nurse assures the mother that the girl can eat:
1. Pretzels
2. Tortilla chips
3. Oatmeal cookies
4. Peanut butter crackers

216. In young children with cystic fibrosis, frequent stools and tenacious mucus often produce:
1. Anal fissures
2. Intussusception
3. Rectal prolapse
4. Meconium ileus

217. The foul-smelling, frothy characteristic stool in cystic fibrosis results from the presence of large amounts of:
1. Undigested fat
2. Sodium and chloride
3. Lipase, trypsin, and amylase
4. Partially digested carbohydrates

218. Which medications are usually used in the therapeutic regimen for a child with cystic fibrosis?
1. Steroids and antimetabolites
2. Pancreatic enzymes and antibiotics
3. Antihistamines and fat-soluble vitamins
4. Multivitamin preparations and aerosol mist

219. At what time should the nurse teach a parent to perform a cellophane-tape test for pinworms?
1. Immediately after meals
2. At bedtime before bathing
3. Early morning before arising
4. Following a bowel movement

220. Pinworms cause a number of symptoms besides anal itching. A complication of pinworm infestation, although rare, that the nurse should be aware of is:
1. Hepatitis
2. Stomatitis
3. Pneumonitis
4. Appendicitis

221. Mebendazole (Vermox) is ordered for a child with pinworms. It is advisable that this drug also be administered to:
1. The child's infant brother
2. People using the same toilet facilities as the child
3. Members of the child's family who test positive
4. The child's mother, father, and siblings even if they are symptom-free

222. The mother of a 14-month-old toddler asks the nurse about how to proceed with her child's bowel training. What should the nurse recommend to optimize success?
1. Place the child on the toilet every 2 hours
2. Start by having her child sit on a potty chair
3. Avoid bowel training until her child is 2 years old
4. Begin while the child is still drinking from a bottle

223. Obesity in children is an ever-increasing problem. Before confronting the problem with individual children, the nurse should be aware that:
1. Enjoyment of specific foods is inherited
2. Childhood obesity is not usually a predictor of adult obesity
3. Children with obese parents and siblings are destined for obesity
4. Familial and cultural influences are deciding factors in children's eating habits

224. The nurse is planning for the discharge of a child after a sickle cell vaso-occlusive crisis (pain episode). What is most important for the nurse to emphasize?
1. A high-calorie diet
2. A rigorous exercise regimen
3. An increased intake of fluids
4. An increase in the hours spent sleeping

225. A child is to receive a blood transfusion. If an allergic reaction to the blood transfusion occurs, what should the nurse do first?
1. Call the practitioner
2. Shut off the infusion
3. Slow the rate of flow
4. Administer the prescribed antihistamine

226. When counseling the parents of children with anemia related to inadequate diets, the nurse explains that several different nutrients are involved. These nutrients include proteins, iron, vitamin B_{12}, and:
1. Calcium
2. Thiamine
3. Folic acid
4. Riboflavin

227. The nurse is developing a teaching plan for an 8-year-old child who has anemia related to inadequate nutrition. In addition to iron, which nutrients are necessary for RBC synthesis?
1. Calcium and vitamin A
2. Vitamin D and riboflavin
3. Proteins and ascorbic acid
4. Carbohydrates and thiamine

228. A pale, lethargic 1 year old weighs 12.6 kg (28 lb) and has a hemoglobin level of 9 g/dL. The mother tells the nurse that her infant refuses solid food when it is offered by spoon and drinks between four and six full bottles of milk per day. The nurse should encourage the mother to:
1. Begin the weaning process immediately
2. Take the infant to the metabolic clinic for an examination

3. Give the infant finger foods such as dry cereal and chopped meat
4. Puncture a large hole in the nipple and add baby foods to the milk

229. A child with β-thalassemia (Cooley's anemia) is admitted to the ambulatory care unit for a transfusion. What instructions should the nurse include in the discharge plan?
1. Encourage fluids
2. Restrict activity
3. Protect from infections
4. Offer small meals frequently

230. A client is to have a sickle-turbidity tube test to screen for sickle cell anemia. The nurse explains to the parents that this test screens for:
1. HbS
2. HbA
3. HCV
4. HBV

231. A child with sickle cell disease has a sequestration crisis. The nurse understands that this type of crisis is characterized by:
1. Peripheral ischemia and pain
2. Diminished RBC production and anemia
3. Accelerated RBC destruction and anemia
4. Decreased blood volume and signs of shock

232. The nurse is caring for a child with sickle cell anemia. What is the priority nursing intervention to prevent thrombus formation in capillaries, and the stasis and clotting of blood that occurs in the sickling process?
1. Administer O_2
2. Encourage bed rest
3. Increase oral fluid intake
4. Give prescribed anticoagulants

233. A 6-year-old child is admitted with severe anemia (hemoglobin level of 6.4 g/dL). What should be the nurse's priority assessment?
1. Elevated bilirubin level
2. Increased white cell count
3. Presence of hemoglobinuria
4. Signs of cardiac decompensation

234. An adolescent in sickle cell crisis (pain episode) is complaining of right knee pain. What is the most appropriate nursing intervention?
1. Decreasing amount of IV fluids
2. Applying a warm soak to the knee
3. Wrapping the right knee in a cold pack
4. Administering the prescribed 0.5 mg of morphine sulfate

235. What nursing care is the same for children with sickle cell anemia and celiac disease that might prevent a crisis?
1. Limit activity
2. Protect from infection
3. Document color and consistency of stools
4. Offer a low-carbohydrate, high-protein, and low-fat diet

236. A 6-year-old child with sickle cell disease is admitted with a vasoocclusive crisis. What are the priority nursing concerns?
1. Hydration and nutrition
2. Pain management and hydration
3. Nutrition and prevention of infection
4. Prevention of infection and pain management

NURSING CARE OF PRESCHOOLERS

237. A 4-year-old girl is brought to the emergency department after falling on the handlebars of her tricycle. She is guarding her abdomen, crying, and not allowing anyone to touch her. Which action best enables the nurse to initiate the assessment process?
1. Medicate the child for pain before proceeding
2. Allow the child to guide the examiner's hand to the area that hurts
3. Have the parents restrain the child while the abdomen is auscultated
4. Suggest the practitioner order a CAT scan. because a child this age is unable to cooperate

238. Two second-graders are brought to the school health office after a fight during gym class. How should the school nurse respond to the situation?
1. "Why did you do this?"
2. "Tell me what happened."
3. "You are both in a lot of trouble."
4. "How many fights have you two had?"

239. As a child with nephrotic syndrome gets older and has repeated relapses, what is most important for the nurse to help the child develop?
1. A positive body image
2. The ability to test urine
3. Fine muscle coordination
4. Acceptance of possible sterility

240. A 3 year old with nephrotic syndrome is being treated with corticosteroid therapy. The nurse evaluates that treatment has been successful when the child has decreased:
1. Polyuria
2. Hematuria
3. Glycosuria
4. Proteinuria

241. A 4-year-old boy being admitted for surgery arrives on the ambulatory surgical unit crying and pulling at his hospital gown while clutching a teddy bear. What is the nurse's best response?
1. "Please stop crying. Nobody will hurt you"
2. "Hello, I'm your nurse. Let's go and see your room"
3. "I know you feel scared. This must be your special teddy bear"
4. "Hi young man. Let me show you the playroom and then we can play"

242. As a preschooler, a 4-year-old child's response to hospitalization is influenced by:
    1. Fear of separation
    2. Fear of bodily harm
    3. Belief in death's finality
    4. Belief in the supernatural

243. The best approach to use when preparing a 4 year old for an otoscopic examination is to say: "I'm going to look in your ear with this tube and:
    1. There won't be any pain."
    2. It will feel like a pencil in your ear."
    3. Please try to sit very still while I'm looking."
    4. You can help by holding it while I get ready."

244. When the nurse brings a dinner tray to a 4-year-old girl hospitalized with pneumonia, the child says, "I'm too sick to feed myself." How should the nurse respond?
    1. "Try to eat as much as you can."
    2. "You can eat later when you feel better."
    3. "Wait a few minutes and I will be back to help you."
    4. "You're a big girl now and you are able to feed yourself."

245. The best way for the nurse to meet a 3-year-old child sitting in the waiting room of the pediatric clinic is to:
    1. Walk into the waiting room and greet the child
    2. Call the child by name at the waiting room door
    3. Ask the receptionist to bring the child into the examining room
    4. Stand at the examining room door while the child walks down the hall

246. A child recovering from a severe asthma attack is given prednisone, 15 mg po twice daily. What is the priority nursing intervention?
    1. Prevent exposing the child to infection
    2. Have the child rest as much as possible
    3. Check the child's eosinophil count daily
    4. Keep the child NPO except for medications

247. A child with acute lymphoid leukemia (ALL) is started on chemotherapy, including prednisone. What side effect of prednisone may be exhibited?
    1. Alopecia
    2. Anorexia
    3. Weight loss
    4. Mood changes

248. Methotrexate (Rheumatrex) is prescribed as part of a child's cancer therapy. The nurse is aware this chemotherapeutic agent accomplishes its action by:
    1. Acting as an antibiotic, thus controlling the spread of infected WBCs
    2. Depressing bone marrow function, thus decreasing WBC production
    3. Interfering with mitosis, thus inhibiting the growth of the malignant cells
    4. Competing for essential structural components, thus inhibiting WBC production

249. The primary reason for using prednisone in the treatment of acute lymphoid leukemia in children is it:
    1. Decreases inflammation
    2. Suppress mitosis in lymphocytes
    3. Increases appetite and a sense of well-being
    4. Reduces irradiation skin irritation and edema

250. A combination of drugs, including vincristine (Oncovin) and prednisone, is prescribed for a child with leukemia. What adverse effects should the nurse expect attributable to the toxicity of vincristine?
    1. GI problems
    2. Hemolytic anemia
    3. Irreversible alopecia
    4. Neurologic complications

251. A young child with acute nonlymphoid leukemia is admitted to the hospital with a fever and neutropenia. What are the most appropriate nursing interventions to minimize the complications associated with neutropenia?
    1. Placing the child in a private room, restricting ill visitors, and using strict handwashing techniques
    2. Encouraging a well-balanced diet, including iron-rich foods, and helping the child avoid overexertion
    3. Avoiding rectal temperatures, limiting injections, and applying direct pressure for 5 to 10 minutes after venipuncture
    4. Offering a moist, bland, soft diet; using toothettes rather than a toothbrush; and providing frequent saline mouthwashes

252. A nurse who works in the parent-child center of a large city hospital shares with the parents of one of the children that it is most challenging to perform a physical examination on a child who is:
    1. From 1 to 4 years of age
    2. Between 6 and 8 years old
    3. Between 6 and 12 months old
    4. From birth to 6 months of age

253. Preschool children engage in role-playing. This is an important part of socialization because it:
    1. Encourages expression of concerns
    2. Helps children think about careers
    3. Teaches children about stereotypes
    4. Provides guidelines for adult behavior

254. The nurse observes that a 4 year old is having difficulty relating with some of the children in the playroom. The nurse understands that it is expected for a child this age to:
    1. Engage only in parallel play
    2. Be extremely dependent on parents
    3. Exaggerate and boast to impress others
    4. Have fierce temper tantrums and negativism

255. A mother expresses her concern to the nurse that her 4-year-old child is spending a large amount of time playing with an imaginary playmate. How should the nurse respond?
    1. "Perhaps your child needs more interaction with friends."
    2. "You have reason to be concerned. This is not typical behavior"
    3. "Imaginary playmates are an important part of a young child's life."
    4. "This is a sign of social immaturity. I recommend psychological counseling."

256. When providing nursing care to a preschooler, the nurse should remember that a child this age has a fear of:
    1. Pain
    2. Death
    3. Isolation
    4. Mutilation

257. The nurse should attempt to involve a hospitalized preschooler in therapeutic play to give the child the opportunity to:
    1. Meet other children on the unit
    2. Work out ways of coping with fears
    3. Learn to accept the hospital situation
    4. Forget the reality of the situation for a while

258. The nurse, teaching a group of mothers whose children are about to enter kindergarten, explains that the average 5 year old is not capable of:
    1. Tying shoelaces
    2. Abstract thought
    3. Making decisions
    4. Hand-eye coordination

259. A toddler is admitted to the emergency department because of sudden hoarseness and unintelligible speech. During assessment what should particularly concern the nurse?
    1. A retropharyngeal abscess
    2. A respiratory tract obstruction
    3. An acute respiratory tract infection
    4. An undetected laryngeal abnormality

260. A 2-year-old child is admitted to the pediatric intensive care unit with a diagnosis of acute asthma. A blood sample is obtained to measure the child's arterial blood gases. What should the nurse expect?
    1. An elevated pH
    2. A raised O_2 level
    3. An increased CO_2 level
    4. A decreased bicarbonate level

261. When planning discharge teaching for the parents of a child with asthma, what information should the nurse include?
    1. Avoid foods high in fat
    2. Stay in the house for at least 2 weeks
    3. Increase the protein and calorie intake
    4. Minimize exertion and exposure to cold

262. When preparing a child with asthma for discharge, what must the nurse emphasize to the family? Check all that apply.
    1. ☐ Eliminate allergens in the home
    2. ☐ Avoid placing limits on the child's behavior
    3. ☐ Maintain a cold, dry environment for the child
    4. ☐ Continue the medications even if the child is asymptomatic
    5. ☐ Prevent exposure to infection by having the child tutored at home

263. Which nursing intervention is most effective in alleviating the fretfulness of a hospitalized 5-year-old girl?
    1. Reading a story to her
    2. Giving her a jigsaw puzzle
    3. Placing her in a room by herself
    4. Encouraging her to play with a doll

264. After a tonsillectomy, which assessment should cause the nurse to suspect hemorrhage?
    1. Noisy snoring
    2. Frequent swallowing
    3. Complaints of thirst
    4. Gradual onset of pallor

265. A 17-year-old high school student with a history of asthma is brought to the emergency department experiencing an acute exacerbation of asthma. Which nursing assessments support this conclusion? Select all that apply.
    1. ☐ Fever
    2. ☐ Crackles
    3. ☐ Wheezing
    4. ☐ Tachycardia
    5. ☐ Hypotension

266. What is the most important nursing intervention for a 3-year-old child with a diagnosis of nephrotic syndrome?
    1. Encouraging fluids
    2. Regulating the diet
    3. Preventing infection
    4. Maintaining bed rest

267. A child with nephrotic syndrome comes to the clinic for a follow-up visit. During the visit the child complains of feeling tired and not wanting to eat. The nurse identifies that the child has a muddy, pale complexion. The nurse concludes that the child is:
    1. In impending renal failure
    2. Being too active in school
    3. Developing a viral infection
    4. Not taking the prescribed medication

268. The practitioner lists orders for a young child with a tentative diagnosis of Wilms' tumor. Which procedure order should the nurse question?
    1. An MRI
    2. A CT scan
    3. A renal biopsy
    4. An abdominal ultrasound

269. A 14 year old who has been on prolonged steroid therapy develops a cushingoid appearance. A nursing assessment of this child would probably reveal:
    1. Increased linear growth
    2. Loss of hair on head and body
    3. Hypotension with hyponatremia
    4. Thin extremities and truncal obesity

270. A 3-year-old preschooler has been hospitalized with nephrotic syndrome. What is the best way for the nurse to evaluate fluid retention or loss?
    1. Have the child urinate in a bedpan
    2. Test the child's urine for proteinuria
    3. Measure the child's abdominal girth daily
    4. Weigh the child at the same time every day

271. A child has been admitted to the pediatric unit with a severe asthma attack. What type of acid-base

imbalance should the nurse expect the child to develop?

1. Metabolic alkalosis caused by excessive production of acid metabolites
2. Respiratory alkalosis caused by accelerated respirations and loss of CO_2
3. Respiratory acidosis caused by impaired respirations and increased formation of carbonic acid
4. Metabolic acidosis caused by the kidneys' inability to compensate for increased carbonic acid formation

272. The nurse caring for a child with acute lymphoblastic leukemia (ALL) should not expect the child to have:

1. Marked fatigue and pallor
2. Multiple bruises and petechiae
3. Enlarged lymph nodes and spleen
4. Marked jaundice and generalized edema

273. A 4 year old, newly diagnosed with leukemia, is admitted for chemotherapy. While assisting with morning care, the nurse notes bloody expectorant after the child has brushed the teeth. How should the nurse respond to this occurrence?

1. Secure a smaller toothbrush for the child to use.
2. Document the incident without alarming the child.
3. Tell the child to be more careful when brushing the teeth.
4. Rinse the child's mouth with half-strength hydrogen peroxide.

274. A 3-year-old child who has acute lymphoblastic leukemia (ALL) is scheduled to receive cranial radiation. The nurse should explain to the parents that it will:

1. Improve the quality of life
2. Prevent CNS involvement
3. Reduce the risk for systemic infection
4. Avoid metastasis to the lymphatic system

NURSING CARE OF SCHOOL-AGE CHILDREN

275. A 6-year-old girl begins thumb-sucking after surgery. This was not the child's behavior preoperatively. What is the best action for the nurse to take?

1. Accept the thumb-sucking
2. Distract her by playing checkers
3. Report this behavior to the practitioner
4. Tell her that thumb-sucking causes buckteeth

276. An 8-year-boy, who has been receiving chemotherapy, will soon return to school after a prolonged absence. His classmates are aware that he is being treated for cancer. To help prepare the class for his return the school nurse should:

1. Encourage the students to think about how they feel toward their classmate
2. Explain to the students why it is important to tolerate those who are different
3. Ask the students not to make fun of their classmate because he has lost weight and has no hair

4. Initiate a discussion with the students about cancer treatments and the side effects of chemotherapy

277. An 11-year-old child with juvenile idiopathic arthritis will be receiving continued nonsteroidal antiinflammatory drug (NSAID) therapy at home. Which important adverse effect of NSAIDs must be included in the discharge instructions for this family?

1. Diarrhea
2. GI bleeding
3. Hypothermia
4. Increased activity

278. If an adolescent with diabetes takes Novolin N insulin at 7:30 AM, what is the time of day that an insulin reaction is likely to occur?

1. 8:30 AM
2. 2:30 PM
3. 7:30 PM
4. 1:30 AM

279. A 6-year-old child is admitted to the hospital with a diagnosis of leukemia. When planning play activities for this 6-year-old child, the nurse should include:

1. Large jigsaw puzzles
2. Simple card games and crayons
3. Action toys such as a hula hoop
4. A CD player and children's magazines

280. What play material should the nurse offer two 6-year-old boys in the playroom?

1. Clay
2. Checkers
3. A board game
4. A building set

281. A 9 year old who is receiving IV antibiotic therapy becomes bored and irritable. What activity for school-age children should the nurse suggest? Check all that apply.

1. ☐ Play solitaire
2. ☐ Start a collection
3. ☐ Do arithmetic puzzles
4. ☐ Make a model airplane
5. ☐ Watch game shows on TV

282. The fifth grader who the nurse should appoint as a health office monitor to promote the child's social development is the student who:

1. Is reserved but is strong academically
2. Has been identified as the class clown
3. Comes to the health office daily for medication
4. Participates in a variety of school-related activities

283. What nursing intervention would be most effective to help relieve the anxiety of a young school-age child during the postoperative period?

1. Allow the child time to talk about feelings
2. Tell a story about a child with a similar surgery
3. Have the child and mother room together for a few days
4. Provide the child with sterile dressing equipment and a doll

284. The school nurse is planning to teach a class about nutrition. Which age-group would be most receptive to this information?
    1. 6 year olds
    2. 8 year olds
    3. 11 year olds
    4. 15 year olds

285. An 11-year-old boy has gained weight. His mother is concerned that her son, who loves sports, may become obese. What is the nurse's most appropriate response?
    1. Suggest an increase in activity
    2. Encourage a decreased caloric intake
    3. Explain this is expected during preadolescence
    4. Discuss the influence of genetics on weight gain

286. A 7 year old is admitted for surgery. What is an essential preoperative nursing intervention?
    1. Provide the child with a favorite toy
    2. Document the child's ASO titer and C-reactive protein level
    3. Inspect the child's mouth for loose teeth and report the findings
    4. Encourage a parent to stay until the child leaves for the operating room

287. A child is admitted with a diagnosis of acute post streptococcal glomerulonephritis (APSGN). When performing a physical assessment, the nurse expects to observe:
    1. Anorexia, hematuria, proteinuria (+1), and decreased blood pressure
    2. Normal blood pressure, anorexia, proteinuria (+1), and glycosuria (+3)
    3. Lowered blood pressure, periorbital edema, proteinuria (+1), and decreased specific gravity (1.001)
    4. Moderately elevated blood pressure, periorbital edema, hematuria, and increased specific gravity (1.030)

288. When planning nursing care for a 5 year old with acute post streptococcal glomerulonephritis, what should the nurse emphasize that the child and family maintain?
    1. A bland diet high in protein
    2. Bed rest for at least 4 weeks
    3. A daily dose of IM penicillin
    4. Isolation from children with infections

289. The parents of a child with acute post streptococcal glomerulonephritis are concerned about activity restrictions after discharge. How should the nurse respond?
    1. Activity must be limited for 1 month
    2. The child should not play active games
    3. The child must remain in bed for 2 weeks
    4. Activity does not affect the course of the disease

290. The mother of a child with acute post streptococcal glomerulonephritis asks why the child is being weighed every morning. What is the nurse's best response?
    1. "It is the best way to measure your child's fluid balance."
    2. "When weight loss stops it indicates the disease process is over."
    3. "It gives the doctors a good idea of how much protein is being lost."
    4. "Plans for the daily caloric intake are made according to the daily weight change."

291. A 7 year old is admitted for a diagnostic work-up because of general malaise, severe headaches, and hematuria. The admission vital signs are as follows: T, 98.2° F; P, 96 beats/min; R, 26 breaths/min; BP, 136/84 mm Hg. A diagnosis of acute post streptococcal glomerulonephritis (APSGN) is made. The mother asks why her child has severe headaches. The nurse explains that the headache probably is caused by the:
    1. Rapid respirations
    2. Elevated blood pressure
    3. Anemia associated with the hematuria
    4. Autoimmune response associated with APSGN

292. A 7-year-old girl has recently been diagnosed with juvenile idiopathic arthritis. The parents are concerned about the lifelong effects of the disorder and are investigating other therapies to use with the medications. What referral should the nurse recommend?
    1. Physical therapy
    2. Special education
    3. Herbal supplements
    4. Nutritional therapy

293. The nurse teaches the parents of a child with idiopathic juvenile arthritis that to prevent loss of joint function the child should avoid:
    1. Riding a bicycle
    2. Walking to school
    3. Swimming in the community pool
    4. Playing computer games for after-school activity

294. Range-of-motion exercises are prescribed for a child with idiopathic juvenile arthritis. What criterion should the nurse use to evaluate the effectiveness of the exercises?
    1. Pain is relieved
    2. Pedal and radial pulses are diminished
    3. Subcutaneous nodules at the joints recede
    4. Affected joints can be flexed and extended

295. The nurse is aware that steroids, usually effective in adult clients with rheumatoid arthritis, will not be administered as a first-choice drug to a preadolescent with juvenile idiopathic arthritis because of their adverse effects on:
    1. Growth
    2. Sexuality
    3. Emotions
    4. Body image

296. When planning a teaching program for a child who has recently been diagnosed with type 1 diabetes, the nurse's first concern is that the child and parents:
    1. Understand their feelings about diabetes
    2. Learn how to administer insulin injections
    3. Understand why activities must be limited
    4. Learn how to monitor blood glucose levels

297. An evening snack is planned for a child receiving NPH (Novolin N) insulin. The nurse understands that this will provide:
1. Energy for immediate utilization
2. Calories to help the child gain weight
3. Encouragement for the child to stay on a diet
4. Nourishment to counteract late insulin activity

298. Before developing a teaching plan for an 8-year-old child who has recently been diagnosed with type 1 diabetes, what developmental characteristic of a child this age should the nurse consider?
1. Child is in the abstract level of cognition
2. Child's dependence on peer influence has reached its peak
3. Child will welcome opportunities for participation in self-care
4. Child's developmental stage involves achieving a sense of identity

299. A 16 year old, recently diagnosed with type 1 diabetes, will receive NPH (Novolin N) insulin subcutaneously. When teaching about this insulin and the potential for hypoglycemia, the nurse should include that its peak effect occurs in:
1. 1 to 2 hours
2. 2 to 4 hours
3. 5 to 10 hours
4. 4 to 12 hours

300. When teaching an adolescent with type 1 diabetes about dietary management, what should the nurse include?
1. Meals should be eaten at home
2. Food should be weighed on a gram scale
3. Food in the form of concentrated glucose should be available
4. Meals should be prepared separately from the rest of the family

301. At 7 AM, the nurse receives the information that an adolescent with diabetes has a 6 AM fasting blood glucose level of 180 mg/dL. What is the priority nursing action at this time?
1. Encourage the adolescent to start exercising
2. Ask the adolescent to obtain an immediate glucometer reading
3. Inform the adolescent that a complex carbohydrate such as cheese should be eaten
4. Tell the adolescent that the prescribed dose of regular insulin should be administered

302. What treatment should the nurse suggest to a male adolescent with type 1 diabetes if an insulin reaction is experienced while at a basketball game?
1. Call his parents immediately
2. Buy a soda and hamburger to eat
3. Administer regular insulin as soon as possible
4. Leave the arena and rest in a quiet place until his symptoms subside

303. One principle to be followed for children with type 1 diabetes is to provide for the variability of the child's activity. What should the nurse teach the child about how to compensate for increased physical activity?
1. Take oral, not injectable insulin, on days of heavy exercise
2. Take the insulin in the morning when extra exercise is anticipated
3. Eat more food when there is a plan to exercise more than usual
4. Eat more foods that contain sugar to compensate for the extra exercise

304. A skin infection caused by streptococci or staphylococci with the possible sequela of glomerulonephritis is:
1. Herpes
2. Scabies
3. Impetigo
4. Intertrigo

305. A mother receives a note from school that a child in her daughter's class has head lice. The mother calls the school nurse to ask how to check her child for head lice. What instructions should the nurse provide?
1. "Ask the child where it itches."
2. "Check to see if your dog has ear mites."
3. "Look along the scalp line for white dots."
4. "Observe between the fingers for red lines."

306. The mother of a 6-year-old boy has arrived at school to take her child home because the school nurse has verified that he has an inflamed throat. The nurse urges his mother to seek treatment because if the causative agent is beta-hemolytic streptococcus he may develop a disorder characterized by inflamed joints, fever, and the possibility of endocarditis. The disorder is:
1. Tetanus
2. Influenza
3. Scarlet fever
4. Rheumatic fever

307. A toddler has been diagnosed with classic hemophilia. The child's mother is taught to administer replacement factor VIII 3 times a week through a venous port. What is the most effective administration schedule?
1. Whenever a bleed is suspected
2. In the morning on scheduled days
3. At bedtime while the child is lying quietly in bed
4. On a regular schedule at the mother's convenience

308. What medication should the nurse expect to administer to control bleeding in a child with hemophilia A?
1. Albumin
2. Fresh frozen plasma
3. Factor VIII concentrate
4. Factors II, VII, IX, X complex

309. What explanation should the nurse include when discussing hemophilia with the parents of a child recently diagnosed with this disorder?
1. Hemophilia follows the Mendelian law of inherited disorders
2. Hemophilia is an autosomal dominant disorder in which the woman carries the trait

3. Hemophilia carriers can be either males or females but the disorder occurs in the sex opposite that of the carrier
4. Hemophilia is an X-linked disorder in which the mother is the carrier of the disorder but is not affected by it

310. The mother of a toddler with hemophilia has just told the nurse, "If my son hurts himself, is it alright if I give him two baby aspirins? How should the nurse respond?
    1. "You seem concerned about giving drugs to your child."
    2. "It is alright to give him aspirin when he hurts himself."
    3. "Aspirin may cause more bleeding. Give him acetaminophen instead."
    4. "He should be given acetaminophen every day. It will prevent bleeding."

311. The parents of a 10-year-old boy with hemophilia are worried about their younger children, two girls and another boy. They want to know what their chances are of having the disorder or being carriers. What is the most appropriate answer to this question?
    1. "Neither of the girls will be affected, but your other son is a carrier."
    2. "Both of the girls will be carriers, but only one of the boys will be affected."
    3. "Each son has a 50% chance of being affected, and each daughter has a 50% chance of being a carrier."
    4. "Each son has a 50% chance of being either affected or a carrier, and the girls will all be carriers."

NURSING CARE OF ADOLESCENTS

312. A 15-year-old male, who has type 1 diabetes, arrives with his mother at the diabetic outpatient clinic. He sits back in his chair with his arms folded and a frown on his face and displays an "I don't care" attitude toward his diabetes. He and his mother argue in front of the nurse. What approach is best for the nurse to use in working with this adolescent and his mother?
    1. Persuade them to work out their differences together before returning to the clinic
    2. Ask the mother to wait in the waiting room while her son meets with the clinic's staff members
    3. Encourage the adolescent to take more interest in and responsibility for treatment because he is almost an adult
    4. Speak separately with the adolescent and the mother, encouraging each of them to recognize and vent their anger

313. The nurse is teaching growth and development to a group of parents. When discussing puberty, one mother asks at what age her daughter will have her first period. The nurse should respond that for most girls the first period occurs:
    1. Before the pubic hair appears
    2. About the same time the breasts develop
    3. At the end of the prepubertal growth spurt
    4. Near the age their mothers had their first periods

314. An adolescent is started on a chemotherapeutic drug regimen for cancer that includes prednisone, vincristine (Oncovin), and L-asparaginase (Elspar). Which side effect of these drugs requires early preparation of the adolescent?
    1. Alopecia
    2. Constipation
    3. Retarded growth in height
    4. Generalized short-term paralysis

315. The nurse can best accomplish therapeutic communication with an adolescent by:
    1. Using teen language
    2. Relating on a peer level
    3. Dealing in concrete terms
    4. Establishing a relationship over time

316. The nurse is aware that an adolescent's approach to illness and treatment is often affected by the fact that adolescents are:
    1. In touch with their feelings and concerns
    2. Striving for industry as a developmental goal
    3. Involved more with the present than the future
    4. Using thinking that is both concrete and reality oriented

317. The nurse teaching a group of parents about developmental expectations explains that one of the earliest signs of sexual maturity in young girls that occurs about the age of 10 years is:
    1. Attention to grooming
    2. Interest in the opposite sex
    3. The first menstrual period or menarche
    4. The appearance of axillary and pubic hair

318. A male adolescent sustains a sports' related fracture of the femur, and an open reduction and internal fixation with a rod insertion is performed. After the surgery, the adolescent is very upset. Considering the client's developmental level, what is the most likely explanation for his concern?
    1. The need to navigate in a wheelchair
    2. The inability to participate in sports for several years
    3. The perception that the rod is an intrusion on his body
    4. The relief of pain will necessitate medication until the bone heals

319. A 12 year old is diagnosed as having idiopathic scoliosis. Because exercise and avoidance of fatigue are essential components of care, which sport should the nurse suggest that would be most therapeutic for this preadolescent?
    1. Golf
    2. Bowling
    3. Swimming
    4. Badminton

320. To slow the progression of the curvature, the preadolescent with scoliosis is fitted with a brace. How should the nurse respond to the parent's questions about when the brace will no longer be needed?
1. When the iliac crests are at equal levels
2. When there is no more pain after prolonged standing
3. After the curvature of the spine has completely straightened
4. After the cessation of bone growth at the time of physical maturity

321. A 14-year-old adolescent, receiving chemotherapy for the treatment of bone cancer, is at risk for mouth lesions from the chemotherapy. What should the nurse include when teaching the child about oral hygiene?
1. Brush with a soft toothbrush
2. Rinse frequently with mouthwash
3. Brush 3 times a day with a toothbrush
4. Rinse frequently with hydrogen peroxide

322. The nurse on the adolescent unit is planning to discuss smoking prevention. The most effective approach for the nurse to use is:
1. Sharing personal experiences with a smoking cessation program
2. Showing pictures of the effects of smoking on the cardiopulmonary system
3. Citing statistics about the relationship between smoking and cardiopulmonary diseases
4. Presenting information on how smoking affects their appearance and the odor of their breath

323. An adolescent girl with a serious health problem refuses to wear a medical alert bracelet. The nurse can foster compliance by encouraging the teen to:
1. Hide the bracelet under long-sleeved clothes
2. Wear the bracelet when engaging in contact sports
3. Ask her friends to wear bracelets that look like hers
4. Select a bracelet that is similar to those worn by her peers

324. A 13-year-old boy tells the school nurse that he is getting breasts. The nurse responds:
1. "This is normal at your age; let's talk about it."
2. "You should see your doctor; I'll make an appointment for you."
3. "There is nothing to worry about; this happens to a lot of boys your age."
4. "Wear a tight undershirt inside a button down shirt; that should hide them."

325. A 17-year-old adolescent with a history of asthma is brought to the emergency department because of respiratory distress. The nurse immediately places the client in a bed with the head of the bed elevated and administers oxygen via a facemask. The practitioner performs a physical assessment, writes orders, and admits the adolescent to the pediatric unit (see client chart below). What is the nurse's priority intervention based on the chart below?
1. Administering the nebulizer treatment to facilitate breathing
2. Obtaining a blood specimen to send to the laboratory for tests
3. Notifying the respiratory therapist to perform chest physiotherapy
4. Sending a requisition to central supply for an incentive spirometer

CLIENT CHART
Practitioner Orders
Bed rest
Complete blood count
SMA 12
Albuterol (Proventil) 2.5 mg via nebulizer, one dose
Chest physical therapy bid
Incentive spirometer
Referral to allergist
Oxygen via mask @ 8 L
Physical Assessment
Respiratory rate 30/min, dyspnea, flaring of nares, productive cough (frothy, clear, gelatinous sputum), wheezing. Child indicates shortness of breath, chest discomfort, headache, and feeling tired.

ANSWERS AND RATIONALES

FOUNDATIONS OF CHILD HEALTH NURSING

1. **2** The nurse should obtain clarification as to the mother's specific concerns regarding the child's behavior. **1** Although this may be true, it cuts off communication; further communication should be encouraged. **3** This response assumes the mother has been inconsistent; the nurse needs more information. **4** This is inappropriate because the nurse is explaining a developmental factor without exploring what the mother means.
Client Need: Health Promotion and Maintenance; **Cognitive Level:** Analysis; **Integrated Process:** Communication/Documentation; **Nursing Process:** Planning/Implementation; **Reference:** Ch 29, Nursing Care Related to Meeting the Needs of the Family of a Child With Special Needs

2. **1** This helps and encourages parents to put their fears and feelings into words. Once these sentiments are expressed, they can then be examined and addressed. **2** This would not assist the parents in coping with the problem; neither would it demonstrate the supportive, empathetic role of the nurse. **3** This response lacks insight. Parents will worry about their infant anyway. **4** This may or may not be helpful.
Client Need: Psychosocial Integrity; **Cognitive Level:** Application; **Integrated Process:** Caring; **Nursing Process:** Planning/Implementation; **Reference:** Ch 29, Nursing Care Related to Meeting the Needs of the Family of a Child With Special Needs

3. **4** Hypersensitivity reactions such as skin rash, erythema, fever, and pruritus occur with much greater frequency in children and adults with AIDS. **1** Hepatic side effects, such as jaundice, may occur but are not common. **2** CNS side effects, such as headache, are rare adverse reactions. **3** This is a rare side effect.
Client Need: Pharmacological and Parenteral Therapies; **Cognitive Level:** Application; **Nursing Process:** Evaluation/Outcomes; **Reference:** Ch 29, Related Pharmacology, Child Health Nursing

4. **Answer: 9.5 mg**
Since there are 2.2 pounds per kilogram, the child's weight of 28 lb is equal to 12.7 kg. The safe dose is determined by multiplying the child's weight in kilograms by 35 (12.7 × 35), which is 444.5 mg/24 hours. To calculate the child's dose in 24 hours, multiply the ordered dose (145 mg) by 3, which equals 435 mg in 24 hours. Subtract 435 from 444.5, which equals 9.5 mg. Because the ordered daily dose is 9.5 mg less than the maximum safe daily dose of 444.5 mg, it is safe to administer this medication as ordered.
Client Need: Pharmacological and Parenteral Therapies; **Cognitive Level:** Application; **Nursing Process:** Assessment/Analysis; **Reference:** Ch 29, Related Pharmacology, Child Health Nursing

5. **4** To maintain the desired blood level, the drug must be given in the exact amount at the times directed. If the blood level of the drug falls, the organisms have an opportunity to build resistance to the drug. **1** Weighing is important with drugs that affect fluid balance. **2** Giving medication with milk or meals is important with drugs that cause GI distress. **3** Monitoring temperature would be important with antipyretic drugs.
Client Need: Pharmacological and Parenteral Therapies; **Cognitive Level:** Application; **Nursing Process:** Planning/Implementation; **Reference:** Ch 29, Related Pharmacology, Child Health Nursing

6. **2** The purpose of digoxin (Lanoxin) is to slow and strengthen the apical rate. The apical rate for a healthy child of 5 years is 70 to 110 beats/min. If the apical rate is slow (10 to 20 beats below normal), administration of the drug may lower the apical rate to an unsafe level. **1** This rate is well below that which necessitates withholding Lanoxin for children; it is the correct rate for withholding Lanoxin in adults. **3, 4** This is within the normal range of the heart rate of 5 year olds and does not necessitate withholding Lanoxin.
Client Need: Pharmacological and Parenteral Therapies; **Cognitive Level:** Application; **Nursing Process:** Planning/Implementation; **Reference:** Ch 29, Characteristics of Growth

7. **Answer: 4.5 mL**
To determine the ordered dose, multiply 15 mg × 9.6 kg = 144 mg. Solve for x by using ratio and proportion:

$$\frac{\text{Desired}}{\text{Have}} \quad \frac{44 \text{ mg}}{160 \text{ mg}} \times \frac{x \text{ mL}}{5 \text{ mL}}$$
$$160x = 144 \times 5$$
$$160x = 720$$
$$x = 720 \div 160$$
$$x = 4.5 \text{ mL}$$

Client Need: Pharmacological and Parenteral Therapies; **Cognitive Level:** Application; **Integrated Process:** Teaching/Learning; **Nursing Process:** Planning/Implementation; **Reference:** Ch 29, Related Pharmacology, Child Health Nursing

8. **4** A specific dose per kilogram of body weight prevents overdose; there is a large range in weight for specific ages, and a uniform dose based on age could be unsafe or ineffective. **1** This could result in an inadequate dose. **2** Medication is important; the child has a fever. **3** This would be unsafe because of the wide range of weights for a specific age-group.
Client Need: Pharmacological and Parenteral Therapies; **Cognitive Level:** Analysis; **Integrated Process:** Teaching/Learning; **Nursing Process:** Planning/Implementation; **Reference:** Ch 29, Related Pharmacology, Child Health Nursing

9. **1** Teaching methods in each age-group are different depending on the children's cognitive ability; individual differences depend on a variety of factors including intelligence and emotional status; the child's readiness to learn must be assessed before developing a teaching plan that will bring success.

2, 3, 4 This would be important later, but not initially. **Client Need:** Health Promotion and Maintenance; **Cognitive Level:** Application; **Integrated Process:** Teaching/Learning; **Nursing Process:** Assessment/Analysis; **Reference:** Ch 29, Principles of Growth

10. **4** In children younger than 3 years old the eustachian tube is shorter, wider, and straighter. Pulling the auricle down and back facilitates passage of fluid to the eardrum.

    1 Pulling the auricle down and back, not forward, helps straighten the canal. **2** Pulling the auricle up and back is used for older children and adults. **3** Pulling the auricle straight back does not help to straighten the canal.

    Client Need: Pharmacological and Parenteral Therapies; **Cognitive Level:** Application; **Integrated Process:** Teaching/Learning; **Nursing Process:** Planning/Implementation; **Reference:** Ch 29, Related Pharmacology, Child Health Nursing

11. **1** The nurse can best evaluate teaching by asking the learner for a demonstration. Behavior, rather than words, more readily shows what a child has learned.

    2 The child may be too young to know if there are any questions. **3** A demonstration rather than an explanation can be evaluated more readily. **4** This would be difficult for 5 year olds; their vocabularies are still growing.

    Client Need: Pharmacological and Parenteral Therapies; **Cognitive Level:** Application; **Integrated Process:** Teaching/Learning; **Nursing Process:** Evaluation/Outcomes; **Reference:** Ch 29, Related Pharmacology, Child Health Nursing

12. Answer: 250 mL/hr

    Volume control devices function on the concept of mL/hr; since the 125 mL must infuse in 30 minutes, the rate should be set at 250 mL/hr to infuse 125 mL in 30 minutes.

    Client Need: Pharmacological and Parenteral Therapies; **Cognitive Level:** Application; **Nursing Process:** Planning/Implementation; **Reference:** Ch 29, Related Pharmacology, Child Health Nursing

13. **4** When taking a health history, all areas of concern should be explored fully before deciding how to address the problem.

    1 The nurse should gather more data to determine the basis for the problem. **2** More data are needed before recommendations can be made. **3** The data are inadequate to focus on nutrition.

    Client Need: Health Promotion and Maintenance; **Cognitive Level:** Analysis; **Integrated Process:** Communication/Documentation; **Nursing Process:** Planning/Implementation; **Reference:** Ch 29, Age-Related Responses to Pain

14. **3** A respiratory rate below 30 breaths/min in the young infant is not within the expected range of 30 to 60 breaths/min; a drop below 30 per minute is a significant change and should be documented.

    1 Respirations will accelerate when there is discomfort. **2** Any significant change should be reported immediately. **4** The respiratory tract is fully developed at birth, and the respiratory rate is a cardinal sign of the infant's well-being.

Client Need: Management of Care; **Cognitive Level:** Application; **Integrated Process:** Communication/Documentation; **Nursing Process:** Evaluation/Outcomes; **Reference:** Ch 29, Characteristics of Growth

15. **4** The nurse made the assessment that the medication was ineffective in relieving the adolescent's pain for the duration ordered. This information should be communicated to the practitioner for evaluation.

    1 The practitioner's order is for administration every 3 hours; legally it can be given only within these guidelines. **2** There are no data to support this; the amount of medication was probably inadequate for the adolescent's pain tolerance level. **3** The nurse should not ignore the adolescent's need for pain relief.

    Client Need: Management of Care; **Cognitive Level:** Analysis; **Integrated Process:** Communication/Documentation; **Nursing Process:** Planning/Implementation; **Reference:** Ch 29, Age-Related Responses to Pain

16. Answer: 5 mL

    For a 500-mL bag, 10 mEq of potassium chloride is needed to equal a concentration of 20 mEq/L. Use ratio and proportion to solve the problem:

    $$\frac{\text{Desired}}{\text{Have}} \quad \frac{10\ mEq}{2\ mEq} \times \frac{x\ mL}{1\ mL}$$
    $$2x = 10$$
    $$x = 10 \div 2$$
    $$x = 5\ mL$$

    Client Need: Pharmacological and Parenteral Therapies; **Cognitive Level:** Application; **Nursing Process:** Planning/Implementation; **Reference:** Ch 29, Related Pharmacology, Child Health Nursing

17. **4** The extracellular body fluid represents 45% at birth, 25% at 2 years of age, and 20% at maturity. Another measurement is percentage of total body weight, which is 80% at birth, 63% at 3 years, and approximately 60% at 12 years.

    1 Cellular metabolism in children is stable, but its rate is higher than that in adults. **2** The proportion of total body water in children (up to 2 years) is greater than it is in adults. **3** Renal function is immature during infancy only.

    Client Need: Physiological Adaptation; **Cognitive Level:** Analysis; **Nursing Process:** Assessment/Analysis; **Reference:** Ch 29, Characteristics of Growth

18. **4** The correct rate is 50 mL/hr. Divide the total volume to be infused (400 mL) by the number of hours it is to be infused (8): 400 ÷ 8 = 50.

    1, 2, 3 This is too slow to administer the fluid ordered.

    Client Need: Pharmacological and Parenteral Therapies; **Cognitive Level:** Application; **Nursing Process:** Planning/Implementation; **Reference:** Ch 29, Related Pharmacology, Child Health Nursing

19. **3** Infants are not protected from water loss because they ingest and excrete a relatively greater daily water volume than adults; therefore the proportion of total body water is higher.

    1 Their metabolic rate is more rapid. **2** Infants have a rapid glomerular filtration rate; a decreased rate is

common in the older adult. **4** Infants and children have a rapid generalized response to insensible fluid loss.
Client Need: Basic Care and Comfort; **Cognitive Level:** Analysis; **Nursing Process:** Planning/Implementation; **Reference:** Ch 29, Characteristics of Growth

20. **2** The aorta bifurcates into the left and right femoral arteries in the lower abdomen. The left femoral pulse can be palpated in the left inguinal area.
1 The brachial pulse is palpated in the antecubital fossa and inner aspect of the upper arm. **3** The popliteal pulse is palpated behind the knee. **4** The dorsalis pedis pulse is palpated on the upper surface of the foot between and behind the first two toes.
Client Need: Health Promotion and Maintenance; **Cognitive Level:** Application; **Nursing Process:** Assessment/Analysis; **Reference:** Ch 29, Characteristics of Growth

21. **2** The protocol of the Centers for Disease Control and Prevention (CDC) for administering parenteral medications requires standard precautions, which include the use of gloves.
1 It is the nurse's responsibility to maintain standard precautions within the clinic environment. **3** Gloves are needed and must be worn when children receive parenteral medications. **4** The child's appearance is not a factor; the CDC protocol for administering parenteral medications requires standard precautions.
Client Need: Safety and Infection Control; **Cognitive Level:** Application; **Integrated Process:** Teaching/Learning; **Nursing Process:** Planning/Implementation; **Reference:** Ch 29, Related Pharmacology, Child Health Nursing

22. **4** The peripheral line must be used until the placement of the central venous line is confirmed by radiography or fluoroscopy; this prevents fluid from entering the lung or interstitial space if the catheter is misplaced.
1, 3 The central line should not be used until placement is confirmed. **2** Drugs and fluids can be administered through central venous lines; most devices have multiple ports.
Client Need: Pharmacological and Parenteral Therapies; **Cognitive Level:** Analysis; **Nursing Process:** Planning/Implementation; **Reference:** Ch 29, Related Pharmacology, Child Health Nursing

23. Answer: 44 pounds
The child's daily dose is 40 mg (10 mg × 4 times a day). Divide the daily dose of 40 mg by 2 mg/kg/day, which equals 20 kg. Since 1 kg is equal to 2.2 lb, multiply 20 × 2.2, which equals 44 lb.
Client Need: Pharmacological and Parenteral Therapies; **Cognitive Level:** Analysis; **Nursing Process:** Planning/Implementation; **Reference:** Ch 29, Related Pharmacology, Child Health Nursing

24. **4** Based on the family's decision, extraordinary care does not have to be employed; the infant's basic needs are met, and nature is allowed to take its course.
1 If the infant's physical needs are met and comfort is provided, the infant's rights are not ignored; "extraordinary," not "all," care is being withheld. **2** Euthanasia is a deliberate intervention to cause

death. **3** It is not illegal to withhold extraordinary treatment; once such treatment is started, it may become a legal issue.
Client Need: Management of Care; **Cognitive Level:** Analysis; **Nursing Process:** Evaluation/Outcomes; **Reference:** Ch 29, Nursing Care Related to Meeting the Needs of the Family of a Child With Special Needs

25. **3** The family members are more inclined to share problems with the nurse if they are not feeling pressured; in addition, it aids in the development of a productive relationship.
1 The father should be included in the visit if at all possible. **2** This may be an inconvenient time for the mother and interfere with productivity. **4** This may be at a time that is inconvenient for the family and thus interfere with productive interaction.
Client Need: Management of Care; **Cognitive Level:** Application; **Integrated Process:** Caring; **Nursing Process:** Planning/Implementation; **Reference:** Ch 29, Nursing Care Related to Meeting the Needs of the Family of a Child With Special Needs

NURSING CARE OF INFANTS

26. **3** A pacifier should be given during the feeding to help the infant associate sucking with feeding and meet oral needs.
1 This will cause complications if the tube is not in the stomach. **2** This should be done after placement of the tube and a residual return are ascertained. **4** Upright positioning is essential to prevent regurgitation or reflux and subsequent aspiration.
Client Need: Health Promotion and Maintenance; **Cognitive Level:** Application; **Integrated Process:** Caring; **Nursing Process:** Planning/Implementation; **Reference:** Ch 30, Hospitalization of Infants, General Nursing Care of Infants

27. **2** Peak crying times are early evening and night, which exhaust the mother. She needs time away from her baby and should be encouraged to make some arrangements for time for herself.
1 Providing warmth through a hot-water bottle or heating pad over the abdomen may be helpful for some children but not for others. **3** Many treatments, including this one, may not be effective; children do outgrow colic, so parents need support to help them manage until that time. **4** Treatment is usually based on relieving abdominal cramping by stimulating peristalsis; a quiet environment may help prevent, not treat, the problem.
Client Need: Psychosocial Integrity; **Cognitive Level:** Application; **Integrated Process:** Caring, Teaching/Learning; **Nursing Process:** Planning/Implementation; **Reference:** Ch 30, Colic, Nursing Care

28. **1** Sucking is a primary need of infancy. It decreases anxiety and does not interfere with gastric decompression.
2 This would be more helpful if the child were a toddler. **3** Usually this does not help to calm the infant. **4** This will probably increase the pain from abdominal distention; 3-month-old infants are not

developmentally ready to crawl; infants should not be placed on their abdomens because this practice is associated with SIDS.
Client Need: Health Promotion and Maintenance; **Cognitive Level:** Application; **Integrated Process:** Caring; **Nursing Process:** Planning/Implementation; **Reference:** Ch 30, Hospitalization of Infants, General Nursing Care of Infants

29. 4 Diphenhydramine (Benadryl) is an antihistamine that prevents histamine from reaching its site of action by competing for the receptors.
   1 Nitrofurazone is a bactericidal agent used especially for burns. 2 Hyaluronidase is a mucolytic enzyme that promotes diffusion and absorption of injected fluids, exudates, and transudates. 3 This is a salicylate.
Client Need: Pharmacological and Parenteral Therapies; **Cognitive Level:** Analysis; **Nursing Process:** Planning/Implementation; **Reference:** Ch 30, Eczema, Data Base

30. 1 The American Academy of Pediatrics and the Centers for Disease Control and Prevention are now recommending the IM polio vaccine because of the danger of acquiring vaccine-associated polio paralysis (VAPP).
   2 Both vaccines are not equally safe; the intramuscular one is safer. 3 Cost is not the issue—safety is. The oral vaccine is less expensive. 4 If the infant is immunocompromised, the primary provider will discuss with the parents whether the vaccine should be administered.
Client Need: Health Promotion and Maintenance; **Cognitive Level:** Application; **Integrated Process:** Teaching/Learning; **Nursing Process:** Planning/Implementation; **Reference:** Ch 30, Health Promotion of Infants, Immunizations

31. 2 This child is 2 inches shorter than expected. At 1 year of age a child should have increased his or her birth length by 50%; 50% of 20 inches is 10 inches; 10 inches added to the birth length of 20 inches equals 30 inches.
   1 This is too short. 3, 4 This is too tall.
Client Need: Health Promotion and Maintenance; **Cognitive Level:** Application; **Nursing Process:** Assessment/Analysis; **Reference:** Ch 30, Growth and Development, Ten to Twelve Months

32. 1 Sucking meets oral needs, which are primary during infancy.
   2 An infant a few days old is too young to focus well on a mobile; in addition, the newborn will be placed in a side-lying position postoperatively and thus would not be able to see the mobile. 3 A 2-day-old infant is not developmentally capable of enjoying a soft, cuddly toy. 4 This is not a developmental need.
Client Need: Health Promotion and Maintenance; **Cognitive Level:** Application; **Integrated Process:** Caring; **Nursing Process:** Planning/Implementation; **Reference:** Ch 30, Hospitalization of Infants, General Nursing Care of Infants

33. 4 Turner's syndrome results from a missing X chromosome; these females have an XO configuration rather than XX.
   1 This occurs when there is a thyroid deficiency. 2 This will result from an autosomal recessive single gene disorder. 3 This will result from an extra chromosome 21.
Client Need: Physiological Adaptation; **Cognitive Level:** Analysis; **Nursing Process:** Assessment/Analysis; **Reference:** Ch 30, Turner's Syndrome, Data Base

34. 2 Play during infancy (solitary play) promotes physical development; mobiles strengthen eye movement, rattles promote fine finger movement, and soft toys encourage tactile sense.
   1 Although social development is important, it requires human interaction. 3 The infant is too young to use play for cognition. 4 Although emotional development is important, it requires human interaction.
Client Need: Health Promotion and Maintenance; **Cognitive Level:** Comprehension; **Nursing Process:** Assessment/Analysis; **Reference:** Ch 30, Play During Infancy

35. 3 Infants who have experienced maternal deprivation usually exhibit failure to thrive (i.e., weight below 3rd percentile, developmental deficit, clinical signs of deprivation, and malnutrition). These physical and emotional factors predispose the infant to a variety of illnesses.
   1 Their weight is usually below the 3rd percentile. 2 Infants who have experienced maternal deprivation are usually quiet and lethargic. 4 Responsiveness to stimuli is limited or nonexistent.
Client Need: Psychosocial Integrity; **Cognitive Level:** Application; **Nursing Process:** Assessment/Analysis; **Reference:** Ch 30, Failure to Thrive, Data Base

36. 3 By 4 months of age, infants are able to turn over and can easily fall from an inadequately guarded height.
   1 Although infants are capable of putting small things in their mouth, they are not yet able to crawl and would probably not be placed on the floor. 2 At 3 months of age infants are not yet able to explore the environment to the point that electric outlets pose a problem. 4 At 3 months of age infants are still too small and have not yet developed motor capabilities to get into containers of poison.
Client Need: Safety and Infection Control; **Cognitive Level:** Application; **Integrated Process:** Teaching/Learning; **Nursing Process:** Planning/Implementation; **Reference:** Ch 30, Injury Prevention During Infancy

37. 2 Muscular coordination and perception are developed enough at 6 months for the infant to roll over. If unaware of this ability, the mother could leave the infant unattended for a moment to reach for something and the infant could roll off an elevated surface.
   1 Sitting up unsupported is accomplished by most infants at 7 to 8 months. 3 Crawling takes place at about 9 months of age. 4 Standing by holding on to furniture is accomplished by most infants between 8 and 10 months of age.

Client Need: Safety and Infection Control; **Cognitive Level:** Comprehension; **Integrated Process:** Teaching/Learning; **Nursing Process:** Planning/Implementation; **Reference:** Ch 30, Injury Prevention During Infancy

38. **4** The 7-month-old infant is accustomed to having the perineal area exposed and cared for and is not in a developmental stage where fears related to sexuality are present.

   1 A "clean catch" at this age is often contaminated; a catheterization has been ordered. **2** The mother does have the right to refuse, but her concerns are not realistic for this age infant. **3** The mother's concern is not appropriate for the developmental age of the infant.

   Client Need: Health Promotion and Maintenance; **Cognitive Level:** Analysis; **Integrated Process:** Teaching/Learning; **Nursing Process:** Planning/Implementation; **Reference:** Ch 30, Hospitalization of Infants, Data Base

39. **2** The bottom incisors are the first teeth to erupt at about 6 to 8 months of age.

   1 The canine teeth appear at about 18 months. **3, 4** The first molars, both upper and lower, appear at about 20 months.

   Client Need: Health Promotion and Maintenance; **Cognitive Level:** Knowledge; **Nursing Process:** Assessment/Analysis; **Reference:** Ch 30, Growth and Development, Six to Seven Months

40. **2** These positions offer the lowest risk for SIDS.

   1, 3 This position has been associated with the incidence of SIDS and should be avoided. **4** These positions are safe, but lying on their backs is also safe and using the three positions offers more variety.

   Client Need: Safety and Infection Control; **Cognitive Level:** Application; **Integrated Process:** Teaching/Learning; **Nursing Process:** Planning/Implementation; **Reference:** Ch 30, Sudden Infant Death Syndrome, Data Base

41. **1** The priority is to assess the throat to determine the extent of inflammation. Significant swelling can create the potential for airway obstruction.

   2, 3, 4 Assessment of the child's problem must be done before initiating any other actions.

   Client Need: Reduction of Risk Potential; **Cognitive Level:** Application; **Nursing Process:** Assessment/Analysis; **Reference:** Ch 30, Respiratory Tract Infections, Nursing Care

42. **2** A common sign of shaken baby syndrome (SBS) is apnea without stridor or adventitious sounds, resulting from CNS trauma.

   1 The age of the infant is beyond the time that respiratory distress caused by immaturity would occur. **3** Short periods of apnea of less than 15 seconds are expected at any age. **4** These are indicative of laryngotracheobronchitis, which is common in children under 5 years of age, but would not be expected at 3 months.

   Client Need: Physiological Adaptation; **Cognitive Level:** Analysis; **Nursing Process:** Assessment/Analysis; **Reference:** Ch 30, Shaken Baby Syndrome, Data Base

43. **3** Grunting and rapid respirations are signs of respiratory distress in an infant. Grunting is a compensatory mechanism whereby the infant attempts to keep air in the alveoli to increase arterial oxygenation; increased respirations increase O_2 and CO_2 exchange.

   1 Sweating in infants is usually scanty because of immature functioning of the exocrine glands; profuse sweating is rarely seen in the sick infant. **2** This is not necessarily a sign of illness. **4** This is not necessarily indicative of illness.

   Client Need: Physiological Adaptation; **Cognitive Level:** Application; **Integrated Process:** Teaching/Learning; **Nursing Process:** Planning/Implementation; **Reference:** Ch 30, Respiratory Tract Infections, Data Base

44. **2** Choanal atresia is a lack of an opening between one or both of the nasal passages and the nasopharynx.

   1 Rectal atresia involves the rectum ending in a pouch and the anal canal opening into the other (nonconnected) end of the rectum. **3** Atresias associated with the GI tract include esophageal and intestinal atresia involving the ileum, jejunum, or colon. **4** An atresia involving the pharynx and larynx is not commonly seen.

   Client Need: Physiological Adaptation; **Cognitive Level:** Knowledge; **Nursing Process:** Assessment/Analysis; **Reference:** Ch 30, Nasopharyngeal and Tracheoesophageal Anomalies, Data Base

45. **1** There is little or no opening between the nasal passages and the nasopharynx; therefore the infant can breathe only through the mouth. When feeding, the infant cannot breathe without aspirating some of the fluid; this causes choking.

   2 The swallowing reflex is present in these infants. **3** Because it is difficult if not impossible to suck, the infant will be hungry. **4** If choanal atresia is unilateral, there may be no symptoms and the infant will be able to feed; if bilateral, sucking will be almost impossible.

   Client Need: Physiological Adaptation; **Cognitive Level:** Application; **Nursing Process:** Evaluation/Outcomes; **Reference:** Ch 30, Nasopharyngeal and Tracheoesophageal Anomalies, Data Base

46. **2** A patent airway and adequate pulmonary ventilation are always priorities after surgery.

   1, 3 This is important, but adequate ventilation is the priority. **4** The IV lines would be checked once the airway, breathing, and circulation are determined to be functioning.

   Client Need: Reduction of Risk Potential; **Cognitive Level:** Application; **Nursing Process:** Evaluation/Outcomes; **Reference:** Ch 30, Cardiac Malformations, General Nursing Care of Children With Cardiac Malformations

47. **2** These infants frequently have difficulty swallowing secretions as well as difficulty breathing after surgery. Nursing measures, such as placing the infant in a partial side-lying position or gently aspirating secretions from the mouth or nasopharynx, may be necessary to prevent aspiration and respiratory complications.

1 Although this is important, maintaining a patent airway is essential. **3** Fluids are usually administered carefully by mouth. **4** This is not necessary.
Client Need: Physiological Adaptation; **Cognitive Level:** Application; **Nursing Process:** Planning/Implementation; **Reference:** Ch 30, Cleft Lip (CL) and Cleft Palate (CP), Nursing Care

48. **4** The priority is a patent airway, and necessary equipment must be immediately available.
1 Although this would be helpful, it is not the priority. **2** This is unnecessary; it may be done if the child has a high fever or a history of febrile seizures. **3** Although appropriate, this is not the priority.
Client Need: Reduction of Risk Potential; **Cognitive Level:** Application; **Nursing Process:** Planning/Implementation; **Reference:** Ch 30, Respiratory Tract Infections, Nursing Care

49. **3** Laryngeal spasms can occur abruptly; patency of the airway is determined by constant assessment for signs of respiratory distress.
1, 2, 4 This is important, but maintenance of respirations has priority.
Client Need: Reduction of Risk Potential; **Cognitive Level:** Application; **Nursing Process:** Planning/Implementation; **Reference:** Ch 30, Respiratory Tract Infections, Nursing Care

50. **3** When the causative organism is isolated, it is tested for antimicrobial susceptibility (sensitivity) to various antimicrobial agents. When an organism is sensitive to a medication, the medication is capable of destroying the organism.
1 The tolerance of the child to the particular antibiotic is unknown since up to this time the child has not developed any allergies. **2** Bacteria are not selective. **4** Although the practitioner may have a preference for a particular antibiotic, it first must be determined if the bacteria have exhibited sensitivity to it.
Client Need: Pharmacological and Parenteral Therapies; **Cognitive Level:** Application; **Nursing Process:** Assessment/Analysis; **Reference:** Ch 30, Respiratory Tract Infections, Data Base

51. **2** Often the infant will have decreased pulmonary reserve and the clustering of care is essential to provide for periods of rest.
1 Antiviral therapy is controversial for this age-group and is not given unless there are complications. **3** Antitussive agents are not used; nasal secretions are aspirated with a bulb syringe, PRN. **4** IV fluids are given during the acute phase to prevent dehydration.
Client Need: Basic Care and Comfort; **Cognitive Level:** Analysis; **Nursing Process:** Planning/Implementation; **Reference:** Ch 30, Respiratory Tract Infections, Nursing Care

52. **1** Rest reduces the need for O_2 and minimizes metabolic needs during the acute, febrile stage of the disease.
2 The child requiring hospitalization for pneumonia is usually confined to bed and needs to reduce activity to conserve O_2. **3** This is not a priority; the child is expected to be anorectic during the febrile phase. **4** Elimination is not usually a problem, except as a result of immobility.

Client Need: Basic Care and Comfort; **Cognitive Level:** Application; **Nursing Process:** Planning/Implementation; **Reference:** Ch 30, Respiratory Tract Infections, Nursing Care

53. **3** Respiratory syncytial virus (RSV) is highly contagious. The infant should be isolated or placed with other infants with RSV. Standard and contact precautions are instituted to limit the spread of pathogens to others.
1 The infant should receive cool, humidified O_2 either by nasal cannula, by mask, or in a croup tent. **2** Because RSV is extremely contagious, the number of visitors should be limited, uninfected children should not be allowed near the infant, and as few personnel as possible should care for the infant. **4** Antibiotics are not effective and their use is contraindicated.
Client Need: Safety and Infection Control; **Cognitive Level:** Application; **Integrated Process:** Communication/Documentation; **Nursing Process:** Planning/Implementation; **Reference:** Ch 30, Respiratory Tract Infections, Nursing Care

54. **2** The bladder membrane is exposed; it must remain moist and, as far as possible, sterile.
1, 3 The exposed membrane would dry and there would be an increased risk for infection. **4** The jelly would adhere to the membrane, causing trauma.
Client Need: Safety and Infection Control; **Cognitive Level:** Application; **Nursing Process:** Planning/Implementation; **Reference:** Ch 30, Exstrophy of the Bladder, Nursing Care

55. **4** The pubic bone and the bladder form during the same time of embryonic development.
1, 2, 3 This defect is not associated with exstrophy of the bladder.
Client Need: Physiological Adaptation; **Cognitive Level:** Comprehension; **Nursing Process:** Assessment/Analysis; **Reference:** Ch 30, Exstrophy of the Bladder, Data Base

56. **1** The greatest problem facing this infant is infection of the bladder mucosa and excoriation of the surrounding tissue; meticulous hygiene is necessary both preoperatively and postoperatively.
2 Dehydration is not a problem because intake and output are not affected. **3** Urinary retention is not a problem because the urine drains continuously. **4** The congenital abnormality involves the genitourinary system, not the intestines.
Client Need: Physiological Adaptation; **Cognitive Level:** Application; **Nursing Process:** Assessment/Analysis; **Reference:** Ch 30, Exstrophy of the Bladder, Nursing Care

57. **2** This is the transplantation of the ureters to a resected section of the colon with one end attached to the abdominal wall as an ileostomy.
1 This is an opening into the bladder through the abdominal wall that allows urine to flow out. **3** This is when the ureter is transplanted into the colon with urine excreted through the rectum. **4** This is when the ureter is transplanted through the abdomen and attached to the skin.
Client Need: Physiological Adaptation; **Cognitive Level:** Knowledge; **Integrated Process:** Teaching/Learning; **Nursing Process:** Planning/Implementation; **Reference:** Ch 30, Exstrophy of the Bladder, Data Base

58. 1 Mumps can cause orchitis (inflammation of the testes) in males and oophoritis (inflammation of the ovaries) in females. Although rare, both can render the postpubescent child sterile.
2, 3, 4 This is not associated with mumps.
Client Need: Safety and Infection Control; **Cognitive Level:** Application; **Integrated Process:** Teaching/Learning; **Nursing Process:** Planning/Implementation; **Reference:** Ch 30, Immunizations

59. 2 Cardiac anomalies often accompany genetic problems such as Down syndrome; 30% to 40% of these infants have congenital heart defects.
1 These infants do not have increased intracranial pressure; the fontanels should be flat. **3** The extremities will more likely be relaxed. **4** They have the usual pupillary reactions to light.
Client Need: Physiological Adaptation; **Cognitive Level:** Application; **Nursing Process:** Assessment/Analysis; **Reference:** Ch 30, Trisomy 21 (Down Syndrome), Data Base

60. 3 Touching the palms of the hands causes flexion of the fingers (grasp reflex); this usually lessens after 3 months of age. An unexpected loud noise causes abduction of the extremities and then flexion of the elbows (startle reflex); this usually disappears by 4 months of age. Persistence of primitive reflexes usually is indicative of a developmental delay.
1 It is not necessary to gather more data because these changes are consistent with expected growth and development. **2** The data do not support making this comment; this would cause needless concern. **4** Sensory stimulation at this age is directed toward experiences to add new motor, language, and social skills.
Client Need: Health Promotion and Maintenance; **Cognitive Level:** Application; **Integrated Process:** Teaching/Learning; **Nursing Process:** Planning/Implementation; **Reference:** Ch 30, Growth and Development, Two to Three Months

61. 3 The Hib vaccine may cause a low-grade fever.
1 Lethargy is not expected. **2** Urticaria is more likely to occur with the tetanus and pertussis vaccines. **4** There may be a mild reaction at the injection site, but a generalized rash is not expected.
Client Need: Health Promotion and Maintenance; **Cognitive Level:** Application; **Nursing Process:** Evaluation/Outcomes; **Reference:** Ch 30, Immunizations

62. 1 Febrile seizures usually are not associated with major neurologic problems. From 95% to 98% of these children do not develop epilepsy or other neurologic problems.
2 The cause of febrile seizures is still uncertain. **3** Most febrile seizures occur after 6 months of age and before age 3 years, with the average age of onset between 18 and 22 months. **4** Boys are affected about twice as often as girls.
Client Need: Health Promotion and Maintenance; **Cognitive Level:** Comprehension; **Integrated Process:** Teaching/Learning; **Nursing Process:** Planning/Implementation; **Reference:** Ch 30, Febrile Seizures, Data Base

63. 1 Shivering increases the metabolic rate, which intensifies the body's need for O_2 and raises the body temperature.
2 Restricting fluids is contraindicated because of the risk for dehydration; fluids should be given to the child. **3** Although monitoring output will provide information about the child's level of hydration, it is more important to take action to prevent increases in fever. **4** Monitoring vital signs is not as important as taking action to prevent increases in fever.
Client Need: Reduction of Risk Potential; **Cognitive Level:** Application; **Nursing Process:** Planning/Implementation; **Reference:** Ch 30, Febrile Seizures, Nursing Care

64. 3 Because the child is in a crib, the nurse should remain, observe, and protect the child from injury to the head or extremities during the seizure activity.
1 This is useless until the seizure is over; the child is apneic during the seizure. **2** Attempts at inserting an airway are futile; this could damage the child's teeth and jaws. **4** An individual should never be restrained during a seizure; fractured bones or torn muscles and ligaments can result.
Client Need: Safety and Infection Control; **Cognitive Level:** Application; **Nursing Process:** Planning/Implementation; **Reference:** Ch 30, Febrile Seizure, Nursing Care

65. 3 This limits the danger of falling and striking the head.
1 Protecting the child is the priority; assistance at this time is futile. **2** This is unsafe; attempting to open the jaw could result in injury. **4** This may cause airway occlusion by forcing the chin onto the neck.
Client Need: Safety and Infection Control; **Cognitive Level:** Application; **Nursing Process:** Planning/Implementation; **Reference:** Ch 30, Febrile Seizure, Nursing Care

66. 1 Bradycardia is a classic sign of increased intracranial pressure.
2 With increased intracranial pressure, there would be decreased alertness or loss of consciousness. **3** The pulse pressure increases with increased intracranial pressure. **4** Systolic BP increases with increased intracranial pressure.
Client Need: Physiological Adaptation; **Cognitive Level:** Application; **Nursing Process:** Assessment/Analysis; **Reference:** Ch 30, Meningitis, Data Base

67. 4 This is what occurs in communicating hydrocephalus.
1 This is often caused by a choroid plexus tumor and does not interfere with the flow of CSF through the ventricles. **2** This is an inaccurate answer; brain cells and the spinal cord are not involved. **3** This reflects the pathophysiologic process of noncommunicating hydrocephalus.
Client Need: Physiological Adaptation; **Cognitive Level:** Comprehension; **Integrated Process:** Teaching/Learning; **Nursing Process:** Planning/Implementation; **Reference:** Ch 30, Hydrocephalus, Data Base

68. 4 Cellular destruction occurs as the brain is pressed against the unyielding skull. This occludes blood vessels and deprives the cells of O_2.
1 The increased CSF does not dilute the blood supply; pressure on vessels diminishes the blood supply, causing atrophy and death of cells. 2 Hydrocephalus results when CSF is produced in too great quantities or is not adequately circulated or absorbed; there is no change in the concentration of CSF or plasma. 3 O_2 deprivation occurs when blood vessels are occluded secondary to the pressure in the skull caused by hydrocephalus.
Client Need: Physiological Adaptation; **Cognitive Level:** Comprehension; **Nursing Process:** Assessment/Analysis; **Reference:** Ch 30, Hydrocephalus, Data Base

69. 2 Elevation of the head helps decrease intracranial pressure by using gravity.
1 This would be done after the insertion of a shunt; if the infant is in the intensive care unit, this would be done routinely. 3 This may be disturbing to the infant and impair the ability to rest. 4 Frequent stimulation may cause further irritability to an already traumatized CNS.
Client Need: Reduction of Risk Potential; **Cognitive Level:** Application; **Nursing Process:** Planning/Implementation; **Reference:** Ch 30, Hydrocephalus, Nursing Care

70. 1 Shunts are revised and the length of the tubing is increased as the child grows. Shunts are prone to malfunction and may need revision.
2 Although treatment of hydrocephalus by shunt replacement is quite successful, there is danger of malfunction and infection of the shunt. 3 Damage to brain cells is irreversible. 4 Hydrocephalus necessitates treatment for the life of the child.
Client Need: Management of Care; **Cognitive Level:** Application; **Integrated Process:** Teaching/Learning; **Nursing Process:** Planning/Implementation; **Reference:** Ch 30, Hydrocephalus, Nursing Care

71. 4 The shunt may obstruct and lead to an accumulation of CSF in the head; the accumulated fluid raises the intracranial pressure, which leads to brainstem hypoxia.
1 Although pain management is essential to minimize an increase in intracranial pressure, sedation is contraindicated because it would mask the infant's level of consciousness (LOC). 2 Positioning the infant flat helps prevent complications resulting from too rapid reduction of intracranial fluid. 3 The infant is positioned on the opposite side from the shunt to prevent pressure on the valve and incisional area.
Client Need: Reduction of Risk Potential; **Cognitive Level:** Application; **Nursing Process:** Evaluation/Outcomes; **Reference:** Ch 30, Hydrocephalus, Nursing Care

72. 3 The affected limbs should be exercised to promote circulation and prevent atrophy.
1 Development should be encouraged; the infant's movements should not be restricted. 2 Fluids should be encouraged to provide adequate kidney function and prevent constipation. 4 The infant needs stimulation to develop mentally and socially.
Client Need: Reduction of Risk Potential; **Cognitive Level:** Application; **Integrated Process:** Teaching/Learning; **Nursing Process:** Planning/Implementation; **Reference:** Ch 30, Hydrocephalus, Nursing Care

73. 4 An infectious process could cause meningitis that would result in a stiff neck.
1 Irritability rather than lethargy would result; lethargy is more often associated with increased intracranial pressure. 2 The pulse rate would increase with an infection; a decreased pulse rate is associated with increased intracranial pressure. 3 Headache is associated with increased intracranial pressure.
Client Need: Physiological Adaptation; **Cognitive Level:** Analysis; **Nursing Process:** Evaluation/Outcomes; **Reference:** Ch 30, Meningitis, Data Base

74. 4 The anterior fontanel would be widened and tense because of the increased volume of CSF.
1 The reflexes would be hyperactive with increased intracranial pressure. 2 The BP would be higher with increased intracranial pressure. 3 The pulse rate would be lower with increased intracranial pressure.
Client Need: Physiological Adaptation; **Cognitive Level:** Application; **Nursing Process:** Evaluation/Outcomes; **Reference:** Ch 30, Hydrocephalus, Nursing Care

75. 2 The meningomyelocele is thinly covered and fragile; trauma to the sac can damage functioning neural tissue; an intact sac reduces a potential portal of entry for microorganisms.
1 Although this is always an important nursing measure, care of the sac is even more important because an intact sac reduces a portal of entry for microorganisms. 3 Although observation of paralysis is an important nursing measure, care of the meningomyelocele sac is of primary importance. 4 The extent of a meningomyelocele will influence the child's ability to control these functions, but control is not developed until the toddler and preschool years.
Client Need: Safety and Infection Control; **Cognitive Level:** Application; **Nursing Process:** Planning/Implementation; **Reference:** Ch 30, Defects of Neural Tube Closure (Spina Bifida), Nursing Care

76. 2 This is the best position for preventing pressure on the sac.
1 Diapers should not be applied because they might irritate or contaminate the sac. 3 Assessment of the area below the defect is essential to determine motor and sensory function. 4 There is no indication for the use of an antiseptic.
Client Need: Safety and Infection Control; **Cognitive Level:** Application; **Nursing Process:** Planning/Implementation; **Reference:** Ch 30, Defects of Neural Tube Closure (Spina Bifida), Nursing Care

77. 3 The surgical closure of the sac decreases absorptive surface and eliminates a route by which the spinal fluid drains. Since the cranial sutures have not closed, the skull will expand if fluid increases, causing hydrocephalus.

1 The lower extremities of most infants with meningomyelocele are partially or completely paralyzed; performing careful range-of-motion exercise is an important part of nursing care. **2** There is no reason to decrease environmental stimuli for infants who have had surgical correction of a meningomyelocele unless they also have seizures. **4** This is not expected, because damage to the meninges of the brain is not a factor in the surgical treatment of meningomyelocele.

Client Need: Reduction of Risk Potential; **Cognitive Level:** Application; **Nursing Process:** Evaluation/Outcomes; **Reference:** Ch 30, Defects of Neural Tube Closure (Spina Bifida), Nursing Care

78. **4** Infections of cranial structures can cause meningitis because bacteria travel by direct anatomic route to the meninges and CSF.

1, 2, 3 This part of the body does not come into contact with CSF.

Client Need: Physiological Adaptation; **Cognitive Level:** Comprehension; **Nursing Process:** Assessment/Analysis; **Reference:** Ch 30, Meningitis, Data Base

79. **4** Most children are no longer contagious after 24 to 48 hours of receiving IV antibiotics.

1 This time period would be inadequate even if antibiotics were started immediately. **2, 3** This would involve an excessive time period.

Client Need: Safety and Infection Control; **Cognitive Level:** Application; **Nursing Process:** Evaluation/Outcomes; **Reference:** Ch 30, Meningitis, Nursing Care

80. **2** The blood-brain barrier is affected, which permits the passage of protein into the CSF.

1 The cell count would be increased. **3** Glucose levels are decreased in proportion to the duration of the disease. **4** Spinal fluid pressure would be increased.

Client Need: Reduction of Risk Potential; **Cognitive Level:** Analysis; **Nursing Process:** Assessment/Analysis; **Reference:** Ch 30, Meningitis, Data Base

81. **2** Meningococcal meningitis is identified by its epidemic nature and purpuric skin rash.

1, 4 This is not characteristic of meningococcal meningitis. **3** The fever of meningitis is usually high.

Client Need: Physiological Adaptation; **Cognitive Level:** Application; **Nursing Process:** Assessment/Analysis; **Reference:** Ch 30, Meningitis, Data Base

82. **2** Increased intracranial pressure can cause headaches. Irritation of cerebral tissue can cause seizures, and pressure on vital centers can cause vomiting.

1 Although the child may be restless and anorectic, pressure on the respiratory center results in a decreased respiratory rate. **3** Although the child may be anorectic and irritable, the inflammatory process of meningitis causes an elevated temperature. **4** BP and temperature will be elevated; a toddler's fontanels are closed, so bulging fontanels are not a sign of increased intracranial pressure.

Client Need: Physiological Adaptation; **Cognitive Level:** Analysis; **Nursing Process:** Assessment/Analysis; **Reference:** Ch 30, Meningitis, Data Base

83. **3** Peripheral circulatory collapse (Waterhouse-Friderichsen syndrome) is a serious complication of meningococcal meningitis caused by bilateral adrenal hemorrhage. The resultant acute adrenocortical insufficiency causes profound shock, petechiae, ecchymotic lesions, vomiting, prostration, and hypotension.

1 Although this may occur, it is controllable and not as serious as peripheral circulatory collapse. **2** Although this may occur, it is not as serious a complication as peripheral circulatory collapse. **4** Although this may occur, it is rare and not as serious as peripheral circulatory collapse.

Client Need: Physiological Adaptation; **Cognitive Level:** Application; **Nursing Process:** Assessment/Analysis; **Reference:** Ch 30, Meningitis, Data Base

84. **4** Water in the ears after a myringotomy may be a source of infection.

1 This will clog the ear canal and serves no purpose. **2** These may be used occasionally in the outer ear but should not be inserted into the inner ear. **3** There is no reason that the child cannot be around other children, because there is no infectious process.

Client Need: Safety and Infection Control; **Cognitive Level:** Application; **Integrated Process:** Teaching/Learning; **Nursing Process:** Planning/Implementation; **Reference:** Ch 30, Otitis Media, Nursing Care

85. **4** Asymmetry of the gluteal dorsal surface of the thighs and inguinal folds indicates developmental dysplasia of the hip; folds on the affected side appear higher than those on the unaffected side.

1 An inguinal hernia is evidenced by protrusion of the intestine into the inguinal sac. **2** Impaired reflex behavior and a shrill cry indicate CNS damage. **3** Peripheral nervous system damage is manifested by limpness or flaccidity of extremities.

Client Need: Physiological Adaptation; **Cognitive Level:** Application; **Nursing Process:** Assessment/Analysis; **Reference:** Ch 30, Developmental Dysplasia of the Hip, Data Base

86. **3** A foul smell emanating from the cast indicates development of an infection and requires immediate treatment.

1 Soiling of the cast with excreta, although problematic, is not a serious complication. **2** This is not necessary nor is it desirable. **4** The infant's position should be changed frequently.

Client Need: Safety and Infection Control; **Cognitive Level:** Application; **Integrated Process:** Teaching/Learning; **Nursing Process:** Planning/Implementation; **Reference:** Ch 30, Developmental Dysplasia of the Hip, Nursing Care

87. **1** Standard seat belts and car seats are not readily adapted for use by children in spica casts; specially designed devices are available to meet safety requirements.

2 This is inadequate; the child's position should be changed at least every 2 hours. **3** Other strategies in

addition to diapers will be necessary to keep the cast clean. **4** Using the abduction bar for lifting or turning could weaken the cast; the abduction bar is designed to keep the hips in alignment.
Client Need: Safety and Infection Control; **Cognitive Level:** Application; **Integrated Process:** Teaching/Learning; **Nursing Process:** Planning/Implementation; **Reference:** Ch 30, Developmental Dysplasia of the Hip, Nursing Care

88. **4** When elevation of the head is desired, the entire mattress or crib should be raised at the head of the crib.
1 Pillows under the head or shoulders of a child in a spica cast will thrust the chest forward against the cast, causing discomfort and respiratory distress. **2** There is no reason to place a time limit on this position. **3** This will not help elevate the infant's head.
Client Need: Safety and Infection Control; **Cognitive Level:** Application; **Nursing Process:** Planning/Implementation; **Reference:** Ch 30, Developmental Dysplasia of the Hip, Nursing Care

89. **2** Congenital hypothyroidism is the result of insufficient secretion by the thyroid gland because of an embryonic defect. Decreased thyroid hormone affects the fetus before birth during cerebral development, so it is likely that there will be some cognitive impairments at birth. Treatment before 3 months will prevent further damage.
1 Congenital hypothyroidism does not become myxedema. **3** This could only occur if the infant had cerebral palsy. **4** Thyrotoxicosis is another term for hyperthyroidism; it is not expected but it can occur with an overdose of exogenous thyroid hormone.
Client Need: Physiological Adaptation; **Cognitive Level:** Comprehension; **Nursing Process:** Assessment/Analysis; **Reference:** Ch 30, Congenital Hypothyroidism, Data Base

90. **4** The goiter associated with Hashimoto's disease is usually transient and regresses spontaneously in 1 or 2 years. The child usually is euthyroid but may show signs of hypothyroidism or hyperthyroidism.
1 This is not a chronic disease. **2** There seems to be a strong genetic predisposition, but no mode of inheritance has been identified. **3** This is not an untreatable or fatal disorder; it can be controlled with a medical regimen.
Client Need: Physiological Adaptation; **Cognitive Level:** Comprehension; **Integrated Process:** Teaching/Learning; **Nursing Process:** Planning/Implementation; **Reference:** Ch 30, Hypothyroidism, Data Base

91. **2** Diaper dermatitis is caused by prolonged repetitive contact with an irritant (e.g., urine, feces, soaps, detergents, ointments, and friction).
1 Both cloth and disposable diapers can cause diaper dermatitis if not changed frequently. **3** A change in diet may contribute, but there is no evidence that this is directly related. **4** An increased pH or alkaline urine can contribute to diaper dermatitis.
Client Need: Basic Care and Comfort; **Cognitive Level:** Comprehension; **Integrated Process:** Teaching/Learning; **Nursing**

Process: Planning/Implementation; **Reference:** Ch 30, Diarrhea, Data Base

92. **2** Varicella (chickenpox) is caused by a virus and may be followed by encephalitis. It is characterized by skin lesions.
1 Pertussis (whooping cough) is caused by a bacterium and does not result in encephalitis. **3** Scarlet fever is caused by a bacterium and does not result in encephalitis. **4** Although poliomyelitis is caused by a virus, it does not result in encephalitis.
Client Need: Safety and Infection Control; **Cognitive Level:** Analysis; **Integrated Process:** Teaching/Learning; **Nursing Process:** Planning/Implementation; **Reference:** Ch 30, Immunizations

93. **1** The signs and symptoms of rubeola (measles) include a high fever, photophobia, Koplik spots (white patches on mucous membranes of the oral cavity), and a rash. Rubella (German measles) usually does not cause a high fever, runs a 3- to 6-day course, and never causes Koplik spots.
2 The rash of rubeola (measles) spreads over most of the body. **3** These symptoms are vague and occur with many illnesses. **4** Some signs may be similar to those of a severe cold, but rubeola is associated with high fever.
Client Need: Safety and Infection Control; **Cognitive Level:** Application; **Integrated Process:** Teaching/Learning; **Nursing Process:** Planning/Implementation; **Reference:** Ch 30, Immunizations

94. **2** Steroids have an immunosuppressive effect. It is thought that resistance to certain viral diseases, including varicella, is greatly decreased when a child takes steroids regularly.
1 There is no known correlation between varicella and insulin. **3** Because varicella is a viral disease, antibiotics would have no effect. **4** There is no known correlation between varicella and anticonvulsants.
Client Need: Pharmacological and Parenteral Therapies; **Cognitive Level:** Application; **Integrated Process:** Teaching/Learning; **Nursing Process:** Planning/Implementation; **Reference:** Ch 30, Immunizations

95. **3** Varicella (chickenpox) begins with a slight fever, malaise, and anorexia. After 24 hours a highly pruritic rash begins with a macule, progressing to papules and then vesicles that break easily. The rash spreads in a centripedal manner from the trunk to the face and proximal extremities. Secondary bacterial complications—encephalitis, pneumonia, and hemorrhagic varicella—are potential complications.
1 This is a benign childhood communicable disease; complications are rare; women of childbearing age should be vaccinated because rubella, contracted in early pregnancy, can cause congenital anomalies in the newborn. **2** Rubeola (measles) produces coldlike respiratory symptoms and, after 3 or 4 days, a dark-red macular or maculopapular skin rash.

4 Yellow fever does not cause respiratory complications.
Client Need: Physiological Adaptation; **Cognitive Level:** Analysis; **Nursing Process:** Assessment/Analysis; **Reference:** Ch 30, Immunizations

96. **4** Chalasia is an incompetent cardiac sphincter, which allows a reflux of gastric contents into the esophagus and eventual regurgitation. Placing the infant in an upright position keeps the gastric contents in the stomach by gravity and limits the pressure against the cardiac sphincter.
1 This will promote regurgitation; it is an unsafe position because of the danger of SIDS. **2** This will probably have little effect on chalasia. **3** This will promote vomiting because it is too much formula for a 1-week-old infant.
Client Need: Safety and Infection Control; **Cognitive Level:** Application; **Integrated Process:** Teaching/Learning; **Nursing Process:** Planning/Implementation; **Reference:** Ch 30, Nasopharyngeal and Tracheoesophageal Anomalies, Nursing Care

97. **3** Offering a new food after giving some formula associates this activity with eating and takes advantage of the infant's unsatisfied hunger.
1 Offering food after the regular feeding decreases the chance of success, because the infant's hunger is already satisfied. **2** New foods should be initiated one at a time and continued for 4 to 5 days to assess for an allergic reaction. **4** Solid food should be introduced by spoon to acquaint the infant with new tastes and textures, as well as the use of the spoon.
Client Need: Health Promotion and Maintenance; **Cognitive Level:** Application; **Integrated Process:** Teaching/Learning; **Nursing Process:** Planning/Implementation; **Reference:** Ch 30, Guidelines for Infant Nutrition

98. **1** Crying should be prevented because it places tension on the suture line. Frequently an appliance called a Logan bow is taped to the cheeks to relax the operative site, which helps prevent trauma.
2 The infant may be positioned on the side and on the back with surveillance. **3** This is not necessary or desirable. **4** The feeding method of choice is by a rubber-tipped syringe or dropper.
Client Need: Physiological Adaptation; **Cognitive Level:** Application; **Nursing Process:** Planning/Implementation; **Reference:** Ch 30, Cleft Lip (CL) and Cleft Palate (CP), Nursing Care

99. **4** Infants with a cleft lip breathe through their mouths, bypassing the natural humidification provided by the nose. As a result, the mucous membranes become dry and cracked and are easily infected.
1 Feeding can be adequate with special equipment and a patient approach. **2** Circulation in the area is unimpaired. **3** The area can be kept clean by washing with water after each feeding.
Client Need: Physiological Adaptation; **Cognitive Level:** Application; **Nursing Process:** Assessment/Analysis; **Reference:** Ch 30, Cleft Lip (CL) and Cleft Palate (CP), Data Base

100. **3** Because the infant with a cleft lip and palate is unable to form the vacuum needed for sucking, a rubber-tipped syringe or dropper is used. This allows formula to flow along the sides and back of the mouth, minimizing the danger of aspiration.
1 Feeding can be accomplished with special equipment; IV fluids are not necessary. **2** A soft cross-cut nipple may be used with some infants, but rapid flow can cause aspiration. **4** Feeding is not different; neither infant can form a vacuum when sucking, and both need special feeding equipment.
Client Need: Basic Care and Comfort; **Cognitive Level:** Application; **Nursing Process:** Planning/Implementation; **Reference:** Ch 30, Cleft Lip (CL) and Cleft Palate (CP), Data Base

101. **4** A child with a cleft palate has distinctive speech because the airflow required for speech cannot be controlled; although speech therapy is usually needed after surgery, surgery is scheduled before the child starts to speak because correct speech is easier to achieve.
1 Although this may be true, this is not the reason why the repair is made at this age; these children may need multiple surgeries as the palate develops. **2** This is not the reason the surgery is done at this age. **3** Children with a cleft palate require orthodontic and prosthodontic treatment for many years because of the malformed palate and the malposition of the teeth; the eruption of the teeth may be considered relative to the timing of surgery throughout childhood, but the 2-year molars are of little importance when considering the overall problem.
Client Need: Reduction of Risk Potential; **Cognitive Level:** Comprehension; **Integrated Process:** Teaching/Learning; **Nursing Process:** Planning/Implementation; **Reference:** Ch 30, Cleft Lip (CL) and Cleft Palate (CP), Data Base

102. **3** The olivelike mass is caused by the thickened muscle (hypertrophy) of the pyloric sphincter.
1 The obstruction is above the intestinal area; the colon is not involved. **2** There is no significant tenderness in the abdomen. **4** There is little or no peristalsis in the intestines.
Client Need: Physiological Adaptation; **Cognitive Level:** Application; **Nursing Process:** Assessment/Analysis; **Reference:** Ch 30, Hypertrophic Pyloric Stenosis (HPS), Data Base

103. **1** Hypertrophy of the pyloric sphincter causes partial and then complete obstruction. Nonprojectile vomiting progresses to projectile vomiting, which rapidly leads to dehydration.
2 The infant's cry is not affected by hypertrophic pyloric stenosis (HPS); there does not appear to be pain associated with this condition, except for the pain of hunger. **3** This can be expected with a tracheoesophageal fistula, but not with HPS. **4** The character of the stool is not relevant when assessing an infant with HPS.
Client Need: Physiological Adaptation; **Cognitive Level:** Application; **Nursing Process:** Assessment/Analysis; **Reference:** Ch 30, Hypertrophic Pyloric Stenosis, Nursing Care

104. **3** Initial feedings of glucose and electrolytes in water or breast milk are given 4 to 6 hours after surgery. When clear fluids are retained, formula feedings are begun within 24 hours.

1 Regular formula should be started within 24 hours after surgery in an attempt to gradually return the infant to a full feeding schedule. **2, 4** This is not necessary.

Client Need: Basic Care and Comfort; **Cognitive Level:** Application; **Nursing Process:** Planning/Implementation; **Reference:** Ch 30, Hypertrophic Pyloric Stenosis, Nursing Care

105. **3** Assessment of the IV site is a priority. The infant will need IV fluids until able to feed orally.

1 Restraints are not needed. **2, 4** This is not the priority action.

Client Need: Pharmacological and Parenteral Therapies; **Cognitive Level:** Application; **Nursing Process:** Planning/ Implementation; **Reference:** Ch 30, Hypertrophic Pyloric Stenosis, Nursing Care

106. **2** An elevated position allows gravity to aid in preventing vomiting.

1 Movement increases the chance of vomiting. **3** This would not prevent reflux and could result in aspiration. **4** Activity increases the chance of vomiting.

Client Need: Basic Care and Comfort; **Cognitive Level:** Application; **Integrated Process:** Teaching/Learning; **Nursing Process:** Planning/Implementation; **Reference:** Ch 30, Hypertrophic Pyloric Stenosis, Nursing Care

107. **4** A strangulated hernia occurs when abdominal tissue is so constricted as it protrudes through the abdominal musculature that the blood supply is interrupted; gangrene will result unless the herniation is reduced.

1 A hiatal hernia is the intrusion of an abdominal structure, usually the stomach, through the esophageal hiatus. **2** An incarcerated hernia is one that cannot be reduced manually. **3** An omphalocele is the protrusion of intraabdominal tissue through a defect in the abdominal wall at the umbilicus; the sac may be covered with peritoneum, not skin.

Client Need: Physiological Adaptation; **Cognitive Level:** Knowledge; **Nursing Process:** Assessment/Analysis; **Reference:** Ch 30, Intestinal Obstruction, Data Base

108. **2** Human milk has a laxative effect that promotes a soft stool; breastfed infants rarely become constipated.

1 There are no data to indicate that this infant has an allergy to milk. **3, 4** This is unnecessary.

Client Need: Basic Care and Comfort; **Cognitive Level:** Application; **Integrated Process:** Teaching/Learning; **Nursing Process:** Planning/Implementation; **Reference:** Ch 30, Anorectal Anomalies (Imperforate Anus), Data Base

109. **3** Hepatitis B virus is in the blood during the late incubation and acute stages of the disease. It may persist in the carrier state for years. It is transmitted when the blood of an infected individual comes in contact with the blood or mucous membranes of another individual.

1 Hepatitis A is transferred principally through oral-fecal routes. **2** Ventilating systems do not transmit this virus. **4** This is unrelated to hepatitis B.

Client Need: Safety and Infection Control; **Cognitive Level:** Application; **Nursing Process:** Assessment/Analysis; **Reference:** Ch 30, Immunizations

110. **4** Because phenylalanine is an essential amino acid, it must be provided in quantities sufficient for promoting growth while maintaining safe blood levels.

1 All proteins do not contain phenylalanine. **2** An enriched protein diet would contain an increased amount of proteins, including phenylalanine, which should be ingested in limited amounts. **3** Phenylalanine is an essential amino acid and cannot be totally removed from the diet.

Client Need: Basic Care and Comfort; **Cognitive Level:** Application; **Nursing Process:** Planning/Implementation; **Reference:** Ch 30, Phenylketonuria (PKU), Data Base

111. **1** In PKU the absence of the hepatic enzyme phenylalanine hydroxylase prevents metabolism (hydroxylation to tyrosine) of the amino acid phenylalanine. The increased fluid levels of phenylalanine in the body and the alternate metabolic by-products (phenylketones) are associated with severe mental retardation if not identified and treated early.

2 Testing for PKU cannot be done until after several days of milk ingestion. **3** Medications are not part of therapy. **4** PKU is transmitted by an autosomal recessive gene.

Client Need: Physiological Adaptation; **Cognitive Level:** Comprehension; **Integrated Process:** Teaching/Learning; **Nursing Process:** Planning/Implementation; **Reference:** Ch 30, Phenylketonuria (PKU), Data Base

112. **4** A diet that maintains low phenylalanine levels is recommended until brain growth is completed, usually by adulthood.

1 The age when dietary restrictions are no longer mandatory is known, and it is the nurse's responsibility to give this information to the parents. **2** Dietary restrictions are necessary until the child reaches adulthood. **3** When adulthood is reached, a regular diet can be resumed; if a woman plans to become pregnant, she should return to a low-phenylalanine diet.

Client Need: Basic Care and Comfort; **Cognitive Level:** Application; **Integrated Process:** Teaching/Learning; **Nursing Process:** Planning/Implementation; **Reference:** Ch 30, Phenylketonuria (PKU), Data Base

113. **1** Obesity is a common nutritional problem of children with Down syndrome. It is thought to be related to excessive caloric intake and impaired growth.

2 This is the most common nutritional problem in children (iron deficiency anemia); it is not usually encountered in these children. **3** This is a nutritional

disorder related to vitamin D deficiency; it is not usually encountered in these children. **4** This is an eating disorder of infancy characterized by repeated regurgitation without gastrointestinal illness; it is not usually encountered in these children.
Client Need: Basic Care and Comfort; **Cognitive Level:** Application; **Nursing Process:** Planning/Implementation; **Reference:** Ch 30, Trisomy 21 (Down Syndrome), Data Base

114. 4 Paroxysmal pain is related to peristaltic action associated with intestinal obstruction. Abdominal distention pushes the diaphragm upward, causing respiratory distress characterized by grunting respirations.
1 These usually do not accompany intestinal obstruction. **2** The pain of intestinal obstruction is paroxysmal. **3** These are not characteristic of intestinal obstruction.
Client Need: Physiological Adaptation; **Cognitive Level:** Application; **Nursing Process:** Assessment/Analysis; **Reference:** Ch 30, Intestinal Obstruction, Data Base

115. 2 The traditional efforts to explain and treat colic center on the paroxysmal pain.
1 Peristalsis is effective because these infants thrive physically and gain weight. **3, 4** The etiology of colic is unknown at this time.
Client Need: Basic Care and Comfort; **Cognitive Level:** Application; **Integrated Process:** Teaching/Learning; **Nursing Process:** Planning/Implementation; **Reference:** Ch 30, Colic, Data Base

116. 2 A suction biopsy removes some rectal tissue, which is examined microscopically for the absence of ganglion cells.
1 A diagnosis cannot be made by inserting a rectal tube; it releases gas pressure but does not relieve the obstruction. **3** Saline enemas may relieve the obstruction but they are not a definitive diagnostic tool; a barium enema may be used for diagnosis after the age of 2 months. **4** This is not used to diagnose the cause of an intestinal obstruction in infants.
Client Need: Reduction of Risk Potential; **Cognitive Level:** Application; **Nursing Process:** Assessment/Analysis; **Reference:** Ch 30, Hirschsprung's Disease (Megacolon), Data Base

117. 2 Tap-water enemas are hypotonic and are contraindicated; they may cause increased absorption of fluid via the bowel and may upset the balance of fluid in the body. There also is interference with potassium ion balance; this electrolyte can be lost via the large intestine.
1 The enema would remove only waste products from the bowel. **3** Fear of intrusive procedures is typical of preschoolers, not infants. **4** The temperature of the water would be regulated so this is not a concern.
Client Need: Basic Care and Comfort; **Cognitive Level:** Application; **Nursing Process:** Evaluation/Outcomes; **Reference:** Ch 30, Hirschsprung's Disease (Megacolon), Data Base

118. 3 No more than 360 mL of solution should be administered to a young child unless ordered, because fluid and electrolyte balance in infants and children is easily disturbed.
1 This quantity may be ordered for a small infant. **2** This quantity may be ordered for an older or larger infant. **4** This quantity is too much for a toddler.
Client Need: Basic Care and Comfort; **Cognitive Level:** Comprehension; **Nursing Process:** Assessment/Analysis; **Reference:** Ch 30, Hirschsprung's Disease (Megacolon), Data Base

119. 4 If the circulation is overloaded with too much fluid or the rate is too rapid, the stress on the heart becomes too great and cardiac overload may occur.
1 Increased output is not the primary consideration. **2** Although fluid replacement is important, prevention of cardiac problems from fluid overload is critical. **3** This is important, but an infiltrated IV is not as serious as a cardiac complication.
Client Need: Pharmacological and Parenteral Therapies; **Cognitive Level:** Application; **Nursing Process:** Evaluation/Outcomes; **Reference:** Ch 30, Dehydration, Nursing Care

120. 2 Weight is the best indicator of fluid loss or gain if measured each day at the same time, on the same scale, and with the same amount of clothing.
1 Oral rehydration therapy (ORT) is employed first; IV therapy is instituted only if there is severe dehydration and it requires an order. **3** This is not a concern at this time; fluid and electrolyte replacement is more important. **4** This temperature is not unusual in infants.
Client Need: Basic Care and Comfort; **Cognitive Level:** Application; **Nursing Process:** Evaluation/Outcomes; **Reference:** Ch 30, Diarrhea, Nursing Care

121. 2 Excessive vomiting causes an increased loss of hydrogen ions (hydrochloric acid), which leads to metabolic alkalosis, an excess of base bicarbonate.
1 This is caused by retention of hydrogen ions and a loss of base bicarbonates, which is more likely to occur with diarrhea. **3** Hypokalemia, not hyperkalemia, will occur. **4** With the loss of chloride ions, hyponatremia is more likely to occur.
Client Need: Physiological Adaptation; **Cognitive Level:** Analysis; **Nursing Process:** Planning/Implementation; **Reference:** Ch 30, Vomiting, Data Base

122. 3 An infant's intravascular compartment is limited and cannot accommodate a large volume of fluid administered in a short time. Equipment such as an infusion pump with a volume-control chamber should be used because it controls the prescribed amount of fluid to be infused.
1 This is important for everyone receiving IV fluids, not just infants. **2** This is the practitioner's role. **4** IV fluids are administered at room temperature.
Client Need: Pharmacological and Parenteral Therapies; **Cognitive Level:** Application; **Nursing Process:** Planning/Implementation; **Reference:** Ch 30, Diarrhea, Nursing Care

123. 1 Tachycardia in infants is often a sign of a heart defect. This infant should be examined for the presence of a heart defect.

2 This does not warrant immediate attention, but the infant should be reevaluated at the next visit. **3** This is frequently seen in infants; it is related to immature muscle control and does not require intervention unless it persists into toddlerhood. **4** This finding at this age does not require immediate attention; however, the infant should be monitored for the attainment of this and other developmental milestones at future visits.

Client Need: Management of Care; **Cognitive Level:** Application; **Integrated Process:** Communication/Documentation; **Nursing Process:** Planning/Implementation; **Reference:** Ch 30, Cardiac Malformations, Data Base

124. **3** Heart failure is characterized by a decrease in the blood flow to the kidneys, causing sodium and water reabsorption, resulting in peripheral edema. The peripheral edema indicates severe cardiac decompensation.

1, 2 This is an early attempt by the body to compensate for decreased cardiac output. **4** This occurs most noticeably in children with post streptococcal glomerulonephritis.

Client Need: Physiological Adaptation; **Cognitive Level:** Application; **Nursing Process:** Assessment/Analysis; **Reference:** Ch 30, Cardiac Malformations, Data Base

125. **3** Children with cardiac malformations often use increased energy in activities of daily living; decreased O_2 utilization and increased energy output in the developing child result in a slow growth rate.

1 Mental retardation is not a common finding in children with congenital heart disease. **2** Cardiac anomalies are more often a result of prenatal, rather than genetic, factors. **4** Clubbing is not characteristic of most children with cardiac anomalies, only of those with more severe hypoxia.

Client Need: Physiological Adaptation; **Cognitive Level:** Application; **Nursing Process:** Assessment/Analysis; **Reference:** Ch 30, Cardiac Malformations, Data Base

126. **3** Polycythemia, reflected in an elevated hematocrit, is a direct attempt of the body to compensate for the decrease in O_2 to all body cells caused by the mixture of oxygenated and unoxygenated circulating blood.

1 This is not characteristic of heart malformations that cause a right-to-left shunting of blood. **2** Edema is not a common finding with heart malformations associated with a right-to-left shunting of blood. **4** This is characteristic of coarctation of the aorta, an obstructive malformation.

Client Need: Reduction of Risk Potential; **Cognitive Level:** Application; **Nursing Process:** Assessment/Analysis; **Reference:** Ch 30, Cardiac Malformations, Data Base

127. **3** Antibiotic prophylaxis can prevent subacute bacterial endocarditis, which can occur in children with abnormal heart structures.

1, 2 This is not generally associated with congenital heart defects in children. **4** Avoidance of exposure, not antibiotics, is recommended to prevent upper respiratory tract infections.

Client Need: Reduction of Risk Potential; **Cognitive Level:** Application; **Integrated Process:** Teaching/Learning; **Nursing Process:** Planning/Implementation; **Reference:** Ch 30, Cardiac Malformations, Data Base

128. **2** The intrapleural space must be drained of fluid and air to facilitate the reestablishment of negative pressure in the intrapleural space.

1 The tidal volume increases as the lung reexpands, but it is not the reason for the insertion of chest tubes. **3** Intrapleural pressure should be negative, not positive; positive intrapleural pressure would cause collapse of the lung. **4** Closed chest drainage is related to intrapleural pressure, not pericardial and chest wall pressure.

Client Need: Physiological Adaptation; **Cognitive Level:** Application; **Integrated Process:** Teaching/Learning; **Nursing Process:** Planning/Implementation; **Reference:** Ch 30, Cardiac Malformations, General Nursing Care of Children With Cardiac Malformations

129. **3** Before birth fetal oxygenated blood is shunted directly into the systemic circulation via the ductus arteriosus, a connection between the pulmonary artery and the aorta. After birth the increased O_2 tension causes a functional closure of the ductus arteriosus. Occasionally, particularly in preterm infants, this vessel remains open and is known as patent ductus arteriosus.

1 This is not the problem in patent ductus arteriosus. **2** This describes pulmonic stenosis. **4** This describes a ventricular septal defect.

Client Need: Physiological Adaptation; **Cognitive Level:** Comprehension; **Nursing Process:** Planning/Implementation; **Reference:** Ch 30, Defects with Increased Pulmonary Blood Flow, Patent Ductus Arteriosus (PDA)

130. **3** With a left-to-right shunt, blood flows through a defect in the ventricular wall of the heart, and is shunted from the higher pressure left side to the lower pressure right side. The increased blood flow from the right ventricle results in an increased blood flow to the lungs.

1 This is not common in children with a left-to-right shunt; tissue perfusion is usually adequate. **2** Clubbing is a more common finding in children with a right-to-left shunt. **4** This is not common in children with a left-to-right shunt.

Client Need: Physiological Adaptation; **Cognitive Level:** Application; **Nursing Process:** Assessment/Analysis; **Reference:** Ch 30, Cardiac Malformations, Data Base

131. **4** Coarctation of the aorta is a narrowing of the aorta, usually in the thoracic segment, causing decreased blood flow below the constriction and increased blood volume above it.

1 The radial pulses are bounding. **2** This is not related to coarctation of the aorta. **3** The femoral pulses are weak or absent.

Client Need: Physiological Adaptation; **Cognitive Level:** Application; **Nursing Process:** Planning/Implementation; **Reference:** Ch 30, Obstructive Defects, Coarctation of the Aorta

132. 3 Compromised heart functioning caused decreased cardiac output; this often results in cyanosis and fatigue from ineffective sucking and swallowing.
1 When a feeding problem persists in a neonate, it is generally an indication of some pathology.
2 Inadequate sucking is never insignificant; it may be indicative of many problems, such as CNS involvement or immaturity as well as heart disease.
4 Generally most newborns are free from mucus within 24 to 48 hours after birth.
Client Need: Physiological Adaptation; **Cognitive Level:** Application; **Integrated Process:** Teaching/Learning; **Nursing Process:** Planning/Implementation; **Reference:** Ch 30, Defects with Increased Pulmonary Blood Flow, Ventricular Septal Defect (VSD)

133. 2 Hemorrhage is a major life-threatening complication, because arterial blood is under pressure and a catheter has been inserted into an artery.
1 The child is kept in bed for 6 to 8 hours after an arterial catheterization. **3** Fluids may be given as soon as tolerated. **4** Pulses, not BP, must be compared for quality and symmetry.
Client Need: Reduction of Risk Potential; **Cognitive Level:** Application; **Nursing Process:** Planning/Implementation; **Reference:** Ch 30, Cardiac Malformations, General Nursing Care of Children With Cardiac Malformations

134. 1 Children with Down syndrome have a high incidence of congenital heart defects as indicated by altered heart sounds. Without treatment the heart defect may become life-threatening.
2, 3, 4 This is expected and is not life-threatening.
Client Need: Physiological Adaptation; **Cognitive Level:** Application; **Nursing Process:** Assessment/Analysis; **Reference:** Ch 30, Trisomy 21 (Down Syndrome), Data Base

135. 3 Tetralogy of Fallot consists of four defects. Three of them are anatomic: ventricular septal defect, pulmonic stenosis, and overriding aorta. The fourth defect, right ventricular hypertrophy, is secondary to increased resistance to blood flow in that ventricle.
1, 4 Although there is right ventricular hypertrophy, the other defects are not associated with tetralogy of Fallot. **2** These are the characteristics of transposition of the great vessels.
Client Need: Physiological Adaptation; **Cognitive Level:** Comprehension; **Nursing Process:** Assessment/Analysis; **Reference:** Ch 30, Defects With Decreased Pulmonary Blood Flow, Tetralogy of Fallot

136. 1 Decreased tissue oxygenation stimulates erythropoiesis, resulting in excessive production RBCs.
2, 4 This is not a direct cause of polycythemia.
3 This may or may not affect the production of RBCs.
Client Need: Reduction of Risk Potential; **Cognitive Level:** Application; **Nursing Process:** Assessment/Analysis; **Reference:** Ch 30, Defects With Decreased Pulmonary Blood Flow, Tetralogy of Fallot

137. 2 Hypoxia leads to poor peripheral circulation; clubbing develops over time as a result of tissue hypertrophy and additional capillary development in the fingers.
1 The respirations are generally rapid to compensate for O_2 deprivation. **3** This is not an adaptation that occurs in children with tetralogy of Fallot. **4** These children have polycythemia.
Client Need: Physiological Adaptation; **Cognitive Level:** Application; **Nursing Process:** Assessment/Analysis; **Reference:** Ch 30, Defects With Decreased Pulmonary Blood Flow, Tetralogy of Fallot

138. 3 Forceful evacuation results in the child taking a deep breath, holding it, and straining (Valsalva maneuver). This increases intrathoracic pressure, which puts excessive strain on the heart sutures.
1 Crying is not a problem after cardiac surgery; it may, in fact, help prevent respiratory complications.
2 Coughing and deep breathing are essential for the prevention of postoperative respiratory complications. **4** Activity is gradually increased.
Client Need: Physiological Adaptation; **Cognitive Level:** Application; **Nursing Process:** Planning/Implementation; **Reference:** Ch 30, Cardiac Malformations, Data Base

139. 2 This is a priority because inadequate antibiotic therapy may predispose the infant to the development of bacterial endocarditis.
1, 3, 4 This is not a priority because instructions are usually printed on the label.
Client Need: Pharmacological and Parenteral Therapies; **Cognitive Level:** Application; **Integrated Process:** Teaching/Learning; **Nursing Process:** Planning/Implementation; **Reference:** Ch 30, Cardiac Malformations, Data Base

140. 4 Gavage feeding is preferred for weak infants, those with respiratory distress or ineffective sucking-swallowing coordination, and those who are easily fatigued because of physical stress such as surgery.
1 This is not a reason for instituting gavage feedings for an infant with CHD; however, vomiting may be lessened because the amount and rapidity of feeding can be controlled. **2** Feeding the infant quickly is not desirable; vomiting with aspiration may occur.
3 The amount can be regulated with oral formula feeding as well.
Client Need: Basic Care and Comfort; **Cognitive Level:** Application; **Integrated Process:** Teaching/Learning; **Nursing Process:** Assessment/Analysis; **Reference:** Ch 30, Cardiac Malformations, Data Base

141. 3 Antibodies received in utero through the placenta and in the newborn via mother's milk provide the infant with immunity against most viral, bacterial, and fungal infections during the first several weeks after birth. Then, as the titer of maternal antibodies drops and is not replaced by the infant's own antibodies, prolonged and repeated infections occur.
1 This is not enough to prevent infections in these infants. **2** Bacteria do not produce antibodies.

4 This probably does not occur in infants born without an immune system.
Client Need: Health Promotion and Maintenance; **Cognitive Level:** Application; **Nursing Process:** Assessment/Analysis, **Reference:** Ch 30, Immunizations

142. **2** This is the expected hematocrit range for a 1 year old.
1 This would be too low; it would only occur with a problem such as prolonged blood loss. **3** This is too high; this would be expected for an adult female. **4** This is too high; this would be expected for a newborn.
Client Need: Health Promotion and Maintenance; **Cognitive Level:** Knowledge; **Nursing Process:** Assessment/Analysis; **Reference:** Ch 30, Growth and Development, Ten to Twelve Months

143. **2** Toxoids are modified toxins that stimulate the body to form antibodies that last up to 10 years against the specific disease.
1 Passive immunity, even the natural type derived from the mother, does not last longer than the first year of life. **3** Only having had the disease can provide lifelong natural immunity. **4** This is provided by tetanus immune globulin.
Client Need: Health Promotion and Maintenance; **Cognitive Level:** Comprehension; **Integrated Process:** Teaching/Learning; **Nursing Process:** Planning/Implementation; **Reference:** Ch 30, Immunizations

144. **1** Corticosteroids depress the immune response. Antineoplastic drugs or high-energy radiation preferentially destroys tissues with high mitotic rates, including lymphatic tissue and bone marrow, where antibody production and other immune responses take place.
2, 4 This is no more valid for these children than for other children. **3** This is not a reason to withhold immunizations.
Client Need: Safety and Infection Control; **Cognitive Level:** Application; **Nursing Process:** Evaluation/Outcomes; **Reference:** Ch 30, Immunizations

145. **2** Scheduled immunizations for preschool children include DTaP, IPV, and MMR at 4 to 6 years (usually required by law).
1 Hepatitis immunization is given in three doses between birth and 9 months; tetanus/diphtheria vaccine is given at 7 to 10 years of age with subsequent doses based on the age when the vaccine was first received. **3** Hepatitis B immunization is not required once immunity is established; a subsequent dose of tetanus/diphtheria vaccine is given based on the age when first received. **4** *Haemophilus influenzae* vaccine is given at 12 to 15 months.
Client Need: Health Promotion and Maintenance; **Cognitive Level:** Application; **Integrated Process:** Teaching/Learning; **Nursing Process:** Planning/Implementation; **Reference:** Ch 30, Immunizations

146. **2** The recommended immunization schedule for infants is administration of the combined diphtheria, pertussis, and tetanus vaccine and the polio virus vaccine at ages 2, 4, and 6 months.

1 Measles vaccine is not usually administered until the child is a minimum of 12 months old. **3** Rubella vaccine is not usually given until a minimum of 12 months of age; there is no tuberculosis vaccine. **4** Measles, mumps, and rubella vaccines are not given until a minimum of 12 months; there is no tuberculosis vaccine.
Client Need: Health Promotion and Maintenance; **Cognitive Level:** Application; **Nursing Process:** Evaluation/Outcomes, **Reference:** Ch 30, Immunizations

147. **3** Immunoglobulin-coated B lymphocytes recognize an antigen (foreign protein) and stimulate antibody production. Antigen-antibody reactions involve the binding of antigens to antibodies to form complexes that may render the toxic antigen harmless, or agglutinizing antigens on the surface of microorganisms stimulate the complement system of the body, resulting in lysis of the antigenic cells.
1 Antibodies are protein substances. **2** Antibodies are produced to fight antigens. **4** Antigens are harmful to the body.
Client Need: Health Promotion and Maintenance; **Cognitive Level:** Application; **Integrated Process:** Teaching/Learning; **Nursing Process:** Planning/Implementation; **Reference:** Ch 30, Immunizations

148. **2** MMR vaccine is composed of live viruses, and its administration could be life-threatening for an immunosuppressed child.
1 When the infant reaches 12 months of age and the blood values return to normal, the MMR vaccine should be given regardless of age. **3** At discharge the parents need information about immunizations, because MMR vaccine is generally given at 12 to 15 months of age. **4** Because the MMR vaccine is composed of live viruses, giving it while the infant is immunosuppressed can be as life-threatening as actually having the disease.
Client Need: Safety and Infection Control; **Cognitive Level:** Application; **Integrated Process:** Teaching/Learning; **Nursing Process:** Planning/Implementation; **Reference:** Ch 30, Immunization

149. **1** The blue-white spots in the mouth are Koplik spots, which appear before the rash and subside about 2 days after the rash is visible. They are a cardinal sign of rubeola (measles).
2 The rash of varicella (chickenpox) is distinctive because the papules become vesicles. There are no Koplik spots. **3** Erythema infectiosum (fifth disease) has a characteristic erythematous rash that appears first on the face and then spreads to the extremities. There are no Koplik spots. **4** Scarlet fever is caused by the group A beta-hemolytic streptococcus bacteria. Although the mouth is affected as evidenced by the typical "strawberry tongue," there are no Koplik spots.
Client Need: Physiological Adaptation; **Cognitive Level:** Analysis; **Nursing Process:** Assessment/Analysis; **Reference:** Ch 30, Immunizations

NURSING CARE OF TODDLERS

150. 1 When unexplained injuries are found, further assessment is required because it is the nurse's legal responsibility to report suspected child abuse.

2 This is just one aspect of assessment for child abuse. 3 This is not related to scars on the child's back. 4 Although chickenpox may leave scars, there are no welts.

Client Need: Psychosocial Integrity; **Cognitive Level:** Application; **Integrated Process:** Communication/Documentation; **Nursing Process:** Assessment/Analysis; **Reference:** Ch 31, Child Maltreatment, Nursing Care

151. 2 It is the nurse's legal responsibility to report child abuse to the appropriate agency.

1 Although the police may be notified, this is not the nurse's responsibility at this time. 3 The nurse has not yet verified the girl's pregnancy; at this time it is most important to protect her and her siblings. 4 This may be done later, but it is not the priority.

Client Need: Management of Care; **Cognitive Level:** Application; **Integrated Process:** Communication/Documentation; **Nursing Process:** Planning/Implementation; **Reference:** Ch 31, Child Maltreatment, Data Base

152. 4 A child who exhibits signs of abuse needs close supervision, especially when members of the family visit.

1 The child needs close monitoring and should not be left alone. 2 This may be desirable, but the priority is for the child to be placed near the nurses' desk. 3 An older child who exhibits signs of friendliness may be threatening to this child.

Client Need: Management of Care; **Cognitive Level:** Application; **Integrated Process:** Caring; **Nursing Process:** Planning/Implementation; **Reference:** Ch 31, Child Maltreatment, Nursing Care

153. 2 If able to handle personal anxiety and give comfort to the child, parents can be helpful to the staff as well as the child. If, however, the parents have moderate to severe anxiety, their anxiety can be transmitted to the child.

1 It is how the parents cope with the situation, rather than the situation itself, that helps determine how helpful their presence may be. 3 Developmentally, toddlers fear separation from their parents; also they are cognitively unable to make decisions of this nature. 4 Parents usually want to participate in their child's care despite the child's response to pain.

Client Need: Psychosocial Integrity; **Cognitive Level:** Application; **Integrated Process:** Caring; **Nursing Process:** Assessment/Analysis; **Reference:** Ch 31, Hospitalization of Toddlers, General Nursing Care of Toddlers

154. 3 Excessive crying and clinging are the usual responses of a toddler who expects to be comforted, not one who has experienced prolonged separation from a parent because of illness.

1 Prolonged hospitalization and separation from parenting can cause delayed growth or even death. 2 Withdrawing active attention is the toddler's way to "turn off" and may be learned from multiple failures in interactions with stimuli. 4 Inattentiveness may be learned from failure to gain response from humans in previous experiences.

Client Need: Health Promotion and Maintenance; **Cognitive Level:** Comprehension; **Nursing Process:** Evaluation/Outcomes; **Reference:** Ch 31, Hospitalization of Toddlers, Data Base

155. 4 A 2-year-old toddler is still attached to and dependent on the parents. Fear of separation is a great stress.

1 This is neither possible nor desirable. 2 These probably will not be remembered accurately. 3 This is not possible in a health care setting.

Client Need: Health Promotion and Maintenance; **Cognitive Level:** Application; **Integrated Process:** Caring; **Nursing Process:** Planning/Implementation; **Reference:** Ch 31, Hospitalization of Toddlers, General Nursing Care of Toddlers

156. 2 The second stage of separation anxiety is despair, in which the child is depressed, lonely, and disinterested in the surroundings.

1 The third stage of separation, denial or detachment, occurs later than that demonstrated in the situation. 3 The child is suffering from separation anxiety, which does not include a stage of mistrust. 4 The child is suffering from separation anxiety, which does not include a stage of rejection.

Client Need: Health Promotion and Maintenance; **Cognitive Level:** Application; **Nursing Process:** Evaluation/Outcomes; **Reference:** Ch 31, Hospitalization of Toddlers, Data Base

157. 2 Detachment is the result of trying to escape the emotional pain of desiring the mother by repressing feelings for her.

1 This interpretation is not appropriate to the situation cited. 3 This conclusion cannot be drawn from the situation cited. 4 This response lacks insight.

Client Need: Health Promotion and Maintenance; **Cognitive Level:** Application; **Integrated Process:** Teaching/Learning; **Nursing Process:** Planning/Implementation; **Reference:** Ch 31, Hospitalization of Toddlers, Data Base

158. 1 Three year olds are entering the developmental stage of creative and imaginative play. Using clay to make shapes both with and without a mold enhances their creativity and improves their fine motor coordination.

2 Stuffed animals that are made of cloth or "fur" cannot be wiped clean; they should be barred from the playroom. Also, stuffed animals are more appropriate for infants. 3 A 3 year old is too young to manipulate a pen or pencil and may cause self-injury or an injury to others. 4 A 3-year-old child does not have the cognitive ability or the fine motor coordination to play even simple video games.

Client Need: Health Promotion and Maintenance; **Cognitive Level:** Application; **Nursing Process:** Planning/Implementation; **Reference:** Ch 31, Play During Toddlerhood (Parallel Play)

159. 4 This is the expected response because medication causes death of the worms.

1 Transient diarrhea, not constipation, could occur. 2 Hypertension does not occur as a result of this medication. 3 Neither the drug nor the worms cause intestinal bleeding. The medication can turn the stool red.

Client Need: Pharmacological and Parenteral Therapies; **Cognitive Level:** Application; **Integrated Process:** Teaching/ Learning; **Nursing Process:** Evaluation/Outcomes; **Reference:** Ch 31, Pinworms, Nursing Care

160. 4 Fewer side effects are desirable. Rapid elimination of the lead prevents further irreversible damage.

1 The combination is preferred because it removes lead more effectively from the brain rather than from bone marrow. 2 There is no marked difference in the rate of urinary elimination when these agents are used together. 3 Each drug is able to accomplish this, but, given alone, each can cause more side effects.

Client Need: Pharmacological and Parenteral Therapies; **Cognitive Level:** Comprehension; **Nursing Process:** Assessment/ Analysis; **Reference:** Ch 31, Lead Poisoning, Data Base

161. 2 At 15 months, strength and balance have improved, and the toddler can stand and walk alone.

1 This usually occurs when the child is 2 years old. 3 Infants are very capable of throwing toys. 4 Infants 9 to 12 months of age can stand with support.

Client Need: Health Promotion and Maintenance; **Cognitive Level:** Application; **Nursing Process:** Assessment/Analysis; **Reference:** Ch 31, Growth and Development, Fifteen Months

162. 2 The psychosocial need during the early toddler age is the development of autonomy. The toddler objects strongly to discipline.

1 Excessive discipline leads to feelings of shame and self-doubt, the major crisis at this stage of development. 3 The sense of initiative is attained during the preschool age, not during the toddler age. 4 It is frightening for a child to be left alone; it leaves the child with feelings of rejection, isolation, and insecurity; a toddler would not understand the reason for the punishment.

Client Need: Health Promotion and Maintenance; **Cognitive Level:** Application; **Integrated Process:** Teaching/Learning; **Nursing Process:** Planning/Implementation; **Reference:** Ch 31, Growth and Development, Eighteen Months

163. 4 Children who are expressing negativism need to have a feeling of control. One way of achieving this within reasonable limits is for the parent or caregiver to provide a choice of two items, rather than force one on the child.

1 This will not achieve the goal of giving fluids. 2 This will probably not be successful with a toddler. 3 This will complicate the situation and further inhibit the child's willingness to take fluids.

Client Need: Health Promotion and Maintenance; **Cognitive Level:** Application; **Integrated Process:** Teaching/Learning;

Nursing Process: Planning/Implementation; **Reference:** Ch 31, Childhood Nutrition

164. 3 The nurse recognizes the child's protest over the mother's absence and tries to comfort him by staying near until the child feels more relaxed. The bathing can be postponed until the child has had time to test the environment and is less anxious.

1 This action does not attempt to relieve the child's anxiety and will probably cause it to increase. 2 This may frighten the child more because the nurse is a stranger who may harm him. 4 This is probably true, but the nurse has not attempted to reduce anxiety.

Client Need: Health Promotion and Maintenance; **Cognitive Level:** Application; **Integrated Process:** Caring; **Nursing Process:** Planning/Implementation; **Reference:** Ch 31, Hospitalization of Toddlers, General Nursing Care of Toddlers

165. 3 Appropriate limit setting and discipline are necessary for children to develop self-control while learning the boundaries of their abilities.

1 Learning to share occurs during the preschool years. 2 Roles within society are learned by the school-age child. 4 Superego control begins in the preschool years.

Client Need: Health Promotion and Maintenance; **Cognitive Level:** Application; **Integrated Process:** Teaching/Learning; **Nursing Process:** Planning/Implementation; **Reference:** Ch 31, Growth and Development, Major Learning Events

166. 1 ☒ Common developmental norms of the toddler, who is struggling for independence, are inability to share easily, egotism, egocentrism, and possessiveness.

2 ☒ Toddlers have a basic understanding of language and the cognitive ability to follow simple directions.

3 ☐ This task is too advanced for toddlers.

4 ☐ This is true of preschool children.

5 ☐ Same as answer 4.

Client Need: Health Promotion and Maintenance; **Cognitive Level:** Analysis; **Nursing Process:** Assessment/Analysis; **Reference:** Ch 31, Growth and Development, Two Years

167. 2 The child should be taken to the dentist between 2 and 3 years of age, when most of the 20 deciduous teeth have erupted.

1, 3 This is too late. 4 This is too indefinite.

Client Need: Health Promotion and Maintenance; **Cognitive Level:** Application; **Integrated Process:** Teaching/Learning; **Nursing Process:** Planning/Implementation; **Reference:** Ch 31, Growth and Development, Thirty Months

168. 4 The toddler is in Erikson's stage of acquiring a sense of autonomy. The negativism is the result of the child's need to express her will and test her environment.

1 This is the developmental goal achieved in infancy. 2 Although this is a factor, toddlers assert themselves in an attempt to attain more autonomy. 3 Children do not assert themselves to obtain discipline.

Client Need: Health Promotion and Maintenance; **Cognitive Level:** Comprehension; **Integrated Process:** Teaching/Learning; **Nursing Process:** Planning/Implementation; **Reference:** Ch 31, Growth and Development, Two Years

169. 1 Toddlers are easily distracted. Taking the child to another part of the store without acknowledging the tantrum will distract the child and avoid embarrassment.

2 Allowing the tantrum to continue will not help the mother cope with the embarrassing situation. 3 It is unreasonable to ask the mother to spend money, which she may not have, on a baby sitter. 4 Giving the child the item acknowledges the tantrum and reinforces the behavior.

Client Need: Health Promotion and Maintenance; **Cognitive Level:** Application; **Integrated Process:** Teaching/Learning; **Nursing Process:** Planning/Implementation; **Reference:** Ch 31, General Nursing Care of Toddlers

170. 4 These are foods that a toddler enjoys and can handle; in addition they are nutritious.

1 Grapes are dangerous because toddlers may choke on the skins. 2 These fried foods have a high fat content and if eaten regularly can lead to obesity. 3 The skin of a hot dog may cause choking, and potato chips are not nutritious.

Client Need: Basic Care and Comfort; **Cognitive Level:** Analysis; **Nursing Process:** Planning/Implementation; **Reference:** Ch 31, Childhood Nutrition

171. 3 Bed-wetting accidents are not uncommon in this age group, especially during hospitalization when regression may occur. Therefore the best approach is to ignore the event.

1 The child may interpret this as punishment; punishment for regressive behavior is inappropriate. 2 Because skin breakdown is a concern, rubber sheets are contraindicated; they would hold moisture close to the skin. 4 This may make the child feel guilty for the behavior.

Client Need: Health Promotion and Maintenance; **Cognitive Level:** Application; **Integrated Process:** Caring; **Nursing Process:** Planning/Implementation; **Reference:** Ch 31, Hospitalization of Toddlers, General Nursing Care of Toddlers

172. 4 This is a task expected of 3-year-old children.

1 This is a task expected of 4- or 5-year-old children. 2, 3 This is a task expected of 4-year-old children.

Client Need: Health Promotion and Maintenance; **Cognitive Level:** Application; **Nursing Process:** Assessment/Analysis; **Reference:** Ch 31, Growth and Development, Thirty Months

173. 2 Of these foods and fluids, an apple provides the best nutrition for a toddler.

1 This is unsafe; a toddler could choke on the skins of the grapes. 3 Cookies are high in fat and sugar and are not as healthy as fruit. 4 Cold fluid may cause bronchospasms.

Client Need: Basic Care and Comfort; **Cognitive Level:** Application; **Integrated Process:** Teaching/Learning; **Nursing Process:** Planning/Implementation; **Reference:** Ch 31, Childhood Nutrition

174. 1 The toddler is still dependent on the mother, is narcissistic, and plays alone, but is aware of others playing nearby.

2 Solitary play or onlookers' play is characteristic of infants. 3 Competitive play is seen in school-age children. 4 Cooperative play starts in the preschool years.

Client Need: Health Promotion and Maintenance; **Cognitive Level:** Comprehension; **Nursing Process:** Assessment/Analysis; **Reference:** Ch 31, Play During Toddlerhood

175. 3 It is not until 2 years of age that toddlers are able to use their feet to walk upstairs instead of crawling.

1 At 18 months the inability of the toddler to use the feet to go upstairs is not a problem; it is expected. 2 Talipes equinovarus is identified using other criteria. 4 Developmental dysplasia of the hip (DDH) is identified using other criteria.

Client Need: Health Promotion and Maintenance; **Cognitive Level:** Application; **Nursing Process:** Assessment/Analysis; **Reference:** Ch 31, Growth and Development, Eighteen Months

176. 4 Play-Doh is age-appropriate and nontoxic; manipulating, rolling, and pounding it may help work out anger at being hospitalized.

1 An infant will enjoy a mobile. 2 This is too advanced for a 2-year-old child. 3 This may be too complicated for a toddler.

Client Need: Health Promotion and Maintenance; **Cognitive Level:** Application; **Nursing Process:** Assessment/Analysis; **Reference:** Ch 31, Play During Toddlerhood

177. 3 More information is needed; developmental delays suggest some milestones for age are not being met at the average time; it is not synonymous with cognitive impairment.

1 This would be inappropriate as more information must be obtained. 2 Although the physician may help, it is not yet known if such a program is needed. 4 The nurse does not know this without more information.

Client Need: Health Promotion and Maintenance; **Cognitive Level:** Analysis; **Integrated Process:** Communication/Documentation; **Nursing Process:** Planning/Implementation; **Reference:** Ch 31, Cognitive Impairment (Mental Retardation), Nursing Care

178. 3 Echolalia in a 2 year old may be a sign of autism; imitation of sounds begins at about 6 months and may continue for several more months; the average 2 year old has a 300-word vocabulary and uses 2- to 3-word phrases.

1 It is not until 30 months of age that the toddler is able to stand on 1 foot. 2 Building a tower of 5 to 6 blocks is expected at age 2. 4 Although the pincer grasp is achieved at 11 months, it is not until age 30 months that the toddler is expected to hold crayons with the fingers rather than the fists.

Client Need: Health Promotion and Maintenance; **Cognitive Level:** Application; **Nursing Process:** Assessment/Analysis; **Reference:** Ch 31, Growth and Development, Two Years

179. 3 The parents' attitude, approach, and understanding of the child's physical and psychologic readiness are essential to letting the child proceed at his or her own pace with appropriate parental intervention.

1 This is not the major motivation for toilet training. 2 Although this is definitely a factor, it is not a major one. 4 This, of course, is a factor, but the major factor is the child, who is strongly influenced by the parents' attitudes and approach.

Client Need: Health Promotion and Maintenance; **Cognitive Level:** Comprehension; **Integrated Process:** Teaching/Learning; **Nursing Process:** Assessment/Analysis; **Reference:** Ch 31, Growth and Development, Major Learning Events

180. 4 A pounding board with pegs to hammer into holes is a safe toy for toddlers, because it is fairly large, easy to manipulate, and sturdy. A pounding board provides an acceptable way for anger to be expressed.

1 The child's motor and hand-eye coordination is too immature for using these. 2 This is not as effective for releasing anger; it may be thrown about, causing injury or damage. 3 This is appropriate for an older child with more mature motor coordination to compensate for a moving object.

Client Need: Health Promotion and Maintenance; **Cognitive Level:** Application; **Integrated Process:** Teaching/Learning; **Nursing Process:** Planning/Implementation; **Reference:** Ch 31, Hospitalization of Toddlers, General Nursing Care of Toddlers

181. 4 Until trust has been reestablished, the child will be unable to develop an emotional tie to the mother.

1 After trust has been reestablished, the child may then test the parents' love by being very demanding. 2 At this stage of separation anxiety, the child would be too detached to be hostile. 3 The child will be despairing and withdrawn.

Client Need: Health Promotion and Maintenance; **Cognitive Level:** Analysis; **Integrated Process:** Teaching/Learning; **Nursing Process:** Planning/Implementation; **Reference:** Ch 31, Hospitalization of Toddlers, Data Base

182. 3 Mucus secretions increase in viscosity and precipitate or coagulate to form concentrations in glands and ducts, which in turn cause obstructions.

1 The eccrine (sweat) glands are not hyperactive, but there is an increased concentration of sweat electrolytes—namely, sodium and chloride. 2 The autonomic nervous system does not play a role in the pathology of cystic fibrosis. 4 There is no alteration in the mucosal lining of the intestines; decreased amounts of pancreatic enzymes cause impairment in the digestion and absorption of nutrients.

Client Need: Physiological Adaptation; **Cognitive Level:** Comprehension; **Nursing Process:** Assessment/Analysis; **Reference:** Ch 31, Cystic Fibrosis, Data Base

183. 3 Both parents are carriers; however, the gene for cystic fibrosis is recessive and the parents do not have the disease.

1 The gene for cystic fibrosis is not located on the X or Y chromosome. 2 The gene for cystic fibrosis is not a mutant gene. 4 The gene for cystic fibrosis is inherited as a recessive, not dominant, gene.

Client Need: Physiological Adaptation; **Cognitive Level:** Comprehension; **Nursing Process:** Assessment/Analysis; **Reference:** Ch 31, Cystic Fibrosis, Data Base

184. 4 Usually the first indication of cystic fibrosis is meconium ileus. The small intestine is blocked with thick, tenacious, mucilaginous meconium, usually near the ileocecal valve. This causes intestinal obstruction with abdominal distention, vomiting, and fluid and electrolyte imbalance.

1 This does not have special significance in cystic fibrosis. 2, 3 This is not an early sign of cystic fibrosis.

Client Need: Physiological Adaptation; **Cognitive Level:** Application; **Nursing Process:** Assessment/Analysis; **Reference:** Ch 31, Cystic Fibrosis, Data Base

185. 2 This regimen will give the child an opportunity to rest before eating.

1 The child should be encouraged to cough; if it is not effective, suctioning can be done after chest percussion and postural drainage. 3 Chest percussion and drainage should be done after aerosol therapy. 4 This could cause the child to vomit.

Client Need: Reduction of Risk Potential; **Cognitive Level:** Application; **Nursing Process:** Planning/Implementation; **Reference:** Ch 31, Cystic Fibrosis, Nursing Care

186. 2 Because the mucous glands secrete thick mucoid secretions that accumulate, reducing ciliary action and mucus flow, the nurse should perform postural drainage, which promotes the removal of mucopurulent secretions by means of gravity.

1 Coughing should be encouraged. 3 Although the nurse should encourage activities appropriate for the child's physical capacity, the child's energy should be conserved during acute phases of illness. 4 This is not necessary; the child with cystic fibrosis can eat regular meals at the usual times.

Client Need: Reduction of Risk Potential; **Cognitive Level:** Application; **Nursing Process:** Planning/Implementation; **Reference:** Ch 31, Cystic Fibrosis, Nursing Care

187. 3 Cystic fibrosis is characterized by an overproduction of viscous mucus by exocrine glands in the lungs. The mucus traps bacteria and foreign debris that adhere to the lining and cannot be expelled by the cilia, thus obstructing the airway and favoring growth of microorganisms and infection.

1 Cardiac defects are not associated with cystic fibrosis. 2 Neuromuscular irritability of the bronchi does not occur in cystic fibrosis. 4 Although there is increased sodium and chloride in the saliva, it does not irritate or inflame the mucous membranes.

Client Need: Physiological Adaptation; **Cognitive Level:** Application; **Nursing Process:** Planning/Implementation; **Reference:** Ch 31, Cystic Fibrosis, Data Base

188. 1 Because children with cystic fibrosis do not absorb the fat-soluble vitamins effectively, they should be given in a water-miscible form.

2 These vitamins can be given with other vitamins once a day; pancreatic enzymes are administered with meals and snacks. 3 The nurse does not have to calibrate a dose of these vitamins based on the child's height and weight. 4 There is no reason to select juice over milk when administering these vitamins.

Client Need: Pharmacological and Parenteral Therapies; **Cognitive Level:** Application; **Integrated Process:** Teaching/ Learning; **Nursing Process:** Planning/Implementation; **Reference:** Ch 31, Cystic Fibrosis, Data Base

189. 1 Hearing is a sense that is not greatly influenced by emotional response in the young child.

2 The emotional trauma of prolonged hospitalization influences the child's cognitive development.

3 The trauma of prolonged hospitalization may also result in speech and other expressive delays.

4 Neuromuscular development may lag because of fewer physical, emotional, and cognitive stimuli.

Client Need: Reduction of Risk Potential; **Cognitive Level:** Application; **Nursing Process:** Assessment/Analysis; **Reference:** Ch 31, Hospitalization of Toddlers, Data Base

190. 3 A 15-month-old toddler would have difficulty complying with directions to remain still and may be extremely frightened by the equipment.

1 This is not necessary; the head must remain still but need not be shaved. 2 This is not necessary unless a contrast medium is being used. 4 The child is too young to understand even a simple explanation of the procedure.

Client Need: Reduction of Risk Potential; **Cognitive Level:** Application; **Nursing Process:** Planning/Implementation; **Reference:** Ch 31, Hospitalization of Toddlers, General Nursing Care of Toddlers

191. 2 Braces are worn to enable the spastic child to control movement. They also prevent deformities that can occur from misalignment.

1 Early ambulation is promoted by maintaining muscle strength and tone, but it is not the reason for applying braces. 3 Exercises, not braces, are used to stretch ligaments and improve muscle strength and tone. 4 Because the child is at the age when self-reliance is important (Erikson's stage of industry versus inferiority) and depends on the braces for self-care, it is unlikely that they would be rejected.

Client Need: Basic Care and Comfort; **Cognitive Level:** Application; **Integrated Process:** Teaching/Learning; **Nursing Process:** Planning/Implementation; **Reference:** Ch 31, Cerebral Palsy, Nursing Care

192. 3 Individuals whose thermoreceptive senses are impaired are unable to detect changes or degrees of temperature. They must be taught to first test the temperature in any water-related activity to prevent scalding and burning.

1 Over-tightening brace straps may lead to circulatory impairment and/or skin breakdown. 2 The child with cerebral palsy has uncontrolled movement of voluntary muscles and does not need to change positions at night to prevent skin breakdown. 4 This is dangerous because this action alters the center of gravity; with practice the child will be able to place the legs in the appropriate position for walking without looking down.

Client Need: Safety and Infection Control; **Cognitive Level:** Application; **Integrated Process:** Teaching/Learning; **Nursing Process:** Planning/Implementation; **Reference:** Ch 31, Cerebral Palsy, Nursing Care

193. 1 The damage is fixed. It does not progressively worsen.

2 Cerebral palsy (CP) is a nonprogressive chronic condition and its effects are predictable. 3 Although mental retardation may be present in some children with cerebral palsy, all children with this disorder are not mentally retarded. 4 A variety of prenatal, perinatal, and postnatal factors contribute to the development of cerebral palsy. It is estimated that the cause of CP is unknown in as many as 80% of people with the disorder.

Client Need: Physiological Adaptation; **Cognitive Level:** Knowledge; **Nursing Process:** Assessment/Analysis; **Reference:** Ch 31, Cerebral Palsy, Data Base

194. 2 Lead poisoning is caused by lead in the environment: sources of lead may be deteriorating paint in a home (inhaled or ingested); lead in products that are used daily, such as batteries, pottery, and glass (ingested); and lead in the atmosphere (which can be inhaled or fall on food that is then ingested).

1 Unless the fat has been exposed to lead, it is not a causative factor. 3 The role of the mother is not an identified factor. 4 This is just one causative factor; there are many others.

Client Need: Safety and Infection Control; **Cognitive Level:** Comprehension; **Nursing Process:** Assessment/Analysis; **Reference:** Ch 31, Lead Poisoning (Plumbism), Data Base

195. 4 Damaged nerve cells do not regenerate. Once mental retardation has occurred, it is not reversible.

1 Damage to kidneys is reversible with treatment. 2 Skeletal changes are not significant and are reversible as lead leaves the body. 3 Effects of lead in bone marrow are reversible when lead is mobilized for excretion in urine or deposition in bone by chelation therapy.

Client Need: Physiological Adaptation; **Cognitive Level:** Application; **Nursing Process:** Assessment/Analysis; **Reference:** Ch 31, Lead Poisoning (Plumbism), Data Base

196. 2 Irreversible neurologic and intellectual damage is the most serious consequence of lead poisoning because of cortical atrophy and encephalopathy.

1 Although there may be a nutritional deficit, it is not the priority. 3, 4 These do occur, but they are reversible.

Client Need: Physiological Adaptation; **Cognitive Level:** Application; **Nursing Process:** Assessment/Analysis; **Reference:** Ch 31, Lead Poisoning (Plumbism), Data Base

197. 3 The child should be given an outlet for tension, and therapeutic play using the equipment needed for the injections is the most appropriate activity.
1 This may ease discomfort, but an outlet for feelings should be provided. 2 Fear is not directed at unfamiliar adults but at the painful treatments. 4 This is part of the preparation, but is not the most important; the child must be allowed to express feelings.
Client Need: Psychosocial Integrity; **Cognitive Level:** Application; **Nursing Process:** Planning/Implementation; **Reference:** Ch 31, Lead Poisoning (Plumbism), Nursing Care

198. 3 Amblyopia is reduced visual acuity that may occur when an eye weakened by strabismus is not forced to function.
1 The lack of binocularity could result in impaired depth and spatial perceptions, not dyslexia. 2 Depth and spatial perceptions are impaired when vision in one eye is severely impaired. 4 Only vision in the affected eye will be diminished.
Client Need: Health Promotion and Maintenance; **Cognitive Level:** Application; **Integrated Process:** Teaching/Learning; **Nursing Process:** Planning/Implementation; **Reference:** Ch 31, Visual Impairment, Data Base

199. 4 If the strabismus is not corrected, sight in the affected eye would be lost because of lack of use.
1 Cataracts do not result from strabismus. 2 Glaucoma is caused by increased intraocular pressure, not strabismus. 3 Refractive errors are related to visual acuity rather than strabismus.
Client Need: Health Promotion and Maintenance; **Cognitive Level:** Application; **Integrated Process:** Teaching/Learning; **Nursing Process:** Planning/Implementation; **Reference:** Ch 31, Visual Impairment, Data Base

200. 2 By 3 to 4 months of age, an infant should localize sound by looking in the direction of the sound.
1 The nurse's observation does not provide information about the infant's ability to see. 3 This response is not within the norm for this age group. 4 This response indicates that that the infant's hearing is not developmentally appropriate.
Client Need: Health Promotion and Maintenance; **Cognitive Level:** Analysis; **Nursing Process:** Assessment/Analysis; **Reference:** Ch 31, Hearing Impairment, Data Base

201. 2 Tinnitus in adolescents is usually related to hearing loud music, especially via headphones.
1 Tinnitus is a concrete occurrence; it is doubtful that it would emerge when there are emotional upsets. 3 Long-resolved ear infections usually have no sequelae, such as buzzing in the ears. 4 Familial deafness is not related to the recent development of an adolescent's tinnitus.
Client Need: Health Promotion and Maintenance; **Cognitive Level:** Analysis; **Nursing Process:** Assessment/Analysis; **Reference:** Ch 31, Hearing Impairment, Data Base

202. 4 This degree of hearing loss causes the child to miss approximately 25% to 40% of conversations. This loss may result in speech deficits if not corrected. Hearing aids usually help improve functioning.
1 The significance of the hearing loss requires further analysis and intervention. 2 There is no evidence that this hearing loss is progressive. 3 The child is missing approximately 25% to 40% of conversations, which would interfere with the educational process unless corrected.
Client Need: Health Promotion and Maintenance; **Cognitive Level:** Application; **Integrated Process:** Teaching/Learning; **Nursing Process:** Planning/Implementation; **Reference:** Ch 31, Hearing Impairment, Data Base

203. 4 Abusive parents may "shop" for hospitals that do not have a previous record of their child; the skeletal survey would provide a revealing injury history if there were abuse.
1 Pinpointing the exact location of a fracture is necessary to plan appropriate treatment and can be done by a single x-ray film of the area; a skeletal survey is more extensive and helpful when abuse is suspected. 2 Cost-effectiveness is not the primary concern if abuse is suspected. 3 A CT scan and MRI would not be required unless internal injuries are suspected.
Client Need: Management of Care; **Cognitive Level:** Analysis; **Nursing Process:** Planning/Implementation; **Reference:** Ch 31, Child Maltreatment, Nursing Care

204. 1 ☐ This is not significant; it may be related to increased fluid intake.
2 ☒ A cast is not flexible and can inhibit circulation. Cold toes, loss of sensation in toes, pain, and inability to move toes should be reported to the physician immediately.
3 ☐ The expected pulse rate for a 9-year-old child ranges from 70 to 110 beats/min.
4 ☒ A tingling sensation in the foot may indicate excessive pressure on the nerves and circulatory system in the casted extremity.
5 ☐ A fiberglass cast dries within minutes; if it remains damp it should be reported before 4 hours have elapsed.
Client Need: Basic Care and Comfort; **Cognitive Level:** Analysis; **Integrated Process:** Communication/Documentation; **Nursing Process:** Evaluation/Outcomes; **Reference:** Ch 31, Fractures, Nursing Care

205. 2 This is the safest way to dry the cast evenly.
1 Besides the danger of burning the child, the cast may dry on the outside and remain damp within. 3 This would impede the circulation of air and delay drying. 4 This may create a draft and be uncomfortable for the child.
Client Need: Basic Care and Comfort; **Cognitive Level:** Application; **Nursing Process:** Planning/Implementation; **Reference:** Ch 31, Fractures, Nursing Care

206. 1 ☐ Rest with elevation of the extremity is recommended; strenuous activity should be avoided for several days.

2 ☒ When swelling of the fingers occurs, the cast can become too tight, resulting in neurovascular damage; permanent damage can occur in 6 to 8 hours.

3 ☒ The casted arm should be in a sling when the child is upright and elevated when resting to promote venous return.

4 ☐ Joints above and below the cast should be moved to maintain flexibility.

Client Need: Basic Care and Comfort; **Cognitive Level:** Analysis; **Integrated Process:** Teaching/Learning; **Nursing Process:** Planning/Implementation; **Reference:** Ch 31, Fractures, Nursing Care

207. 1 The immediate postburn period is marked by dramatic changes in fluid and electrolyte balance. Alterations in electrolyte balance can produce confusion, weakness, cardiac irregularities, and seizures. Secondary to large fluid losses through the denuded skin, vasodilation, and edema formation, hypovolemic shock may develop.

2 Pneumonia would be a later complication associated with immobility. 3 Contractures are a later complication associated with scarring and aggravated by improper positioning and splinting. 4 Hypotension, not hypertension, occurs with hypovolemic shock.

Client Need: Physiological Adaptation; **Cognitive Level:** Application; **Nursing Process:** Planning/Implementation; **Reference:** Ch 31, Burns, Data Base

208. 2 Inhalation burns are usually present with facial burns, regardless of the depth; the immediate threat to life is asphyxia from irritation and edema of the respiratory passages and lungs.

1 Although wound sepsis is a possible complication, it would not be evident until the third to fifth day. 3 Although the child is probably fearful, maintaining a patent airway is the priority. This child is too old for separation anxiety; however, complications related to stress can occur later. 4 Fluid losses can be extremely high but reach their maximum about the fourth day; the initial priority is maintaining a patent airway.

Client Need: Physiological Adaptation; **Cognitive Level:** Application; **Nursing Process:** Assessment/Analysis; **Reference:** Ch 31, Burns, Nursing Care

209. 3 Intramuscular medications are avoided when possible to avoid tissue absorption problems.

1 This is not a consideration in this situation. 2, 4 The mode of administration does not alter the effectiveness of the drug.

Client Need: Pharmacological and Parenteral Therapies; **Cognitive Level:** Comprehension; **Nursing Process:** Assessment/Analysis; **Reference:** Ch 31, Burns, Nursing Care

210. 4 The early school-age child has become a cooperative member of the family and will mimic parents' attitudes and food habits readily.

1 This does not have a major influence on later eating habits. 2 This certainly has some influence, though not major, on later eating habits. 3 The peer group does not become influential until later school age and during adolescence.

Client Need: Psychosocial Integrity; **Cognitive Level:** Application; **Nursing Process:** Assessment/Analysis; **Reference:** Ch 31, Childhood Nutrition

211. 2 Positioning on the right side after feeding facilitates digestion because the pyloric sphincter is on this side and gravity aids in emptying the stomach.

1 The feeding may begin immediately after opening the tube. 3 If the gastrostomy tube is flushed before or after a feeding, water, not normal saline, is used. 4 The usual height for elevation of the gastrostomy tube when feeding an infant is 6 to 8 inches above the stomach.

Client Need: Basic Care and Comfort; **Cognitive Level:** Application; **Nursing Process:** Planning/Implementation; **Reference:** Ch 31, Burns, Nursing Care

212. 3 It is the nurse's responsibility to assess tube placement before each feeding; withdrawing gastric contents before each feeding ensures that the tip of the tube is in the stomach.

1, 2, 4 This is not frequent enough; the tube could be displaced between feedings.

Client Need: Basic Care and Comfort; **Cognitive Level:** Application; **Nursing Process:** Planning/Implementation; **Reference:** Ch 31, Burns, Nursing Care

213. 1 Pinworms emerge nocturnally to lay eggs in the perianal area; eggs are caught on transparent tape in the morning before toileting.

2 A culture will not reveal the presence of parasites. 3 Ova cannot be seen with the naked eye; the parasite is rarely observed in the stool. 4 This is not a test to diagnose pinworms.

Client Need: Reduction of Risk Potential; **Cognitive Level:** Application; **Integrated Process:** Teaching/Learning; **Nursing Process:** Planning/Implementation; **Reference:** Ch 31, Pinworms, Data Base

214. 3 Children with celiac disease have a gluten-induced enteropathy and are unable to absorb fats from the intestinal tract.

1 Stools are large and fatty or frothy, not mucoid. 2 Although stools are large and frothy, they are pale in color because of their high fat content. 4 Stools are large and foul-smelling, and have little color.

Client Need: Basic Care and Comfort; **Cognitive Level:** Comprehension; **Nursing Process:** Assessment/Analysis; **Reference:** Ch 31, Celiac Disease, Data Base

215. 2 Products composed of corn, rice, and millet do not contain gluten and are permitted on a low-gluten diet; tortilla chips are made from corn flour.

1 Pretzels contain wheat flour, which is not permitted on a low-gluten diet; products containing rye, oats, and barley are also restricted. 3 Oatmeal cookies contain oats, which are not permitted on a

low-gluten diet. **4** Peanut butter crackers contain wheat flour, which is not permitted on a low-gluten diet.
Client Need: Basic Care and Comfort; **Cognitive Level:** Analysis; **Integrated Process:** Teaching/Learning; **Nursing Process:** Planning/Implementation; **Reference:** Ch 31, Celiac Disease, Nursing Care

216. **3** Rectal prolapse is a common GI complication of cystic fibrosis and results from wasting of perirectal supporting tissues, secondary to malnutrition.
1 Anal fissures may or may not occur with cystic fibrosis. **2** Intussusception is not associated with cystic fibrosis. **4** Meconium ileus is associated with cystic fibrosis in newborns; it prevents the passage of meconium.
Client Need: Physiological Adaptation; **Cognitive Level:** Comprehension; **Nursing Process:** Assessment/Analysis; **Reference:** Ch 31, Cystic Fibrosis; Data Base

217. **1** Because of a lack of the pancreatic enzyme lipase, fats remain unabsorbed and are excreted in excessive amounts in the stool.
2, 4 This does not cause the typical characteristics of the stools. **3** These are the pancreatic enzymes, whose passage into the intestine is prevented by blocked pancreatic ducts.
Client Need: Physiological Adaptation; **Cognitive Level:** Comprehension; **Nursing Process:** Assessment/Analysis; **Reference:** Ch 31, Cystic Fibrosis, Data Base

218. **2** Thick secretions block the pancreatic ducts, leading to acini dilation and degeneration and producing progressive diffuse fibrosis. Essential pancreatic enzymes are blocked from reaching the duodenum; therefore pancreatic enzymes are administered with meals to assist with digestion. Antibiotics are prescribed to treat respiratory tract infections.
1 These are not indicated in the treatment of cystic fibrosis. **3** Fat-soluble vitamins are necessary in CF secondary to the decreased absorption of fat. Antihistamines are not used because of the drying effect on the already tenacious mucus secretions. **4** These may be used but are not specific for cystic fibrosis. Certain medications may be given via nebulizer.
Client Need: Pharmacological and Parenteral Therapies; **Cognitive Level:** Comprehension; **Nursing Process:** Assessment/Analysis; **Reference:** Ch 31, Cystic Fibrosis, Nursing Care

219. **3** The adult pinworm lives in the rectum or colon and emerges onto the perirectal skin during the hours of sleep, depositing its eggs during this time.
1, 2, 4 Pinworms attach to the bowel wall and do not emerge from the rectum at this time.
Client Need: Reduction of Risk Potential; **Cognitive Level:** Comprehension; **Integrated Process:** Teaching/Learning; **Nursing Process:** Planning/Implementation; **Reference:** Ch 31, Pinworms, Data Base

220. **4** Pinworms attache to the bowel wall in the cecum and appendix and can damage the mucosa, causing appendicitis.
1 Pinworms do not migrate to the liver. **2** Although pinworms (and their ova) are ingested by mouth, they do not attach there; inflammation of the mouth is not a complication of pinworm infestation. **3** Pinworms do not migrate to the respiratory system.
Client Need: Physiological Adaptation; **Cognitive Level:** Comprehension; **Nursing Process:** Assessment/Analysis; **Reference:** Ch 31, Pinworms, Data Base

221. **4** All household members should be treated at the same time unless they are younger than 2 years or pregnant.
1 This drug is not recommended for children under the age of 2 years. **2** This is not a significant criterion for administration of medication because eggs are airborne. **3** Positive testing is not a criterion for administration to family members.
Client Need: Pharmacological and Parenteral Therapies; **Cognitive Level:** Application; **Nursing Process:** Planning/Implementation; **Reference:** Ch 31, Pinworms, Nursing Care

222. **2** The use of a potty chair allows the child to display its contents with pride; sitting on top of a toilet seat is frightening for many children. Potty chairs also allow the child to place feet on the floor for an effective Valsalva maneuver for bowel evacuation.
1 Sitting on a toilet seat can be frightening for a toddler; timing of bowel training should coincide with the gastrocolic reflex. **3** Bowel training should begin when the child shows readiness. **4** A diet consisting mainly of solid foods will make stools more bulky and easier to control.
Client Need: Health Promotion and Maintenance; **Cognitive Level:** Application; **Integrated Process:** Teaching/Learning; **Nursing Process:** Planning/Implementation; **Reference:** Ch 31, Growth and Development, Major Learning Events

223. **4** Studies have shown that culture and family eating habits have an impact on a child's eating habits.
1 Inheritance is not known to influence eating habits, although it is believed that there may be hereditary factors associated with obesity. **2** Childhood obesity is a known predictor of adult obesity. **3** Although there is a trend toward this, with intervention it can be prevented.
Client Need: Psychosocial Integrity; **Cognitive Level:** Application; **Nursing Process:** Assessment/Analysis; **Reference:** Ch 31, Childhood Nutrition

224. **3** Dehydration promotes the sickling of erythrocytes. Increased fluid intake minimizes the chance that a sickle cell pain episode will reoccur.
1 This is not necessary or helpful for a child with sickle cell anemia. **2** Rigorous exercise is contraindicated because the decrease in oxygenation may cause sickling. **4** This is not necessary.

Client Need: Reduction of Risk Potential; **Cognitive Level:** Application; **Nursing Process:** Planning/Implementation; **Reference:** Ch 31, Sickle Cell Anemia, Nursing Care

225. **2** The child is having an allergic reaction, and the infusion must be stopped immediately to prevent serious complications.

1 The primary care practitioner should be notified after the infusion has been stopped. **3** Slowing the rate of infusion will not halt the allergic reaction to the transfused blood. **4** This is dangerous as an initial action because the degree of allergic reaction cannot be determined at this time.

Client Need: Pharmacological and Parenteral Therapies; **Cognitive Level:** Application; **Nursing Process:** Planning/ Implementation; **Reference:** Ch 31, β-Thalassemia (Cooley's Anemia), Nursing Care

226. **3** Folic acid acts as a necessary coenzyme in the formation of heme, the iron-containing protein in hemoglobin.

1 Calcium is not involved in the production of red blood cells. **2** This is a coenzyme in carbohydrate metabolism. **4** This is a control agent for energy production and tissue formation.

Client Need: Basic Care and Comfort; **Cognitive Level:** Comprehension; **Integrated Process:** Teaching/Learning; **Nursing Process:** Planning/Implementation; **Reference:** Ch 31, Iron Deficiency Anemia, Nursing Care

227. **3** Proteins are essential for the synthesis of the blood proteins, albumin, fibrinogen, and hemoglobin. Ascorbic acid influences the removal of iron from ferritin (making more iron available for production of heme) and influences the conversion of folic acid to folinic acid.

1, 2, 4 These are not involved in the synthesis of red blood cells.

Client Need: Basic Care and Comfort; **Cognitive Level:** Comprehension; **Integrated Process:** Teaching/Learning; **Nursing Process:** Planning/Implementation; **Reference:** Ch 31, Iron Deficiency Anemia, Nursing Care

228. **3** A diet of only milk is not sufficient to meet the infant's iron needs. Meat and fortified cereals are high in iron. Finger foods are appropriate for older infants.

1 At this age weaning from the bottle is not the issue—supplementary iron intake is. **2** Although health care and monitoring will be required, the metabolic clinic is not the appropriate referral. **4** Although this would increase iron intake, it is not appropriate for a 1 year old, nor is it desirable.

Client Need: Basic Care and Comfort; **Cognitive Level:** Application; **Integrated Process:** Teaching/Learning; **Nursing Process:** Planning/Implementation; **Reference:** Ch 31, Iron Deficiency Anemia, Nursing Care

229. **3** Children with a chronic illness, such as hemolytic anemia, should not be exposed to the additional stress of infection.

1 A regular intake of fluid is recommended. **2** Activity is not restricted, although the child may self-restrict activity because of anemia-induced fatigue. **4** Regular meals with the family should be encouraged.

Client Need: Safety and Infection Control; **Cognitive Level:** Application; **Integrated Process:** Teaching/Learning; **Nursing Process:** Planning/Implementation; **Reference:** Ch 31, β-Thalassemia (Cooley's Anemia), Nursing Care

230. **1** HbS is the abbreviation for sickle cell hemoglobin, a genetic defect. This hemoglobin assumes a crescent shape when deoxygenated.

2 HbA is the abbreviation for expected adult hemoglobin. **3** HCV is the abbreviation for the hepatitis C. **4** HBV is the abbreviation for the hepatitis B virus.

Client Need: Reduction of Risk Potential; **Cognitive Level:** Analysis; **Integrated Process:** Teaching/Learning; **Nursing Process:** Planning/Implementation; **Reference:** Ch 31, Sickle Cell Anemia, Data Base

231. **4** In this type of episode there is a pooling of blood in the liver and spleen with a decreased circulating blood volume and subsequent shock.

1 Painful episodes are characteristic of vaso-occlusive crisis. **2** Decreased RBC production and the profound anemia that ensues are characteristics of aplastic crisis. **3** Increased RBC destruction and concomitant anemia, jaundice, and reticulocytosis are characteristics of hyperhemolytic crisis.

Client Need: Physiological Adaptation; **Cognitive Level:** Application; **Nursing Process:** Assessment/Analysis; **Reference:** Ch 31, Sickle Cell Anemia, Data Base

232. **3** RBCs change to the sickle shape when deoxygenated because of polymerization of the abnormal hemoglobin. This process damages the RBC membrane, and can cause the cells to become entangled in the blood vessels. This deprives the tissues that are downstream from the occlusion of O_2 and causes ischemia and infarction, which can result in organ damage. Dehydration, stress, infection, and electrolyte imbalance can cause this sickling process.

1 This will not prevent thrombus formation. **2** The child's condition determines the activity level; although bed rest may be required during a pain episode, at other times it is rarely necessary. **4** Anticoagulants do not help prevent thrombus formation in sickle cell anemia.

Client Need: Reduction of Risk Potential; **Cognitive Level:** Application; **Nursing Process:** Planning/Implementation; **Reference:** Ch 31, Sickle Cell Anemia, Nursing Care

233. **4** Cardiac decompensation results because the heart attempts to maintain tissue oxygenation by increasing its workload.

1 Although an elevated bilirubin level can occur with hemolytic anemia, this is not the priority assessment. **2** An elevated WBC count indicates that there is an infection; however, the data do not indicate the presence of an infection. **3** Hemoglobin in the urine suggests hemolytic anemia. Although it is important

to assess for the cause of the anemia, it is not the priority.
Client Need: Physiological Adaptation; **Cognitive Level:** Application; **Nursing Process:** Assessment/Analysis; **Reference:** Ch 31, Iron Deficiency Anemia, Data Base

234. **2** Warmth causes vasodilation, which will lessen the pain of the vaso-occlusive crisis.
1 IV fluids should be increased to dilute the blood and prevent further sickling. **3** Cold will cause more vasoconstriction and increase pain. **4** This is an inadequate dose for an adolescent.
Client Need: Basic Care and Comfort; **Cognitive Level:** Application; **Nursing Process:** Planning/Implementation; **Reference:** Ch 31, Sickle Cell Anemia, Nursing Care

235. **2** Children with both illnesses have inadequate resistance to infection. Sickling results from low oxygen levels; celiac crisis results from malnourishment and immunologic defects.
1 Activity need not be limited in celiac disease; strenuous activity should be limited in sickle cell anemia. **3** This is important for children with celiac disease; it is not necessary for children with sickle cell anemia. **4** This diet is not particularly helpful for children with sickle cell anemia or celiac disease.
Client Need: Reduction of Risk Potential; **Cognitive Level:** Application; **Nursing Process:** Planning/Implementation; **Reference:** Ch 31, Sickle Cell Anemia, Nursing Care

236. **2** Pain in the area of involvement is a major problem in pain episodes and demands priority care; hydration is necessary to promote and maintain hemodilution.
1 Although hydration is a major concern, nutrition is not. **3** Neither of these are priority concerns during a pain episode. **4** Prevention of infection is not a major concern during a crisis; the major concern is pain management.
Client Need: Basic Care and Comfort; **Cognitive Level:** Application; **Nursing Process:** Planning/Implementation; **Reference:** Ch 31, Sickle Cell Anemia, Nursing Care

NURSING CARE OF PRESCHOOLERS

237. **2** The child will move her hand to the abdomen; the nurse can then engage the child's cooperation and do a general assessment.
1 Further assessment is necessary; it should be determined whether the crying is due to pain or fear. **3** The parents may hold the child, but they should not restrain her because this could increase anxiety. **4** This is not an initial intervention; the child's cooperation will be needed for this procedure.
Client Need: Health Promotion and Maintenance; **Cognitive Level:** Application; **Integrated Process:** Caring; **Nursing Process:** Assessment/Analysis; **Reference:** Ch 32, Hospitalization of Preschoolers, Data Base

238. **2** The nurse is seeking clarification while encouraging each child to communicate verbally, rather than expressing their differences physically.

1 This is accusatory and nontherapeutic. **3** This is a threatening response. **4** This is not relevant; the nurse should be concerned with the present situation.
Client Need: Health Promotion and Maintenance; **Cognitive Level:** Application; **Integrated Process:** Communication/ Documentation; **Nursing Process:** Planning/Implementation; **Reference:** Ch 32, Play (Cooperative Play)

239. **1** Children with nephrotic syndrome are treated with immunosuppressive agents including steroids. During exacerbations they may have a characteristic pale, overweight appearance from edema. Steroid side effects include growth retardation, cataracts, obesity, and hirsutism. Children may become very sensitive about these changes as they grow older.
2 Although this may be indicated, body-image problems pose a greater threat. **3** Engaging in usual childhood activities between attacks should promote the development of fine muscle coordination. **4** Sterility is not associated with nephrotic syndrome.
Client Need: Psychosocial Integrity; **Cognitive Level:** Application; **Integrated Process:** Caring; **Nursing Process:** Planning/ Implementation; **Reference:** Ch 32, Nephrotic Syndrome, Nursing Care

240. **4** A classic sign of nephrotic syndrome is gross proteinuria; a decrease indicates that treatment has been successful.
1 A child with nephrotic syndrome has gross edema and oliguria; increased urine output is the desired outcome. **2** Children with glomerulonephritis have hematuria; it is not expected in children with nephrotic syndrome. **3** Children with diabetes mellitus have glycosuria; it is not expected in children with nephrotic syndrome.
Client Need: Physiological Adaptation; **Cognitive Level:** Analysis; **Nursing Process:** Evaluation/Outcomes; **Reference:** Ch 32, Nephrotic Syndrome, Data Base

241. **3** This focuses on the child's feelings and a familiar object of security.
1 The child may experience pain as part of the treatment, so the statement is untruthful. **2, 4** Diverting the child will not alleviate fear and anxiety.
Client Need: Psychosocial Integrity; **Cognitive Level:** Application; **Integrated Process:** Caring; **Nursing Process:** Planning/ Implementation; **Reference:** Ch 32, Hospitalization of Preschoolers, General Nursing Care of Preschoolers

242. **2** Fear of mutilation is typical of the preschooler because they have vague views of body boundaries.
1 Toddlers are more likely to fear separation from parents. **3** Preschoolers do not view death as final. **4** Although preschoolers do indulge in magical thinking, they have not yet developed the concept of supernatural beliefs.
Client Need: Health Promotion and Maintenance; **Cognitive Level:** Comprehension; **Nursing Process:** Assessment/Analysis; **Reference:** Ch 32, Hospitalization of Preschoolers, Data Base

243. **4** The anxiety that occurs in 4 year olds regarding invasive procedures will be lessened when the child holds the scope and realizes how it will be used.

1 Stating the word pain may increase anxiety; a 4-year-old child thinks in concrete terms and probably will not believe the nurse until experiencing the procedure. **2** This is suggesting an unsafe activity. **3** This request will more likely be instituted after the child has handled the scope and recognizes what to expect.

Client Need: Health Promotion and Maintenance; **Cognitive Level:** Application; **Nursing Process:** Planning/Implementation; **Reference:** Ch 32, Hospitalization of Preschoolers, Data Base

244. **3** A few minutes will be enough time for the child to begin self-feeding. The nurse should provide both physical and emotional support, because the child's request for help indicates regression and the need for dependence during a period of stress.

1 This does not provide the child the help that may be needed. **2** It may be a while until the child feels better; in the meantime, adequate nourishment to provide for healing is needed. **4** This can cause stress, feelings of guilt, and embarrassment to a sick child.

Client Need: Health Promotion and Maintenance; **Cognitive Level:** Analysis; **Integrated Process:** Caring; **Nursing Process:** Planning/Implementation; **Reference:** Ch 32, Hospitalization of Preschoolers, Data Base

245. **1** The child may be fearful of the examining room experience. If the nurse greets the child while in the safety of the waiting room, it might help to make the experience less threatening.

2 Calling the child without entering the room is an authoritarian approach that will not limit the child's anxiety. **3** Having someone else bring the child into the examining room is an authoritarian approach that may make the child more fearful. **4** Standing at the examining room door while the child walks down the hall is an authoritarian approach that may increase the child's anxiety.

Client Need: Health Promotion and Maintenance; **Cognitive Level:** Application; **Integrated Process:** Caring; **Nursing Process:** Planning/Implementation; **Reference:** Ch 32, Hospitalization of Preschoolers, General Nursing Care of Preschoolers

246. **1** Prednisone reduces the individual's resistance to certain infectious processes. Also prednisone is an antiinflammatory drug that masks infection.

2 The child will self-limit activity based on the respiratory status. **3** Eosinophil counts are often consistently elevated in children with asthma. **4** The child will need adequate hydration to assist with loosening and removing mucus.

Client Need: Pharmacological and Parenteral Therapies; **Cognitive Level:** Application; **Nursing Process:** Planning/Implementation; **Reference:** Ch 32, Asthma, Nursing Care

247. **4** Euphoria and mood swings may result from steroid therapy.

1 Alopecia does not result from steroid therapy. **2** An increased appetite, not anorexia, results from steroid therapy. **3** Weight gain, not weight loss, results from steroid therapy.

Client Need: Pharmacological and Parenteral Therapies; **Cognitive Level:** Application; **Nursing Process:** Evaluation/Outcomes; **Reference:** Ch 32, Leukemia, Nursing Care

248. **3** Generally, antineoplastic drugs act by interfering with, or inhibiting, synthesis of DNA in malignant cells.

1 Malignant cells are not infected, in the normal sense of the term; therefore this drug does not act in this manner. **2** Bone marrow depression is a side effect of this drug, not a desired action. **4** This is the activity of the malignant cells themselves.

Client Need: Pharmacological and Parenteral Therapies; **Cognitive Level:** Comprehension; **Nursing Process:** Assessment/Analysis; **Reference:** Ch 32, Leukemia, Data Base

249. **1** Prednisone is a synthetic glucocorticoid that has an active antiinflammatory effect by stabilizing lysosomal membranes and thus inhibiting proteolytic enzyme release.

2 Prednisone does not affect mitosis, but inhibits proteolytic enzyme release. **3** Although prednisone increases the appetite and creates a sense of well-being, these are not the reasons it is administered. **4** There is no indication the child is receiving radiation.

Client Need: Pharmacological and Parenteral Therapies; **Cognitive Level:** Application; **Nursing Process:** Planning/Implementation; **Reference:** Ch 32, Leukemia, Data Base

250. **4** Vincristine is highly neurotoxic, causing paresthesias, muscle weakness, ptosis, diplopia, paralytic ileus, vocal cord paralysis, and loss of deep tendon reflexes.

1 The most severe problems associated with vincristine are neurologic and neuromuscular. **2** Hematologic effects are rare with vincristine. **3** Alopecia is reversible with cessation of the drug.

Client Need: Pharmacological and Parenteral Therapies; **Cognitive Level:** Application; **Nursing Process:** Evaluation/Outcomes; **Reference:** Ch 32, Leukemia, Nursing Care

251. **1** Children with leukemia most often die of infection; a lowered neutrophil count is associated with myelosuppressant therapy.

2 These measures are not appropriate to prevent infection resulting from neutropenia; they are appropriate for treating the anemia. **3** These measures are not appropriate to prevent infection resulting from neutropenia; they are more appropriate for preventing hemorrhage. **4** These measures are not appropriate to prevent infection resulting from neutropenia; they are used to treat stomatitis.

Client Need: Pharmacological and Parenteral Therapies; **Cognitive Level:** Analysis; **Nursing Process:** Planning/Implementation; **Reference:** Ch 32, Leukemia, Nursing Care

252. **1** The child from 1 to 4 years of age is learning to use the body and manipulate and experiment with all aspects of the environment; these abilities

challenge the examiner and may require modifications when doing a physical examination. **2** The school-age child is able to cooperate and understand during the examination; however, modesty should be respected. **3** From 6 to 12 months of age it is usually easier for the examination to be done with the infant held on the parent's lap to limit stranger anxiety. **4** The infant often enjoys having clothing removed and is easily distracted with sounds and smiles.

Client Need: Health Promotion and Maintenance; **Cognitive Level:** Application; **Nursing Process:** Assessment/Analysis; **Reference:** Ch 32, Hospitalization of Preschoolers, Data Base

253. **1** Role-playing encourages expression of concerns through behavior, since children's ability to verbalize feelings is limited.

2 The preschooler is too young to think about careers. **3** This may occur, but it is not a purpose of role-playing. **4** Although preschoolers try to imitate adults, providing guidelines for adult behavior is premature.

Client Need: Health Promotion and Maintenance; **Cognitive Level:** Comprehension; **Nursing Process:** Assessment/Analysis; **Reference:** Ch 32, Play (Cooperative Play)

254. **3** It is common for 4 year olds to boast and exaggerate and to be impatient, noisy, and selfish.

1 More advanced, cooperative play is expected of 4 year olds. **2** This is unusual for 4 year olds since they are striving toward more initiative and less dependence. **4** The toddler's tendency toward tantrums and negativism should have waned by 4 years of age.

Client Need: Health Promotion and Maintenance; **Cognitive Level:** Application; **Nursing Process:** Assessment/Analysis; **Reference:** Ch 32, Play (Cooperative Play)

255. **3** Most 4 year olds are imaginative; because the line between fantasy and reality is blurred, imaginary playmates are common at this age. Generally, they are given up when the child starts school.

1 This assumption is not relevant at this age; it becomes a concern when the child reaches school age. **2, 4** This response would cause unnecessary concern; it provides false information.

Client Need: Health Promotion and Maintenance; **Cognitive Level:** Analysis; **Integrated Process:** Teaching/Learning; **Nursing Process:** Planning/Implementation; **Reference:** Ch 32, Play (Cooperative Play)

256. **4** Fear of mutilation and intrusive procedures is most common at this age because of fantasies and active imagination. These children also connect illness with being bad and view intrusion as punishment.

1 A child this age usually has little previous contact with pain and therefore little experience on which to base fear. **2** Death is seen as reversible and not final. **3** Fear of isolation from peers is a problem for school-age children and adolescents.

Client Need: Health Promotion and Maintenance; **Cognitive Level:** Comprehension; **Integrated Process:** Caring; **Nursing Process:** Assessment/Analysis; **Reference:** Ch 32, Hospitalization of Preschoolers, Data Base

257. **2** Because their verbal ability is still limited, preschool children act out their feelings via play.

1 Therapeutic play does not necessarily involve other children. **3** Acceptance of hospitalization will not occur until the child has coped with fears. **4** The child needs to cope with feelings rather than forget them.

Client Need: Psychosocial Integrity; **Cognitive Level:** Application; **Integrated Process:** Caring; **Nursing Process:** Planning/Implementation; **Reference:** Ch 32, Hospitalization of Preschoolers, General Nursing Care of Preschoolers

258. **2** Piaget stresses that age 7 is the turning point in mental development. New forms of organization appear at this age that mark the beginning of logic, symbolism, and abstract thought.

1 A 5-year-old is capable of tying laces. **3** A toddler is capable of making simple decisions. **4** An infant is capable of hand-eye coordination.

Client Need: Health Promotion and Maintenance; **Cognitive Level:** Application; **Integrated Process:** Teaching/Learning; **Nursing Process:** Planning/Implementation; **Reference:** Ch 32, Growth and Development, Five Years

259. **2** A respiratory tract obstruction usually occurs in the larynx, trachea, or major bronchi (usually right bronchus). Hoarseness may indicate vocal cord injury. Unintelligible speech may indicate an interference in the flow of air out of the respiratory tract and/or obstruction or injury to the larynx.

1 A retropharyngeal abscess would not produce these clinical signs. **3** An acute respiratory tract infection would not immediately cause these clinical signs. **4** Because of the sudden onset of these clinical signs and the age of the child, this is unlikely.

Client Need: Physiological Adaptation; **Cognitive Level:** Analysis; **Nursing Process:** Assessment/Analysis; **Reference:** Ch 32, Aspiration of Foreign Objects, Data Base

260. **3** Gas exchange is limited because of narrowing and swelling of the bronchi; the Pco_2 level rises.

1 The pH would decrease; the child is in respiratory acidosis, not alkalosis. **2** The O_2 level would be decreased, not increased. **4** This would be increased to compensate for acidosis.

Client Need: Physiological Adaptation; **Cognitive Level:** Application; **Nursing Process:** Assessment/Analysis; **Reference:** Ch 32, Asthma, Data Base

261. **4** Cold can precipitate bronchospasm, and increased exercise depletes O_2.

1 Treatment of asthma does not involve a low-fat diet. **2** Asthma is a chronic condition. Return to usual activities after the acute stage is essential for growth and development. **3** Although increased protein and calories may be needed to support the child during a coexisting bacterial infection in the

acute stage, a return to usual eating habits is indicated by the time of discharge.
Client Need: Reduction of Risk Potential; **Cognitive Level:** Application; **Nursing Process:** Planning/Implementation; **Reference:** Ch 32, Asthma, Nursing Care

262. 1 ⊠ Parents should be taught to limit allergens in the home that can precipitate asthma attacks (e.g., no carpets, no down pillows, wet-mop floors, vacuum when the child is not in the home, no scented household products).
2 ☐ Consistent limits should be placed on the child's behavior regardless of the illness; a chronic illness does not eliminate the need for limit setting.
3 ☐ Environmental moisture is necessary for these children; cold environments should be avoided.
4 ⊠ Medications to control inflammation including inhaled corticosteroids and long-acting beta$_2$-agonists must be continued to suppress exacerbations of asthma.
5 ☐ The child should return to school and continue to interact with schoolmates and friends.
Client Need: Health Promotion and Maintenance; **Cognitive Level:** Analysis; **Integrated Process:** Teaching/Learning; **Nursing Process:** Planning/Implementation; **Reference:** Ch 32, Asthma, Nursing Care

263. 1 Nonstrenuous, diversional activities involving interpersonal relationships with another person provide better support and resting conditions than does more active play.
2 A jigsaw puzzle is too complicated for a 5-year-old child and does not provide the human contact needed. 3 This will probably increase the child's fretfulness and does not provide the human contact needed. 4 Although a doll is appropriate for a 5-year-old child, it does not provide the human contact needed.
Client Need: Psychosocial Integrity; **Cognitive Level:** Analysis; **Integrated Process:** Caring; **Nursing Process:** Planning/Implementation; **Reference:** Ch 32, Hospitalization of Preschoolers, General Nursing Care of Preschoolers

264. 2 The seepage of blood from the operative site fills the oral cavity, causing the child to swallow frequently.
1 Snoring can be expected after a tonsillectomy. 3 Because the child has been NPO for an extended time and is not able to swallow fluids easily, there will probably be complaints of thirst. 4 This may be a later sign of hemorrhage; frequent swallowing would be an initial sign.
Client Need: Physiological Adaptation; **Cognitive Level:** Application; **Nursing Process:** Evaluation/Outcomes; **Reference:** Ch 32, Tonsillectomy and Adenoidectomy, Nursing Care

265. 1 ☐ An elevated temperature is a characteristic of sepsis, not asthma.
2 ☐ Crackles are associated with pulmonary edema, not asthma.

3 ⊠ Bronchial constriction with mucus production causes wheezing.
4 ⊠ With the decrease in arterial oxygenation associated with asthma, the heart rate will increase.
5 ☐ Hypertension, not hypotension, may occur with asthma.
Client Need: Physiological Adaptation; **Cognitive Level:** Analysis; **Nursing Process:** Assessment/Analysis; **Reference:** Ch 32, Asthma, Data Base

266. 3 Infection is a constant threat because of a poor general state of nutrition, a tendency toward skin breakdown in edematous areas, corticosteroid therapy, and lowered immunoglobulin levels.
1 Fluid monitoring is important in determining whether restriction is indicated. 2 The nurse should encourage intake of foods with high nutritional value and restrict salt during massive edema; the priority is preventing infection. 4 Bed rest may be needed for severe edema, but generally ambulation is preferred.
Client Need: Safety and Infection Control; **Cognitive Level:** Application; **Nursing Process:** Planning/Implementation; **Reference:** Ch 32, Nephrotic Syndrome, Nursing Care

267. 1 Poor appetite and decreased energy are associated with the accumulation of toxic waste; anemia accounts for the pallor.
2 Activity would not cause these signs and symptoms. 3 An elevated temperature probably would be present but an infection would not cause a muddy pallor. 4 Discontinuing the corticosteroids and diuretics that are usually prescribed would probably result in recurrence of edema in steroid-dependent children.
Client Need: Physiological Adaptation; **Cognitive Level:** Analysis; **Nursing Process:** Assessment/Analysis; **Reference:** Ch 32, Nephrotic Syndrome, Nursing Care

268. 3 A renal biopsy is an invasive procedure. In the early stages, Wilms' tumor is encapsulated. Any disruption of the tumor capsule could precipitate metastasis.
1 An MRI is helpful in making a diagnosis. 2 A CT scan is helpful in making a diagnosis. 4 An abdominal ultrasound is helpful in making a diagnosis.
Client Need: Reduction of Risk Potential; **Cognitive Level:** Application; **Integrated Process:** Communication/Documentation; **Nursing Process:** Planning/Implementation; **Reference:** Ch 32, Wilms' Tumor (Nephroblastoma), Nursing Care

269. 4 There is an increased appetite with increased deposition of fat on the abdomen and trunk and muscle wasting, which results in thin extremities.
1 Increased excretion of calcium causes a retarded linear growth with a short stature. 2 Because of the excess production of androgens, virilization and hirsutism occur. 3 Increased salt and water retention cause hypertension and hypernatremia.

Client Need: Pharmacological and Parenteral Therapies; **Cognitive Level:** Application; **Nursing Process:** Evaluation/ Outcomes; **Reference:** Ch 32, Nephrotic Syndrome, Nursing Care

270. **4** Comparison of daily weights is the most accurate way to assess fluid retention or loss.

1 This would be difficult for a child this age and would not be accurate. **2** Assessment of urine for protein gives information about the disease process but not about the amount of fluid retention. **3** This is a measure for the degree of ascites; it would only measure fluid retention indirectly.

Client Need: Basic Care and Comfort; **Cognitive Level:** Application; **Nursing Process:** Evaluation/Outcomes; **Reference:** Ch 32, Nephrotic Syndrome, Nursing Care

271. **3** The restricted ventilation accompanying an asthma attack limits the body's ability to blow off CO_2. As CO_2 accumulates in the body fluids, it reacts with water to produce carbonic acid (H_2CO_3); the result is respiratory acidosis.

1 The problem basic to asthma is respiratory, not metabolic. **2** Respiratory alkalosis is caused by exhaling large amounts of CO_2; asthma attacks cause CO_2 retention. **4** Asthma is a respiratory problem, not a metabolic one; metabolic acidosis can result from an increase of nonvolatile acids or a loss of base bicarbonate.

Client Need: Physiological Adaptation; **Cognitive Level:** Analysis; **Nursing Process:** Assessment/Analysis; **Reference:** Ch 32, Asthma, Data Base

272. **4** Jaundice usually indicates liver damage or excessive hemolysis and is not a sign of leukemia unless hepatic damage from late effects of the disease or drugs has occurred. Edema is not a manifestation of the disease, because the pathophysiology does not involve transport of fluids.

1 Marked fatigue and pallor are the result of anemia associated with leukemia. **2** Multiple bruises and petechiae are the result of thrombocytopenia associated with leukemia. **3** Enlarged lymph nodes, spleen, and liver are the result of the infiltration of these organs with leukemic cells.

Client Need: Physiological Adaptation; **Cognitive Level:** Application; **Nursing Process:** Assessment/Analysis; **Reference:** Ch 32, Leukemia, Data Base

273. **2** Because of the increased capillary fragility and decreased platelet count that accompany leukemia, even the slightest trauma can cause hemorrhage. Brushing the teeth has caused gingival hemorrhage and the incident should be documented; this information may also assist in defining the treatment plan.

1 It would be wiser to eliminate the use of a toothbrush and use a sponge-type applicator. **3** It cannot be assumed that a 4 year old would or could follow such a direction. **4** This can irritate the gums, causing more trauma. If oral ulcers develop, the mouth should be rinsed with an isotonic solution such as normal saline.

Client Need: Safety and Infection Control; **Cognitive Level:** Application; **Integrated Process:** Communication/ Documentation; **Nursing Process:** Planning/Implementation; **Reference:** Ch 32, Leukemia, Nursing Care

274. **2** Radiation is used to destroy leukemic cells in the brain because chemotherapeutic agents are inadequately absorbed through the blood-brain barrier.

1 This is not the primary reason for the treatment; it is a curative measure. **3** Radiation does not reduce the risk for infection. **4** Cranial radiation has no effect on the systemic leukemic process.

Client Need: Physiological Adaptation; **Cognitive Level:** Comprehension; **Integrated Process:** Teaching/Learning; **Nursing Process:** Planning/Implementation; **Reference:** Ch 32, Leukemia, Data Base

NURSING CARE OF SCHOOL-AGE CHILDREN

275. **1** Regression is expected in times of stress. It is a transient need that should be accepted, because it helps reduce anxiety.

2 Distraction works only as long as it is employed. **3** It is the nurse's responsibility to understand the child's response to hospitalization and address the child's needs at this time. **4** Cause (thumb-sucking) and future effect (buckteeth) will not be meaningful to a 6 year old; furthermore, thumb-sucking may or may not cause malocclusion.

Client Need: Health Promotion and Maintenance; **Cognitive Level:** Application; **Integrated Process:** Caring; **Nursing Process:** Planning/Implementation; **Reference:** Ch 33, Hospitalization of School-Age Children, General Nursing Care of School-Age Children

276. **4** According to Piaget's cognitive development theory, school-age children use concrete operational thinking; a general discussion in concrete terms will be understood and transferred to the actual situation.

1, 2 This requires conceptual thinking, which is just beginning to develop during the school-age years; 8 year olds are not ready for this thought process. **3** These children are capable of understanding a concrete explanation; this request belittles them.

Client Need: Health Promotion and Maintenance; **Cognitive Level:** Application; **Integrated Process:** Teaching/Learning; **Nursing Process:** Planning/Implementation; **Reference:** Ch 33, Growth and Development

277. **2** GI bleeding may result from prolonged use of NSAIDs because of their irritating effect on the mucosa.

1 This can occur but is not a sign of toxicity. **3** This does not occur with NSAIDs. **4** Drowsiness, not hyperactivity, may occur.

Client Need: Pharmacological and Parenteral Therapies; **Cognitive Level:** Application; **Nursing Process:** Evaluation/ Outcomes; **Reference:** Ch 33, Juvenile Idiopathic Arthritis, Nursing Care

278. 2 The peak action of Novolin N insulin is 6 to 8 hours.
1 This is the peak time for regular insulin, not Novolin N insulin. **3, 4** The peak action of Novolin N insulin is 6 to 8 hours; this is too late.
Client Need: Pharmacological and Parenteral Therapies; **Cognitive Level:** Application; **Nursing Process:** Evaluation/Outcomes; **Reference:** Ch 33, Diabetes Mellitus, Nursing Care

279. 2 School-age children enjoy competition, have manipulative skills, and are creative.
1 This is more appropriate for the toddler or preschooler, who is developing fine motor skills. **3** This activity is inappropriate during an acute illness because it requires too much energy. **4** These activities are passive and ignore the 6-year-old child's developmental needs.
Client Need: Health Promotion and Maintenance; **Cognitive Level:** Application; **Nursing Process:** Planning/Implementation; **Reference:** Ch 33, Hospitalization of School-Age Children, Play

280. 4 6 year olds are aware of their hands as tools and enjoy building simple structures.
1 This is more appropriate for preschoolers. **2, 3** This is more useful for an older school-age child, with a longer attention span and a better ability to follow instructions.
Client Need: Health Promotion and Maintenance; **Cognitive Level:** Application; **Nursing Process:** Planning/Implementation; **Reference:** Ch 33, Hospitalization of School-Age Children, Play

281. 1 ☐ This could increase his boredom.
2 ☒ School-age children have an interest in hobbies or collections of various kinds as a means of gathering information and knowledge about the world in which they live.
3 ☐ This would not interest the average 9 year old.
4 ☒ School-age children are industrious and making a model airplane is an appropriate age-related activity.
5 ☐ These probably would not interest a 9 year old.
Client Need: Health Promotion and Maintenance; **Cognitive Level:** Analysis; **Nursing Process:** Planning/Implementation; **Reference:** Ch 33, Hospitalization of School-Age Children, Play

282. 1 The reserved student should be given the opportunity to interact with peers.
2 The class clown may not be able to accept the responsibility needed for a leadership role. **3** The child who has an established nurse-client relationship may have difficulty interacting with the nurse in a new role. **4** Although the outgoing child probably would be able to take on added responsibility, the child does not need help with social interaction.
Client Need: Psychosocial Integrity; **Cognitive Level:** Analysis; **Nursing Process:** Planning/Implementation; **Reference:** Ch 33, Hospitalization of School-Age Children, Play

283. 4 Because young children have difficulty verbalizing their fears or anxiety, play is a therapeutic way for these feelings to be expressed.
1 A child this age is unable to express feelings entirely through words. **2** Young school-age children are still somewhat egocentric and therefore interested in their own experiences and sensations. **3** This may be helpful for a toddler or preschooler; school-age children need to act out their fears.
Client Need: Psychosocial Integrity; **Cognitive Level:** Application; **Integrated Process:** Caring; **Nursing Process:** Planning/Implementation; **Reference:** Ch 33, Hospitalization of School-Age Children, General Nursing Care of School-Age Children

284. 2 Eight year olds are beginning to achieve a sense of industry and accomplishment. They are in Piaget's stage of concrete operations wherein they are able to use their thought processes to experience actions. Their growing independence enables them to make decisions based on what they have learned.
1 Six year olds are just beginning to experience the developmental goals of the school-age child. They are not ready to make choices based upon what they have learned. **3** Preadolescents are beginning to assert their independence and probably would rebel if taught what they should eat. **4** Adolescents need to conform to their peer group. What is learned in a nutrition class probably would be ignored in favor of preestablished preferences.
Client Need: Health Promotion and Maintenance; **Cognitive Level:** Analysis; **Integrated Process:** Teaching/Learning; **Nursing Process:** Assessment/Analysis; **Reference:** Ch 33, Growth and Development

285. 3 There may be a weight gain caused by the influence of hormones before the growth spurt. Most 10- to 12-year-old children can eat an adult-size meal without becoming obese.
1 Before advising increased activity, the nurse should assess the child's present activity level. **2** An adequate caloric intake is needed for the growth spurt that will occur during adolescence. **4** Family eating patterns appear to have more effect on weight than do genetics.
Client Need: Health Promotion and Maintenance; **Cognitive Level:** Application; **Integrated Process:** Teaching/Learning; **Nursing Process:** Planning/Implementation; **Reference:** Ch 33, Growth and Development

286. 3 School-age children lose their primary teeth, which could be aspirated during surgery. The anesthesiologist must take special precautions to maintain safety. **1** This is a comforting gesture, but it is not essential. **2** There is no reason to obtain an antistreptolysin O (ASO) titer or a C-reactive protein level. **4** This is important but not always possible.
Client Need: Safety and Infection Control; **Cognitive Level:** Application; **Integrated Process:** Communication/Documentation; **Nursing Process:** Planning/Implementation; **Reference:** Ch 33, Hospitalization of School-Age Children, General Nursing Care of School-Age Children

287. 4 The glomerular filtration rate is reduced, resulting in sodium retention; there is bleeding as evidenced by hematuria, and fluid accumulation as evidenced by edema.
1, 2, 3 Not all of these support the diagnosis of glomerulonephritis.

Client Need: Physiological Adaptation; **Cognitive Level:** Analysis; **Nursing Process:** Assessment/Analysis; **Reference:** Ch 33, Acute Post Streptococcal Glomerulonephritis (APSGN), Data Base

288. **4** During the acute stage, anorexia and general malaise lower the child's resistance to infection.

1 A bland diet is not necessary, but high-protein and high-sodium foods should be avoided. **2** Bed rest is not a necessary restriction. It is encouraged when the child is easily fatigued. **3** Antibiotics are not necessary for all children with acute glomerulonephritis, only those with persistent streptococcal infections. The intramuscular route would not be used.

Client Need: Safety and Infection Control; **Cognitive Level:** Application; **Nursing Process:** Planning/Implementation; **Reference:** Ch 33, Acute Post Streptococcal Glomerulonephritis (APSGN), Nursing Care

289. **4** When urinary findings are normal, such as no evidence of hematuria or proteinuria, the child may resume preillness activities.

1, 2 This restriction is unnecessary. **3** Bed rest is unnecessary.

Client Need: Health Promotion and Maintenance; **Cognitive Level:** Application; **Integrated Process:** Teaching/Learning; **Nursing Process:** Planning/Implementation; **Reference:** Ch 33, Acute Post Streptococcal Glomerulonephritis (APSGN), Nursing Care

290. **1** Daily changes in weight are indicators of fluid changes; loss or gain of muscle and fat do not cause daily fluctuations in weight.

2 When fluid weight gain, not loss, stops, the disease is being controlled. **3** Protein molecules do not weigh enough to be reflected in the child's weight on a daily basis. **4** It is not beneficial to plan the child's daily caloric intake on fluid weight loss or gain.

Client Need: Reduction of Risk Potential; **Cognitive Level:** Application; **Integrated Process:** Teaching/Learning; **Nursing Process:** Planning/Implementation; **Reference:** Ch 33, Acute Post Streptococcal Glomerulonephritis (APSGN), Nursing Care

291. **2** The child has an elevated BP that can cause hypertensive encephalopathy, resulting in hyperperfusion of the brain and cerebral edema; one of the early signs of encephalopathy is a severe headache.

1 Rapid respirations do not cause a severe headache. **3** Anemia does not cause a severe headache. **4** The autoimmune response associated with APSGN is not the cause of the severe headache.

Client Need: Physiological Adaptation; **Cognitive Level:** Application; **Integrated Process:** Teaching/Learning; **Nursing Process:** Planning/Implementation; **Reference:** Ch 33, Acute Post Streptococcal Glomerulonephritis (APSGN), Data Base

292. **1** A physical therapist can prescribe an exercise protocol to keep the joints as mobile as possible; a routine can be developed to help the child alleviate morning stiffness.

2 Although this might be necessary in the future, there is no evidence that it is needed at this time. **3** Over-the-counter medications should not be used

without the supervision of the practitioner. **4** Although nutrition is an appropriate part of therapy, it is the physical therapy program that can most directly influence movement.

Client Need: Management of Care; **Cognitive Level:** Application; **Integrated Process:** Teaching/Learning; **Nursing Process:** Planning/Implementation; **Reference:** Ch 33, Juvenile Idiopathic Arthritis, Nursing Care

293. **4** Prolonged sitting or lying in one position can lead to stiffness and flexion contractures and should be avoided.

1 This helps maintain joint mobility. **2** This promotes functional movement. **3** This helps maintain muscle tone while providing freedom of movement.

Client Need: Health Promotion and Maintenance; **Cognitive Level:** Application; **Integrated Process:** Teaching/Learning; **Nursing Process:** Planning/Implementation; **Reference:** Ch 33, Juvenile Idiopathic Arthritis, Nursing Care

294. **4** The exercises are done to preserve joint function.

1 Exercises do not necessarily relieve pain. **2** Circulation is not affected by the arthritic process. **3** Exercising does not affect the subcutaneous nodules.

Client Need: Basic Care and Comfort; **Cognitive Level:** Application; **Nursing Process:** Evaluation/Outcomes; **Reference:** Ch 33, Juvenile Idiopathic Arthritis, Nursing Care

295. **1** Preadolescence is a critical period of growth, and steroids could lead to growth retardation.

2 The effect of steroids on sexuality is unclear. **3** Although mood changes have been documented, this is not the reason why steroids are avoided during preadolescence. **4** Poor body image is a result of many variables, not just medications.

Client Need: Pharmacological and Parenteral Therapies; **Cognitive Level:** Comprehension; **Nursing Process:** Assessment/Analysis; **Reference:** Ch 33, Juvenile Idiopathic Arthritis, Data Base

296. **1** Helping families understand their feelings about diabetes is essential in assisting them to develop positive attitudes; these attitudes will motivate them to achieve optimal control of the disease and promote a healthy lifestyle for the child.

2 This is important; however, if feelings are not addressed first, compliance with insulin administration is less likely. Also, the age and developmental level of the child must be considered before teaching can begin. **3** The child should participate in age-appropriate activities; adequate exercise is an important part of the treatment regimen for children who have diabetes. **4** This is important; however, if feelings are not addressed first, compliance with glucose monitoring is less likely. Also, the age and developmental level of the child must be considered before teaching can begin.

Client Need: Psychosocial Integrity; **Cognitive Level:** Application; **Integrated Process:** Caring; Teaching/Learning; **Nursing Process:** Planning/Implementation; **Reference:** Ch 33, Diabetes Mellitus, Nursing Care

297. **4** A bedtime snack is needed for the evening. NPH insulin is intermediate-acting insulin, which peaks 4 to 12 hours later and lasts for 16 to 24 hours. Protein and carbohydrate ingestion before sleep prevents hypoglycemia during the night, when the NPH insulin is still active.

1 The snack must contain mainly protein-rich foods, not simple carbohydrates, to help cover the intermediate-acting insulin during sleep. **2** There are no data to indicate such a need; a bedtime snack is routinely provided to help cover intermediate-acting insulin during sleep. **3** The snack is important for diet/insulin balance during the night, not encouragement.

Client Need: Pharmacological and Parenteral Therapies; **Cognitive Level:** Application; **Nursing Process:** Assessment/Analysis; **Reference:** Ch 33, Diabetes Mellitus, Nursing Care

298. **3** An 8-year-old child is in the stage of industry and strives to complete assigned tasks.

1 This is true of an older child (adolescent). **2** Peer influences increase as the child enters the preadolescent and adolescent years. **4** This stage occurs during adolescence.

Client Need: Health Promotion and Maintenance; **Cognitive Level:** Application; **Integrated Process:** Teaching/Learning; **Nursing Process:** Assessment/Analysis; **Reference:** Ch 33, Hospitalization of School-Age Children, Data Base

299. **4** NPH insulin peaks in 4 to 12 hours; it has an onset of 1 to 2 hours and a duration of 16 to 24 hours.

1 This is the onset of action of NPH insulin. **2** This is the peak action of regular insulin. **3** The peak hours for NPH insulin start sooner and last longer.

Client Need: Pharmacological and Parenteral Therapies; **Cognitive Level:** Knowledge; **Integrated Process:** Teaching/Learning; **Nursing Process:** Planning/Implementation; **Reference:** Ch 33, Diabetes Mellitus, Nursing Care

300. **3** A client with type 1 diabetes must carry a source of concentrated glucose (e.g., glucose tablets, Insta-Glucose, sugar-containing candy such as Life Savers) as a rapid source of carbohydrate if there are signs of hypoglycemia. This should be followed by a complex carbohydrate and a protein.

1 This is an unrealistic and unnatural pattern for an adolescent. **2** This is an unnecessary and time-consuming procedure. **4** The adolescent should be made to feel a part of the family; the recommended diet is nutritious and no different from that of the rest of the family; the timing of when food is eaten in relation to insulin dosage is important.

Client Need: Reduction of Risk Potential; **Cognitive Level:** Application; **Integrated Process:** Teaching/Learning; **Nursing Process:** Planning/Implementation; **Reference:** Ch 33, Diabetes Mellitus, Nursing Care

301. **4** A blood glucose level of 180 mg/dL is above the average range, and regular insulin, which is fast-acting, is needed.

1 Although exercise does decrease insulin requirements and does lower blood glucose levels, the immediate action of regular insulin is needed. **2** This action will not correct the problem; the blood glucose level is already known. **3** Food intake at this time would raise the level of blood glucose.

Client Need: Pharmacological and Parenteral Therapies; **Cognitive Level:** Application; **Nursing Process:** Planning/Implementation; **Reference:** Ch 33, Diabetes Mellitus, Nursing Care

302. **2** The adolescent needs immediate and easily absorbable glucose, such as soda, and long-lasting complex carbohydrates and protein, which are supplied by the bun and hamburger.

1 This can be done after some glucose has been ingested; otherwise, the adolescent's hypoglycemia can become severe. **3** Extra insulin will further aggravate the problem. **4** This may not be necessary if the symptoms subside quickly after the adolescent eats.

Client Need: Reduction of Risk Potential; **Cognitive Level:** Analysis; **Integrated Process:** Teaching/Learning; **Nursing Process:** Planning/Implementation; **Reference:** Ch 33, Diabetes Mellitus, Data Base

303. **3** By increasing the child's caloric intake, thereby increasing the protein and carbohydrate intake, a hypoglycemic reaction caused by exercise is less likely to occur.

1 An oral hypoglycemic is an inappropriate treatment for individuals with type 1 diabetes. **2** This would not prevent a hypoglycemic reaction when the child exercises more vigorously than usual. **4** This type of intake is less effective than other nutrients, such as protein, that are absorbed more slowly and provide a more consistent blood glucose level.

Client Need: Reduction of Risk Potential; **Cognitive Level:** Application; **Integrated Process:** Teaching/Learning; **Nursing Process:** Planning/Implementation; **Reference:** Ch 33, Diabetes Mellitus, Nursing Care

304. **3** Impetigo is a bacterial infection of the skin caused by streptococci or staphylococci. An illness caused by group A hemolytic streptococci can result in rheumatic fever and glomerulonephritis.

1 This is a viral condition; it is not associated with rheumatic fever or glomerulonephritis. **2** This infectious condition of the skin is a result of infestation by mites; it is not associated with rheumatic fever or glomerulonephritis. **4** Intertrigo is a superficial dermatitis in the folds of the skin; it is not associated with rheumatic fever or glomerulonephritis.

Client Need: Safety and Infection Control; **Cognitive Level:** Analysis; **Nursing Process:** Assessment/Analysis; **Reference:** Ch 33, Impetigo, Data Base

305. **3** The white dots are nits, the eggs of head lice *(Pediculosis capitis);* they can be seen along the scalp line, behind the ears, and at the nape of the neck.

1 This is too vague; objective visualization would confirm the presence of nits. **2** Canine ear mites are not transferable to humans. **4** This would be a sign of scabies, which is the *Sarcoptes scabiei* mite.

Client Need: Safety and Infection Control; **Cognitive Level:** Application; **Integrated Process:** Teaching/Learning; **Nursing Process:** Planning/Implementation; **Reference:** Ch 33, Pediculosis (Lice), Data Base

306. 4 Rheumatic fever is an inflammatory disease involving the joints, heart, CNS, and subcutaneous tissue. It is thought to be an autoimmune process that causes connective tissue damage.

1 Tetanus is not caused by a streptococcal infection. 2 The disorder described in the question is not influenza. 3 The disorder described in the question is not scarlet fever.

Client Need: Physiological Adaptation; **Cognitive Level:** Analysis; **Nursing Process:** Assessment/Analysis; **Reference:** Ch 33, Rheumatic Fever (RF), Data Base

307. 2 Factor VIII has a short half-life; therefore the prophylactic treatment involves administering the factor on the scheduled days in the morning so that the child will get the most benefit during the day when he is most active.

1 Prophylactic treatment is done on a scheduled basis to prevent a bleed from occurring. 3 Administering the drug at bedtime will limit its effectiveness as bleeds are more common when the child is active. 4 This does not take into consideration the properties of the drug.

Client Need: Pharmacological and Parenteral Therapies; **Cognitive Level:** Application; **Integrated Process:** Teaching/Learning; **Nursing Process:** Planning/Implementation; **Reference:** Ch 33, Hemophilia, Nursing Care

308. 3 Factor VIII is the missing plasma component necessary to control bleeding in a child with hemophilia A.

1, 4 Factor VIII, the missing component, would not be provided by this blood derivative. 2 Although fresh frozen plasma does contain factor VIII, there is an insufficient amount in a plasma transfusion; a higher volume is required.

Client Need: Pharmacological and Parenteral Therapies; **Cognitive Level:** Comprehension; **Nursing Process:** Planning/Implementation; **Reference:** Ch 33, Hemophilia, Data Base

309. 4 The hemophilia gene is carried on the X chromosome but is recessive. Therefore the female is the carrier (an unaffected XO and an affected XH). If the male receives the affected XH (XHYO), the disorder is manifested.

1 Hemophilia is carried by the female; the Mendelian laws of inheritance are not sex-specific. 2 Hemophilia is a sex-linked recessive disorder. 3 Only females carry the trait; males are usually affected.

Client Need: Physiological Adaptation; **Cognitive Level:** Comprehension; **Nursing Process:** Planning/Implementation; **Reference:** Ch 33, Hemophilia, Data Base

310. 3 Aspirin is an anticoagulant and it could harm a child with bleeding problems; in addition, aspirin is contraindicated for all children because of its relationship to Reye's syndrome.

1 This response does not answer the mother's question; it could cause the mother to feel defensive.

2 Aspirin is contraindicated. 4 Acetaminophen cannot prevent bleeding episodes; it is an analgesic.

Client Need: Pharmacological and Parenteral Therapies; **Cognitive Level:** Application; **Integrated Process:** Teaching/Learning; **Nursing Process:** Planning/Implementation; **Reference:** Ch 33, Hemophilia, Nursing Care

311. 3 The children of a carrier female (XOXH) and an unaffected male (XOYO) have the probability of being a carrier female (XOXH), an unaffected female (XOXO), an unaffected male (XOYO), or an affected male (XHYO).

1 For each child there is a 50% chance of not being affected. 2 For each child there is a 50% chance of being affected. 4 Males cannot carry the trait; females have a 50% chance of being carriers.

Client Need: Physiological Adaptation; **Cognitive Level:** Analysis; **Integrated Process:** Teaching/Learning; **Nursing Process:** Planning/Implementation; **Reference:** Ch 33, Hemophilia, Data Base

NURSING CARE OF ADOLESCENTS

312. 4 Anger interferes with communication; recognition and ventilation of anger help to resolve it and can help increase productive communication.

1 They are too angry with each other to work this out alone; they may continue to express anger to each other, which probably will escalate the conflict in their relationship. 2 The mother should be involved with the therapy and therefore must be present when treatment is discussed. 3 Anger is interfering with the acceptance of responsibility and must be addressed first.

Client Need: Psychosocial Integrity; **Cognitive Level:** Analysis; **Integrated Process:** Communication/Documentation; **Nursing Process:** Planning/Implementation; **Reference:** Ch 34, Hospitalization of Adolescents, General Nursing Care of Adolescents

313. 3 The menarche occurs when the prepubertal growth spurt is almost completed and after the primary and secondary sexual characteristics are almost fully developed.

1 Pubic hair is seen about 6 months after the breasts begin to develop. 2 The breasts are the first secondary sexual characteristics to develop early during the prepubertal growth and development period. 4 Although there may be a familial tendency to reach the menarche at the same age, there are too many variables to use this as a guideline.

Client Need: Health Promotion and Maintenance; **Cognitive Level:** Comprehension; **Integrated Process:** Teaching/Learning; **Nursing Process:** Planning/Implementation; **Reference:** Ch 34, Growth and Development

314. 1 A side effect of vincristine is alopecia. To adolescents, who are very concerned with identity, this represents a tremendous threat to their self-image.

2 Constipation, although very serious, does not require early preparation. 3 This will not be

immediately obvious. **4** Although neurologic side effects are serious, the adolescent need not be prepared this early.

Client Need: Pharmacological and Parenteral Therapies; **Cognitive Level:** Application; **Integrated Process:** Teaching/Learning; **Nursing Process:** Planning/Implementation; **Reference:** Ch 34, Bone Tumors, Nursing Care

315. **4** Several meetings with an adolescent provide an opportunity to develop trust and establish a relationship.

1 This is not necessary and may not help in establishing a relationship. **2** This is not realistic because the nurse is not the teenager's peer. **3** It is not necessary to deal in concrete terms, because the average adolescent is past this level.

Client Need: Psychosocial Integrity; **Cognitive Level:** Application; **Integrated Process:** Caring; Communication/Documentation; **Nursing Process:** Planning/Implementation; **Reference:** Ch 34, Hospitalization of Adolescents, General Nursing Care of Adolescents

316. **3** The future seems far away, and immediate gratification takes priority.

1 Adolescents are often confused about their feelings. **2** This is the developmental stage of children 6 to 12 years of age; identity is the developmental stage of the adolescent. **4** School-age children (7 to 11 years) use concrete operational reasoning; adolescents are learning to think abstractly and use formal operational reasoning.

Client Need: Health Promotion and Maintenance; **Cognitive Level:** Application; **Nursing Process:** Assessment/Analysis; **Reference:** Ch 34, Growth and Development

317. **4** The hypothalamic-pituitary-gonadal-adrenal mechanism is responsible for the physiologic and structural changes that occur at puberty. In girls the adrenal glands secrete androgens that are responsible for the appearance of axillary and pubic hair. Menarche usually occurs 2 years after initial pubescent changes.

1 This is not an indicator of sexual maturity. **2** This is not a reliable indicator of sexual maturity. **3** The first menstrual period (menarche) occurs at or toward the end of puberty; ovulation usually begins within a year after the first menstrual period.

Client Need: Health Promotion and Maintenance; **Cognitive Level:** Comprehension; **Integrated Process:** Teaching/Learning; **Nursing Process:** Planning/Implementation; **Reference:** Ch 34, Growth and Development

318. **3** Adolescents are concerned about body image and fitting in with a peer group; the stabilizing rod may be viewed as an insult to the intactness of his body.

1 Weight-bearing can be prevented with crutches, which provide greater mobility than a wheelchair. **2** After open reduction and internal fixation with a rod insertion, adolescents generally return to activities after several months. **4** The need for pain medication will decrease as the trauma from the injury and surgery subsides.

Client Need: Health Promotion and Maintenance; **Cognitive Level:** Application; **Nursing Process:** Assessment/Analysis; **Reference:** Ch 34, Hospitalization of Adolescents, Data Base

319. **3** The hyperextension required in swimming aids in strengthening back muscles and increases deeper respirations, both of which are necessary before surgery and/or before wearing a brace or cast.

1, 2, 4 This involves twisting the back muscles, which is not therapeutic for a child with this condition.

Client Need: Basic Care and Comfort; **Cognitive Level:** Application; **Integrated Process:** Teaching/Learning; **Nursing Process:** Planning/Implementation; **Reference:** Ch 34, Scoliosis, Nursing Care

320. **4** Continuing growth causes changes in muscle, bone structure, and position. The brace is worn for 6 months after physical maturity, which is confirmed by radiographic examination showing cessation of bone growth.

1 This is not an appropriate criterion for removal of the brace. **2** Pain is not usually a symptom of scoliosis. **3** The brace is used to halt the progression of the curvature, not correct it.

Client Need: Basic Care and Comfort; **Cognitive Level:** Application; **Integrated Process:** Teaching/Learning; **Nursing Process:** Planning/Implementation; **Reference:** Ch 34, Scoliosis, Data Base

321. **1** A soft toothbrush or soft-tipped applicator should be used to reduce trauma to the oral mucosa.

2 This may irritate the oral mucosa and should be diluted, if used at all. **3** This will injure the oral mucosa. **4** This will irritate the mucosa.

Client Need: Safety and Infection Control; **Cognitive Level:** Application; **Integrated Process:** Teaching/Learning; **Nursing Process:** Planning/Implementation; **Reference:** Ch 34, Bone Tumors, Nursing Care

322. **4** Establishing an identity is the major developmental task of the adolescent; to achieve this task there is a need to conform to group norms that include appearance and acceptance; appealing to this need may achieve more success than other teaching strategies.

1 This teaching strategy may be successful with an older, more secure group of people. **2** Adolescents tend to believe that they are invincible and probably would not relate to this teaching strategy. **3** Because adolescents believe they are invincible, they would not relate to this teaching strategy.

Client Need: Health Promotion and Maintenance; **Cognitive Level:** Application; **Integrated Process:** Teaching/Learning; **Nursing Process:** Planning/Implementation; **Reference:** Ch 34, Growth and Development

323. **4** Because adolescents have a developmental need to conform to their peers, the child should be able to select a bracelet with a similar configuration to those worn by her peers.

1 Hiding the bracelet under long-sleeved clothes might be acceptable in cool weather, but not when it is warm and friends are wearing sleeveless t-shirts.

2 The bracelet should be worn at all times when not with responsible family members. **3** This would be difficult, especially if the girl does not wish to tell her friends why she needs the bracelet.
Client Need: Health Promotion and Maintenance; **Cognitive Level:** Application; **Integrated Process:** Caring; **Nursing Process:** Planning/Implementation; **Reference:** 34, Hospitalization of Adolescents, General Nursing Care of Adolescents

324. **1** Although the child should be told that this is a common occurrence at this age, to relieve his anxiety he should be helped to understand and expect both this and other changes that occur during puberty.
2 This response will increase the child's anxiety because it implies that he has a problem. **3** This response is not sensitive to the child's concern; it does not offer follow-up discussion, education, or counseling. **4** This response will increase the child's anxiety because it implies that he has a problem.
Client Need: Psychosocial Integrity; **Cognitive Level:** Analysis; **Integrated Process:** Communication/Documentation; Teaching/Learning; **Nursing Process:** Planning/Implementation; **Reference:** Ch 34, Growth and Development

325. **1** Albuterol (Proventil) relaxes smooth muscles in the respiratory tract, resulting in bronchodilation. The priority is to facilitate respirations. This intervention follows the ABCs of emergency care—Airway, Breathing, Circulation.
2 This is not the priority. The results will not influence the priority intervention. **3** This is not the priority. Chest physical therapy is performed after the respiratory airways are opened. In many facilities chest physical therapy is the responsibility of the nurse, not a respiratory therapist. **4** The use of an incentive spirometer can be taught after the acute episode of respiratory distress. It will take time to receive the device and teach the child regarding its use. It should be used after the respiratory airways are opened.
Client Need: Reduction of Risk Potential; **Cognitive Level:** Analysis; **Nursing Process:** Planning/Implementation; **Reference:** Ch 32, Asthma, Nursing Care

Study Worksheet for the Comprehensive Examination

INTRODUCTION

The questions in the following comprehensive examination have been developed to reflect the current NCLEX-RN® CAT. Their purpose is to provide an opportunity for test takers to experience a testing situation that approximates the NCLEX-RN examination. These questions cross clinical disciplines and require the test taker to respond to individual and specific needs associated with common health problems and nursing responsibilities. Answers and Rationales are provided for each question. The rationales for correct and incorrect options introduce or reinforce the theories, principles, concepts, and information contained within the practice of nursing. Questions are classified further according to the NCLEX-RN examination test plan to provide a guide for identifying those nursing activities that are essential to the safe practice of nursing. A second 265-question Comprehensive Examination is included on the Companion CD accompanying this book. This test provides the student with an opportunity to take computerized version of a comprehensive examination.

CLASSIFICATION OF QUESTIONS

Each question in both Comprehensive Tests is classified by the following categories.

CLIENT NEEDS

These categories reflect nursing activities most frequently performed by entry level nurses.
- *Safe and Effective Care Environment*
  - *Management of Care:* These questions provide or direct nursing activities that promote the delivery of care to clients, family members, significant others, and other health care personnel.
  - *Safety and Infection Control:* These questions address the protection of clients, family members, significant others, and health care personnel from health and environmental hazards.
- *Health Promotion and Maintenance:* These questions provide or direct nursing care of the client, family members, and significant others. They include knowledge of the principles of growth and development, prevention and/or detection of health problems, and interventions to achieve optimum health.
- *Psychosocial Integrity:* These questions provide or direct nursing care that supports and promotes the emotional, mental, and social well-being of the client, family members, and significant others who are experiencing stressful events, as well as clients with acute or chronic mental health illness.
- *Physiologic Integrity*
  - *Basic Care and Comfort:* These questions address the provision of comfort and support in the performance of activities of daily living.
  - *Pharmacologic and Parenteral Therapies:* These questions address the provision of care related to the administration of medications, parenteral therapies, and blood products.
  - *Reduction of Risk Potential:* These questions address nursing care that may limit the likelihood that the client will develop complications or health problems related to existing disorders, treatments, or procedures.
  - *Physiologic Adaptation:* These questions address the provision and management of nursing care for clients with acute, chronic, or life-threatening physical health problems.

COGNITIVE LEVELS

This category reflects the thinking processes required to answer the question.
- *Knowledge:* These questions require the test taker to recall information from memory. They involve knowledge of facts, principles, generalizations, terminology, trends, and so forth.
- *Comprehension:* These questions require the test taker to understand information. They involve interpretation, paraphrasing, and summarization of information, as well as determination of the implications and consequences of information.
- *Application:* These questions require the test taker to use information, principles, or concepts. They involve identifying, manipulating, changing, or modifying information and performing mathematical calculations.
- *Analysis:* These questions require the test taker to interpret a variety of information. They involve the recognition of commonalities, differences, and interrelationships among data, concepts, principles, and situations.

INTEGRATED PROCESSES

Integrated processes are fundamental components that are critical to the practice of nursing. These include the nursing process, caring, communication and documentation, and teaching and learning. Because the nursing process (a scientific problem-solving process that involves critical thinking) is essential to all nursing care, it subsequently is presented in detail.

- *Caring:* These questions reflect interactions between the nurse and client/significant others that demonstrate mutual trust and respect. They involve nursing care thath provides support, encouragement, hope, and compassion.
- *Communication and Documentation:* These questions involve verbal and nonverbal interactions between the nurse and client, significant others, and members of the health care team. Client status, events, and interventions are communicated and documented according to rights, responsibilities, and standards of care.
- *Teaching and Learning:* These questions include nursing assessments and interventions that relate to the attainment of knowledge, skills, or attitudes that meet client needs.

PHASES OF THE NURSING PROCESS

This category reflects the problem-solving process used by nurses to identify client needs, plan and implement nursing care, and evaluate client responses to care.

- *Assessment/Analysis:* This phase requires the nurse to obtain objective and subjective data from primary and secondary sources, to identify and group significant data, and to communicate this information to other members of the health care team. This phase also requires the nurse to interpret data gathered through assessment for the purpose of making nursing decisions. Client and family needs are identified, and short-term and long-term goals/outcomes are set.
- *Planning/Implementation:* This phase requires the nurse to design and implement a regimen with the client, family, and other health care team members to achieve goals/outcomes set during the assessment/analysis phase. It also requires setting priorities for intervention. The client may be given total care or may be assisted and encouraged to perform activities of daily living or to follow the regimen prescribed by the practitioner. In addition, it involves activities such as counseling, teaching, and supervising health care team members.
- *Evaluation/Outcomes:* This phase requires the nurse to determine the effectiveness of nursing care. Care is reviewed, the client's response to intervention is identified, and a determination is made as to whether the client has achieved the predetermined outcomes and goals. It also includes appraisal of the client's ability to implement and fulfill the health care plan.

REFERENCE

Each question refers the test taker to the section where, within *Mosby's Comprehensive Review of Nursing for the NCLEX-RN Examination*, related content concerning the question can be found. This promotes a review of specific information as it relates to the question and permits a more thorough review of related information.

HOW TO MAXIMIZE USE OF THE COMPREHENSIVE TESTS

To achieve maximum learning from the experience of taking these examinations, we have divided each Comprehensive Test into two sections. Part A contains 75 questions, which is the minimum number of questions every candidate must answer on the NCLEX-RN®. Part B contains 190 questions. Part B and Part A together total 265 questions, the maximum number of questions on the NCLEX-RN examination.

With Comprehensive Test 1, we recommend that you review the answers and rationales and the classifications of questions for each part as you complete it. In Comprehensive Test 2, which appears on the Companion CD, you must wait until you have completed both parts before checking the answers and rationales and classifications of questions. We have made these recommendations so that Test 1 will reinforce your immediate learning, and so that Test 2, although it also reinforces learning, will better reflect the actual situation that you will experience when you take the computerized NCLEX-RN examination.

To help you analyze your mistakes on the comprehensive examinations and to provide a database for making study plans, Focus for Study worksheets have been included for each test. These worksheets are designed to assist you in identifying and recording errors in the way you process information, and to help you identify and record gaps in knowledge. Follow the directions that appear below under HOW TO DEVELOP A FOCUS FOR STUDY. As you review material in class notes or in this book, pay attention to correcting your most common problems and identifying the topics you should review further. It might be helpful to set priorities; review the most difficult topics first so that you will have time to review them more than once. The worksheets can be used to focus your future study. Remember, if you study the proper subject matter, the knowledge you gain will provide you with the ability to answer questions, regardless of the medium used to ask the question, because the required knowledge of the subject matter does not change.

HOW TO DEVELOP A FOCUS FOR STUDY

At the end of each Comprehensive Exam, you will find two Focus for Study Worksheets.

- **Focus for Study Worksheet—Adapted NCLEX-RN® Test Plan**
- **Focus for Study Worksheet—Content Areas**

These Focus for Study Worksheets should be used at the completion of each Comprehensive Test to analyze each question that you answered incorrectly. It is important that you take the time to complete the worksheets carefully. The resulting information will assist you in identifying areas of strength and weakness and will help you to use your study time effectively and efficiently.

FOCUS FOR STUDY WORKSHEET: ADAPTED NCLEX-RN® TEST PLAN

This worksheet has 19 columns cross the top. The first column lists the number of the question that you answered incorrectly. Eight columns are the subclassifications of Client Need; six columns are the subclassifications of Integrated Processes (including the Nursing Process); and four columns are the subclassifications of the Cognitive Level of the question.

To develop a meaningful focus of study, simply follow these directions.

1. In the Comprehensive Test, reread the question that you missed.
2. In the Answers and Rationales section, read the rationale for the correct answer and the rationales for all the incorrect options.
3. Reread the answer you chose, and read the reason your answer was incorrect.
4. Place the number of the question you got wrong in its own box in the first column.
5. Look at the classifications for the question that accompany the answers and rationales for the question. Place an X in the box on the Focus for Study Worksheet–Adapted NCLEX-RN Test Plan that relates to Client Need, Integrated Processes (including Nursing Process), and Cognitive Level for the question.
6. Perform steps 1 through 5 for each question that you got wrong.

At the completion of this process, you will have an overview of where you made mistakes in relation to the NCLEX-RN test plan. You may see a pattern of errors that will provide a direction for studying.

FOCUS FOR STUDY WORKSHEET REFERENCE/CHAPTER

This worksheet has 8 columns. The first column lists Content Areas that reflect a broad classification of information essential to the practice of nursing. These content areas mirror the chapters in *Mosby's Comprehensive Review of Nursing for the NCLEX-RN® Examination*. The other seven columns reflect specific information that crosses clinical disciplines: Pathophysiology, Pharmacology, Nutrition, Diagnostic Studies, Developmental Factors, Physical Care, and Emotional Care.

To develop a meaningful focus of study, simply follow these directions.

1. In the Comprehensive Test, reread the question that you missed.
2. In the Answers and Rationales section, read the rationale for the correct answer, as well as the rationales for all incorrect options.
3. Reread the answer you chose, and read the reason your answer was incorrect.
4. Identify the Reference for the question by looking at the group of classifications that accompanies the rationale for the question. Next to Reference will be the chapter and the headings under which the information in the question is reviewed in this book. Find this content area in column one of the worksheet, Reference/Chapter.
5. Look at the question you missed, and decide where the subject matter that is being tested best fits under one of the headings in the first horizontal row of the worksheet (Pathophysiology & Basic Sciences, Pharmacology, Nutrition, Diagnostic Studies, Developmental Factors, Physical Care, and Emotional Care).
6. Write the number of the question you got wrong in the box that intersects the content area row and the appropriate heading in the vertical column of the worksheet. Make your numbers small, so that more than one question number can fit in a box if necessary.
7. Perform steps 1 through 6 for each question you got wrong.

At the completion of this process, you will be able to identify the areas of knowledge in which you missed the greatest number of questions. These gaps require additional study. You can access a review of the information tested in the question by going to the appropriate chapter and heading in *Mosby's Comprehensive Review of Nursing for the NCLEX-RN® Examination* that is listed next to Reference in the classifications that follow each question's answers and rationales. Also, the topics in the worksheets can be found in the index of most nursing textbooks. Therefore, you can use whatever text or resource material is available to you and with which you are already familiar.

As you review material in class notes or in this book, pay attention to correcting your most common problems and identifying the topics you should review further. It might be helpful to set priorities; review the most difficult topics first, so that you will have time to review them more than once. Remember, if you study the proper subject matter, the knowledge you gain will provide you with the ability to answer questions, regardless of the medium used to ask the question, because the required knowledge of the subject matter does not change.

FOCUS FOR STUDY WORKSHEET—ADAPTED NCLEX-RN® TEST PLAN

Number of the Question	CLIENT NEED							
	SAFE & EFFECTIVE CARE ENVIRONMENT		Health Promotion & Maintenance	Psychosocial Integrity	PHYSIOLOGICAL INTEGRITY			
	Management of Care	Safety & Infection Control			Basic Care & Comfort	Pharmacological & Parenteral Therapies	Reduction of Risk Potential	Physiological Adaptation

FOCUS FOR STUDY WORKSHEET—ADAPTED NCLEX-RN® TEST PLAN (Continued)

	INTEGRATED PROCESSES			NURSING PROCESS			COGNITIVE LEVEL			
Emotional Care (Caring)	Communication & Documentation	Teaching & Learning	Assessment & Analysis	Planning & Implementation	Evaluation & Outcomes	Knowledge	Comprehension	Application	Analysis

FOCUS FOR STUDY WORKSHEET—CONTENT AREAS

Reference/Chapter	Pathophysiology & Basic Sciences	Pharmacology	Nutrition
Foundations of Nursing Practice (Ch 1, 2, & 3)			
Growth & Development of the Adult (Ch 5)			
Circulatory System Disorders (Ch 6)			
Respiratory System Disorders (Ch 7)			
Gastrointestinal System Disorders (Ch 8)			
Endocrine System Disorders (Ch 9)			
Integumentary System Disorders (Ch 10)			
Neuromusculo-skeletal System Disorders (Ch 11)			
Urinary/Reproductive System Disorders (Ch 12)			
Infectious Diseases (Ch 13)			
Foundations & the Practice of Mental Health Nursing (Ch 15 & 16)			
Disorders First Evident During Infancy, Childhood, & Adolescence (Ch 17)			
Disorders Related to Alterations in Cognition & Perception (Ch 18)			
Disorders Related to Anxiety & Alterations in Mood (Ch 19)			
Disorders Related to Alterations in Behavior (Ch 20)			
Sexual & Gender Identity Disorders (Ch 21)			
Nursing Care to Promote Childbearing & Women's Health (Ch 23)			
Major Disorders Affecting Women's Health (Ch 24)			
Uncomplicated Pregnancy, Labor, Childbirth, & the Postpartum Period (Ch 25)			
Women at Risk During Pregnancy, Labor, Childbirth, & the Postpartum Period (Ch 26)			
Nursing Care of the Newborn (Ch 27)			
Foundations of Child Health Nursing (Ch 29)			
Nursing Care of Infants (Ch 30)			
Nursing Care of Toddlers (Ch 31)			
Nursing Care of Preschoolers (Ch 32)			
Nursing Care of School-Age Children (Ch 33)			
Nursing Care of Adolescents (Ch 34)			

Diagnostic Studies	Developmental Factors	Physical Care	Emotional Care

Comprehensive Test 1

1. To assess the neurovascular status of an extremity casted from the ankle to the thigh the nurse should:
   1. Palpate the femoral artery of the affected leg
   2. Assess the affected leg for a positive Homans' sign
   3. Compress and release the toenails of the affected foot
   4. Instruct the client to flex and extend the knee of the affected leg

2. The nurse is caring for a 52-year-old woman who is experiencing postmenopausal bleeding, and endometrial cancer is suspected. Which information about the client is a risk factor associated with endometrial cancer?
   1. Obesity
   2. Multiparity
   3. Cigarette smoking
   4. Early onset of menopause

3. A client who has breast cancer has received chemotherapy and a lumpectomy. She is now scheduled for radiation on an outpatient basis. The nurse should:
   1. Assess the radiated site daily for redness or irritation
   2. Rinse the radiated site once a day with an antibacterial solution
   3. Encourage the client to wear a snug-fitting bra between treatments
   4. Instruct the client to apply lotion twice daily to the skin at the radiated site

4. A client's problem with ineffective control of type 1 diabetes is pinpointed as a sudden decrease in blood glucose level followed by rebound hyperglycemia. The nurse identifies this as:
   1. Diabetic ketoacidosis
   2. Somogyi phenomenon
   3. Diabetic hypoinsulinemia
   4. Hyperosmolar nonketotic coma

5. To avoid lipodystrophy in a client on insulin therapy, the nurse should teach the client to:
   1. Exercise regularly
   2. Rotate injection sites
   3. Use the Z-track technique
   4. Avoid massaging the injection site

6. A client with type 1 diabetes asks, "Why can't I take insulin by mouth? I have a cousin who takes pills." The nurse's response is based on the fact that:
   1. The cousin probably does not have diabetes
   2. Oral hypoglycemics predispose diabetic clients to lipodystrophy
   3. Insulin taken by mouth is destroyed by gastric juices in the stomach
   4. Oral hypoglycemics and insulin are the same, but oral agents are used for mild diabetes

7. The nurse identifies that additional teaching about the diet appropriate for a person with type 2 diabetes mellitus is needed when the following statement is made by the client:
   1. "I can eat as much dietetic fruit as I want."
   2. "I can have a lettuce salad whenever I want it."
   3. "I know that half of my diet should be carbohydrates."
   4. "I need to reduce the amounts of saturated fats in my diet."

8. When reviewing an appropriate diet for a client with type 2 diabetes, the client expresses a dislike for sweet potatoes. The nurse teaches the client that a safe equivalent is:
   1. White bread
   2. A cup of milk
   3. A slice of avocado
   4. Mayonnaise on salad

9. A client on the psychiatric unit who begins a regimen of haloperidol (Haldol) is observed pacing and shifting weight from one foot to another. The nurse identifies that this may indicate:
   1. Akathisia
   2. Parkinsonism
   3. Tardive dyskinesia
   4. Acute dystonic reaction

10. A client on the psychiatric unit continually talks about delusional material. It is most therapeutic for the nurse to:
    1. Ask the client to explain the delusion
    2. Allow the client to maintain the delusion
    3. Encourage the client to focus on reality issues
    4. Explain to the client why the thoughts are not true

11. A female client has a tonic-clonic seizure. What is the priority nursing intervention during the tonic-clonic stage of the seizure?
    1. Turn her on her side
    2. Protect her from injury
    3. Call for additional help
    4. Establish a patent airway

12. An infant is born with a myelomeningocele. When answering the parents' questions, the nurse understands that this condition is a:
    1. Herniation of brain and meninges through a defect in the base of the skull
    2. Fusion failure of the vertebral arches without herniation of cord or meninges

3. Membrane-covered sac of meninges filled with spinal fluid that protrudes through a defect in the spine

4. Saclike cyst of meninges, containing a portion of spinal cord and fluid, that protrudes through a defect in the spine

13. Immediate nursing care for an infant with a myelomeningocele should include:
1. Changing the diaper immediately when it is moist
2. Positioning the infant prone with the legs adducted
3. Applying sterile, moist nonadherent dressings to the sac
4. Placing the infant in the reverse Trendelenburg position

14. Oxytocin (Pitocin) augmentation via IVPB is ordered for a client in labor after a period of ineffective uterine contractions. If strong contractions that last 90 seconds or longer should occur, the nurse should:
1. Stop the infusion and turn the client on her side
2. Slow the infusion and give oxygen to prevent fetal hypoxia
3. Continue the infusion and notify the client's physician
4. Apply a fetal monitor to verify the length of contractions

15. A client in labor is dilated 8 cm, has a desire to push, and is becoming increasingly uncomfortable. She requests pain medication. The nurse should:
1. Help her to take panting breaths
2. Prepare the birthing bed for the birth
3. Assist her out of bed to the bathroom
4. Administer meperidine HCl (Demerol) as ordered

16. The nurse administers an intramuscular injection of vitamin K to a newborn. The purpose of the injection is to:
1. Maintain the intestinal floral count
2. Promote proliferation of intestinal flora
3. Stimulate vitamin K production in the baby
4. Provide protection until intestinal flora is established

17. A new mother asks the nurse how to care for her baby's umbilical cord stump. The nurse should teach the mother to:
1. Expect a moderate amount of drainage
2. Keep the area moist with normal saline
3. Apply a small sterile dressing twice a day
4. Sponge-bathe the baby until the cord stump falls off

18. A client complains of nausea, dyspnea, and right upper quadrant pain unrelieved by antacids. The pain occurs most often after eating in fast-food restaurants. Which diet should the nurse instruct the client to follow?
1. Low fat
2. Low carbohydrate
3. Soft textured and bland
4. High protein and kilocalories

19. After an abdominal cholecystectomy, a client has a T-tube attached to a collection device. On the day of surgery, at 10:30 PM, 300 mL of bile is emptied from the collection bag. At 6:30 AM the next day, the bag contains 60 mL of bile. The nurse's intervention is guided by the knowledge that:
1. The T-tube may have to be irrigated
2. The bile is now draining into the duodenum
3. Mechanical problems may develop with the T-tube
4. Suction must be reestablished in the portable drainage system

20. A 39-year-old divorced man has a history of gambling. He is involved in legal difficulties for embezzling money and is required to obtain counseling. During an intake interview, he says, "I never would have done this if I had been paid what I am worth." The greatest difficulty the nurse will have in assisting this client to develop insight is his:
1. Grandiosity related to his abilities
2. Feelings of boredom and emptiness
3. Anger toward those in authority positions
4. Tendency to project responsibility for his difficulties

21. When working with a client who has the diagnosis of borderline personality disorder with antisocial behavior, the nurse should expect the client to be:
1. Retiring and devious
2. Engaging and rejecting
3. Suspicious and withdrawn
4. Indecisive and perfectionistic

22. A client is diagnosed with an antisocial personality disorder. A realistic initial intervention should be that the client will:
1. Explore job possibilities with the nurse
2. Acknowledge resentment of authority figures
3. Initiate discussion of feelings of being victimized
4. Spend 15 minutes twice a day discussing problems with the nurse

23. A client with the diagnosis of personality disorder with antisocial behavior is hospitalized. He openly discusses his history, which includes problems in his relationships with his ex-wife, children, and employer, from whom he has stolen money. He is presently facing criminal charges. Behavior that indicates that the client is ready for discharge with continued care in a clinic is:
1. Expression of feelings of resentment toward his employer
2. Discussion of plans for each of the possible outcomes of his trial
3. Expression of resignation over the outcome of his marriage and his relationship with his children
4. Discussion of his decision to file a grievance against his boss after he is discharged from the hospital

24. An adolescent who is pregnant comes to the clinic at 10 weeks' gestation. The nutrition interview indicates that her dietary intake consists mainly of soft drinks, candy, French fries, and potato chips. This diet is considered inadequate because the:
1. Caloric content of this diet will make her gain too much weight
2. Ingredients in soft drinks and candy can be teratogenic in early pregnancy

3. Salt in this diet will contribute to the development of gestational hypertension

4. Nutritional composition of the diet places her at risk for a low-birth-weight infant

25. At 34 weeks' gestation, the nurse identifies a client's BP as 166/100 mm Hg and her urine as 3+ for protein. The client complains of a severe headache and occasional blurred vision. Her baseline BP was 100/62 mm Hg. The nurse identifies that this client is exhibiting signs of:
1. Eclampsia
2. Mild preeclampsia
3. Severe preeclampsia
4. Gestational hypertension

26. A client with severe preeclampsia is hospitalized. What should the nurse do first to ensure her physical safety?
1. Decrease environmental stimuli
2. Administer sedatives as ordered
3. Place her on seizure precautions
4. Strictly monitor her intake and output

27. The nurse should assist a client with glaucoma to accept the need for treatment of the disease because:
1. Total blindness is inevitable
2. Lost vision cannot be restored
3. Use of both eyes usually is restricted
4. Surgery will help the problem only temporarily

28. After an amputation, the nurse can help a client prepare the residual limb for a prosthesis by encouraging the client to:
1. Abduct the residual limb when ambulating
2. Dangle the residual limb off the bed frequently
3. Soak the residual limb in warm water twice a day
4. Periodically press the end of the residual limb against a pillow

29. A client is admitted to the hospital with a diagnosis of bronchial asthma. The nurse understands that this client may have difficulty breathing because of:
1. A too rapid expulsion of air
2. Spasms of the bronchi, which trap the air
3. Hyperventilation due to an anxiety reaction
4. An increase in the vital capacity of the lungs

30. The physician orders daily sputum specimens to be collected from a client. It is most appropriate for the nurse to collect this specimen from the client:
1. After activity
2. Before meals
3. On awakening
4. Before a respiratory treatment

31. A child is found to be allergic to dust. The nurse is preparing a teaching plan for the parents. The nurse should include that:
1. Housework must be done by professional house cleaners
2. Damp-dusting the house will help limit dust particles in the air
3. The condition must be accepted because dust cannot be limited
4. The house must be redecorated because the environment must be dust-free

32. After surgery, a client is extubated in the postanesthesia unit. For which common adaptation should the nurse be alert when monitoring a client for acute respiratory distress?
1. Bradycardia
2. Restlessness
3. Constricted pupils
4. Clubbing of the fingers

33. When assessing a child with croup, the nurse expects certain adaptations. Select all that apply.
1. ☐ Fever
2. ☐ Crackles
3. ☐ Bronchospasm
4. ☐ Barking cough
5. ☐ Inspiratory stridor

34. The physician orders magnesium sulfate for a client with severe preeclampsia. The dose ordered is twice the usual adult dose. The physician insists that it is the desired dose and directs the nurse to administer the medication. The nurse should:
1. Give the dose and observe the client closely
2. Withhold the dose and notify the nursing supervisor
3. Give the dose and document the situation on the chart
4. Administer the usual dose and notify the director of the obstetric department

35. A client who is lying in the supine position while in active labor has an IV oxytocin (Pitocin) drip and external monitors in place. Using the monitoring strips below, identify the appropriate nursing interventions. Select all that apply.
1. ☐ Provide oxygen
2. ☐ Give ampicillin
3. ☐ Turn Pitocin off
4. ☐ Increase IV fluids
5. ☐ Reposition mother

36. A nursing action to be included in the plan of care for a child with acute poststreptococcal glomerulonephritis is:
1. Encouraging fluids
2. Checking the pupils
3. Measuring abdominal girth
4. Monitoring for seizure activity

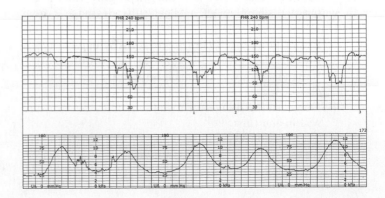

37. A child with acute poststreptococcal glomerulonephritis requests a snack. The most therapeutic selection of food the nurse could provide should include:
    1. Peanuts
    2. Pretzels
    3. Bananas
    4. Applesauce

38. An adolescent is admitted to the psychiatric unit with the diagnosis of anorexia nervosa. The nurse understands that the primary gain a client with anorexia achieves from this disorder is:
    1. Reduction of anxiety via control over food
    2. Separation from parents via hospitalization
    3. Release from school responsibilities via illness
    4. Parental overattentiveness via massive weight loss

39. The nurse is caring for an adolescent girl who has developed anorexia nervosa. In addition to being underweight, a characteristic that is typical of girls with this disorder is:
    1. Pyrexia
    2. Tachycardia
    3. Heat intolerance
    4. Secondary amenorrhea

40. The nurse anticipates that initial treatment of an adolescent with anorexia nervosa should specifically include:
    1. Medications to reduce anxiety
    2. Family psychotherapy sessions
    3. Separation from family members
    4. Correction of electrolyte imbalances

41. During the first trimester, a pregnant client complains of frequently feeling nauseated. The nurse should teach that nausea and vomiting may best be reduced by:
    1. Eating small but frequent meals
    2. Taking an antacid between meals
    3. Eating a pat of butter before rising
    4. Drinking large amounts of hot or cold tea until nausea subsides

42. When a client has a history of COPD, the nurse must be able to identify the most common complications, which generally involve:
    1. Kidney function
    2. Cardiac function
    3. Joint inflammation
    4. Peripheral neuropathy

43. The nurse understands that the purpose of water in the water seal chamber of a chest tube drainage system is to:
    1. Foster removal of chest secretions by capillarity
    2. Prevent the entrance of air into the pleural cavity
    3. Facilitate emptying of bloody drainage from the chest
    4. Decrease the danger of a sudden change in pressure within the tube

44. After resection of a lower lobe of the lung, a client has excessive respiratory secretions. In addition to encouraging the client to cough, independent nursing care should include:
    1. Postural drainage
    2. Turning and positioning
    3. Administration of an expectorant
    4. Percussion and vibration techniques

45. The physician plans a cystectomy and an ileal conduit for a male client with invasive carcinoma of the bladder. After the procedure is described, the client expresses concerns about the offensiveness of the odor. The best response that the nurse can provide is:
    1. "Tell me more about what you are thinking."
    2. "Products are available to limit this problem."
    3. "This is a problem, but the surgery is necessary."
    4. "Most people who have this surgery share this same concern."

46. Using Piaget's theory of cognitive development, the nurse should expect a 6-month-old infant to be demonstrating:
    1. Early traces of memory
    2. Beginning sense of time
    3. Repetitious reflex responses
    4. Beginning of object permanence

47. A client in labor is placed on an internal fetal monitor. The nurse should tell the client that while she is on the monitor, she:
    1. Should detach the monitor leads when using the toilet
    2. May feel free to assume any position that is comfortable for her
    3. Must maintain a side-lying position to ensure more accurate monitoring
    4. Should maintain a supine position to avoid dislodging of the internal electrode

48. It is suspected that a newborn may be developing respiratory distress when the nurse observes:
    1. Flaring nares
    2. Acrocyanosis
    3. Abdominal respirations
    4. Respirations of 48 breaths/min

49. On the third postpartum day, a woman who is breast-feeding calls the clinic complaining of tight, swollen breasts. The nurse explains that engorgement of the breasts on the third postpartum day is due to:
    1. An overabundance of milk
    2. Ineffective nursing of the baby
    3. Lack of adequate breast support
    4. Congestion of the lymphatic system

50. When a client sustains a deep partial-thickness burn because of severe sunburn, the nurse teaches that the best first-aid measure is:
    1. Cool, moist towels
    2. Dry, sterile dressings
    3. Analgesic sunburn spray
    4. Vitamin A and D ointment

51. A client sustains deep partial-thickness burns but refuses to seek medical attention. The nurse should advise this individual to go to the hospital or to see a physician if:
    1. Blisters appear
    2. Urinary output decreases
    3. Edema and redness occur
    4. Low-grade fever develops

52. When assessing older adults, the nurse understands that aging usually does not affect their:
    1. Sense of taste or smell
    2. Gastrointestinal motility
    3. Muscle or motor strength
    4. Strategies to handle life's stresses

53. Nurses who care for the terminally ill apply the theories of Kübler-Ross in planning care. According to Kübler-Ross, individuals who experience a terminal illness go through a grieving process. Place the stages of this process in the order identified by Kübler-Ross.
    _____ Anger
    _____ Denial
    _____ Bargaining
    _____ Depression

54. A client has a urinary catheter in place after surgery. When planning for the client's safety needs in relation to this device, the nurse should:
    1. Empty the bag every 6 hours
    2. Keep the system closed at all times
    3. Maintain the tension on the tubing
    4. Attach the bag to the side rail of the bed

55. After transurethral resection of the prostate, the client's nursing care should include:
    1. Maintaining patency of the cystostomy tube
    2. Keeping the abdominal dressing clean and dry
    3. Observing the wound for hemorrhage and infection
    4. Promoting the patency of the three-way indwelling catheter

56. A client is to receive 125 mL of IV fluid every hour. The drop factor of the IV tubing is 10 gtt/mL. How many drops per minute should the nurse administer?
    1. Answer: _____ gtt/min.

57. A client on a psychiatric unit who has been hearing voices is receiving a neuroleptic medication for the first time. The client takes the cup of water and the pill and stares at them. The most therapeutic statement the nurse can make is:
    1. "You have to take your medicine."
    2. "This is the medication that your doctor ordered."
    3. "Your doctor wants you to have this medicine. Swallow it."
    4. "There must be a reason why you don't want to take your medicine."

58. After a therapy session with the psychologist in the mental health clinic, a client tells the nurse that the therapist is uncaring and impersonal. The nurse's best response is:
    1. "Your therapist is really very good."
    2. "I hope that the rest of the staff is caring."
    3. "The therapist is there to help you; try to cooperate."
    4. "You have strong feelings about your therapy session and your therapist."

59. A client who just had a kidney transplant is transferred from the postanesthesia care unit to the intensive care unit (ICU). The nurse in the ICU should monitor the urinary output every:
    1. Hour
    2. 2 hours
    3. 15 minutes
    4. 30 minutes

60. The most important test the nurse should check to determine whether a transplanted kidney is working is:
    1. WBC cell count
    2. Renal ultrasound
    3. Serum creatinine level
    4. Twenty-four hour urinary output

61. Three weeks after a kidney transplant, a client develops leukopenia. The nurse understands that this client's leukopenia is probably caused by:
    1. Bacterial infection
    2. High creatinine levels
    3. Rejection of the kidney
    4. Antirejection medications

62. The nurse is caring for a 4-year-old child who has just been diagnosed with cystic fibrosis. He has been passing loose, bulky, foul-smelling stools and his weight is now less than the third percentile for his age. Which statement best explains the growth failure?
    1. Impaired digestion and absorption because of the lack of pancreatic enzymes
    2. Dyspnea and shortness of breath, which cause anorexia and disinterest in food
    3. Increased bowel motility and diarrhea, which lead to inadequate absorption of nutrients
    4. Pulmonary obstruction, which has caused an oxygen deficit and inadequate tissue nourishment

63. A child has cystic fibrosis. The nurse evaluates that the parents understand the dietary regimen for their child when they say they will:
    1. Restrict fluids during mealtimes
    2. Discontinue use of salt when cooking
    3. Provide high-calorie foods between meals
    4. Eliminate milk and milk products from the diet

64. The parent of a 2-year-old child who was just diagnosed with cystic fibrosis expresses concern about the child's frailty and low weight. What is the nurse's most appropriate reply?
    1. "Digestive enzymes will be given to help your child digest food."
    2. "Your child's appetite will improve once respiratory therapy is initiated."
    3. "Your child's coughing and shortness of breath prevent adequate chewing of food."
    4. "I suggest that you offer baby foods to your child because they are more easily digested."

65. During the first well-baby visit after discharge from the hospital, the mother informs the nurse that her baby has difficulty sucking and swallowing and tires easily. What should the nurse consider when assessing this infant?
    1. Feeding problems are fairly common in newborns
    2. Decreased sucking is insignificant in the absence of cyanosis
    3. Poor feeding may be an early indications of a heart defect
    4. Many babies retain mucus that may interfere with feeding for several days

66. When assessing a child with chronic hypoxia, the nurse should monitor for:
    1. Clubbing of fingers
    2. Decreased RBC count
    3. Slow, irregular respirations
    4. Subcutaneous hemorrhages

67. The nurse understands that Buck's extension may be ordered initially for clients with a fracture of the head of the femur primarily to:
    1. Prevent soft tissue edema
    2. Reduce the need for cast application
    3. Prevent damage to the surrounding nerves
    4. Reduce muscle spasms around the fracture site

68. A client has a total hip arthroplasty. After surgery, the nurse should:
    1. Log-roll the client when turning
    2. Elevate the client's affected limb on a pillow
    3. Place a trochanter roll along the entire extremity
    4. Keep an abduction pillow between the legs at all times

69. The client in a psychiatric unit who needs immediate therapeutic intervention from the nurse is a:
    1. 45-year-old man who sits quietly in the corner of the room watching the movements of other clients
    2. 25-year-old man who is making sounds and actions like a machine gun in front of the nurse's station
    3. 50-year-old woman who is pacing back and forth across the dayroom and picking fights with other clients
    4. 33-year-old woman who wanders aimlessly around the unit saying, "I just don't know what to do. I feel so lost."

70. A client in a psychiatric hospital with the diagnosis of major depression is tearful and refuses to eat dinner after a visit with a friend. It is most therapeutic for the nurse to:
    1. Allow the client to skip the meal
    2. Provide adequate quiet thinking time
    3. Reinforce the importance of adequate nutrition
    4. Offer the client the opportunity to discuss the visit

71. A person with a history of alcoholism states, "I have been drinking since last Friday to celebrate my son's graduation from college." Before responding, the nurse understands that this person's statement is an example of the defense mechanism of:
    1. Denial
    2. Projection
    3. Identification
    4. Rationalization

72. When the nurse evaluates whether the unit environment is conducive to psychologic safety for a confused client with dementia, which factor is essential?
    1. Nursing care is flexible
    2. Client's needs are met entirely
    3. Realistic limits and controls are set
    4. Physical surroundings are clean and orderly

73. A client who uses ritualistic behavior taps other clients on the shoulders three times while going through the ritual. The inference made by the nurse that is most appropriate is that this client has a:
    1. Blurred personal identity
    2. Poor control of sudden urges
    3. Disturbance in spatial boundaries
    4. Reduced ability to adapt to life's stresses

74. After surgery for a colostomy, the most effective way the nurse can initially help a client to accept the colostomy is to:
    1. Provide literature containing factual data about colostomies
    2. Ask a member of a support group to come to speak with the client
    3. Point out the number of important people who have had colostomies
    4. Begin to teach self-care of the colostomy by introducing equipment

75. When planning care for a child with autism, the nurse understands that given a choice, the child with autism usually enjoys playing:
    1. On a jungle gym
    2. With a cuddly toy
    3. With a small yellow block
    4. On a playground merry-go-round

REVIEW QUESTIONS: PART B

76. A client who is 6 months pregnant arrives at the clinic for her scheduled examination. Her BP is 150/86, and she states that she has gained 2.27 kg (5 lb) in the last 2 weeks. The nurse should:
    1. Take the client's body temperature
    2. Prepare the client for a vaginal examination
    3. Give the client another appointment in 2 weeks
    4. Test the client's urine for the presence of albumin

77. A pregnant client with preeclampsia is receiving magnesium sulfate. What should the nurse keep at the bedside to prepare for the possibility of magnesium sulfate toxicity?
    1. Nalline
    2. Oxygen
    3. Calcium gluconate
    4. Suction equipment

78. A client who has a phobia about dogs is about to begin systematic desensitization. The client asks what the treatment will involve. The nurse should reply," You will:
    1. "Be rewarded for not becoming anxious around dogs."
    2. "Be exposed to dogs until you no longer feel anxious."
    3. "Increase your contact with dogs while using relaxation techniques."
    4. "Discuss with me in depth what caused your phobia and how it affects your life."

79. A client who is recovering from an acute episode of colitis is receiving a high-protein diet. The nurse should teach the client that this diet primarily will:
    1. Repair tissues
    2. Slow peristalsis
    3. Correct the anemia
    4. Improve muscle tone

80. Nursing management for a client with an acute episode of bronchial asthma should be directed toward:
    1. Curing the condition permanently
    2. Raising mucous secretions from the chest
    3. Limiting pulmonary secretions by decreasing fluid intake
    4. Convincing the client that the condition is emotionally based

81. The nurse administers beclomethasone (Vanceril) by inhalation to a client with asthma. The nurse understands that the purpose of this therapy is to:
    1. Promote comfort
    2. Reduce respiratory bacteria
    3. Stimulate smooth muscle relaxation
    4. Decrease inflammatory cell responses

82. When a new mother refuses to look at her baby, who has a severe birth defect, the nursing approach that is most therapeutic is to:
    1. Explain to the family why she needs to be distracted

    2. Gently tell her that she should stop blaming herself for the child's handicap
    3. Reinforce the explanation of the handicap and allow time for the mother to discuss her fears
    4. Wait until she has sufficiently recovered from the stress of birth before bringing the baby to her again

83. When teaching a class about parenting, the nurse asks the participants what they do when their toddlers have a temper tantrum. Which statement demonstrates one father's understanding of the origin of temper tantrums?
    1. After a temper tantrum, he disciplines his child by restricting a favorite food or activity
    2. When a temper tantrum begins, he isolates and ignores his child until the behavior improves
    3. During a temper tantrum, he partially gives in to his child before the tantrum becomes excessive
    4. He tries to prevent a temper tantrum by allowing his child to choose between two reasonable alternatives

84. If the nurse interrupts a client with obsessive-compulsive disorder during the performance of a ritual, the client most likely will react with:
    1. Anxiety
    2. Hostility
    3. Aggression
    4. Withdrawal

85. When a nurse is working with a client with psychiatric problems, a primary goal is the establishment of a therapeutic nurse-client relationship. The major purpose of this relationship is to:
    1. Increase nonverbal communication
    2. Provide an outlet for suppressed hostile feelings
    3. Assist the client in acquiring more effective behavior
    4. Provide the client with someone who can make decisions

86. An African American woman is diagnosed with primary hypertension. She asks, "Is hypertension a disease of black people?" The nurse's best response is:
    1. "The higher-risk population is composed of black men and women."
    2. "The highest-risk population consists of older white men and women."
    3. "The prevalence of hypertension is about equal for women of all races."
    4. "The prevalence of hypertension is greater for black women than for black men."

87. The physician prescribes a diuretic for a client with hypertension. When providing client teaching, the nurse explains that diuretics reduce BP by:
    1. Facilitating vasodilation
    2. Promoting smooth muscle relaxation
    3. Reducing the circulating blood volume
    4. Blocking the sympathetic nervous system

88. The nurse is caring for a client who is receiving a thiazide diuretic for hypertension. Based on this information,

when guiding the client to select foods from the daily menu, the nurse should explain that a good food choice is:

1. Apples
2. Broccoli
3. Cherries
4. Cauliflower

89. A 20-year-old college student comes to the college health clinic complaining of increasing anxiety, loss of appetite, and an inability to concentrate. An appropriate response by the nurse is:

1. "With whom have you shared your feelings of anxiety?"
2. "What have you identified as the cause of your anxiety?"
3. "It has been difficult for you. How long has this been going on?"
4. "Let's talk about your problems. Are you having difficulty adjusting?"

90. When a client attempts suicide, the nurse identifies that the immediate short-term goal during this crisis situation should be, "The client will:

1. Strengthen coping skills."
2. Establish a no-suicide contract."
3. Learn problem-solving techniques."
4. Recognize why suicide was attempted."

91. A 3½-year-old child is admitted to the hospital for an appendectomy. What should the nurse use to best prepare the child for the hospital experience?

1. A diagram
2. Puppet play
3. A storybook
4. Therapeutic play

92. The nurse understands that a preschooler's concept of death includes the belief that it is:

1. Not a permanent condition
2. The result of certain illnesses
3. Something that happens in the hospital
4. An event that eventually happens to everyone

93. A client is admitted to the hospital with a diagnosis of chronic kidney failure. When assessing this client, the nurse should monitor for the occurrence of:

1. Hypokalemia
2. Hypocalcemia
3. Hyperglycemia
4. Hypernatremia

94. During her sixth month of pregnancy, a woman comes to the prenatal clinic for the first time. As part of the obstetric workup, a CBC and a urinalysis are performed. The nurse identifies that further assessment is required if laboratory findings reveal a:

1. WBC count of 9000/mm^3
2. Trace of glucose in the urine
3. Hemoglobin level of 10 g/dL
4. Urine specific gravity of 1.020

95. Two hours after an uneventful labor and birth, a client's uterus is 4 fingerbreadths above the umbilicus, BP is 80/40 mm Hg, and TPR is 98/100/22. After urinary catheterization, the fundus remains firm and 4 fingerbreadths above the umbilicus. The nurse should:

1. Notify the client's physician immediately
2. Palpate the client's fundus every 2 hours
3. Recheck the client's vital signs again in 30 minutes
4. Catheterize the client again in 1 hour for residual urine

96. During labor and birth, a client receives spinal anesthesia. Twenty-four hours later, the woman complains of a headache. The nurse identifies that this is a reaction to the anesthesia when the client states:

1. "My headache improves when I sit up."
2. "My headache gets better as soon as I walk a while."
3. "My head hurts worse when I am resting flat in the bed."
4. "My head hurts worse when I am sitting up feeding the baby."

97. A client has a history of myxedema. When performing a physical assessment, the nurse expects the client's skin to be:

1. Dry
2. Moist
3. Flushed
4. Smooth

98. After open reduction and internal fixation of a fractured hip, the nursing assessment of the affected leg should include checking the:

1. Femoral pulse
2. Toes for mobility
3. Condition of the pin
4. Range of motion of the knee

99. The nurse is caring for a client with myxedema who has undergone abdominal surgery. When administering opioids, the nurse understands that:

1. Tolerance to the drug develops readily
2. Opioids may interfere with the thyroid hormone
3. Sedation will have a paradoxical effect, causing hyperactivity
4. One-third to one-half the usual dose of the opioid should be prescribed

100. The nurse is caring for a child with spasmodic croup. The nurse knows that immediate nursing intervention is required for which adaptation?

1. Irritability
2. Hoarseness
3. Barking cough
4. Rapid respirations

101. What must the nurse emphasize to the family when preparing a child with persistent asthma for discharge?

1. A cold, dry environment is best for the child
2. Limits should not be placed on the child's behavior
3. When the child is asymptomatic, the health problem is gone
4. Medications must be continued even if the child is asymptomatic

102. The parents of a child with croup ask why their child is receiving humidified oxygen. The nurse should explain that humidified oxygen is given to:
    1. Minimize tissue edema
    2. Provide a mode for giving inhalant drugs
    3. Increase the surface tension of the respiratory tract
    4. Provide an environment free of pathogenic organisms

103. The nurse teaches the parents of a child with fever, headache, and a stiff neck that the test used to confirm the diagnosis of meningitis in a child is a:
    1. Blood culture
    2. Lumbar puncture
    3. Meningiomyelogram
    4. Peripheral skin smear

104. When caring for a client following a left pneumonectomy for cancer, the nurse should palpate the client's trachea at least once a day because:
    1. A mediastinal shift may have occurred
    2. Nodular lesions may demonstrate metastasis
    3. Tracheal edema may lead to an obstructed airway
    4. The cuff of the endotracheal tube may be overinflated

105. CBC, urinalysis, and x-ray examination of the chest are ordered for a client before surgery. The client asks why these tests are done. Which is the best reply by the nurse?
    1. "I don't know; the doctor ordered them."
    2. "Don't worry, these tests are strictly routine."
    3. "They are done to identify other health risks."
    4. "They determine whether surgery will be safe."

106. A client is scheduled for an abdominal resection. The first priority of preoperative nursing care is directed toward:
    1. Recording accurate vital signs
    2. Alleviating the client's anxiety
    3. Teaching about early ambulation
    4. Maintaining proper nutritional status

107. An infant born with hydrocephalus is to be discharged after insertion of a ventriculoperitoneal shunt. Which common complication of this type of surgery should the nurse explain to the parents to prepare them for their child's discharge?
    1. Violent involuntary muscle contractions
    2. Eyes with sclerae visible above the irises
    3. Excessive fluid accumulation in the abdomen
    4. Fever accompanied by decreased responsiveness

108. The parents are considering a bone marrow transplant for their child who has recurrent leukemia. The parents ask the nurse for clarification about the procedure. What is the most appropriate answer for the nurse to give the parents?
    1. "It is rarely performed in children."
    2. "The hematopoietic stem cells are surgically implanted in the bone marrow."
    3. "Your child's immune system must be destroyed before the transplantation can take place."

    4. "It is a simple procedure with little preparation needed, and the stem cells are infused as in a blood transfusion."

109. When helping a new mother on the postpartum unit develop her parenting role, the nurse should first:
    1. Give care to the baby in the mother's presence
    2. Provide enough time for her and the baby to be together
    3. Demonstrate baby bathing and care before discharge
    4. Find out what she knows about babies and proceed from there

110. A newborn develops a cephalhematoma. The nurse should plan to explain to the mother that:
    1. The swelling may cross a suture line
    2. The soft sac will bulge when the infant cries
    3. This will resolve spontaneously in several weeks
    4. This condition is unusual when a client has a vaginal birth

111. The physician orders famotidine (Pepcid) for a client with dyspepsia. The nurse should teach the client that this drug acts by:
    1. Lowering the stress level
    2. Neutralizing gastric acidity
    3. Decreasing gastrointestinal peristalsis
    4. Diminishing secretions in the stomach

112. Although the nurse is unable to identify any obvious signs or symptoms of bleeding, the client repeatedly has tested positive for occult blood in the stool. The nurse understands that continuous loss of a small amount of blood over a long period often results in:
    1. Iron depletion
    2. Shock syndrome
    3. Pernicious anemia
    4. Thrombocytopenia

113. The nurse is caring for a client with severe gastritis who has vomited a large amount of blood. A lavage is ordered. The nurse uses a room temperature irrigating solution to produce:
    1. Coagulation of blood
    2. Neutralization of acids
    3. Constriction of blood vessels
    4. Stimulation of the vagus nerve

114. After emergency surgery, a client requires a blood transfusion. When the client develops fever, chills, and low back pain, the nurse's first intervention is to:
    1. Call the physician immediately
    2. Stop the blood and infuse saline
    3. Relieve the symptoms with the ordered antihistamine
    4. Slow the rate of the transfusion and notify the blood bank

115. When entering a room, the nurse finds a new mother looking at her newborn, who is lying in the bassinet with eyes wide open. In response to this infant's behavior, the nurse:
    1. Turns on the lights in the room
    2. Positions the baby on the abdomen

3. Begins the baby's physical assessment

4. Encourages the mother to talk to her baby

116. The postpartum nurse notes that a client is gravida 1 and para 1. Her blood type is B negative, and her baby's blood type is O positive. The nurse identifies that the client's plan of care should include:
    1. Obtaining an order for RhoGAM
    2. Observing for ABO incompatibility
    3. Determining the father's blood type
    4. Immediate typing and cross-matching of her blood

117. While changing her baby's diaper, a client expresses concern about a small spot of red vaginal discharge on the diaper. The nurse should:
    1. Assess for other signs of bleeding
    2. Obtain an order for vaginal cultures
    3. Explain that this is an expected finding
    4. Apply a urine specimen bag to the perineum

118. When assessing a client with hyperthyroidism, the nurse should expect:
    1. Lethargy
    2. Weight gain
    3. Constipation
    4. Exophthalmos

119. A client with a small nodule of the thyroid gland is to have a subtotal thyroidectomy. When teaching the client about the surgery, the nurse explains that:
    1. The entire thyroid gland is removed
    2. A small part of the gland is left intact
    3. One parathyroid gland is also removed
    4. A portion of the thyroid and four parathyroids are removed

120. When assessing for the presence of affective behaviors associated with major depression, the nurse should monitor the client for:
    1. Echolalia
    2. Delusions
    3. Confusion
    4. Hopelessness

121. The most therapeutic nursing intervention for a client with major depression shortly after admission to the hospital is:
    1. Introducing the client to one other client
    2. Requiring participation in therapy sessions
    3. Encouraging interaction with others in small groups
    4. Conveying an attitude of concern that is not intrusive

122. A person who is hospitalized for alcoholism becomes boisterous and belligerent and verbally threatens the nurse. It is most appropriate for the nurse to:
    1. Place the client in restraints to prevent accidental self-injury
    2. Sedate and place the client in a quiet, controlled environment
    3. Allow the client to use excess energy by playing cards and visiting
    4. Set firm limits on the client's behavior and enforce adherence to them

123. A client with a history of alcohol abuse says to the nurse, "Drinking is a way out of my depression." Which strategy probably is most effective for the client at this time?
    1. A self-help group
    2. Psychoanalytic therapy
    3. A visit with a religious advisor
    4. Talking with an alcoholic friend

124. The nurse explores the possibility of joining Narcotics Anonymous (NA) with a client who has a history of drug abuse. This is based on the concept that NA is helpful in treating addictive behavior because:
    1. More change will take place within the group
    2. Group members share a common background and history
    3. Group members are supportive of each other's problems
    4. Addiction problems are dealt with more effectively in a group

125. The most important nursing action after a client undergoes cardiac catheterization via the femoral artery is to:
    1. Provide a bed cradle
    2. Check for a pulse deficit
    3. Elevate the head of the bed
    4. Assess the groin for bleeding

126. A client with heart failure is on a drug regimen of digoxin (Lanoxin) and furosemide (Lasix). The client dislikes oranges and bananas. Therefore the nurse should encourage the intake of:
    1. Apples
    2. Grapes
    3. Apricots
    4. Cranberries

127. A client in whom sexual dysfunction is diagnosed comments to the nurse, "Well, I guess my sex life is over." The most appropriate response by the nurse is:
    1. "I'm sorry to hear that."
    2. "Oh, you have a lot of good years left."
    3. "You are concerned about your sex life?"
    4. "Have you asked your doctor about that?"

128. A hospitalized client hurriedly approaches the nurse, saying that it sounds like there is a roaring fire in the bathroom. In reality, the client's roommate has just turned the shower on full force. The term that best describes this experience is:
    1. Illusion
    2. Delusion
    3. Dissociation
    4. Hallucination

129. The nurse understands that newborns with acquired herpes simplex virus type 2 infection often exhibit deficits in:
    1. Visual clarity
    2. Renal function
    3. Long bone growth
    4. Glucose metabolism

130. A newborn weighing 5 pounds 6 ounces is admitted to the newborn nursery after a cesarean birth. The nurse identifies that the respiratory rate is within expected limits if it is within the range of:
    1. 20 and 40/min
    2. 30 and 50/min
    3. 60 and 80/min
    4. 70 and 90/min

131. When the nurse assesses a newborn, a finding that indicates a need for follow-up care is:
    1. Babinski reflex is positive
    2. Head circumference is 33 cm
    3. Hips are abducted 30 degrees
    4. Umbilical cord has three vessels

132. A client is to be discharged with her newborn, who was just circumcised. The nurse, who is planning discharge instructions on postcircumcision care, should include telling the mother to:
    1. Apply diapers loosely
    2. Withhold feeding for 6 hours
    3. Cleanse the site with alcohol daily
    4. Expect some bleeding for 48 hours

133. A client in the psychiatric hospital with the diagnosis of bipolar disorder, manic phase, is argumentative, domineering, and exhibitionistic. Another visitor reports that this client is running down the hall scaring people. The nurse should initially:
    1. Ask the client the reason for running down the hall
    2. Assess the client's behavior in a nonthreatening manner
    3. Gather several staff members and approach the client together
    4. Contact the physician for seclusion and medication orders for the client

134. The nurse, caring for a 3-year-old child with meningitis, assesses for signs and symptoms of increased intracranial pressure. Select all that apply.
    1. ☐ Vomiting
    2. ☐ Headache
    3. ☐ Irritability
    4. ☐ Tachypnea
    5. ☐ Hypotension

135. A 65-year-old client is admitted to a nursing home with the diagnosis of dementia. When the nurse is assessing this client's mental status, the question that best tests ability for abstract thinking is:
    1. "Can you give me today's complete date?"
    2. "How are a television set and a radio alike?"
    3. "What would you do if you fell and hurt yourself?"
    4. "Can you repeat the following numbers: 8, 3, 7, 1, 5?"

136. An older adult with dementia is admitted to a nursing home. The client is confused, agitated, and at times unaware of the presence of others. To help this client initially adapt to the unit, the best nursing approach is to:
    1. Initiate a program of planned interaction
    2. Explain the nature and routines of the unit
    3. Explore in depth the reasons for the admission

4. Provide for the continuous presence of a staff member

137. An older adult male with dementia is admitted to a nursing home. His wife appears frail, tired, and angry when she first visits her husband. She remarks to the unit nurse in a sarcastic tone, "Let's see what you can do with him." The nurse's most therapeutic response to this comment is:
    1. "It has been very difficult to care for him."
    2. "I don't understand what you mean by that comment."
    3. "I know how to care for clients such as your husband."
    4. "It's too bad you didn't get some help to care for him at home."

138. A client is admitted to the hospital with myasthenia gravis. Because of the involvement of the ocular muscles, a common early adaptation for which the nurse should monitor the client is:
    1. Tearing
    2. Blurring
    3. Diplopia
    4. Nystagmus

139. The nurse teaches a client who is undergoing a neurologic evaluation that the test that might be ordered to help confirm the diagnosis of myasthenia gravis involves the use of the medication:
    1. Prednisolone
    2. Disodium EDTA
    3. Phenytoin (Dilantin)
    4. Edrophonium (Tensilon)

140. A hospitalized client is receiving neostigmine bromide (Prostigmin) for control of myasthenia gravis. In the middle of the night, the nurse finds the client weak, unable to move, and barely breathing. Signs that would identify the problems as being related to neostigmine bromide are:
    1. Distention of the bladder
    2. High-pitched gurgling bowel sounds
    3. Fine tremor of the fingers and eyelids
    4. Rapid pulse and occasional ectopic beats

141. The family of a client with myasthenia gravis asks the nurse whether the client will be an invalid. Given the individuality of response to myasthenia gravis, the nurse's best response is:
    1. "Medications will mask the signs of the disease."
    2. "With continuous treatment, the progression of the disease can usually be controlled."
    3. "The progression is slow, so people with myasthenia will spend their younger life with few problems."
    4. "There will be periods when bed rest will be necessary and times when regular activity will be possible."

142. The diversional activity that best meets the nursing objectives for a client with myasthenia gravis during periods of remission is:
    1. Hiking
    2. Swimming

3. Sewing classes

4. Watching television

143. A mother whose newborn infant son has a cleft lip and palate asks how to feed her baby, since he cannot suck properly. What information should the nurse provide concerning safe feeding technique for this infant?

1. "Since he tires easily, it is best to have him lying in bed while he is being fed."

2. "He should be held in a horizontal position and fed slowly to avoid aspiration."

3. "Try using a soft nipple with an enlarged opening, so he can get the milk through a chewing motion."

4. "Give him brief rest periods and frequent burpings during feedings, so he can get rid of swallowed air."

144. A client in her fourth month of pregnancy calls the nurse and states that her husband just told her he has genital herpes. When teaching about sexual activity, the nurse should include the fact that:

1. It will be necessary to refrain from all sexual contact during pregnancy

2. The use of condoms by her husband during sexual activity will be required

3. Sexual abstinence should be practiced during the last 6 weeks of a pregnancy

4. Meticulous cleaning of the hands and vaginal area after intercourse is essential

145. Early in the ninth month of pregnancy, a client experiences painless vaginal bleeding and is admitted to the hospital. The nursing care plan for this client should include:

1. Giving vitamin K to promote clotting

2. Performing a rectal examination to assess cervical dilation

3. Administering an enema to prevent contamination during birth

4. Placing her in a semi-Fowler's position to increase cervical pressure

146. Which criterion should the nurse use when assessing the gestational age of a preterm infant?

1. Simian creases

2. Reflex stability

3. Breast bud size

4. Fingernail length

147. The initial nursing action after the birth of a preterm baby with an Apgar score of 8 should be to:

1. Check, clamp, and dress the umbilical cord

2. Assist the physician with resuscitative measures

3. Obtain a footprint and apply an identification band

4. Quickly dry the baby and place in a controlled, warm environment

148. About 1 hour after birth, the nurse can expect a neonate to be:

1. Crying and cranky

2. Hyperresponsive to stimuli

3. Relaxed and sleeping quietly

4. Intensely alert with eyes wide open

149. When caring for clients with atherosclerosis, the nurse understands that atherosclerosis is:

1. Development of atheromas in the myocardium

2. Mobilization of free fatty acid from adipose tissue

3. Accumulation of fatty deposits within the intima of the arteries

4. Loss of elasticity in and thickening and hardening of the arteries

150. The nurse's initial approach to creating a therapeutic environment for any client should give priority to:

1. Providing for the client's safety

2. Accepting the client's individuality

3. Promoting the client's independence

4. Explaining to the client what is being done

151. The nurse raises three of the four side rails on the bed of a 73-year-old client who has had surgery for a fractured hip, specifically:

1. As a safety measure because of the client's age

2. Because clients older than 65 years of age should use side rails

3. To be used as handholds to facilitate the client's ability to move in bed

4. Because older adults often are disoriented for several days after anesthesia

152. A 4½-year-old child is brought to the emergency department with a fractured tibia. The nurse knows that in children of this age, the most frequently encountered type of fracture is classified as:

1. Greenstick

2. Transverse

3. Compound

4. Comminuted

153. The parents of a 4½-year-old child are concerned about the effects of hospitalization on their child. Based on an understanding of expected preschool behavior during hospitalization, the nurse should explain that the child probably will:

1. Refuse to cooperate with the nurses during their absence

2. Demonstrate despair if they do not visit at least once a day

3. Cry when they leave and return but not during their absence

4. Be unable to relate to children in the playroom if other parents are present

154. When caring for preschoolers, the nurse should understand that they think of death as a:

1. Cessation of life

2. Reversible separation

3. Happening that affects old people

4. Being who takes one away from the family

155. A client is in the intensive care unit after sustaining a T2 spinal cord injury. Which priority interventions should the nurse include in the client's plan of care? Select all that apply.

1. ❑ Minimizing environmental stimuli

2. ❑ Assessing for respiratory complications

3. ❑ Monitoring and maintaining blood pressure

4. ❏ Initiating a bowel and bladder training program
5. ❏ Discussing long-term treatment plans with the family

156. A client is scheduled for a vacuum aspiration abortion to terminate an unwanted pregnancy. The nurse's teaching plan should include telling her that:
1. It is a lengthy procedure that will cause no pain
2. Both she and her husband must sign the consent
3. An elevated temperature of 100.4° F or more should be reported immediately
4. She will experience a heavy menstrual flow for 1 to 2 weeks following the procedure

157. A client asks for and receives instruction regarding birth control methods. She elects to use a diaphragm with a spermicide. The nurse understands that a disadvantage of using a diaphragm is:
1. Its failure rate is 50% when used alone
2. It is physically uncomfortable when in place
3. It can lead to thrombus formation and pulmonary embolus
4. Insertion and removal sometimes are found to be objectionable

158. A client's sputum smears for acid-fast bacillus (AFB) are positive, and transmission-based precautions are instituted. The nurse plans to instruct the family to:
1. Avoid contact with objects in the room
2. Limit contact with nonexposed family members
3. Put on a gown and gloves before going into the room
4. Wear a high-efficiency particulate respirator when visiting

159. A 2-year-old child who has been restricted to bed rest because of a diagnosis of meningitis is now allowed out of bed. When the nurse suggests going to the playroom, the child, shaking the head vigorously from side to side, states, "No! Won't!" However, the child is trying to climb out of the crib at the same time. The nurse interprets this to mean that the child is:
1. Attempting to assert independence
2. Eager to resume regular play activities
3. Unsure of the difference between yes and no
4. Confused because of increased intracranial pressure

160. The nurse explains to a client with heart failure that sodium restriction is an effective therapeutic tool because it:
1. Allows excess tissue fluid to be excreted
2. Helps to control food intake and thus weight
3. Aids the weakened heart muscle to contract and improves cardiac output
4. Helps to prevent the potassium accumulation that occurs when sodium intake is high

161. When assisting a client to ambulate after repair of a fractured right hip, the nurse should stand:
1. Behind the client
2. In front of the client
3. On the client's left side
4. On the client's right side

162. A preschool-age boy has been restricted to bed rest since he was admitted to the hospital. As he begins to recover, he becomes interested in playing. Based on his developmental level and activity restriction, the nurse should provide him with:
1. Television viewing time
2. Squeaky stuffed animals
3. Little cars and a shoebox garage
4. Simple three- or four-piece wooden puzzles

163. A newborn is Rh-positive, and the mother is Rh-negative. The infant is to receive an exchange transfusion. The nurse understands that the baby will receive Rh-negative blood because:
1. It is the same as the mother's blood
2. It is neutral and will not react with the baby's blood
3. It eliminates the possibility of a transfusion reaction
4. Its RBCs will not be destroyed by maternal anti-Rh antibodies

164. An emergency tracheotomy is performed on a child with croup, and the child is receiving humidified air via a tracheotomy collar. When caring for this child, the nurse should suction the tracheotomy as soon as the child:
1. Is agitated, diaphoretic, and cyanotic
2. Tells the nurse of difficulty with breathing
3. Has severe substernal retractions and stridor
4. Becomes restless and pale, and the pulse increases

165. When caring for a client with a spinal cord injury during the immediate postinjury period, the nurse has the initial responsibility of:
1. Inhibiting urinary tract infections
2. Preventing contractures and atrophy
3. Avoiding flexion or hyperextension of the spine
4. Preparing the client for vocational rehabilitation

166. Three days after birth, a newborn is slightly jaundiced. The nurse understands that this is due primarily to:
1. Immature liver function
2. An inability to synthesize bile
3. An elevated maternal hemoglobin level
4. High hemoglobin with low hematocrit levels

167. During phototherapy, the nurse should apply eye patches to the newborn's eyes to:
1. Be sure the eyes are closed
2. Reduce overstimulation from bright lights
3. Prevent injury to the conjunctiva and retina
4. Limit excessive rapid eye movements and anxiety

168. When a developmental appraisal is performed on a 6-month-old infant, which observation is most important to the nurse in light of a diagnosis of hydrocephalus?
1. Head lag
2. Inability to sit unsupported
3. Absence of the grasp reflex
4. Presence of the Babinski reflex

169. When an infant with hydrocephalus is assessed, which assessment causes the nurse to suspect increasing intracranial pressure?
    1. Sunken eyes
    2. Projectile vomiting
    3. Depressed fontanels
    4. Narrowing pulse pressure

170. In the immediate postoperative period after a gastrectomy, the client's nasogastric tube is draining a light-red liquid. When assessing this client, the nurse expects this drainage for:
    1. 1 to 2 hours
    2. 3 to 4 hours
    3. 10 to 12 hours
    4. 24 to 48 hours

171. The nurse administers a parenteral preparation of potassium slowly and cautiously to prevent:
    1. Acidosis
    2. Cardiac arrest
    3. Psychotic-like reactions
    4. Edema of the extremities

172. The nurse is assessing a newborn. Which characteristic is unexpected in a full-term newborn?
    1. Few testicle rugae
    2. Multiple sole creases
    3. Pinna that stay flat when folded
    4. Angle of the wrist and forearm of 90 degrees

173. The nurse is caring for a client who is scheduled for a gastric bypass to treat morbid obesity. The nurse teaches the client that dumping syndrome can be avoided by maintaining a:
    1. Low-residue, bland diet
    2. Fluid intake below 500 mL
    3. Small, frequent feeding schedule
    4. Low-protein, high-carbohydrate diet

174. Nursing care for a client on the evening of surgery after a below-the-knee amputation should include:
    1. Elevating the foot of the bed
    2. Reapply the elastic bandage q2h
    3. Having the client walk in the room
    4. Assisting the client out of bed to a chair

175. A pregnant client complains of constipation. The nurse should explain that constipation frequently occurs during pregnancy because of:
    1. Changes in the metabolic rate
    2. Slowing of peristalsis in the GI tract
    3. Pressure of the growing uterus on the anus
    4. Increased intake of milk as recommended during pregnancy

176. The nurse identifies that the transition phase of labor has probably begun when the client:
    1. Complains of pain in the back
    2. Assumes the lithotomy position
    3. Perspires and has a flushed face
    4. States that her pains have lessened and contractions are less frequent

177. Shortly after giving birth, a client says she feels that she is bleeding. When checking the fundus, the nurse notes a steady trickling of blood from the vagina. The nurse's first action should be to:
    1. Call the physician immediately
    2. Check the client's BP and pulse
    3. Hold the fundus firmly and gently massage it
    4. Recognize the trickling of blood is a common occurrence

178. A postoperative client is diagnosed as having atelectasis. Which nursing assessment on auscultation of the client's lungs supports this diagnosis?
    1. Productive cough
    2. Clubbing of the fingertips
    3. Crackles at the height of inhalation
    4. Areas of diminished breath sounds

179. What is important nursing care for children with acute lymphocytic leukemia (ALL) on chemotherapeutic protocols?
    1. Preventing physical activity
    2. Checking their vital signs q2h
    3. Having them avoid contact with infected persons
    4. Reducing unnecessary stimuli in their environment

180. A child is receiving vincristine (Oncovin). What should the nurse expect the dietary plan to include to minimize the side effects of vincristine?
    1. Low in fat
    2. High in iron
    3. High in fluids
    4. Low in residue

181. The nurse is caring for a child with a very low platelet count related to chemotherapy. The nurse should monitor this child's urine for the presence of:
    1. Protein
    2. Glucose
    3. Erythrocytes
    4. Lymphocytes

182. The parents of a child with leukemia ask the nurse why irradiation of the spine and skull is necessary. What is the most accurate response by the nurse?
    1. "Radiation retards growth of cells in bone marrow of the cranium."
    2. "This therapy decreases cerebral edema preventing increased intracranial pressure."
    3. "Leukemic cells may invade the nervous system, but the usual drugs are ineffective in the brain."
    4. "Neoplastic drug therapy without radiation is effective in most cases, but this is a precautionary treatment."

183. The father of a child who is dying of cancer asks the nurse whether he should tell his 7-year-old son that his sister is dying. What is the most appropriate response by the nurse?
    1. "Your child cannot comprehend the real meaning of death, so don't tell him until the last moment."
    2. "You should talk this over with your doctor, who probably knows best what is happening in terms of your daughter's prognosis."

3. "Your son probably fears separation most and wants to know that you will care for him, rather than what will happen to his sister."

4. "Your son probably doesn't understand death as we do but fears it just the same. He should be told the truth to let him prepare for his sister's possible death."

184. During a routine prenatal visit, a client complains of leg cramps. The nurse suspects:
1. Hypercalcemia and tells her to increase her activity
2. Hypocalcemia and tells her to increase her intake of milk
3. Hyperkalemia and tells her to see a physician immediately
4. Hypokalemia and tells her to increase her intake of green, leafy vegetables

185. The nurse finds a 4½-year-old hospitalized girl, who has several siblings, crying and shouting at her teddy bear, "There! You bad girl! Don't be mad at your brother! Go to the hospital!" An understanding of preschooler development leads the nurse to believe that this behavior is based on the fact that the child:
1. Believes the parents love the brother more
2. Is mad at the brother and wishes he were sick
3. Misses the brother and wishes that they could be together
4. Thinks that being sick is related to bad thoughts about the brother

186. What gross motor skill should the nurse expect a developmentally appropriate 3-year-old child to perform?
1. Skipping on alternate feet
2. Riding alone on a small bicycle
3. Standing on one foot for a few seconds
4. Jumping rope by lifting both feet simultaneously

187. Methylphenidate hydrochloride (Ritalin) has been prescribed for a 7-year-old child with attention deficit/hyperactivity disorder (ADHD) to be taken with meals. What rationale should the nurse provide for the parents about the timing of medication administration?
1. Ritalin depresses the appetite
2. This will ensure proper absorption
3. It is an oral mucous membrane irritant
4. Children tend to forget to take it before meals

188. A client with acute respiratory distress syndrome is intubated and placed on a ventilator. Considering the purpose, operation, and complications associated with mechanical ventilators, the nurse should:
1. Regulate the PEEP according to the rate and depth of the client's respirations
2. Deflate the cuff on the endotracheal tube for a few minutes every one to two hours
3. Assess the need for suctioning when the high-pressure alarm of the ventilator is activated
4. Adjust the temperature of fluid in the humidification chamber depending on the volume of gas delivered

189. A client who has had thoracic surgery is admitted to the postanesthesia care unit. After the chest tubes are attached to a closed drainage system, the nurse should:
1. Check that the fluid in the water seal compartment rises with expiration
2. Ensure the security of the connections from the client to the drainage unit
3. Verify that there is vigorous bubbling in the wet suction control compartment
4. Empty the drainage container, measure and record the amount, and send a sample for analysis once a day

190. A client with schizophrenia has been experiencing hallucinations. The nurse should expect the hallucinations to be more frequent when the client is:
1. Trying to rest
2. Playing sports
3. Watching television
4. Interacting with others

191. The nurse determines that a person with schizophrenia, undifferentiated type, is improving when the client:
1. Stays away from other clients
2. Express negative feelings freely
3. Verbalizes better-developed delusions
4. Communicates in an organized manner

192. During the first prenatal visit of a woman who is 5 months pregnant, the nurse identifies that the client has a history of pica. The most appropriate nursing action is to:
1. Obtain an order for an iron supplement
2. Seek a psychologic referral for the client
3. Inform her of the danger this poses to her baby
4. Determine whether her diet is nutritionally adequate

193. During a prenatal visit, a client at 36 weeks' gestation complains of discomfort with irregular contractions. The nurse should instruct her to:
1. Lie down until they stop
2. Time them for at least 1 hour
3. Walk around until they subside
4. Take 10 grains of aspirin for the discomfort

194. A client is admitted to the hospital in active labor. After an amniotomy, the nurse should expect:
1. Increased fetal heart rate
2. Diminished vaginal bleeding
3. Less discomfort with contractions
4. Progressive dilation and effacement

195. During the postpartum period, the nurse identifies that a client's rubella titer is negative. The nurse should plan to:
1. Check for allergies to penicillin
2. Alert the nursing staff in the newborn nursery
3. Obtain an order for immunization at discharge
4. Assure the client that she has an active immunity

196. An infant with hydrocephalus has a ventriculoperitoneal (VP) shunt surgically inserted. What nursing care is essential during the first 24 hours after this procedure?
1. Medicating the infant for pain
2. Placing the infant in a high-Fowler's position

3. Positioning the infant on the side that has the shunt

4. Monitoring the infant for increasing intracranial pressure

197. An older adult is hospitalized for weight loss and dehydration because of nutritional deficits. When caring for this client, the nurse understands that in the older adult:

1. The daily fluid intake must be markedly increased

2. Financial resources usually are unrelated to nutritional status

3. Except for decreased caloric needs, the nutritional needs are unchanged

4. The individual's diet should be high in carbohydrates and low in proteins

198. Calcium EDTA (edetate calcium disodium) is to be used intravenously as the chelating agent for a child with plumbism (lead poisoning) who has not responded to succimer (Chemet). Which nursing intervention is most important to minimize the side effects of this therapy?

1. Testing the stool for occult blood

2. Assessing the diet because no junk food is allowed

3. Monitoring the urine output for adequate hydration

4. Administering the medication at night to reduce associated pain

199. The nurse explains to a client with arthritis that the prescribed steroid medication should be taken at mealtime because:

1. This will decrease gastric irritation

2. This will serve as a reminder to take the drug

3. The presence of food will enhance absorption

4. The medication is ineffective in an acid medium

200. The priority nursing intervention on admission of a primigravida in labor is:

1. Monitoring the fetal heart

2. Taking an obstetric history

3. Asking the client when she ate last

4. Determining whether the membranes have ruptured

201. An external monitor is placed on the abdomen of a client admitted in active labor. The nurse identifies that during each contraction, the fetal heart rate decelerates as the contraction peaks. The nurse should:

1. Notify the physician because of possible head compression

2. Place the client in a knee-chest position to avoid cord compression

3. Monitor the fetal heart rate until it returns to baseline when the contraction ends

4. Put the client in a semi-Fowler's position to prevent compression of the vena cava

202. When caring for a client with the diagnosis of bulimia nervosa, the nurse should understand that individuals with bulimia use food to:

1. Control others

2. Gain attention

3. Avoid growing up

4. Meet emotional needs

203. The nurse is admitting a client with a history of bipolar disorder. The nurse determines that the client is in the manic phase. Which signs and symptoms contribute to the nurse's conclusion? Select all that apply.

1. ☐ Irritability

2. ☐ Grandiosity

3. ☐ Pressured speech

4. ☐ Thought blocking

5. ☐ Psychomotor retardation

204. A client is admitted with a diagnosis of chronic adrenal insufficiency. Because of this condition, it is unwise for the nurse to place this client in a room:

1. With a middle-aged client who has pneumonia

2. Next to an adolescent client with a fractured leg

3. With an older adult who has had a brain attack

4. Away from the nurses' station in a private room

205. A client with adrenal insufficiency complains of weakness and dizziness, especially in the morning. The nurse understands that probably this is caused by:

1. A lack of potassium

2. Postural hypertension

3. A hypoglycemic reaction

4. Increased extracellular fluid volume

206. When teaching a client with Addison's disease about an appropriate diet, the nurse should instruct the client to:

1. Add extra salt to food

2. Limit intake to 1200 calories

3. Omit protein foods at each meal

4. Restrict the daily intake of fluids to 1 liter

207. When observing a client for side effects of long-term cortisone therapy, the nurse is particularly alert for:

1. Hypoglycemia

2. Severe anorexia

3. Anaphylactic shock

4. Behavioral changes

208. The nurse is caring for a 12-month-old infant with a diagnosis of failure to thrive. The infant's weight is below the third percentile, and development is delayed. Which behaviors of the child might suggest to the nurse the possibility of parental neglect?

1. Stiff, unpliable, and uncomforted by touch

2. Cuddly, responsive to touch, and seeks to be held

3. Able to sleep soundly, easily satisfied, but a poor eater

4. Responsive to adults, rarely cries, but shows little interest in the environment

209. The nurse observes that an infant has head control and can roll over, but can neither sit up without support nor transfer an object from one hand to the other. What developmental age should the nurse estimate based on these observations?

1. 2 to 3 months

2. 3 to 4 months

3. 4 to 6 months
4. 6 to 8 months

210. When selecting toys for a 5-month-old infant, the nurse should avoid giving the infant:
1. Large snap beads
2. Brightly colored mobiles
3. Rattles that the infant can hold
4. Soft stuffed animals that the infant can hold

211. The nurse plans care for a client with a somatoform disorder based on the knowledge that the disorder is:
1. A physiologic response to stress
2. A conscious defense against anxiety
3. An intentional attempt to gain attention
4. An unconscious means of reducing stress

212. During a group therapy session, some members accuse a client of intellectualizing to avoid discussing feelings. The client asks whether the nurse agrees with the others. The nurse's best response is:
1. "It seems that way to me, too."
2. "What is your perception of my behavior?"
3. "Are you uncomfortable with what you were told?"
4. "I'd rather not give my personal opinion at this time."

213. A client who was in an automobile accident is admitted to the hospital with multiple injuries. Approximately 14 hours after admission, the client begins to experience signs and symptoms of withdrawal from alcohol. Which of these signs and symptoms should the nurse relate to alcohol withdrawal? Select all that apply.
1. ☐ Fatigue
2. ☐ Anxiety
3. ☐ Runny nose
4. ☐ Diaphoresis
5. ☐ Psychomotor agitation

214. A client is admitted to the postanesthesia care unit after an abdominal hysterectomy. Which assessment should the nurse report to the physician immediately?
1. Apical pulse of 90
2. Decreased urinary output
3. Increased drainage from the nasogastric tube
4. Sero sanguineous drainage on the perineal pad

215. A client was rescued from a burning building and suffered partial- and full-thickness burns over 40% of the body. The initial physiologic change that the nurse expects is:
1. An increase in blood volume
2. An increase in serum potassium
3. A decrease in capillary permeability
4. A decrease in urinary specific gravity

216. The nurse is caring for a newly admitted male client, with the diagnosis of bipolar disorder, who has a history of hyperactivity and combativeness. Later in the evening, a commotion is heard, and this client is found beating another client. Legally:
1. The client should have been placed in restraints on admission
2. A client who is known to have been combative should have been kept sedated

3. A client with bipolar disorder who is in contact with reality does not require supervision
4. Because it was known that the client was frequently combative, close observation by the nursing staff was indicated

217. While the nurse is talking to a hypermanic client, the client's conversation becomes embarrassingly vulgar. The nurse should respond to the client's behavior by:
1. Tactfully teasing the client about the use of such vulgarity
2. Restricting the client's contact with staff members until the behavior stops
3. Asking the client to limit the use of vulgarity while continuing the conversation
4. Discreetly refusing to talk to the client when the client is speaking in this manner

218. A client who is recovering from an acute myocardial infarction complains about the lack of salt in the food. The nurse should explain that the salt must be limited to:
1. Prevent any rise in blood pressure from tissue edema
2. Reduce the circulating blood volume via a diuretic effect
3. Reduce the amount of edema present, which interferes with heart action
4. Prevent further accumulation of fluid, which increases the workload of the heart

219. The practitioner diagnoses that a client has acute cholecystitis with biliary colic. In addition to pain in the right upper quadrant, the nurse expects the client to exhibit:
1. Diarrhea with melena
2. Intolerance to foods high in lipids
3. Vomiting of coffee-ground emesis
4. Gnawing pain when the stomach is empty

220. After a cholecystectomy, the nurse should assess the client for signs of bleeding or hemorrhage. The nurse makes these observations because:
1. Prostaglandins are released at the surgical site
2. Inflammation interferes with platelet formation
3. Diaphragmatic excursion places pressure on the suture line
4. Blood clotting may be hindered by lack of vitamin K absorption

221. A client has a T-tube in place after an abdominal cholecystectomy and a choledochostomy. The nurse teaches the client that a T-tube is inserted primarily to:
1. Drain bile from the cystic duct
2. Keep the common bile duct patent
3. Prevent abscess formation at the surgical site
4. Provide a port for contrast dye in a cholangiogram

222. The nurse is assessing a client 8 hours after the creation of a colostomy. Which assessment finding should the nurse expect?
1. Presence of hyperactive bowel sounds
2. Absence of drainage from the colostomy
3. Dusky-colored, edematous-appearing stoma
4. Bright bloody drainage from the nasogastric tube

223. When admitting a client who is in labor to the birthing unit, the nurse asks the client about her marital status.

The client refuses to answer and becomes very agitated, telling the nurse to leave. The nurse should:

1. Refer the client to a social service organization for help
2. Question the family about the marital status of the client
3. Obtain this information to complete the client's history
4. Have restricted questions to those relevant to the situation

224. A 5-week-old infant is admitted to the hospital with a tentative diagnosis of a congenital heart defect. The infant tires easily and has difficulty breathing and feeding. In what position should the nurse place this infant?

1. Supine with the knees flexed
2. Orthopneic with pillows for support
3. Prone with the head supported by pillows
4. Side-lying with the upper body elevated

225. Anorexia nervosa follows a cyclic pattern. List the following statements in order of progression through this cycle. Number 1 is the first step and Number 4 is the fourth step in the cycle.

_____ Self-esteem increases as weight is lost
_____ Dieting is an attempt to maintain control
_____ Secondary gains reinforce the anorectic client's behaviors
_____ Sociocultural attitudes exert pressure for people to attain an idolized body

226. A client is admitted to the psychiatric unit with a history of agitation and difficulty sleeping. The client frequently reports, "The president is sending me secret microwave messages." The nurse repeatedly tells the client that this is not true and urges the client to forget about it and join the other clients in the dayroom. The client becomes more agitated and needs sedation. The situation may have been addressed more appropriately if the nurse recalled that:

1. The client's delusions should be accepted without rebuff or argument
2. Clients should be given antidepressants before incidents such as this occur
3. The client's sleeplessness and agitation should have been treated as symptoms
4. Clients need to be encouraged and often gently pushed into relating to other clients

227. Nutritional management is most important for the pregnant woman with cardiac problems. The nurse should advise these clients to eat a balanced diet with:

1. Limited fats
2. Moderate protein
3. Increased sodium
4. Controlled calories

228. A new father tells the nurse that he is anxious about feeling like a father. To meet the father's needs, the priority nursing action should be to:

1. Encourage the father's participation in a fathering class

2. Provide time for the father to be alone with and get to know the baby
3. Offer the father a demonstration on newborn diapering, feeding, and bathing
4. Allow time for the father to ask questions after viewing a film about a new baby

229. On a 6-week postpartum visit, a new mother tells the nurse she wants to feed her baby whole milk after 2 months because she will be returning to work. The nurse should plan to teach her that whole milk does not meet this infant's nutritional requirements because it is low in:

1. Fat and calcium
2. Vitamin C and iron
3. Thiamine and sodium
4. Protein and carbohydrates

230. The nurse is caring for a client who is receiving a unit of packed RBCs. Which finding leads the nurse to suspect a transfusion reaction caused by incompatible blood?

1. Dyspnea
2. Cyanosis
3. Backache
4. Bradycardia

231. As a result of a transfusion reaction, a client develops kidney damage. What is the most significant clinical response that the nurse should assess when determining kidney damage?

1. Glycosuria
2. Blood in the urine
3. Decreased urinary output
4. Acute pain over the kidney

232. A client with acute kidney failure complains of nausea, pain in the abdomen, diarrhea, and muscular weakness. Also, the nurse notes an irregularity in pulse. Based on this assessment data, the nurse concludes that the client most likely has:

1. Hyperkalemia
2. Hyponatremia
3. Hypouricemia
4. Hypercalcemia

233. To control uremia in a client with kidney failure, the nurse should teach the client to limit intake of:

1. Fluid
2. Protein
3. Sodium
4. Potassium

234. When caring for a client who is receiving peritoneal dialysis, the nurse should:

1. Position the client from side to side if fluid is not draining adequately
2. Notify the physician if there is a deficit of 200 mL in the drainage fluid
3. Maintain the client in a flat, supine position during the entire procedure
4. Remove the cannula at the end of the procedure, applying a dry, sterile dressing

235. Children with special needs have the same needs as those without special needs, although their means of

satisfying these needs may be limited. The nurse expects that these limitations will frequently cause:

1. Frustration
2. Overcompensation
3. Feelings of rejection
4. Emotional dysfunction

236. A nursing assessment of a client recently admitted to an alcohol-detoxification unit will probably reveal:
1. Nausea
2. Euphoria
3. Bradycardia
4. Hypotension

237. After a weight gain of 5 pounds in the past week, proteinuria of 3+, and a pronounced rise in blood pressure, a client at 38 weeks' gestation is admitted to the high-risk prenatal unit with a diagnosis of severe preeclampsia. Appropriate nursing care for this client should include:
1. Administering calcium gluconate
2. Preparing her for an immediate cesarean birth
3. Instituting IV therapy to facilitate renal emptying
4. Providing a dark, quiet room to minimize stimuli

238. When assessing a client who has been beaten and sexually assaulted, the emergency department nurse understands that emotional care for this client at this time should focus on:
1. The client's feelings of social isolation
2. Her inability to cope with the situation
3. The family's feelings about the attack
4. Disturbance in the client's thought processes

239. The physician orders oxygen therapy via nasal cannula at 2 L/min for an older, confused client with heart failure. The nursing action that takes priority is:
1. Maintaining the client on bed rest
2. Determining whether the client is agitated
3. Investigating whether the client has COPD
4. Obtaining a cannula of appropriate size for the client

240. The physician orders oropharyngeal suctioning as needed for a client in a coma. Which assessment made by the nurse indicates the need for suctioning?
1. Gurgling sounds with each breath
2. Fine crackles at the base of the lungs
3. Cyanosis in the nail beds of the fingers
4. Dry cough at increasingly frequent intervals

241. A father of three young children has contracted tuberculosis. Members of his family who have a positive reaction to the tuberculin test are candidates for treatment with:
1. Isoniazid (INH)
2. Multiple puncture tests (MPTs)
3. Bacille Calmette-Guèrin (BCG)
4. Purified protein derivative (PPD)

242. The nurse is caring for a client with a diagnosis of varicose veins. Which finding can the nurse expect to identify?
1. Discolored toenails
2. Complaints of leg fatigue
3. Localized heat in the calves
4. Reddened areas on the legs

243. When teaching a client about the causes of varicose veins, the nurse should include the occurrence of:
1. Repeated venous inflammatory episodes
2. Increased hydrostatic pressure in the veins
3. Obstruction of blood flow to the heart by the valves
4. Hereditary weakness in the surrounding leg muscles

244. The nurse understands that clients with AIDS are at risk for fungal and protozoal infections primarily because of the:
1. Autoimmune nature of the disease
2. Destruction of T4 cells by the AIDS virus
3. Invasion of vital organs by the AIDS virus
4. Associated high-risk sexual behaviors and drug-related practices

245. A client with AIDS is receiving a treatment protocol that includes a protease inhibitor. When assessing the client's response to this drug, which common side effect associated with this classification of drugs should the nurse expect?
1. Diarrhea
2. Hypoglycemia
3. Paresthesias of the extremities
4. Seeing yellow halos around lights

246. The nurse identifies that teaching about Coumadin (warfarin) is effective when the client states, "I must not drink:
1. Apple juice."
2. Grape juice."
3. Orange juice."
4. Cranberry juice."

247. Medication is prescribed for a 7-year-old child with attention deficit hyperactivity disorder (ADHD). When discussing this child's treatment with the parents, the school nurse emphasizes that it is important for them to:
1. Tutor their child in the subjects that are troublesome
2. Monitor the effects of the drug on their child's behavior
3. Explain to their child that the behavior can be controlled if desired
4. Avoid imposing too many rules because these will frustrate the child

248. The nurse performs preoperative teaching for a client who is to have cataract surgery. The nurse should include that after surgery, it is most important to:
1. Remain flat for 3 hours
2. Eat a soft diet for 2 days
3. Breathe and cough deeply
4. Avoid bending from the waist

249. A client receiving hemodialysis has an external shunt for circulatory access. With which life-threatening complication associated with external cannulas should the nurse be most concerned?
1. Infection
2. Hemorrhage

3. Skin breakdown

4. Impaired circulation

250. A male client receiving hemodialysis undergoes surgery to create an arteriovenous fistula. Before discharge, the nurse discusses care at home with the client and his wife. Which statement by the client's wife indicates that further teaching is required?
    1. "I must touch the shunt several times a day to feel for the bruit."
    2. "I have to take his blood pressure every day in the arm with the fistula."
    3. "He will have to be very careful at night not to lie on the arm with the fistula."
    4. "We really should check the fistula every day for signs of redness and swelling."

251. The practitioner diagnoses that a pale, listless, and tired 14-month-old child with a depressed appetite has acute nonlymphoid leukemia. The child is admitted to the hospital. In addition to the symptoms reported by the mother, what signs of the disease should the nurse expect?
    1. Oliguria
    2. Hypoblastemia
    3. Inability to swallow
    4. Depressed bone marrow

252. A 7-year-old child with juvenile idiopathic arthritis has difficulty getting ready for school in the morning because of joint pain and stiffness. Which recommendation should the nurse make to the family?
    1. Administer acetaminophen before bedtime
    2. Ice the joints that are painful in the evening
    3. Encourage a program of active exercise after awakening
    4. Provide warm, moist heat to the affected joints before arising

253. Which action should the nurse implement to prevent a secondary bladder infection in a client who has just had a suprapubic prostatectomy?
    1. Observe for signs of uremia
    2. Attach the catheter to suction
    3. Clamp off the connecting tube
    4. Change the dressings frequently

254. The nurse is caring for a client who just had a suprapubic prostatectomy. Which is the initial response of the nurse when this client complains of pain in the operative area?
    1. Administer the prescribed analgesic
    2. Inspect the drainage tubing for occlusion
    3. Encourage intake of fluids to dilute urine
    4. Assess vital signs before administering an analgesic

255. The nurse is discussing weight loss with an obese individual with Ménière's disease. Which suggestion by the nurse is most important?
    1. Limit intake to 900 calories a day
    2. Enroll in an exercise class at the local high school
    3. Get involved in diversionary activities when there is an urge to eat

4. Keep a diary of all foods eaten each day, making certain to list everything

256. A 3-year-old child is to receive a liquid iron preparation. The nurse should teach the mother to:
    1. Explain that loose stools are common with iron
    2. Administer the iron at least an hour before meals
    3. Have the child take the diluted iron preparation through a straw
    4. Avoid giving the child orange or other citrus juices with the iron preparation

257. When attempting to meet the emotional needs of a 4-year-old child who is receiving daily injections, the nurse should:
    1. Allow the child to play with a needle and syringe, and encourage acting out
    2. Provide the child with a doll and other equipment and observe what happens
    3. Encourage the child to draw pictures about what is happening and associated feelings
    4. Explain the procedure to the child in simple terms and allow at least 1 hour before an injection is scheduled

258. In addition to the usual problems associated with receiving multiple transfusions, the nurse should anticipate that a child with anemia has an increased risk for developing:
    1. Serum hepatitis
    2. Allergic response
    3. Pulmonary edema
    4. Hemolytic reaction

259. The school nurse understands that children with attention deficit problems may be learning disabled. This means that they:
    1. Probably will not be self-sufficient as adults
    2. Have intellectual deficits that interfere with learning
    3. Usually are performing two grade levels below their age norm
    4. Experience perceptual difficulties that make learning problematic

260. The nurse is evaluating the practice of a home health aide who is caring for a client who has paraplegia. Which behavior of the home health aide indicates understanding about the nursing team's responsibility in relation to pressure ulcers?
    1. Inspecting the client's skin daily
    2. Having the client sit on a rubber cushion
    3. Massaging body lotion over reddened areas
    4. Applying a heating pad to bony prominences

261. The occurrence of a pattern of behavior that uses physical symptoms in response to stress can be reduced if the nurse:
    1. Provides client teaching regarding medical care
    2. Teaches the client how to eliminate stress at home
    3. Assists the client in developing new coping mechanisms
    4. Decreases anxiety by limiting discussion of problems with the client

262. When assessing the oral cavity of a client with acquired immunodeficiency syndrome, the nurse identifies areas of white plaque on the client's tongue and palate. What is the nurse's initial response?
    1. Scrape an area of one of the lesions and send the specimen for a biopsy
    2. Instruct the client to perform meticulous oral hygiene at least once daily
    3. Document the presence of the lesions, describing their size, location, and color
    4. Realize that these lesions are almost universally found in clients with AIDS and require no special treatment

263. Three days after surgery for cancer of the colon, the nurse introduces the client to colostomy care. Which action should the nurse teach the client about skin care around the stoma?
    1. Rinse the area with peroxide before applying fresh gauze bandages
    2. Apply liberal amounts of Vaseline for 3 inches around the stoma
    3. Pour saline over the stoma and rub the area to remove hard fecal matter
    4. Wash the area with soap and water and then apply a protective ointment

264. Before discharge, a client with a colostomy questions the nurse about resuming prior activities. What is the nurse's best response?
    1. "Most sport activities, except for swimming, can be resumed based on your overall physical condition."
    2. "With counseling and medical guidance, a near normal lifestyle, including complete sexual function, is possible."
    3. "Activities of daily living should be resumed as quickly as possible to avoid depression and further dependency."
    4. "After surgery, changes in lifestyle must be made to accommodate the physiologic changes caused by the operation."

265. After surgical clipping of a cerebral aneurysm, the client develops the syndrome of inappropriate secretion of antidiuretic hormone. For which manifestation of excessive levels of antidiuretic hormone (ADH) should the nurse assess?
    1. Increased BUN
    2. Decreased urine output
    3. Decreased specific gravity
    4. Increased serum sodium level

ANSWERS AND RATIONALES: PART A

1. **3** Capillary refill based on the blanch test is an accurate assessment for neurovascular integrity; immediate refill is expected.

   1 Palpation of the pedal pulse, which is distal to the injury, is more appropriate than palpation of the femoral artery. **2** The pain associated with Homans' sign indicates thrombophlebitis, not compromise of blood flow or innervation. **4** Flexion and extension of the affected knee is impossible with this cast.

   Client Need: Reduction of Risk Potential; **Cognitive Level:** Application; **Nursing Process:** Evaluation/Outcomes; **Reference:** Ch 11, Fractures of the Extremities, Nursing Care

2. **1** Obesity is a risk factor for endometrial cancer because adipose cells store estrogen; the extent of exposure to estrogen is the most significant risk factor.

   2 Nulliparity, not multiparity, is a risk factor for endometrial cancer because of the increased exposure to estrogen. **3** Cigarette smoking is not identified as a risk factor for endometrial cancer. **4** Late, not early, onset of menopause is a risk factor for endometrial cancer because of the increased exposure to estrogen.

   Client Need: Physiological Adaptation; **Cognitive Level:** Application; **Nursing Process:** Assessment/Analysis; **Reference:** Ch 24, Uterine Neoplasms, Data Base

3. **1** Radiation is damaging to the skin and may cause it to become sensitive and friable.

   2 A radiated site should be cleaned only with water. **3** A snug-fitting bra can irritate delicate, irradiated skin and should be avoided until the irradiated area has healed. **4** This is contraindicated; lotion may contain compounds that alter the direction of x-rays.

   Client Need: Physiological Adaptation; **Cognitive Level:** Application; **Nursing Process:** Evaluation/Outcomes; **Reference:** Ch 3, Radiation, Major Side Effects

4. **2** This is a paradoxical situation in which sudden falls in blood glucose are followed by rebound hyperglycemia; this can result from insulin therapy.

   1 This is associated only with hyperglycemia; no sudden hypoglycemia occurs initially. **3** An insulin deficiency will result in hyperglycemia and ketoacidosis. **4** This occurs with hyperglycemia and hyperosmolarity, usually in clients who have type 2 diabetes.

   Client Need: Pharmacological and Parenteral Therapies; **Cognitive Level:** Analysis; **Nursing Process:** Evaluation/Outcomes; **Reference:** Ch 9, Diabetes Mellitus, Data Base

5. **2** Fibrous scar tissue can result from the trauma of repeated injections at the same site.

   1 Exercise is unrelated to lipodystrophy but it reduces blood glucose, which lowers insulin requirements. **3** Insulin is given subcutaneously; Z-track technique is used with some intramuscular injections. **4** Gentle pressure around the injection site after insulin administration promotes absorption.

   Client Need: Pharmacological and Parenteral Therapies; **Cognitive Level:** Application; **Integrated Process:** Teaching/Learning; **Nursing Process:** Planning/Implementation; **Reference:** Ch 9, Diabetes Mellitus, Nursing Care

6. **3** To be effective, insulin must be administered subcutaneously, where it can be absorbed; gastric juices destroy insulin taken by mouth.

   1 The other person has type 2 diabetes, which may be controlled with oral hypoglycemics, as well as by diet and exercise. **2** Oral hypoglycemics are not related to lipodystrophy; repeated injections of insulin cause lipodystrophies. **4** Oral hypoglycemics are not insulin; they either increase insulin secretion from the islet cells of the pancreas or increase the insulin sensitivity of extrapancreatic tissues in clients with type 2 diabetes.

   Client Need: Pharmacological and Parenteral Therapies; **Cognitive Level:** Application; **Integrated Process:** Teaching/Learning; **Nursing Process:** Planning/Implementation; **Reference:** Ch 9, Related Pharmacology, Antidiabetic Agents

7. **1** The client needs further teaching; dietetic fruit is not sugar-free and must be calculated in a diabetic individual's diet.

   2 Lettuce is considered a free food in the diet of a diabetic person. **3** It is suggested that the caloric intake of a diabetic person's diet should be 50% carbohydrate, 20% protein, and 30% fat. **4** Saturated fats should be limited to 10% of the fat intake; 90% should be unsaturated fats.

   Client Need: Basic Care and Comfort; **Cognitive Level:** Analysis; **Integrated Process:** Teaching/Learning; **Nursing Process:** Evaluation/Outcomes; **Reference:** Ch 9, Diabetes Mellitus, Data Base

8. **1** A sweet potato is equivalent to a serving of bread.

   2 One cup of skim or nonfat milk is a serving of milk. **3** A slice of avocado is equivalent to a serving of fat. **4** One teaspoon of mayonnaise is equivalent to a serving of fat.

   Client Need: Basic Care and Comfort; **Cognitive Level:** Analysis; **Integrated Process:** Teaching/Learning; **Nursing Process:** Planning/Implementation; **Reference:** Ch 9, Diabetes Mellitus, Data Base

9. **1** Akathisia (restlessness or desire to keep moving) can occur within 6 hours of the first dose of Haldol. This side effect is noted with most neuroleptics.

   2 This side effect of Haldol resembles Parkinson's disease, with masklike facies, characteristic tremor, and shuffling gait. **3** This most severe, largely irreversible, extrapyramidal side effect occurs after prolonged treatment with phenothiazines. **4** These reactions are characterized by severe, bizarre muscle contractions and would occur in the first few days of treatment.

   Client Need: Pharmacology and Parenteral Therapies; **Cognitive Level:** Application; **Nursing Process:** Evaluation/Outcomes; **Reference:** Ch 16, Neuroleptics (Antipsychotic Agents), Precautions

10. 3 Discussing reality-based issues helps decrease delusional and hallucinatory activity by reducing feelings of isolation and competition for sensory awareness.

1, 2 This will support and reinforce delusions and tend to validate them; the nurse should foster reality. 4 This is a judgmental response that may decrease the client's trust and increase anxiety.

Client Need: Psychosocial Integrity; **Cognitive Level:** Application; **Nursing Process:** Planning/Implementation; **Reference:** Ch 18, Schizophrenic Disorders, Nursing Care

11. 2 This, together with observation and documentation of the seizure activity, is the primary nursing care for a client with a tonic-clonic seizure.

1 This will assist with establishing an airway after the seizure, but it is an unsafe action during a seizure. 3 The client should not be left unattended; calling out for help may frighten the other clients. The nurse should remain with and protect the client. 4 This is done after the seizure; the mouth should not be pried open to insert an airway during a seizure, because injury may occur.

Client Need: Safety and Infection Control; **Cognitive Level:** Application; **Nursing Process:** Planning/Implementation; **Reference:** Ch 11, Epilepsy (Seizure Disorders), Nursing Care

12. 4 This is a description of a myelomeningocele, a neural tube defect in which the meninges and spinal nerves come through the opening in the spinal column. Nerve damage can occur at and below the level of the defect.

1 This is a description of an encephalocele, in which a portion of the brain, not the spinal cord, is involved. 2 This is a description of spina bifida occulta; this requires no intervention, because no break in the skin or protrusion of any structure has occurred. 3 This is a description of a meningocele; usually, no nerve damage is associated. Individuals may have minor disabilities.

Client Need: Physiological Adaptation; **Cognitive Level:** Comprehension; **Integrated Process:** Teaching/Learning; **Nursing Process:** Assessment/Analysis; **Reference:** Ch 30, Defects of Neural Tube Closure (Spina Bifida), Data Base

13. 3 This is done to prevent drying and breakage of the sac, because any opening increases the risk for infection to the central nervous system.

1 Diapering is contraindicated until the defect is repaired; the diaper may irritate the sac and cause rupture, predisposing to infection. 2 The legs are abducted to counteract subluxation, since the infant is unable to move the legs. 4 The baby generally is placed in a neutral position to reduce pressure on the affected area.

Client Need: Reduction of Risk Potential; **Cognitive Level:** Application; **Nursing Process:** Planning/Implementation; **Reference:** Ch 30, Defects of Neural Tube Closure (Spinal Bifida), Nursing Care

14. 1 Discontinuing the Pitocin lessens uterine stimulation and decreases intrauterine pressure; continuing the Pitocin may lead to fetal hypoxia, placental separation, or uterine rupture; turning the client onto the side increases oxygen perfusion to the fetus.

2 Although oxygen may be administered, continuing the administration of Pitocin may precipitate obstetric emergencies. 3 This is unsafe because it may precipitate complications such as placental separation or uterine rupture. 4 Pitocin should not be administered until the client is on a monitor.

Client Need: Pharmacology and Parenteral Therapies; **Cognitive Level:** Application; **Nursing Process:** Planning/Implementation; **Reference:** Ch 25, Intrapartum Period (Labor and Birth), Data Base

15. 1 This is the appropriate breathing technique for the transitional phase; it prevents the client from pushing too early.

2 The client is not fully dilated and is not ready to give birth. 3 The client is in active labor; she should be offered a bed pan if she requests to go to the bathroom. 4 Meperidine HCl (Demerol) should not be used in this phase of labor; the infant may be born with respiratory depression.

Client Need: Health Promotion and Maintenance; **Cognitive Level:** Application; **Nursing Process:** Planning/Implementation; **Reference:** Ch 25, Intrapartum Period (Labor and Birth), Nursing Care

16. 4 Vitamin K prevents hemorrhagic disease of the newborn because it activates coagulation factors in the liver. Intestinal flora, which synthesizes vitamin K, is absent in the newborn because the GI tract is sterile. With feeding and adaptation to the environment, intestinal flora become established.

1 The intestinal tract of the newborn is considered sterile. 2 Vitamin K substitutes for the action of intestinal flora. 3 Vitamin K does not stimulate further production of this vitamin; eventually, the bacterial flora of the intestine stimulates the production of vitamin K.

Client Need: Pharmacology and Parenteral Therapies; **Cognitive Level:** Comprehension; **Nursing Process:** Assessment/Analysis; **Reference:** Ch 27, Foundations of Nursing Care for Newborns, Adaptation to Extrauterine Life

17. 4 This is done instead of immersing the baby in a tub of water because the moisture will retard drying of the cord stump and will delay its falling off.

1 Drainage is indicative of infection; the cord stump should be dry. 2 Drying is desirable; moisture slows the drying process and promotes bacterial growth. 3 Keeping the cord stump covered delays drying.

Client Need: Health Promotion and Maintenance; **Cognitive Level:** Application; **Integrated Process:** Teaching/Learning; **Nursing Process:** Planning/Implementation; **Reference:** Ch 27, Foundations of Nursing Care for Newborns, Nursing Care Common to all Newborns

18. 1 The presence of fat in the duodenum stimulates painful contractions of the gallbladder to release bile; fat intake should be restricted.

2 Carbohydrates do not have to be restricted. 3 A reduction in spices and bulk is not necessary.

4 Although this diet might be desirable as long as the protein is not high in saturated fat, a high-calorie diet generally is not ordered.
Client Need: Basic Care and Comfort; **Cognitive Level:** Analysis; **Integrated Process:** Teaching/Learning; **Nursing Process:** Planning/Implementation; **Reference:** Ch 8, Cholelithiasis/Cholecystitis, Data Base

19. 3 This amount of drainage is inadequate; 1000 mL of bile is expected in 24 hours via this surgically implanted tube; the presence of a mechanical obstruction (tube compression or kinking) should be determined.
1 This is unlikely; also, this is not an independent nursing function. 2 This is unlikely; common bile duct edema takes several days to subside. 4 A T-tube drains by gravity, not by suction.
Client Need: Physiological Adaptation; **Cognitive Level:** Analysis; **Nursing Process:** Evaluation/Outcomes; **Reference:** Ch 8, Cholelithiasis/Cholecystitis, Nursing Care

20. 4 The development of insight is impeded by the client's unwillingness or inability to face his own contribution to a problem.
1 This will not impede the development of insight. Grandiosity is often a cover for feelings of inadequacy, which are threatening to the client; these feelings usually disappear with insight. 2 These will not impede the development of insight. These feelings are common in clients with borderline personality disorders. 3 This will not impede the development of insight. It is not the anger itself, but how the anger contributes to interpersonal difficulty, that the client must recognize.
Client Need: Psychosocial Integrity; **Cognitive Level:** Analysis; **Nursing Process:** Assessment/Analysis; **Reference:** Ch 15, Anxiety and Coping Behaviors, Defense Mechanisms

21. 2 Clients with borderline personality disorders initially tend to be engaging and to establish intense relationships, which they then test for signs of rejection. They tend to make others feel that they are not helpful and never could be.
1 These clients may be manipulative, but they rarely are devious or retiring. 3 These clients have a pronounced intolerance for being alone and usually are quite social. 4 These clients often are opinionated; they are not perfectionistic.
Client Need: Psychosocial Integrity; **Cognitive Level:** Application; **Nursing Process:** Assessment/Analysis; **Reference:** Ch 20, Personality Disorders, Data Base

22. 4 This action helps to establish a mutual relationship, which individuals with borderline personality disorders have difficulty maintaining on an ongoing basis.
1 Exploration of this topic in a meaningful manner can occur only after an ongoing relationship has been established. 2 Difficulty with authority figures often results from poor impulse control and a tendency to act out rather than to discuss problems; establishing a working relationship must precede this long-term goal. 3 Feeling victimized is a frequent theme among

clients with this disorder; however, they rarely have the insight to initiate discussion of these feelings and usually show resistance when the topic is mentioned.
Client Need: Psychosocial Integrity; **Cognitive Level:** Application; **Integrated Process:** Communication/Documentation; **Nursing Process:** Planning/Implementation; **Reference:** Ch 20, Personality Disorders, Nursing Care

23. 2 Since his legal difficulties were a precipitating event for hospitalization, if the client can realistically examine the possible outcomes of the trial, then some benefit has been gained from the therapy.
1 The client has been freely expressing resentment and victimization by his employer and authority figures; this would not show improvement or insight. 3 The client has been discussing his problems since admission, so this would not indicate the development of insight into his own behavior. 4 This would indicate unrealistic planning and would not demonstrate the development of insight into his own behavior.
Client Need: Psychosocial Integrity; **Cognitive Level:** Analysis; **Integrated Process:** Communication/Documentation; **Nursing Process:** Evaluation/Outcomes; **Reference:** Ch 20, Personality Disorders, Nursing Care

24. 4 There is no indication of adequate nutrition, especially of protein; an adequate caloric intake may also be missing. Both factors are necessary for the birth of a healthy full-term infant whose weight is appropriate for gestational age.
1 The caloric content of these foods is not high if small amounts are consumed; in addition, the weight gain of the client may not be reflective of an adequate weight gain in the developing fetus. 2 No data are available to support this. 3 Unrestricted salt intake does not contribute to the development of gestational hypertension.
Client Need: Basic Care and Comfort; **Cognitive Level:** Analysis; **Nursing Process:** Assessment/Analysis; **Reference:** Ch 25, Prenatal Period: Physical, Physiologic, and Emotional Changes During Pregnancy

25. 3 Severe preeclampsia develops suddenly with a blood pressure of 160/110 or higher and proteinuria of 2+ to 3+ or more. Severe headache, blurred vision, and photophobia may be present.
1 This is characterized by seizures. 2 In mild preeclampsia, the systolic pressure is 30 mm Hg above baseline, and the diastolic pressure is 15 mm Hg above baseline; proteinuria may be 2+; headaches may be absent or transient, and blurred vision is not present. 4 Gestational hypertension occurs after mid-pregnancy as an elevation of blood pressure without proteinuria.
Client Need: Physiological Adaptation; **Cognitive Level:** Analysis; **Nursing Process:** Assessment/Analysis; **Reference:** Ch 26, Hypertensive Disorders of Pregnancy, Data Base

26. 3 This client can become eclamptic suddenly and have a seizure; seizure precautions are necessary to protect her from injuring herself and the fetus.

1 This is important, but the client's safety should be ensured first by placing her on seizure precautions. **2** Administering sedatives will help to reduce nervous system irritability; it will not ensure safety if the client has a seizure. **4** This will be required when the client is placed on magnesium sulfate therapy.

Client Need: Safety and Infection Control; **Cognitive Level:** Application; **Nursing Process:** Planning/Implementation; **Reference:** Ch 26, Hypertensive Disorders of Pregnancy, Nursing Care

27. **2** Retinal damage caused by the increased intraocular pressure of glaucoma is permanent and is progressive if the disease is not controlled.

1 Early treatment may prevent blindness. **3** One eye may be affected, and there is no restriction on the use of either eye. **4** Surgery can open up drainage and permanently reduce pressure.

Client Need: Physiological Adaptation; **Cognitive Level:** Comprehension; **Integrated Process:** Teaching/Learning; **Nursing Process:** Planning/Implementation; **Reference:** Ch 11, Glaucoma, Data Base

28. **4** The client usually is instructed to do this to toughen the limb for weight bearing. This process is begun by pushing the residual limb against increasingly harder surfaces.

1 Abduction of the residual limb does not maintain functional alignment and should be avoided; it does not prepare the end of the residual limb for a prosthesis. **2** Dangling the residual limb does not help prepare it for a prosthesis and may impede venous return, which prolongs healing. **3** This may macerate the residual limb and hinder the use of a prosthesis.

Client Need: Reduction of Risk Potential; **Cognitive Level:** Application; **Integrated Process:** Teaching/Learning; **Nursing Process:** Planning/Implementation; **Reference:** Ch 11, Amputation, Nursing Care

29. **2** Asthma involves spasms of the bronchi and bronchioles, as well as increased production of mucus. This decreases the size of the lumina, interfering with inhalation and exhalation.

1 This is not a mechanism involved in asthma, in which interference with both inhalation and exhalation occurs. **3** The client cannot hyperventilate because of mucosal edema, bronchoconstriction, and secretions, all of which cause airway obstruction. Emotional stress is only one of many precipitating factors, such as allergens, temperature changes, odors, and chemicals. **4** A decrease in the vital capacity of the lungs will occur.

Client Need: Physiological Adaptation; **Cognitive Level:** Comprehension; **Nursing Process:** Assessment/Analysis; **Reference:** Ch 7, Obstructive Airway Diseases, Data Base

30. **3** During sleep, mucous secretions in the respiratory tract move slowly toward the throat. On awakening, increased ciliary motion raises these secretions more vigorously, thus facilitating expectoration and the collection of sputum specimens.

1 Although activity mobilizes secretions, no secretions may be present at the time of activity; sputum is most plentiful upon arising. **2** The sputum may leave an unpleasant taste in the mouth, which may interfere with appetite. **4** Sputum more likely would be collected after respiratory treatment, because this mobilizes secretions.

Client Need: Reduction of Risk Potential; **Cognitive Level:** Application; **Nursing Process:** Planning/Implementation; **Reference:** Ch 7, Pneumonia, Nursing Care

31. **2** Although dust cannot be avoided completely, use of a damp cloth helps eliminate the quantity of airborne particles that might be inhaled.

1 This is unnecessary and unrealistic. **3** There are ways to limit the quantity of airborne particles. **4** Redecorating will not eliminate dust; it is part of our environment.

Client Need: Health Promotion and Maintenance; **Cognitive Level:** Application; **Integrated Process:** Teaching/Learning; **Nursing Process:** Planning/Implementation; **Reference:** Ch 32, Asthma, Nursing Care

32. **2** Inadequate oxygenation of the brain may produce restlessness or behavioral changes.

1 The pulse increases with cerebral hypoxia. **3** The pupils dilate with cerebral hypoxia. **4** This is the result of increased vascularization and reflects an adaptation to prolonged hypoxia.

Client Need: Physiological Adaptation; **Cognitive Level:** Application; **Nursing Process:** Evaluation/Outcomes; **Reference:** Ch 3, Perioperative Care, General Nursing Care of Clients During the Postoperative Period

33. 1. ☒ Fever is a common finding in croup.
2. ☐ Crackles are not characteristic of croup.
3. ☐ Bronchospasm is not characteristic of croup.
4. ☒ The cough is tight, with a barking, metallic sound due to laryngeal edema.
5. ☒ Children with croup experience inspiratory stridor because of laryngeal edema.

Client Need: Physiological Adaptation; **Cognitive Level:** Analysis; **Nursing Process:** Assessment/Analysis; **Reference:** Ch 30, Respiratory Tract Infections, Data Base

34. **2** To follow the physician's order would result in an act of negligence that may endanger the client. If the dosage is not changed after the physician is questioned, the nurse should contact the supervisor.

1 The dose should be withheld because it may result in respiratory depression and may endanger both the woman and the fetus. **3** The nurse is at risk for negligence, since giving this medication can endanger the woman and the fetus. **4** The nurse does not have an order for the usual dose and should notify the nursing supervisor before calling the director of obstetrics.

Client Need: Management of Care; **Cognitive Level:** Application; **Integrated Process:** Communication/Documentation; **Nursing Process:** Planning/Implementation; **Reference:** Ch 26, Hypertensive Disorders of Pregnancy, Data Base

35.
1. ☒ Increased oxygen safeguards the fetus.
2. ☐ There is no infection present and therefore there is no reason for an antibiotic to be administered.
3. ☒ This will decrease uterine activity. Five contractions in 8 minutes does not allow enough time for uterine relaxation and reperfusion between contractions.
4. ☒ This improves umbilical circulation by increasing cardiac output.
5. ☒ Repositioning the mother on the side decreases cord compression, which improves circulation to the fetus.

Client Need: Pharmacological and Parenteral Therapies; **Cognitive Level:** Analysis; **Nursing Process:** Planning/Implementation; **Reference:** Ch 25, Intrapartum Period (Labor and Birth), Data Base

36. 4 Cerebral edema from hypertension or cerebral ischemia may occur and may cause seizures.
1 Increasing fluid intake may lead to an increase in blood pressure and edema. **2** Glomerulonephritis will not alter pupillary action. **3** This is appropriate for children with nephrotic syndrome, in which the child has hypoalbuminemia that causes fluid to shift from plasma to the abdominal cavity.

Client Need: Safety and Infection Control; **Cognitive Level:** Application; **Nursing Process:** Planning/Implementation; **Reference:** Ch 33, Acute Post Streptococcal Glomerulonephritis, Nursing Care

37. 4 Applesauce provides nutrition without large additional amounts of potassium and sodium.
1 Peanuts are high in sodium, which increases fluid retention. **2** Pretzels are high in sodium, which increases fluid retention. **3** Bananas are high in potassium, which is contraindicated.

Client Need: Basic Care and Comfort; **Cognitive Level:** Analysis; **Nursing Process:** Planning/Implementation; **Reference:** Ch 33, Acute Post Streptococcal Glomerulonephritis, Data Base

38. 1 The client controls anxiety by maintaining a childlike body build and by demonstrating mastery over food intake.
2 Families of anorectic persons usually are fused, so separation from parents is not a desirable gain. **3** Anorectic persons generally excel in academic areas and receive attention and praise as the perfect child; they will not gain from having this source of attention removed. **4** Maintenance of an immature body build, not the resulting overattention of parents, is the primary gain.

Client Need: Psychosocial Integrity; **Cognitive Level:** Application; **Nursing Process:** Assessment/Analysis; **Reference:** Ch 20, Eating Disorders, Overview

39. 4 This occurs because of endocrine imbalance resulting from starvation; it is thought that severe starvation damages the hypothalamus.
1 Many of these clients have lowered body temperature. **2** These clients have bradycardia. **3** These clients are cold intolerant.

Client Need: Physiological Adaptation; **Cognitive Level:** Application; **Nursing Process:** Assessment/Analysis; **Reference:** Ch 20, Anorexia Nervosa, Data Base

40. 4 Starvation or inadequate/inappropriate nutrition can lead to electrolyte imbalances, which are life threatening.
1, 2 This will be a later therapy; the priority is to correct electrolyte imbalances. **3** Client independence, not separation from family members, is supported.

Client Need: Physiological Adaptation; **Cognitive Level:** Application; **Nursing Process:** Planning/Implementation; **Reference:** Ch 20, Anorexia Nervosa, Data Base

41. 1 Alteration in the hormone hCG may cause nausea and vomiting during the first trimester; the stomach should be neither too full nor too empty. Small, more frequent meals usually are suggested.
2 This will not help the nausea and vomiting associated with the first trimester of pregnancy; it may be prescribed during the second trimester when pyrosis and acid indigestion occur because progesterone slows GI tract motility. **3** This is not a treatment for nausea. **4** Ingestion of large amounts of fluids, combined with prolonged emptying of the stomach during pregnancy, may increase nausea; small sips of fluid are recommended.

Client Need: Basic Care and Comfort; **Cognitive Level:** Application; **Integrated Process:** Teaching/Learning; **Nursing Process:** Planning/Implementation; **Reference:** Ch 25, Prenatal Period: Physical, Physiological, and Emotional Changes During Pregnancy

42. 2 COPD causes increased pressure in the pulmonary circulation. The right side of the heart hypertrophies (cor pulmonale), causing right ventricular heart failure.
1 This system is not as closely related to the pulmonary system as is the cardiac system; kidney problems usually do not occur because of COPD. **3** The skeletal system is not directly related to the pulmonary system; joint inflammation does not occur because of COPD. **4** Peripheral nerves are not as closely related to the pulmonary system as to the cardiac system; peripheral neuropathy does not occur because of COPD.

Client Need: Physiological Adaptation; **Cognitive Level:** Application; **Nursing Process:** Assessment/Analysis; **Reference:** Ch 7, Obstructive Airway Diseases, Data Base

43. 2 Atmospheric pressure is greater than pressure inside the pleural space. If a chest tube is not attached to a drainage system closed by a water seal, air will enter the pleural space and will collapse the lung (pneumothorax).
1 Capillarity is the tendency of cohesive liquid molecules to rise in a tube; this is not the purpose of water in a chest tube drainage system. **3** This is the purpose of the drainage collection chamber and suction working together, not the water seal chamber. **4** The concern is not primarily to prevent pressure within the tube itself, but to prevent atmospheric pressure from collapsing the lung.

Client Need: Physiological Adaptation; **Cognitive Level:** Comprehension; **Nursing Process:** Planning/Implementation; **Reference:** Ch 7, Related Procedures, Chest Tubes

44. **2** This action does not require a physician's order and is an independent action.

1, 3, 4 This is a dependent nursing function, which requires a physician's order.

Client Need: Physiological Adaptation; **Cognitive Level:** Application; **Nursing Process:** Planning/Implementation; **Reference:** Ch 7, Malignant Lung Tumors, Nursing Care

45. **1** This open-ended statement focuses on the client's concerns and allows further verbalization of feelings.

2, 4 This moves the focus away from the client and minimizes the client's concerns. **3** Although true, this response may increase anxiety and may cut off communication.

Client Need: Psychosocial Integrity; **Cognitive Level:** Analysis; **Integrated Process:** Caring; Communication/Documentation; **Nursing Process:** Planning/Implementation, **Reference:** Ch 12, Bladder Tumors; Nursing Care

46. **4** The concept of object permanence begins to develop around 6 months of age.

1, 2 This occurs at between 13 and 24 months. **3** This occurs during the first several months of life.

Client Need: Health Promotion and Maintenance; **Cognitive Level:** Application; **Nursing Process:** Assessment/Analysis; **Reference:** Ch 30, Health Promotion of Infants, Play During Infancy

47. **2** Because electrodes are placed internally (on the fetal scalp, not on the mother's abdomen), position does not affect the monitor.

1 Constant monitoring provides continuous ongoing assessment of fetal status; there is no reason to detach the leads. **3** It is not the position but the internal placement of electrodes on the fetal scalp that ensures accurate monitoring. **4** This position can cause hypotension because the gravid uterus causes decreased venous return, leading to reduced cardiac output.

Client Need: Basic Care and Comfort; **Cognitive Level:** Application; **Integrated Process:** Teaching/Learning; **Nursing Process:** Planning/Implementation; **Reference:** Ch 25, Intrapartum Period (Labor and Birth), Nursing Care

48. **1** According to the Silverman-Anderson Index for respiratory function, flaring of the nares indicates respiratory distress.

2 Acrocyanosis (blue color of hands and feet) is common in all newborns at birth because of inadequate circulation to the extremities. **3** These are expected in the neonate; respiratory function is largely a matter of diaphragmatic contraction; expansion of the rib cage is limited in the neonate. **4** The expected respiratory rate for neonates ranges between 30 and 60/min; therefore 48 indicates that there is no distress.

Client Need: Reduction of Risk Potential; **Cognitive Level:** Application; **Nursing Process:** Assessment/Analysis; **Reference:** Ch 27, Foundations of Nursing Care for Newborns, Nursing Care Common to All Newborns

49. **3** This occurs prior to lactation; it is an exaggeration of venous and lymphatic circulation caused by prolactin.

1 Engorgement occurs before lactation or milk production. **2** Effective breastfeeding does not prevent engorgement; a lag between the production of milk and the efficiency of the ejection reflex often causes engorgement. **4** This does not cause engorgement, but support may relieve some of the discomfort.

Client Need: Health Promotion and Maintenance; **Cognitive Level:** Application; **Integrated Process:** Teaching/Learning; **Nursing Process:** Planning/Implementation; **Reference:** Ch 25, Postpartum Period, Data Base

50. **1** This will decrease edema and minimize pain.

2 Dry dressings, when removed, may further damage the burn site. **3** Although pain is temporarily alleviated, removal of the spray is necessary before medical treatment can be instituted; removal may cause injury. **4** Ointments are contraindicated on burns because they have an oil base.

Client Need: Physiological Adaptation; **Cognitive Level:** Application; **Integrated Process:** Teaching/Learning; **Nursing Process:** Planning/Implementation; **Reference:** Ch 10, Burns, Nursing Care

51. **2** Decreasing urinary output indicates hypovolemia that results from a fluid shift from the vascular space to the burned area.

1, 3, 4 This is expected with deep partial-thickness burns.

Client Need: Physiological Adaptation; **Cognitive Level:** Application; **Integrated Process:** Teaching/Learning; **Nursing Process:** Planning/Implementation; **Reference:** Ch 10, Burns, Data Base

52. **4** Although older adults may be faced with multiple stressors as they age, how people cope with stress remains fairly constant throughout life.

1 Decreases in the senses of taste and smell are noted as people age. **2** GI motility decreases slightly with aging; sedentary lifestyles and lack of dietary fiber compound the problem. **3** Muscle strength decreases with aging.

Client Need: Psychosocial Integrity; **Cognitive Level:** Analysis; **Nursing Process:** Assessment/Analysis; **Reference:** Ch 15, Anxiety and Coping Behaviors, Overview

53. **2, 1, 3, 4**

____1____ When negating the diagnosis is unsuccessful, the client becomes angry and negative.

____2____ The initial response is shock, disbelief, and denial, and the client seeks additional opinions to negate the diagnosis.

____3____ Bargaining for wellness follows in an attempt to prolong life.

____4____ As the reality of the situation becomes more apparent, depression sets in and the client may become withdrawn.

Client Need: Psychosocial Integrity; **Cognitive Level:** Analysis; **Nursing Process:** Assessment/Analysis; **Reference:** Ch 1, Grieving Process, Theorists: Stages of Grieving

54. **2** A closed, sterile drainage system reduces the likelihood that microorganisms will be introduced into the bladder.

1 The bag usually is emptied according to hospital protocol or if it becomes full. **3** Tension on the tubing should be avoided because this may injure the mucous membranes of the urinary tract. **4** This is unsafe because if the side rail is put down abruptly, it may pull out the catheter.

Client Need: Basic Care and Comfort; **Cognitive Level:** Application; **Nursing Process:** Planning/Implementation; **Reference:** Ch 12, Related Procedures, Urinary Catheterization

55. **4** Patency promotes bladder decompression, which prevents distention and bleeding; continuous flow of an irrigant limits clot formation and promotes hemostasis.

1 This is not associated with a transurethral resection of the prostate (TURP); a cystostomy tube is a catheter that is placed directly into the bladder through a suprapubic incision. **2** No abdominal incision is made because the resection is performed via the urethra. **3** Although hemorrhage and infection may occur, no wound is observed because the surgery was performed via the urethra.

Client Need: Basic Care and Comfort; **Cognitive Level:** Application; **Nursing Process:** Planning/Implementation; **Reference:** Ch 12, Benign Prostatic Hyperplasia, Nursing Care

56. Answer: 21 gtt/min

Multiply the amount to be infused (125) by the drop factor (10) and divide the result by the amount of time in minutes (60 minutes):

$$\frac{125}{60} \times 10 = 20.8$$

20.8 must be rounded up to 21 gtt/min.

Client Need: Pharmacological and Parenteral Therapies; **Cognitive Level:** Application; **Nursing Process:** Planning/Implementation; **Reference:** Ch 3, Fluid, Electrolyte, and Acid-Base Balance; General Nursing Care of Clients With Fluid and Electrolyte Problems

57. **3** This presents reality and simply states expected behavior.

1 This is an authoritarian, not a therapeutic, statement. **2** This does not tell the client what behavior is expected. **4** This assumes that the client does not want to take medication, whereas the client may not understand what to do.

Client Need: Pharmacology and Parenteral Therapies; **Cognitive Level:** Application; **Integrated Process:** Communication/Documentation; **Nursing Process:** Planning/Implementation; **Reference:** Ch 18, Schizophrenic Disorders, Nursing Care

58. **4** The use of reflection assists the client in expressing feelings, which is the major goal of therapy.

1, 3 This is a defensive response by the nurse that tends to cut off communication and limit the expression of feelings. **2** This response avoids discussion of the client's feelings about the therapist.

Client Need: Psychosocial Integrity; **Cognitive Level:** Analysis; **Integrated Process:** Communication/Documentation;

Nursing Process: Planning/Implementation; **Reference:** Ch 16, Therapeutic Nurse-Client Relationship, Overview

59. **1** Hourly output is critical when kidney function is assessed; decreasing urinary output is a sign of rejection.

2 This is too long an interval between assessments of urinary output after a kidney transplant. **3, 4** This is too short an interval between assessments of urinary output after a kidney transplant.

Client Need: Reduction of Risk Potential; **Cognitive Level:** Application; **Nursing Process:** Planning/Implementation; **Reference:** Ch 12, Chronic Kidney Failure/End-Stage Renal Disease, Nursing Care

60. **3** Serum creatinine concentration measures the kidney's ability to excrete metabolic wastes. Creatinine, a nitrogenous product of protein breakdown, is elevated in renal insufficiency.

1 WBC does not measure kidney function; white blood cells usually are depressed because of immunosuppressive therapy to prevent rejection. **2** This test is more valuable for assessing structure than function. **4** Although this should be considered, it is not as definitive as the serum creatinine level.

Client Need: Reduction of Risk Potential; **Cognitive Level:** Analysis; **Nursing Process:** Evaluation/Outcomes; **Reference:** Ch 12, Chronic Kidney Failure/End-Stage Renal Disease, Nursing Care

61. **4** Immunosuppressants such as azathioprine (Imuran) and cyclosporine (Sandimmune) are given to prevent rejection and depress WBCs.

1 Elevated WBC is associated with bacterial infection; leukopenia is associated with immunosuppressive therapy. **2** High creatinine levels do not cause leukopenia; elevated creatinine levels are caused by kidney failure. **3** Rejection of the kidney does not cause leukopenia; signs of rejection include decreased urine output, elevated serum creatinine, hypertension, and edema.

Client Need: Pharmacological and Parenteral Therapies; **Cognitive Level:** Analysis; **Nursing Process:** Evaluation/Outcomes; **Reference:** Ch 12, Chronic Kidney Failure/End-Stage Renal Disease, Nursing Care

62. **1** Obstruction of the pancreatic duct and the absence of enzymes (trypsin, amylase, and lipase) to aid fat digestion and absorption lead to wasting of tissues and failure to thrive. Currently, it is recommended that children with CF consume 150% to 200% of the calories recommended for their body weight.

2 Despite dyspnea and shortness of breath, when feeling well, these children have voracious appetites; the difficulty involves poor digestion and malabsorption of fats and fat-soluble vitamins. **3** Increased bowel motility and diarrhea are not associated with cystic fibrosis. **4** The pulmonary disease process leads to localized respiratory dysfunction, not to retarded physical growth.

Client Need: Physiological Adaptation; **Cognitive Level:** Comprehension; **Nursing Process:** Assessment/Analysis; **Reference:** Ch 31, Cystic Fibrosis, Data Base

63. **3** The caloric intake should be 150% to 200% more than the expected intake for size and age, because absorption of fats and nutrients is compromised by the disease process.

1 Fluids are encouraged, to keep bronchial secretions from becoming too thick and tenacious. **2** Salt is added to the diet to compensate for excessive sodium losses in saliva and perspiration. **4** Whole milk may not be tolerated because of its high fat content; skim milk or other milk products should be substituted.

Client Need: Basic Care and Comfort; **Cognitive Level:** Analysis; **Integrated Process:** Teaching/Learning; **Nursing Process:** Evaluation/Outcomes; **Reference:** Ch 31, Cystic Fibrosis, Data Base

64. **1** Because the pancreatic ducts are blocked and fibrotic, oral pancreatic enzymes must be given to make the nutrients digestible and absorbable.

2 Children with cystic fibrosis have good, even voracious, appetites despite respiratory impairment. **3** Chewing of food is adequate despite coughing and shortness of breath; undernourishment results from inadequate nutrient absorption. **4** It is not the consistency of the foods that leads to inadequate digestion and absorption, but the lack of enzymes from the pancreatic duct.

Client Need: Basic Care and Comfort; **Cognitive Level:** Application; **Integrated Process:** Teaching/Learning; **Nursing Process:** Planning/Implementation; **Reference:** Ch 31, Cystic Fibrosis, Data Base

65. **3** Compromised heart function in the infant often results in cyanosis and fatigue during sucking and swallowing because cardiac output is decreased.

1 When a feeding problem persists in a newborn, this generally is an indication of some pathology. **2** Impaired sucking is never insignificant; it may be indicative of many problems, such as CNS involvement, immaturity, or a congenital defect. **4** Healthy infants are free of mucus within 24 to 48 hours after birth.

Client Need: Physiological Adaptation; **Cognitive Level:** Analysis; **Nursing Process:** Assessment/Analysis; **Reference:** Ch 30, Cardiac Malformations, Data Base

66. **1** Hypoxia leads to poor peripheral circulation; clubbing occurs as a result of tissue hypertrophy and additional capillary development in the fingers.

2 These children have polycythemia. **3** Respirations generally are rapid to compensate for O_2 deprivation. **4** This is not an adaptation of children with chronic hypoxia.

Client Need: Physiological Adaptation; **Cognitive Level:** Application; **Nursing Process:** Assessment/Analysis; **Reference:** Ch 30, Cardiac Malformations, Data Base

67. **4** This traction is used to reduce the fracture, align the bone, and temporarily reduce muscle spasm.

1 Edema occurs because of tissue trauma and will not be prevented by Buck's extension. **2** A fractured head

of the femur is repaired via internal fixation; a cast is unnecessary. **3** Damage already has occurred at the time of trauma and is not prevented by Buck's extension.

Client Need: Basic Care and Comfort; **Cognitive Level:** Comprehension; **Nursing Process:** Assessment/Analysis; **Reference:** Ch 11, Fracture of the Hip, Data Base

68. **4** This ensures abduction of the leg to maintain position of the prosthesis and avoid dislocation.

1 This is not necessary as long as abduction of the limb is maintained. **2** This causes flexion of the hip; it is done only if ordered by the physician. **3** A trochanter roll at the ankle can cause damage to the peroneal nerve along the external malleolus.

Client Need: Basic Care and Comfort; **Cognitive Level:** Application; **Nursing Process:** Planning/Implementation; **Reference:** Ch 11, Fracture of the Hip, Nursing Care

69. **3** This client is demonstrating increased agitation and poses an immediate threat to the safety of other clients. The behavior requires immediate nursing intervention to prevent injury to self or others.

1 Although the client may be suspicious, data given do not indicate that this presents a danger to the self or to others; controlling the client who is threatening others is the priority. **2** Although the client probably is hallucinating, there is no immediate threat to the self or others; controlling the agitated client is the priority. **4** Although anxious, this client does not represent a threat to self or others; controlling the agitated client is the priority.

Client Need: Management of Care; **Cognitive Level:** Analysis; **Nursing Process:** Planning/Implementation; **Reference:** Ch 16, Anger Management, The Nurse's Role in Anger Management Therapy

70. **4** This offers support and provides the client with an opportunity to discuss feelings.

1 This intervention does not address the client's depression. **2** This limits further communication and may imply rejection. **3** Teaching is inappropriate when a client is emotionally distressed.

Client Need: Psychosocial Integrity; **Cognitive Level:** Application; **Integrated Process:** Communication/Documentation; **Nursing Process:** Planning/Implementation; **Reference:** Ch 19, General Nursing Care of Clients With Mood Disorders

71. **4** Rationalization is an unconscious defense mechanism whereby a person finds logical reasons for behavior or feelings while ignoring the illogical or unacceptable real reasons.

1 Denial is an unconscious defense mechanism whereby intolerable situations or events are not acknowledged. **2** Projection is an unconscious defense mechanism whereby an individual attributes or blames personal inadequacies on others. **3** Identification is an unconscious defense mechanism whereby an individual assumes the characteristics, traits, posture, and achievements of another person or group.

Client Need: Psychosocial Integrity; **Cognitive Level:** Analysis; **Nursing Process:** Assessment/Analysis; **Reference:** Ch 15, Anxiety and Coping Behaviors, Defense Mechanisms

72. 3 Confused clients find comfort and security in an environment that provides it, because this reduces the need for self-regulation.

1 This may be confusing and may precipitate anxiety. 2 No environment can meet all of any client's needs. 4 This provides for physical, not psychologic, safety.

Client Need: Psychosocial Integrity; **Cognitive Level:** Application; **Nursing Process:** Planning/Implementation; **Reference:** Ch 18, Dementia, Nursing Care

73. 4 Ineffective coping is the impairment of a person's adaptive behaviors and problem-solving abilities in meeting life's demands; ritualistic behavior fits under this category as a defining characteristic.

1, 2, 3 Not enough information is available to lead to this conclusion.

Client Need: Psychosocial Integrity; **Cognitive Level:** Comprehension; **Nursing Process:** Assessment/Analysis; **Reference:** Ch 19, Obsessive-Compulsive Disorders, Data Base

74. 4 Beginning with equipment is less threatening and may stimulate feelings of mastery.

1 This will provide information but will do little to aid acceptance. 2 This is helpful but may take time and therefore may not meet immediate needs. 3 This will do little to aid acceptance.

Client Need: Health Promotion and Maintenance; **Cognitive Level:** Application; **Integrated Process:** Teaching/Learning; **Nursing Process:** Planning/Implementation; **Reference:** Ch 8, Cancer of Small Intestine, Colon, or Rectum, Nursing Care

75. 4 The rhythmic movement of the merry-go-round provides an opportunity for the child to practice spatial and sensory orientation. This is important in helping the child increase interaction with the environment.

1, 3 This does not provide rhythmic movements that would engage the child. 2 The autistic child rejects cuddling and anything that feels cuddly.

Client Need: Psychosocial Integrity; **Cognitive Level:** Analysis; **Nursing Process:** Assessment/Analysis; **Reference:** Ch 17, Pervasive Developmental Disorders (Including Autism and Asperger's), Data Base

ANSWERS AND RATIONALES: PART B

76. **4** Protein in the urine is a sign of preeclampsia, as are elevated BP and weight gain of more than 1 kg (2.2 lb) per week.

1 Changes in body temperature are not associated with preeclampsia. **2** These signs indicate preeclampsia; treatment does not require a vaginal examination. **3** The signs indicate preeclampsia, and the client should be seen more frequently than every 2 eeks.

Client Need: Reduction of Risk Potential; **Cognitive Level:** Analysis; **Nursing Process:** Planning/Implementation; **Reference:** Ch 26, Hypertensive Disorders of Pregnancy, Data Base

77. **3** The antagonist of magnesium sulfate is calcium gluconate, and it should be at the bedside.

1 This is an opiate antagonist. **2** This is ineffective if the action of magnesium is not reversed. **4** This is not related to the toxic effect of magnesium sulfate; it may be necessary if the client has a seizure.

Client Need: Pharmacological and Parenteral Therapies; **Cognitive Level:** Comprehension; **Nursing Process:** Planning/Implementation; **Reference:** Ch 26, Hypertensive Disorders of Pregnancy, Data Base

78. **3** This accurately describes the behavioral therapy method of systematic desensitization.

1 This is a different behavioral approach called operant conditioning. **2** This is a different behavioral approach called flooding. **4** This is a psychoanalytic type therapy rather than a behavioral approach.

Client Need: Psychosocial Integrity; **Cognitive Level:** Application; **Integrated Process:** Communication/Documentation; **Nursing Process:** Planning/Implementation; **Reference:** Ch 19, Phobic Disorders, Data Base

79. **1** Protein is required for the building and repair of intestinal tissues.

2 Increased protein will not significantly affect peristalsis. **3** Anemia may result from chronic bleeding; usually, it is corrected with increased iron and adequate protein intake. **4** Protein is given to promote healing; once tissues are repaired, muscle tone may improve eventually.

Client Need: Basic Care and Comfort; **Cognitive Level:** Comprehension; **Integrated Process:** Teaching/Learning; **Nursing Process:** Planning/Implementation; **Reference:** Ch 8, Review of Nutrients, Sources of Energy

80. **2** In addition to dilation of bronchi, treatment is aimed at expectoration of mucus. Mucus interferes with gas exchange in the lungs.

1 This is an unrealistic goal; asthma is a chronic illness. **3** Increased fluid intake helps liquefy secretions. **4** Asthma has a psychogenic factor but this is not the only cause; it may occur as an allergic response to an antigen, such as dust.

Client Need: Physiological Adaptation; **Cognitive Level:** Application; **Nursing Process:** Planning/Implementation; **Reference:** Ch 7, Obstructive Airway Diseases, Data Base

81. **4** This drug reduces inflammation and the inflammatory response in bronchial walls.

1 Beclomethasone does not directly promote comfort. **2** Beclomethasone is not an antibiotic. **3** Beclomethasone does not stimulate smooth muscle relaxation.

Client Need: Pharmacological and Parenteral Therapies; **Cognitive Level:** Application; **Nursing Process:** Assessment/Analysis; **Reference:** Ch 7, Related Pharmacology, Bronchodilators and Antiasthmatics

82. **3** This approach allows for ventilation of feelings and clarifies explanations that probably were not heard or understood because of anxiety.

1 This prevents the client from facing the problem, thereby increasing her feelings of loss of control. **2** This closes off communication by not allowing free expression of grief and assumes that the client blames herself. **4** This supports avoidance of the reality of the situation; it does not solve the problem.

Client Need: Psychosocial Integrity; **Cognitive Level:** Application; **Integrated Process:** Teaching/Learning; **Nursing Process:** Planning/Implementation; **Reference:** Ch 29, Nursing Care Related to Meeting the Needs of the Family of a Child With Special Needs

83. **4** This parent's action gives his child more control by allowing the child to make a decision. This demonstrates an understanding of what the toddler can and cannot do safely.

1 Toddlers are too young to understand that this type of punishment is a response to the temper tantrum; it may lead to more frustration and anger. **2** Although tantrums as attention-getting devices largely must be ignored, isolating the child will produce feelings of rejection and insecurity. **3** This may lead to the development of more manipulative tactics, since the action brought a degree of success initially.

Client Need: Health Promotion and Maintenance; **Cognitive Level:** Analysis; **Integrated Process:** Teaching/Learning; **Nursing Process:** Evaluation/Outcomes; **Reference:** Ch 31, Growth and Development, Major Learning Events

84. **1** Because the compulsive ritual is used to control anxiety, any attempt to prevent the action will increase the anxiety.

2 Underlying hostility is considered to be part of the disorder itself, not a reaction to an interruption of the ritual. **3** This is possible only if the anxiety reached panic levels and caused the person to express anger overtly. **4** This is not a pattern of behavior associated with this disorder.

Client Need: Psychosocial Integrity; **Cognitive Level:** Analysis; **Nursing Process:** Evaluation/Outcomes; **Reference:** Ch 19, Obsessive-Compulsive Disorders, Nursing Care

85. **3** The therapeutic nurse-client relationship provides an opportunity for the client to try out different behaviors in an accepting atmosphere and ultimately to replace pathologic responses with more effective responses. **1** Verbal communication, not nonverbal communication, is the objective of the therapeutic relationship. **2** The nurse, although accepting of the client's hostile feelings, uses the therapeutic relationship to redirect hostile feelings into more acceptable behaviors. **4** The nurse provides the support and acceptance that encourage clients to make their own decisions.

Client Need: Psychosocial Integrity; **Cognitive Level:** Comprehension; **Integrated Process:** Communication/ Documentation; **Nursing Process:** Assessment/Analysis; **Reference:** Ch 16, General Nursing Care of Clients with Mental Health/Psychiatric Problems

86. **1** African Americans represent a higher-risk population than Caucasian Americans for hypertension; the reason is unknown. **2** Blacks of both sexes have a higher prevalence than whites of both sexes. **3** Black women are more frequently affected by hypertension than are white women. **4** Black men have a higher risk than black women.

Client Need: Health Promotion and Maintenance; **Cognitive Level:** Application; **Integrated Process:** Teaching/Learning; **Nursing Process:** Planning/Implementation; **Reference:** Ch 6, Hypertension, Data Base

87. **3** Diuretics block sodium reabsorption and promote fluid loss, decreasing blood volume and reducing arterial pressure. **1** Direct relaxation of arteriolar smooth muscle is accomplished by vasodilators, not by diuretics. **2** Vasodilators, not diuretics, act on vascular smooth muscle. **4** Drugs that act on the nervous system, not diuretics, inhibit sympathetic vasoconstriction.

Client Need: Pharmacological and Parenteral Therapies; **Cognitive Level:** Comprehension; **Integrated Process:** Teaching/ Learning; **Nursing Process:** Assessment/Analysis; **Reference:** Ch 6, Related Pharmacology, Diuretics

88. **2** Thiazide diuretics are potassium-depleting agents; broccoli provides 267 mg of potassium per 100 grams. **1** Apples provide 80 to 110 mg of potassium per 100 grams of fruit. **3** Cherries provide 191 mg of potassium per 100 g of fruit. **4** Cauliflower provides 206 mg of potassium per 100 g.

Client Need: Basic Care and Comfort; **Cognitive Level:** Analysis; **Integrated Process:** Teaching/Learning; **Nursing Process:** Planning/Implementation; **Reference:** Ch 8, Review of Nutrients, Minerals

89. **3** This response acknowledges feelings and attempts to collect more data. **1** This will not facilitate data collection about the extent of anxiety. **2** Anxiety is most often a response to a vague, nonspecific threat; the client will not be able to answer this question. **4** It is too early to try to identify the cause of the anxiety; crisis intervention with anxious clients requires a more structured approach than "Let's talk."

Client Need: Psychosocial Integrity; **Cognitive Level:** Analysis; **Integrated Process:** Communication/Documentation; **Nursing Process:** Planning/Implementation; **Reference:** Ch 16, Crisis Intervention, Nursing Care of Clients in Crisis

90. **2** The primary goal is to keep the client safe. A no-suicide contract secures the client's agreement not to attempt suicide for a specified period and to seek help when suicidal ideas increase. **1, 4** This is part of the treatment plan after the immediate crisis is controlled. **3** This is part of the long-range treatment plan after the immediate crisis is controlled.

Client Need: Psychosocial Integrity; **Cognitive Level:** Application; **Nursing Process:** Planning/Implementation; **Reference:** Ch 19, General Nursing Care of Clients With Mood Disorders

91. **4** This allows the child to manipulate unfamiliar equipment; this action tends to reduce the stress of hospitalization. **1** This is appropriate for school-age children and adolescents. **2** Although this is appropriate play for a 3-year-old child, it is somewhat limited because it does not give the child an opportunity to handle unfamiliar hospital equipment. **3** Storytelling is more appropriate for the school-age child.

Client Need: Health Promotion and Maintenance; **Cognitive Level:** Application; **Nursing Process:** Planning/Implementation; **Reference:** Ch 32, Hospitalization of Preschoolers, General Nursing Care of Preschoolers

92. **1** Preschoolers do not have the cognitive ability to understand that death is irreversible. **2** Preschoolers are unable to make logical connections between cause and effect. **3** If a family member died in the hospital, this might be true; however, this is not a predominant belief. **4** Preschoolers do not have an understanding of the inevitability of death.

Client Need: Health Promotion and Maintenance; **Cognitive Level:** Comprehension; **Nursing Process:** Assessment/Analysis; **Reference:** Ch 32, Hospitalization of Preschoolers, Data Base

93. **2** Hypocalcemia, decreased calcium in the blood, occurs because of the reciprocal relationship with phosphorus, which is increased by the decreased glomerular filtration rate. **1** Hyperkalemia, not hypokalemia, is more likely to occur because of decreased kidney function. **3** Hyperglycemia, an elevated serum glucose level, is directly related to kidney function. **4** Hypernatremia, an elevated serum sodium, generally will not be present because fluid will be retained in the same proportion as sodium.

Client Need: Physiological Adaptation; **Cognitive Level:** Analysis; **Nursing Process:** Assessment/Analysis; **Reference:** Ch 12, Chronic Kidney Failure/End-Stage Renal Disease, Data Base

94. **3** This reading suggests a true anemia rather than the physiologic anemia of pregnancy, which occurs because the plasma volume increases to a greater extent than the red blood cells during pregnancy.

1 This is within the expected range of 5000 to 10,000/mm^3; it may rise to 15,000/mm^3 during the second half of pregnancy. **2** This is not unusual during pregnancy; a lowered renal threshold for glucose exists during pregnancy. **4** This is within the expected range of 1.010 to 1.030.
Client Need: Reduction of Risk Potential; **Cognitive Level:** Analysis; **Nursing Process:** Assessment/Analysis; **Reference:** Ch 25, Prenatal Period: Physical, Physiologic, and Emotional Changes During Pregnancy

95. **1** The increased height of the uterus may result from accumulation of blood in the uterus from internal hemorrhaging; vital signs may be indicative of impending shock.
2, 3, 4 The client needs immediate medical intervention; she may be having an intrauterine hemorrhage.
Client Need: Management of Care; **Cognitive Level:** Application; **Integrated Process:** Communication/Documentation; **Nursing Process:** Planning/Implementation; **Reference:** Ch 26, Postpartum Bleeding, Data Base

96. **4** A headache that results from low spinal anesthesia usually occurs 24 to 72 hours after its administration. The headache worsens when the client assumes an upright position.
1 This type of headache will worsen when the head is elevated. **2** This type of headache will worsen when the client is ambulatory. **3** A headache that results from spinal anesthesia improves when the client is lying flat.
Client Need: Pharmacological and Parenteral Therapies; **Cognitive Level:** Analysis; **Nursing Process:** Evaluation/Outcomes; **Reference:** Ch 25, Intrapartum Period (Labor and Birth), Data Base

97. **1** This is caused by decreased function of sebaceous glands; a paucity of thyroid hormones T3 and T4, which control the basal metabolic rate and can alter the function of almost every body system, is evident.
2, 4 This occurs with hyperfunction of the thyroid and an increase in BMR. **3** The skin will not be flushed.
Client Need: Physiological Adaptation; **Cognitive Level:** Application; **Nursing Process:** Assessment/Analysis; **Reference:** Ch 9, Hypothyroidism, Data Base

98. **2** This assesses neural integrity distal to the surgical site.
1 The femoral artery is not assessed because it is not distal to the surgical site. **3** No pin is present because an internal fixation was performed.
4 This assessment may cause flexion of the hip, which is contraindicated.
Client Need: Physiological Adaptation; **Cognitive Level:** Application; **Nursing Process:** Evaluation/Outcomes; **Reference:** Ch 11, Fracture of the Hip, Nursing Care

99. **4** Because of lowered metabolism, the usual adult dose of an opioid may result in an overdose.
1 Hypothyroidism does not alter tolerance. **2** Opioids do not alter the thyroid hormone; a lowered basal metabolic rate prolongs the time for drug detoxification and elimination. **3** Opioids will cause excessive sedation, not hyperactivity.
Client Need: Reduction of Risk Potential; **Cognitive Level:** Application; **Nursing Process:** Planning/Implementation; **Reference:** Ch 9, Hypothyroidism, Nursing Care

100. **4** Rapid respirations may be a sign of impending airway obstruction.
1 Unless irritability is accompanied by severe restlessness, symptomatic care should be given.
2 Unless accompanied by signs of respiratory embarrassment, this needs no immediate intervention. **3** This may sound ominous, but it is not a sign of respiratory embarrassment.
Client Need: Physiological Adaptation; **Cognitive Level:** Application; **Nursing Process:** Planning/Implementation; **Reference:** Ch 30, Respiratory Tract Infections, Data Base

101. **4** Children with persistent asthma must continue taking medications to keep them asymptomatic. Inhaled corticosteroids, long-acting β_2 agonists, and leukotriene modifiers are used as controller medications.
1 Some environmental moisture is necessary for these children. **2** Consistent limits should be placed on the child's behavior regardless of the disease; a chronic illness does not remove the need for limit setting. **3** The child's symptoms are being controlled by medications that are necessary to keep the child asymptomatic.
Client Need: Management of Care; **Cognitive Level:** Analysis; **Integrated Process:** Teaching/Learning; **Nursing Process:** Planning/Implementation; **Reference:** Ch 32, Asthma, Nursing Care

102. **1** Cool mist helps reduce inflammation of the upper respiratory tract.
2 Inhalant drugs are administered through nebulizers. **3** The mist has no effect on surface tension of the respiratory tract. **4** This is not the purpose of humidified oxygen.
Client Need: Physiological Adaptation; **Cognitive Level:** Comprehension; **Integrated Process:** Teaching/Learning; **Nursing Process:** Planning/Implmentation; **Reference:** Ch 30, Respiratory Tract Infections, Nursing Care

103. **2** A culture of cerebrospinal fluid (CSF) would reveal the presence of a causative organism (e.g., pneumococcus, tubercle bacillus, meningococcus, or streptococcus).
1 This is not a definitive test, although it is done because occasionally a blood culture will be positive when a CSF culture is negative. **3** This is used to detect the presence of abnormalities through injection of a contrast medium into the subarachnoid space; it does not identify the organism. **4** This demonstrates the presence of bacteria on the skin; it does not identify organisms in the CSF.
Client Need: Reduction of Risk Potential; **Cognitive Level:** Analysis; **Integrated Process:** Teaching/Learning; **Nursing Process:** Assessment/Analysis; **Reference:** Ch 30, Meningitis, Nursing Care

104. 1 After a pneumonectomy, the mediastinum may shift toward the remaining lung, or the remaining lung may shift toward the empty space, depending on the pressure within the empty space. Either of these shifts will cause the trachea to move from its usual midline position. (The trachea is palpated above the suprasternal notch.)

2 Metastatic lesions do not appear rapidly. 3 Tracheal edema cannot be assessed through palpation. 4 The cuff of the endotracheal tube cannot be assessed through palpation of the trachea.

Client Need: Physiological Adaptation; **Cognitive Level:** Analysis; **Nursing Process:** Evaluation/Outcomes; **Reference:** Ch 7, Malignant Lung Tumors, Nursing Care

105. 3 Certain diagnostic tests (e.g., CBC, urinalysis, chest x-ray examination) are done preoperatively to rule out the existence of health problems that may increase the risks involved with surgery.

1 Lack of knowledge without a statement of plans to obtain the information suggests incompetence on the part of the nurse. 2 Feelings would not be dispelled by this response; it also blocks further communication. 4 Surgery poses a risk despite test results.

Client Need: Reduction of Risk Potential; **Cognitive Level:** Analysis; **Integrated Process:** Teaching/Learning; **Nursing Process:** Planning/Implementation; **Reference:** Ch 3, Perioperative Care, General Nursing Care of Clients During the Preoperative and Intraoperative Periods

106. 2 Anxiety experienced by a preoperative client can be a disruptive force that may affect the client's ability to adapt psychologically and physiologically. For other nursing measures to be effective, anxiety must be alleviated.

1 Vital signs must be recorded, because they will serve as a baseline in postoperative assessment; however, reduction of anxiety is the priority. 3 Learning is hampered by high anxiety levels. 4 The diet is limited before surgery so that residue in the intestines will be decreased.

Client Need: Psychosocial Integrity; **Cognitive Level:** Application; **Integrated Process:** Caring; **Nursing Process:** Planning/Implementation; **Reference:** Ch 3, Perioperative Care, General Nursing Care of Clients During the Preoperative and Intraoperative Periods

107. 4 These are associated with infection. This is the greatest postoperative hazard for children with shunts for hydrocephalus.

1 This may occur as the result of an infected shunt; however, it is not the most common sign of an infectious process. 2 These occur with progressively increasing intracranial pressure, usually before shunt insertion. 3 The peritoneum absorbs cerebrospinal fluid adequately; ascites is not a problem.

Client Need: Physiological Adaptation; **Cognitive Level:** Application; **Integrated Process:** Teaching/Learning; **Nursing Process:** Evaluation/Outcomes; **Reference:** Ch 30, Hydrocephalus, Nursing Care

108. 3 An intensive preparatory regimen is needed to destroy the child's immune system. Once the process is started, no rescue therapy except for the transplant is provided.

1 The procedure is performed in children for recurrent malignancies. 2 The child's bone marrow must be clear of all cells before transfusion of the stem cells is performed. 4 Preparation for the transfusion is accomplished by destroying the immune system; this is not a simple procedure.

Client Need: Health Promotion and Maintenance; **Cognitive Level:** Comprehension; **Integrated Process:** Teaching/Learning; **Nursing Process:** Planning/Implementation; **Reference:** Ch 6, Leukemia, Data Base

109. 2 Parenting can begin only when the baby and the mother get to know each other. To promote development, the nurse should provide time for parent-child interaction.

1 This may make the mother feel incompetent and may delay the development of her mothering skills. 3 Time must be provided for the mother to return demonstrations with the baby and ask questions. 4 Knowledge does not ensure effective mothering; time with the infant is more important.

Client Need: Health Promotion and Maintenance; **Cognitive Level:** Application; **Integrated Process:** Caring; **Nursing Process:** Planning/Implementation; **Reference:** Ch 27, Foundations of Nursing Care for Newborns, Parent-Infant Relationships

110. 3 Cephalhematoma is a collection of blood between the skull bone and its periosteum that results from trauma. It resolves spontaneously in 3 to 6 weeks.

1 Caput succedaneum, rather than cephalhematoma, crosses the suture line. 2 A cephalhematoma is a hard, indurated area that remains immobile even when the infant cries. 4 This trauma is caused by pressure of the head against the birth canal, which occurs during a vaginal birth.

Client Need: Health Promotion and Maintenance; **Cognitive Level:** Analysis; **Integrated Process:** Teaching/Learning; **Nursing Process:** Planning/Implementation; **Reference:** Ch 27, Foundations of Nursing Care for Newborns, Nursing Care Common to All Newborns

111. 4 Famotidine inhibits histamine at H_2-receptor sites in the stomach, inhibiting gastric acid secretion.

1 Famotidine does not affect stress levels. 2 Famotidine inhibits, rather than neutralizes, gastric secretion. 3 Famotidine inhibits gastric secretion, not peristalsis.

Client Need: Pharmacological and Parenteral Therapies; **Cognitive Level:** Comprehension; **Integrated Process:** Teaching/Learning; **Nursing Process:** Planning/Implementation; **Reference:** Ch 8, Related Pharmacology, Antisecretory Agents

112. 1 Intermittent or continuous loss of a small amount of blood over extended periods may lead to depleted hemosiderin (stored iron); hypochromic microcytic anemia may result.

2 Shock results from acute blood loss, which can occur when as little as 10% of the body's total amount of blood is lost quickly. **3** This is caused by lack of the intrinsic factor, not by slow or rapid blood loss. **4** Platelet decrease indicates reduced blood clotting capacity, not blood loss.
Client Need: Physiological Adaptation; **Cognitive Level:** Comprehension; **Nursing Process:** Assessment/Analysis; **Reference:** Ch 8, Peptic Ulcer Disease, Data Base

113. **3** Lavage removes blood from the stomach, and the irrigating solution produces vascular constriction, which helps control bleeding by limiting blood flow to the area.
1 Lavage does not cause the blood to clot. **2** Neutralization of acid by water irrigation will take time; antacids may be instilled to alter the pH. **4** This is not the purpose of a lavage for gastric hemorrhage.
Client Need: Physiological Adaptation; **Cognitive Level:** Comprehension; **Nursing Process:** Assessment/Analysis; **Reference:** Ch 8, Peptic Ulcer Disease, Data Base

114. **2** Fever, chills and low back pain indicate an acute hemolytic reaction, which is potentially life threatening; discontinuing the transfusion immediately limits kidney damage; the vein can be kept open by running the primary bottle of normal saline.
1 This may be done later. The client's safety must be addressed first. **3** This is not an initial action; it may be performed later. **4** This is unsafe because the reaction will continue; although the blood bank generally is notified if a reaction occurs, the nurse still has to first discontinue the blood transfusion, infuse saline, and notify the physician.
Client Need: Pharmacological and Parenteral Therapies; **Cognitive Level:** Application; **Nursing Process:** Planning/Implementation; **Reference:** Ch 6, Related Procedures, Blood Transfusion

115. **4** A quiet, alert state is an optimum time for infant stimulation and interaction with the mother.
1 Bright lights are disturbing to newborns and may impede mother-child interaction. **2** This position places the baby at risk for SIDS and does not increase the opportunity for stimulation and interaction. **3** The physical examination can be delayed.
Client Need: Psychosocial Integrity; **Cognitive Level:** Application; **Integrated Process:** Caring; **Nursing Process:** Planning/Implementation; **Reference:** Ch 27, Foundations of Nursing Care for Newborns, Parent-Infant Relationships

116. **1** RhoGAM will prevent sensitization from Rh incompatibility that may arise between an Rh-negative mother and an Rh-positive infant.
2 ABO incompatibility does not exist; it could if the mother had O positive and the baby had type B blood. **3** Only the mother's and the baby's Rh factors are relevant at this time. **4** Because the baby has type O blood with no ABO incompatibility, neither mother nor child would require a transfusion; this is the mother's first

pregnancy, so the risk for RH incompatibility is minimal.
Client Need: Pharmacological and Parenteral Therapies; **Cognitive Level:** Analysis; **Integrated Process:** Communication/Documentation; **Nursing Process:** Planning/Implementation; **Reference:** Ch 27, Hemolytic Disorders, Data Base

117. **3** This is temporary; it is related to the influence of maternal hormones.
1 This is unrelated to problems with bleeding. **2** This finding is not related to infection. **4** This finding is unrelated to urinary elimination.
Client Need: Health Promotion and Maintenance; **Cognitive Level:** Application; **Integrated Process:** Teaching/Learning; **Nursing Process:** Planning/Implementation; **Reference:** Ch 27, Foundations of Nursing Care for Newborns, Adaptation to Extrauterine Life

118. **4** This adaptation is associated with hyperthyroidism and results from accumulation of fluid behind the eyeball.
1 This is associated with hypothyroidism; hyperactivity occurs with hyperthyroidism. **2** Weight gain occurs with hypothyroidism; weight loss occurs with hyperthyroidism because of the high metabolic rate. **3** This is associated with hypothyroidism; frequent loose stools occur with hyperthyroidism.
Client Need: Physiological Adaptation; **Cognitive Level:** Application; **Nursing Process:** Assessment/Analysis; **Reference:** Ch 9, Hyperthyroidism (Graves' Disease, Thyrotoxicosis), Data Base

119. **2** The remaining thyroid tissue may provide enough hormone for adequate function.
1 The entire gland is not removed; a small portion is left in the hope that it will provide enough hormone for adequate function. **3, 4** The parathyroids are not removed.
Client Need: Health Promotion and Maintenance; **Cognitive Level:** Comprehension; **Integrated Process:** Teaching/Learning; **Nursing Process:** Planning/Implementation; **Reference:** Ch 9, Hyperthyroidism, Data Base

120. **4** Feelings of hopelessness are symptomatic of depression; the individual feels unable to find any solution to problems and thus feels overwhelmed.
1 Echolalia is the pathologic meaningless repetition of another's words or phrases and is associated with schizophrenia, not with depression. **2** Delusions are false fixed beliefs that are resistant to logical reasoning and are commonly associated with schizophrenia, not with depression. **3** Confusion is not common, in that these individuals are in contact with reality.
Client Need: Psychosocial Integrity; **Cognitive Level:** Application; **Nursing Process:** Assessment/Analysis; **Reference:** Ch 19, Major Depression, Data Base

121. **4** This approach allows the client to control the pace of development of the nurse-client relationship.
1 Depressed clients are unable to move into relationships with other clients. **2** It is too early for

therapy sessions; the first thing that must be established is a trusting nurse-client relationship. **3** Depressed clients are unable to move into group situations.
Client Need: Psychosocial Integrity; **Cognitive Level:** Application; **Nursing Process:** Planning/Implementation; **Reference:** Ch 19, General Nursing Care of Clients With Mood Disorders

122. **2** The client is out of control and is dangerous to self and others. Safety requires sedation and a controlled environment.
1 Restraining a disturbed, belligerent client can cause injury because restraints generally increase anxiety and acting out. **3** The client's attention span is too short for either of these activities. **4** Any measures directed at verbal or physical correction of the client's behavior will be taken to no avail.
Client Need: Safety and Infection Control; **Cognitive Level:** Application; **Nursing Process:** Planning/Implementation; **Reference:** Ch 20, Alcohol Abuse, Nursing Care

123. **1** Members of self-help groups, particularly Alcoholics Anonymous, are living with the problem themselves; therefore, problem identification and self-responsibility are emphasized, and manipulation is limited.
2 Long-term therapy tends to increase anxiety until resolution occurs; level of commitment and duration of therapy render it a less desirable choice for substance abusers. **3** Depending on the client's feelings about religion, this may be traumatic. **4** This depends on the friend's drinking status; it may be helpful or harmful. These variables negate the effectiveness of this choice.
Client Need: Management of Care; **Cognitive Level:** Application; **Nursing Process:** Planning/Implementation; **Reference:** Ch 20, Alcohol Abuse, Data Base

124. **3** Although members of the group may become impatient with each other's problems at times, the group usually is supportive. Members share common goals, and the opportunity is available to test out new patterns of behavior.
1 This statement is too universal; the rate and amount of change are individually based variables. **2** People with addiction problems have varied backgrounds. **4** This statement is too universal; although many clients function well in a group, some clients cannot.
Client Need: Psychosocial Integrity; **Cognitive Level:** Comprehension; **Nursing Process:** Assessment/Analysis; **Reference:** Ch 20, Drug Abuse, Data Base

125. **4** Most complications after cardiac catheterization involve the puncture site; included are localized hemorrhage and hematomas, as well as thrombosis of the femoral artery.
1 This is not necessary after cardiac catheterization. **2** This is important but secondary to assessment of the femoral puncture site. **3** The client should remain supine to avoid disturbing the insertion site.
Client Need: Reduction of Risk Potential; **Cognitive Level:** Application; **Nursing Process:** Evaluation/Outcomes; **Reference:** Ch 6, Related Procedures, Cardiac Catheterization

126. **3** Lasix is potassium depleting; apricots have more than 440 mg of potassium per 100 g.
1 Apples have about 80 to 110 mg of potassium per 100 g. **2** Grapes have about 80 to 160 mg of potassium per 100 g, depending on the variety. **4** Cranberries have about 65 mg of potassium per 100 g.
Client Need: Basic Care and Comfort; **Cognitive Level:** Analysis; **Integrated Process:** Teaching/Learning; **Nursing Process:** Planning/Implementation; **Reference:** Ch 8, Review of Nutrients, Minerals

127. **3** This explores the meaning of the statement and allows further expression of concern.
1 This does not allow an explanation of feelings and cuts off communication. **2** This response lacks both empathy and understanding; it also cuts off communication. **4** This shirks responsibility; the client may be embarrassed to ask the physician and needs the nurse to act as facilitator.
Client Need: Psychosocial Integrity; **Cognitive Level:** Analysis; **Integrated Process:** Communication/Documentation; **Nursing Process:** Planning/Implementation; **Reference:** Ch 21, General Nursing Care of Clients With Sexual and Gender Identity Disorders

128. **1** An illusion is a misperception of an actual stimulus.
2 A delusion is a fixed false belief that is unrelated to an external stimulus. **3** Dissociation is a disturbance in the integrative functions of the client. **4** A hallucination is a false perception with no actual external stimulus.
Client Need: Psychosocial Integrity; **Cognitive Level:** Analysis; **Nursing Process:** Assessment/Analysis; **Reference:** Ch 18, Delirium, Data Base

129. **1** These infants may have retinal dysplasia.
2 This does not affect renal function. **3** This does not affect long bone growth. **4** This does not affect glucose metabolism.
Client Need: Physiological Adaptation; **Cognitive Level:** Application; **Nursing Process:** Assessment/Analysis; **Reference:** Ch 27, TORCH, Data Base

130. **2** This is the expected respiratory rate for a healthy newborn.
1 This is too slow. **3, 4** This is too fast, unless the infant is active or crying; the rate should not be assessed at these times.
Client Need: Reduction of Risk Potential; **Cognitive Level:** Knowledge; **Nursing Process:** Assessment/Analysis; **Reference:** Ch 27, Foundations of Nursing Care for Newborns, Adaptation to Extrauterine Life

131. **3** This is limited hip abduction and is indicative of developmental dysplasia of the hip.
1 This is an expected newborn reflex. **2** This is an expected measurement for a newborn at term. **4** This is an expected finding.
Client Need: Physiological Adaptation; **Cognitive Level:** Application; **Nursing Process:** Assessment/Analysis; **Reference:** Ch 30, Developmental Dysplasia of the Hip, Data Base

132. **1** Applying the diaper loosely for 2 or 3 days lessens pressure on the penis.

2 Bleeding is not expected; the newborn should be monitored for signs of bleeding. **3** The newborn can be fed as usual. **4** This will be painful and irritating to the wound.

Client Need: Health Promotion and Maintenance; **Cognitive Level:** Application; **Integrated Process:** Teaching/Learning; **Nursing Process:** Planning/Implementation; **Reference:** Ch 27, Foundations of Nursing Care for Newborns, Nursing Care Common to All Newborns

133. **2** The nurse needs to make the assessment; the nurse cannot rely on a visitor's observations.

1 The client probably will be unable to answer. **3** The nurse is intervening without first assessing the client; this may be threatening if the client is not out of control. **4** This might be done later, after the client has been assessed.

Client Need: Psychosocial Integrity; **Cognitive Level:** Application; **Nursing Process:** Assessment/Analysis; **Reference:** Ch 19, Manic Episode of a Bipolar Disorder, Nursing Care

134. 1. ☒ Increased intracranial pressure can precipitate vomiting because of its effect on the chemoreceptor trigger zone in the medulla.
2. ☒ Because the cranial sutures are closed by this age, increased pressure can cause headache.
3. ☒ Irritability results from increased pressure in the cranium and as a response to related discomforts.
4. ☐ Pressure on the respiratory center in the brain results in a decreased, not increased, respiratory rate.
5. ☐ Blood pressure is increased, not decreased, in the toddler who has closed fontanels.

Client Need: Physiological Adaptation; **Cognitive Level:** Analysis; **Nursing Process:** Assessment/Analysis; **Reference:** Ch 30, Meningitis, Data Base

135. **2** This forces the client to find a common characteristic of two things, an ability that is a criterion for abstract thinking.

1 This tests orientation, not abstract thinking. **3** This tests judgment, not abstract thinking. **4** This tests short-term memory, not abstract thinking.

Client Need: Psychosocial Integrity; **Cognitive Level:** Analysis; **Integrated Process:** Communication/Documentation; **Nursing Process:** Assessment/Analysis; **Reference:** Ch 18, Dementia, Data Base

136. **4** The presence of staff members will give the client support and will provide an opportunity for staff to distract and reassure the client.

1 Although this intervention has value as a general measure, it is too soon to initiate this; it will not decrease the client's level of anxiety at this time. **2** This will be ineffective because it is unlikely the client will comprehend or remember explanations. **3** The client does not have the capacity to explore concerns; in fact, this can be counterproductive and anxiety producing.

Client Need: Psychosocial Integrity; **Cognitive Level:** Application; **Integrated Process:** Caring; **Nursing Process:** Planning/

Implementation; **Reference:** Ch 18, General Nursing Care of Clients With Disorders Related to Alterations in Cognition and Perception

137. **1** Acknowledgment of the client's behavior will help lower the spouse's anxiety, reduce guilt, and encourage discussion of feelings.

2 Lack of understanding by the nurse can be interpreted as uncaring and can incite the spouse to make more angry remarks. **3** This is insensitive; it implies that the spouse did not know how to care for the client. **4** This is insensitive; it suggests inadequate judgment on the spouse's part.

Client Need: Psychosocial Integrity; **Cognitive Level:** Analysis; **Integrated Process:** Caring; Communication/Documentation; **Nursing Process:** Planning/Implementation; **Reference:** Ch 18, Dementia, Nursing Care

138. **3** In myasthenia gravis, the sensitivity of the end plates at the postsynaptic junction to acetylcholine is reduced, thus interfering with muscle contraction. Inadequate contraction of the ocular muscles results in double vision (diplopia).

1, 2 This is not an adaptation associated with myasthenia gravis. **4** This is not an adaptation associated with myasthenia gravis; it is associated with multiple sclerosis.

Client Need: Physiological Adaptation; **Cognitive Level:** Application; **Nursing Process:** Assessment/Analysis; **Reference:** Ch 11, Myasthenia Gravis, Data Base

139. **4** Tensilon is an anticholinesterase compound that increases muscle strength when administered to an individual with myasthenia gravis.

1 Prednisolone is a steroid; it is not used to diagnose this disease. **2** Disodium EDTA is a calcium-chelating agent; it is not used to diagnose this disease. **3** Dilantin is an anticonvulsant; it is not used to diagnose this disease.

Client Need: Pharmacological and Parenteral Therapies; **Cognitive Level:** Analysis; **Integrated Process:** Teaching/Learning; **Nursing Process:** Planning/Implementation; **Reference:** Ch 11, Related Pharmacology, Cholinesterase Inhibitors

140. **2** Neostigmine bromide (Prostigmin) is an anticholinergic that increases the peristaltic activity of the intestines. The result is hyperactive bowel sounds.

1 Bladder distention is not associated with neostigmine. **3** These are not side effects associated with neostigmine. **4** Bradycardia and hypotension may occur with neostigmine.

Client Need: Pharmacological and Parenteral Therapies; **Cognitive Level:** Application; **Nursing Process:** Evaluation/Outcomes; **Reference:** Ch 11, Related Pharmacology, Cholinesterase Inhibitors

141. **4** This response is as optimistic as is possible while still being realistic.

1 This is false reassurance; the client's status will depend on individual response. **2** Medication does not affect progression of the disease; it only treats the adaptations. **3** This gives false reassurance; individual responses vary.

Client Need: Physiological Adaptation; **Cognitive Level:** Analysis; **Integrated Process:** Teaching/Learning; **Nursing Process:** Planning/Implementation; **Reference:** Ch 11, Myasthenia Gravis, Data Base

142. **2** Swimming helps keep the muscles supple, without requiring fine motor activity.

1 This might prove too rigorous for the client. **3** Sewing requires fine motor activity and would be difficult for the client. **4** Sedentary activities are not helpful in maintaining muscle tone.

Client Need: Health Promotion and Maintenance; **Cognitive Level:** Application; **Nursing Process:** Planning/Implementation; **Reference:** Ch 11, Myasthenia Gravis, Nursing Care

143. **4** The congenital defect prevents the infant from creating a tight seal with the lips to promote sucking. As a result, the infant swallows large amounts of air when feeding. The mother should be taught to provide frequent rest periods and to burp the infant often to expel excess air in the stomach.

1, 2 Infants with cleft lip and palate should be held upright during feedings. **3** Newborn infants cannot chew.

Client Need: Basic Care and Comfort; **Cognitive Level:** Application; **Integrated Process:** Teaching/Learning; **Nursing Process:** Planning/Implementation; **Reference:** Ch 30, Cleft Lip (CL) and Cleft Palate (CP), Nursing Care

144. **3** Abstinence 4 to 6 weeks before term is the best way to avoid contracting the virus and having an outbreak before the birth.

1 Abstinence is necessary only when disease symptoms are present in the partner and during the last 4 to 6 weeks. **2** Because the herpes virus is smaller than the pores of a condom, this type of protection has limited effectiveness. **4** Washing is not sufficient to prevent contraction of this virus; contact already has been made.

Client Need: Safety and Infection Control; **Cognitive Level:** Application; **Integrated Process:** Teaching/Learning; **Nursing Process:** Planning/Implementation, **Reference:** Ch 27, TORCH, Data Base

145. **4** Placing the client in a semi-Fowler's position forces the heavy uterus to put temporary pressure on the blood vessels at the site of the separating placenta. This controls bleeding to some extent.

1 There is no indication that the clotting mechanism is disturbed. **2** This is contraindicated with placenta previa; it may further dislodge the placenta. **3** This is contraindicated in any client admitted with vaginal bleeding.

Client Need: Physiological Adaptation; **Cognitive Level:** Analysis; **Nursing Process:** Planning/Implementation; **Reference:** Ch 26, Placenta Previa, Data Base

146. **3** The size of the breast bud is an indication of gestational age. Small, underdeveloped nipples reflect prematurity.

1 This is a clinical manifestation of Down syndrome, not of prematurity. **2** This is not a reliable indicator

of gestational age; also, reflexes may be impaired in full-term infants. **4** This is not related to gestational age.

Client Need: Health Promotion and Maintenance; **Cognitive Level:** Application; **Nursing Process:** Assessment/Analysis; **Reference:** Ch 27, Preterm Infant, Data Base

147. **4** Cold stress produces hypoxia and acidemia. Because of physiologic factors, such as lack of brown fat, the preterm infant is more vulnerable to cool temperatures.

1 These are not a priority; keeping the infant warm is more important. **2** This is necessary only if the infant had an Apgar of 0 to 3. **3** Proper identification is important when the infant is separated from the mother.

Client Need: Health Promotion and Maintenance; **Cognitive Level:** Application; **Nursing Process:** Planning/Implementation; **Reference:** Ch 27, Foundations of Nursing Care for Newborns, Nursing Care Common to All Newborns

148. **3** It is expected that a newborn will enter a sleep phase about 30 minutes after birth.

1 After the initial cry, the baby will settle down and become quiet and alert. **2** This occurs after the first sleep. **4** This occurs during the first period of reactivity.

Client Need: Health Promotion and Maintenance; **Cognitive Level:** Comprehension; **Nursing Process:** Assessment/Analysis; **Reference:** Ch 27, Foundations of Nursing Care of Newborns, Adaptation to Extrauterine Life

149. **3** Atherosclerosis begins with the accumulation of fatty deposits (plaques) within the inner lining (intima) of the arteries, leading to narrowing of the lumen. Later, the plaques enlarge, causing occlusion, and harden through deposition of calcium (atheroarteriosclerosis), eventually increasing the work of the heart.

1 Atheromas develop within the intima of arteries, not in cardiac muscle. **2** Although atheromas or plaques are deposited from circulating fat, mobilization from adipose storage is not a prerequisite. **4** This is arteriosclerosis.

Client Need: Physiological Adaptation; **Cognitive Level:** Comprehension; **Nursing Process:** Assessment/Analysis; **Reference:** Ch 6, Coronary Artery Disease: Atherosclerosis, Data Base

150. **1** Safety is the priority before any other intervention is provided.

2 This is important, but less of a priority. **3** This is a later nursing action. **4** It is important that the client understand what is happening; however, individuality must be considered first.

Client Need: Safety and Infection Control; **Cognitive Level:** Application; **Nursing Process:** Planning/Implementation; **Reference:** Ch 16, General Nursing Care of Clients With Mental Health/Psychiatric Problems

151. **3** Side rails can help clients increase their movement in bed. They are immovable objects that provide a handhold for leverage when changing positions.

1, 2, 4 The need to use side rails for safety must be evaluated for each individual on the basis of mental and physical status and hospital regulations.

Client Need: Basic Care and Comfort; **Cognitive Level:** Application; **Nursing Process:** Planning/Implementation; **Reference:** Ch 11, Brain Attack/Cerebral Vascular Accident (CVA), Nursing Care

152. 1 Ossification of the long bones is incomplete in childhood; children's bones can flex to about a 45-degree angle before breaking. When the bone is angulated beyond 45 degrees, the compressed side bends and the torsion side breaks (greenstick fracture).

2 This usually is a complete fracture seen in blunt trauma; it occurs in adults because bone ossification is complete. 3 This is a fracture with an open wound from which the bone protrudes; it seldom is seen in children. 4 This is a fracture in which small fragments of bone are broken from the fracture site and lie in the surrounding tissue; it is seen rarely in children.

Client Need: Physiological Adaptation; **Cognitive Level:** Comprehension; **Nursing Process:** Assessment/Analysis; **Reference:** Ch 31, Fractures, Data Base

153. 3 Preschoolers generally have learned to cope with parents' absence; however, emotions associated with separation are difficult to hide when parents arrive or leave. Anger at being left also may account for the emotional outburst.

1 Preschoolers enjoy social interaction and probably will be cooperative. 2 Preschoolers have learned to cope with their parents' absence. 4 They have developed social skills with peers and will be able to interact with them even when their parents are present.

Client Need: Health Promotion and Maintenance; **Cognitive Level:** Application; **Integrated Process:** Teaching/Learning; **Nursing Process:** Assessment/Analysis; **Reference:** Ch 32, Hospitalization of Preschoolers, Data Base

154. 2 Preschoolers view death as a separation; they believe the deceased will return to life; this is part of their fantasy world.

1 Preschoolers view death as a separation, or possibly a kind of sleep, and expect the deceased to return or wake up. 3 The preschooler does not yet have the understanding that older people are more likely to die. 4 The preschooler believes that the separation was initiated by the deceased, not by another force.

Client Need: Health Promotion and Maintenance; **Cognitive Level:** Comprehension; **Nursing Process:** Assessment/Analysis; **Reference:** Ch 32, Hospitalization of Preschoolers, Data Base

155. 1. ☐ Environmental stimuli do not have to be reduced.

2. ☒ Individuals with spinal cord injury, particularly injury higher in the vertebral column, remain unstable for several weeks after the injury. Maintaining a patent airway is a priority.

3. ☒ Physiologic instability during the first several weeks after injury results in fluctuating vital signs, including blood pressure readings.

4. ☐ This is too early to institute a bowel and bladder training program.

5. ☐ This is inappropriate because family members are coping in the present; also, it is too early to determine how much function the client may recover.

Client Need: Reduction of Risk Potential; **Cognitive Level:** Analysis; **Nursing Process:** Planning/Implementation; **Reference:** Ch 11, Spinal Cord Injury, Nursing Care

156. 3 The elevated temperature may be indicative of the presence of infection; if so, the abortion should not be done until the infection clears.

1 The procedure is a short one; there is some pain or discomfort. 2 The woman's signature is all that is required in most states. 4 A light menstrual flow is expected for several days.

Client Need: Reduction of Risk Potential; **Cognitive Level:** Application; **Integrated Process:** Teaching/Learning; **Nursing Process:** Planning/Implementation; **Reference:** Ch 23, Induced Abortion, Nursing Care

157. 4 This is a complaint of some women that must be considered.

1 The failure rate is 4% to 35% when used without a spermicide; effectiveness increases with the use of a spermicide. 2 No complaints have been documented. 3 These can be side effects of oral contraceptives.

Client Need: Health Promotion and Maintenance; **Cognitive Level:** Comprehension; **Integrated Process:** Teaching/Learning; **Nursing Process:** Assessment/Analysis; **Reference:** Ch 23, Contraceptive Methods, Nursing Care

158. 4 Tubercle bacilli are transmitted through airborne droplets; therefore respiratory isolation with an Ultra-Filter mask is necessary.

1 Transmission occurs through the airborne route, not via fomites. 2 Contact does not have to be limited as long as isolation precautions are employed. 3 Transmission occurs through the airborne route; gowns and gloves are unnecessary.

Client Need: Safety and Infection Control; **Cognitive Level:** Analysis; **Integrated Process:** Teaching/Learning; **Nursing Process:** Planning/Implementation; **Reference:** Ch 7, Pulmonary Tuberculosis, Nursing Care

159. 1 The toddler is exhibiting typical behavior for this developmental level; most toddlers will say "no" as a means of asserting their independence.

2 Although the child may be eager to resume playing, the behavior described is related to the child's assertion of autonomy. 3 A toddler who is attempting to assert independence will say "no" even if meaning yes. 4 This does not indicate confusion; the child's behavior is typical of 2-year-old children; they will say "no" to most things as a means of asserting their independence.

Client Need: Health Promotion and Maintenance; **Cognitive Level:** Application; **Nursing Process:** Assessment/Analysis; **Reference:** Ch 31, Growth and Development, Two Years

160. 1 A lowered concentration of extracellular sodium causes a decrease in the release of ADH. This leads to increased excretion of urine.

2 Sodium restriction does not control the volume of food intake; weight is controlled by a low-calorie

diet, exercise (if permitted), and prevention of fluid retention. **3** The resulting elimination of excess fluid reduces the workload of the heart but does not improve contractility. **4** Potassium is inefficiently retained by the body; an adequate intake of potassium is needed.
Client Need: Basic Care and Comfort; **Cognitive Level:** Application; **Integrated Process:** Teaching/Learning; **Nursing Process:** Planning/Implementation; **Reference:** Ch 6, Heart Failure, Data Base

161. **3** When ambulating a client, the nurse walks on the client's stronger or unaffected side. This provides a wide base of support and therefore increases stability during the phase of ambulation that calls for weight bearing on the affected side as the unaffected limb moves forward.
1, 2 This tends to change the center of gravity from directly above the feet and may cause instability.
4 This will not support the client as the strong leg moves forward and weight bearing is on the affected side.
Client Need: Basic Care and Comfort; **Cognitive Level:** Application; **Nursing Process:** Planning/Implementation; **Reference:** Ch 11, Fracture of the Hip, Nursing Care

162. **3** This allows an active preschooler to move within restrictions and encourages use of the imagination.
1 Unless carefully selected, many television shows are inappropriate and uninteresting for a 4-year-old.
2 Although a 4-year-old child may still cling to a security toy, it would not stimulate the child's imagination. **4** This may provide the child with rest, but this activity is too simple for a child of this age and will not promote development.
Client Need: Health Promotion and Maintenance; **Cognitive Level:** Application; **Nursing Process:** Planning/Implementation; **Reference:** Ch 32, Health Promotion of Preschoolers, Play (Cooperative Play)

163. **4** Giving Rh-positive cells would lead to further hemolysis; Rh-negative cells are not attacked by maternal antibodies in the infant's blood.
1 This is irrelevant because the blood cells usually do not come from the mother. **2** Rh-negative blood is not neutral; it provides a temporary safeguard from further hemolysis. **3** A reaction to other antigens in the cross-matched blood may occur.
Client Need: Pharmacological and Parenteral Therapies; **Cognitive Level:** Comprehension; **Nursing Process:** Planning/Implementation; **Reference:** Ch 27, Hemolytic Disorders, Data Base

164. **4** These are some of the first signs of hypoxia; the airway must be kept patent to promote oxygenation.
1 These are late signs of respiratory difficulty; suctioning and other measures should have been done before this time. **2** The child will not be able to communicate verbally after a tracheotomy. **3** These are late signs of hypoxia; suctioning should have been done before this time.

Client Need: Physiological Adaptation; **Cognitive Level:** Application; **Nursing Process:** Evaluation/Outcome; **Reference:** Ch 30, Respiratory Tract Infections, Nursing Care

165. **3** The priority of care at this time is to protect the spine from additional damage to the traumatized area while it heals.
1 Infection can result from prolonged immobility; although important, it is not the immediate priority.
2 Although important, it is not the priority in the immediate postinjury period. **4** Survival and safety take priority; vocational rehabilitation will assume greater importance after the client's condition stabilizes.
Client Need: Basic Care and Comfort; **Cognitive Level:** Application; **Nursing Process:** Planning/Implementation; **Reference:** Ch 11, Spinal Cord Injury, Data Base

166. **1** Jaundice occurs because of the expected physiologic breakdown of fetal red blood cells and the inability of the newborn's immature liver to conjugate the resulting bilirubin.
2 Conjugation and excretion, not synthesis of bile, are compromised because of the immature liver.
3 This is unrelated to the newborn's hemoglobin level; the mother and the fetus have separate circulations. **4** Newborns usually have high hemoglobin and high hematocrit levels.
Client Need: Health Promotion and Maintenance; **Cognitive Level:** Comprehension; **Nursing Process:** Assessment/Analysis; **Reference:** Ch 27, Foundations of Nursing Care for Newborns, Adaptation to Extrauterine Life

167. **3** Eye patches are applied to prevent drying of the conjunctiva, injury to the retina, and alterations in biorhythms.
1 The infant will close the eyes automatically in response to bright lights and application of a patch.
2 The infant should be exposed to bright lights periodically, so circadian rhythms will become established. **4** These movements are automatic during different phases of sleep and will not be affected by eye patches.
Client Need: Physiological Adaptation; **Cognitive Level:** Comprehension; **Nursing Process:** Planning/Implementation; **Reference:** Ch 27, Hemolytic Disorders, Data Base

168. **1** Head lag in an infant who is 6 months old is abnormal and is frequently a sign of cerebral damage.
2 The ability to sit unsupported is achieved at 7 to 8 months. **3** The grasp reflex usually disappears by 3 months. **4** The Babinski reflex may be present until 2 years of age.
Client Need: Physiological Adaptation; **Cognitive Level:** Application; **Nursing Process:** Assessment/Analysis; **Reference:** Ch 30, Hydrocephalus, Data Base

169. **2** Increased intracranial pressure exerts pressure on the vomiting center in the brain, resulting in projectile vomiting unrelated to feeding.
1 The eyeballs will show signs of increased fluid volume in the skull and will be pushed forward, pulling the lids taut. **3** The fontanels will show signs

of increased fluid volume in the skull and therefore will bulge. **4** Systolic pressure is elevated and diastolic pressure is the same or lower, creating a widening, not narrowing, pulse pressure.

Client Need: Physiological Adaptation; **Cognitive Level:** Application; **Nursing Process:** Assessment/Analysis; **Reference:** Ch 30, Hydrocephalus, Data Base

170. **3** The trauma of surgery results in some seeping or oozing of blood into the remaining gastric area for 10 to 12 hours until coagulation takes place.

1, 2 The trauma of surgery will result in some blood loss, which will continue until coagulation takes place; this is too short a time for this to occur. **4** Light-red drainage 24 to 48 hours after surgery is abnormal; the physician should be notified.

Client Need: Physiological Adaptation; **Cognitive Level:** Comprehension; **Nursing Process:** Evaluation/Outcomes; **Reference:** Ch 8, Peptic Ulcer Disease, Nursing Care

171. **2** Too rapid administration can cause hyperkalemia, which contributes to a long refractory period in the cardiac cycle, resulting in cardiac dysrhythmias and arrest.

1 Although acidosis can cause hyperkalemia, hyperkalemia will not lead to acidosis. **3** These reactions do not occur with hyperkalemia. **4** Hyperkalemia usually causes nausea, vomiting, and diarrhea, which may result in dehydration; in this instance, fluid would shift from interstitial spaces to the intravascular compartment. With edema, the fluid shift occurs in the opposite direction.

Client Need: Pharmacological and Parenteral Therapies; **Cognitive Level:** Analysis; **Nursing Process:** Evaluation/ Outcomes; **Reference:** Ch 3, Fluid and Electrolyte Balance, Major Ions (Electrolytes)

172. **4** The angle the wrist forms with the forearm decreases as gestation increases.

1 Preterm male infants' testes are undescended; rugae develop progressively and cover the entire scrotum of the full-term male newborn. **2** Sole creases develop progressively, covering the entire foot at term. **3** Preterm infants' ears contain little cartilage and are very springy when folded; at term, the ears contain cartilage and the pinnae are firm.

Client Need: Health Promotion and Maintenance; **Cognitive Level:** Application; **Nursing Process:** Assessment/Analysis; **Reference:** Ch 27, Preterm Infant, Data Base

173. **3** Small feedings reduce the amount of bulk passing into the jejunum and therefore reduce the fluid that shifts into the jejunum.

1 Although a diet high in roughage may be avoided, a low-residue, bland diet is not necessary. **2** Total fluid intake does not have to be restricted; however, fluids should not be taken immediately before, during, or after a meal because they promote rapid stomach emptying. **4** Concentrated sweets pass rapidly out of the stomach and increase fluid shifts; the diet should be low in carbohydrates. Protein is needed to promote tissue repair.

Client Need: Basic Care and Comfort; **Cognitive Level:** Application; **Integrated Process:** Teaching/Learning; **Nursing Process:** Planning/Implementation; **Reference:** Ch 8, Peptic Ulcer Disease, Nursing Care

174. **1** The residual limb is elevated for the first 24 hours after surgery to reduce edema and then is placed flat on the bed to prevent hip flexion contractures.

2 The dressing applied in the operating room should not be disturbed at this time. **3, 4** This is too soon; the residual limb is elevated in bed for the first 24 hours.

Client Need: Physiological Adaptation; **Cognitive Level:** Application; **Nursing Process:** Planning/Implementation; **Reference:** Chapter 11, Amputation, Nursing Care

175. **2** The growing uterus exerts pressure on the mesentery, thereby slowing peristalsis; more water is reabsorbed from the colon and constipation results.

1 The metabolism increases; the bowel is not affected. **3** The growing uterus tends to exert pressure on the bladder and intestines, not on the anus. **4** The bowel is not affected by increased intake of milk.

Client Need: Basic Care and Comfort; **Cognitive Level:** Comprehension; **Integrated Process:** Teaching/Learning; **Nursing Process:** Planning/Implementation; **Reference:** Ch 25, Prenatal Period: Physical, Physiologic, and Emotional Changes During Pregnancy

176. **3** As cervical dilation nears completion, labor is intensified with an increase in pain and energy expenditure.

1 Back pain usually indicates a posterior-lying position of the fetus' head. **2** The client usually is very restless and thrashes about, assuming no particular position. **4** Pain is increased, because contractions are more frequent and intense and they last longer.

Client Need: Health Promotion and Maintenance; **Cognitive Level:** Application; **Nursing Process:** Assessment/Analysis; **Reference:** Ch 25, Intrapartum Period (Labor and Birth), Data Base

177. **3** A relaxed uterus is the most frequent cause of bleeding in the early postpartum period. The uterus can be returned to a state of firmness via intermittent gentle fundal massage.

1 Immediate action is directed toward the client's safety; the physician is called if uterine massage does not control bleeding. **2** Assessment of the uterus and massage take priority; then the vital signs are checked. **4** Steady bleeding is a complication that must be attended to immediately.

Client Need: Health Promotion and Maintenance; **Cognitive Level:** Application; **Nursing Process:** Planning/Implementation; **Reference:** Ch 25, Intrapartum Period (Labor and Birth), Nursing Care

178. **4** Atelectasis refers to the collapse of alveoli; breath sounds over the area are diminished.

1 A productive cough most often is associated with inflammation or infection, not with atelectasis. **2** This is not specific to atelectasis. Clubbing of the fingertips is a late sign of chronic hypoxia related to prolonged obstructive lung disease. **3** Crackles are associated with fluid in the alveoli, which occurs with heart failure and pulmonary edema.

Client Need: Physiological Adaptation; **Cognitive Level:** Application; **Nursing Process:** Evaluation/Outcomes; **Reference:** Ch 3, Perioperative Care, Nursing Care of Clients During the Postoperative Period

179. **3** Chemotherapy and ALL cause immunosuppression (low WBCs), thus increasing the risk for infection.

1 The child should maintain physical activity that can be tolerated. **2** Although vital signs must be checked to assess for changes in pulse or BP, unless there is clinical evidence of bleeding, it is not necessary to take readings every 2 hours. **4** Children need stimulation that is appropriate for their developmental level except when acutely ill.

Client Need: Reduction of Risk Potential; **Cognitive Level:** Application; **Nursing Process:** Planning/Implementation; **Reference:** Ch 32, Leukemia, Nursing Care

180. **3** A common side effect of vincristine is a paralytic ileus that results in constipation. Preventative measures include high-fiber foods and fluids that exceed minimum requirements. These will keep the stool bulky and soft, thereby promoting evacuation.

1, 2, 4 This will not provide the roughage and fluids needed to minimize the constipation associated with vincristine.

Client Need: Pharmacological and Parenteral Therapies; **Cognitive Level:** Analysis; **Nursing Process:** Planning/Implementation; **Reference:** Ch 32, Leukemia, Nursing Care

181. **3** A low platelet count predisposes to bleeding, which may be evident in the urine. Red blood cells are seen microscopically in the sediment.

1 Protein is not found in the urine when the platelet count is low. **2** Glucose is not found in the urine when the platelet count is low. **4** Lymphocytes usually are not found in the urine.

Client Need: Pharmacological and Parenteral Therapies; **Cognitive Level:** Analysis; **Nursing Process:** Evaluation/Outcome; **Reference:** Ch 32, Leukemia, Nursing Care

182. **3** The protective blood-brain barrier initially screens leukemic cells from the CNS. However, in advanced stages, leukemic infiltration occurs. Chemotherapeutic agents, also screened out by the blood-brain barrier, are ineffective.

1 Radiation destroys, not just retards, malignant cells. **2** Radiation does not decrease cerebral edema. **4** Irradiation of the cranium is needed because chemotherapy does not pass the blood-brain barrier.

Client Need: Physiological Adaptation; **Cognitive Level:** Comprehension; **Integrated Process:** Teaching/Learning; **Nursing Process:** Planning/Implementation; **Reference:** Ch 32, Leukemia, Nursing Care

183. **4** Children at early school age are not yet able to comprehend death's universality and inevitability; they fear it, often personifying death as a

"bogeyman" or "death angel." They need an opportunity to prepare for this.

1 A child this age needs to know the seriousness of the illness and that recovery may not be possible. **2** This response only avoids the question. **3** Children of this age interpret death as separation and punishment; they fear this, in addition to death itself.

Client Need: Psychosocial Integrity; **Cognitive Level:** Analysis; **Integrated Process:** Communication/Documentation; **Nursing Process:** Planning/Implementation; **Reference:** Ch 33, Hospitalization of School-Age Children, Data Base

184. **2** The most likely cause is a disturbance in the ratio of calcium to phosphorus, with the amount of serum calcium reduced and the serum phosphorus increased; milk is an excellent source of calcium.

1 Leg cramps are related to hypocalcemia, not to hypercalcemia. **3** An elevated potassium level is manifested by muscle weakness. **4** A low potassium level is evidenced by fatigue and muscle weakness.

Client Need: Physiological Adaptation; **Cognitive Level:** Analysis; **Nursing Process:** Assessment/Analysis; **Reference:** Ch 25, Prenatal Period: Physical, Physiological, and Emotional Changes During Pregnancy

185. **4** The magical and egocentric thinking of preschoolers results in the belief that their sickness is a punishment for bad thoughts.

1 The egocentric thinking of the preschooler would not lead the child to think this way. **2** This is not indicative of the current behavior. **3** More likely, the child will feel that she has gotten sick because she has bad feelings toward her sibling.

Client Need: Health Promotion and Maintenance; **Cognitive Level:** Application; **Nursing Process:** Assessment/Analysis; **Reference:** Ch 32, Hospitalization of Preschoolers, Data Base

186. **3** This can be expected; usually, it is accomplished by 3 years of age.

1 This usually is accomplished at 5 years of age. **2** This requires balance that is not present until 4 or 5 years of age; the 3-year-old child usually can ride a tricycle. **4** This is not accomplished until later in the school-age years.

Client Need: Health Promotion and Maintenance; **Cognitive Level:** Application; **Nursing Process:** Assessment/Analysis; **Reference:** Ch 32, Growth and Development, Three Years

187. **1** A side effect of Ritalin is anorexia; it should be given during or immediately after breakfast and lunch.

2 The absorption rate is not affected by the timing of when it is given. **3** This is not a side effect of Ritalin. **4** At this age, the parents are responsible for administering medications.

Client Need: Pharmacological and Parenteral Therapies; **Cognitive Level:** Application; **Integrated Process:** Teaching/Learning; **Nursing Process:** Planning/Implementation; **Reference:** Ch 17, General Nursing Care of Children With Disorders First Evident in Infancy, Childhood, or Adolescence

188. **3** The high-pressure alarm signifies increased pressure in the tubing or the respiratory tract;

obstruction usually is caused by excessive secretions.

1 This is a dependent function of the nurse. **2** High-volume low-pressure cuffs make this unnecessary; it will decrease the effectiveness of the ventilator and compromise respiratory status. **4** The temperature can remain constant, usually at about 5° F to 10° F below normal body temperature.

Client Need: Physiological Adaptation; **Cognitive Level:** Analysis; **Nursing Process:** Planning/Implementation; **Reference:** Ch 7, Related Procedures, Mechanical Ventilation

189. **2** The system must remain airtight (closed) to prevent collapse of the lung.

1 The water will rise with inspiration and fall with expiration; this is known as tidaling. **3** It should bubble but not vigorously; vigorous bubbling will not increase the suction but will cause the fluid to evaporate more rapidly. **4** The system is kept closed; a record of drainage is kept by marking the outside of the container or chamber.

Client Need: Physiological Adaptation; **Cognitive Level:** Analysis; **Nursing Process:** Planning/Implementation; **Reference:** Ch 7, Related Procedures, Chest Tubes

190. **1** Hallucinations occur most often when sensory stimulation is diminished because there is less competition for attention.

2, 3, 4 Although this may stimulate delusional thoughts, it frequently competes for sensory attention and thereby diminishes hallucinations.

Client Need: Psychosocial Integrity; **Cognitive Level:** Application; **Nursing Process:** Assessment/Analysis; **Reference:** Ch 18, Schizophrenic Disorders, Nursing Care

191. **4** The presence of loosely associated, tangential thinking is one of the cardinal symptoms of schizophrenia; its lessening will demonstrate improvement.

1 This behavior may reflect withdrawal from reality and would not necessarily signal improvement. **2** Most clients with schizophrenia are able to express negative feelings freely because control by the ego is ineffective. **3** This does not demonstrate an improvement; paranoid delusions usually are well organized and on the surface often seem logical.

Client Need: Psychosocial Integrity; **Cognitive Level:** Application; **Nursing Process:** Evaluation/Outcomes; **Reference:** Ch 18, Schizophrenic Disorders, Nursing Care

192. **4** The primary concern in the practice of pica is that other intake will be nutritionally inadequate.

1 This is ordered routinely; it is ordered specifically to address the practice of pica. **2** Pica does not indicate a psychologic/emotional disturbance; frequently, it is influenced by the client's culture. **3** If not toxic to the mother, it is generally not fetotoxic.

Client Need: Basic Care and Comfort; **Cognitive Level:** Application; **Nursing Process:** Assessment/Analysis; **Reference:** Ch 25, Prenatal Period: Physical, Physiological, and Emotional Changes During Pregnancy

193. **3** Ambulation decreases irregular contractions (preparatory contractions, Braxton Hicks contractions).

1 Preparatory contractions increase when the client is resting. **2** These contractions are not indicative of true labor and need not be timed. **4** Medications should not be recommended by the nurse; this is a dependent nursing function.

Client Need: Health Promotion and Maintenance; **Cognitive Level:** Application; **Integrated Process:** Teaching/Learning; **Nursing Process:** Planning/Implementation; **Reference:** Ch 25, Intrapartum Period (Labor and Birth), Data Base

194. **4** An amniotomy allows for more effective pressure of the fetal head on the cervix, enhancing dilation and effacement.

1 This should not affect the fetal heart rate. **2** Vaginal bleeding may increase because of the progression of labor. **3** Discomfort may become greater because contractions usually become more intense after an amniotomy.

Client Need: Reduction of Risk Potential; **Cognitive Level:** Application; **Nursing Process:** Evaluation/Outcomes; **Reference:** Ch 25, Intrapartum Period (Labor and Birth), Nursing Care

195. **3** A negative rubella titer indicates no immunity. Immunizations are given safely during the immediate postpartum period.

1 Penicillin will not affect the client's immune status. **2** The mother's negative rubella titer does not affect the infant. **4** A client with a negative titer has no immunity to rubella.

Client Need: Management of Care; **Cognitive Level:** Application; **Integrated Process:** Communication/Documentation; **Nursing Process:** Planning/Implementation; **Reference:** Ch 25, Postpartum Period, Nursing Care

196. **4** The shunt may obstruct, leading to accumulation of CSF and increased intracranial pressure.

1 Although providing pain relief for the infant is an important part of postsurgical care, monitoring for potentially severe complications such as increased intracranial pressure takes precedence. **2** Positioning the infant flat helps prevent complications that may result from too rapid reduction of intracranial fluid. **3** The infant is positioned off the shunt to prevent pressure on the valve and incisional area.

Client Need: Physiological Adaptation; **Cognitive Level:** Application; **Nursing Process:** Evaluation/Outcomes; **Reference:** Ch 30, Hydrocephalus, Nursing Care

197. **3** A well-balanced diet with fewer calories because of decreased metabolism is suggested for older adults.

1 Fluid needs do not increase. An older client who becomes dehydrated probably is not maintaining a minimum fluid intake. **2** Limited financial resources are one cause of malnutrition in the older adult. **4** High carbohydrates would provide excessive calories, which may result in obesity. Balance should be maintained among the food groups according to dietary guidelines advocated by the U.S. Department of Agriculture and the U.S. Department of Health and Human Services; protein is needed for tissue repair.

Client Need: Health Promotion and Maintenance; **Cognitive Level:** Comprehension; **Nursing Process:** Assessment/Analysis; **Reference:** Ch 5, The Middle-Older Adult (Aged 75 to 84 Years) and Old-Older Adult (Aged 85 Years)

198. 3 Urinary output must be sufficient to excrete the lead and the metabolized chelating agent. In addition, EDTA can damage kidney tissue.

1 Calcium EDTA is not irritating to intestinal mucosa because it is excreted by the kidneys. 2 A regular diet with some junk food is permitted. 4 Calcium EDTA does not cause pain when given intravenously.

Client Need: Pharmacological and Parenteral Therapies; **Cognitive Level:** Application; **Nursing Process:** Planning/Implementation; **Reference:** Ch 31, Lead Poisoning (Plumbism), Nursing Care

199. 1 The presence of food limits the irritating effect of steroids on the gastric mucosa.

2 It may help the client remember to take the medication, but it is not the reason for taking it with meals. 3 Food does not increase or decrease absorption of steroids. 4 The medication is not affected by acid media.

Client Need: Pharmacological and Parenteral Therapies; **Cognitive Level:** Application; **Integrated Process:** Teaching/Learning; **Nursing Process:** Planning/Implementation; **Reference:** Ch 9, Related Pharmacology, Adrenocorticoids

200. 1 Determining fetal well-being supersedes all other measures; if the fetal heart rate (FHR) is absent or is persistently decelerating, immediate intervention is required.

2, 3, 4 This is important, but it is not the priority.

Client Need: Health Promotion and Maintenance; **Cognitive Level:** Application; **Nursing Process:** Assessment/Analysis; **Reference:** Ch 25, Intrapartum Period (Labor and Birth), Nursing Care

201. 3 The fetal heart rate (FHR) is expected to decelerate when the head is compressed during a contraction. If the FHR returns to baseline at the end of the contraction, fetal well-being is indicated.

1 This needs no medical intervention; this is an expected occurrence as long as the FHR returns to baseline at the end of the contraction. 2 Cord compression is a common occurrence; no intervention is necessary if the FHR returns to baseline at the end of the contraction. 4 This position will increase pressure on the vena cava.

Client Need: Health Promotion and Maintenance; **Cognitive Level:** Analysis; **Nursing Process:** Planning/Implementation; **Reference:** Ch 25, Intrapartum Period (Labor and Birth), Nursing Care

202. 4 Clients with bulimia eat to blunt emotional pain because they frequently feel unloved, inadequate, and/or unworthy; purging is precipitated to relieve feelings of guilt for bingeing and/or to limit the fear of obesity.

1 Clients with bulimia often feel out of control and perform their behaviors in secret. 2 The bingeing and purging usually are done alone and in secret. 3 This is one of the psychodynamic theories related to anorexia nervosa, not to bulimia nervosa.

Client Need: Psychosocial Integrity; **Cognitive Level:** Comprehension; **Nursing Process:** Assessment/Analysis; **Reference:** Ch 20, Eating Disorders, Overview

203. 1. ☒ Irritability and emotional lability, fluctuating between euphoria and anger, are common moods associated with mania.

2. ☒ An inflated self-esteem and delusions of grandeur represent mood-congruent psychotic features of mania; clients believe that they possess extraordinary talents, that they are famous, or that they know someone famous.

3. ☒ They are extremely talkative and their speech is rapid with an urgent quality; they rapidly change subjects and have flight of ideas and racing thoughts.

4. ☐ This occurs most often with schizophrenia; the client loses the train of thinking and is unable to retrieve the previous thought.

5. ☐ This is related to depression; clients with mania move fast, pace, fidget, and rarely are still.

Client Need: Psychosocial Integrity; **Cognitive Level:** Analysis; **Nursing Process:** Assessment/Analysis; **Reference:** Ch 19, Manic Episode of a Bipolar Disorder, Data Base

204. 1 Circulatory collapse can be caused by exposure to an infection or a cold or by overexertion of a client with chronic adrenocortical insufficiency (Addison's disease).

2, 3, 4 This is an appropriate room assignment.

Client Need: Safety and Infection Control; **Cognitive Level:** Analysis; **Nursing Process:** Planning/Implementation; **Reference:** Ch 9, Addison's Disease (Primary Adrenal Insufficiency), Nursing Care

205. 3 Deficiency of the glucocorticoids causes hypoglycemia in the client with Addison's disease. Signs of hypoglycemia include nervousness; weakness; dizziness; cool, moist skin; hunger; and tremors.

1 Hypokalemia is evidenced by nausea, vomiting, muscle weakness, and dysrhythmias. 2 Weakness with dizziness on arising is postural hypotension, not hypertension. 4 This is evidenced by edema, increased BP, and crackles.

Client Need: Physiological Adaptation; **Cognitive Level:** Analysis; **Nursing Process:** Assessment/Analysis; **Reference:** Ch 9, Addison's Disease (Primary Adrenal Insufficiency), Data Base

206. 1 Because of diminished mineralocorticoid secretion, clients with Addison's disease are prone to development of hyponatremia. Therefore the addition of salt to the diet is advised.

2 Intake of calories and fluid is determined on an individual basis, not because the client has Addison's disease. 3 Protein is not omitted from the diet;

ingestion of essential amino acids is necessary for optimum metabolism. **4** Fluids are not restricted for clients with Addison's disease.

Client Need: Basic Care and Comfort; **Cognitive Level:** Analysis; **Integrated Process:** Teaching/Learning; **Nursing Process:** Planning/Implementation; **Reference:** Ch 9, Addison's Disease (Primary Adrenal Insufficiency), Nursing Care

207. **4** Development of mood swings and psychosis is possible during long-term therapy with glucocorticoids because of fluid and electrolyte alterations.

1, 2, 3 This is not a sign of long-term glucocorticoid therapy.

Client Need: Pharmacological and Parenteral Therapies; **Cognitive Level:** Application; **Nursing Process:** Evaluation/ Outcomes; **Reference:** Ch 9, Related Pharmacology, Adrenocorticoids

208. **1** These infants have difficulty reaching out to the environment and tend to be withdrawn. They get little response from parents and do not learn how to respond to others.

2 The infant with failure to thrive usually is nonresponsive or minimally responsive to human contact. **3** These infants show little satisfaction and are very difficult to comfort. **4** These infants do not respond readily to human contact.

Client Need: Psychosocial Integrity; **Cognitive Level:** Application; **Nursing Process:** Assessment/Analysis; **Reference:** Ch 30, Failure to Thrive (FTT), Data Base

209. **3** Head control and rolling over are achieved at 4 and 5 months, respectively. Transferring objects from one hand to another and sitting unsupported are achieved at 7 and 8 months.

1, 2 This is too young; the ability to roll over is achieved by approximately 5 months of age. **4** This is too old; transferring objects from hand to hand usually is achieved at approximately 7 months.

Client Need: Health Promotion and Maintenance; **Cognitive Level:** Comprehension; **Nursing Process:** Assessment/Analysis; **Reference:** Ch 30, Growth and Development, Developmental Timetable

210. **1** Fine motor coordination is developed inadequately for manipulation of snap toys. Also, small beads are a choking hazard.

2 These are appropriate to stimulate visual attention. **3** The voluntary grasp will allow the child to hold the toy, and the rattling sound will stimulate the auditory system. **4** These stimulate the sense of touch, and since voluntary grasp appears at about 3 to 4 months, they would be handled satisfactorily.

Client Need: Health Promotion and Maintenance; **Cognitive Level:** Application; **Nursing Process:** Planning/Implementation; **Reference:** Ch 30, Health Promotion of Infants, Play During Infancy

211. **4** When emotional stress overwhelms an individual's ability to cope, the unconscious seeks to reduce stress. A conversion reaction removes the client from the stressful situation, and the conversion reaction's physical/sensory manifestation causes little or no anxiety in the individual. This lack of concern is called la belle indifference.

1 No physiologic changes are involved with this unconscious resolution of a conflict. **2, 3** The conversion of anxiety to physical symptoms operates on an unconscious level.

Client Need: Psychosocial Integrity; **Cognitive Level:** Comprehension; **Nursing Process:** Assessment/Analysis; **Reference:** Ch 19, Conversion Disorders, Data Base

212. **3** This helps the client identify behavior and feelings in a nonthreatening manner.

1 This judges the client, indicating a lack of acceptance. **2** The nurse's behavior is not the issue; the situation should be turned back to the client's behavior. **4** This evasion and refusal to answer will have the psychologic effect of removing the nurse from the group.

Client Need: Psychosocial Integrity; **Cognitive Level:** Analysis; **Integrated Process:** Communication/Documentation; **Nursing Process:** Planning/Implementation; **Reference:** Ch 16, Group Therapy, The Nurse's Role in Group Therapy

213. 1. ☐ Fatigue is associated with withdrawal from caffeine or stimulants.

2. ☒ Anxiety is a symptom that is commonly associated with withdrawal from alcohol.

3. ☐ A runny nose and tearing of the eyes are associated with withdrawal from opioids.

4. ☒ When a person is withdrawing from alcohol, associated autonomic hyperactivity causes an increased heart rate and diaphoresis.

5. ☒ Excited motor activity is associated with alcohol withdrawal.

Client Need: Psychosocial Integrity; **Cognitive Level:** Analysis; **Nursing Process:** Assessment/Analysis; **Reference:** Ch 20, Alcohol Abuse, Nursing Care

214. **2** Accidental ligation of a ureter is a serious complication of total abdominal hysterectomy. A decrease in urine output should be reported immediately to the surgeon.

1 An apical rate of 90 falls within normal limits but should be evaluated in relation to the client's previous vital signs. **3** A nasogastric tube is not inserted routinely. **4** This is to be expected.

Client Need: Physiological Adaptation; **Cognitive Level:** Application; **Nursing Process:** Evaluation/Outcomes; **Reference:** Ch 24, Uterine Neoplasms, Nursing Care

215. **2** Because of tissue destruction, potassium ions are liberated from the injured cells. The result is hyperkalemia.

1 Blood volume decreases, and hypovolemic shock may occur. **3** Capillary permeability is increased as a result of the inflammatory response. **4** Because of the fluid shift, glomerular filtration is decreased, leading to increased specific gravity.

Client Need: Physiological Adaptation; **Cognitive Level:** Analysis; **Nursing Process:** Assessment/Analysis; **Reference:** Ch 10, Burns, Data Base

216. **4** The nurse, knowing the client was combative, was negligent in not providing close supervision; a reasonable, prudent nurse should have observed the client closely to protect against self-imposed injury and to protect others.

1 A client can be placed in restraints only because of current unsafe behaviors, not because of past history. **2** It is unrealistic to keep a client sedated at all times. **3** All clients should be supervised, especially those who have a history of combativeness.

Client Need: Management of Care; **Cognitive Level:** Analysis; **Nursing Process:** Evaluation/Outcomes; **Reference:** Ch 19, Manic Episode of a Biopolar Disorder, Nursing Care

217. **3** This sets appropriate limits for the client who cannot set self-limits; it rejects the behavior but accepts the client.

1 This may have the effect of reinforcing the behavior rather than decreasing it. **2** This does not show acceptance of the client, nor does it help the client control behavior. **4** This does not address the problem directly; the nurse's response can confuse the client because the client may not be aware of why the nurse is refusing to talk.

Client Need: Psychosocial Integrity; **Cognitive Level:** Application; **Integrated Process:** Communication/Documentation; **Nursing Process:** Planning/Implementation; **Reference:** Ch 19, Manic Episode of a Bipolar Disorder, Nursing Care

218. **4** An increase in total body fluid increases intravascular volume and cardiac workload. Salt in the diet contributes to fluid retention and edema.

1 Fluid in the interstitial compartment will not increase blood pressure. Excess fluid in the intravascular compartment will increase blood pressure. **2** Limiting sodium will not have a diuretic effect; it will reduce additional fluid retention. **3** This is the action of diuretics, not of a sodium-restricted diet.

Client Need: Basic Care and Comfort; **Cognitive Level:** Comprehension; **Integrated Process:** Teaching/Learning; **Nursing Process:** Planning/Implementation; **Reference:** Ch 6, Coronary Artery Disease (CAD): Myocardial Infarction (MI), Nursing Care

219. **2** Interference with bile flow into the intestine will lead to an increasing inability to tolerate fatty foods. The unemulsified fat remains in the intestine for prolonged periods, and the result is an inhibition of stomach emptying with possible gas formation.

1 These are not associated with cholecystitis. Melena is tarry stools associated with upper GI bleeding; diarrhea is associated with increased intestinal motility. **3** This is indicative of gastric bleeding; it is not associated with cholecystitis. **4** This is associated with duodenal ulcers, not with cholecystitis.

Client Need: Physiological Adaptation; **Cognitive Level:** Application; **Nursing Process:** Assessment/Analysis; **Reference:** Ch 8, Cholelithiasis/Cholecystitis, Data Base

220. **4** Bleeding disorders are common when bile does not flow through the intestine. Vitamin K, a fat-soluble vitamin synthesized in the small intestine, requires bile salts for its absorption; vitamin K is used by the liver to synthesize prothrombin.

1 Prostaglandins regulate platelet aggregation and control inflammation and vascular permeability. **2** Platelets aggregate at the site of injury; inflammation does not interfere with this process. **3** Diaphragmatic excursion does not put pressure on the suture line.

Client Need: Physiological Adaptation; **Cognitive Level:** Analysis; **Nursing Process:** Evaluation/Outcomes; **Reference:** Ch 8, Cholelithiasis/Cholecystitis, Nursing Care

221. **2** Exploration of the common bile duct may cause edema; a T-tube prevents edema from obstructing the duct.

1 The cystic duct is ligated when the gallbladder is removed. **3** The T-tube will not prevent the formation of an abscess. **4** A T-tube can be used to inject dye for a cholangiogram, but it is not inserted for that purpose.

Client Need: Reduction of Risk Potential; **Cognitive Level:** Comprehension; **Integrated Process:** Teaching/Learning; **Nursing Process:** Planning/Implementation; **Reference:** Ch 8, Cholelithiasis/Cholecystitis, Nursing Care

222. **2** A colostomy does not function for 2 to 4 days postoperatively because of the lack of peristalsis.

1 Bowel sounds will be absent until peristaltic activity returns. **3** This indicates a problem with circulation to the stoma; it should be cherry red. **4** This indicates gastric bleeding, which is abnormal.

Client Need: Physiological Adaptation; **Cognitive Level:** Application; **Nursing Process:** Evaluation/Outcomes; **Reference:** Ch 8, Cancer of Small Intestine, Colon, or Rectum, Nursing Care

223. **4** This is an invasion of privacy. The marital status has no bearing on the needs of the client at this time.

1 There is no indication at this time that the client requires this referral. **2** This action is an invasion of privacy. **3** Although this information may be obtained at the first prenatal visit, the client's marital status has no bearing on the course of labor.

Client Need: Psychosocial Integrity; **Cognitive Level:** Application; **Integrated Process:** Communication/Documentation; **Nursing Process:** Planning/Implementation; **Reference:** Ch 2, Communication, The Nurse-Client Relationship

224. **4** With the head and chest elevated, gravity promotes respiratory excursion; alternating side-lying positions allows for pulmonary drainage and expansion. Placing the infant in an infant seat helps to maintain these positions.

1 This causes the abdominal viscera to put pressure on the diaphragm, thereby impeding lung expansion. **2** It is difficult to maintain a 5-week-old infant in this position; in addition, this position will not promote rest. **3** This position will make it difficult for the lungs to expand, causing difficulty

in breathing. The prone position is contraindicated for all infants because of its relationship to SIDS.
Client Need: Physiological Adaptation; **Cognitive Level:** Application; **Nursing Process:** Planning/Implementation; **Reference:** Ch 30, Cardiac Malformations, General Nursing Care of Children With Cardiac Malformations

225. 3, 2, 4, 1

    __3__ As weight is lost, the individual feels a sense of accomplishment, and self-esteem increases.

    __2__ Dieting, exercise, purging, and laxatives are used to lose weight, with the resulting primary gain of a feeling of control over one's life.

    __4__ Finally, secondary gains such as attention from parents and peers reinforce the behaviors associated with anorexia nervosa.

    __1__ Sociocultural (fashion, "superwoman" issues, and the diet and fitness industry), biologic, psychologic, and familial factors all influence the development of anorexia nervosa.

Client Need: Psychosocial Integrity; **Cognitive Level:** Analysis; **Nursing Process:** Assessment/Analysis; **Reference:** Ch 20, Anorexia Nervosa, Data Base

226. **1** Clients use delusions as a defense and cannot be argued out of them. The nurse's response did not demonstrate acceptance and only added to the client's anxiety and agitation.

2 Maximum clinical effectiveness of antidepressants takes approximately 4 to 6 weeks; therefore psychotropic drug therapy must be combined with psychotherapy and the therapeutic milieu on an inpatient unit. **3** No data indicate that treatment had not been started toward relieving these symptoms. **4** The client should have a one-to-one relationship with staff before being encouraged to relate to other clients on the unit.

Client Need: Psychosocial Integrity; **Cognitive Level:** Application; **Nursing Process:** Evaluation/Outcomes; **Reference:** Ch 18, Schizophrenic Disorders, Nursing Care

227. **4** This is recommended to attempt to keep weight gain to no more than 25 lb, so that the increased cardiac workload that occurs during pregnancy can be somewhat controlled.

1 Fats specifically are not limited; however, they should be eaten in moderation to control the total quantity of calories consumed. **2** Decreasing protein intake is not advised for clients with cardiac problems. **3** Increasing sodium intake is not advised for clients with cardiac problems.

Client Need: Basic Care and Comfort; **Cognitive Level:** Application; **Integrated Process:** Teaching/Learning; **Nursing Process:** Planning/Implementation; **Reference:** Ch 26, Heart Disease, Nursing Care

228. **2** This provides the opportunity for paternal-infant bonding. Handling the infant may reduce some of the father's anxiety.

1 Although helpful, this does not meet the need for paternal-infant bonding. **3** This does not acknowledge the father's anxiety; also, he may not be ready to absorb this information. **4** This is a

simplistic approach to the father's emotional needs and does not address the father's concerns.
Client Need: Psychosocial Integrity; **Cognitive Level:** Application; **Integrated Process:** Caring; **Nursing Process:** Planning/Implementation; **Reference:** Ch 27, Foundations of Nursing Care for Newborns, Parent-Infant Relationships

229. **2** Whole milk does not meet the infant's need for vitamin C and iron. Also, it contains large amounts of protein and sodium, which may be harmful.

1 Whole milk contains adequate fats; the calcium content is 3½ times that of human milk. **3** Whole milk contains adequate thiamine; the sodium content is 3 times that of human milk. **4** Whole milk contains adequate carbohydrates; the protein content is 3 times that of human milk.

Client Need: Basic Care and Comfort; **Cognitive Level:** Comprehension; **Integrated Process:** Teaching/Learning; **Nursing Process:** Planning/Implementation; **Reference:** Ch 30, Nutrition During Infancy, Guidelines for Infant Nutrition

230. **3** Mismatched blood cells are attacked by antibodies, and the hemoglobin released from ruptured erythrocytes plugs the kidney tubules; such kidney involvement results in backache.

1, 2, 4 This symptom is not common to transfusion reactions.

Client Need: Pharmacological and Parenteral Therapies; **Cognitive Level:** Application; **Nursing Process:** Evaluation/Outcomes; **Reference:** Ch 6, Related Procedures, Blood Transfusion

231. **3** Diminished renal function usually is evidenced by a decrease in output to less than 400 mL/24 hours.

1 Glycosuria is unrelated to a transfusion reaction. **2, 4** Although this symptom is related to the renal system and is a sign of an acute hemolytic reaction, its presence does not necessarily indicate kidney damage.

Client Need: Physiological Adaptation; **Cognitive Level:** Application; **Nursing Process:** Evaluation/Outcomes; **Reference:** Ch 12, Acute Kidney Failure, Data Base

232. **1** Hyperkalemia occurs in kidney failure. Because the kidneys are damaged, they are unable to excrete potassium.

2 Hyponatremia generally is not associated with acute renal failure; hyponatremia is associated with headache, muscle weakness, apathy, and abdominal cramps, not with an irregular pulse or diarrhea. **3** Hypouricemia will not occur, because uric acid is excessive in the blood of clients with kidney failure. **4** Hypercalcemia is not associated with the assessment data listed in the scenario; hypocalcemia is associated with renal calculi and with pathologic fracture.

Client Need: Basic Care and Comfort; **Cognitive Level:** Application; **Nursing Process:** Assessment/Analysis; **Reference:** Ch 12, Acute Kidney Failure, Data Base

233. **2** The waste products of protein metabolism are the main cause of uremia. The degree of protein restriction is determined by the severity of the disease.

1 Fluid restriction may be necessary to prevent edema, heart failure, or hypertension; fluid intake does not directly influence uremia. **3** Sodium is restricted to control fluid retention, not uremia. **4** Potassium is restricted to prevent hyperkalemia, not uremia.

Client Need: Basic Care and Comfort; **Cognitive Level:** Analysis; **Integrated Process:** Teaching/Learning; **Nursing Process:** Planning/Implementation; **Reference:** Ch 12, Acute Kidney Failure, Data Base

234. **1** If fluid is not draining adequately, the client should be positioned from side to side or with the head raised, or manual pressure should be applied to the lower abdomen to facilitate drainage with the use of external pressure and gravity.

2 This deficit is not enough to require notifying the physician. **3** A supine position does not facilitate drainage by gravity. **4** The physician, not the nurse, removes the cannula.

Client Need: Physiological Integrity; **Cognitive Level:** Application; **Nursing Process:** Planning/Implementation; **Reference:** Ch 12, Chronic Kidney Failure/End-Stage Renal Disease, Nursing Care

235. **1** When one's efforts toward meeting a goal are blocked or thwarted, frustration results. The child with special needs may be repeatedly thwarted when trying to meet developmental needs, especially in an environment where certain achievements beyond the child's ability are expected.

2 This does not occur. **3** This is an external factor that has little to do with the child's ability to cope with limitations. **4** This is not a frequent occurrence.

Client Need: Psychosocial Integrity; **Cognitive Level:** Comprehension; **Nursing Process:** Assessment/Analysis; **Reference:** Ch 29, The Family; Nursing Care Related to Meeting the Needs of the Family of a Child With Special Needs

236. **1** During the first stage of alcohol detoxification, nausea and anorexia are experienced.

2 Irritability, not euphoria, is experienced during this stage. **3** Tachycardia, not bradycardia, is experienced during this stage. **4** Hypertension, not hypotension, is experienced during this stage.

Client Need: Physiological Adaptation; **Cognitive Level:** Application; **Nursing Process:** Assessment/Analysis; **Reference:** Ch 20, Alcohol Abuse, Nursing Care

237. **4** Increasing cerebral edema may predispose the client to seizures; therefore, stimuli of any kind should be minimized.

1 Magnesium sulfate is used; calcium gluconate is its antidote. **2** A cesarean birth may not be needed. **3** The client probably will receive intravenous magnesium sulfate to prevent a seizure; diuresis is secondary to seizure prevention.

Client Need: Reduction of Risk Potential; **Cognitive Level:** Application; **Nursing Process:** Planning/Implementation; **Reference:** Ch 26, Hypertensive Disorders of Pregnancy, Nursing Care

238. **2** The situation is so traumatic that the individual may be unable to use past coping behaviors to comprehend what occurred.

1 Social isolation is not an immediate concern. **3** This may be a later concern. The client should be the focus of care at this time. **4** Coping skills, not thought processes, are challenged at this time.

Client Need: Psychosocial Integrity; **Cognitive Level:** Application; **Integrated Process:** Caring; **Nursing Process:** Planning/Implementation; **Reference:** Ch 16, Rape Counseling, Nursing Care

239. **2** Maintaining the cannula in place may be compromised if the client is confused or agitated, thus interfering with the consistent delivery of oxygen; also, agitation is an indication of hypoxia.

1 Although rest should be encouraged (the client could rest in a chair), the priority is that the client receives the oxygen. **3** Two liters of oxygen per minute is not contraindicated for a client with chronic obstructive pulmonary disease (COPD); if the client has COPD, levels above 2 L should be avoided to prevent CO_2 narcosis. **4** In the adult, nasal cannulas do not come in a variety of sizes; the elastic strap is adjustable.

Client Need: Physiological Adaptation; **Cognitive Level:** Application; **Nursing Process:** Planning/Implementation; **Reference:** Ch 7, Related Procedures, Oxygen Therapy

240. **1** Secretions in the upper airway produce gurgling sounds that interfere with the free flow of air with each breath.

2 Oropharyngeal suction will not address this problem. **3** Cyanosis can result from a variety of problems unrelated to the presence of secretions; suctioning should be done only when secretions are blocking the airway. **4** Suctioning is not needed in the absence of accumulated oropharyngeal secretions.

Client Need: Physiological Adaptation; **Cognitive Level:** Analysis; **Nursing Process:** Assessment/Analysis; **Reference:** Ch 7, Related Procedures, Suctioning of Airway

241. **1** Isoniazid (INH) is used as a prophylactic agent for people who have been exposed to tuberculosis; also, it is one of several drugs used to treat the disease.

2 Multiple puncture tests (MPTs), such as the tine test, are used to test for TB; these are no longer recommended. **3** Bacille Calmette-Guérin (BCG) is a vaccine that provides limited immunity; it is not recommended for use in the United States. **4** Purified protein derivative (PPD), the Mantoux test, is a widely used skin test for detecting tuberculosis.

Client Need: Pharmacological and Parenteral Therapies; **Cognitive Level:** Analysis; **Nursing Process:** Planning/Implementation; **Reference:** Ch 7, Pulmonary Tuberculosis (TB), Data Base

242. 2 Leg fatigue is a common clinical manifestation caused by venous stasis and poor tissue oxygenation.

1 This results from a fungus under the nail or chronic hypoxia. 3, 4 This is indicative of thrombophlebitis.

Client Need: Physiological Adaptation; **Cognitive Level:** Application; **Nursing Process:** Assessment/Analysis; **Reference:** Ch 6, Vascular Disease: Varicose Veins, Data Base

243. 2 As valves become incompetent, they allow blood to pool in the veins, which increases hydrostatic pressure and leads to further valve destruction.

1 Inflammation is specific to thrombophlebitis, not to varicose veins. 3 Valves promote, not obstruct, the flow of blood to the heart. 4 No hereditary diseases are known to affect only the leg muscles surrounding the veins.

Client Need: Physiological Adaptation; **Cognitive Level:** Comprehension; **Integrated Process:** Teaching/Learning; **Nursing Process:** Planning/Implementation; **Reference:** Ch 6, Review of Anatomy and Physiology, Regulatory Mechanisms Affecting Circulation

244. 2 This is the manner in which the AIDS virus interferes with the individual's immunity to other infections.

1 AIDS is not an autoimmune process. 3 This is not related to opportunistic infections associated with AIDS; these infections result from the immune deficiency caused by the HIV infection. 4 This is not related to the presence of opportunistic infections or illnesses associated with AIDS; it is associated with the immune deficiency caused by human immunodeficiency virus (HIV) infection.

Client Need: Physiological Adaptation; **Cognitive Level:** Comprehension; **Nursing Process:** Assessment/Analysis; **Reference:** Ch 13, Acquired Immunodeficiency Syndrome (AIDS), Data Base

245. 1 Diarrhea, nausea, and vomiting are common side effects; clients should take these medications with a meal or light snack.

2 These drugs may cause hyperglycemia, not hypoglycemia. 3 Circumoral (perioral), not peripheral, paresthesias may occur with protease inhibitors; peripheral paresthesias may occur with nucleoside reverse transcriptase inhibitors. 4 This does not occur with protease inhibitors; it may occur with digoxin toxicity.

Client Need: Pharmacological and Parenteral Therapies; **Cognitive Level:** Application; **Nursing Process:** Evaluation/Outcomes; **Reference:** Ch 13, Acquired Immunodeficiency Syndrome (AIDS), Data Base

246. 4 Antioxidants in cranberry juice may inhibit the mechanism that metabolizes Coumadin (warfarin), causing elevations in the international normalized ratio (INR) and resulting in hemorrhage.

1, 2, 3 This juice is not contraindicated when Coumadin (warfarin) is taken.

Client Need: Pharmacological and Parenteral Therapies; **Cognitive Level:** Analysis; **Integrated Process:** Teaching/Learning; **Nursing Process:** Evaluation/Outcomes; **Reference:** Ch 6, Related Pharmacology, Anticoagulants

247. 2 By monitoring and reporting changes in the child's behavior, the physician can determine the effectiveness of the medication and the optimum dosage.

1 Parents should not be encouraged to tutor their children because there may be too much emotional interaction. 3 Children need more structure and rules than adults do. 4 This child's behavior is not deliberate or easily controllable; this type of statement may lead to diminished self-esteem in the child if control does not occur.

Client Need: Pharmacological and Parenteral Therapies; **Cognitive Level:** Application; **Integrated Process:** Teaching/Learning; **Nursing Process:** Planning/Implementation; **Reference:** Ch 17, General Nursing Care of Children With Disorders First Evident in Infancy, Childhood, or Adolescence

248. 4 Bending increases intraocular pressure and must be avoided.

1, 2 This is not necessary. 3 Coughing deeply increases intraocular pressure and is contraindicated.

Client Need: Reduction of Risk Potential; **Cognitive Level:** Application; **Integrated Process:** Teaching/Learning; **Nursing Process:** Evaluation/Outcomes; **Reference:** Ch 11, Cataract, Nursing Care

249. 2 Exsanguination can occur in a matter of minutes if cannulas are dislodged.

1, 3, 4 This is not a life-threatening situation; preventing exsanguination takes priority.

Client Need: Physiological Adaptation; **Cognitive Level:** Analysis; **Nursing Process:** Evaluation/Outcomes; **Reference:** Ch 12, Chronic Kidney Failure/End-Stage Renal Disease, Nursing Care

250. 2 Taking the blood pressure in the affected arm may injure the fistula.

1 The presence of a bruit indicates that the circulation is not obstructed by a thrombus. 3 Exsanguination can occur in a matter of minutes if the cannula is dislodged. 4 These are signs of infection, which is a complication of cannulization.

Client Need: Safety and Infection Control; **Cognitive Level:** Application; **Integrated Process:** Teaching/Learning; **Nursing Process:** Evaluation/Outcomes; **Reference:** Ch 12, Chronic Kidney Failure/End-Stage Renal Disease, Nursing Care

251. 4 The major problem that occurs with leukemia is depressed bone marrow production of formed elements of blood, which leads to neutropenia and increased susceptibility to infection.

1 Urine output will be within normal limits; no kidney involvement is noted at this stage of the disease. 2 Excessive, not lesser, quantities of "blasts" are found in the peripheral blood and bone marrow. 3 The swallowing reflex is not affected.

Client Need: Physiological Adaptation; **Cognitive Level:** Application; **Nursing Process:** Assessment/Analysis; **Reference:** Ch 32, Leukemia, Data Base

252. 4 Warm, moist heat will reduce inflammation and pain, thus promoting mobility.

1 Acetaminophen administered at night will not decrease pain experienced the following morning. 2 Ice will not be beneficial regardless of the time it is administered. 3 Gentle stretching, not active exercise, should be employed.

Client Need: Physiological Adaptation; Cognitive Level: Application; Integrated Process: Teaching/Learning; Nursing Process: Planning/Implementation; Reference: Ch 33, Juvenile Idiopathic Arthritis, Nursing Care

253. 4 After a suprapubic prostatectomy, leakage of urine generally is noted around the suprapubic tube. This creates an environment in which bacteria can flourish if the dressing is not changed frequently.

1 Uremia is caused by inadequate kidney function; it is not directly related to bladder infection. 2 Negative pressure on the bladder may traumatize the delicate tissue; urine should flow because of gravity. 3 Clamping off the tube causes urinary stasis, which increases the risk for infection.

Client Need: Physiological Adaptation; Cognitive Level: Application; Nursing Process: Planning/Implementation; Reference: Ch 12, Benign Prostatic Hyperplasia, Nursing Care

254. 2 Pain after a suprapubic prostatectomy may denote retention of urine as a result of blocked drainage tubes or infection, or it may be a normal response to surgery. The possibility of any complication must be investigated.

1 Analgesics can be administered after the cause of pain has been investigated. 3 Encouraging fluids without a patent drainage tube will increase pressure and discomfort; assessment should occur before implementation. 4 The need to measure vital signs is dependent upon the analgesic ordered; assessing the cause of pain takes priority.

Client Need: Physiological Adaptation; Cognitive Level: Application; Nursing Process: Evaluation/Outcomes; Reference: Ch 12, Benign Prostatic Hyperplasia, Nursing Care

255. 4 Keeping a record of what one eats helps to limit unconscious and nervous eating by making the individual aware of intake.

1 Limiting calories to 900 per day is a severe restriction that requires a physician's order. 2 Exercise causes rapid head movements, which may precipitate a Ménière's attack. 3 Although this is a therapeutic intervention, the nurse first should make suggestions that help increase the client's awareness of personal eating habits.

Client Need: Basic Care and Comfort; Cognitive Level: Application; Integrated Process: Teaching/Learning; Nursing Process: Planning/Implementation; Reference: Ch 8, Obesity, Nursing Care

256. 3 Liquid iron preparations may stain tooth enamel; therefore these should be diluted and administered through a straw.

1 Constipation, rather than loose stools, often results from the administration of iron. 2 To avoid gastric irritation, iron should be given with food. 4 To improve absorption, iron may be given with orange juice.

Client Need: Pharmacological and Parenteral Therapies; Cognitive Level: Application; Integrated Process: Teaching/Learning; Nursing Process: Planning/Implementation; Reference: Ch 31, Health Promotion of Toddlers, Childhood Nutrition

257. 2 The 4-year-old can express feelings better through play than with words.

1 A needle is dangerous; a play syringe would focus the child's attention on only one aspect of treatment. 3 This may help the nurse understand emotional problems; however, it is not as helpful as therapeutic play in meeting the child's emotional needs. 4 Understanding explanations requires abstract thinking; 4-year-olds think in a concrete manner and have little concept of time.

Client Need: Psychosocial Integrity; Cognitive Level: Application; Integrated Process: Caring; Nursing Process: Planning/Implementation; Reference: Ch 32, Hospitalization of Preschoolers, General Nursing Care of Preschoolers

258. 3 The added cardiac workload of individuals with anemia who are receiving transfusions increases the risk for heart failure that leads to pulmonary edema.

1, 2, 4 This problem occurs with frequent transfusions, but anemia does not increase the risk for its occurrence.

Client Need: Pharmacological and Parenteral Therapies; Cognitive Level: Analysis; Nursing Process: Evaluation/Outcomes; Reference: Ch 31, β-Thalassemia, Nursing Care

259. 4 This disorder interferes with the ability to perceive and respond to sensory stimuli, which causes a deficit in interpreting new sensory data, makes learning difficult, and results in learning disabilities.

1, 3 This is not necessarily true. 2 It is not an intellectual deficit that prevents learning but rather a perceptual difficulty; these children may have superior intelligence.

Client Need: Psychosocial Integrity; Cognitive Level: Comprehension; Nursing Process: Assessment/Analysis; Reference: Ch 17, Attention Deficit Hyperactivity Disorder, Data Base

260. 1 Because the client is paralyzed and movement is compromised, daily inspection to determine the presence of reddened areas or lesions is necessary so that treatment can be initiated quickly.

2 This may contribute to circumscribed pressure, which can lead to skin breakdown. 3 Massage of reddened areas may cause further damage and should be avoided. 4 Because sensation may be compromised, a heating pad should not be used.

Client Need: Basic Care and Comfort; Cognitive Level: Application; Nursing Process: Planning/Implementation;

Reference: Ch 10, Pressure Ulcers (Decubitus Ulcers), Nursing Care

261. 3 Until the client learns new ways of coping with anxiety, this pattern of behavior will continue. Learning new ways to operate will break the pattern.

1 This will reinforce the sick role. 2 A certain amount of stress is present in everyday family situations; the client must learn new coping mechanisms. 4 This will avoid the problem; the client must learn to cope with problems.

Client Need: Psychosocial Integrity; **Cognitive Level:** Application; **Nursing Process:** Planning/Implementation; **Reference:** Ch 19, General Nursing Care of Clients With Anxiety Disorders

262. 3 Documentation of nursing findings during assessment is a nursing function. This facilitates early treatment.

1 This medical intervention is beyond the scope of nursing practice. 2 Inadequate oral hygiene has not been identified as a cause of plaques; once-daily treatment is insufficient for anyone. 4 *Candida* is a frequent secondary infection in clients with AIDS; it is treated when present.

Client Need: Physiological Adaptation; **Cognitive Level:** Application; **Integrated Process:** Communication/Documentation; **Nursing Process:** Planning/Implementation; **Reference:** Ch 13, Acquired Immunodeficiency Syndrome (AIDS), Data Base

263. 4 Using soap and water and ointment helps maintain skin integrity and prevent infection.

1 Soap and water are adequate unless peroxide is specifically prescribed by the physician; gauze bandages generally are not applied around or over a stoma. 2 Applying an ointment to this extent is contraindicated because it will interfere with adherence of the appliance. 3 Rubbing may be irritating and may promote conditions that contribute to infection.

Client Need: Physiological Adaptation; **Cognitive Level:** Application; **Integrated Process:** Teaching/Learning; **Nursing Process:** Planning/Implementation; **Reference:** Ch 8, Related Procedures, Colostomy Irrigation

264. 2 Few physical restraints on activity are required postoperatively, but the client may have emotional problems as a result of body image changes.

1 Swimming is not prohibited because water does not harm the stoma. 3 ADLs are resumed 6 to 8 weeks after surgery. 4 No changes in lifestyle are necessary.

Client Need: Health Promotion and Maintenance; **Cognitive Level:** Analysis; **Integrated Process:** Teaching/Learning; **Nursing Process:** Planning/Implementation; **Reference:** Ch 8, Cancer of Small Intestine, Colon, or Rectum, Nursing Care

265. 2 Antidiuretic hormone (ADH) causes water retention, resulting in decreased urine output.

1 Blood volume may increase, causing dilution of nitrogenous wastes in the blood. 3 ADH acts on nephrons to cause water to be reabsorbed from glomerular filtrate, leading to an increased specific gravity of urine. 4 The client is overhydrated so that serum sodium is decreased.

Client Need: Physiological Adaptation; **Cognitive Level:** Application; **Nursing Process:** Assessment/Analysis; **Reference:** Ch 9, Syndrome of Inappropriate Antidiuretic Hormone Secretion, Data Base

Index

Page numbers followed by f indicate figures; t, tables.